T0252624

FOURTH EDITION

Biomedical Engineering Fundamentals

THE BIOMEDICAL ENGINEERING HANDBOOK

FOURTH EDITION

Biomedical Engineering Fundamentals

Edited by

Joseph D. Bronzino
Founder and President
Biomedical Engineering Alliance and Consortium (BEACON)
Hartford, Connecticut, U.S.A.

Donald R. Peterson
Professor of Engineering
Dean of the College of Science, Technology, Engineering, Mathematics, and Nursing
Texas A&M University – Texarkana
Texarkana, Texas, U.S.A.

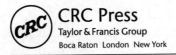

CRC Press
Taylor & Francis Group
Boca Raton London New York

CRC Press is an imprint of the
Taylor & Francis Group, an **informa** business

MATLAB® is a trademark of The MathWorks, Inc. and is used with permission. The MathWorks does not warrant the accuracy of the text or exercises in this book. This book's use or discussion of MATLAB® software or related products does not constitute endorsement or sponsorship by The MathWorks of a particular pedagogical approach or particular use of the MATLAB® software.

CRC Press
Taylor & Francis Group
6000 Broken Sound Parkway NW, Suite 300
Boca Raton, FL 33487-2742

First issued in paperback 2017

© 2015 by Taylor & Francis Group, LLC
CRC Press is an imprint of Taylor & Francis Group, an Informa business

No claim to original U.S. Government works

ISBN-13: 978-1-4398-2518-1 (hbk)
ISBN-13: 978-1-138-74807-1 (pbk)

This book contains information obtained from authentic and highly regarded sources. Reasonable efforts have been made to publish reliable data and information, but the author and publisher cannot assume responsibility for the validity of all materials or the consequences of their use. The authors and publishers have attempted to trace the copyright holders of all material reproduced in this publication and apologize to copyright holders if permission to publish in this form has not been obtained. If any copyright material has not been acknowledged please write and let us know so we may rectify in any future reprint.

Except as permitted under U.S. Copyright Law, no part of this book may be reprinted, reproduced, transmitted, or utilized in any form by any electronic, mechanical, or other means, now known or hereafter invented, including photocopying, microfilming, and recording, or in any information storage or retrieval system, without written permission from the publishers.

For permission to photocopy or use material electronically from this work, please access www.copyright.com (http://www.copyright.com/) or contact the Copyright Clearance Center, Inc. (CCC), 222 Rosewood Drive, Danvers, MA 01923, 978-750-8400. CCC is a not-for-profit organization that provides licenses and registration for a variety of users. For organizations that have been granted a photocopy license by the CCC, a separate system of payment has been arranged.

Trademark Notice: Product or corporate names may be trademarks or registered trademarks, and are used only for identification and explanation without intent to infringe.

Library of Congress Cataloging-in-Publication Data

Biomedical engineering fundamentals / edited by Joseph D. Bronzino and Donald R. Peterson.
   p. ; cm.
   Preceded by The biomedical engineering handbook / edited by Joseph D. Bronzino. 3rd. 2006.
   Includes bibliographical references and index.
   ISBN 978-1-4398-2518-1 (hardcover : alk. paper)
   I. Bronzino, Joseph D., 1937- , editor. II. Peterson, Donald R., editor.
   [DNLM: 1. Biomedical Engineering. 2. Bioengineering. 3. Biomechanical Phenomena. 4. Biomedical Technology. QT 36]

   R856
   610.28--dc23
                               2014035623

Visit the Taylor & Francis Web site at
http://www.taylorandfrancis.com

and the CRC Press Web site at
http://www.crcpress.com

Contents

Preface...ix

Editors... xv

Contributors xvii

MATLAB Statement xxv

SECTION I Physiologic Systems

Herbert F. Voigt

1 An Outline of Cardiovascular Structure and Function..................................... 1-1
   Daniel J. Schneck

2 Kidney Structure and Physiology 2-1
   Joel M. Henderson and Mostafa Belghasem

3 Nervous System..3-1
   Evangelia Micheli-Tzanakou

4 Vision System 4-1
   Aaron P. Batista and George D. Stetten

5 Auditory System 5-1
   Ben M. Clopton and Herbert F. Voigt

6 Gastrointestinal System...6-1
   Berj L. Bardakjian

7 Respiratory System... 7-1
   Arthur T. Johnson, Christopher G. Lausted, and Joseph D. Bronzino

SECTION II Biomechanics

Donald R. Peterson

8 Mechanics of Hard Tissue...8-1
   J. Lawrence Katz, Anil Misra, Orestes Marangos, Qiang Ye, and Paulette Spencer

9 Musculoskeletal Soft-Tissue Mechanics..9-1
   Richard L. Lieber, Samuel R. Ward, and Thomas J. Burkholder

10 Joint-Articulating Surface Motion **10-1**
Kenton R. Kaufman and Kai-Nan An

11 Joint Lubrication... **11-1**
Michael J. Furey

12 Analysis of Gait.. **12-1**
Roy B. Davis III, Sylvia Õunpuu, and Peter A. DeLuca

13 Mechanics of Head/Neck **13-1**
Albert I. King and David C. Viano

14 Biomechanics of Chest and Abdomen Impact **14-1**
David C. Viano and Albert I. King

15 Cardiac Biomechanics... **15-1**
Andrew D. McCulloch and Roy C. P. Kerckhoffs

16 Heart Valve Dynamics... **16-1**
Choon Hwai Yap, Erin Spinner, Muralidhar Padala, and Ajit P. Yoganathan

17 Arterial Macrocirculatory Hemodynamics.. **17-1**
Baruch B. Lieber

18 Mechanics of Blood Vessels.. **18-1**
Thomas R. Canfield and Philip B. Dobrin

19 The Venous System **19-1**
Artin A. Shoukas and Carl F. Rothe

20 The Microcirculation Physiome.. **20-1**
Aleksander S. Popel and Roland N. Pittman

21 Mechanics and Deformability of Hematocytes.. **21-1**
Richard E. Waugh and Robert M. Hochmuth

22 Mechanics of Tissue/Lymphatic Transport.. **22-1**
Geert W. Schmid-Schönbein and Alan R. Hargens

23 Modeling in Cellular Biomechanics.. **23-1**
Alexander A. Spector and Roger Tran-Son-Tay

24 Cochlear Mechanics **24-1**
Charles R. Steele and Sunil Puria

25 Inner Ear Hair Cell Bundle Mechanics.. **25-1**
Jong-Hoon Nam and Wally Grant

26 Exercise Physiology... **26-1**
Cathryn R. Dooly and Arthur T. Johnson

27 Factors Affecting Mechanical Work in Humans.. **27-1**
Ben F. Hurley and Arthur T. Johnson

SECTION III   Biomaterials

Joyce Y. Wong

28 Metallic Biomaterials **28-1**
Joon B. Park and Young Kon Kim

29 Ceramic Biomaterials 29-1
    W. G. Billotte

30 Polymeric Biomaterials 30-1
    Hai Bang Lee, Gilson Khang, and Jin Ho Lee

31 Composite Biomaterials 31-1
    Roderic S. Lakes

32 Biodegradable Polymeric Biomaterials: An Updated Overview 32-1
    C. C. Chu

33 Biologic Biomaterials: Tissue-Derived Biomaterials (Collagen) 33-1
    Shu-Tung Li

34 Biologic Biomaterials: Silk 34-1
    Biman Mandal and David L. Kaplan

35 Biofunctional Hydrogels 35-1
    Melissa K. McHale and Jennifer L. West

36 Soft Tissue Replacements 36-1
    K. B. Chandran, K. J. L. Burg, and S. W. Shalaby

37 Hard Tissue Replacements 37-1
    Sang-Hyun Park, Adolfo Llinás, and Vijay K. Goel

SECTION IV   Bioelectric Phenomena

Roger C. Barr

38 Basic Electrophysiology 38-1
    Roger C. Barr

39 Volume Conductor Theory 39-1
    Robert Plonsey

40 Electrical Conductivity of Tissues 40-1
    Bradley J. Roth

41 Cardiac Microimpedances 41-1
    Andrew E. Pollard

42 Membrane Models 42-1
    Anthony Varghese

43 Computational Methods and Software for Bioelectric
    Field Problems 43-1
    Christopher R. Johnson

44 The Potential Fields of Triangular Boundary Elements 44-1
    A. van Oosterom

45 Principles of Electrocardiography 45-1
    Edward J. Berbari

46 Electrodiagnostic Studies 46-1
    Sanjeev D. Nandedkar

47 Principles of Electroencephalography...47-1
    Joseph D. Bronzino

48 Biomagnetism...48-1
    Jaakko Malmivuo

49 Electrical Stimulation of Excitable Tissue.......................................49-1
    Dominique M. Durand

SECTION V   Neuroengineering

Daniel J. DiLorenzo

50 History and Overview of Neural Engineering..................................50-1
    Daniel J. DiLorenzo and Robert E. Gross

51 Theory and Physiology of Electrical Stimulation of the Central
    Nervous System...51-1
    Warren M. Grill

52 Transcutaneous FES for Ambulation: The Parastep System..............52-1
    Daniel Graupe

53 Comparing Electrodes for Use as Cortical Control Signals: Tines,
    Wires, or Cones on Wires—Which Is Best?......................................53-1
    Philip R. Kennedy

54 Development of a Multifunctional 22-Channel Functional Electrical
    Stimulator for Paraplegia..54-1
    Ross Davis, T. Johnston, B. Smith, R. Betz, T. Houdayer, and A. Barriskill

55 An Implantable Bionic Network of Injectable Neural Prosthetic
    Devices: The Future Platform for Functional Electrical Stimulation
    and Sensing to Restore Movement and Sensation...........................55-1
    J. Schulman, P. Mobley, J. Wolfe, Ross Davis, and I. Arcos

56 Visual Prostheses..56-1
    Robert J. Greenberg

57 Interfering with the Genesis and Propagation of Epileptic Seizures
    by Neuromodulation...57-1
    *Ana Luisa Velasco, Francisco Velasco, Marcos Velasco, Bernardo Boleaga,
    Mauricio Kuri, Fiacro Jiménez, and José María Núñez*

58 Transcranial Magnetic Stimulation of Deep Brain Regions 58-1
    Yiftach Roth and Abraham Zangen

Index...Index-1

Preface

During the past eight years since the publication of the third edition—a three-volume set—of *The Biomedical Engineering Handbook*, the field of biomedical engineering has continued to evolve and expand. As a result, the fourth edition has been significantly modified to reflect state-of-the-field knowledge and applications in this important discipline and has been enlarged to a four-volume set:

- Volume I: *Biomedical Engineering Fundamentals*
- Volume II: *Medical Devices and Human Engineering*
- Volume III: *Biomedical Signals, Imaging, and Informatics*
- Volume IV: *Molecular, Cellular, and Tissue Engineering*

More specifically, this fourth edition has been considerably updated and contains completely new sections, including

- Stem Cell Engineering
- Drug Design, Delivery Systems, and Devices
- Personalized Medicine

as well as a number of substantially updated sections, including

- Tissue Engineering (which has been completely restructured)
- Transport Phenomena and Biomimetic Systems
- Artificial Organs
- Medical Imaging
- Infrared Imaging
- Medical Informatics

In addition, Volume IV contains a chapter on ethics because of its ever-increasing role in the biomedical engineering arts.

Nearly all the sections that have appeared in the first three editions have been significantly revised. Therefore, this fourth edition presents an excellent summary of the status of knowledge and activities of biomedical engineers in the first decades of the twenty-first century. As such, it can serve as an excellent reference for individuals interested not only in a review of fundamental physiology but also in quickly being brought up to speed in certain areas of biomedical engineering research. It can serve as an excellent textbook for students in areas where traditional textbooks have not yet been developed and as an excellent review of the major areas of activity in each biomedical engineering sub-discipline, such as biomechanics, biomaterials, bioinstrumentation, medical imaging, and so on. Finally, it can serve as the "bible" for practicing biomedical engineering professionals by covering such topics as historical perspective of medical technology, the role of professional societies, the ethical issues associated with medical technology, and the FDA process.

Biomedical engineering is now an important and vital interdisciplinary field. Biomedical engineers are involved in virtually all aspects of developing new medical technology. They are involved in the design, development, and utilization of materials, devices (such as pacemakers, lithotripsy, etc.), and techniques (such as signal processing, artificial intelligence, etc.) for clinical research and use, and they serve as members of the healthcare delivery team (clinical engineering, medical informatics, rehabilitation engineering, etc.) seeking new solutions for the difficult healthcare problems confronting our society. To meet the needs of this diverse body of biomedical engineers, this handbook provides a central core of knowledge in those fields encompassed by the discipline. However, before presenting this detailed information, it is important to provide a sense of the evolution of the modern healthcare system and identify the diverse activities biomedical engineers perform to assist in the diagnosis and treatment of patients.

Evolution of the Modern Healthcare System

Before 1900, medicine had little to offer average citizens, since its resources consisted mainly of physicians, their education, and their "little black bag." In general, physicians seemed to be in short supply, but the shortage had rather different causes than the current crisis in the availability of healthcare professionals. Although the costs of obtaining medical training were relatively low, the demand for doctors' services also was very small, since many of the services provided by physicians also could be obtained from experienced amateurs in the community. The home was typically the site for treatment and recuperation, and relatives and neighbors constituted an able and willing nursing staff. Babies were delivered by midwives, and those illnesses not cured by home remedies were left to run their natural, albeit frequently fatal, course. The contrast with contemporary healthcare practices in which specialized physicians and nurses located within hospitals provide critical diagnostic and treatment services is dramatic.

The changes that have occurred within medical science originated in the rapid developments that took place in the applied sciences (i.e., chemistry, physics, engineering, microbiology, physiology, pharmacology, etc.) at the turn of the twentieth century. This process of development was characterized by intense interdisciplinary cross-fertilization, which provided an environment in which medical research was able to take giant strides in developing techniques for the diagnosis and treatment of diseases. For example, in 1903, Willem Einthoven, a Dutch physiologist, devised the first electrocardiograph to measure the electrical activity of the heart. In applying discoveries in the physical sciences to the analysis of the biological process, he initiated a new age in both cardiovascular medicine and electrical measurement techniques.

New discoveries in medical sciences followed one another like intermediates in a chain reaction. However, the most significant innovation for clinical medicine was the development of x-rays. These "new kinds of rays," as W. K. Roentgen described them in 1895, opened the "inner man" to medical inspection. Initially, x-rays were used to diagnose bone fractures and dislocations, and in the process, x-ray machines became commonplace in most urban hospitals. Separate departments of radiology were established, and their influence spread to other departments throughout the hospital. By the 1930s, x-ray visualization of practically all organ systems of the body had been made possible through the use of barium salts and a wide variety of radiopaque materials.

X-ray technology gave physicians a powerful tool that, for the first time, permitted accurate diagnosis of a wide variety of diseases and injuries. Moreover, since x-ray machines were too cumbersome and expensive for local doctors and clinics, they had to be placed in healthcare centers or hospitals. Once there, x-ray technology essentially triggered the transformation of the hospital from a passive receptacle for the sick to an active curative institution for all members of society.

For economic reasons, the centralization of healthcare services became essential because of many other important technological innovations appearing on the medical scene. However, hospitals remained institutions to dread, and it was not until the introduction of sulfanilamide in the mid-1930s and penicillin in the early 1940s that the main danger of hospitalization, that is, cross-infection among patients, was significantly reduced. With these new drugs in their arsenals, surgeons were able to perform their operations without prohibitive morbidity and mortality due to infection. Furthermore, even though the different blood groups and their incompatibility were discovered in 1900 and sodium citrate was used in 1913 to prevent clotting, full development of blood banks was not practical until the 1930s, when technology provided adequate refrigeration. Until that time, "fresh" donors were bled and the blood transfused while it was still warm.

Once these surgical suites were established, the employment of specifically designed pieces of medical technology assisted in further advancing the development of complex surgical procedures. For example, the Drinker respirator was introduced in 1927 and the first heart–lung bypass in 1939. By the 1940s, medical procedures heavily dependent on medical technology, such as cardiac catheterization and angiography (the use of a cannula threaded through an arm vein and into the heart with the injection of radiopaque dye) for the x-ray visualization of congenital and acquired heart disease (mainly valve disorders due to rheumatic fever) became possible, and a new era of cardiac and vascular surgery was established.

In the decades following World War II, technological advances were spurred on by efforts to develop superior weapon systems and to establish habitats in space and on the ocean floor. As a by-product of these efforts, the development of medical devices accelerated and the medical profession benefited greatly from this rapid surge of technological finds. Consider the following examples:

1. Advances in solid-state electronics made it possible to map the subtle behavior of the fundamental unit of the central nervous system—the neuron—as well as to monitor the various physiological parameters, such as the electrocardiogram, of patients in intensive care units.
2. New prosthetic devices became a goal of engineers involved in providing the disabled with tools to improve their quality of life.
3. Nuclear medicine—an outgrowth of the atomic age—emerged as a powerful and effective approach in detecting and treating specific physiological abnormalities.
4. Diagnostic ultrasound based on sonar technology became so widely accepted that ultrasonic studies are now part of the routine diagnostic workup in many medical specialties.
5. "Spare parts" surgery also became commonplace. Technologists were encouraged to provide cardiac assist devices, such as artificial heart valves and artificial blood vessels, and the artificial heart program was launched to develop a replacement for a defective or diseased human heart.
6. Advances in materials have made the development of disposable medical devices, such as needles and thermometers, a reality.
7. Advancements in molecular engineering have allowed for the discovery of countless pharmacological agents and to the design of their delivery, including implantable delivery systems.
8. Computers similar to those developed to control the flight plans of the Apollo capsule were used to store, process, and cross-check medical records, to monitor patient status in intensive care units, and to provide sophisticated statistical diagnoses of potential diseases correlated with specific sets of patient symptoms.
9. Development of the first computer-based medical instrument, the computerized axial tomography scanner, revolutionized clinical approaches to noninvasive diagnostic imaging procedures, which now include magnetic resonance imaging and positron emission tomography as well.
10. A wide variety of new cardiovascular technologies including implantable defibrillators and chemically treated stents were developed.
11. Neuronal pacing systems were used to detect and prevent epileptic seizures.
12. Artificial organs and tissue have been created.
13. The completion of the genome project has stimulated the search for new biological markers and personalized medicine.
14. The further understanding of cellular and biomolecular processes has led to the engineering of stem cells into therapeutically valuable lineages and to the regeneration of organs and tissue structures.

15. Developments in nanotechnology have yielded nanomaterials for use in tissue engineering and facilitated the creation and study of nanoparticles and molecular machine systems that will assist in the detection and treatment of disease and injury.

The impact of these discoveries and many others has been profound. The healthcare system of today consists of technologically sophisticated clinical staff operating primarily in modern hospitals designed to accommodate the new medical technology. This evolutionary process continues, with advances in the physical sciences such as materials and nanotechnology and in the life sciences such as molecular biology, genomics, stem cell biology, and artificial and regenerated tissue and organs. These advances have altered and will continue to alter the very nature of the healthcare delivery system itself.

Biomedical Engineering: A Definition

Bioengineering is usually defined as a basic research-oriented activity closely related to biotechnology and genetic engineering, that is, the modification of animal or plant cells or parts of cells to improve plants or animals or to develop new microorganisms for beneficial ends. In the food industry, for example, this has meant the improvement of strains of yeast for fermentation. In agriculture, bioengineers may be concerned with the improvement of crop yields by treatment of plants with organisms to reduce frost damage. It is clear that future bioengineers will have a tremendous impact on the quality of human life. The potential of this specialty is difficult to imagine. Consider the following activities of bioengineers:

- Development of improved species of plants and animals for food production
- Invention of new medical diagnostic tests for diseases
- Production of synthetic vaccines from clone cells
- Bioenvironmental engineering to protect human, animal, and plant life from toxicants and pollutants
- Study of protein–surface interactions
- Modeling of the growth kinetics of yeast and hybridoma cells
- Research in immobilized enzyme technology
- Development of therapeutic proteins and monoclonal antibodies

Biomedical engineers, on the other hand, apply electrical, mechanical, chemical, optical, and other engineering principles to understand, modify, or control biological (i.e., human and animal) systems as well as design and manufacture products that can monitor physiological functions and assist in the diagnosis and treatment of patients. When biomedical engineers work in a hospital or clinic, they are more aptly called clinical engineers.

Activities of Biomedical Engineers

The breadth of activity of biomedical engineers is now significant. The field has moved from being concerned primarily with the development of medical instruments in the 1950s and 1960s to include a more wide-ranging set of activities. As illustrated below, the field of biomedical engineering now includes many new career areas (see Figure P.1), each of which is presented in this handbook. These areas include

- Application of engineering system analysis (physiological modeling, simulation, and control) to biological problems
- Detection, measurement, and monitoring of physiological signals (i.e., biosensors and biomedical instrumentation)
- Diagnostic interpretation via signal-processing techniques of bioelectric data
- Therapeutic and rehabilitation procedures and devices (rehabilitation engineering)
- Devices for replacement or augmentation of bodily functions (artificial organs)

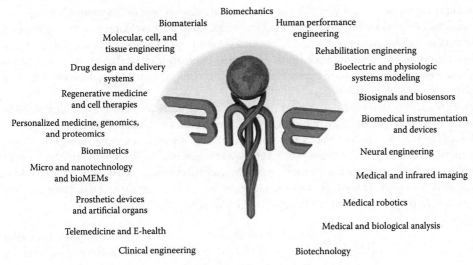

FIGURE P.1 The world of biomedical engineering.

- Computer analysis of patient-related data and clinical decision making (i.e., medical informatics and artificial intelligence)
- Medical imaging, that is, the graphic display of anatomic detail or physiological function
- The creation of new biological products (e.g., biotechnology and tissue engineering)
- The development of new materials to be used within the body (biomaterials)

Typical pursuits of biomedical engineers, therefore, include

- Research in new materials for implanted artificial organs
- Development of new diagnostic instruments for blood analysis
- Computer modeling of the function of the human heart
- Writing software for analysis of medical research data
- Analysis of medical device hazards for safety and efficacy
- Development of new diagnostic imaging systems
- Design of telemetry systems for patient monitoring
- Design of biomedical sensors for measurement of human physiological systems variables
- Development of expert systems for diagnosis of disease
- Design of closed-loop control systems for drug administration
- Modeling of the physiological systems of the human body
- Design of instrumentation for sports medicine
- Development of new dental materials
- Design of communication aids for the handicapped
- Study of pulmonary fluid dynamics
- Study of the biomechanics of the human body
- Development of material to be used as a replacement for human skin

Biomedical engineering, then, is an interdisciplinary branch of engineering that ranges from theoretical, nonexperimental undertakings to state-of-the-art applications. It can encompass research, development, implementation, and operation. Accordingly, like medical practice itself, it is unlikely that any single person can acquire expertise that encompasses the entire field. Yet, because of the interdisciplinary nature of this activity, there is considerable interplay and overlapping of interest and effort between them. For example, biomedical engineers engaged in the development of biosensors may interact with those interested in prosthetic devices to develop a means to detect and use the same bio-electric signal to power a prosthetic device. Those engaged in automating clinical chemistry laboratories may collaborate with those developing expert systems to assist clinicians in making decisions based on specific laboratory data. The possibilities are endless.

Perhaps, a greater potential benefit occurring from the use of biomedical engineering is identification of the problems and needs of our present healthcare system that can be solved using existing engineering technology and systems methodology. Consequently, the field of biomedical engineering offers hope in the continuing battle to provide high-quality care at a reasonable cost. If properly directed toward solving problems related to preventive medical approaches, ambulatory care services, and the like, biomedical engineers can provide the tools and techniques to make our healthcare system more effective and efficient and, in the process, improve the quality of life for all.

Joseph D. Bronzino
Donald R. Peterson
Editors-in-Chief

Editors

Joseph D. Bronzino is currently the president of the Biomedical Engineering Alliance and Consortium (BEACON; www.beaconalliance.org), which is a nonprofit organization dedicated to the promotion of collaborative research, translation, and partnership among academic, medical, and industry people in the field of biomedical engineering to develop new medical technologies and devices. To accomplish this goal, Dr. Bronzino and BEACON facilitate collaborative research, industrial partnering, and the development of emerging companies. Dr. Bronzino earned a BSEE from Worcester Polytechnic Institute, Worcester, Massachusetts, in 1959, an MSEE from the Naval Postgraduate School, Monterey, California, in 1961, and a PhD in electrical engineering from Worcester Polytechnic Institute in 1968. He was recently the Vernon Roosa Professor of Applied Science and endowed chair at Trinity College, Hartford, Connecticut.

Dr. Bronzino is the author of over 200 journal articles and 15 books, including *Technology for Patient Care* (C.V. Mosby, 1977), *Computer Applications for Patient Care* (Addison-Wesley, 1982), *Biomedical Engineering: Basic Concepts and Instrumentation* (PWS Publishing Co., 1986), *Expert Systems: Basic Concepts* (Research Foundation of State University of New York, 1989), *Medical Technology and Society: An Interdisciplinary Perspective* (MIT Press and McGraw-Hill, 1990), *Management of Medical Technology* (Butterworth/Heinemann, 1992), *The Biomedical Engineering Handbook* (CRC Press, 1st Edition, 1995; 2nd Edition, 2000; 3rd Edition, 2006), *Introduction to Biomedical Engineering* (Academic Press, 1st Edition, 1999; 2nd Edition, 2005; 3rd Edition, 2011), *Biomechanics: Principles and Applications* (CRC Press, 2002), *Biomaterials: Principles and Applications* (CRC Press, 2002), *Tissue Engineering* (CRC Press, 2002), and *Biomedical Imaging* (CRC Press, 2002).

Dr. Bronzino is a fellow of IEEE and the American Institute of Medical and Biological Engineering (AIMBE), an honorary member of the Italian Society of Experimental Biology, past chairman of the Biomedical Engineering Division of the American Society for Engineering Education (ASEE), a charter member of the Connecticut Academy of Science and Engineering (CASE), a charter member of the American College of Clinical Engineering (ACCE), a member of the Association for the Advancement of Medical Instrumentation (AAMI), past president of the IEEE-Engineering in Medicine and Biology Society (EMBS), past chairman of the IEEE Health Care Engineering Policy Committee (HCEPC), and past chairman of the IEEE Technical Policy Council in Washington, DC. He is a member of Eta Kappa Nu, Sigma Xi, and Tau Beta Pi. He is also a recipient of the IEEE Millennium Medal for "his contributions to biomedical engineering research and education" and the Goddard Award from WPI for Outstanding Professional Achievement in 2005. He is presently editor-in-chief of the Academic Press/Elsevier BME Book Series.

Donald R. Peterson is a professor of engineering and the dean of the College of Science, Technology, Engineering, Mathematics, and Nursing at Texas A&M University in Texarkana, Texas, and holds a joint appointment in the Department of Biomedical Engineering (BME) at Texas A&M University in College Station, Texas. He was recently an associate professor of medicine and the director of the

Biodynamics Laboratory in the School of Medicine at the University of Connecticut (UConn) and served as chair of the BME Program in the School of Engineering at UConn as well as the director of the BME Graduate and Undergraduate Programs. Dr. Peterson earned a BS in aerospace engineering and a BS in biomechanical engineering from Worcester Polytechnic Institute, in Worcester, Massachusetts, in 1992, an MS in mechanical engineering from the UConn, in Storrs, Connecticut, in 1995, and a PhD in biomedical engineering from UConn in 1999. He has 17 years of experience in BME education and has offered graduate-level and undergraduate-level courses in the areas of biomechanics, biodynamics, biofluid mechanics, BME communication, BME senior design, and ergonomics, and has taught subjects such as gross anatomy, occupational biomechanics, and occupational exposure and response in the School of Medicine. Dr. Peterson was also recently the co-executive director of the Biomedical Engineering Alliance and Consortium (BEACON), which is a nonprofit organization dedicated to the promotion of collaborative research, translation, and partnership among academic, medical, and industry people in the field of biomedical engineering to develop new medical technologies and devices.

Dr. Peterson has over 21 years of experience in devices and systems and in engineering and medical research, and his work on human–device interaction has led to applications on the design and development of several medical devices and tools. Other recent translations of his research include the development of devices such as robotic assist devices and prosthetics, long-duration biosensor monitoring systems, surgical and dental instruments, patient care medical devices, spacesuits and space tools for NASA, powered and non-powered hand tools, musical instruments, sports equipment, computer input devices, and so on. Other overlapping research initiatives focus on the development of computational models and simulations of biofluid dynamics and biomechanical performance, cell mechanics and cellular responses to fluid shear stress, human exposure and response to vibration, and the acoustics of hearing protection and communication. He has also been involved clinically with the Occupational and Environmental Medicine group at the UConn Health Center, where his work has been directed toward the objective engineering analysis of the anatomic and physiological processes involved in the onset of musculoskeletal and neuromuscular diseases, including strategies of disease mitigation.

Dr. Peterson's scholarly activities include over 50 published journal articles, 2 textbook chapters, 2 textbook sections, and 12 textbooks, including his new appointment as co-editor-in-chief for *The Biomedical Engineering Handbook* by CRC Press.

Contributors

Kai-Nan An
Mayo Clinic
Rochester, Minnesota

I. Arcos
Alfred Mann Foundation for Scientific
   Research
Valencia, California

Berj L. Bardakjian
University of Toronto
Toronto, Ontario, Canada

Roger C. Barr
Department of Biomedical Engineering
and
Department of Pediatrics
Duke University
Durham, North Carolina

A. Barriskill
Neopraxis Pty. Ltd.
North South Wales, Australia

Aaron P. Batista
Department of Bioengineering
Swanson School of Engineering
University of Pittsburgh
and
Carnegie Mellon University
Pittsburgh, Pennsylvania

Mostafa Belghasem
Department of Pathology and Laboratory
   Medicine
Boston University School of Medicine
Boston, Massachusetts

Edward J. Berbari
Indiana University–Purdue University,
   Indianapolis
Indianapolis, Indiana

R. Betz
Shriners Hospital for Children
Philadelphia, Pennsylvania

W. G. Billotte
Department of Biology
University of Dayton
Dayton, Ohio

Bernardo Boleaga
CTScanner de México
Mexico City, Mexico

Joseph D. Bronzino
Trinity College
Hartford, Connecticut

K. J. L. Burg
Department of Bioengineering
Clemson University
Clemson, South Carolina

Thomas J. Burkholder
School of Applied Physiology
Georgia Institute of Technology
Atlanta, Georgia

Thomas R. Canfield
Argonne National Laboratory
Argonne, Illinois

K. B. Chandran
Department of Biomedical Engineering
University of Iowa
Iowa City, Iowa

C. C. Chu
Department of Fiber Science and Apparel
 Design
Cornell University
Ithaca, New York

Ben M. Clopton
Advanced Cochlear Systems
Snoqualmie, Washington

Ross Davis
Florida Institute of Technology
Melbourne, Florida

Roy B. Davis III
Motion Analysis Laboratory
Shriners Hospitals for Children
Greenville, South Carolina

Peter A. DeLuca
Center for Motion Analysis
Connecticut Children's Medical Center
Farmington, Connecticut

Daniel J. DiLorenzo
Neurosurgery Department
University of Texas Medical Branch
Galveston, Texas

and

NeuroVista Corporation
and
DiLorenzo Biomedical, LLC
Seattle, Washington

Philip B. Dobrin
Hines VA Hospital
Hines, Illinois

and

Loyola University Medical Center
Maywood, Illinois

Cathryn R. Dooly
Department of Physical Education
Lander University
Greenwood, South Carolina

Dominique M. Durand
Department of Biomedical Engineering
Case Western Reserve University
Cleveland, Ohio

Michael J. Furey
Department of Mechanical Engineering
Virginia Polytechnic Institute and
 State University
Blacksburg, Virginia

Vijay K. Goel
Department of Bioengineering
University of Toledo
Toledo, Ohio

Wally Grant
Department of Biomedical Engineering
and
Department of Engineering Science and
 Mechanics
College of Engineering
Virginia Polytechnic Institute and State
 University
Blacksburg, Virginia

Daniel Graupe
University of Illinois at Chicago
Urbana, Illinois

Robert J. Greenberg
Second Sight Inc.
Sylmar, California

Warren M. Grill
Department of Biomedical Engineering
Duke University
Durham, North Carolina

Robert E. Gross
Emory University
Atlanta, Georgia

Alan R. Hargens
Department of Orthopaedic Surgery
UCSD Medical Center
University of California, San Diego
San Diego, California

Joel M. Henderson
Department of Pathology and Laboratory
    Medicine
Boston University School of Medicine
Boston Medical Center
and
Department of Biomedical Engineering
Boston University College of Engineering
Boston, Massachusetts

Robert M. Hochmuth
Department of Mechanical Engineering and
    Materials Science
Duke University
Durham, North Carolina

T. Houdayer
Neural Engineering Clinic
Augusta, Maine

Ben F. Hurley
University of Maryland
Baltimore, Maryland

Fiacro Jiménez
Mexico City General Hospital
Stereotaxic and Functional Neurosurgery Unit
Mexico City, Mexico

Arthur T. Johnson
University of Maryland
Baltimore, Maryland

Christopher R. Johnson
Scientific Computing and Imaging
    Institute
University of Utah
Salt Lake City, Utah

T. Johnston
Shriners Hospital for Children
Philadelphia, Pennsylvania

David L. Kaplan
Department of Biomedical
    Engineering
Tufts University
Medford, Massachusetts

J. Lawrence Katz (deceased)
Department of Biomedical
    Engineering
Case School of Engineering and School of Medicine
and
Department of Oral and Maxillofacial
    Surgery
School of Dental Medicine
Case Western Reserve University
Cleveland, Ohio

and

Department of Mechanical Engineering
    and Surgery, Orthopedics
Schools of Engineering and
    Medicine
University of Kansas
Lawrence, Kansas

Kenton R. Kaufman
Mayo Clinic
Rochester, Minnesota

Philip R. Kennedy
Neural Signals Inc
Duluth, Georgia

Roy C. P. Kerckhoffs
School of Bioengineering
Institute of Engineering in Medicine
University of California, San Diego
La Jolla, California

Gilson Khang
Department of BIN Fusion
    Technology
Chonbuk National University
Jeonju, South Korea

Young Kon Kim
Inje University
Gimhae, South Korea

Albert I. King
Wayne State University
Detroit, Michigan

Mauricio Kuri
CTScanner de México
Mexico City, Mexico

Roderic S. Lakes
Departments of Engineering Physics, Materials
    Science, and Biomedical Engineering
University of Wisconsin
Madison, Wisconsin

Christopher G. Lausted
Institute for Systems Biology
Seattle, Washington

Hai Bang Lee
Biomaterials Laboratory
Korea Research Institute of Chemical Technology
Daejeon, South Korea

Jin Ho Lee
Department of Advanced Materials
Hannam University
Daejeon, South Korea

Shu-Tung Li
Collagen Matrix Inc.
Oakland, New Jersey

Baruch B. Lieber
Department of Neurosurgery
State University of New York at Stony Brook
Stony Brook, New York

Richard L. Lieber
Departments of Orthopaedics, Radiology and
    Bioengineering
Biomedical Sciences Graduate Group
University of California, San Diego
and
Veterans Administration Medical Centers
La Jolla, California

Adolfo Llinás
Department of Orthopaedics and Traumatology
Fundacion Santafe de Bogota University
    Hospital
Fundacion Cosme and Damian
and
Universidad de los Andes
Bogota, Colombia

Jaakko Malmivuo
Aalto University
Helsinki, Finland

Biman Mandal
Department of Biomedical Engineering
Tufts University
Medford, Massachusetts

Orestes Marangos
Bioengineering Research Center
School of Engineering
University of Kansas
Lawrence, Kansas

Andrew D. McCulloch
School of Bioengineering
Institute of Engineering in Medicine
University of California, San Diego
La Jolla, California

Melissa K. McHale
Department of Bioengineering
Rice University
Houston, Texas

Evangelia Micheli-Tzanakou (deceased)
Department of Biomedical Engineering
Rutgers University
Piscataway, New Jersey

Anil Misra
Department of Civil Engineering
School of Engineering
University of Kansas
Lawrence, Kansas

P. Mobley
Alfred Mann Foundation for Scientific
    Research
Valencia, California

Jong-Hoon Nam
Department of Biomedical Engineering
and
Department of Mechanical Engineering
Hajim School of Engineering and Applied
    Sciences
University of Rochester
Rochester, New York

Sanjeev D. Nandedkar
Natus Medical Inc.
New York

José María Núñez
Mexico City General Hospital
Stereotaxic and Functional
    Neurosurgery Unit
Mexico City, Mexico

Sylvia Õunpuu
Center for Motion Analysis
Connecticut Children's Medical Center
Farmington, Connecticut

Muralidhar Padala
Division of Cardiothoracic Surgery
Emory University School of Medicine
Atlanta, Georgia

Joon B. Park
Department of Biomedical
    Engineering
University of Iowa
Iowa City, Iowa

Sang-Hyun Park
Tissue Healing Laboratory
Orthopedic Hospital
and
Department of Orthopaedics
University of California, Los Angeles
Los Angeles, California

Roland N. Pittman
Department of Physiology and Biophysics
Medical College of Virginia Campus
Virginia Commonwealth University
Richmond, Virginia

Robert Plonsey
Department of Biomedical Engineering
Duke University
Durham, North Carolina

Andrew E. Pollard
Department of Biomedical Engineering
University of Alabama at Birmingham
Birmingham, Alabama

Aleksander S. Popel
Department of Biomedical Engineering
School of Medicine
Johns Hopkins University
Baltimore, Maryland

Sunil Puria
Department of Mechanical Engineering
and
Department of Otolaryngology-HNS
Stanford University
Stanford, California

Bradley J. Roth
Department of Physics
Oakland University
Rochester, Michigan

Yiftach Roth
New Advanced Technology Center
Sheba Medical Center
Tel-Hashomer, Israel

Carl F. Rothe
Department of Cellular and Integrative
    Physiology
School of Medicine
Indiana University
Indianapolis, Indiana

Geert W. Schmid-Schönbein
Department of Bioengineering
University of California, San Diego
La Jolla, California

Daniel J. Schneck
Virginia Polytechnic Institute and State
    University
Blacksburg, Virginia

J. Schulman
Alfred Mann Foundation for Scientific
    Research
Valencia, California

S. W. Shalaby (deceased)
Poly-Med, Inc.
Anderson, South Carolina

Artin A. Shoukas
Department of Biomedical Engineering
School of Medicine
Johns Hopkins University
Baltimore, Maryland

B. Smith
Shriners Hospital for Children
Philadelphia, Pennsylvania

Alexander A. Spector
Department of Biomedical Engineering
School of Medicine
Johns Hopkins University
Baltimore, Maryland

Paulette Spencer
Department of Mechanical Engineering
Bioengineering Research Center
School of Engineering
University of Kansas
Lawrence, Kansas

Erin Spinner
School of Biomedical Engineering
Georgia Institute of Technology
Atlanta, Georgia

Charles R. Steele
Department of Mechanical Engineering
Stanford University
Stanford, California

George D. Stetten
University of Pittsburgh
and
Carnegie Mellon University
Pittsburgh, Pennsylvania

Roger Tran-Son-Tay
University of Florida
Gainesville, Florida

A. van Oosterom
Radboud University Nijmegen
Nijmegen, The Netherlands

Anthony Varghese
Department of Computer Science
University of Wisconsin, River Falls
River Falls, Wisconsin

Ana Luisa Velasco
Mexico City General Hospital
Stereotaxic and Functional
    Neurosurgery Unit
Mexico City, Mexico

Francisco Velasco
Mexico City General Hospital
Stereotaxic and Functional Neurosurgery Unit
Mexico City, Mexico

Marcos Velasco
Mexico City General Hospital
Stereotaxic and Functional Neurosurgery Unit
Mexico City, Mexico

David C. Viano
Wayne State University
Detroit, Michigan

Herbert F. Voigt
Boston University
Boston, Massachusetts

Samuel R. Ward
Departments of Orthopaedics, Radiology and
    Bioengineering
Biomedical Sciences Graduate Group
University of California, San Diego
and
Veterans Administration Medical Centers
La Jolla, California

Richard E. Waugh
Department of Biomedical Engineering
University of Rochester
Rochester, New York

Jennifer L. West
Department of Bioengineering
Rice University
Houston, Texas

J. Wolfe
Alfred Mann Foundation for Scientific
    Research
Valencia, California

Choon Hwai Yap
School of Biomedical Engineering
Georgia Institute of Technology
Atlanta, Georgia

Qiang Ye
Bioengineering Research Center
School of Engineering
University of Kansas
Lawrence, Kansas

Ajit P. Yoganathan
School of Biomedical Engineering
Georgia Institute of Technology
Atlanta, Georgia

Abraham Zangen
Department of Neurobiology
Weizmann Institute of Science
Rehovot, Israel

MATLAB Statement

MATLAB® and Simulink® are registered trademarks of The MathWorks, Inc. For product information, please contact:

The MathWorks, Inc.
3 Apple Hill Drive
Natick, MA 01760-2098 USA
Tel: 508 647 7000
Fax: 508-647-7001
E-mail: info@mathworks.com
Web: www.mathworks.com

I

Physiologic Systems

Herbert F. Voigt
Boston University

1 An Outline of Cardiovascular Structure and Function *Daniel J. Schneck* 1-1
Working Fluid: Blood • Pumping Station: The Heart • Piping Network: Blood
Vessels • Cardiovascular Control • Defining Terms • Acknowledgments • References

2 Kidney Structure and Physiology *Joel M. Henderson and Mostafa Belghasem* 2-1
Introduction • Kidney Anatomy • Vasculature of the Kidney • Architecture
of the Nephron • Structure of the Glomerulus and the Glomerular
Filtration Barrier • Mechanical Properties of the Glomerulus • Glomerular
Filtration • Factors Governing Glomerular Filtration • Permselectivity of the
Glomerular Barrier • Tubulo-Interstitial Structure and Organization • Solute Recovery
from the Ultrafiltrate • Water Reabsorption and Its Regulation • Endocrine Function of
Kidney • Assessment of Kidney Function • References

3 Nervous System *Evangelia Micheli-Tzanakou* 3-1
Definitions • Functions of the Nervous System • Representation of Information
in the Nervous System • Lateral Inhibition • Higher Functions of the Nervous
System • Abnormalities of the Nervous System • References

4 Vision System *Aaron P. Batista and George D. Stetten* 4-1
Fundamentals of Vision Research • A Modular View of the Vision System • Eye
Movements • Defining Terms • References • Further Reading

5 Auditory System *Ben M. Clopton and Herbert F. Voigt* 5-1
Overview • Peripheral Auditory System • Central Auditory
System • Pathologies • Further Topics • References

6 Gastrointestinal System *Berj L. Bardakjian* 6-1
Introduction • GI Electrical Oscillations • A Historical
Perspective • The Stomach • The Small Intestine • The
Colon • Epilogue • Acknowledgments • References

7 Respiratory System *Arthur T. Johnson, Christopher G. Lausted,*
and Joseph D. Bronzino 7-1
Respiration Anatomy • Lung Volumes and Gas Exchange • Perfusion of the Lung • Gas
Partial Pressure • Pulmonary Mechanics • Respiratory Control • Pulmonary Function
Laboratory • Defining Terms • References • Further Reading

An Outline of Cardiovascular Structure and Function

1.1 Working Fluid: Blood... 1-1
1.2 Pumping Station: The Heart 1-3
1.3 Piping Network: Blood Vessels... 1-7
1.4 Cardiovascular Control 1-11
Defining Terms 1-12
Acknowledgments.. 1-13
References.. 1-13

Daniel J. Schneck
Virginia Polytechnic Institute and State University

Since not every cell in the human body is near enough to the environment to easily exchange its mass (including nutrients, oxygen, carbon dioxide, and the waste products of metabolism), energy (including heat), and momentum, the physiologic system is endowed with a major highway network—organized to make available thousands of miles of access tubing for the transport to and from a different neighborhood (on the order of 10 μm or less) of any given cell whatever it needs to sustain life. This highway network, called the *cardiovascular system* (Schneck, 1990; Tortora and Grabowski, 1993), includes a pumping station, the heart; a working fluid, blood; a complex branching configuration of distributing and collecting pipes and channels, blood vessels; and a sophisticated means for both intrinsic (inherent) and extrinsic (autonomic and endocrine) control.

1.1 Working Fluid: Blood

Accounting for about $8 \pm 1\%$ of the total body weight, averaging 5200 mL, blood is a complex, heterogeneous suspension of formed elements—the *blood cells*, or *hematocytes*—suspended in a continuous, straw-colored fluid called *plasma*. Nominally, the composite fluid has a mass density of 1.057 ± 0.007 g/cm^3, and it is 3–6 times as viscous as water. The hematocytes (Table 1.1) include three basic types of cells: red blood cells (erythrocytes, totaling nearly 95% of the formed elements), white blood cells (leukocytes, averaging <0.15% of all hematocytes), and platelets (thrombocytes, on the order of 5% of all blood cells). All hematocytes are derived in the active ("red") bone marrow (about 1500 g) of adults from undifferentiated stem cells called *hemocytoblasts*, and all reach ultimate maturity via a process called *hematocytopoiesis*.

The primary function of erythrocytes is to aid in the transport of blood gases—about 30–34% (by weight) of each cell consisting of the oxygen- and carbon dioxide-carrying protein hemoglobin ($64,000 \leq$ MW $\leq 68,000$) and a small portion of the cell containing the enzyme carbonic anhydrase, which catalyzes the reversible formation of carbonic acid from carbon dioxide and water. The primary function of leukocytes is to endow the human body with the ability to identify and dispose of foreign

TABLE 1.1 Hematocytes

Cell Type	Number Cells per mm³ Blood[a]	Corpuscular Diameter (μm)[a]	Corpuscular Surface Area (μm²)[a]	Corpuscular Volume (μm³)[a]	Mass Density (g/cm³)[a]	Percent Water[a]	Percent Protein[a]	Percent Extractives[a,b]
Erythrocytes (red blood cells)	4.2–5.4 × 10⁶ ♀ 4.6–6.2 × 10⁶ ♂ (5 × 10⁶)	6–9 (7.5) Thickness 1.84–2.84 "Neck" 0.81–1.44	120–163 (140)	80–100 (90)	1.089–1.100 (1.098)	64–68 (66)	29–35 (32)	1.6–2.8 (2)
Leukocytes (white blood cells)	4000–11,000 (7500)	6–10	300–625	160–450	1.055–1.085	52–60 (56)	30–36 (33)	4–18 (11)
Granulocytes								
Neutrophils: 55–70% WBC (65%)	2–6 × 10³ (4875)	8–8.6 (8.3)	422–511 (467)	268–333 (300)	1.075–1.085 (1.080)	—	—	—
Eosinophils: 1–4% WBC (3%)	45–480 (225)	8–9 (8.5)	422–560 (491)	268–382 (321)	1.075–1.085 (1.080)	—	—	—
Basophils: 0–1.5% WBC (1%)	0–113 (75)	7.7–8.5 (8.1)	391–500 (445)	239–321 (278)	1.075–1.085 (1.080)	—	—	—
Agranulocytes								
Lymphocytes: 20–35% WBC (25%)	1000–4800 (1875)	6.75–7.34 (7.06)	300–372 (336)	161–207 (184)	1.055–1.070 (1.063)	—	—	—
Monocytes: 3–8% WBC (6%)	100–800 (450)	9–9.5 (9.25)	534–624 (579)	382–449 (414)	1.055–1.070 (1.063)	—	—	—
Thrombocytes (Platelets)	(1.4 ♂) 2.14 (♀) –5 × 10⁵ (2.675#10⁵)	2–4 (3) Thickness 0.9–1.3	16–35 (25)	5–10 (7.5)	1.04–1.06 (1.05)	60–68 (64)	32–40 (36)	Negligible

[a] Normal physiologic range, with "typical" value in parentheses.
[b] Extractives mostly include minerals (ash), carbohydrates, and fats (lipids).

substances (such as infectious organisms) that do not belong there—agranulocytes (lymphocytes and monocytes) essentially doing the "identifying" and granulocytes (neutrophils, basophils, and eosinophils) essentially doing the "disposing" (Beall et al., 1993). The primary function of platelets is to participate in the blood-clotting process.

The removal of all hematocytes from blood by centrifugation or other separating techniques leaves behind the aqueous (91% water by weight, 94.8% water by volume), saline (0.15 N) suspending medium called *plasma*, which has an average mass density of 1.035 ± 0.005 g/cm³ and a viscosity that is $1\frac{1}{2}$ times that of water. Some 6.5–8% by weight of plasma consists of the plasma proteins, of which there are three major types—albumin, the globulins, and fibrinogen—and several others of lesser prominence (Table 1.2) (Bhagavan, 1992).

The primary functions of albumin are to help maintain the osmotic (oncotic) transmural pressure differential that ensures proper mass exchange between the blood and the interstitial fluid at the capillary level and to serve as a transport-carrier molecule for several hormones and other small biochemical constituents (such as some metal ions). The primary function of the globulin class of proteins is to act as transport-carrier molecules (mostly of the α and β class) for large biochemical substances, such as fats (lipoproteins) and certain carbohydrates (muco- and glycoproteins) and heavy metals (mineraloproteins), and to work together with leukocytes in the body's immune system. The latter function is primarily the responsibility of the γ class of immunoglobulins, which have antibody activity. The primary function of fibrinogen is to work with thrombocytes in the formation of a blood clot—a process also aided by one of the most abundant of the lesser proteins, prothrombin (MW $\simeq$ 62,000).

Of the remaining 2% or so (by weight) of plasma, just under half (0.95%, or 983 mg/dL plasma) consists of minerals (inorganic ash), trace elements, and electrolytes, mostly the cations sodium, potassium, calcium, and magnesium and the anions chlorine, bicarbonate, phosphate, and sulfate—the latter three helping as buffers to maintain the fluid at a slightly alkaline pH between 7.35 and 7.45 (average 7.4) (Frausto da Silva and Williams, 1993). What is left, about 1087 mg of material per deciliter of plasma, includes (1) mainly (0.8% by weight) three major types of fat, that is, cholesterol (in a free and esterified form), phospholipid (a major ingredient of cell membranes), and triglyceride, with lesser amounts of the fat-soluble vitamins (A, D, E, and K), free fatty acids, and other lipids, and (2) "extractives" (0.25% by weight), of which about two-thirds includes glucose and other forms of carbohydrate, the remainder consisting of the water-soluble vitamins (B-complex and C), certain enzymes, nonnitrogenous and nitrogenous waste products of metabolism (including urea, creatine, and creatinine), and many smaller amounts of other biochemical constituents—the list seeming virtually endless (Lentner, 1984).

The removal of all hematocytes from the blood and the protein fibrinogen (by allowing the fluid to completely clot before centrifuging) leaves behind a clear fluid called *serum*, which has a density of about 1.018 ± 0.003 g/cm³ and a viscosity up to $1\frac{1}{2}$ times that of water. A glimpse of Tables 1.1 and 1.2, together with the very brief summary presented above, nevertheless gives the reader an immediate appreciation for why blood is often referred to as the "river of life." This river is made to flow through the vascular piping network by two central pumping stations arranged in series: the left and right sides of the human heart (Lentner, 1990).

1.2 Pumping Station: The Heart

Barely the size of the clenched fist of the individual in whom it resides—an inverted, conically shaped, and hollow muscular organ measuring 12–13 cm from the base (top) to the apex (bottom) and 7–8 cm at its widest point and weighing just under 0.75 lb (about 0.474% of the individual's body weight, or some 325 g)—the human heart occupies a small region between the third and sixth ribs in the central portion of the thoracic cavity of the body. It rests on the diaphragm, between the lower part of the two lungs, its base-to-apex axis leaning mostly toward the left side of the body and slightly forward. The heart is divided by a tough muscular wall—the interatrial–interventricular septum—into a somewhat crescent-shaped right side and cylindrically shaped left side (Figure 1.1), each being one

TABLE 1.2 Plasma

Constituent	Concentration Range (mg/dL Plasma)	Typical Plasma Value (mg/dL)	Molecular Weight Range	Typical Value	Typical Size (nm)
Total protein, 7% by weight	6400–8300	7245	21,000–1,200,000	—	—
Albumin (56% TP)	2800–5600	4057	66,500–69,000	69,000	15 × 4
α_1-Globulin (5.5% TP)	300–600	400	21,000–435,000	60,000	5–12
α_2-Globulin (7.5% TP)	400–900	542	100,000–725,000	200,000	50–500
β-Globulin (13% TP)	500–1230	942	90,000–1,200,000	100,000	18–50
γ-Globulin (12% TP)	500–1800	869	150,000–196,000	150,000	23 × 4
Fibrinogen (4% TP)	150–470	290	330,000–450,000	390,000	(50–60) × (3–8)
Other (2% TP)	70–210	145	70,000–1,000,000	200,000	(15–25) × (2–6)
Inorganic ash, 0.95% by weight	930–1140	983	20–100	—	—
(Radius)					
Sodium	300–340	325	—	22.98977	0.102 (Na^+)
Potassium	13–21	17	—	39.09800	0.138 (K^+)
Calcium	8.4–11.0	10	—	40.08000	0.099 (Ca^{2+})
Magnesium	1.5–3.0	2	—	24.30500	0.072 (Mg^{2+})
Chloride	336–390	369	—	35.45300	0.181 (Cl^-)
Bicarbonate	110–240	175	—	61.01710	0.163 (HCO_3^-)

Phosphate	2.7–4.5	3.6	—	95.97926	0.210 (HPO_4^{2-})
Sulfate	0.5–1.5	1.0	—	96.05760	0.230 (SO_4^{2-})
Other	0–100	80.4	20–100	-	0.1–0.3
Lipids (fats), 0.80% by weight	541–1000	828	44,000–3,200,000	= Lipoproteins	Up to 200 or more
Cholesterol (34% TL)	12–105 "free"	59	386.67	Contained mostly in intermediate to low-density lipoprotein (LDL) β-lipoproteins; higher in women	
	72–259 esterified	224			
	84–364 "total"	283			
Phospholipid (35% TL)	150–331	292	690–1010	Contained mainly in high-density lipoprotein (HDL) to very high-density lipoprotein (VHDL) α_1-lipoproteins	
Triglyceride (26% TL)	65–240	215	400–1370	Contained mainly in VLDL α_2-lipoproteins and chylomicrons	
Other (5% TL)	0–80	38	280–1500	Fat-soluble vitamins, prostaglandins, and fatty acids	
Extractives, 0.25% by weight	200–500	259	—	—	
Glucose	60–120, fasting	90	—	180.1572	0.86 D
Urea	20–30	25	—	60.0554	0.36 D
Carbohydrate	60–105	83	180.16–342.3	0.74–0.108 D	
Other	11–111	61	—	—	

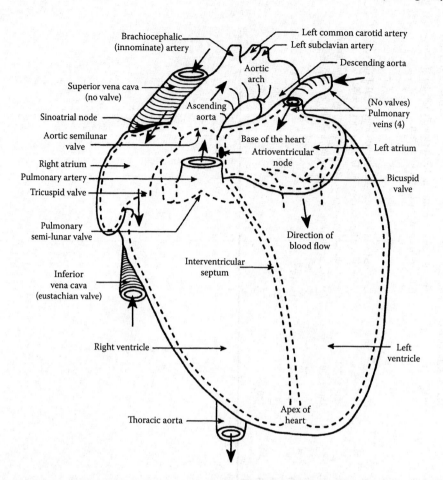

FIGURE 1.1 Anterior view of the human heart showing the four chambers, the inlet and outlet valves, the inlet and outlet major blood vessels, the wall separating the right side from the left side, and the two cardiac pacing centers—the sinoatrial node and the atrioventricular node. The boldface arrows show the direction of flow through the heart chambers, the valves, and the major vessels.

self-contained pumping station, but the two being connected in series. The left side of the heart drives oxygen-rich blood through the aortic semilunar outlet valve into the *systemic circulation*, which carries the fluid to within a differential neighborhood of each cell in the body—from which it returns to the right side of the heart low in oxygen and rich in carbon dioxide. The right side of the heart then drives this oxygen-poor blood through the pulmonary semilunar (pulmonic) outlet valve into the *pulmonary circulation*, which carries the fluid to the lungs—where its oxygen supply is replenished and its carbon dioxide content is purged before it returns to the left side of the heart to begin the cycle all over again. Because of the anatomic proximity of the heart to the lungs, the right side of the heart does not have to work very hard to drive blood through the pulmonary circulation; so, it functions as a low-pressure ($P \leq 40$ mmHg gauge) pump compared with the left side of the heart, which does most of its work at a high pressure (up to 140 mmHg gauge or more) to drive blood through the entire systemic circulation to the furthest extremes of the organism.

Each cardiac (heart) pump is further divided into two chambers: a small upper receiving chamber, or atrium (auricle), separated by a one-way valve from a lower discharging chamber, or ventricle, which is about twice the size of its corresponding atrium. In order of size, the somewhat spherically shaped left atrium is the smallest chamber—holding about 45 mL of blood (at rest), operating at pressures on the order of 0–25 mmHg gauge, and having a wall thickness of about 3 mm. The pouch-shaped right atrium is next (63 mL of blood, 0–10 mmHg gauge of pressure, and 2 mm wall thickness), followed by the conical/cylindrically shaped left ventricle (100 mL of blood, up to 140 mmHg gauge of pressure, and variable wall thickness up to 12 mm), and the crescent-shaped right ventricle (about 130 mL of blood, up to 40 mmHg gauge of pressure, and a wall thickness on the order of one-third that of the left ventricle, up to about 4 mm). Altogether, then, the heart chambers collectively have a capacity of some 325–350 mL, or about 6.5% of the total blood volume in a "typical" individual—but these values are nominal, since the organ alternately fills and expands, contracts, and then empties as it generates a *cardiac output* (CO).

During the 480 ms or so filling phase—diastole—of the average 750 ms cardiac cycle, the inlet valves of the two ventricles (3.8-cm-diameter tricuspid valve from the right atrium to the right ventricle, 3.1-cm-diameter bicuspid or mitral valve from the left atrium to the left ventricle) are open, and the outlet valves (2.4-cm-diameter pulmonary valve and 2.25-cm-diameter aortic semilunar valve, respectively) are closed—the heart ultimately expanding to its end-diastolic volume (EDV), which is on the order of 140 mL of blood for the left ventricle. During the 270 ms emptying phase—systole—an electrically induced vigorous contraction of the cardiac muscle drives the intraventricular pressure up, forcing the one-way inlet valves to close and the unidirectional outlet valves to open as the heart contracts to its end-systolic volume (ESV), which is typically on the order of 70 mL of blood for the left ventricle. Thus, the ventricles normally empty about half their contained volume with each heartbeat, the remainder being termed the *cardiac reserve volume*. More generally, the difference between the *actual* EDV and the *actual* ESV, called the *stroke volume* (SV), is the volume of blood expelled from the heart during each systolic interval, and the ratio of SV to EDV is called the *cardiac ejection fraction*, or *ejection ratio* (0.5–0.75 is normal, 0.4–0.5 signifies mild cardiac damage, 0.25–0.40 implies moderate heart damage, and <0.25 warns of severe damage to the heart's pumping ability). If the SV is multiplied by the number of systolic intervals per minute, or heart rate (HR), one obtains the total CO:

$$CO = HR \times (EDV - ESV) \tag{1.1}$$

Dawson (1991) has suggested that the CO (in milliliters per minute) is proportional to the weight W (in kilograms) of an individual according to the equation

$$CO = 224W^{3/4} \tag{1.2}$$

and that "normal" HR obeys very closely the relation

$$HR = 229W^{-1/4} \tag{1.3}$$

For a "typical" 68.7-kg individual (blood volume = 5200 mL), Equations 1.1 through 1.3 yield CO = 5345 mL/min, HR = 80 beats/min (cardiac cycle period = 754 ms), and SV = CO/HR = $224W^{3/4}$/$229W^{-1/4}$ = $0.978W$ = 67.2 mL/beat, which are very reasonable values. Furthermore, assuming this individual lives about 75 years, his or her heart will have cycled over 3.1536 billion times, pumping a total of 0.2107 billion liters of blood (55.665 million gallons, or 8134 quarts per day)—all of it emptying into the circulatory pathways that constitute the vascular system.

1.3 Piping Network: Blood Vessels

The vascular system is divided by a microscopic capillary network (Kaley and Altura, 1977, 1978, 1980) into an upstream, high-pressure, efferent arterial side (Table 1.3)—consisting of relatively thick-walled, viscoelastic tubes that carry blood away from the heart—and a downstream, low-pressure, afferent venous side (Table 1.4)—consisting of correspondingly thinner (but having a larger

TABLE 1.3 Arterial System[a]

Blood Vessel Type	(Systemic) Typical Number	Internal Diameter Range	Length Range[b]	Wall Thickness	Systemic Volume (mL)	(Pulmonary) Typical Number	Pulmonary Volume (mL)
Aorta	1	1.0–3.0 cm	30–65 cm	2–3 mm	156	—	—
Pulmonary artery	—	2.5–3.1 cm	6–9 cm	2–3 cm	—	1	52
Wall morphology: Complete tunica adventitia, external elastic lamina, tunica media, internal elastic lamina, tunica intima, subendothelium, endothelium, and vasa vasorum vascular supply							
Main branches	32	5 mm–2.25 cm	3.3–6 cm	≃2 mm	83.2	6	41.6
(Along with the aorta and pulmonary artery, the largest, most well developed of all blood vessels)							
Large arteries	288	4.0–5.0 mm	1.4–2.8 cm	≃1 mm	104	64	23.5
(A well-developed tunica adventitia and vasa vasorum although the wall layers are gradually thinning)							
Medium arteries	1152	2.5–4.0 mm	1.0–2.2 cm	≃0.75 mm	117	144	7.3
Small arteries	3456	1.0–2.5 mm	0.6–1.7 cm	≃0.50 mm	104	432	5.7
Tributaries	20,736	0.5–1.0 mm	0.3–1.3 cm	≃0.25 mm	91	5184	7.3
(A well-developed tunica media and external elastic lamina, but tunica adventitia is virtually nonexistent)							
Small rami	82,944	250–500 μm	0.2–0.8 cm	≃125 μm	57.2	11,664	2.3
Terminal branches	497,664	100–250 μm	1.0–6.0 mm	≃60 μm	52	139,968	3.0
(A well-developed endothelium, subendothelium, and internal elastic lamina, plus about two to three 15-μm-thick concentric layers forming just a very thin tunica media but no external elastic lamina)							
Arterioles	18,579,456	25–100 μm	0.2–3.8 mm	≃20–30 μm	52	4,094,064	2.3
Wall morphology: More than one smooth muscle layer (with nerve association in the outermost muscle layer), a well-developed internal elastic lamina, gradually thinning in 25- to 50-μm vessels to a single layer of smooth muscle tissue, connective tissue, and scant supporting tissue							
Metarterioles	238,878,720	10–25 μm	0.1–1.8 mm	≃5–15 μm	41.6	157,306,536	4.0
(A well-developed subendothelium, discontinuous contractile muscle elements, and one layer of connective tissue)							
Capillaries	16,124,431,360	3.5–10 μm	0.5–1.1 mm	≃0.5–1 μm	260	3,218,406,696	104
(Simple endothelial tubes devoid of smooth muscle tissue; one-cell-layer-thick walls)							

[a] Values are approximate for a 68.7-kg individual having a total blood volume of 5200 mL.

[b] Average uninterrupted distance between the branch origins (except the aorta and the pulmonary artery, which are total length).

TABLE 1.4   Venous System

Blood Vessel Type	(Systemic) Typical Number	Internal Diameter Range	Length Range	Wall Thickness	Systemic Volume (mL)	(Pulmonary) Typical Number	Pulmonary Volume (mL)
Postcapillary venules	4,408,161,734	8–30 μm	0.1–0.6 mm	1.0–5.0 μm	166.7	306,110,016	10.4
(The wall consists of thin endothelium exhibiting occasional pericytes (pericapillary connective tissue cells) that increase in number as the vessel's lumen gradually increases)							
Collecting venules	160,444,500	30–50 μm	0.1–0.8 mm	5.0–10 μm	161.3	8,503,056	1.2
(One complete layer of pericytes, one complete layer of veil-like cells [veil-like cells forming a thin membrane], and occasional primitive smooth muscle tissue fibers that increase in number with vessel size)							
Muscular venules	32,088,900	50–100 μm	0.2–1.0 mm	10–25 μm	141.8	3,779,136	3.7
(Relatively thick wall of smooth muscle tissue)							
Small collecting veins	10,241,508	100–200 μm	0.5–3.2 mm	≈30 μm	329.6	419,904	6.7
(Prominent tunica media of continuous layers of smooth muscle cells)							
Terminal branches	496,900	200–600 μm	1.0–6.0 mm	30–150 μm	206.6	34,992	5.2
(A well-developed endothelium, subendothelium, and internal elastic lamina; a well-developed tunica media but fewer elastic fibers than the corresponding arteries and much thinner walls)							
Small veins	19,968	600 μm–1.1 mm	2.0–9.0 mm	≈0.25 mm	63.5	17,280	44.9
Medium veins	512	1–5 mm	1–2 cm	≈0.50 mm	67.0	144	22.0
Large veins	256	5–9 mm	1.4–3.7 cm	≈0.75 mm	476.1	48	29.5
(Well-developed wall layers comparable to large arteries but about 25% thinner)							
Main branches	224	9.0 mm–2.0 cm	2.0–10 cm	≈1.00 mm	1538.1	16	39.4
(Along with the vena cava and pulmonary veins, the largest, most well-developed of all blood vessels)							
Vena cava	1	2.0–3.5 cm	20–50 cm	≈1.50 mm	125.3	—	—
Pulmonary veins	—	1.7–2.5 cm	5–8 cm	≈1.50 mm	—	4	52

Wall morphology: Essentially the same as comparable major arteries but a much thinner tunica intima, a much thinner tunica media, and a somewhat thicker tunica adventitia; contains a vasa vasorum

Total systemic blood volume: 4394 mL—84.5% of the total blood volume; 19.5% in arteries (~3:2 large:small), 5.9% in capillaries, and 74.6% in veins (~3:1 large:small); 63% of the volume is in vessels greater than 1 mm internal diameter.

Total pulmonary blood volume: 468 mL—9.0% of the total blood volume; 31.8% in arteries, 22.2% in capillaries, and 46% in veins; 58.3% of the volume is in vessels greater than 1 mm internal diameter; the remainder of the blood in the heart, about 338 mL (6.5% of the total blood volume).

caliber) elastic conduits that return blood back to the heart (Chandran, 1992). Except for their differences in thickness, the walls of the largest arteries and veins consist of the same three distinct, well-defined, and well-developed layers (Kessel and Kardon, 1979). From the innermost to the outermost, these layers are (1) the thinnest *tunica intima*, a continuous lining (the vascular endothelium) consisting of a single layer of simple squamous (thin, sheetlike) endothelial cells "glued" together by a polysaccharide (sugar) intercellular matrix, surrounded by a thin layer of subendothelial connective tissue interlaced with a number of circularly arranged elastic fibers to form the subendothelium, and separated from the next adjacent wall layer by a thick elastic band called the *internal elastic lamina*, (2) the thickest *tunica media*, composed of numerous circularly arranged elastic fibers, especially prevalent in the largest blood vessels on the arterial side (allowing them to expand during systole and to recoil passively during diastole), a significant amount of smooth muscle cells arranged in spiraling layers around the vessel wall, especially prevalent in medium-sized arteries and arterioles (allowing them to function as control points for blood distribution), and some interlacing collagenous connective tissue, elastic fibers, and intercellular mucopolysaccharide substance (extractives), all separated from the next adjacent wall layer by another thick elastic band called the *external elastic lamina*, and (3) the medium-sized *tunica adventitia*, an outer vascular sheath consisting entirely of connective tissue.

The largest blood vessels, such as the aorta, the pulmonary artery, the pulmonary veins, and others, have such thick walls that they require a separate network of tiny blood vessels—the vasa vasorum—just to service the vascular tissue itself. As one moves toward the capillaries from the arterial side (see Table 1.3), the vascular wall keeps thinning, as if it were shedding 15-μm-thick, onion-peel-like concentric layers and while the percentage of water in the vessel wall stays relatively constant at 70% (by weight), the ratio of elastin to collagen decreases (actually reverses)—from 3:2 in large arteries (9% elastin, 6% collagen, by weight) to 1:2 in small tributaries (5% elastin, 10% collagen)—and the amount of smooth muscle tissue increases from 7.5% by weight of large arteries (the remaining 7.5% consisting of various extractives) to 15% in small tributaries. By the time one reaches the capillaries, one encounters single-cell-thick endothelial tubes—devoid of any smooth muscle tissue, elastin, or collagen—downstream of which the vascular wall gradually "reassembles itself," layer by layer, as it directs blood back to the heart through the venous system (Table 1.4).

The blood vessel structure is directly related to function (Caro et al., 1978; Duck, 1990). The thick-walled large arteries and the main *distributing branches* are designed to withstand the pulsating 80–130 mmHg blood pressures that they must endure. The smaller elastic *conducting vessels* only need to operate under steadier blood pressures in the range 70–90 mmHg, but they must be thin enough to penetrate and course through organs without unduly disturbing the anatomic integrity of the mass involved. The controlling arterioles operate at blood pressures between 45 and 70 mmHg but are heavily endowed with smooth muscle tissue (hence, they are referred to as *muscular vessels*) so that they may be actively shut down when flow to the capillary bed they service is to be restricted (for whatever reason), and the smallest capillary *resistance vessels* (which operate at blood pressures on the order of 10–45 mmHg) are designed to optimize conditions for transport to occur between blood and the surrounding interstitial fluid. Traveling back up the venous side, one encounters relatively steady blood pressures continuously decreasing from around 30 mmHg all the way down to near zero; so, these vessels can be thin walled without disease consequence. However, the low blood pressure, slower, steady (time-independent) flow, thin walls, and larger caliber that characterize the venous system cause the blood to tend to "pool" in veins, allowing them to act somewhat like reservoirs. It is not surprising, then, that at any given instant, one normally finds about two-thirds of the total human blood volume residing in the venous system, the remaining one-third being divided among the heart (6.5%), the microcirculation (7% in the systemic and pulmonary capillaries), and the arterial system (19.5–20%).

In a global sense, then, one can think of the human cardiovascular system—using an electrical analogy—as a voltage source (the heart), two capacitors (a large venous system and a smaller arterial system), and a resistor (the microcirculation taken as a whole). Blood flow and the dynamics of the system represent electrical inductance (inertia), and useful engineering approximations can be derived from such a simple model. The cardiovascular system is designed to bring blood to within a capillary size of each and every one of the more than 10^{14} cells of the body—but *which* cells receive blood at any given time, *how much* blood they get, the *composition* of the fluid coursing by them, and related physiologic considerations are all matters that are not left up to chance.

1.4 Cardiovascular Control

Blood flows through organs and tissues either to nourish and sanitize them or to be itself processed in some sense—for example, to be oxygenated (pulmonary circulation), stocked with nutrients (splanchnic circulation), dialyzed (renal circulation), cooled (cutaneous circulation), filtered of dilapidated red blood cells (splenic circulation), and so on. Thus, any given vascular network normally receives blood according to the metabolic needs of the region it perfuses and/or the function of that region as a blood treatment plant and/or a thermoregulatory pathway (Schneck, 1990). However, it is not feasible to expect that our physiologic transport system can be "all things to all cells all of the time"—especially when resources are scarce and/or time is a factor. Thus, the distribution of blood is further prioritized according to three basic criteria: (1) how essential the perfused region is to the maintenance of life itself (e.g., we can survive without an arm, a leg, a stomach, or even a large portion of our small intestine but not without a brain, a heart, and at least one functioning kidney and lung, (2) how essential the perfused region is in allowing the organism to respond to a life-threatening situation (e.g., digesting a meal is among the least of the body's concerns in a "fight or flight" circumstance), and (3) how well the perfused region can function and survive on a decreased supply of blood (e.g., some tissues—such as striated skeletal and smooth muscle—have significant anaerobic capability; others—such as several forms of the connective tissue—can function quite effectively at a significantly decreased metabolic rate when necessary; some organs—such as the liver—are larger than they really need to be; and some anatomic structures—such as the eyes, ears, and limbs—have duplicates, giving them a built-in redundancy).

Within this generalized prioritization scheme, control of the cardiovascular function is accomplished by mechanisms that are based either on the inherent physicochemical attributes of the tissues and organs themselves—the so-called intrinsic control—or on responses that can be attributed to the effects on cardiovascular tissues of other organ systems in the body (most notably the autonomic nervous system and the endocrine system (Tortora and Grabowski, 1993))—the so-called extrinsic control. For example, both the accumulation of wastes and depletion of oxygen and nutrients that accompany the increased rate of metabolism in an active tissue lead to an *intrinsic* relaxation of the local precapillary sphincters (rings of the muscle)—with a consequent widening of the corresponding capillary entrances—which reduces the local resistance to flow and thereby allows more blood to perfuse the active region. On the other hand, the *extrinsic* innervation by the autonomic nervous system of smooth muscle tissues in the walls of arterioles allows the central nervous system to completely shutdown the flow to the entire vascular beds (such as the cutaneous circulation) when this becomes necessary (such as during exposure to extremely cold environments).

In addition to prioritizing and controlling the *distribution* of blood, the physiologic regulation of cardiovascular function is directed mainly at four other variables: CO, blood pressure, blood volume, and blood composition. From Equation 1.1, we see that CO can be increased by increasing the HR (a chronotropic effect), increasing the EDV (allowing the heart to fill longer by delaying the onset of systole), decreasing the ESV (an inotropic effect), or doing all three things at once. Indeed, under the extrinsic influence of the sympathetic nervous system and the adrenal glands, HR can triple—to some 240 beats/min if necessary—EDV can increase by as much as 50%—to around 200 mL or more of blood—and ESV can decrease a comparable amount (the cardiac reserve)—to about 30–35 mL or less. The combined result of all three effects can lead to over a sevenfold increase in CO—from the normal 5 to 5.5 L/min to as much as 40 to 41 L/min or more for very brief periods of strenuous exertion.

The control of blood pressure is accomplished mainly by adjusting the downstream resistance to flow at the arteriolar level—an increased resistance leading to a rise in arterial backpressure and vice versa. This effect is conveniently quantified by a fluid-dynamic analog to Ohm's famous $E = IR$ law in electromagnetic theory, voltage drop E being equated to fluid pressure drop ΔP, electric current I corresponding to flow—CO—and electric resistance R being associated with an analogous vascular "peripheral resistance" (PR). Thus, one may write

$$\Delta P = (CO)(PR) \qquad\qquad (1.4)$$

Normally, the total systemic PR is 15–20 mmHg/L/min of flow but can increase significantly under the influence of the vasomotor center located in the medulla of the brain, which controls arteriolar muscle tone.

The control of blood volume is accomplished mainly through the excretory function of the kidney. For example, antidiuretic hormone (ADH) secreted by the pituitary gland acts to prevent renal fluid loss (excretion via urination) and thus increases plasma volume, whereas perceived extracellular fluid overloads such as those that result from the peripheral vasoconstriction response to cold stress leading to a sympathetic/adrenergic receptor-induced renal diuresis (urination) that tends to decrease the plasma volume—if not checked, to sometimes dangerously low dehydration levels. Blood composition too is maintained primarily through the activity of endocrine hormones and enzymes that enhance or repress specific biochemical pathways. Since these pathways are too numerous to itemize here, suffice it to say that in the body's quest for homeostasis and stability, virtually nothing is left to chance, and every biochemical end can be arrived at through a number of alternative means. In a broader sense, as the organism strives to maintain life, it coordinates a wide variety of different functions, and central to its ability to do just that is the role played by the cardiovascular system in transporting mass, energy, and momentum (Schneck, 1990).

Defining Terms

Atrioventricular (AV) node: A highly specialized cluster of neuromuscular cells at the lower portion of the right atrium leading to the interventricular septum; the AV node delays sinoatrial (SA), node-generated electrical impulses momentarily (allowing the atria to contract first) and then conducts the depolarization wave to the bundle of His and its bundle branches.

Autonomic nervous system: The functional division of the nervous system that innervates most glands, the heart, and the smooth muscle tissue to maintain the internal environment of the body.

Cardiac muscle: Involuntary muscle possessing much of the anatomic attributes of the skeletal voluntary muscle and some of the physiologic attributes of the involuntary smooth muscle tissue; SA node-induced contraction of its interconnected network of fibers allows the heart to expel blood during systole.

Chronotropic: Affecting the periodicity of a recurring action, such as the slowing (bradycardia) or speeding up (tachycardia) of the heartbeat that results from extrinsic control of the SA node.

Endocrine system: The system of ductless glands and organs secreting substances directly into the blood to produce a specific response from another "target" organ or body part.

Endothelium: Flat cells that line the innermost surfaces of blood and lymphatic vessels and the heart.

Homeostasis: A tendency to uniformity or stability in an organism by maintaining within narrow limits certain variables that are critical to life.

Inotropic: Affecting the contractility of the muscular tissue, such as the increase in cardiac *power* that results from extrinsic control of the myocardial musculature.

Precapillary sphincters: Rings of smooth muscle surrounding the entrance to capillaries where they branch off from the upstream metarterioles. Contraction and relaxation of these sphincters close and open the access to downstream blood vessels, thus controlling the irrigation of different capillary networks.

Sinoatrial (SA) node: Neuromuscular tissue in the right atrium near where the superior vena cava joins the posterior right atrium (the sinus venarum); the SA node generates electrical impulses that initiate the heartbeat; hence, its nickname the cardiac "pacemaker."

Stem cells: A generalized parent cell spawning descendants that become individually specialized.

Acknowledgments

The author gratefully acknowledges the assistance of Professor Robert Hochmuth in the preparation of Table 1.1 and the Radford Community Hospital for their support of the Biomedical Engineering Program at Virginia Tech.

References

Beall, H.P.T., Needham, D., and Hochmuth, R.M. 1993. Volume and osmotic properties of human neutrophils. *Blood* 81: 2774–2780.

Bhagavan, N.V. 1992. *Medical Biochemistry*. Boston, Jones and Bartlett.

Caro, C.G., Pedley, T.J., Schroter, R.C., and Seed, W.A. 1978. *The Mechanics of the Circulation*. New York, Oxford University Press.

Chandran, K.B. 1992. *Cardiovascular Biomechanics*. New York, New York University Press.

Dawson, T.H. 1991. *Engineering Design of the Cardiovascular System of Mammals*. Englewood Cliffs, NJ, Prentice-Hall.

Duck, F.A. 1990. *Physical Properties of Tissue*. San Diego, Academic Press.

Frausto da Silva, J.J.R. and Williams, R.J.P. 1993. *The Biological Chemistry of the Elements*. New York, Oxford University Press/Clarendon.

Kaley, G. and Altura, B.M. (eds.). *Microcirculation*, Vol. I (1977), Vol. II (1978), Vol. III (1980). Baltimore, University Park Press.

Kessel, R.G. and Kardon, R.H. 1979. *Tissue and Organs—A Text-Atlas of Scanning Electron Microscopy*. San Francisco, WH Freeman.

Lentner, C. (ed.). 1984. *Geigy Scientific Tables, Vol 3: Physical Chemistry, Composition of Blood, Hematology and Somatometric Data*, 8th ed. New Jersey, Ciba-Geigy.

Lentner, C. 1990. *Heart and Circulation*, 8th ed., Vol. 5. New Jersey, Ciba-Geigy.

Schneck, D.J. 1990. *Engineering Principles of Physiologic Function*. New York, New York University Press.

Tortora, G.J. and Grabowski, S.R. 1993. *Principles of Anatomy and Physiology*, 7th ed. New York, Harper Collins.

2

Kidney Structure and Physiology

2.1   Introduction 2-1
2.2   Kidney Anatomy 2-2
2.3   Vasculature of the Kidney 2-4
2.4   Architecture of the Nephron 2-4
2.5   Structure of the Glomerulus and the Glomerular Filtration Barrier 2-5
2.6   Mechanical Properties of the Glomerulus 2-7
2.7   Glomerular Filtration 2-8
2.8   Factors Governing Glomerular Filtration 2-9
     Hydraulic Permeability of the Glomerular Barrier • Surface Area of the Glomerular Barrier • Ultrafiltration Coefficient • Intraluminal Hydrostatic Pressure of the Glomerular Capillary
2.9   Permselectivity of the Glomerular Barrier 2-11
2.10   Tubulo-Interstitial Structure and Organization 2-12
2.11   Solute Recovery from the Ultrafiltrate 2-14
     Mechanisms of Solute Transport • Regulation of Solute Transport • Recovery of Sodium • Recovery of Other Small Solutes and Regulation of pH
2.12   Water Reabsorption and Its Regulation 2-16
2.13   Endocrine Function of Kidney 2-18
     Renin • Erythropoietin • Vitamin D
2.14   Assessment of Kidney Function 2-19
References 2-20

Joel M. Henderson
Boston University School of Medicine

Boston University College of Engineering

Mostafa Belghasem
Boston University School of Medicine

2.1 Introduction

The kidney regulates body fluid composition and distribution. To accomplish this, it separates wastes from the blood, controls the total volume of body fluid (water), manages blood pressure, plays a role in the regulation of body fluid pH and solute concentration, and secretes or modifies certain hormones that relate to its other physiologic roles (Guyton and Hall 2006). With the exception of its role as an endocrine organ, most of these functions are accomplished via selective and actively adjusted filtration of the blood.

The adjustment of blood composition in the kidney involves three processes: (1) *filtration*—the selective filtration of small solutes from blood plasma, along with water, to form an ultrafiltrate, (2) *reabsorption*—the recovery of water and valuable solutes from the ultrafiltrate, which are too small to be retained by the filter, and (3) *secretion*—the addition of waste products to the ultrafiltrate by secretion from specialized cells. All these processes take place along the *nephron*, which is the basic functional unit of the kidney. An individual nephron is in some ways analogous to a single-channel microfluidic device. Each nephron is essentially a long microscopic tube, several centimeters long but only a few micrometers in diameter, into which an ultrafiltrate of blood is collected and processed. Blood is initially filtered through a microscopic, globular tuft of capillaries called a *glomerulus*. The ultrafiltrate then travels along the tube (the *tubule*), which is entirely lined by specialized cells, capable of active adjustment of the composition of the fluids moving through it. Passive transport processes across the wall of the tubule also play an important role. At the end of the tubule, the processed ultrafiltrate, now called *urine*, is collected for expulsion from the body.

The fundamental structural and functional organization of the nephron is conserved in the vertebrate kidney, and tissues with similar structure and function are observed throughout the animal kingdom (Weavers et al. 2009). The total number of nephrons present in a given species is proportional to its body mass; human kidneys are composed of roughly 1 million nephrons. In the simplest terms, a kidney is a compact structure composed of many nephrons arranged in parallel, with optimized networks serving all the nephrons to facilitate blood distribution, waste fluid collection, and neural signaling.

2.2 Kidney Anatomy

The kidneys are embedded in connective tissues in the dorsal aspect of the trunk in the retroperitoneal space behind the abdominal cavity. Human kidneys are bean-shaped organs, approximating a prolate spheroid with a concave indentation of one surface midway between the poles (Figure 2.1a). In humans, they are roughly the size of fists, weighing about 150 g each and measuring approximately 12 cm in maximum dimension. They are dense, firmly rubbery, and somewhat friable organs with a smooth, glistening reddish-brown external surface. Each kidney is composed of individually functioning segments or *lobes* that have merged together to form one organ; this is reflected in the lobulated surface, which is apparent during fetal development. A tough, thin, and sac-like fibrous capsule surrounds the outer

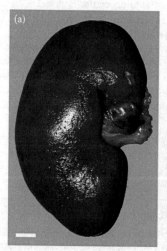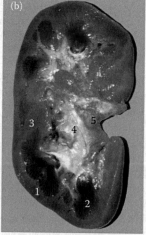

FIGURE 2.1 (a) Adult human kidney, decapsulated. In this image, the renal artery, vein, and ureter emanate from the hilum at the right edge of the kidney. (b) Cut surface of bisected kidney; same specimen as in (a). A continuous rim of cortex (1), about 8 mm thick, encircles the outer aspect of the cut surface. The medulla, evident as fan-like arrays of alternating dark and light stripes composing individual medullary pyramids (2), exhibits a distinctive lobar organization. Individual lobes are often separated by penetrating columns of the cortical tissue called septae or columns of Bertin (3). The plane of the cut surface is outside the cavity of the renal pelvis; so, the central region shows the connective tissue and vasculature that surrounds the exterior of the pelvis (4). The renal vein can be seen exiting at the hilum (5). Bar = 1 cm for both images. (Images kindly provided by Dr. Mark Flomenbaum, Boston University Medical Center.)

surface of each kidney. The kidneys are cushioned by a surrounding layer of a connective tissue and fat called *Gerota's fascia*. Each kidney is capped by a closely approximated *adrenal gland*, each of which produces several important steroid hormones, including epinephrine and aldosterone.

The kidney parenchyma is organized in layers, based upon the nephron components present in each layer (Figures 2.1b and 2.2a). The outermost layer, the *cortex*, is primarily defined by the presence of glomeruli, but also includes portions of the tubules, vasculature, and the interstitial fibrous tissue that

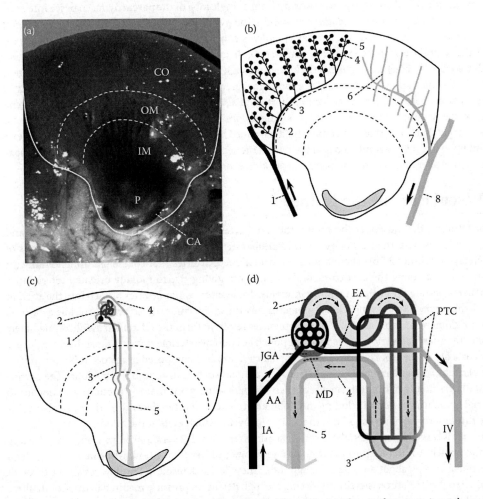

FIGURE 2.2 (a) An individual renal lobe, from Figure 2.1b. The solid white line is the approximate boundary with adjacent renal lobes. CO, cortex; OM, outer medulla; IM, inner medulla; P, papilla; CA, calyx. (b) Diagram of the vascular organization in an individual lobe of the kidney. For clarity, arterial vasculature is represented on the left and venous vasculature is represented on the right, although both occur concurrently in all areas of the kidney (not to scale; see text). (1) Interlobar artery, (2) arcuate artery, (3) interlobular artery, (4) afferent arteriole, (5) glomerulus, (6) interlobular veins, (7) arcuate vein, and (8) interlobar vein. The solid arrows indicate blood flow in vasculature. The efferent arterioles and peritubular capillary bed are not shown. (c) Diagram of the organization of a typical individual nephron within a lobe of the kidney (not to scale; see text). (1) Glomerulus, (2) proximal convoluted tubule, (3) loop of Henle, (4) distal convoluted tubule, and (5) collecting duct. (d) Schematic representation of the organization and spatial relationships of nephron structures (not to scale; see text). Compare the numbered structures to those represented in (c). Additional structures represented in (d): IA, interlobular artery; AA, afferent arteriole; EA, efferent arteriole; PTC, peritubular capillary bed; IV, interlobular vein; MD, macula densa; JGA, juxtaglomerular apparatus. The arrows indicate the direction of fluid flow, solid arrows indicate blood flow in the vasculature, and dashed arrows indicate the flow of the ultrafiltrate in the tubular system.

binds the structures together. This is where ultrafiltration and initial adjustment of ultrafiltrate composition take place. The segments of the tubules present in this layer are quite tortuous or convoluted. The next layer is the *medulla*, which is composed of radially oriented tubular and vascular structures responsible for recovering water from the ultrafiltrate and thereby increasing urine concentration. The medulla is composed of the outer medulla, just deep to the cortex, which is composed of thick-walled segments of the tubules, and the inner medulla, where thin-walled segments of the tubules are more prominent. Groups of adjacent nephrons arising from a single lobe of the parenchyma coalesce into subdivisions of the medulla called *medullary pyramids*. The pyramids converge to form a rounded *papilla* that projects into an associated cup-like cavity called a *calyx*. Each calyx is continuous with the *pelvis*, which is the central cavity of the kidney where urine collects for transport out of the body.

Fluids (blood and urine) enter and exit the kidney through the *hilum* at the concave aspect of each organ. In the body, the hilum is oriented toward the abdominal great vessels. Each kidney is typically served by a single *renal artery* arising from the abdominal aorta and a single *renal vein* that adjoins the inferior vena cava. The kidneys are only a few centimeters from the abdominal great vessels and so the renal branches are correspondingly short. The excess interstitial fluid is drained by multiple small lymphatic vessels, which exit via the hilum to drain into lymph nodes in the retroperitoneum. Microscopic nerve fibers from the sympathetic autonomic nervous system also penetrate the kidney on the surface of the renal artery.

2.3 Vasculature of the Kidney

Upon penetrating the kidney at the hilum, the renal artery immediately branches into anterior and posterior divisions, and then arborizes into interlobar arteries that course radially between lobes of the parenchyma (Figure 2.2b). These branch to form arcuate arteries that course circumferentially (in the form of an arc) along the cortico-medullary junction, giving rise to radially oriented interlobular arteries that penetrate the cortex at regular intervals. These interlobular arteries branch into the afferent arterioles that carry blood to individual glomeruli. At the glomerulus, the afferent arteriole arborizes to form the glomerular capillary tuft. These capillaries rejoin to form the efferent arteriole immediately adjacent to the afferent arteriole at the vascular pole. The efferent arteriole travels a short distance deeper into the cortex to again arborize into a less compact capillary bed composed of the peritubular capillaries. The peritubular capillary bed extends from the cortical surface deep into the medulla. The peritubular capillaries finally rejoin to form a sequence of venules and veins that is structurally analogous to the arterial branching pattern, including interlobular, arcuate, and interlobar veins. The interlobar veins coalesce through regional veins to form the main renal vein, which exits at the hilum.

The kidney is served by an arterial network that arborizes several generations from a single renal artery into approximately 1 million arterioles over a short distance of less than 10 cm, while increasing in total cross-sectional area by about an order of magnitude. These features result in low flow resistance through the renal arterial vasculature, thereby preserving the high perfusion pressure required to drive both ultrafiltration at the glomeruli and perfusion of the distal peritubular capillary bed. Studies in rodents indicate that the central arterial pressure (typically 110 mm Hg) is maintained in the interlobular arteries. The hydrostatic pressure drops about 60% through the afferent arterioles and into the glomerular capillaries, but is nevertheless maintained at an unusually high value for a capillary bed. Typical direct micropuncture measurements of mean hydrostatic pressure in the glomerular capillaries are about 50 mm Hg. The hydrostatic pressure drops further across the efferent arterioles, so that the hydrostatic pressure in peritubular capillaries is typically less than 10 mm Hg (Brenner 2008). Thus, most of the resistance to flow in the kidney is encountered between the afferent and efferent arterioles serving the glomerulus.

2.4 Architecture of the Nephron

Individual nephrons are radially oriented throughout the kidney, with their proximal ends oriented outward (Figure 2.2c and d). Filtration is accomplished at the proximal end of the nephron by the glomerulus. Blood flows into the glomerulus via the afferent arteriole and enters the glomerular capillaries. The glomerular capillary walls are highly permeable to water and small solutes, and a substantial proportion of the fluid flowing through the glomerulus (about 20%) crosses this barrier. The resulting ultrafiltrate accumulates in the space surrounding the glomerular capillary tuft, called *Bowman's space*, and is collected by a cup-like structure that surrounds and closely approximates the tuft called *Bowman's capsule*. Bowman's space is continuous with the lumen of the tubule, thus accumulating ultrafiltrate flows into the tubular lumen. The flow continues radially inward along the tubule, where the ultrafiltrate is processed further through reabsorption and secretion by the tubular epithelial cells. The initial tubular segment, the *proximal convoluted tubule,* meanders in the vicinity of its associated glomerulus. As the tubule continues, it becomes directed toward the deeper kidney and transitions into a thin-walled tube with flattened epithelium, which penetrates the medulla. In nephrons arising deep in the cortex, this tube penetrates the medullary pyramids and is responsible for establishing the countercurrent flow needed to recover the filtered water. This thin tube, the *loop of Henle,* eventually turns 180° and reemerges in the cortex. There, the tubule redevelops a thickened cuboidal epithelium, and again meanders in the vicinity of its corresponding glomerulus, becoming the *distal convoluted tubule.* This portion of the tubule passes next to the vascular pole of the glomerulus at one point, where a small patch of specialized tubular epithelial cells called the *macula densa* are positioned. The basal aspect of these cells makes contact with a small collection of cells adjacent to the arterioles at the glomerular vascular pole, called the *juxtaglomerular apparatus.* These structures play an important role in the regulation of glomerular perfusion through the regulation of constriction of the arterioles serving the glomerulus. The distal convoluted tubule continues toward the medulla, and eventually coalesces with other tubules to form larger *collecting ducts.* The collecting ducts continue radially through the medullary pyramid to the papilla, where they open into the adjacent calyx. The processed ultrafiltrate, now called *urine,* flows out of the collecting ducts at the papilla into the calyx, and the adjoining renal pelvis.

Although all nephrons share this same general structural and functional arrangement, there is regional variation among the nephrons with regard to physical parameters, including glomerular size, relative lengths of the various tubular segments, and the pattern of organization of the nephron in the kidney parenchyma. These structural and functional differences among the nephrons vary depending upon the location of their glomeruli in the cortex, and the corresponding distance blood must travel to reach them. Blood travels the least distance to perfuse glomeruli closest to the medulla; therefore, the perfusion pressure in these *juxtamedullary glomeruli* is somewhat higher than that of the glomeruli closer to the capsular surface. Juxtamedullary glomeruli are also larger than superficial glomeruli, and their corresponding tubules include thin segments that penetrate more deeply into the inner medulla than those of superficial glomeruli. These differences result in corresponding variations in functional contribution.

2.5 Structure of the Glomerulus and the Glomerular Filtration Barrier

The glomerulus is composed of a compact tuft of capillaries branching from a single afferent arteriole (Figure 2.3a). These capillaries intertwine to form a compact ball, the glomerular tuft, about 200 μm in diameter. The afferent and efferent arterioles enter and exit the glomerular capillary tuft adjacent to each other, at the *vascular pole.* The afferent arteriole immediately branches into several capillaries that follow a tortuous pathway around the tuft surface, approaching the opposite tip of the capillary tuft, called the *tubular pole.* From this point, the capillaries penetrate the center of the tuft and coalesce near the vascular pole to form the efferent arteriole. Throughout their path, the capillaries are supported centrally by the connective tissue and the cells known as the *mesangium* (Figure 2.3b). Although the central aspect of each capillary abuts and is continuous with the mesangial tissue, the peripheral aspect of each capillary projects freely into Bowman's space. This exposed capillary wall forms the filtration barrier of the glomerulus. From the capillary lumen outward, this barrier is physically composed of

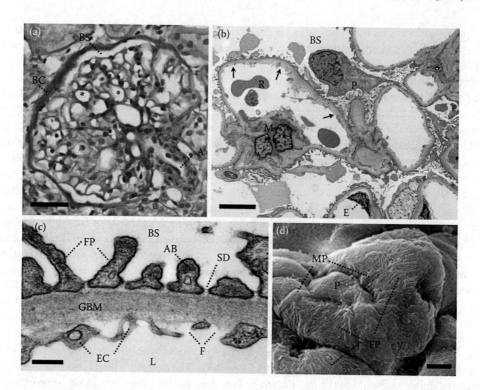

FIGURE 2.3 (a) Photomicrograph of a human glomerulus from a section of formalin-fixed, paraffin-embedded tissue. Many cross sections of glomerular capillaries ("capillary loops") are evident (asterisks). The Bowman's capsule (BC) surrounds the glomerular tuft and defines the Bowman's space between these two structures (BS). An arteriole (A) enters the vascular pole on the lower right. Periodic acid-Schiff; bar = 50 μm. (b) Transmission electron micrograph (TEM) of a segment of a human glomerulus. The wall of a single capillary in cross section is demarcated by arrows from within the lumen. Note the cell body of a podocyte (P) protruding into the Bowman's space (BS), red blood cell (R) within the lumen of a capillary, mesangium with a mesangial cell (M), and cell body of an endothelial cell (E) lining a capillary wall. Bar = 5 μm. (c) High magnification TEM of a section of a glomerular capillary wall. In this image, water and small solutes move across this filtration barrier from the capillary lumen at the bottom (L) to the Bowman's space at the top (BS). FP, podocyte foot processes (seen in cross section); AB, actin bundle (seen in cross section); SD, filtration slit diaphragm; GBM, glomerular basement membrane; EC, endothelial cell; and F, endothelial cell fenestrae. Bar = 300 nm. (d) Scanning electron micrograph of the exterior of a glomerular capillary segment. The surface of the capillary is covered with interlocking podocyte foot processes (FP), which are branching off of major processes (MP). The major processes, in turn, arise from the podocyte cell body (P). Bar = 5 μm.

the *endothelium*, the *glomerular basement membrane* (GBM), and the *glomerular visceral epithelium* or *podocytes* (Figure 2.3c). These three layers combined about 1 μm thick.

The endothelium is a thin monolayer of flat cells about 100 nm thick, which are heavily perforated or *fenestrated* (Figure 2.3c). These fenestrations, which are continuous channels connecting the apical and basal aspects of the cell, are unique to the glomerular endothelium and a few other specialized capillary beds throughout the body. The exterior surface of the endothelial plasma membrane and the lumina of the fenestrations are covered with a glycocalyx composed of complex carbohydrates linked to cell membrane proteins. This glycocalyx carries a net negative charge and plays an important role in modulating filtration by sieving and repelling negatively charged plasma proteins and preventing them from crossing the barrier.

The GBM is analogous to epithelial basement membranes throughout the body but has unique characteristics. It is essentially the fused basement membrane of the endothelium and podocytes, and is therefore unusually thick (mean thickness 350 nm in adult humans). It is composed of a dense mesh-work of proteins, most notably collagen IV and laminin, and complex carbohydrates. The GBM contrib-utes to the glomerular barrier function by sieving proteins and presenting an additional net negative charge. It also provides structural support to the glomerular capillary wall and ligands for cell adhesion. Alterations in certain GBM proteins are known causes of kidney disease.

The podocytes are arranged around the external surface of the glomerular capillaries (Figure 2.3d). A central cell body projects outward from the capillary surface into Bowman's space. Several *major pro-cesses* emanate from the cell body and wrap around adjacent capillaries. These major processes give rise to an intricate layer of interlocking cytoplasmic projections, the *foot processes*, which wrap around and entirely cover the external surface of the GBM. The foot processes are about 300 nm wide and several micrometers long when sitting on the basement membrane. The adjacent foot processes are connected by a specialized cell–cell junction called the *slit diaphragm*, which is composed of a complex of proteins of which some are specific to the podocyte, such as nephrin and podocin. The slit diaphragm maintains a 40 nm spacing between adjacent foot processes (the *filtration slits*), and has a porous, zipper-like struc-ture when viewed en-face. The pores in the slit diaphragm are highly permeable to water, but the overall proportion of the total glomerular capillary wall surface area that is occupied by filtration slits is likely to be an important determinant of water transport through the glomerular capillary wall (Deen et al. 2001).

2.6 Mechanical Properties of the Glomerulus

The intricate structure of the glomerular capillary wall must be maintained in the presence of a demand-ing mechanical environment. Direct measurements in animals have revealed that the hydrostatic pres-sure gradient across the glomerular capillary wall is normally about 45 mm Hg (Brenner 2008). This outward hydrostatic pressure gradient creates tensile forces in the glomerular capillary wall. Therefore, the components of the glomerular capillary wall that compose the filtration barrier must also serve as structural members that resist these forces. Most of the glomerular capillary wall components have adapted structural features that are likely to contribute to this dual role. Mesangial cells exhibit con-tractile properties and project fibers that blend into the GBM, and may contract to resist glomerular capillary wall tension or alter the surface area of the glomerular filtration barrier (Kriz et al. 1995). Mechanical testing of basement membrane samples from kidney tubules indicates that this structure exhibits nonlinear mechanical properties, becoming stiffer as the strain is increased (Welling et al. 1995). The GBM is up to an order of magnitude thicker than most epithelial basement membranes, and exhibits increased electron density, suggesting a more robust structure with increased stiffness. The cytoskeletal components of the podocyte are similarly robust and include dense longitudinal bundles of actin microfilaments along each foot process, and numerous microtubules and actin microfilaments in the major processes (Figure 2.3c) (Kriz 1995). Podocytes also exhibit contractile properties and have been shown to respond to applied forces in a variety of ways, including actin cytoskeleton reorganization (Endlich and Endlich 2006). These capabilities may indicate the presence of adaptive responses tending to structurally reinforce the glomerular capillary wall in the presence of increased luminal hydrostatic pressure. Glomerular endothelial cells do not feature a comparably robust cytoskeletal structure and are therefore not as likely to play an important structural role in the glomerular capillary.

It is likely that the mechanical properties of the glomerular capillary wall are anisotropic. The varying orientation of podocyte processes along the capillaries (see Figure 2.3d) and the varying geometry of the glomerular capillaries themselves make it possible that the mechanical properties of the glomerular capillary wall are spatially varying as well. This spatial variation could explain the segmental nature of many glomerular diseases. Evidence suggests that disease states affecting structural components of the glomerular capillary do indeed alter the mechanical properties of this structure, potentially increasing the vulnerability of the glomerulus to mechanically mediated dam-age (Wyss et al. 2011).

2.7 Glomerular Filtration

The filtration function of the kidney involves the separation of small solutes from the blood through bulk convection of blood plasma (the noncellular fluid component of blood) across the glomerular capillary wall, which serves as a semipermeable filtration barrier. The physical structure of the glomerular filter differs from the more familiar paradigm of a filtration barrier composed of a flat sheet, instead consisting of many compact bundles of intertwining microscopic tubes (the glomerular tufts). In this way, a large filtration surface area is efficiently contained within a relatively small volume. The process of filtration takes place within each nephron on an individual basis, but the overall kidney function results from the sum total of the contributions of all the individual nephrons. Filtration function is expressed as a volume of fluid that crosses the glomerular barrier per unit time. This may be expressed for all functioning nephrons in sum, as the *total glomerular filtration rate* (GFR), or for an individual nephron as the *single-nephron glomerular filtration rate* (snGFR).

In adult humans, approximately 25% of the entire cardiac output, or about 1.2 L/min of blood, perfuses the kidneys. Thus, about 600 mL of filterable blood plasma (the liquid, noncellular component of blood) passes through the kidneys each minute (the *renal plasma flow*). Essentially all this fluid is directed to the glomeruli, but only a small fraction of this volume (the *filtration fraction*), about 20%, actually passes across the permeability barrier. Therefore, the volume flow rate of fluid actually crossing the glomerular barrier (the GFR) is about 125 mL/min. The remaining plasma fluid continues through the kidney (with essentially all the accompanying blood cells) to perfuse the peritubular capillary bed and continue on to the venous circulation. Most of the fluid that crosses the glomerular barrier is also reabsorbed in the tubules, as discussed below. As a result, although approximately 180 L/day of fluid crosses the glomerular barrier over the entire kidney mass, only about 1 L/day is excreted as urine.

The process of glomerular filtration is governed by Starling's law of capillary filtration, which states that filtration through a capillary is proportional to the net pressure balance between the (outwardly directed) hydraulic pressure imparted by the blood within the capillary and the (inward) oncotic pressure resulting from the dissolved proteins in the blood, which tend to attract water molecules. This is expressed mathematically as follows:

$$GFR = LpS \, (\Delta \text{ hydraulic pressure} - \Delta \text{ oncotic pressure}) = LpS \, [(P_{gc} - P_{bs}) - s(\Pi_p - \Pi_{bs})]$$

where Lp is the unit hydraulic permeability of the capillary wall, S is the total surface area of the capillary wall through which filtration is occurring, P_{gc} and Π_p are the hydraulic and oncotic pressures within the glomerular capillary, respectively, P_{bs} and Π_{bs} are the hydraulic and oncotic pressures in Bowman's space, respectively, and s is the reflection coefficient of oncotically active proteins across the filtration barrier. The reflection coefficient ranges from 0 (entirely permeable) to 1 (entirely impermeable). Under normal conditions, s is 1 and Π_{bs} is 0, since essentially no oncotically active proteins cross the glomerular barrier, and the ultrafiltrate therefore contains no oncotically active proteins. Thus

$$GFR = LpS \, (P_{gc} - P_{bs} - \Pi_p)$$

All three pressure components contribute significantly to GFR, and P_{gc} generally exceeds P_{bs} and Π_p combined, resulting in a net outward driving force for ultrafiltration, from the capillary lumen to Bowman's space. The glomerular capillary and Bowman's space hydraulic pressures are generally constant regardless of the position in the glomerulus or along the glomerular capillaries. Typical values for P_{gc} and P_{bs} are, as measured in rodent models, 45 and 10 mm Hg, respectively. In contrast, the oncotic pressure likely increases along the length of the glomerular capillary, as water crosses the glomerular filtration barrier and the concentration of oncotically active proteins in the lumen increases. In rodents, the plasma oncotic pressure increases from 20 to 35 mm Hg along the length of the glomerular capillary, thereby achieving "filtration equilibrium" with hydrostatic pressure before exiting the glomerular tuft. There is considerable variation in this tendency across species and it is not known if filtration equilibrium is achieved in human glomeruli.

The parameters most likely to result in changes in GFR are the hydraulic permeability and surface area of the glomerular barrier, and the intraluminal pressure in the glomerular capillary. These parameters, particularly the intraluminal pressure, can be actively adjusted under normal conditions to maintain an appropriate level of glomerular filtration. Further, all these parameters may be altered in disease states, leading to abnormally low levels of glomerular filtration.

2.8 Factors Governing Glomerular Filtration

2.8.1 Hydraulic Permeability of the Glomerular Barrier

The hydraulic permeability (Lp) is a proportionality constant relating a given pressure difference across the glomerular barrier to a corresponding flow rate of the ultrafiltrate (the GFR), and it indicates how easily this fluid permeates the glomerular barrier. It is dependent upon the geometric properties of the barrier, including the proportion of the barrier surface through which the fluid can flow, also known as the porosity, and the tortuosity of the fluid path through each of the component layers of the glomerular capillary wall (see Figure 2.3c). The cell membranes of the endothelium and podocyte foot processes are generally impermeable to water; therefore, the ultrafiltrate must cross these cellular layers through cell–cell junctions or fenestrae that cross the cells. Despite this, the endothelium as a whole is highly permeable due to the relatively large proportion of the endothelial surface occupied by fenestrae. The GBM is analogous to a woven matrix of protein filaments and fluid flows between these filaments. The path taken by water across the GBM layer is highly tortuous, and so, this layer is less permeable. The fluid crosses the podocyte foot process layer through the extracellular pathway of the filtration slits. At the foot process layer, the proportion of the surface area occupied by the filtration slits is relatively small; therefore, this layer is also relatively impermeable. Mathematical modeling has been used to estimate the relative contributions of the individual components of the glomerular barrier to hydraulic permeability (Drummond and Deen 1994; Deen 2001). These studies, which estimated the hydraulic resistance of each layer (inversely related to hydraulic permeability), suggest that the endothelium presents very little resistance to fluid flux, contributing only about 2% of the hydraulic resistance, whereas the GBM and podocyte foot process layer present about 50% each. Overall, the glomerular capillary wall is 50–100 times more permeable than capillaries elsewhere in the body.

Since the components of the glomerular barrier impede the fluid movement in series, any of the components (endothelium, GBM, and podocyte foot processes) could play a role in modulating barrier permeability. On the basis of its structure, location, and relative contribution to hydraulic resistance, it is plausible that the podocyte may be the most important of these three components. It has been speculated that the filtration slits between foot processes may be involved in active modulation of hydraulic permeability, through adjustment of the filtration slit geometry, potentially in response to local hemodynamic stresses. This response could involve slit diaphragm structures as sensors of mechanical stress. Podocytes also appear to be sensitive to fluid shear stress across their cell membrane surface; thus, changes in ultrafiltrate flow through the filtration slits or across the podocyte membrane surface could provide another mechanism for such a response (Friedrich et al. 2006).

2.8.2 Surface Area of the Glomerular Barrier

Mechanisms may exist by which the total surface area of the glomerular barrier available for filtration can be modulated in physiologic states. It has been proposed that mesangial cells may actively adjust capillary dimensions through contraction, to modulate the surface area of the glomerular barrier presented for filtration (Stockand and Sansom 1997). This effect may result from the direct alteration of the circumference of a capillary through mesangial contraction and retraction of the GBM, or from the redirection of fluid flow away from capillaries by the constriction of entrances to capillary segments through the contraction of adjacent mesangium. In pathologic conditions, kidney damage associated with glomerular loss will result in a permanent decrease in the available filtration surface area and an attendant decrease in GFR.

2.8.3 Ultrafiltration Coefficient

Although the podocyte may hold unique importance as an intrinsic regulator of barrier permeability, it is clinically observed that *pathologic* alteration of *any* of the barrier components can alter the hydraulic permeability or the available surface area of the glomerular barrier. This is reflected in clinical assessment of GFR, where GFR is decreased despite pharmacologic glomerular capillary pressure support, in association with morphologic changes in components of the glomerular capillary wall revealed in biopsy material. It is not clinically possible to distinguish the effect of altered barrier permeability from changes in total barrier surface area, and pathologic conditions often alter both these barrier properties simultaneously. In view of this, the product of the hydraulic permeability and the total surface area, the *glomerular ultrafiltration coefficient, Kf* (= LpS), is often used to indicate the overall transport properties of the glomerular filtration barrier.

2.8.4 Intraluminal Hydrostatic Pressure of the Glomerular Capillary

Systemic arterial blood pressure varies throughout the day. Despite this, the perfusion pressure in the kidney is tightly regulated via several mechanisms to maintain the pressure gradient required to drive glomerular filtration at an optimal level. The glomerular capillary pressure driving filtration is dependent upon the upstream hemodynamic pressure in the renal arterial system, and the resistances imparted by the afferent and efferent arterioles. Contraction of the afferent arteriole increases the resistance proximal to the glomerulus, thereby reducing blood pressure within the glomerular capillaries. The resistance due to the contraction of the efferent arteriole raises the glomerular capillary blood pressure. These two arterioles respond differentially to various stimuli, as discussed below. The two most important mechanisms modulating glomerular capillary hemodynamics are *autoregulation* and *tubuloglomerular feedback*.

2.8.4.1 Autoregulation

Autoregulation is a feedback mechanism that exists in various capillary beds throughout the body. It is the tendency for arteriolar smooth muscle to constrict the arteriolar lumen in response to decreased luminal pressure, thereby increasing resistance to flow and driving up blood pressure proximal to the arteriole. A corresponding opposite response occurs when arteriolar luminal pressure increases. This may involve a direct response of arteriolar smooth muscle to stretch via mechanoreceptors. In the glomerulus, the responses of the afferent and efferent arterioles are distinct. If systemic blood pressure increases, afferent arteriolar resistance increases so that glomerular capillary pressure is held constant. This protects the glomerulus from damage and prevents the tubular system from being overwhelmed by an excessive flow rate of the ultrafiltrate. In contrast, a significant decrease in the perfusion pressure stimulates smooth muscle contraction in both glomerular arterioles (efferent > afferent), in concert with the activation of the renin–angiotensin hormone system (discussed below). This differential arteriolar smooth muscle contraction increases efferent arteriolar resistance preferentially, which increases glomerular capillary pressure and thereby maintains sufficient plasma filtration. These autoregulatory responses, which increase flow resistance through the kidney, have a cost: in both cases, the renal plasma flow to the kidney is decreased, which reduces the functional capacity of the kidney, and the perfusion of the peritubular capillary bed is decreased, which places the tubules at risk of hypoperfusion and ischemic injury. Thus, over the long term, optimal renal function requires arterial perfusion pressures that are usually in the normal range.

2.8.4.2 Tubuloglomerular Feedback

The distal tubular reabsorptive capacity is limited; so, a closed-loop feedback mechanism has evolved to govern the production of ultrafiltrate based upon the flow rate of the (processed) ultrafiltrate reaching the distal tubule. In this system, the distal tubular flow rate sensor is composed of specialized distal tubular epithelial cells called the macula densa. These cells are located where the distal tubule, returning from the medulla, abuts the vascular pole of its corresponding upstream glomerulus. The macula densa cells respond to the rate at which chloride ions in the tubular luminal fluid are presented and reabsorbed at their apical surface by the $Na^+–K^+–2Cl^-$ cotransporter. In response to decreased chloride ion delivery (corresponding to a decrease in distal tubular fluid flow), macula densa cells stimulate glomerular afferent arteriolar dilatation by an as yet unknown mechanism, thereby increasing glomerular capillary pressure and GFR.

The macula densa cells also stimulate the release of the hormone renin by the specialized juxtaglomerular cells immediately adjacent to them (discussed in more detail below). The effect of renin release into the circulation is to cause arteriolar constriction in certain vascular beds, including the glomerular efferent arteriole. Constriction of the efferent arteriole also acts to increase the glomerular capillary pressure by increasing the resistance to the flow distal to the glomerulus. Thus, the macula densa cells mediate two distinct responses that modulate glomerular capillary pressure, in response to deviations in distal tubular flow rate.

Other mechanisms play a minor role in glomerular perfusion pressure regulation. As mentioned previously, glomeruli adjacent to the medulla are perfused at higher pressures. These glomeruli appear to maintain a somewhat higher perfusion pressure in part because they respond differently to changes in perfusion pressure, as compared to the more superficial glomeruli. These differences suggest that juxtamedullary glomeruli are functionally distinct from superficial glomeruli. Sympathetic autonomic nerve fibers have a role in modulating vascular tone within the kidney; when stimulated, arterial vessels contract, thereby reducing blood flow to the kidney.

2.9 Permselectivity of the Glomerular Barrier

Permselectivity refers to the mechanism by which the glomerular barrier filters small molecules out of the blood while retaining large molecules. The primary barrier to large molecules appears to be the glycocalyx that covers the surface of the endothelium and projects into the fenestrae and the gap between adjacent cells. The glycocalyx is in direct contact with blood, and therefore deflects large molecules from entering and becoming trapped within the deeper layers of the glomerular barrier. Some of the permselectivity results from the mechanical resistance (low porosity and high tortuosity) of the glycocalyx. Additionally, the glycocalyx presents a negative charge and this negative charge contributes to the permselectivity by repelling anionic molecules, including most larger soluble proteins in the blood, particularly albumin, which also carries a net negative charge.

The ease with which a particular substance can cross the glomerular barrier is represented by the fractional clearance of the molecule, which ranges from 1 (entirely permeable) to 0 (entirely impermeable). The fractional clearance is a property that is molecule specific and depends upon the size (molecular weight), conformation (shape), and electrical charge of the molecule. The effect of size and conformation combined may be represented by the *effective molecular diameter*. Neutral molecules with an effective molecular diameter up to about 4 nm are freely filtered through the glomerular barrier, and therefore, their fractional clearance is 1 (Figure 2.4). Fractional clearance for neutral molecules steadily decreases between 4 and 8 nm, and approaches zero for molecules greater than about 8 nm of effective molecular diameter. Anionic molecules larger than 6 nm are almost entirely excluded from the ultrafiltrate. This includes albumin, which has a molecular weight of approximately 67 kDa and an effective molecular diameter of 7 nm. Cationic molecules pass through the negatively charged components of the barrier more easily and are freely filtered up to about 6 nm of effective molecular diameter.

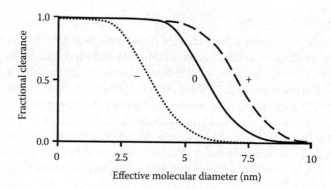

FIGURE 2.4 Fractional clearance of molecules through the glomerular barrier as a function of molecular size (effective molecular diameter) and charge. The fractional clearance as a function of size for negatively charged molecules is represented by the dotted line ("–"), neutral molecules are represented by the solid line ("0"), and positively charged molecules are represented by the dashed line ("+"). The negatively charged molecules are impeded by the fixed negative charge in the endothelial glycocalyx and GBM; the passage of positively charged molecules is enhanced.

The glomerular ultrafiltrate in Bowman's space is similar in composition to blood plasma, with the exception that plasma proteins larger than approximately 60 kDa are excluded from the ultrafiltrate. Upon moving out of Bowman's space and into the proximal tubule, the ultrafiltrate is immediately altered by tubular reabsorption and secretion.

2.10 Tubulo-Interstitial Structure and Organization

The nephron distal to the glomerulus is responsible for the reabsorption of useful solutes that cross the glomerular barrier, and water. In general, most components of the ultrafiltrate are reabsorbed in the proximal tubule, with fine adjustments occurring distally in the nephron. The structural complexity of the distal nephron is required to accomplish these fine adjustments. Some substances are secreted from the tubule into the ultrafiltrate as well. Although an individual nephron distal to the glomerulus is a single tubular channel, this tubule can be subdivided based upon spatial, structural, and functional differences. In particular, the cells that line the tubule are structurally and functionally diverse, and this diversity defines the tubular segments. The function of the renal tubules is highly dependent upon the spatial organization and relationships between the tubular segments. Like the glomeruli, the tubulo-interstitium has evolved to form an optimally efficient and compact structure, while maintaining these important spatial relationships.

The proximal tubule, about 70 μm in diameter, exhibits a convoluted path in the cortex for 1–1.5 cm in the vicinity of its associated glomerulus (Figures 2.2c and 2.5a). Ultrafiltrate flows directly from Bowman's space into the lumen of the proximal tubule. The tubules are surrounded by a network of peritubular capillaries and are separated from them by a minimal layer of interstitial connective tissue. The proximal tubular epithelium consists of the cells that line this initial segment of the tubule. As with all cells along the length of the tubule, these cells are situated upon a well-formed basement membrane. The apical surface of the proximal tubular epithelium (the surface facing the tubular lumen) is lined by dense microvilli. This *brush border*, visible by light microscopy, is a distinctive feature of proximal tubular epithelial cells. The microvilli serve to increase the cell surface area in contact with the ultrafiltrate by over an order of magnitude, and in doing so, increase the reabsorptive capacity of these cells. The cytoplasm of the proximal tubular epithelium contains a large number of mitochondria, which serve as a source of energy to facilitate transcellular active transport processes. The basolateral surface of the epithelial cells is characterized by an interdigitating network of deep intercellular channels, referred to as

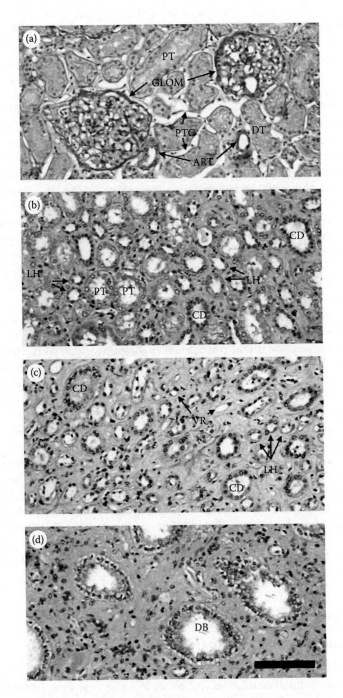

FIGURE 2.5 Light micrographs of circumferential sections of kidney parenchyma, perpendicular to the "long axis" of the nephron. Key for all annotations: PT, proximal tubule; GLOM, glomeruli; PTC, peritubular capillaries; ART, arterioles; DT, distal tubule; LH, loop of Henle; CD, collecting duct; VR, vasa recta; DB, duct of Bellini. All the images are periodic acid-Schiff; bar = 100 μm. (a) Cortex. Note the distal tubule, seen approaching the vascular pole. (b) Outer medulla. The straight segments of the proximal tubule are present in this superficial section. (c) Inner medulla. Most thick-walled tubular structures are superficial to this section. (d) Papilla. Several ducts of Bellini are present.

the basal labyrinth. This feature serves to increase cell membrane surface area at the basolateral aspect, which also increases the transport capacity of the cells. The proximal tubule ultimately turns inward to dive deep into the cortex and penetrate the medulla. This straight segment of the proximal tubule is characterized by epithelial cells with a less-dense brush border and fewer mitochondria.

Upon entering the medulla, the robust epithelium of the proximal tubule abruptly transitions into a simplified, thin layer of flattened (squamous) epithelium, and becomes the descending thin limb of the loop of Henle (Figures 2.2c, 2.5b and c). The thin limb of the loop of Henle is a radially oriented straight segment of the tubule about 20 μm in diameter, and penetrates up to 1.5 cm into the medulla. This straight segment continues into the medulla, and at some point dependent upon the depth of the associated glomerulus in the cortex (loops of Henle of juxtamedullary glomeruli penetrate the farthest), the loop of Henle turns 180° and proceeds back toward the cortex as the ascending thin limb. The epithelial cells of the loop of Henle are connected to each other at their apical surface by tight junctions, forming impermeable barriers between neighboring epithelial cells. Compared to proximal tubular epithelium, the cells of the loop of Henle have few microvilli and few mitochondria. Although the epithelial cells in the descending and ascending limbs of the loop of Henle are structurally similar, they are functionally distinct, particularly with respect to their transport properties. The loops of Henle are surrounded by peritubular capillaries arising from efferent arterioles in the cortex (as with the cortical peritubular capillaries). The peritubular capillaries adjacent to the deeply penetrating loops of Henle assume a similar hairpin structure, with descending and ascending limbs, and are known as the *vasa recta*. The loops of Henle and the vasa recta play an important role in the recovery of water from the ultrafiltrate.

As the loop of Henle ascends toward the cortex, another abrupt transition takes place, and the epithelium develops into a thicker layer of cuboidal epithelium. This thick ascending limb has dimensions similar to the proximal tubule, but does not have well-developed microvilli. As the thick ascending limb enters the cortex, it becomes the structurally similar distal convoluted tubule and it approaches and passes close to its associated glomerulus at its vascular pole. At the point of approximation, a patch of specialized epithelium called the *macula densa* forms, as discussed previously. The distal convoluted tubule continues in the adjacent cortex with a tortuous path similar to the proximal tubule (Figures 2.2c and 2.5a). Although the entire distal convoluted tubule has a similar cuboidal epithelial lining, the distal tubules are functionally subdivided into early and late segments, which have different reabsorption selectivity.

The distal tubules gradually transition into the collecting ducts, which are relatively straight segments lined with a further simplified cuboidal epithelium (Figures 2.2c, 2.5b and c). Although simplified, these epithelial cells have an important role in the fine adjustment of the ultrafiltrate composition. The collecting ducts turn toward the medulla and successively converge, ultimately becoming the ducts of Bellini (Figure 2.5d). These radially oriented large ducts up to 200 μm in diameter are located in the papilla and empty into the calyx.

2.11 Solute Recovery from the Ultrafiltrate

2.11.1 Mechanisms of Solute Transport

The mechanisms of reabsorption and transport of filtered solutes from the tubular lumen are widely varied and specific to each reabsorbed solute. Many solutes require energy expenditure to accomplish reabsorption. The routes taken by various solutes between the tubular lumen and the peritubular capillary lumen also depend upon the solute and the location in the nephron where reabsorption takes place. Solutes transported from the tubular lumen through the epithelial cell membranes are said to utilize a *transcellular route*, whereas solutes moving through the intercellular space (the potential space between cells) utilize a *paracellular route*. Regional variation throughout the nephron in the utilization of paracellular transport is often dependent upon the structure of intercellular junctions in that region.

Several important solutes, most notably ionic sodium, are transported via active (energy-expending) mechanisms. Primary active transport requires a transmembrane transporter protein, and hydrolysis of adenosine triphosphate (ATP) for a substance to be transported against its electrochemical gradient across the cell membrane. The primary active transporters in the tubules are sodium–potassium ATPase, calcium ATPase, hydrogen ATPase, and hydrogen–potassium ATPase. Secondary active transport mechanisms are not directly dependent upon the hydrolysis of ATP, but instead rely on the existing electrochemical gradient of one substance developed by an ATPase transporter, to facilitate movement of one or more other solutes, coupled via a carrier molecule on the cell membrane. These secondary transporters move passenger molecules either with the concentration gradient of the driving substance (cotransporter) or opposite to this gradient (countertransporter). Other solutes diffuse passively via paracellular or transcellular routes. Some larger solutes such as peptide hormones and proteins are reabsorbed via endocytosis in the proximal tubules.

Solutes recovered from the tubular lumen, regardless of the mechanism of transepithelial transport, must cross the tubular epithelial cell layer, its basement membrane, the interstitial connective tissue, the peritubular capillary basement membrane, and endothelial cell to return to the circulation through peritubular capillary uptake. This movement is generally a convective process, whereby solutes are carried with water as it returns to the circulation. The tubular epithelial layer presents the most significant resistance to fluid movement across this tissue, and as a result, water movement across the tubular epithelium is an energy-dependent process requiring active transport of oncotically active solutes across the barrier. Once across the epithelial layer, Starling forces govern the fluid movement (and convection of the solute) into the peritubular capillary

$$\text{Uptake} \propto (\Delta \text{ hydrostatic pressure} - \Delta \text{ oncotic pressure}) \propto (P_I - P_C) - (\Pi_I - \Pi_C)$$

where P_I and P_C are the interstitial and peritubular capillary hydrostatic pressures, respectively, and Π_I and Π_C are the interstitial and peritubular capillary oncotic pressures, respectively. From this, it is evident that in the peritubular capillaries, increased peritubular capillary hydrostatic pressure or decreased peritubular capillary oncotic pressure will have an adverse effect on the overall solute uptake by the peritubular capillary network.

2.11.2 Regulation of Solute Transport

The reabsorption and excretion of important solutes are regulated in response to their physiologic levels in body fluids. Some of these mechanisms are discussed below for certain key solutes. A general mechanism affecting solutes reabsorbed by the proximal tubule, termed *glomerulo-tubular balance*, is the intrinsic ability of the nephron to increase tubular reabsorption in response to tubular overload associated with increased glomerular filtration. As the GFR increases, the absolute tubular reabsorption rate increases. This mechanism appears to be completely independent from hormonal and neural influence, and to be primarily governed by the effect of altered GFR on filtration fraction and the resulting peritubular capillary oncotic pressure.

2.11.3 Recovery of Sodium

Sodium reabsorption is critical not only for the normal physiologic function throughout the body but also for its role as a transport facilitator for other solutes and water throughout the nephron. Most sodium is recovered in the proximal tubule. The proximal tubule is highly permeable to sodium ions in both directions. Sodium enters the tubular epithelial cells along a negative electrochemical gradient of 70 mV, usually in exchange for H^+ ions via a countertransporter. No energy is required and the transfer rate is linear, depending upon the solute concentration gradients. The sodium–potassium ATPase pump, a transmembrane protein located on the basolateral side of the epithelial cells, actively transports sodium out of the cell through the basal or paracellular aspects of the cell. The resulting low intracellular sodium concentration forms a chemical gradient, which, in addition to the electrochemical gradient, favors the passive diffusion of sodium into the cell from the tubular lumen across the apical (luminal) cell membrane. Usually, the tubular sodium concentration is 10-fold higher than the intracellular sodium concentration.

In contrast to sodium, the electrochemical gradient is not favorable for chloride transport in the proximal tubular epithelium. Thus, chloride ions are usually transported across the tubular epithelium in exchange for other ions, such as bicarbonate or formate. Distally in the proximal tubule, as chloride ion concentration builds in the tubular lumen, the resulting concentration gradient drives passive paracellular transport of chloride and sodium together. This latter mechanism is generally seen only in superficial nephrons.

The result of these processes is the accumulation of an isotonic sodium chloride and sodium bicarbonate solution in the interstitium. Most of this returns to the tubular lumen but a significant fraction, about 20%, enters the peritubular capillaries and returns to the circulation. Some additional sodium is recovered in the ascending limb of the loop of Henle, or in the distal tubule, via active transport processes.

2.11.4 Recovery of Other Small Solutes and Regulation of pH

Most other filtered small solutes are transported out of the proximal tubular lumen by mechanisms driven by sodium transport or by passive paracellular transport. For instance, molecules such as glucose and amino acids are reabsorbed primarily in the proximal tubular epithelium via a cotransport mechanism with sodium, and return to the blood along a concentration gradient that builds in the interstitium. Phosphate is also cotransported with sodium, but its uptake is regulated by parathyroid hormone and vitamin D. Urea, a by-product of protein catabolism, is reabsorbed passively in the proximal tubule along its concentration gradient, but only a portion of the filtered load of urea is reabsorbed (the remainder is excreted in urine). Potassium ions are reabsorbed with water through the paracellular route between the cells.

As mentioned previously, H^+ is exchanged for sodium as sodium is absorbed at the apex of the proximal tubular epithelial cell. Upon entering the tubular lumen, the H^+ reacts with filtered bicarbonate to form CO_2 and water, catalyzed by carbonic anhydrase at the proximal tubular brush border. The CO_2 is reabsorbed by the cells and is rapidly converted back to bicarbonate. In this way, some bicarbonate is effectively reabsorbed, acid is excreted, and body fluid pH is modulated.

2.12 Water Reabsorption and Its Regulation

About 180 L of water crosses the glomerular barrier each day, to excrete the solute load required to maintain homeostasis. Almost all of this water is recovered by the tubular system of the nephron, so that only 1 L of urine is normally excreted per day. The kidney can adjust the excretion of water depending upon the water intake, while continuing to filter 180 L of water at the glomerulus as required to handle solute filtration and to maintain the body fluid volume. For instance, during dehydration, the kidney increases the reabsorption of water in the tubules, and as a result, the kidney produces concentrated urine, up to 5 times the normal plasma solute concentration of 300 mOsm/kg water. In contrast, when excess water is consumed, the kidney produces diluted urine by limiting water reabsorption in the distal part of the nephron, to excrete excess water and avoid fluid overload. Each segment of the nephron contributes to this adjustment process. Hormones secreted in remote parts of the body also play an important role in tightly regulating water balance.

Most of the water that crosses the glomerular barrier, about 70%, is reabsorbed in the proximal tubules. The active reabsorption of sodium by the Na–K ATPase, which is coupled with chloride ion transport, creates an osmotic gradient between the tubular lumen and the renal interstitium as the sodium and chloride concentrations decrease in the tubular lumen. This osmotic gradient is the driving force for water reabsorption from the lumen, and therefore, water reabsorption in the proximal tubule is a passive process. However, there is indirect energy expenditure, consumed by the Na–K ATPase, which creates the osmotic force. Water is absorbed by the paracellular route, through the tight junctions between adjacent epithelial cells, and by the transcellular route, through the apical and basolateral cell membranes. To cross the cell membranes, water diffuses through transmembrane protein channels termed *aquaporins*, and to a lesser degree directly through the lipid bilayer. Although most filtered water is reabsorbed in the proximal tubule, it remains isosmotic upon entering the loop of Henle, since water passively moves across the tubular epithelium along the solute concentration gradient established by the ionic pumps.

Concentrated urine is produced by a mechanism known as a *countercurrent multiplier system*. This system establishes a hyperosmotic interstitium deep in the medulla, which can act to pull the water out of the medullary collecting duct and produce a highly concentrated urine. The hairpin arrangement of the loop of Henle and vasa recta in the deep medulla, as well as the functional distinctions between the epithelium of the descending and ascending loops of Henle, are key to the operation of this mechanism (Figure 2.6). The descending limb of the loop of Henle is permeable to water and NaCl, but does not actively transport NaCl across the cell. In contrast, the ascending limb is not permeable to water, but a Na–K ATPase pump is present on the basolateral membrane of these cells. As isotonic urine enters the descending thin loop from the proximal tubule, it establishes osmotic equilibrium with the surrounding interstitium. This occurs because water passively moves out of the tubule and NaCl passively moves in, in the face of a preexisting hypertonic interstitium deep in the medulla. Thus, the fluid at the hairpin turn of the loop of Henle becomes highly concentrated. As this concentrated urine moves into the ascending limb, water is prevented from following sodium as it is pumped across the epithelium, and the increased osmolality of the interstitium is maintained. Some of the NaCl recovered from the ascending limb moves into the freely permeable descending limb, and is carried back into the medulla, such that

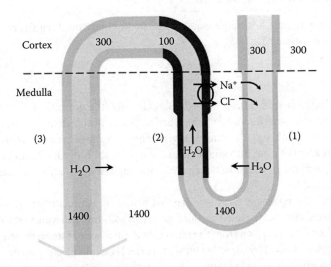

FIGURE 2.6 Countercurrent multiplication mechanism in the kidney. The numbers indicate osmolality (solute concentration) at various locations in the vicinity of the nephron in milliosmoles per kilogram water. (1) Water enters the water- and NaCl-permeable descending loop of Henle, and comes into osmotic equilibrium with the interstitium, reaching a high concentration at the hairpin. (2) Fluid returns up the water-impermeable ascending loop of Henle (indicated in black), where NaCl is actively transported across the wall into the interstitium, thereby reducing the solute concentration in the ascending limb while increasing it in the interstitium. (3) Fluid proceeds through the distal tubule in the cortex and into the water- permeable collecting duct in the medulla, where it equilibrates with the hyperosmotic interstitium, and concentrates the final urine product that exits the nephron. The recovered water returns to the body via the vasa recta, although this does not alter the solute concentration in the medulla due to the countercurrent arrangement of the vasa recta (not shown).

the highest interstitial concentrations are maintained near the hairpin of the loop of Henle. The interstitium in the deep medulla surrounds the collecting ducts and ducts of Bellini (see Figure 2.5c and d); thus, fluid in these collecting ducts will osmotically equilibrate with the high solute concentration in this region, under conditions where the walls of the collecting ducts are permeable to water.

Antidiuretic hormone (ADH), also known as *vasopressin*, participates in the maintenance of body fluid homeostasis. The principal action of ADH is to increase the renal collecting duct permeability to water. ADH is synthesized in the hypothalamus and is transferred to the posterior pituitary where it is stored to be released into the systemic circulation. The secretion of ADH occurs in response to hemodynamic signals, including plasma hyperosmolality (increased solute concentration), hypovolumia and hypotension, increased sympathetic activity, and by the direct effect of angiotensin II on the hypothalamus. However, the primary stimulus of ADH secretion is hyperosmolality. The hormone binds to its receptors, V2 receptors, located on the basal membrane of the collecting tubules, resulting in the insertion of aquaporin channels into the collecting duct epithelial cell membrane, increased water reabsorption, increased urine concentration, and decreased urine volume. ADH also causes arterial vasoconstriction, increasing the systemic blood pressure when released in large amounts.

Aldosterone, a steroid hormone secreted by the adrenal cortex, acts on the distal convoluted tubules causing increased sodium reabsorption and potassium secretion. As a result of increased sodium reabsorption, concomitant water reabsorption also occurs, resulting in increased blood volume and elevated blood pressure. Aldosterone acts by the activation of the Na–K ATPase pump on the basolateral membrane of the distal convoluted tubular epithelium, and by increasing the luminal membrane permeability to sodium. Aldosterone is released from the adrenal cortex in response to decreased plasma sodium and increased plasma potassium concentrations, through a direct effect on the adrenal cortex.

2.13 Endocrine Function of Kidney

Certain cells in the kidney secrete hormones generally related to body fluid regulation. These include renin, erythropoietin, and vitamin D.

2.13.1 Renin

Renin is a zymogen released by specialized juxtaglomerular cells (the granular cells) when perfusion pressures decrease (detected via mechanoreceptors), when sodium chloride delivery to the distal tubules is decreased, or due to neurogenic signals. Renin converts angiotensinogen, a circulating serum globulin produced and released by the liver, into angiotensin I. Angiotensin I, in turn, is further modified by angiotensin-converting enzyme in the pulmonary and renal capillaries by an endothelial cell surface enzyme to form angiotensin II.

Angiotensin II is a circulating vasoactive hormone that primarily stimulates arteriolar contraction, but has several other related effects. Angiotensin II is a powerful sodium- and water-retaining hormone. It directly increases sodium reabsorption from the renal tubules in response to decreased total body fluids. Angiotensin II exhibits its effect by directly stimulating the Na–K ATPase pump on the basolateral membrane of the tubular epithelium. Angiotensin II also directly affects the adrenal cortex, by stimulating the secretion of aldosterone hormone. This further increases sodium and water reabsorption. Angiotensin II is a potent vasoconstrictor and increases the systemic vascular resistance. Thus, angiotensin II increases the systemic blood pressure and maintains the extracellular fluid volume in the body.

2.13.2 Erythropoietin

The kidney secretes erythropoietin, a hormone that stimulates the production of red blood cells in the bone marrow. Most circulating erythropoietin is produced by the mesangial cells and renal tubular cells in the kidney, whereas the remainder is produced by the liver. Erythropoietin secretion is stimulated by hypoxia. The target cells are the bone marrow stem cells, which are activated by erythropoietin to increase the production of erythrocytes, thereby increasing the oxygen-carrying capacity of the blood. Patients with chronic renal failure are prone to developing anemia due to the lack of erythropoietin. Therefore, these individuals usually receive erythropoietin supplementation to prevent and treat anemia.

2.13.3 Vitamin D

The kidney plays an important role in the metabolism of vitamin D, by converting the inactive form obtained through diet or skin production into the active form of the vitamin. Vitamin D precursors, either dietary or produced by the skin, undergo a series of modifications in the liver and the kidney to form its active form, calcitriol. Initially, vitamin D precursors are hydroxylated in the liver to form 25-hydroxycholecalciferol. This circulating intermediate undergoes further hydroxylation in the proximal tubular epithelial cells of the kidney by a mitochondrial oxygenase, 25-hydroxyvitamin D_3 1-α-hydroxylase. This reaction forms 1,25-dihydroxylcholecalciferol, or calcitriol, the active form of vitamin D. Calcitriol plays an essential role in calcium and phosphorus metabolism and maintains their serum levels. It facilitates bone mineralization and increases the intestinal absorption of calcium.

2.14 Assessment of Kidney Function

Clinical measures of glomerular function monitor filtration efficiency and barrier integrity. The efficiency of filtration is indicated by the concentration in the urine of freely filtered solutes that are generated by the body at a constant rate and are not reabsorbed from or secreted into the urine after filtration. The primary solutes that are monitored clinically include blood urea nitrogen (pronounced "B-U-N") and serum creatinine. Urea nitrogen is a metabolic by-product of protein metabolism and it is produced at a constant rate except in certain forms of systemic disease where protein (muscle) metabolism is increased. Serum creatinine concentration is the primary clinical measure of renal function. It is produced at a relatively constant rate by the breakdown of the muscle and is freely filtered by the glomerulus with minimal tubular processing (except in extreme instances of renal failure). Clinically, these two measures are usually obtained and reported together, in view of the possibility that baseline values in an individual may be shifted as described above. These measures require obtainment of a small blood sample via phlebotomy.

Urinalysis is the assessment of the composition of the urine. Many parameters are routinely measured, including protein concentration, specific gravity (dimensionless ratio of the density of urine to the density of pure water, and representing solute concentration), osmolality (osmotically active solute concentration), presence of blood (hematuria), evidence of bacterial infection, presence of expelled material, including crystals and tubular "casts," and concentrations of molecules and ions modulated by the kidney (sodium, potassium, and creatinine). These parameters may indicate abnormalities in the glomerular or tubular function, or provide direct evidence of a specific disease process. Urinalysis may be performed on a "spot" sample (collected at one instance in time) or on a sample of all urine excreted over 24 h. The latter is used specifically to measure protein excretion, since protein levels may vary in spot samples throughout the day.

Kidney biopsy is used to evaluate the morphologic appearance of the kidney tissue. Most known and common kidney diseases exhibit specific morphologic features in the kidney parenchyma that allow for diagnosis and formulation of an appropriate treatment plan (Jennette and Heptinstall 2007). Kidney biopsies are performed when there is clinical evidence of intrinsic kidney disease, including acute or chronic renal failure, hematuria, proteinuria, nephritic syndrome, or the nephrotic syndrome. Biopsy is also useful to assess the extent of chronic, irreversible damage to the kidney in cases where the disease process has been identified (Figure 2.7). The kidney tissue is routinely evaluated using light (brightfield) microscopy, immuno-epifluorescence microscopy, and transmission electron microscopy (see Figure

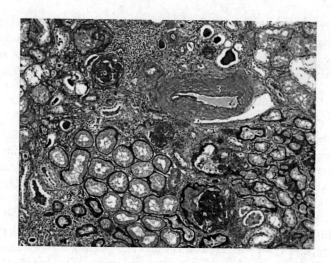

FIGURE 2.7 Photomicrograph of a periodic acid-Schiff-stained section of a human kidney biopsy, showing features of chronic damage in the kidney. (1) Globally sclerosed (scarred) glomeruli, (2) atrophic and nonfunctional tubules, (3) artery with sclerosis (fibrosis) of the intima, and (4) proteinaceous casts in atrophic tubules. The width of the image corresponds to a region that is 1.5 mm wide.

2.3b and c). Transmission electron microscopy is particularly valuable for evaluating the ultrastructure of the glomerulus, as features of a variety of disease processes affecting the glomerulus may only be confidently distinguished by examination at the ultrastructural level.

References

Brenner, B. M. 2008. *The Kidney*, 8th ed. Philadelphia: Saunders.

Deen, W. M., M. J. Lazzara, and B. D. Myers. 2001. Structural determinants of glomerular permeability. *American Journal of Physiology: Renal Physiology* 281:F579–96.

Drumond, M. C. and W. M. Deen. 1994. Structural determinants of glomerular hydraulic permeability. *American Journal of Physiology: Renal Physiology* 266:F1–12.

Endlich, N. and K. Endlich. 2006. Stretch, tension and adhesion—Adaptive mechanisms of the actin cytoskeleton in podocytes. *European Journal of Cell Biology* 85:229–34.

Friedrich, C., N. Endlich, W. Kriz, and K. Endlich. 2006. Podocytes are sensitive to fluid shear stress *in vitro*. *American Journal of Physiology: Renal Physiology* 291:F856–65.

Guyton, A. C. and J. E. Hall. 2006. *Textbook of Medical Physiology*, 11th ed. Philadelphia: Elsevier Saunders.

Jennette, J. C. and R. H. Heptinstall. 2007. *Heptinstall's Pathology of the Kidney*, 6th ed. Philadelphia: Lippincott Williams & Wilkins.

Kriz, W., M. Elger, P. Mundel, and K. V. Lemley. 1995. Structure-stabilizing forces in the glomerular tuft. *Journal of the American Society of Nephrology* 5:1731–9.

Stockand, J. D. and S. C. Sansom. 1997. Regulation of filtration rate by glomerular mesangial cells in health and diabetic renal disease. *American Journal of Kidney Disease* 29:971–81.

Weavers, H., S. Prieto-Sánchez, F. Grawe et al. 2009. The insect nephrocyte is a podocyte-like cell with a filtration slit diaphragm. *Nature* 457:322–6.

Welling, L. W., M. T. Zupka, and D. J. Welling. 1995. Mechanical properties of basement membrane. *Physiology* 10:30–35.

Wyss, H.M., J. M. Henderson, F. J. Byfield et al. 2011. Biophysical properties of normal and diseased renal glomeruli. *American Journal of Physiology: Cell Physiology* 300:C397–C405.

3

Nervous System

3.1	Definitions	3-1
3.2	Functions of the Nervous System	3-3
3.3	Representation of Information in the Nervous System	3-5
3.4	Lateral Inhibition	3-6
3.5	Higher Functions of the Nervous System	3-7
	Human Perception and Pattern Recognition • Memory and Learning	
3.6	Abnormalities of the Nervous System	3-11
	Parkinson's Disease • Alzheimer's Disease • Epilepsy • Phantom Limb Sensation/Pain	
	References	3-15

Evangelia
Micheli-Tzanakou*
Rutgers University

The nervous system unlike other organ systems is primarily concerned with signals, information encoding and processing, and control rather than manipulation of energy. It acts like a communication device whose components use substances and energy in processing signals, reorganizing them, choosing and commanding, as well as in developing and learning. A central question that is often asked is how nervous systems work and what governs the principles of their operation. In an attempt to answer this question, we, at the same time, ignore other fundamental questions such as anatomical or neurochemical and moecular aspects. We rather concentrate on relations and transactions between neurons and their assemblages in the nervous system. We deal with neural signals (encoding and decoding), the evaluation and weighting of incoming signals, and the formulation of outputs. A major part of this chapter is devoted to higher aspects of the nervous system such as memory and learning rather than individual systems such as vision and audition, which are treated extensively elsewhere [1]. Finally, some known abnormalities of the nervous system including Parkinson's and Alzheimer's disease, epilepsy, phantom limb sensation, and pain are the subjects we deal with.

3.1 Definitions

Nervous systems can be defined as organized assemblies of nerve cells as well as nonnervous cells. Nerve cells or neurons are specialized in the generation, integration, and conduction of incoming signals from the outside world or from other neurons and deliver them to other excitable cells or to *effectors* such as muscle cells. Nervous systems are easily recognized in higher animals, but not in the lower species, since the defining criteria are difficult to apply.

A central nervous system (CNS) can be easily distinguished from a peripheral nervous system (PNS) since it contains most of the motor and the nucleated parts of neurons that innervate muscles and other effectors. The PNS contains all the sensory nerve cell bodies with some exceptions, plus local *plexuses*, local *ganglia*, and peripheral axons that make up the *nerves*. Most sensory axons go all the way into the

---

* Deceased.

CNS while the remaining sensory axons relay in the peripheral plexuses. Motor axons originating in the CNS innervate effector cells.

The nervous system has two major roles: first, to regulate, acting homeostatically, in restoring some conditions of the organism after some external stimulus, and second, to act to alter a preexisting condition by replacing it or modifying it. In both cases—regulation or initiation of a process—learning can be superimposed. In most species, learning is more or less an adaptive mechanism, combining and timing species-characteristic acts, with a large degree of evolution toward perfection.

The nervous system is a complex structure for which realistic assumptions have led to irrelevant over-simplifications. One can break down the nervous system into four components: sensory transducers, neurons, axons, and muscle fibers. Each of these components gathers processes and transmits information impinging upon them from the outside world, usually in the form of complex stimuli. The processing is carried out by excitable tissues—neurons, axons, sensory receptors, and muscle fibers. Neurons are the basic elements of the nervous system. If put in small assemblies or clusters, they form neuronal assemblies or neuronal networks, communicating with each other either chemically via *synaptic junctions* or electrically via *tight* junctions. The main characteristics of a cell are the *cell body* or *soma*, which contains the *nucleus*, and a number of processes originating from the cell body called the *dendrites*, which reach out to the surroundings to make contacts with other cells. These contacts serve as the incoming information to the cell, while the outgoing information follows a conduction path, the axon. The incoming information is integrated in the cell body and generates the result of this at the *axon hillock*. There are two types of outputs that can be generated and therefore two types of neurons: those generating *grated* potentials that attenuate with distance and those generating *action* potentials. The action potential travels through the axon, a thin, long process that passively passes the action potential or rather a train of action potentials without attenuation (*all-or-none* effect). A series of action potentials is often called a *spike train*. A threshold built into the hillock, and depending on its level, allows or stops the generation of the spike trains. Axons usually terminate on other neurons by means of *synaptic terminals* or *boutons* and have properties similar to those of an electric cable with varying diameters and speeds of signal transmission. Axons can be of two types, namely, *myelinated* and *unmyelinated*. In the former, the axon is surrounded by a thick fatty material, the myelin sheath, which is interrupted at regular intervals by gaps called the *nodes of Ranvier*. These nodes provide for the *saltatory* conduction of the signal along the axon. The axon makes functional connections with other neurons at synapses on the cell body, the dendrites, or the axons. There exist two kinds of synapses: *excitatory* and *inhibitory* and, as the name implies, they either increase the *firing* frequency of the postsynaptic neurons or decrease it, respectively [5].

Sensory receptors are specialized cells that, in response to an incoming stimulus, generate a corresponding electrical signal, a graded receptor potential. Although the mechanisms by which the sensory receptors generate receptor potentials are not exactly known, the most plausible scenario is that an external stimulus alters the membrane permeabilities. Then the neuron's receptor potential is the change in intracellular potential relative to its *resting* potential.

It is important to note here that the term "receptor" is used in physiology to refer not only to sensory receptors but in a different sense to proteins that bind neurotransmitters, hormones, and other substances with great affinity and specificity as a first step in starting up physiological responses. This receptor is often associated with nonneural cells that surround it and form a *sense organ*. The forms of energy converted by the receptors include mechanical, thermal, electromagnetic, and chemical energy. The particular form of energy to which a receptor is most sensitive is called its *adequate stimulus*. The problem of how receptors convert energy into action potentials in the sensory nerves has been the subject of intensive study. In the complex sense organs such as those concerned with hearing and vision, there exist separate receptor cells and synaptic junctions between receptors and afferent nerves. In other cases such as the cutaneous sense organs, the receptors are specialized. Where a stimulus of constant strength is applied to a receptor repeatedly, the frequency of the action potentials in its sensor nerve declines over a period of time. This phenomenon is known as *adaptation*; if the adaptation is very rapid, then the receptors are called *phasic*; otherwise, they are called as *tonic*.

Another important issue is the *coding* of sensory information. Action potentials are similar in all nerves although there are variations in their speed of conduction and other characteristics. But if the action potentials are the same in most cells, then what makes the visual cells sensitive to light and not to sound and what makes the touch receptors sensitive to a sensation of touch and not of smell? And how can we tell if these sensations are strong or not? These sensations depend upon the specific part of the brain called the *doctrine of specific nerve energies* and has been questioned over time by several researchers. No matter where a particular sensory pathway is stimulated along its path of connecting to the brain, the sensation produced is always referred to the location of the receptor site. This is the principle of the *law of projections*. An example of this law is the "phantom limb" where an amputee complains about pain or an itching sensation in that missing limb. This phenomenon is discussed in a greater detail later on in the chapter.

3.2 Functions of the Nervous System

The basic unit of integrated activity is the *reflex arc*. This arc consists of a sense organ, an afferent neuron, one or more synapses in a central integrating station (or sympathetic ganglion), an efferent neuron, as well as an effector. The simplest reflex arc is the *monosynaptic* one, which only has one synapse between the afferent and efferent neuron. With more than one synapse, the reflex arc is called *polysynaptic*. In each of these cases, activity is modified by both spatial and temporal facilitation, occlusion, and other effects [2,3].

In mammals, the connection between afferent and efferent somatic neurons is found either in the brain or the spinal cord. The Bell–Magendie law dictates the fact that in the spinal cord, the dorsal roots are sensory while the ventral roots are motor. The action potential message that is carried by an axon is eventually fed to a muscle, a secretory cell, or the dendrite of another neuron. If an axon is carrying a graded potential, its output is too weak to stimulate a muscle, but it can terminate on a secretory cell or a dendrite. The latter can have as many as 10,000 inputs. If the endpoint is a motor neuron, which has been found experimentally in the case of fibers from the primary endings, then there is a time lag between the time when a stimulus was applied and a response obtained from the muscle. This time interval is called the *reaction time* and in humans, it is approximately 20 ms for a stretch reflex. The distance from the spinal cord can be measured and since the conduction velocities of both the efferent and afferent fibers are known, another important quantity can be calculated, namely, the *central delay*. This delay is the portion of the reaction time that was spent for conduction to and from the spinal cord. It has been found that muscle spindles also make connections that cause muscle contraction via polysynaptic pathways, while the afferents from secondary endings make connections that excite extensor muscles. When a motor neuron sends a burst of action potentials to its skeletal muscle, the amount of contraction depends largely on the discharge frequency and on many other factors as well, such as the history of the load on the muscle and the load itself. *The stretch error* can be calculated from the desired motion minus the actual stretch. If this error is then fed back to the motor neuron, its discharge frequency is modified appropriately. This frequency modification corresponds to one of the three feedback loops that are available locally. Another loop corrects for overstretching beyond the point at which the muscle or tendon may tear. Since a muscle can only contract, it must be paired with another muscle (*antagonist*) to affect the return motion. Generally speaking, a flexor muscle is paired with an extension muscle that cannot be activated simultaneously. This means that the motor neurons that affect each one of these muscles are not activated at the same time. Instead, when one set of motor neurons is active, the other is inhibited and vice versa. When a movement involves two or more muscles that normally cooperate by contracting simultaneously, the excitation of one causes the facilitation of the other *synergistic* members via cross connections. All these networks form feedback loops. An engineer's interpretation of how these loops work would be to assume dynamic conditions, as is the case in all parts of the nervous system. This has little value in dealing with stationary conditions, but it provides for an ability to adjust to changing conditions.

The nervous system, as mentioned in the introduction, is a control system of processes that adjust both internal and external operations. As humans, we have experiences that change our perception of events in our environment. The same is true for higher animals that besides having an internal environment, the status of which is of major importance, also share an external environment of utmost richness and variety. Objects and conditions that have direct contact with the surface of an animal directly affect the future of the animal. The information about changes at some point provides a prediction of possible future. The amount of information required to represent changing conditions increases as the required temporal resolution of detail increases. This creates a vast amount of data to be processed by any finite system. Considering the fact that the information reaching sensory receptors is too extensive and redundant, as well as modified by external interference (noise), the nervous system has a tremendously difficult task to accomplish. Enhanced responsiveness to a particular stimulus can be produced by structures that either increase the energy converging on a receptor or increase the effectiveness of coupling of a specific type of stimulus to the receptor. Different species have sensory systems that respond to stimuli that are important to them for survival. Often, one nervous system responds to conditions that are not sensed by another nervous system [4,5]. The transduction, processing, and transmission of signals in any nervous system produces a survival mechanism for an organism but only after these signals have been further modified by effector organs. Although the nerve impulses that drive a muscle are discrete events as explained earlier, a muscle twitch takes much longer to happen, a fact that allows for responses to overlap and produce a much smoother output. The neural control of the motor activity of the skeletal muscle is accomplished entirely by the modification of the muscle excitation, which involves changes in velocity, length, stiffness, and heat production. The importance of accurate timing of inputs, and the maintenance of this timing across several synapses, is obvious in sensory pathways of the nervous system. The cells are located next to other cells that have overlapping or adjacent receptive or motor fields. The dendrites provide important and complicated sites of interactions as well as channels of variable effectiveness for excitatory inputs, depending on their position relative to the cell body. Among the best examples are the cells of the medial superior olive in the auditory pathway. These cells have two major dendritic trees extending from opposite poles of the cell body. One receives synaptic inhibitory input from the ipsilateral cochlear nucleus and the other receives synaptic inhibitory input from the contralateral, which normally is an excitatory input. These cells deal with the determination of the azimuth of a sound. When a sound is present at the contralateral side, most cells are excited while ipsilateral sounds cause inhibition. It has been shown that the cells can go from complete excitation to full inhibition with a difference of only a few hundred milliseconds in arrival time of the two inputs.

The question then arises: how does the nervous system put together the signals available to it so that a determination of our output takes place? To arrive at an understanding of how the nervous system integrates the incoming information at a given moment of time, we must understand that the processes that take place depend both on cellular forms and a topological architecture as well as on the physiological properties that relate input to output. That is, we have to know the *transfer* functions or *coupling* functions. Integration depends on the weighting of inputs. One of the important factors determining weighting is the area of synaptic contact. The extensive dendrites are the primary integrating structures. Electronic spread is the means of mixing, smoothing, attenuating, delaying, and summing postsynaptic potentials. The spatial distribution of input is often not random but is systematically restricted. Also, the wide variety of characteristic geometries of synapses is, no doubt, important not just for the weighting of different combinations of inputs. When repeated stimuli are presented at various intervals at different junctions, higher-amplitude synaptic potentials are generated, if the intervals between them are not too short or too long. This increase in amplitude is due to a phenomenon called *facilitation*. If the response lasts longer than the interval between impulses, so that the second response rises from the residue of the first, then it is called *temporal summation*. If in addition, the response increment due to the second stimulus is larger than the previous one, then it is facilitation. Facilitation is an important function of the nervous system and is found in quite different forms and durations, ranging from a few milliseconds to tenths of seconds. Facilitation may grade from forms of sensitization to learning, especially at long intervals. A special case is the so-called *posttetanic potentiation*, which is the result of high-frequency stimulation for long periods of time (about 10 s). The latter is an interesting case since no effects can be seen during the stimulation but afterward, any test stimulus at various intervals creates a marked increase in response up to many times more than the "tetanic" stimulus. *Antifacilitation* is the phenomenon where a decrease of response from the neuron is observed at certain junctions, due to successive impulses. Its mechanism is less understood than facilitation. Both facilitation and antifacilitation may be observed on the same neuron but when different functions are performed.

3.3 Representation of Information in the Nervous System

Whenever information is transferred between different parts of the nervous system, some communication paths have to be established, and some parameters of impulse firing relevant to communication must be set up. Since what is communicated is nothing more than impulses—spike trains—the only basic variables in a train of events are the number of spikes and the interval between spikes. With respect to that, the nervous system acts like a pulse-coded analog device since the intervals are continuously graded. There exists a distribution of interval lengths between individual spikes, which in any sample can be expressed by the shape of the interval histogram. If one examines different examples, it will be seen that their distributions differ markedly. Some histograms look like Poisson distributions, some others exhibit Gaussian or bimodal shapes. The coefficient of variation—expressed as the standard deviation over the mean—in some cases is constant while in others, it varies. Some other properties depend on the sequence of longer and shorter intervals than the mean. Some neurons show no linear dependence, some others show positive or negative correlations of successive intervals. If the stimulus is delivered and a discharge from the neuron is observed, a *poststimulus time histogram* can be used using the onset of the stimulus as a reference point and average many responses to reveal certain consistent features of temporal patterns. Coding of information can then be based on the average frequency, which can represent relevant gradations of the input. Mean frequency is the code in most cases, although no definition of it has been given with respect to measured quantities such as averaging time, weighting functions, and forgetting functions. The characteristic transfer functions have been found that suggest that there are several distinct coding principles in addition to the mean frequency. Each theoretically possible code becomes a candidate code as long as there exists some evidence that is readable by the system under investigation. So, one has to first test for the availability of the code by imposing a stimulus that is considered normal. After a response has been observed, the code is considered to be available. If the input is changed to different levels of one parameter and changes are observed at the postsynaptic level, the code is called *readable*. However, only if both are formed in the same preparation and no other parameter is available and readable, can the code be said to be the *actual* code employed. Some such parameters are

- Time of firing
- Temporal pattern
- Number of spikes in the train
- Variance of interspike intervals
- Spike delays or latencies
- Constellation code

The latter is a very important one, especially when used in conjunction with the concept of *receptive fields* of units in different sensory pathways. The unit receptors do not need to have highly specialized abilities to permit encoding of a large number of distinct stimuli. Receptive fields are topographic and overlap extensively. Any given stimulus will excite a certain constellation of receptors and is therefore encoded in the particular set that is activated. A large degree of uncertainty prevails and requires the brain to operate probabilistically. In the nervous system, there exists a large amount of *redundancy* although neurons might have different thresholds. It is questionable, however, if these units are entirely equivalent although they share parts of their receptive fields. The nonoverlapping parts might be of importance and are critical to sensory function. On the other hand, redundancy does not necessarily mean unspecified or random connectivity. It rather allows for greater sensitivity and resolution, improvement of signal-to-noise ratio, while at the same time, it provides stability of performance.

The integration of large numbers of converging inputs to give a single output can be considered as an averaging or probabilistic operation. The "decisions" made by a unit depend on its inputs or some intrinsic states and on its reaching a certain threshold. This way, every unit in the nervous system can make a decision, when it changes from one state to a different one. A theoretical possibility also exists that a mass of randomly connected neurons may constitute a trigger unit and that activity with a sharp threshold can spread through such a mass redundancy. Each part of the nervous system and in particular the receiving side can be thought of as a filter. Higher-order neurons do not merely pass that information on, but instead, they use convergence from different channels, as well as divergence of the same channels and other processes, to modify incoming signals. Depending on the structure and coupling functions of the network, what gets through is determined. Similar networks exist at the output side. They also act as filters but since they formulate decisions and commands with precise *spatiotemporal* properties, they can be thought of as *pattern generators*.

3.4 Lateral Inhibition

Our discussion will be incomplete without the description of a very important phenomenon in the nervous system. This phenomenon called *lateral inhibition* is used by the nervous system to improve spatial resolution and contrast. The effectiveness of this type of inhibition decreases with distance. In the retina, for example, lateral inhibition is used extensively to improve contrast. As the stimulus approaches a certain unit, it first excites neighbors of the recorded cell. Since these neighbors inhibit that unit, its response is a decreased firing frequency. If the stimulus is exactly over the recorded unit, this unit is excited and fires above its normal rate, and as the stimulus moves out again, the neighbors are excited while the unit under consideration fires less. If we now examine the output of all the units as a whole and at once, while half of the considered array is stimulated and the other half is not, we will notice that at the point of discontinuity of the stimulus going from stimulation to nonstimulation, the firing frequencies of the two halves have been differentiated to the extreme at the stimulus edge, which has been enhanced. The neuronal circuits responsible for lateral shifts are relatively simple. Lateral inhibition can be considered to give the negative of the second spatial derivative of the input stimulus. A second layer of neurons could be constructed to perform this spatial differentiation on the input signal to detect only the edge. It is probably lateral inhibition that explains the psychophysical illusion known as *Mach bands*. It is probably the same principle that operates widely in the nervous system to enhance the sensitivity to contrast in the visual system in particular and in all other modalities in general. Through the years, different models have been developed to describe lateral inhibition mathematically and various methods of analysis have been employed. These models include both one-dimensional examination of the phenomenon and two-dimensional treatment, where a two-dimensional array is used as a stimulus. This two-dimensional treatment is justified since most of the sensory receptors of the body form two-dimensional maps (receptive fields). In principle, if a one-dimensional lateral inhibition system is linear, one can extend the analysis to two dimensions by means of superposition. The objective is the same as that of the nervous system: to improve image sharpness without introducing too much distortion. This technique requires storage of each picture element (pixel) and lateral "inhibitory" interactions between adjacent pixels. Since a picture may contain millions of pixels, high-speed computers with large-scale memories are required.

At a higher level, similar algorithms can be used to evaluate decision-making mechanisms. In this case, many inputs from different sensory systems are competing for attention. The brain evaluates each one of the inputs as a function of the remaining ones. One can picture a decision-making mechanism resembling a "locator" of stimulus peaks. The final output depends on what weights are used at the inputs of a push–pull mechanism. Thus, a decision can be made depending on the weights an individual's brain is applying to the incoming information about the situation under consideration. The most important information is heavily weighted while the rest is either totally masked or weighted very lightly.

3.5 Higher Functions of the Nervous System

3.5.1 Human Perception and Pattern Recognition

One way of understanding human perception is to study the mechanisms of information processing in the brain. The recognition of patterns of sensory input is one function of the brain, a task accomplished by neuronal circuits, the *feature extractors*. Although such neuronal information is more likely to be processed globally, by a large number of neurons, in animals, single-unit recording is one of the most powerful tools in the hands of a physiologist. Most often, the concept of the *receptive field* is used as a method of understanding the sensory information processing. In the case of the visual system, we would call the receptive field a well-defined region of the visual field, which when stimulated will change the firing rate of a neuron in the visual pathway. The neuron's response will usually depend on the distribution of light in the receptive field. Therefore, the information collected by the brain from the outside world is transformed into spatial as well as temporal patterns of neural activity.

The question often asked is how do we perceive and recognize faces, objects, and scenes. Even in those cases where only noisy representations exist, we are still able to make some inference as to what the pattern represents. Unfortunately, in humans, single-unit recording, as mentioned earlier, is impossible. As a result, one has to use other kinds of measurements, such as evoked potentials (EPs) or functional imaging techniques such as functional magnetic resonance imaging (fMRI) and positron emission tomography (PET). Although physiological in nature, EPs are still far away from giving us information at the neuronal level. All these methods, however, have been used extensively as a way of probing the human (and animal) brains because of their noninvasive character. EPs can be considered to be the result of integrations of the neuronal activity of many neurons somewhere in the brain. These gross potentials can be used as a measure of the response of the brain to sensory inputs.

The question then arises: Can we use this response to influence the brain in producing patterns of activity that we want? None of the efforts of the past closed that loop. Then, how do we explain the phenomenon of selective attention by which we selectively direct our attention to something of interest and discard the rest? And what happens with the evolution of certain species that change appearance according to their everyday needs? All these questions tend to lead to the fact that somewhere in the brain there is a loop where previous knowledge or experience is used as a feedback to the brain itself. This feedback modifies the ability of the brain to respond in a different way to the same stimulus the next time it is presented. In a way then, the brain creates mental "images" independent of the stimulus, which tends to modify the representation of the stimulus in the brain [1].

This section describes some efforts in which different methods have been used in trying to address the difficult task of feedback loops in the brain. No attempt, however, will be made to explain or even postulate where these feedback loops might be located. If one considers the brain as a huge set of neural networks, then one question has been debated for many years: what is the role of the individual neuron in the net and what is the role of each network in the global processes of the brain? More specifically, does the neuron act as an analyzer or a detector of specific features or does it merely reflect the characteristic response of a population of cells of which it happens to be a member? What invariant relationships exist between sensory input and the response of a single neuron and how much can be "read" about the stimulus parameters from the record of a single EP? In turn, then, how much feedback can one use from a single EP to influence the stimulus and how successful can that influence be? Many physiologists express doubts that simultaneous observations of a large number of individual neuronal activities can be readily interpreted. In other words, can then a feedback process influence and modulate the stimulus patterns so that they appear as being optimal? If this was proven to be true, it would mean that we can reverse the

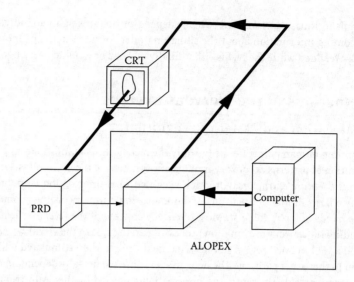

FIGURE 3.1 An ALOPEX system. The stimulus is presented on the cathode ray tube (CRT). The observer or any pattern-recognition device (PRD) faces the CRT; the subject's response is sent to the ALOPEX interface unit where it is recorded and integrated and the final response is sent to the computer. The computer calculates the values of the new pattern to be presented on the CRT according to the ALOPEX algorithm and the process continues until the desired pattern appears on the CRT. At this point, the response is considered to be optimal and the process stops.

pattern-recognition process, and instead of recognizing a pattern, we would be able to create a pattern from a vast variety of possible patterns. It would be like creating a link between our brain and a computer, equivalent to a brain–computer system network. Figure 3.1 is a schematic representation of such a process involved in what we call the feedback loop of the system. The *pattern-recognition device* (PRD) is connected to an ALOPEX system (a computer algorithm and an image processor in this case) and faces a display monitor where different intensity patterns can be shown. In this figure, the thin arrows represent response information and heavy arrows represent detailed pattern information generated by the computer and relayed by an ALOPEX system to the monitor. (ALOPEX is a set of algorithms described in detail elsewhere in the author's publications.) If this kind of arrangement is used for the determination of visual-receptive fields of neurons, then the PRD is nothing more than the brain of the experimental animal or human. This way, the neuron under investigation does its own selection of the best stimulus or trigger feature, and reverses the role of the neuron from being a feature extractor to becoming a feature generator as mentioned earlier. The idea is to find the response of the neuron to a stimulus and use this response as a positive feedback in the directed evaluation of the initially random pattern. Thus, the cell filters out the key trigger features from the stimulus and reinforces them with the feedback.

As a generalization of this process, we might consider that a neuron, N, receives a visual input from a pattern, P, which is transmitted in a modified form P′ to an analyzer neuron AN (or even a complex of such neurons) as shown in Figure 3.2. The analyzer responds with a scalar variable, R, that is then fed back to the system and the pattern is modified accordingly. The process continues in small steps (iterations) until there is an almost perfect correlation between the original pattern (template) and the one that the neuron, N, indirectly created. This integrator sends the response back to the original modifier. The integrator need not be a linear one. It could take any nonlinear form, a fact that is a more realistic representation of the visual cortex. We can envision the input patterns as templates preexisting in the memory of the system, a situation that might come about with visual experience. For a "naive" system, any initial pattern will do. As experience is gained, the patterns become less random. If one starts with a pattern that has some resemblance to one of the preexisting patterns, evolution will take its course. In nature, there might exist a mechanism similar to that of ALOPEX [1]. By filtering the characteristics that

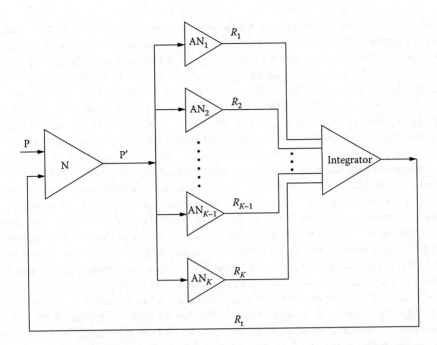

FIGURE 3.2 Schematic representation of the ALOPEX "inverse" pattern-recognition scheme. Each neuron represents a feature analyzer, which responds to the stimulus with a scalar quantity R called the *response*. R is then fed back to the system and the pattern is modified accordingly. This process continues until there is an almost perfect correlation between the desired output and the original pattern.

are most important for the survival of the species, changes would be triggered. *Perception*, therefore, could be considered to be an interaction between sensory inputs and past experience in the form of templates stored in the memory bank of the perceiver and is specific to the perceiver's needs. These templates are modifiable with time and are adjusted accordingly to the input stimuli. With this approach, the neural nets and ensembles of nets generate patterns that describe their thinking and memory properties. Thus, the normal flow of information is *reversed* and controls the afferent systems.

Perception processes as well as feature extraction or suppression of images or objects can be ascribed to specific neural mechanisms due to some sensory input, or even due to some "wishful thinking" of the PRD. If it is true that the association cortex is affecting the sensitivity of the sensory cortex, then an ALOPEX mechanism is what one needs to close the loop for memory and learning.

3.5.2 Memory and Learning

If we try to define what memory is, we will face the fact that memory is not a single mental faculty but it is rather composed of multiple abilities mediated by separate and distinct brain systems. Memory for a recent event can be expressed *explicitly* as a conscious recollection, or *implicitly*, as a facilitation of test performance without conscious recollection. The major distinction between these two memories is that explicit or *declarative* memory depends on limbic and diencephalic structures and provides the basis for recollection of events, while implicit or *nondeclarative* memory supports skills and habit learning, single conditioning, and the well-researched phenomenon of *priming* [7].

Declarative memory refers to memory of recent events and is usually assessed by tests of recall or recognition for specific single items. When the list of items becomes longer, a subject not only learns about each item on the list but also makes associations about what all these items have in common, that is, the subject learns about the category that the items belong to. Learning leads to changes that increase or decrease the effectiveness of impulses arriving at the junctions between neurons and the cumulative effect of these changes constitutes memory. Very often, a particular pattern of neural activity leads to a result that occurs sometime after that activity has ended. Learning then requires some means of relating the activity that is to be changed to the evaluation that can be made only by the delayed consequence. This phenomenon in physics is called *hysteresis* and refers to any modifications of future actions due to past actions. *Learning* then could be defined as a change in any neuronal response resulting from previous experiences due to an external stimulus. *Memory* in turn, would be the maintenance of these changes over time. The collection of neural changes representing memory is commonly known as the *engram* and a major part of recent work has been to identify and locate engrams in the brain, since specific parts of the nervous system are capable of specific types of learning. The view of memory that has recently emerged is that information storage is tied to specific processing areas that are engaged during learning. The brain is organized so that separate regions of the neocortex simultaneously carry out computations on specific features or characteristics of the external stimulus, no matter how complex that stimulus might be. If the brain learns specific properties or features of the stimulus, then we talk about the *nonassociative memory*. Associated with this type of learning is the phenomenon of *habituation* in which, if the same stimulus is presented repeatedly, the neurons respond less and less, while the introduction of a new stimulus increases the sensitization of the neuron. If learning includes two related stimuli, then we talk about associative learning. This type of learning can be of two types: classical conditioning and operant conditioning. The former deals with relationships among stimuli while the latter deals with the relationship of the stimulus to the animal's own behavior. In humans, there exist two types of memory: short- and long-term memories. The best way to study any physiological process in humans (especially memory) is to study its pathology. The study of amnesia has provided strong evidence of distinguishing between these types of memory. Amnesic patients can keep a short list of numbers in mind for several minutes if they pay attention to the task. The difficulty comes when the list becomes longer, especially if the amount to be learned exceeds the brain capacity of what can be held in immediate memory. It could be that this happens because more systems have to be involved and that temporary information storage may occur within each brain area where stable changes in synaptic efficacy can eventually develop. *Plasticity* within existing pathways can account for most of the observations and short-term memory occurs too quickly for it to require any major modifications of neuronal pathways. The capacity of long-term memory requires the integrity of the medial, temporal, and diencephalic regions, in conjunction with neurons for storage of information. Within the domain of long-term memory, amnesic patients demonstrate intact learning and retention of certain motor, perceptual and cognitive skills, and intact priming effects. These patients do not exhibit any learning deficits but have no conscious awareness of prior study sessions or recognition of previously presented stimuli.

Priming effects can be tested by presenting words and then providing either the first few letters of the word or the last part of the word for recognition by the patient. Normal subjects, as expected, perform better than amnesic subjects. But if these patients are instructed to "read" the incomplete word instead of memorizing it, then they perform as well as the normal subjects. Also, amnesic patients perform well if words are cued by category names. Thus, priming effects seem to be independent of the processes of recall and recognition memory, which is also observed in normal subjects. All these evidences support the notion that the brain has organized its memory functions around fundamentally different information storage systems. In perceiving a word, a preexisting array of neurons is activated that has concurrent activities that produce perception and priming is one of these functions.

Memory is not fixed immediately after learning, but continues to grow toward stabilization over a period of time. This stabilization is called *consolidation of memory*. Memory consolidation is a *dynamic* feature of long-term memory, especially the declarative memory, but is neither an automatic process with fixed lifetime nor is it determined at the time of learning. It is rather a process of reorganization of stored information. As time passes, some not yet consolidated memories fade out by remodeling the neural circuitry that is responsible for the original representation or by establishing new representations, since the original one might be forgotten.

The problems of learning and memory are studied continuously and with increased interest in these years, especially because artificial systems such as neural networks can be used to mimic functions of the nervous system.

3.6 Abnormalities of the Nervous System

3.6.1 Parkinson's Disease

Parkinson's disease (PD) is a slowly progressive neurodegenerative disease of the CNS first described in 1817 by James Parkinson. The incidence rates ranges from 4.5 to 21 per 100,000 individuals per year. At least 750,000,000 people are affected in the United States alone. Although most patients affected are over 60 years of age, as many as 10% may be less than 40.

PD occurs due to degeneration of the substantia nigra, a part of the brain involved in motor control, whose cells secretes the neurotransmitter dopamine to other movement-control centers known as the basal ganglia. The basal ganglia circuitry, which utilizes other neurotransmitters such as γ-aminobutyric acid and serotonin among others, is therefore affected. It is due to these other neurotransmitters that patients may develop nonmotor symptoms later in the disease. Some of these symptoms include cognitive problems, psychiatric disorders (e.g., depression), sleep disorders (e.g., restless leg syndrome, rapid eye movement [REM], and behavior disorder), and autonomic nervous system dysfunction among others [8].

A minority of patients may have a genetic disorder. Those patients know of other family members, throughout the different generations, with PD. But what causes the degeneration in the substantia nigra in the majority of the patients is still unknown. Multiple reports were published in the late 1970s and early 1980s of patients who developed Parkinsonism induced by 1-methyl-4-phenyl-1,2,3,6-tetrahydro-pyridine (MPTP), a contaminant of illicit narcotics. Some other culprits include manganese, carbon monoxide, pesticides, and antidopaminergic therapy, but these are implicated only in very few cases.

The diagnosis is made clinically when the characteristic motor deficits appear. These include tremor, bradykinesia (slowed movements), rigidity, and postural instability. The tremor occurs at rest. It occasionally begins with an alternating opposition of the fingers and thumb called "pill-rolling" tremor. The characteristic frequency of the Parkinsonian tremor is of 3–5 cycles/s. The symptoms usually begin on one side of the body and slowly progress over years to decades to include the other side.

The various pharmacological treatments currently available are designed to affect the dopaminergic system. The "gold standard" is levodopa. However, the long-term use of levodopa leads to motor complications, mainly dyskinesias or chorea (involuntary, uncontrolled movements of the body). Dopamine agonists appear to delay the onset of dyskinesias for a few years. Currently under study are a few non-dopaminergic drugs with the hope of improving motor symptoms, avoiding motor complications, and delaying neurodegeneration [10].

In patients with more advanced disease, when medications alone are no longer controlling symptoms, surgical options may be considered as part of PD treatment. The most common surgical option offered to patients is deep brain stimulation (DBS) that uses an implanted electrode to stimulate parts of the brain. The goal is to restore some balance to the activity in the parts of the brain most affected in PD and therefore reduces symptoms. It is particularly good at controlling tremor. The effects of surgical procedures such as this, however, are quite variable, and, like other treatments, is not a cure for the disease.

The stimulator is connected to a pulse generator, a device that controls the electrical stimulation delivered through the electrodes in the brain. The pulse generator is a small metal device that is generally implanted under the skin on the upper chest. When the electrodes deliver electrical stimulation, they cause the cells in the subthalamic nucleus to shut down. This aims to help balance out the imbalance that is caused by PD. The specific location and type of electrical stimulation can be adjusted and are often changed to try to optimize the treatment and maximize symptom resolution while minimizing any side effects.

New, but still experimental procedures are being introduced: (a) the repetitive transcranial magnetic stimulation (rTMS) and (b) the transcranial direct current stimulation (tDCS). Motor cortex stimulation could impact on any station within the cortico-basal ganglia-thalamo-cortical loops that are involved in motor control, providing alleviation of Parkinsonian symptoms. Depending on the target, cortical stimulation might improve motor performance or other symptoms associated with PD, such as depression. The clinical application of rTMS to treat PD patients is limited by the short duration of the effects beyond the time of stimulation, even if long-lasting improvements have been observed after repeated rTMS sessions. In any case, the place of cortical stimulation in the therapeutic management of PD patients remains to be determined, as an alternative or a complementary technique to DBS. The rTMS technique could be used to define better the targets and the parameters of stimulation subsequently applied in chronic epidural stimulation [12,13]. Most studies to date have shown beneficial effects of rTMS or tDCS on clinical symptoms in PD and support the notion of spatial specificity to the effects on motor and nonmotor symptoms. Stimulation parameters have varied widely, however, and some studies are poorly controlled. It remains unclear how to individually adjust rTMS or tDCS factors for the most beneficial effects on symptoms of PD or dystonia. Nonetheless, the noninvasive nature, minimal side effects, positive effects in preliminary clinical studies, and increasing evidence for rational mechanisms make rTMS and tDCS attractive for ongoing investigation [22].

3.6.2 Alzheimer's Disease

Alzheimer's disease (AD) is the most common form of dementia among elders. It is named after Alois Alzheimer, who described both the clinical features and pathologic changes in 1906. Similar to PD, it is also a progressive neurodegenerative disease. The prevalence in the United States in patients aged above 65 years is 10.3%, rising to 47% in those over the age of 80.

AD is primarily the result of degeneration or death of nerve cells in the cerebral cortex and in areas that usually control functions such as memory, personality, logical thinking, and others. As the nerve cells become withered and small, they cause the enlargement of the ventricles of the brain. Recent events are not remembered; the individual is not able to perform calculations or make plans and decisions. Abrupt personality changes alarm family members and friends, thus disabling the person from functioning normally.

The etiology of the majority of the cases still remains unknown, although it appears to be depending on multiple factors. Familial AD, although rare, can be inherited. The patients in this group have an earlier onset (aged 30–60) than the common form of AD. The one risk factor for the more common form is a protein involved in cholesterol transport known as apolipoprotein E (apoE). The allele frequency of an isoform of apoE (apoE4) was found to be 40% in either familial or common form AD compared to 15% in patients without AD [11].

AD is characterized by atrophy of the cerebral cortex, usually more severe in the frontal, parietal, and temporal lobes. The most characteristic microscopic findings are the senile plaques and neurofibrillary tangles. These are mostly found throughout the cerebral cortex and hippocampus. The activity of choline acetyltransferase, the biosynthetic enzyme of acetylcholine, has a 50–90% reduction in the cerebral cortex and hippocampus in AD. Therefore, cholinergic neurons are largely affected.

Amyloid-beta (AB) is the major substance implicated in the progression of AD. Large amounts of this peptide due to overproduction, lack of degradation, or other factors lead to the formation of senile plaques. Their presence may trigger the release of cytochrome C, which is associated with *apoptosis* (cell death) and neurodegeneration. (PD also involves amyloids that aggregate and participate in the direct or indirect loss of synapses and neurons.) Other studies point to excessive amounts of glutamate in the extracellular fluid. Their presence is thought to very rapidly inhibit the transport of molecules from the cell body to the end terminal of the axon, therefore leading to the loss of synapses—the end result of AD. Thus, chemical synaptic input is stopped and the ability of the person to perform certain functions is greatly inhibited.

Since the only definite way to diagnose AD is through histopathology, clinicians can diagnose possible or probable AD depending on signs and symptoms until a brain autopsy confirms the diagnosis. Some of the symptoms include progressive worsening of memory and other cognitive functions and cognitive loss impairing social or occupational functioning and causing a significant decline from a previous level of functioning. The current therapies used for AD include cholinesterase inhibitors, estrogen, nonsteroidal anti-inflammatory drugs, and vitamin E.

At a recent meeting of the Alzheimer's Association (AAICAD 2010) [13], promising investigations were reported and being pursued on a variety of fronts—avenues that could very well lead to significant changes in Alzheimer diagnosis and treatment.

Three long-term, large-scale studies (Framingham Study, Cardiovascular Health Study, and NHANES III) support the association of physical activity and certain dietary elements (tea, vitamin D) with possibly maintaining cognitive ability and reducing dementia risk in older adults. Plus, a new study in an animal model of Alzheimer's reported at AAICAD 2010 suggests that an antioxidant-rich diet with walnuts may benefit brain function. Research has pointed toward a number of factors that may impact our risk of Alzheimer's and cognitive decline, the strongest being reducing cardiovascular risk factors. Experimental immunotherapies are also suggested that target the β-amyloid.

While the role of biomarkers differs in each of the three stages of the disease, much remains to be understood concerning their reliability and validity in diagnosis. This makes it critical that any new recommendations can be thoroughly tested.

Some early reports on a gene known as FTO, which appears to be correlated with obesity, suggest that FTO may have a correlation with increased risk for AD. Two studies also reported at AAICAD 2010 give more information about the TOMM40 gene—a newly identified risk factor.

Alzheimer's patients also run the risk of other disabling health conditions, including seizures and anemia. The common coexistence of Alzheimer's and cerebrovascular disease is now appreciated. Much more is known about dementia resulting from Lewy body disease, and also about Pick's disease and other frontotemporal dementias.

Alzheimer's-driven changes in the brain, as well as the accompanying cognitive deficits, develop slowly over many years with dementia representing the end stage of years of pathology accumulation. At the same time, we know that some people have the brain changes associated with Alzheimer's and yet do not show symptoms of dementia.

A physiological approach in determining the relative severity of the pathological changes in the associative cortex is the use of EPs, mainly visual. These recordings account for the clinical finding of diminished visual interpretation skills with normal visual acuity. The most important finding and consistent abnormality with flash visual-evoked potentials (VEPs) is the delayed latency of the P_{100} component and at the same time, an increase in its amplitude. The later VEP peaks may also be delayed in patients with AD. A sophisticated analysis with β-spline wavelets was performed on data collected from 40 subjects, 14 of them suffering from a degenerative disease such as AD. The scatter plot of Figure 3.3 shows that the VEP complex (N_{70}–P_{100}–N_{130}) in the delta–theta and alpha bands yields a negative wavelet coefficient D_{3-2} in the [−2, −1] region, a positive D_{4-3} in the region [1, 2], and a negative third coefficient in the sixth octave, standing for an alpha discharge, is observed for normal waveforms. Any deviations from these findings may be interpreted as abnormal behavior.

3.6.3 Epilepsy

This is a disease that affects 1% of the world's population and is characterized by a sudden malfunction of the brain. The malfunctioning might reappear and reflects the clinical signs of extensive activity of neurons in synchrony. Two types of epilepsy have been identified: *generalized* and *focal*. The former involves the whole brain whereas the latter involves specific smaller well-defined regions of the brain. The symptoms associated with epilepsy include impairment of consciousness, autonomic or sensory symptoms, motor phenomena, as well as psychic symptoms.

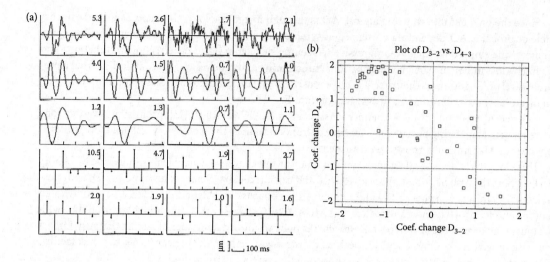

FIGURE 3.3 (a) A normal waveform (leftmost column) and three pathological waveforms. The sixth octave wavelet and residual signals (second and third rows) and their wavelet coefficients (fourth and fifth rows, respectively). The vertical tickmarks indicate the vertical scale of the plots. (b) Scatter plot of D_{3-2} versus D_{4-3}. In the scatter plot, the upper leftmost grid and its immediate right and down neighbors indicate an acceptable range of coefficient changes for the $(N_{70}-P_{100}-N_{130})$ complex of the pattern reversal VEP, analyzed by β-spline wavelets.

When antiepileptic medication stops affecting the patient's symptoms, surgery is recommended. However, the gold standard of the exact localization of the epileptic focus is to use electroencephalography (EEG). Depending on the individual occurrence of seizures, EEG analysis has been proven very valuable. It would be even more valuable if it could give a reliable prediction of when a seizure might occur, a fact that would be of enormous importance to the individual suffering from epilepsy.

In a recent article by Mormann et al. [16], the authors review prediction algorithms that deal with continuous multiday EEG recordings of studies done in the 1990s and early 2000s that yielded results that are promising but not reproducible by others. They critically discuss and address some of the problems involved in the designing and testing of these algorithms and point toward future directions. They also propose methodological guidelines for future studies.

As in many other nervous system disorders, our knowledge of epilepsy comes from animal models. Despite the fact that there exists an enormous amount of literature on the subject, the main mechanisms (both physiological and chemical) are still not well understood. A deeper and more comprehensive understanding of the neurophysiological mechanisms underlying the interictal discharge is crucial to developing more complete models of epileptic activity and more principled and effective methods for controlling seizures [23]. While the morphology of the interictal discharge was highly variable across patients, they selected events such that time zero would be aligned to the peak of the fast component of the interictal discharge. Additionally, these local field potentials were derived from the local microelectrode channel; therefore, this temporal shift in different neuronal firing patterns could not result from a shift between the macroelectrode intracranial EEG recording and the microelectrode local field potential recording. Nevertheless, such preevent changes have also been seen in advance of seizures in an animal model of temporal lobe epilepsy [24].

A lot of work is still needed, especially in terms of understanding the content of EEGs using both linear and nonlinear methods; the latter is used lately more often. So far, research with nonlinear methods of analysis can, at best, predict a seizure only a few seconds before it happens and none of these methods have been adopted clinically.

3.6.4 Phantom Limb Sensation/Pain

Phantom limb pain (PLP) is a term that describes a class of painful phenomena that affect individuals who have undergone a traumatic amputation of a limb. These individuals experience painful sensations that are perceived to be originating from the amputated limb. In subjects with PLP, the painful sensations are generated in the higher cortical areas of the CNS. This is in contrast to the normal condition in which pain signals originate in the PNS and are then passed to the higher-processing centers where these signals are perceived as pain. The fact that PLP is centrally generated means that traditional pain treatments are relatively ineffective in the long-term treatment of PLP, since these treatments act on the pathway between the PNS and the CNS to stop the transmission of painful stimuli.

It has been observed that chronic PLP can lead to significant impairment in areas of daily living. Of the sufferers of PLP, 18% were unable to work, 33.5% report that PLP interferes with their ability to work, 82% have sleep disorders, 43% report that PLP impairs their social activities, and 45% of patients report impairment in their daily activities.

The work performed in my laboratories utilized fMRI to test the hypothesis that there exists a neural construct such that higher-processing areas in the brain responsible for integrating motor, somatosensory, and visual information into a unified somatic perception expect certain cohesive patterns of input from the lower areas of the brain. More specifically, these areas expect that somatosensory and visual feedback is consistent and that it agrees with motor output. Under normal conditions, these expectations are typically met. When a part of the body is amputated, however, the motor cortex is still capable of issuing motor commands to the missing limb but there is erroneous somatosensory and a complete lack of visual feedback. This inconsistency in information pertaining to the limb results in higher-processing centers receiving patterns of input that are not consistent with the neural construct. It is hypothesized that upon receiving patterns of inconsistent information, the higher-associative areas that comprise the hypothetical neural construct conclude that things are not as they should be with the missing limb and that this conclusion leads to the perception of pain originating from the missing limb. One would expect that, if the hypothesis is correct, there might be found a conflict recognition center, or a region or regions of the brain that are active in response to somatosensory sensory conflict. The insula is an area of the brain that is known to be a center of multimodal sensory integration and an area whose activity is correlated with various types of pain. For these reasons, the insula is an area of great interest in the search for the hypothetical conflict recognition center.

The fMRI was used to investigate patterns of neural activation in normal subjects and amputees during experiments involving the movement and visual monitoring of intact and phantom limbs. With amputees, visual feedback was manipulated to bring visual and motor activity into closer agreement. In the normal experiments, visual feedback was manipulated to create disagreement between visual and motor activity. If the hypothesis was correct, one would expect to see different patterns of activation when the motor and sensory systems are in agreement as opposed to when they are not.

The work by other laboratories supports the role of insula as an integrator of information, a region associated with various forms of pain and discomfort and a region whose activity has been found to correlate with conditions being other than what they should be according to the individual [14]. It is suggested here that it is the identification that things are not as they should be that leads to the perception of pain and that this process is mediated, in part, by the insula.

References

1. Micheli-Tzanakou, E. 2000. *Supervised and Unsupervised Pattern Recognition: Feature Extraction and Computational Intelligence*, CRC Press, Boca Raton, FL.
2. McMahon, T.A. 1984. *Muscles, Reflexes and Locomotion*, Princeton University Press, Princeton, NJ.
3. Hartzell, H.C. 1981. Mechanisms of slow postsynaptic potentials. *Nature*, 291, 593.

4. Cowan, W.M. and Cuenod, M. (eds.), 1975. *Use of Axonal Transport for Studies of Neuronal Connectivity*, Elsevier, Amsterdam, pp. 217–248.

5. Shepherd, G.M. 1978. Microcircuits in the nervous system. *Sci. Am.*, 238(2), 93–103.

6. Deutsch, S. and Micheli-Tzanakou, E. 1987. *Neuroelectric Systems*, New York University Press, New York.

7. Partridge, L.D. and Partridge, D.L. 1993. *The Nervous System: Its Function and Interaction with the World*, MIT Press, Cambridge, MA.

8. Ganong, W.F. 1989. *Review of Medical Physiology*, 14th ed., Appleton and Lange, Norwalk, CT.

9. Deutsch, S. and Deutsch, A. 1993. *Understanding the Nervous System: An Engineering Perspective*, IEEE Press, Piscataway, NJ.

10. Watts, R.L. and Koller, W.C. (eds.), 1997. *Movement Disorders Neurologic Principles and Practice*, McGraw-Hill, New York.

11. Rowland, L.P. (ed.), 2000. *Merritt's Textbook of Neurology*, 10th ed., Lippincott Williams & Wilkins, Pennsylvania.

12. Lefaucheur, J.P. 2006. Repetitive transcranial magnetic stimulation (rTMS): Insights into the treatment of Parkinson's disease by cortical stimulation. *Clin. Neurophysiol.*, 36(3), 125–133.

13. del Olmo, M.F., Bello, O., and Cudeiro, J. 2007. Transcranial magnetic stimulation over dorsolateral prefrontal cortex in Parkinson's disease. *Clin. Neurophysiol.*, 118, 131–139.

14. Ostrowsky, K., Magnin, M., Ryvlin, P., Isnard, J., Guenot, M., and Mauguiere, F. 2002. Representation of pain and somatic sensation in the human insula: A study of responses to direct electrical cortical stimulation. *Cereb. Cortex*, 12, 376–385.

15. *Alzheimer's Association's 2010 International Conference on Alzheimer's Disease (AAICAD 2010)*, Honolulu, Hawaii.

16. Mormann, F., Andrzejak, R.G., Elger, C.E., and Lehnertz, K. 2007. Seizure prediction: The long and winding road. *Brain.*, 130(2), 314–333.

17. Ito, S.I. 1998. Possible representation of somatic pain in the rat insular visceral sensory cortex: A field potential study. *Neurosci. Lett.*, 241(2–3), 171–174.

18. Chan, B.L. et al. 2007. Mirror therapy for phantom limb pain. *N. Engl. J. Med.*, 357, 2206.

19. Davis, K.D. 2000. The neural circuitry of pain as explored with functional MRI. *Neurol. Res.*, 22(3), 313–317.

20. Ramachandran, V.S. et al. 2009. The use of visual feedback, in particular mirror visual feedback, in restoring brain function. *Brain*, 32, 1693.

21. Jankovic, J. 2008. Parkinson's disease: Clinical features and diagnosis. *J. Neurol. Neurosurg. Psychiatr.*, 79(4), 368–376.

22. Wu, A.D., Fregni, F., Simon, D.K., Deblieck, C., and Pascual-Leone, A. 2008. Noninvasive brain stimulation for Parkinson's disease and dystonia. *Neurotherapeutics: J. Am. Soc. Exp. Neurother.*, 5, 345–361.

23. Keller, C.J. et al. 2010. Heterogeneous neuronal firing patterns during interictal epileptiform discharges in the human cortex. *Brain*, 133, 1668–1681.

24. Bower, M.R. and Buckmaster, P.S. 2008. Changes in granule cell firing rates precede locally recorded spontaneous seizures by minutes in an animal model of temporal lobe epilepsy. *Neurophysiology*, 99, 2431–2442.

4

Vision System

Aaron P. Batista
University of Pittsburgh
Carnegie Mellon University

George D. Stetten
University of Pittsburgh
Carnegie Mellon University

4.1 Fundamentals of Vision Research...4-1
4.2 A Modular View of the Vision System 4-2
    Eyes • Retina • Optic Chiasm • Lateral Geniculate
    Nucleus • Area V1 • Color • Motion • Higher Cortical Centers
4.3 Eye Movements 4-9
    Types of Eye Movements • Superior Colliculus • Coping with a
    Moving Sensor
Defining Terms 4-10
References...4-10
Further Reading...4-12

David Marr, an early pioneer in computer vision, defined vision as extracting "… from images of the external world, a description that is useful for the viewer and not cluttered with irrelevant information" (Marr, 1982). Advances in computers and video technology in the past decades have created the expectation that artificial vision should be realizable. The nontriviality of the task is evidenced by the continuing proliferation of new and different approaches by computer vision researchers with only recent observable applications in our everyday lives, such as that found in consumer-grade photo management software. Computer vision has actually for some time offered reliable solutions in industrial assembly and inspection, security and military applications, automated reading of hand-written numerals, and so on. However, computer vision has a long way to go to match the vision capabilities of the average 4-year-old human. In this chapter, we explore what is known about how nature has succeeded at this formidable task—that of interpreting the visual world.

4.1 Fundamentals of Vision Research

Research into biological vision systems has followed several distinct approaches. The oldest is psychophysics, in which human and animal subjects are presented with visual stimuli and their responses recorded. Important early insights were also garnered by correlating clinical observations of visual defects with known neuroanatomical injury. In the past 50 years, a more detailed approach to understanding the mechanisms of vision has been undertaken by inserting small electrodes deep within the living brain of animals to monitor the electrical activity of individual neurons and by using dyes and biochemical markers to track the anatomic course of nerve tracts. This research has led to a detailed and coherent, if not complete, theory of a visual system capable of explaining the discrimination of form, color, motion, and depth. This theory has been confirmed by noninvasive radiologic techniques that have been used recently to study the physiologic responses of the visual system, including positron emission tomography (Zeki et al., 1991) and functional magnetic resonance imaging (Belliveau et al., 1992; Cohen and Bookheimer, 1994), although these noninvasive techniques provide far less spatial resolution and thus can only show general regions of activity in the brain.

4.2 A Modular View of the Vision System

4.2.1 Eyes

The eyeball is spherical and therefore free to turn in both the horizontal and vertical directions. Each eye is rotated by three pairs of mutually opposing muscles, innervated by the oculomotor nuclei in the brainstem. The eyes turn in conjunction to find and follow objects, and they move disconjugately (converging inward or diverging outward) to allow adjustment for parallax as objects become closer or further away. The movement of the eyes is essential to vision, allowing rapid location and tracking of objects.

The optical portion of the eye, which puts an image on the retina, is closely analogous to a camera. Light enters the eye, passing through a series of transparent layers—the cornea, the aqueous humor, the lens, and the vitreous body—to eventually project onto the retina.

The cornea, the protective outer layer of the eye, is heavily innervated with sensory neurons, triggering the blink reflex and tear duct secretion in response to irritation. The cornea is also an essential optical element, supplying two-thirds of the total refraction in the eye. Behind the cornea is a clear fluid, the aqueous humor, in which the central aperture of the iris, the pupil, is free to constrict or dilate. The two actions are accomplished by opposing sets of muscles.

The lens, a flexible transparent object behind the iris, provides the remainder of refraction necessary to focus an image on the retina. The ciliary muscles surrounding the lens can increase the lens' curvature, thereby decreasing its focal length and bringing nearer objects into focus. This is called accommodation. When the ciliary muscles are at rest, distant objects are in focus, at least for those of us who are not near-sighted (myopic). There are no contradictory muscles to flatten the lens. This depends simply on the elasticity of the lens, which decreases with age (presbyopia). Behind the lens is the vitreous humor, consisting of a semigelatinous material filling the volume between the lens and the retina.

4.2.2 Retina

The retina coats the back of the eye and is therefore spherical, not flat, making optical *magnification* constant at 3.5° of scan angle per millimeter. The retina is the neuronal front end of the visual system, the image sensor. It performs a biological form of image compression before sending the processed information along the optic nerve to the brain. The retina contains five major classes of cells, organized into a three-layer neural network. The dendrites of any one of these cells, which gather signals from other neurons, occupy no more than 1–2 mm^2 in the retina. This determines the extent of spatial integration from one layer of the retina to the next. Interestingly, the retina is inverted, such that light passes through all the layers before being absorbed by the photoreceptors.

The input layer of the retinal network comprises the photoreceptors, which number approximately 125 million in each eye and contain the light-sensitive pigments responsible for converting photons into chemical energy and subsequently the neural signals. The photopigments that convert the light to chemical energy must be replenished after being bleached by light. An opaque layer of tissue called the pigment epithelium just behind the input layer provides fresh photopigment. This arrangement helps explain why the retina is inverted. Receptor cells are of two varieties: rods and cones. The cones are responsible for the perception of color, and function only in bright light. When the light is dim, only rods are sensitive enough to respond. Exposure to a single photon may result in a measurable increase in the membrane potential of a rod. When psychophysical subjects are fully dark adapted, they can report perceiving that single photon. This sensitivity is the result of a chemical cascade, similar in operation to the photomultiplier tube, in which the single photon generates a cascade of electrons. Exquisite gain control mechanisms tune this cascade and allow us to see over nine orders of magnitude of light intensity (from starlight to bright sunlight). All rods use the same photopigment, whereas three separate kinds of cones exist, each with a different pigment. The differential sensitivity to wavelength among the three cone types is the basis of our color experience.

The examination of the retina with an otoscope reveals its gross topography. The yellow circular area occupying the central 5° of the retina is called the macula lutea, within which a small circular pit called the fovea may be seen. Detailed vision occurs only in the fovea, where a dense packing of cones provides visual activity to the central 1° of the visual field.

The output layer of the retina comprises ganglion cells, whose axons make up the optic nerve. They number approximately 1 million, or less than 1% of the number of receptor cells. Clearly, some data compression has already occurred in the space between the receptors and the ganglion cells. Traversing this space are the bipolar cells, which run from the receptors through the retina to the ganglion cells. Bipolar cells exhibit the first level of information processing in the visual system. Their response to light on the retina demonstrates "center/surround" *receptive fields*, that is, a small dot on the retina elicits a response (excitatory or inhibitory), while the area surrounding the spot elicits the opposite response. If both the center and the surround are illuminated, the net result is no change in the neural activity. Thus, bipolar cells respond only at the border between dark and light areas. Bipolar cells come in two varieties, on-center and off-center, which prefer the center brighter or darker, respectively, than the surround.

The center response of bipolar cells results from direct contact with the receptors. The surround response is supplied by the horizontal cells, which run parallel to the surface of the retina between the receptor layer and the bipolar layer, allowing the surrounding area to oppose the influence of the center. The amacrine cells, a final cell type, also run parallel to the surface but in a different layer, between the bipolar cells and the ganglion cells, and are involved in the detection of motion in lower vertebrates.

Ganglion cells, since they are triggered by bipolar cells, also have center/surround receptive fields and come in two types: on- and off-center. On-center ganglion cells have a receptive field in which illumination of the center increases the firing rate and a surround where it decreases the rate. Off-center ganglion cells display the opposite behavior. Both types of ganglion cells produce little or no change in excitability when the entire receptive field is illuminated because the center and surround cancel each other. Ganglion cells also have temporal responses; they respond maximally when a spot of light first appears (on-center cells) or first disappears (off-center cells). The retina is essentially computing spatial and temporal derivatives of the visual image. An interesting consequence of this is that our eyes make small eye movements (termed *microsaccades*) all the time. If microsaccades are measured in the lab and the visual scene is jittered by the exact amount required to keep the image immobile on the retina, the visual scene rapidly fades to a uniform gray.

Multiple ganglion cells may receive output from the same receptor, since many receptive fields overlap. However, this does not limit the overall spatial resolution, which is maximum in the fovea, where two points separated by 0.5' of arc may be discriminated. This separation corresponds to a distance on the retina of 2.5 μm, which is approximately the center-to-center spacing between cones. If the spacing between lines, rather than points, are distinguished, acuity can improve to 5" s of arc. This phenomenon, termed hyperacuity, is thought to rely on integrating information across coaligned photoreceptors. (The Vernier scale on a caliper relies on hyperacuity). Spatial resolution falls off as one moves away from the fovea into the peripheral vision, where resolution is as low as 1° of visual angle.

Several aspects of this natural design deserve consideration. Why do we have center/surround receptive fields? The ganglion cells, whose axons make up the optic nerve, do not fire unless there is meaningful information, that is, a border, falling within the receptive field. It is the edge of a shape we see rather than its interior. Edges provide rich visual information, as any pen-and-ink artist can attest. This represents a form of data compression: in a sense, the retina transmits spatial and temporal derivatives of the visual scene. Center/surround receptive fields also allow for relative rather than absolute measurements of color and brightness. This is essential for analyzing the image independent of lighting conditions. Why do we have both on- and off-center cells? Evidently, both light and dark are considered information. The same shape is detected whether it is lighter or darker than the background.

4.2.3 Optic Chiasm

All of this preprocessing by the retina is essential because the optic nerve constitutes a bottleneck. Evolution's solution to the need to transmit visual information from the retina to the brain through that narrow pipeline is retinal data compression, a high-acuity fovea, and a moveable sensor. The two optic nerves, from the left and right eyes, join at the optic chiasm, forming a *hemidecussation*, meaning that half the axons cross while the rest proceed uncrossed. The resulting two bundles of axons leaving the chiasm are called the optic tracts. The left optic tract contains only axons from the left half of each retina. Since the images are reversed by the lens, this represents the right side of the visual field. The division between the right and left optic tracts basically splits the retina down the middle, although there is a vertical strip of the visual field that runs through the fovea that is represented in both hemispheres. This overlap accounts for the fact that occipital strokes and trauma often spare the fovea. The segregation of sensory information into the contralateral hemispheres corresponds to the general organization of sensory and motor centers in the brain: the right hemisphere controls the left half of the body, and vice versa.

Each optic tract has two major destinations on its side of the brain: (1) the lateral geniculate nucleus (LGN) and (2) the superior colliculus. The *topographic mapping* present in the retina is preserved in both major destinations so that right, left, up, and down in the image correspond to specific directions within those anatomic structures. We will first discuss the LGN, tracing that major pathway to higher cortical centers, before returning to discuss the superior colliculus in the midbrain and its role in controlling eye movements.

4.2.4 Lateral Geniculate Nucleus

The thalamus is often called "the gateway to the cortex" because it processes much of the sensory information reaching the brain. Within the thalamus, we find the LGN, a peanut-sized structure that contains a single synaptic stage in the major pathway of visual information to higher centers. The LGN also receives enormous feedback information back from the cortex, as well as from the nuclei in the brainstem that control vigilance and arousal. The anatomical connectivity of the LGN indicates that vision is an active process; the brain searches the visual scene to select the information relevant to current goals.

The cells in the LGN are organized into three pairs of layers. Each pair contains two layers, one from each eye. The upper two pairs consist of parvocellular cells (P cells) that respond with preference to different colors and have small dendritic fields. The remaining lower pair of layers consists of magnocellular cells (M cells) with no color preference but with transient responses that contribute to motion perception. These cells have larger dendritic fields, allowing them to integrate information over broader regions, which is required to detect motion. The topographic mapping is identical for all six layers, that is, passing an electrode through the layers at a given point yields neurons responding to a single area of the retina. Neurons in the LGN display the same center/surround response as the retinal ganglion cells. Axons from the LGN proceed to the primary visual cortex in broad bands, called *optic radiations*, preserving the topographic mapping found in the LGN.

4.2.5 Area V1

The LGN contains approximately 1.5 million cells. By comparison, the primary visual cortex, or striate cortex, which receives the visual information from the LGN, contains 200 million cells. It consists of a thin (2-mm) layer of gray matter (neuronal cell bodies) over a thicker collection of white matter and occupies a few square inches of the occipital lobes. The primary visual cortex has been called *area 17* from the days when the cortical areas were first differentiated by their *cytoarchitectonics* (the microscopic architecture of their layered neurons). In modern terminology, the primary visual cortex is often called *visual area 1*, or simply *V1*.

Destroying any small piece of V1 eliminates a small area in the visual field, resulting in scotoma, a local blind spot. Clinical evidence has long been available that a scotoma may result from injury, stroke, or tumor in a local part of V1. Between neighboring cells in V1's gray matter, horizontal connections are at most 2–5 mm in length. Thus, at any given time, the image from the retina is analyzed piecemeal in V1. Topographic mapping from the retina is preserved in great detail. Such mapping is seen elsewhere in the brain, such as in the somatosensory cortex (Mountcastle, 1957). Like all cortical surfaces, V1 is a highly convoluted sheet, with much of its area hidden within its folds. If unfolded, V1 would be roughly pear shaped, with the top of the pear processing information from the fovea and the bottom of the pear processing the peripheral vision. Circling the pear at a given latitude would correspond roughly to circling the fovea at a fixed radius. A disproportionately large number of V1 neurons are dedicated to the central visual field This phenomenon is called *magnification*. The fovea maps to a greater area on the surface of V1 than does the peripheral retina, by as much as 36-fold (Daniel and Whitteridge, 1961). The majority of V1 processes only the central 10° of the visual field.

The primary visual cortex contains six layers, designated 1 (surface) through 6 (deepest). Distinct functional and anatomic types of cells are found in each layer. Layer 4 contains neurons that receive information from the LGN. Beyond the initial synapses, cells demonstrate progressively more complex responses. Information processing chiefly occurs perpendicular to the cortical surface, between cortical layers. This creates a columnar architecture within V1 (as in most other sensory cortical areas).

The outputs of V1 project to an area known as visual area 2 (V2), which surrounds V1, and to higher visual areas in the occipital, temporal, and parietal lobes as well as to the superior colliculus. Feedback projections are present at almost every level of the visual system (Felleman and Van Essen, 1991).

Cells in V1 have been studied extensively in animals by inserting small electrodes into the living brain (which causes surprisingly little damage) and monitoring the individual responses of neurons to visual stimuli. Various categories of cortical cells have thus been identified (Hubel and Wiesel, 1962). One category, the *simple cells*, respond to illuminated edges or bars at specific locations and at specific angular orientations in the visual field. These cells are smoothly tuned to orientation, exhibiting a graded decline in excitability as a bar rotates away from its preferred orientation. All orientations are equally represented. Moving the electrode a short distance parallel to the surface yields a smooth rotation in the orientation of cell responses by about 10° for each 50 μm that the electrode is advanced. It is easy to imagine how a simple cell response might be built up from a small group of LGN cells, by receiving projections from cells with adjacent collinear center–surround receptive fields. Note that simple cells respond best to moving bars and edges; again, it seems to be the changes in the visual scene that are most salient for the brain.

Other cells, more common than simple cells, are termed *complex cells*. Complex cells also respond to bars within their receptive field, but unlike simple cells, they are invariant to the position of the bar within the receptive field. This may contribute in part to the translation invariance of our visual experience. Complex cells will respond to movement perpendicular to the orientation of the edge. Some prefer one direction of movement to its opposite. Some complex and simple cells are end-stopped, meaning they fire only if the illuminated bar or edge terminates within the cell's receptive field. Presumably, these cells detect corners, curves, or discontinuities in borders and lines. End-stopping takes place in layers 2 and 3 of the primary visual cortex. From the LGN through the simple cells and complex cells, there appears to be a sequential processing of the image. A remarkable feature in the organization of V1 is *binocular convergence*, in which a single neuron responds to identical receptive fields in both eyes, including location, orientation, and directional sensitivity to motion. This does not occur in the LGN, where axons from the left and right eyes are still segregated into different layers. Some binocular neurons are equally weighted in terms of responsiveness to both eyes, while others are more sensitive to one eye than to the other. V1 is also organized into columns containing cells in which one eye dominates, called ocular dominance columns. Ocular dominance columns occur in adjacent pairs, one for each eye, and are prominent in predatory animals with forward-facing eyes, such as cats, chimpanzees, and humans. They are nearly absent in rodents and other prey animals whose eyes face outward.

As an electrode is passed down through the cortex perpendicular to the surface, each layer demonstrates receptive fields of characteristic size, the smallest being in layer 4, the input layer. Receptive fields are larger in other layers due to lateral integration of information. Passing the electrode parallel to the surface of the cortex reveals another important uniformity to V1. For example, in layer 3, which sends output fibers to higher cortical centers, one must move the electrode approximately 2 mm to pass from one collection of receptive fields to another that does not overlap. An area approximately 2 mm across thus represents the smallest unit piece of V1, that is, that which can completely process the visual information arising from one portion of the visual field. Indeed, it is just the right size to contain a complete set of orientations and more than enough to contain information from both eyes. It receives a few tens of thousands of fibers from the LGN, produces perhaps 50,000 output fibers, and is fairly constant in cytoarchitectonics whether at the center of vision, where it processes approximately 30' of arc, or at the far periphery, where it processes 7–8° of visual angle.

The topographic mapping of the visual field onto the cortex undergoes an abrupt discontinuity between the left and right hemispheres, and yet our perception of the visual scene suffers no obvious rift in the midline. This is due to the corpus callosum, an enormous tract containing at least 200 million axons, that connects the two hemispheres. The posterior portion of the corpus callosum connects the two halves of V1, linking cells that have similar orientations and whose receptive fields overlap in the vertical midline. Thus, a perceptually seamless merging of left and right visual fields is achieved. Higher levels of the visual system are likewise connected across the corpus callosum. This is demonstrated, for example, by the clinical observation that cutting the corpus callosum prevents a subject from verbally describing objects in the left field of view (the right hemisphere). Speech, which normally involves the left hemisphere, cannot process visual objects in the left visual field (right hemisphere) without the corpus callosum.

By merging the information from both eyes, V1 is capable of analyzing the distance to an object. Many cues for depth are available to the visual system, including occlusion, vergence and accommodation of the eyes, expected size of objects, shape based on perspective, and shadow casting. *Stereopsis*, which uses the parallax between images due to the separation of the eyes, was first enunciated in 1838 by Sir Charles Wheatstone (Wheatstone, 1838). Fixating on an object causes it to fall on the two foveas. Other objects that are nearer become outwardly displaced on the two retinas, while objects that are farther away become inwardly displaced. About 2° of horizontal disparity is tolerated, while still maintaining fusion by the visual system into a single perceived object. Greater horizontal disparity results in double vision. We seldom notice because this generally occurs in the low-resolution visual periphery. Physiologic experiments have revealed a particular class of complex cells in V1 that are disparity tuned. They fall into three general classes. One class fires only when the object is at the fixation distance, another only when the object is nearer, and a third only when it is farther away (Poggio and Talbot, 1981).

When the images arriving at the two retinas cannot be combined, one or the other image is rejected. This phenomenon is known as binocular rivalry, and if a chronic condition, it can lead to blindness in one eye. The general term *amblyopia* refers to the partial or complete loss of eyesight not caused by abnormalities in the eye. The most common form of amblyopia is caused by *strabismus*, in which the eyes are not aimed in a parallel direction, but rather are turned inward (cross-eyed) or outward (wall-eyed). This condition leads to habitual suppression of vision from one of the eyes and sometimes to blindness in that eye or to *alternation*, in which the subject maintains vision in both eyes by using only one eye at a time. Cutting selected ocular muscles in kittens causes strabismus, and the kittens respond by developing alternation, preserving functional vision in both eyes. However, the number of cells in the cortex displaying binocular responses becomes greatly reduced. In humans with long-standing alternating strabismus, surgical repair to make the eyes parallel again does not bring back a sense of depth. Permanent damage has been caused by the subtle condition of the images on the two retinas not coinciding. This may be explained by the Hebbian model for associative learning, in which temporal association between inputs strengthens synaptic connections (Hebb, 1961).

Further evidence that successful development of the visual system depends on proper input comes from clinical experience with children who have cataracts at birth. Cataracts constitute a clouding of the lens, permitting light, but not images, to reach the retina. If surgery to remove the cataracts is delayed until the child is several years old, the child remains blind even though images are restored to the retina. Kittens and monkeys whose eyelids are sewn shut during a critical period of early development stay blind even when the eyes are opened. Physiologic studies in these animals show very few cells responding in the visual cortex. Other experiments depriving more specific elements of an image, such as certain orientations or motion in a certain direction, yield a cortex without the corresponding cell type, and a degradation of the corresponding visual experience.

4.2.6 Color

Cone photoreceptors, which dominate the fovea, can detect light with wavelengths between 400 and 700 nm. Three types of cones exist, each containing a different pigment. This was established by direct microscopic illumination of the retina (Marks et al., 1964; Wald, 1974). The pigments have a bandwidth on the order of 100 nm, with significant overlap, and with peak sensitivities at 560 nm (yellow–green light), 530 nm (blue–green), and 430 nm (blue–violet). These three cone types are commonly known as red, green, and blue, but for reasons made clear below, are more appropriately called L (long wavelength responsive), M (medium), and S (short). Compared with the auditory system, whose array of cochlear sensors are tuned to thousands of different sonic frequencies, the visual system is relatively impoverished with only three receptor types. Remarkably, humans can distinguish millions of hues using just these three receptor types. By having three types of cones sample the illumination at each location on the retina, the light spectrum can be represented by three independent variables, a concept known as trichromacy. Full color vision is rare among mammals; only primates have three cone types (dogs and cats have two), while some insects, birds, lizards, and aquatic animals have more than three different photopigments, which are tuned to the wavelengths that matter most for their survival. Most nocturnal animals lack color vision, since cones are useless in low light.

Three theories about the mechanisms of color vision, originally formulated based on psychophysical evidence, have garnered physiologic evidence. In the nineteenth century, Thomas Young and Hermann Von Helmholtz (Young, 1802; Helmholtz, 1889) proposed the trichromatic theory of color vision. They found that any color could be matched by mixing red, green, and blue light in various intensities. This phenomenon, *metameric color matching* (physically different stimuli that generate the same percept), led Young and Helmholtz to predict that there were three types of color-sensitive detectors in the eye. Their theory was later verified by the identification of the three cone types in the retina.

Soon after, a second, rival, theory of color vision was proposed by Ewald Hering. He suggested that color vision occurred via an *opponent process*: colors occur in opponent pairs that are mutually antagonistic. Evidence for this theory comes from the fact that we see blue afterimages after staring at a yellow object then looking away at a white wall, and in the fact that we never see reddish-green colors or bluish-yellow colors. It turns out this theory is also correct; cells in the visual cortex receive excitatory inputs from one cone type and inhibitory inputs from another. Thus, if the output of long-wavelength cones excites a cell, then the output of medium-wavelength cells will inhibit the same cell, and vice versa. Such cells lead to our perception of red and green. Similarly, perceptions of blue arise from cells that are excited by short-wavelength cones and inhibited by both long- and medium-wavelength cones, and vice versa for yellow. This subtraction of cone outputs may be part of the image compression made necessary by the optic nerve bottleneck. Thus, the trichromacy and opponent process theories of color vision are not rival theories at all. They simply describe different stages in the color processing pathway.

However, opponent cells cannot explain another remarkable trait of color vision: *color constancy*. This is the fact that color experience does not depend on the spectrum of the illuminating light. An apple looks red in bright sunlight, and it also looks red under fluorescent lights, but the spectra reflected from it in these two circumstances differ dramatically. In the twentieth century, Edwin Land, the founder of

Polaroid, proposed an explanation called the *retinex* theory of color vision. It posits that local color experience arises from global computations, over the entire visual scene. Cells have recently been identified in V1 that maintain their color sensitivity despite changes in the overall light level. It is these *double opponent* cells (exhibiting color opponency that is robust to changes in luminance) that might ultimately provide our color experience, as Land predicted. Thus, these three theories help explain how sophisticated biological computations that compare relative activations of just three cone types can generate the rich gamut of color experience we enjoy. Now, it can be seen why calling the long-wavelength cone the "red" cone is a misnomer: the sensation of red actually arises from the relative activations of two cone types.

It makes sense to describe the color vision system as performing a dimensionality reduction on the incoming light spectrum, which has essentially an infinite number of frequencies, into three dimensions. The spectrum is projected onto three axes, the scalar outputs of the three cone types. Further compression within that 3D space is performed by the color opponent and double opponent cells. This fact explains why color reproduction technologies like video displays and printers can do such a remarkable job with only three colors.

4.2.7 Motion

Several higher visual areas are specialized to detect the characteristics of moving stimuli. Chiefly, area MT (the "middle temporal" area, named for its location in squirrel monkeys, where it was discovered) responds to the motion of the objects around us, and area MST (medial superior temporal area) responds to motion generated by our movement through the environment.

Area MT has been used to explore the links between the activity of neurons and visual experience. In rare cases, lesions to MT results in *motion blindness*, an inability to perceive motion. Instead, these patients experience the world as a series of snapshots without continuity between them. In an important series of studies, Bill Newsome and his colleagues trained monkeys to report their perceptions of motion with eye movements. When MT is temporarily inactivated with lidocaine in these animals, the animals temporarily lose the ability to perceive motion. When MT is stimulated by passing current through an electrode, animals report seeing motion that is not actually present in the stimulus. Based on the properties of the neurons near the electrode tip, the researchers could predict the nature of the motion experience the animals would have upon microstimulation. For example, stimulating neurons active for motion to the right leads the animal to report observing rightward motion (Salzman et al., 1990).

This team also showed that individual neurons are exquisitely sensitive to motion; under carefully tailored experimental conditions, some individual neurons are just as accurate at signaling motion as is the entire animal (Britten et al., 1992). In fact, random noise in the activity of MT neurons was found to be correlated to fluctuations in the animal's reported visual experience (Britten et al., 1996).

Area MST responds to moving stimuli that fill the whole visual field. As we move through our environment, the retinas experience an "optic flow" stimulation pattern emanating from the point of visual fixation. Neurons in MST are especially sensitive to this type of stimulus, and from their activities, the direction in which we are headed as we move through the environment can be estimated.

4.2.8 Higher Cortical Centers

How are the primitive elements of image processing discussed so far united into an understanding of the image? Beyond V1 are many higher cortical centers for visual processing throughout the occipital, temporal, and parietal lobes. Those within the occipital lobe have been labeled V3, V4, V5 (also known as MT, already discussed), and so on and provide specialized processing of visual information, such as shape, color, and motion.

A total lesion of V1 results in total blindness. However, some such "blind" patients can actually perform better than random guessing when instructed to point to the location of an object. Even as they deny being able to see anything, they point toward stimuli appearing on a screen. This condition is called *blindsight* (Weiskrantz, 1990). Recall that the LGN projects to the superior colliculus (which, as discussed below, performs visually guided action) as well as to V1. It could be that this area helps mediate the residual "unconscious" visual function.

Beyond the occipital lobe, visual information is elaborated upon for various purposes, including (in the temporal lobe and hippocampus) face and object recognition, memory, and speech; and (in the parietal lobe) spatial perception and action, such as reaching out to pick up an object. This bifurcation of the visual pathway has been termed the "what" versus "where" pathways.

Visual responses in the higher cortical centers become increasingly specialized. In the extreme of specialization, neurobiologists half-jokingly talk about the mythical "grandmother cell," which would respond to the face of your grandmother, but to no other stimulus. Remarkable specificity to faces has actually been reported in the human temporal lobe during neurosurgery (Quian Quiroga et al., 2005). So, a theory that was originally posited as a *reductio ad absurdum* has turned out to be partly true.

4.3 Eye Movements

Evolution's solution to the anatomical bottleneck of the optic nerve was to create a small high-acuity sensor and mount it on an actuator. This means that vision and eye movements are inextricably linked, and it is hard to fully understand one without the other.

4.3.1 Types of Eye Movements

Eye movements are usually classified into five major types. The *saccade* is the quick motion of the eyes over a significant distance that is mediated by the superior colliculus (described below). The saccade is how the eyes explore an image, jumping from landmark to landmark, rarely stopping in featureless areas. We also use *smooth pursuit* to voluntarily track moving objects. While looking out a car's side window, our eyes will smoothly pursue the visual scene to the limit of the orbits, then rapidly saccade back, in a repeating cycle. This is *optokinetic nystagmus*. When our head moves, our eyes counter-roll to stabilize the image, which is the *vestibulo-ocular reflex*. The fifth category of eye movement is *vergence*, the disconjugate introversion and extroversion our eyes perform to look at objects at varying depths.

4.3.2 Superior Colliculus

The superior colliculus comprises a small pair of bumps on the dorsal surface of the midbrain. After the visual cortex, it is the other main recipient of projection from the LGN. Stimulation of the superior colliculus results in a contralateral saccadic eye movement. Output tracts from the superior colliculus run to areas that control eye, neck, and arm movements. The superior colliculus mediates our near-reflexive eye and head movements, for example, our ability to duck a branch while walking at twilight before we even perceive it. The superior colliculus processes information from other sensory modalities as well as vision, allowing the eyes to quickly find and follow targets based on visual, auditory, and tactile cues.

4.3.3 Coping with a Moving Sensor

When gazing at a page of text at arm's length, typically, only the next 5–7 characters are legible. To read, or when examining our environment, we perform saccades 2–3 times each second. In ordinary life, we are completely unaware of this sequential sampling: the whole world seems rendered in high resolution all at once, despite the fact that the image projected onto our retinas is changing suddenly every time we saccade. The brain accomplishes this feat, known as *saccadic stability,* by somehow stitching together snapshots of the visual world taken from different perspectives. It requires that the visual centers know the position of the eyes when each snapshot was taken. Indeed, it can be shown by carefully controlled psychophysical environments that this process of compensating for eye movements is not perfect, but rather that small distortions (shifting and stretching) of the visual world occur around the time of every saccade (Ross et al., 2001).

These fleeting distortions of vision provide researchers a handle on discovering the neural basis for saccadic stability. Whenever the eyes move, the visual centers anticipate the consequence for vision of the eye movement and correct for it. Neurons begin to respond to visual stimuli that will enter their receptive fields after the saccade, even before the eyes have begun to move (Duhamel et al., 1992). This "perisaccadic remapping" shows that visual information can be passed between neurons within higher visual areas, and need not be attained from the retina after each saccade. Doing so is presumably essential to avoid the temporal gaps in our vision that would result if we had to wait for new visual information to arrive from the retina after each saccade. However, predictive remapping means that there are a few milliseconds of time around each eye movement when the visual world is represented twice within our visual areas: at its "old" (presaccadic) and "new" (postsaccadic) locations. This probably creates the subtle perceptual distortions described above.

Perisaccadic remapping is just one example of a ubiquitous neural phenomenon: sensory and motor centers interact in the brain. Sensation guides action, and internal copies of motor commands are used by sensory areas to anticipate the consequences that action will have for sensation. Through this general mechanism, crickets avoid deafening themselves when they chirp, bats locate their prey through echolocation, and songbirds and humans can communicate through complex vocalizations (Crapse and Sommer 1998).

Defining Terms

Binocular convergence: The response of a single neuron to the same location in the visual field of each eye.

Color constancy: The perception that the color of an object remains constant under different lighting conditions. Even though the spectrum reaching the eye from that object can be vastly different other objects in the field of view are used to compare.

Cytoarchitectonics: The organization of neuron types into layers as seen by various staining techniques under the microscope. Electrophysiological responses of individual cells can be correlated with their cell type and individual layer.

Magnification: The variation in amount of retinal area represented per unit area of V1 from the fovea to the visual periphery. The fovea takes up an inordinate percentage of V1 compared with the rest of the visual field; thus, the image from the fovea is, in effect, magnified before processing.

Receptive field: The area in the visual field that evokes a response in a neuron. In addition to its spatial receptive field, a neuron will respond to specific stimuli such as illuminated points, bars, or edges with particular colors, directions of motion, and so on.

Stereopsis: The determination of distance to objects based on relative displacement on the two retinas because of parallax.

Topographic mapping: The one-to-one correspondence between location on the retina and location within a structure in the brain. Topographic mapping further implies that contiguous areas on the retina map to contiguous areas in the particular brain structure.

References

Belliveau J.H., Kwong K.K. et al. 1992. Magnetic resonance imaging mapping of brain function: Human visual cortex. *Invest. Radiol.* 27: S59.

Britten K.H., Newsome W.T., Shadlen M.N., Celebrini S., and Movshon J.A. 1996. A relationship between behavioral choice and the visual responses of neurons in macaque MT. *Vis. Neurosci.* 13: 87–100.

Britten K.H., Shadlen M.N., Newsome W.T., and Movshon J.A. 1992. The analysis of visual motion: A comparison of neuronal and psychophysical performance. *J. Neurosci.* 12: 4745–4765.

Cohen M.S. and Bookheimer S.Y. 1994. Localization of brain function using magnetic resonance imaging. *Trends Neurosci.* 17: 268.

Crapse T.B., and Sommer M.A. 1998. Corollary discharge across the animal kingdom. *Nat. Rev. Neurosci.* 9: 587–600.

Daniel P.M. and Whitteridge D. 1961. The representation of the visual field on the cerebral cortex in monkeys. *J. Physiol.* 159: 203.

Duhamel J.-R., Colby C.L., and Goldberg M.E. 1992. The updating of the representation of visual space in parietal cortex by intended eye movements. *Science* 255: 90–92.

Ennes H.E. 1981. NTSC color fundamentals. In *Television Broadcasting: Equipment, Systems, and Operating Fundamentals*. Indianapolis, Howard W. Sams & Co.

Felleman D.J. and Van Essen D.C. 1991. Distributed hierarchical processing in the primate cerebral cortex. *Cereb. Cortex* 1: 1.

Gross C.G. and Sergen J. 1992. Face recognition. *Curr. Opin. Neurobiol.* 2: 156.

Hebb D.O. 1961. *The Organization of Behavior*. New York, John Wiley & Sons.

Helmholtz H. 1889. *Popular Scientific Lectures*. London, Longmans.

Hering E. 1864. *Outlines of a Theory of Light Sense*. Cambridge, Harvard University Press.

Hubel D.H. 1998. *Eye, Brain, and Vision*. New York, Scientific American Library.

Hubel D.H. and Wiesel T.N. 1962. Receptive fields, binocular interaction and functional architecture in the cat's visual cortex. *J. Physiol.* 160: 106–154.

Land E.H. and McCann J.J. 1971. Lightness and retinex theory. *J. Opt. Soc. Am.* 61: 1.

Livingstone M.S. and Hubel D.H. 1984. Anatomy and physiology of a color system in the primate visual cortex. *J. Neurosci.* 4: 309.

Marks W.B., Dobelle W.H., and MacNichol E.F. 1964. Visual pigments of single primate cones. *Science* 143: 1181.

Marr D. 1982. *Vision*. San Francisco, WH Freeman.

Mountcastle V.B. 1957. Modality and topographic properties of single neurons of cat's somatic sensory cortex. *J. Neurophysiol.* 20: 408.

Poggio G.F. and Talbot W.H. 1981. Mechanisms of static and dynamic stereopsis in foveal cortex of the rhesus monkey. *J. Physiol.* 315: 469.

Quian Quiroga R., Reddy L., Krieman G., Koch C., and Fried I. 2005. Invariant visual representation by single neurons in the human brain. *Nature* 435: 1102–1107.

Ross J., Concetta Morrone M., Goldberg M.E., and Burr D.C. 2001. Changes in visual perception at the time of saccades. *Trends Neurosci.* 24: 113–121.

Salzman C.D., Britten K., and Newsome W.T. 1990. Cortical microstimulation influences perceptual judgements of motion direction. *Nature* 346: 174–177.

Wald G. 1974. Proceedings: Visual pigments and photoreceptors—Review and outlook. *Exp. Eye Res.* 18: 333.

Weiskrantz L. 1990. The Ferrier Lecture: Outlooks for blindsight: Explicit methodologies for implicit processors. *Proc. R. Soc. Lond.* B 239: 247.

Wheatstone S.C. 1838. Contribution to the physiology of vision. *Philosoph. Trans. R. Soc. Lond.* 128: 371–394.

Young T. 1802. The Bakerian Lecture: On the theory of lights and colours. *Philosoph. Trans. R. Soc. Lond.* 92: 12.

Zeki S. 1992. The visual image in mind and brain. *Sci. Am.* September, 69.

Zeki S., Watson J.D., Lueck C.J. et al. 1991. A direct demonstration of functional specialization in human visual cortex. *J. Neurosci.* 11: 641.

Further Reading

An excellent introductory text about the visual system is *Eye, Brain, and Vision*, by the Nobel laureate David H. Hubel (1995, Scientific American Library, New York). A more recent general text with a thorough treatment of color vision, as well as the higher cortical centers, is *A Vision of the Brain*, by Semir Zeki (1993, Blackwell Scientific Publications, Oxford).

Other useful texts with greater detail about the nervous system are *From Neuron to Brain*, by Nicholls, Martin, Wallace, and Kuffler (3rd ed., 1992, Sinauer Assoc., Sunderand Mass.), *The Synaptic Organization of the Brain*, by Shepherd (4th ed., 1998, Oxford Press, New York), and *Fundamental Neuroanatomy*, by Nauta and Feirtag (1986, Freeman, New York).

A classic text that laid the foundation of computer vision was *Vision*, by David Marr (1982, Freeman, New York). Other texts dealing with the mathematics of image processing and image analysis are *Digital Image Processing*, by Pratt (1991, Wiley, New York) and *Digital Imaging Processing and Computer Vision*, by Schalkoff (1989, Wiley, New York).

Two books dealing with perceptual issues are *Visual Perception: Physiology, Psychology and Ecology*, by Bruce, Green, and Georgeson (3rd ed., 1996, Psychology Press, Hove, East Sussex.) and *Sensation and Perception*, by Goldstein (6th ed., 2001, Wadsworth Publishing).

5

Auditory System

5.1	Overview	5-1
5.2	Peripheral Auditory System	5-1
	External and Middle Ear • Inner Ear	
5.3	Central Auditory System	5-7
	Cochlear Nuclei • Superior Olivary Complex • Nuclei of the Lateral Lemniscus • Inferior Colliculi • Thalamocortical System	
5.4	Pathologies	5-14
5.5	Further Topics	5-15
References		5-15

Ben M. Clopton
Advanced Cochlear Systems

Herbert F. Voigt
Boston University

5.1 Overview

Human hearing arises from airborne waves alternating 50–20,000 times a second about the mean atmospheric pressure. These pressure variations induce vibrations of the tympanic membrane, movement of the middle-ear ossicles connected to it, and subsequent displacements of the fluids and tissues of the cochlea in the inner ear. Biomechanical processes in the cochlea analyze sounds to frequency-mapped vibrations along the basilar membrane (BM), and approximately 3500 inner hair cells (IHCs) modulate transmitter release and spike generation in 30,000 spiral ganglion cells (SGCs) whose proximal processes make up the auditory nerve. This neural activity enters the central auditory system and reflects sound patterns as temporal and spatial spike patterns. The nerve branches and synapses extensively in the cochlear nuclei, the first of the central auditory nuclei. Subsequent brainstem nuclei pass auditory information to the medial geniculate and auditory cortex (AC) of the thalamocortical system.

We extract more information from sound than from any other sense. Although primates are described as "visual" animals, speech and music carry more of our cultural and societal meaning than sight or other senses, and we suffer more from deafness than with other sensory losses. Highly effective adaptations of auditory processing occur in many animals, including insects, amphibians, birds, cetaceans, and bats for prey acquisition, predator avoidance, intraspecies signaling, and other tasks. This chapter surveys the current understanding of the hearing process.

5.2 Peripheral Auditory System

5.2.1 External and Middle Ear

As shown in Figure 5.1, ambient sounds are collected by the pinna, the visible portion of the external ear, and guided to the middle ear by the external auditory meatus, or ear canal. Sounds are filtered due to the geometry of the pinna and sound shadowing effects of the head. In species with movable pinnae, selective scanning of the auditory environment is possible for high frequencies (Geisler, 1998; Kinsler et al., 1999).

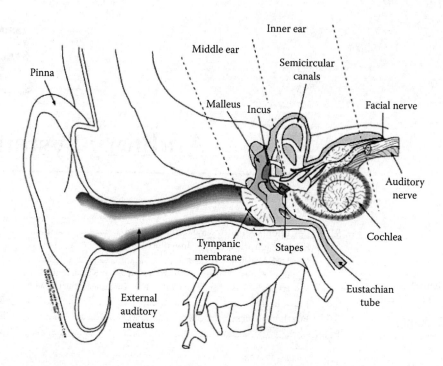

FIGURE 5.1 The peripheral auditory system showing the external-ear structures (pinna and external meatus), the middle ear, and the inner ear. (Courtesy of Virginia Merrill Bloedel Hearing Research Center, Seattle, Washington.)

The bounding interface between the external and middle ear is the tympanic membrane. Pressure variations across the membrane move three ossicles, the malleus (hammer) connected to the membrane, the incus (anvil), and the stapes (stirrup) whose footplate is a piston-like structure fitting into the oval window, an opening to the fluid-filled cavities of the inner ear. Ligaments and muscles suspend the middle-ear ossicles so that they move freely. If the sound reaches the fluids of the inner ear directly, 99.9% of the energy is reflected (Wever and Lawrence, 1954), a 30-dB loss due to the mismatch in acoustic impedance between air and inner-ear fluids. Properties of the external meatus, middle-ear cavity, tympanic membrane, and middle-ear ossicles shape the responsiveness of a species to different frequencies.

The eustachian tube is a bony channel lined with soft tissue extending from the middle ear to the nasopharynx. In humans, it is often closed, except during swallowing, and provides a means by which pressure is equalized across the tympanic membrane. The function is clearly observed with changes in altitude or barometric pressure. A second function of the eustachian tube is to aerate the tissues of the middle ear.

The volume of the air-filled middle-ear cavity inversely determines the stiffness of the tympanic membrane at low frequencies. A reduction of low-frequency impedance for some desert rodents with large middle-ear cavities (Ravicz and Rosowski, 1997) enhances the detection of predators at a distance. However, the mass of the middle-ear ossicles dominates impedance at high frequencies and is related to the head mass (Nummela, 1995). For this reason, small mammals generally have good high-frequency hearing, often extending above 60 kHz. As sound frequency increases, impedances decrease due to eardrum stiffness and increase due to ossicular mass leaving a middle range where sound transmission to the inner ear is most efficient, limited only by resistive forces (Geisler, 1998), resonances of the cavities, and mechanical advantages provided by the tympanic membrane, ossicles, and oval window.

Since the ear canal and middle-ear cavities are, or approximate, closed volumes, they support quarter-wavelength resonances. The human meatus has a broad resonance between 3 and 4 kHz, enhancing sound pressure at the membrane by 12 dB (Weiner and Ross, 1946; von Békésy, 1960). This will be modified by obstructing the meatus with headphones or a hearing aid and must be considered in system designs.

The head and external and middle-ear structures impose a transfer function on sound pressure at the tympanic membrane (Batteau, 1967; Blauert, 1997). The monaural (single-ear) head-related transfer function (HRTF) is a function of sound-source azimuth and elevation relative to pressure waveforms at the tympanic membrane. It is complex, affecting both sound amplitudes and phases over their spectrum. Sound localization, highly dependent on binaural hearing, involves a binaural HRTF combining the left and right monaural HRTFs. Since the structures determining these functions vary, individualized HRTFs combined with head-position sensing are important for computer synthesis of realistic three-dimensional sound experiences delivered through headphones (Wightman and Kistler, 1989). For some source locations, even the shadowing effects of the torso produce HRTF cues (Algazi et al., 2002).

Since the acoustic impedance of the atmospheric source is much less than that of the aqueous medium of the inner ear, a very inefficient energy transfer would exist without the external and middle ears. The ossicles form an impedance transformer with a mechanical advantage that passes the acoustic signal at the tympanic membrane to inner-ear fluids with low loss. Essentially, air-based sounds of low-pressure and high-volume velocity are transformed to fluid displacements in the inner ear having high-pressure and low-volume velocity. Two important mechanisms promote this transfer: the area of the tympanic membrane is about 20 times that of the footplate of the stapes, and the lengths of the malleus and incus form a lever advantage from the eardrum to oval window of about 1.3 in humans (Wever and Lawrence, 1954; Geisler, 1998). The hydraulic piston due to the areal ratio contributes about 26 dB to counteract the impedance mismatch, and the lever mechanism about 2.3 dB. These concepts of middle-ear mechanisms hold at frequencies below about 2 kHz, but the tympanic membrane does not behave as a piston at higher frequencies and can support multiple modes of vibration. Second, the mass of the ossicles becomes significant, contributing to resonances. Third, connections between the ossicles are not lossless, and their stiffness cannot be ignored. Fourth, pressure variations in the middle-ear cavity can change the stiffness of the tympanic membrane, as do reflexive contractions of middle-ear muscles, especially in response to intense sounds. Fifth, the cavity of the middle ear produces resonances at acoustic frequencies. All these factors produce variations in high-frequency acoustic transmission from the external to the inner ear specific to individuals, species, and conditions.

5.2.2 Inner Ear

The acoustic portion of the mammalian inner ear is a spiral structure, the cochlea (snail), containing a central core, the modiolus, where fibers of the auditory nerve collect. The nerve fibers arise from SGCs whose somas form the spiral ganglion in a bony canal around the modiolus. Around the modiolus spiral three fluid-filled chambers or scalae, the scala vestibule (SV), the scala media (SM), and the scala tympani (ST) as shown in Figure 5.2. At the base of the cochlea, the stapes footplate displaces fluid in the SV through the oval window. At the other end of the spiral, the apex of the cochlea, the SV and the ST communicate through the helicotrema. Both are filled with perilymph, similar to extracellular fluid. The SM spirals between them and is filled with endolymph, a medium high in K^+ and low in Na^+ due to active processes in the stria vascularis lining the lateral wall. A positive potential of 80 mV is maintained in the SM by the metabolically driven ionic pumps of the stria vascularis. The SM is separated from the SV by Reissner's membrane, which is impermeable to ions. The SM is separated from the ST by the BM with a length of about 31 mm over 2.5 spiral turns in human (Wever and Lawrence, 1954). Resting on the BM is the organ of Corti consisting of one row of IHCs that transduce acoustic signals into neural signals, three rows of outer hair cells (OHCs) that play an active role in the biomechanics of the cochlea, cells that support the hair cells, and the tectorial membrane overlying the stereocilia of the hair cells.

Stapes displacements for tones above behavioral threshold are very small, estimates of 0.0001 nm being common (Geisler, 1998). This can be compared to 0.1 nm for the diameter of a hydrogen atom. The

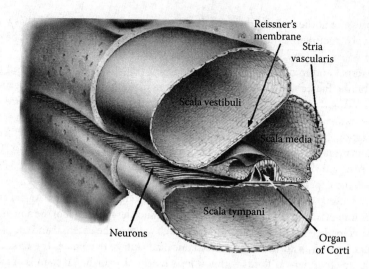

Reissner's
membrane

Stria
vascularis

Scala vestibuli

Scala media

Scala tympani

Neurons

Organ
of Corti

FIGURE 5.2   A cross-sectional representation of one turn of the cochlea.

structures of the inner ear transform these infinitesimal movements to neural discharges that underlie
the detection of sounds.

5.2.2.1 Basilar Membrane

The cochlear partition (BM and organ of Corti) provides the primary passive mechanical filter function
of the inner ear. Alternating fluid displacements at the footplate of the stapes induce pressure differences
across the partition from its base near the oval window to its apex near the helicotrema. The cochlear
partition has graded mechanical properties favoring rapid movement to high frequencies near the base
and slower movement to low frequencies near the apex, resulting in a traveling wave motion in that
order. The membrane's width varies as it traverses the cochlear duct, narrower at its basal end than at
its apical end. It is stiffer at the base than at the apex, with stiffness varying by about two orders of magnitude. Pressure relief is provided for the incompressible fluids of the inner ear by the round window, a
membrane-covered opening from the ST to the middle-ear cavity. A transient pressure increase (condensation) at the stapes displaces its footplate inward, a traveling wave is initiated along the BM, pressure is increased in the ST, and a compensatory outward displacement of the round window membrane
occurs. A rarefaction causes the round window membrane to move inward toward the ST.

Sound decomposition into its frequency components is a major function of the cochlea. Georg von
Békésy observed the traveling wave on the cochlear partitions of cadavers under stroboscopic light synchronized to high-intensity, low-frequency tones. The traveling wave reached a maximum displacement
along the BM depending on the frequency of the tone, indicating a roughly logarithmic mapping of increasing frequencies from the apex to the base. His experiments on the peripheral auditory system are collected
in a book (von Békésy, 1950), and he was awarded the 1961 Nobel Prize in Medicine for his research.

Movements of the BM are very small, in the nanometer range or less for normal hearing, and a
new technique increased the measurement resolution to this level (Johnstone and Boyle, 1967). The
Mössbauer technique uses Doppler shift in γ emissions from a small radioactive particle placed on the
moving tissue being observed. In 1971, Rhode published Mössbauer measurements of tuning in the
basal region of the living cochlea. These tuning curves were remarkably sharp (Q_{10} of 7–8) for pure
tones at low intensities, but they degraded to broad tuning at high intensities. The slopes of the tuning
curve are much greater at the high-frequency edge than at the low-frequency edge. In the absence of an
explanation using passive models, these and subsequent observations came to implicate active tuning
processes in the cochlea, sometimes called the "cochlear amplifier."

Measurements using laser interferometer techniques now allow displacement resolutions of less than a nanometer (Mammano and Ashmore, 1995) and have aided investigations of the cochlea's active tuning mechanisms. It has been discovered that the cochlear amplifier operates primarily in the basal, high-frequency regions and is highly compressive, that is, large increases in high-frequency tone intensity cause small increases in the maximum displacement of the BM (Geisler, 1998).

5.2.2.2 Organ of Corti

As shown in Figure 5.3, the organ of Corti is composed of supporting cells, the hair cells themselves, and the tectorial membrane. The ciliated ends of both OHCs and IHCs are rigidly fixed by supporting cells, for example, Deiter's cells form the reticular lamina, a rigid plate holding the upper ends of the OHCs. Pillar cells form a rigid triangular tunnel whose upper surface extends the reticular lamina. The reticular lamina and upper ends of the pillar cells and other support cells form a barrier to ions, thereby isolating the endolymph of the SM from the perilymph of the ST surrounding the lower parts of the hair cells.

Both IHCs and OHCs have precise patterns of stereocilia at the end held within the rigid plate formed by supporting cells. The tectorial membrane overlies the stereocilia, but while those of OHCs contact the tectorial membrane, the stereocilia of the IHCs do not. At the end opposite the stereocilia, IHCs synapse with the distal processes of SGCs. The proximal processes of SGCs are generally myelinated and form most of the auditory nerve. The nerve is laid down as these fibers collect from the apex and base in an orderly spiral manner. The nerve retains the frequency map of the BM, that is, it is tonotopically organized, a characteristic that carries through much of the auditory system.

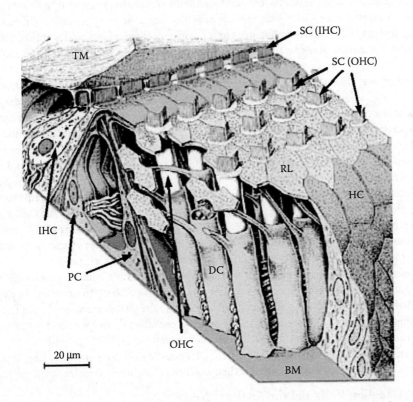

FIGURE 5.3 A depiction of the organ of Corti and its cellular structures. TM: tectorial membrane elevated to show stereocilia, PC: inner and outer pillar cells, DC: Deiter's cells, RL: reticular lamina, SC (IHC): one row of stereocilia for IHCs, SC (OHC): three rows of stereocilia for OHCs, HC: Hensen's cells. Other abbreviations are as used in text. Synapses from SGCs are seen at the bottoms of IHCs with efferent axons to OHCs seen in the tunnel and passing between Deiter's cells.

5.2.2.2.1 *Inner Hair Cells*

The IHCs lie in a single row on the modiolar side of the organ of Corti and number between 3000 and 4000 in human (Nadol, 1988). The IHCs' stereocilia are of graded, increasing length from the modiolar side of the cell. Early in ontogeny, a kinocilium is positioned next to the longest stereocilia, and excitation of hair cells occurs from ciliary displacement in that direction, further opening membrane channels to potassium and depolarizing the cell (Hudspeth, 1987). The positive potential in the endolymph of the SM drives K+ ions through the gating mechanism of IHC stereocilia to the negative intracellular potential. Displacement in the other direction reduces channel opening and produces a relative hyperpolarization (Hudspeth and Corey, 1977). These changes in intracellular potential modulate transmitter release through vesicle exocytosis at the base of the IHCs. The transmitter is related to glutamate but not glutamate itself (Gleich et al., 1990).

The IHCs are not attached to the tectorial membrane, so their response is thought to be responsive to fluid velocity over their stereocilia rather than direct displacement. Hair cells in some species exhibit frequency tuning when isolated (Crawford and Fettiplace, 1985), but mammalian hair cells do not. The tuning of the mammalian auditory system arises from the motions of the cochlear partition, and this is transferred to the IHCs and to the rest of the auditory system through their connection to SGCs. The nature of membrane channels and molecular mechanisms in auditory hair cells is being examined using a number of techniques (Hudspeth, 2000; Ashmore and Mammano, 2001).

5.2.2.2.2 *Outer Hair Cells*

There are about 12,000 OHCs in the human cochlea (Nadol, 1988). They have primarily *efferent* innervation, a puzzling arrangement for many years since the cochlea was a "sensory organ." The discovery of cochlear tuning that was not readily explainable from passive mechanical properties shifted attention to the OHCs where research, over the last few decades, has focused on their cellular and molecular mechanisms.

It was discovered that electrical stimulation of isolated OHCs produced lengthening or shortening (Brownell et al., 1985). It is generally accepted that the motility of OHCs counters viscous drag from fluids and cells of the cochlear partition. Through their contact to the tectorial membrane, they sense the subnanometer displacements of the BM and feedback, in phase, to augment them. This positive feedback occurs at auditory frequencies and is responsible for cochlear amplification. It occurs, or is most obvious, at low sound intensities, so it is responsible for the incredible sensitivity of the ear and for the nonlinear compression of the dynamic range of intensity coding. It was also observed that iontophoretic application of acetylcholine to the synaptic end of OHCs causes them to shorten. Efferents to OHCs release acetylcholine and thereby modulate the mechanical properties of the cochlea. The OHCs appear to affect the response of the auditory system in several ways. They enhance the tuning characteristics of the system to sinusoidal stimuli, decreasing thresholds and narrowing the filter's bandwidth, and they likely influence the damping of the BM dynamically by actively changing its stiffness.

Before the role of OHCs was determined, it was observed that sounds could be measured in the meatus, both spontaneously and in response to other sounds (Wilson, 1986). In humans, they tend to contain spectrally narrow components and vary across individuals. OHCs are strongly implicated as the source for these emissions because sounds in the opposite ear affect them (presumably through the efferent system) and aspirin, known to affect OHCs, reduces them (Geisler, 1998). As with most positive-feedback systems, spontaneous oscillation is suggested. Otoacoustic emissions are becoming important in the clinical evaluation of cochlear function for their potential signaling of cochlear pathologies.

5.2.2.3 Spiral Ganglion Cells and the Auditory Nerve

The auditory nerve of the human contains about 30,000 afferent fibers. Most (93%) are heavily myelinated and arise from Type I SGCs whose distal processes synapse on IHCs. The rest are from smaller, more lightly myelinated Type II SGCs. Each IHC has, on average, a number of Type I SCCs that synapse with it, 8 in the human and 18 in the cat. In contrast, each Type II SGC contacts OHCs at a rate of about

10–60 cells per fiber. The tonotopically organized nerve (low-frequency fibers in the center and high-frequency fibers in the outer layers) exits the modiolus and enters the internal auditory meatus of the temporal bone on its path to the cochlear nuclei.

Discharge spike patterns from the nerve have typically been characterized with repeated tone bursts varied in frequency and intensity (Kiang et al., 1965). Three views of the data are commonly used:

1. The temporal pattern of response to a tone burst is summarized in a peristimulus time histogram (PSTH). Auditory neurons may discharge only a few times during a brief tone burst, but if a histogram of spike events is synchronized to the onset of repeated tone bursts, a PSTH results that is more statistically representative of the neuron's response. Discharge patterns from the nerve have a primary-like pattern (see Figure 5.5).
2. A rate-level function of spike counts versus intensity at one tonal frequency has a threshold level, where counts rise from quiet levels, and a maximum rate, often a plateau holding for further increases in intensity. The range from threshold to the maximum, or saturation, level is called the dynamic range for sound-intensity signaling by response rate changes. A spontaneous rate of discharge, ranging from 50 spikes per second to less than 10, is usually measured for subthreshold stimulus levels.
3. Fiber responses are also characterized with tuning curves, a plot of thresholds for stimulus intensity versus frequency. Tuning curves for auditory nerve fibers have a minimum intensity (maximum sensitivity) at a characteristic frequency.

Sounds are coded in nerve discharges in two major ways: the level of discharge activity within the fiber population reflects the spectrum of sounds (labeled-line or place coding), and the temporal pattern of discharges in a fiber is partially synchronized to the cycle-by-cycle timing of frequencies near its characteristic frequency (temporal synchrony coding). Furthermore, complex sounds undergo nonlinear interactions in the cochlea, an example being two-tone suppression where the introduction of a new tone reduces both the discharge rate and synchrony of a fiber to characteristic frequency tones (Geisler, 1998).

While these coding mechanisms were discovered with tones, Sachs and Young (1979) found that the spectra of lower-intensity vowel sounds are represented as corresponding tonotopic rate peaks in nerve activity, but for higher intensities, this place code is lost as discharge rates saturate. At high intensities, spike synchrony to frequencies near characteristic frequency continues to signal the relative spectral content of vowels, a temporal code. These results hold for high-spontaneous-rate fibers (over 15 spikes per second), which are numerous. Less common, low-spontaneous-rate fibers (<15 spikes per second) appear to maintain the rate code at higher intensities, suggesting different coding roles for these two fiber populations. Furthermore, it has more recently been argued that these results from the cat do not represent the human cochlea. When vowels are spectrally scaled to match the cat's cochlea, the rate code appears to remain at high intensities (Recio et al., 2002).

5.3 Central Auditory System

The central auditory system consists of the cochlear nuclei; groups of brainstem nuclei including the superior olivary complex (SOC), nuclei of the lateral lemniscus (LL), and inferior colliculus (IC); and the auditory thalamocortical system consisting of the medial geniculate in the thalamus and multiple areas of the cerebral cortex. Figure 5.4 schematically indicates the nuclear levels and pathways. Efferent pathways are not shown. Page constraints prevent us from providing uniform detail for all levels of the auditory system.

5.3.1 Cochlear Nuclei

Many studies have focused on the anatomy and physiology of the cochlear nucleus (CN) revealing a wealth of information. It can be subdivided into three regions, the anteroventral CN (AVCN) anterior

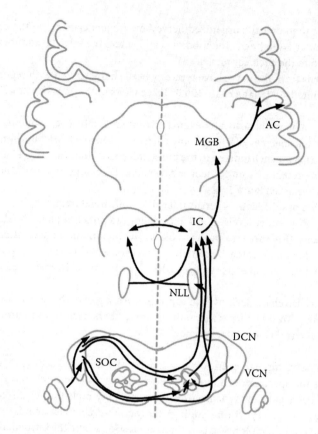

FIGURE 5.4 Schematic of the auditory system. Some of the major pathways and connections have been represented. The system is bilaterally symmetrical (midline as dashed line), and paths are crossed and shown for one side in most cases for clarity.

to the nerve entry, the posteroventral CN (PVCN), and the dorsal CN (DCN), each with one or more distinctive neuron types and connections. The axon from each Type I SGC in the nerve branches to each of the three divisions in an orderly manner so that tonotopic organization is maintained. Neurons with common morphologic classifications are found in all three divisions, especially granule cells, which tend to receive connections from Type II SGCs.

Morphologic categories based on shapes of dendritic trees and somas include spherical bushy cells in the anterior part of the AVCN, both globular bushy cells and spherical bushy in posterior AVCN, stellate cells throughout the AVCN and in the lower layers of the DCN, octopus cells (asymmetrical dendritic tree resembling an octopus) in the PVCN, and fusiform and giant cells in DCN. In AVCN, spherical bushy cells receive input from one Type I ganglion cell through a large synapse formation containing end bulbs of Held, while the globular cells receive inputs from a few afferent fibers. The AVCN is tonotopically organized, and neurons having similar characteristic frequencies form layers called "isofrequency laminae" (Bourk et al., 1981), an organization repeated with variation through most auditory nuclei. The DCN is structurally the most intricate of the CN subnuclei having four or five layers in many species giving it a "cortical" structure comparable to the cerebellum (see Young, 1998; Oertel and Young, 2004). Extracellular recording techniques, including simultaneous recording from pairs of physiologically identified DCN units and responses to tones and noise has allowed the development of conceptual models of DCN neuronal circuitry in cat (Young and Brownell, 1976; Voigt and Young, 1980, 1990; Young and Davis, 2002) and gerbil (Davis and Voigt, 1997). Although some differences between the two species have been noted, these may well be explained by a similar underlying neural circuit model whose parameters are somewhat species specific (as opposed to completely different neuronal architectures) (Davis and Voigt, 1997).

Intracellular recording in slice preparation has identified the membrane characteristics of CN neuronal types (Manis, 1990; Bal and Oertel, 2001). Some of these characteristics have been confirmed *in vivo* (Hancock and Voigt, 2002). The diversity of neuronal morphologic types, their participation in local circuits, and the emerging knowledge of their membrane biophysics are motivating detailed modeling (Babalian et al., 2003).

5.3.1.1 Spike Discharge Patterns

Tone bursts at a cell's characteristic frequency and 40 dB above threshold produce PSTHs with shapes distinctive to different nuclear subdivisions and even different morphologic types. PSTH patterns provide insight into sound features exciting auditory neurons. Figure 5.5 illustrates the major PSTH pattern types obtained from the auditory nerve and CN. Auditory nerve fibers and spherical bushy cells in AVCN have primary-like patterns in their PSTHs, an elevated spike rate after tone onset, falling to a slowly adapting level until the tone burst ends. Globular bushy cells may have primary-like, pri-notch (primary-like with a brief notch after onset), or chopper patterns. Stellate cells have nonprimary-like patterns. Onset response patterns, one or a few brief peaks of discharge at onset with little or no discharges afterward, are observed in the PVCN from octopus cells. Chopper, pauser, and buildup patterns are observed in many cells of the DCN. For most CN neurons, these patterns are not necessarily stable over different stimulus intensities; a primary-like pattern may change to a pauser pattern and then to a chopper pattern as the intensity is raised (Young, 1984).

Because central neurons often have inhibitory inputs, some stimuli reduce discharge probabilities, and so threshold tuning curves are extended to response-field maps. Figure 5.6 shows three response-field patterns, but many variations have been observed on these. Fibers and neurons with primary-like PSTHs generally have response maps with only an excitatory region (Figure 5.6a) although controls must be used to identify two-tone suppression. The lower edges of this region approximate the threshold-tuning curve. Octopus cells often have very broad tuning curves and extended response maps, as suggested by their frequency-spanning dendritic trees. More complex response maps are observed for some neurons, such as those in the DCN. Inhibitory regions alone, a frequency–intensity area of suppressed spontaneous discharge rates, or combinations of excitatory and inhibitory regions have been observed. Some neurons are

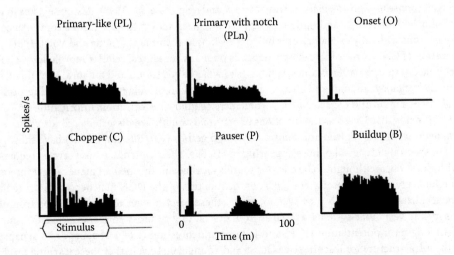

FIGURE 5.5 PSTH categories obtained for neural spike activity in the nerve and cochlear nuclei in response to brief tone bursts (stimulus envelope shown in lower left). Discharges in the nerve have the PL pattern while the others are associated with regions of the VCN and DCN and with specific morphological types.

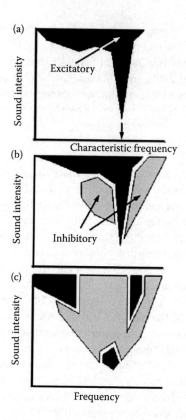

(a)

Sound intensity

Excitatory

Characteristic frequency

(b)

Sound intensity

Inhibitory

(c)

Sound intensity

Frequency

FIGURE 5.6 Response-field maps characteristic of auditory nerve fibers (a) and central neurons. Two-tone suppression in the cochlea, not due to inhibitory synapses, may resemble panel b maps. Maps are extracted from discharge rates sampled over the stimulus intensity–frequency parameter space. The inhibitory areas represent decreases in spontaneous or evoked discharge rates by tone bursts of the frequency and intensity under test.

excited only within islands of frequency–intensity combinations, demonstrating a characteristic frequency but having no response to high-intensity or wide-band sounds (Spirou et al., 1999). Response maps in the DCN containing both excitatory and inhibitory regions have been shown to arise from a convergence of inputs from neurons with only excitatory or inhibitory regions in their maps (Young and Voigt, 1981).

Categorization of CN neurons increasingly depends on many measures: cellular morphology, PSTH and response-field response patterns tones, responses to wide-band stimuli and binaural stimuli, membrane channel physiology, afferent and efferent connectivity, and molecular expressions and responses (Spirou et al., 1999; Fujino and Oertel, 2001). Beyond mere cellular categorization, information processing in the CN is being discovered as the functions of neuronal circuits are dissected.

Principal neurons of cats (Spirou and Young, 1991) and gerbils (Parsons et al., 2001) have shown to be sensitive to spectral notches like those appearing in HRTFs. These notches, whose center frequency changes with elevation, are thought to be cues for sounds localized in the median plane, where interaural time and intensity cues are absent. Thus, part of the function of the DCN may be to aide in median plane sound localization. The DCN, however, integrates these spectral cues with information from the somatosensory and vestibular systems, as well as from descending auditory pathways. The DCN shows signs of both long-term potentiation (LTP) and long-term depression (LTD) of some of its synapses, providing the infrastructure for learning (see Oertel and Young, 2004). Whether these learning mechanisms are used exclusively during development (e.g., when we need to learn to associate specific spectral notch frequencies with specific median plane locations) or if they function in adults navigating within their acoustic environments remains a topic of intense interest.

In addition to the contributions to our understanding of CN function gained through anatomy, physiology, pharmacology, and behavioral approaches, computational modeling of the neuronal circuitry of the CN has also contributed to our understanding of CN function. Auditory nerve models have provided the front ends to CN models (Carney, 1993). Single CN neurons (Kim et al., 1994, Hewitt and Meddis, 1995) as well as neural populations have been modeled (Voigt and Davis, 1996; Hancock and Voigt, 1999). A major reason for computational modeling of the neuronal circuitry is to verify the behavior of the model, compare it to the known physiology, and to predict the behavior of the model to novel stimuli (see Hancock et al., 1997; Nelkin et al., 1997).

5.3.2 Superior Olivary Complex

The SOC contains 10 or more subdivisions in some species. It is the first major site at which connections from the two ears converge and is therefore a center for binaural processing that underlies sound localization. There are large differences in the subdivisions between mammalian groups such as bats, primates, cetaceans, and burrowing rodents that utilize vastly different binaural cues. Binaural cues to the locus of sounds include interaural level differences (ILDs), interaural time differences (ITDs), and detailed spectral differences for multispectral sounds due to head and pinna filtering characteristics. These are summarized in the binaural HRTF (Tollin and Yin, 2001).

The medial superior olive (MSO) and lateral superior olive (LSO) process ITDs and ILDs, respectively. A neuron in the MSO receives projections from spherical bushy cells of the CN from both sides and thereby the precise timing and tuning cues of nerve fibers passed through the large synapses mentioned. The temporal accuracy of the pathways and the comparison precision of MSO neurons permit the discrimination of changes in ITD of a few tens of microseconds. MSO neurons project to the ipsilateral IC through the LL. Globular bushy cells of the CN project to the medial nucleus of the trapezoid body (MNTB) on the contralateral side, where they synapse on one and only one neuron in a large, excitatory synapse, the calyx of Held. MNTB neurons send inhibitory projections to neurons of the LSO on the same side, which also receives excitatory input from spherical bushy cells and probably other neurons in the AVCN on the same side (Doucet and Ryugo, 2003). Sounds reaching the ipsilateral side will excite discharges from an LSO neuron, while those reaching the contralateral side will inhibit its discharge. The relative balance of excitation and inhibition is a function of ILD resulting in this cue being encoded in LSO discharge rates.

One of the subdivisions of the SOC, the dorsomedial periolivary nucleus (DMPO), is a source of efferent fibers that reach the contralateral cochlea in the crossed olivocochlear bundle (COCB). Neurons of the DMPO receive inputs from collaterals of globular bushy cell axons of the contralateral ACVN that project to the MNTB and from octopus cells on both sides. The functional role of the feedback from the DMPO to the cochlea is not well understood.

5.3.3 Nuclei of the Lateral Lemniscus

The LL consists of ascending axons from the CN and LSO. The nuclei of the lateral lemniscus (NLL) lie within this tract, and some, such as the dorsal nucleus LL (DNLL), are known to process binaural information (Burger and Pollak, 2001), but less is known about these nuclei as a group than others, partially due to their relative inaccessibility.

5.3.4 Inferior Colliculi

The ICs are paired structures lying on the surface of the upper brainstem. Each colliculus has a large central nucleus, the ICC, a surface cortex, and paracentral nuclei. Each colliculus receives afferents from a number of lower brainstem nuclei, projects to the medial geniculate body (MGB) through the brachium, and communicates with the other colliculus through a commissure. The ICC is the major division and has distinctive isofrequency laminae formed from cells with disk-shaped dendritic trees and afferent fibers. The terminal endings of afferents form fibrous layers between laminae. The remaining neurons in the ICC are stellate cells that have dendritic trees spanning laminae. Axons from these two cell types make up much of the ascending ICC output.

Both monaural and binaural information converge at the IC through direct projections from the CN and from the SOC and NLL. Crossed CN inputs and those from the ipsilateral MSO are excitatory. Inhibitory synapses in the ICC arise from the DNLL, mediated by gamma-amino-butyric acid (GABA), and from the ipsilateral LSO, mediated by glycine (Faingold et al., 1991).

These connections provide an extensive base for identifying sound direction at this midbrain level, but due to their convergence, it is difficult to determine what binaural processing occurs at the IC as opposed to being passed from the SOC and NLL. Many neurons in the IC respond differently, depending on binaural parameters. Varying ILDs for clicks or high-frequency tones often indicate that contralateral sound is excitatory. Ipsilateral sound may have no effect on responses to contralateral sound, classifying the cell as E0, or it may inhibit responses, in which case the neuron is classified as EI, or maximal excitation may occur for sound at both ears, classifying the neuron as EE. Neurons responding to lower frequencies are influenced by ITDs, specifically the phase difference between sinusoids at the ears. Spatial receptive fields for sounds are not well documented in the mammalian IC, but barn owls, who use the sounds of prey for hunting at night, have sound-based spatial maps in the homologous structure (Knudsen and Knudsen, 1983; Bala et al., 2003). In mammals and owls, the superior colliculus, situated just rostral to the IC and largely visual in function, has spatial auditory receptive field maps.

5.3.5 Thalamocortical System

5.3.5.1 Medial Geniculate

The MGB and AC form the auditory thalamocortical system. As with other sensory systems, extensive projections to and from the cortical region exist in this system. The MGB has three divisions, the ventral, dorsal, and medial. The ventral division is the largest and has the most precise tonotopic organization. Almost all its input is from the ipsilateral ICC through the brachium of the IC. Its large bushy cells have dendrites oriented so as to lie in isofrequency layers, and the axons of these neurons project to the AC.

5.3.5.2 Auditory Cortex

As suggested previously, it is inaccurate to view central auditory pathways as a frequency-mapped sensory conduit to higher centers. The auditory system, and indeed the entire brain, operates to ensure survival by promoting effective behaviors and storing experience in memory for future decisions. In essence, audition identifies critical sound events and associates them with appropriate responses. This is evident in many observations at the cerebral cortex, but examples for bats and human speech suggest the range and complexity of processing in auditory pathways.

5.3.5.2.1 Bat Cortex

Bats of the suborder Microchiroptera use echos from cries they emit to locate and capture prey, usually insects. A well-studied species, the mustached bat (*Pteronotus parnellii*) emits brief sounds with a fundamental continuous frequency (CF) around 30 kHz with a short downward frequency-modulated (FM) sweep at the end. This cry has strong harmonics, so much of the returning energy is at multiples of the fundamental. This CF–FM sound is just one strategy used by various Microchiroptera, but the role of the AC in the mustached bat has been extensively studied. Figure 5.7 shows responsive regions in this bat's cortex. In an expanded region of a tonotopic map is the Doppler-shifted CF (DSCF) area with responses to the second harmonic of the 30-kHz chirp the bat emits. Cochlear specializations in this bat's inner ear greatly emphasize frequency resolution in the 60-kHz region. Specifically, returning CF sounds are mapped so precisely that the Doppler shift produced by insect wing flutters will cause the site

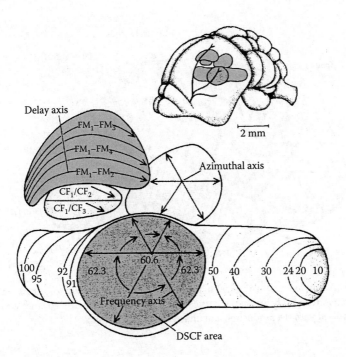

Delay axis

Azimuthal axis

Frequency axis

DSCF area

FIGURE 5.7 Auditory cortical areas of the mustached bat showing selective processing in different cortical areas for the emitted and returning components of the CF–FM echolocation cry. (Adapted from Suga N. 1990. *Sci. Am.* 262: 60–68.)

of maximum activity to vary. Another area, the CF/CF area, compares the frequency of the returning CF signal with that of the emitted signal, a cue for the relative velocity of the prey. The FM–FM region responds to the time difference between the emitted and returning FM cry components as a cue to the distance of the prey (Suga, 1990).

To illustrate the variation in cortical function, it is noted that other species of bats process sound differently in their auditory cortices. The pallid bat uses echolocation for obstacle avoidance and passive listening to locate prey (Razak and Fuzessery, 2002). As with the mustached bat, echolocation uses frequencies above 30 kHz, but prey location uses frequencies below 20 kHz, and neuron responses differ accordingly over the tonotopic map at cortex.

5.3.5.2.2 Human Cortex

The understanding and production of speech have evolved in human-ancestral primates over the last 200,000 years and are mediated by the primary AC and surrounding areas. The primary AC is tonotopically organized, but the surrounding areas implicated in higher-level language functions are not easily analyzed. Studies of stroke and injury have helped differentiate the roles of these areas. In most individuals, these functions are limited to the left side of the brain.

Figure 5.8 shows the major regions of auditory and language processing relative to common cortical landmarks. The primary auditory area is on the upper surface of the temporal lobe (not shown), but supplementary areas are located on the lateral temporal lobe. Broca's area is located in the posterior portion of the frontal lobe near the auditory regions in the temporal lobe. Wernicke's area is in the posterior part of the temporal lobe. Regions surrounding these also participate in language, but it is difficult to define many of the functions involved because they involve mixtures of speech production and understanding with subtle grammatical and logical relationships.

Two clinical conditions arising from stroke or injury have been studied extensively, Broca's and Wernicke's aphasias. Damage to Broca's area will often lead to labored but generally correct speech

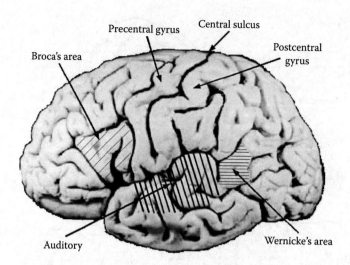

FIGURE 5.8 Cortical areas in human involved with hearing and language. The auditory areas are located on the temporal lobe, the primary area (A1) being on the dorsal surface within the Sylvan sulcus (not visible). Broca and Wernicke's areas are involved with the production and understanding of language.

production, but spoken sentences with complex grammars will not be understood. The concept that Broca's area provides short-term working memory for the comparison of sentence components has been suggested. In contrast, patients with damage to Wernicke's area will often speak effortlessly but with many lexical errors, and they generally do not understand sentences spoken by others. Wernicke's area, once thought to underlie "speech comprehension" is now considered a link between areas for concept and meaning with those for word choice and grammar. Wernicke's area is often grouped with the supramarginal gyrus (SMG) just above it. A third clinical syndrome, conduction aphasia, results from damage to neural pathways linking Wernicke's to the SMG and Broca's area. Speech production and understanding are less affected in conduction aphasia, but it has distinctive features, including an inability to repeat sentences accurately and difficulty in naming things.

Significant variations arise over the range of clinical damage to cortical and white matter surrounding these areas, especially the SMG, and if tissue damage is restricted to a small area, the aphasia may be transient. Auditory input at the cortical level goes far beyond tonotopic organization to complexities of language, and when it is absent, other sensory input may take over. An example of the generality of function is the disruption of signing by a deaf patient during electrical stimulation of these areas during awake brain surgery for temporal lobe epilepsy (Corina et al., 1999). Tissues normally involved with understanding and producing speech switch to visual cues with deafness.

5.4 Pathologies

Hearing loss results from conductive and neural deficits. Conductive hearing loss due to attenuation in the outer or middle ear can often be alleviated by amplification provided by hearing aids and may be subject to surgical correction. Sensorineural loss due to the absence of IHCs results from genetic deficits, biochemical insult, and exposure to intense sound, or aging (presbycusis). For some cases of sensorineural loss, partial hearing function can be restored with the cochlear prosthesis, direct electrical stimulation of remaining SGCs using small arrays of electrodes inserted into the ST. As of 2004, an estimated 70,000 people have received cochlear implants.

Lesions of the nerve and central structures occur due to trauma, tumor growth, and vascular accidents. These may be subject to surgical intervention to prevent further damage and promote functional recovery. In patients having no auditory nerve due to tumor removal, direct electrical stimulation of the CN has been used to provide auditory sensation.

5.5 Further Topics

It is not possible to cover many important topics for the auditory system in a brief survey. Excellent books treat these in detail. A great deal of attention has been and is being paid to plasticity in neural and behavioral mechanisms of hearing (Parks et al., 2004). Likewise, little has been said about perceptual mechanisms and the techniques for assessing the behavioral limits of hearing (Hartmann, 1998).

References

Algazi V.R., Duda R.O., Duraiswami R., Gumerov N.A., and Tang Z. 2002. Approximating the head-related transfer function using simple geometric models of the head and torso. *J. Acoust. Soc. Am.* 112: 2053–2064.

Ashmore J.F. and Mammano F. 2001. Can you still see the cochlea for the molecules? *Curr. Opin. Neurobiol.* 11: 449–454.

Babalian A.L., Ryugo D.K., and Rouiller E.M. 2003. Discharge properties of identified cochlear nucleus neurons and auditory nerve fibers in response to repetitive electrical stimulation of the auditory nerve. *Exp. Brain Res.* 153: 452–460.

Bal R. and Oertel D. 2001. Potassium currents in octopus cells of the mammalian cochlear nucleus. *J. Neurophysiol.* 86: 2299–2311.

Bala A.D.S., Spitzer M.W., and Takahashi T.T. 2003. Prediction of auditory spatial acuity from neuronal images on the owl's auditory space map. *Nature* 424: 771–773.

Batteau D.W. 1967. The role of the pinna in human localization. *Proc. R. Soc. London, Ser. B* 168: 158–180.

Blauert J.P. 1997. *Spatial Hearing.* Cambridge: MIT Press.

Bourk T.R., Mielcarz J.P., and Norris B.E. 1981. Tonotopic organization of the anteroventral cochlear nucleus of the cat. *Hear. Res.* 4: 215.

Brownell W.E., Bader C.R., Bertrand D., and de Ribaupierre Y. 1985. Evoked mechanical responses of isolated cochlear outer hair cells. *Science* 227: 194–196.

Burger R.M. and Pollak G.D. 2001. Reversible inactivation of the dorsal nucleus of the lateral lemniscus reveals its role in the processing of multiple sound sources in the inferior colliculus of bats. *J. Neurosci.* 21: 4830–4843.

Carney L.H. 1993. A model for the responses of low-frequency auditory nerve fibers in cat. *J. Acoust. Soc. Am.* 93: 401–417.

Corina D.P., McBurney S.L., Dodrill C., Hinshaw K., Brinkley J., and Ojeman G. 1999. Functional roles of Broca's area and SMG: Evidence from cortical stimulation mapping in a deaf signer. *NeuroImage* 10: 570–581.

Crawford A.C. and Fettiplace R. 1985. The mechanical properties of ciliary bundles of turtle cochlear hair cells. *J. Physiol.* 364: 359.

Davis K.A. and Voigt H.F. 1997. Evidence of stimulus-dependent correlated activity in the dorsal cochlear nucleus of decerebrate gerbils. *J. Neurophysiol.* 78: 229–247.

Doucet J.R. and Ryugo D.K. 2003. Axonal pathways to the lateral superior olive labeled with biotinylated dextran amine injections in the dorsal cochlear nucleus of rats. *J. Comp. Neurol.* 461: 452–465.

Faingold C.L., Gehlbach G., and Caspary D.M. 1991. Functional pharmacology of inferior colliculus neurons. In: *Neurobiology of Hearing: The Central Auditory System.* Altschuler R.A., Bobbin R.P., Clopton B.M., and Hoffman D.W. (Eds.), New York: Raven Press, pp. 223–251.

Fujino K. and Oertel D. 2001. Cholinergic modulation of stellate cells in the mammalian ventral cochlear nucleus. *J. Neurosci.* 21: 7372–7383.

Geisler C.D. 1998. *From Sound to Synapse: Physiology of the Mammalian Ear.* New York: Oxford University Press.

Gleich O., Johnstone B.M., and Robertson D. 1990. Effects of L-glutamate on auditory afferent activity in view of proposed excitatory transmitter role in the mammalian cochlea. *Hear. Res.* 45: 295–312.

Hancock K.E., Davis K.A., and Voigt H.F. 1997. Modeling inhibition of type II units in the dorsal cochlear nucleus. *Biol. Cybern.* 76: 419–428.

Hancock K.E. and Voigt H.F. 1999. Wideband inhibition of dorsal cochlear nucleus type IV units in cat: A computational model. *Ann. Biomed. Eng.* 27: 73–87.

Hancock K.E. and Voigt H.F. 2002. Intracellularly labeled fusiform cells in dorsal cochlear nucleus of the gerbil. I. Physiological response properties. *J. Neurophysiol.* 87: 2505–2519.

Hartmann W.M. 1998. *Signals, Sound, and Sensation.* New York: Springer-Verlag.

Hewitt M.J. and Meddis R. 1995. A computer model of dorsal cochlear nucleus pyramidal cells: Intrinsic membrane properties. *J. Acoust. Soc. Am.* 97(4): 2405–2413.

Hudspeth A.J. 1987. Mechanoelectrical transduction by hair cells in the acousticolateralis sensory system. *Ann. Rev. Neurosci.* 6: 187.

Hudspeth A.J. 2000. Sensory transduction in the ear. In: *Principles of Neural Science.* Chapter 31, Kandel E.R., Schwartz J.H., and Jessell T.M. (Eds.), New York: McGraw-Hill, pp. 614–624.

Hudspeth A.J. and Corey D.P. 1977. Sensitivity, polarity, and conductance change in the response of vertebrate hair cells to controlled mechanical stimuli. *Proc. Natl Acad. Sci. USA* 74: 2407.

Johnstone B.M. and Boyle A.J.F 1967. Basilar membrane vibration examined with the Mössbauer technique. *Science* 158: 390–391.

Kiang N.Y.-S., Watanabe T., Thomas E.C., and Clark L.F. 1965. *Discharge Patterns of Single Fibers in the Cat's Auditory Nerve.* Cambridge: MIT Press.

Kim D.O., Ghosal S., Khant S.L. and Parham K. 1994. A computational model with ionic conductances for the dorsal cochlear nucleus (DCN) fusiform cell. *J. Acoust. Soc. Am.* 96: 1501–1514.

Kinsler L.E., Frey A.R., Coppens A.B., and Sanders J.V. 1999. *Fundamentals of Acoustics.* New York: Wiley.

Knudsen E.I. and Knudsen P.F. 1983. Space-mapped auditory projections from the inferior colliculus to the optic tectum in the barn owl. *J. Comp. Neurol.* 218: 187–196.

Mammano F. and Ashmore J.F. 1995. A laser interferometer for sub nanometre measurements in the cochlea. *J. Neurosci. Meth.* 60: 89–94.

Manis P.B. 1990. Membrane properties and discharge characteristics of guinea pigs dorsal cochlear nucleus neurons studied *in vitro. J. Neurosci.* 10: 2338–2351.

Nadol J.B. Jr. 1988. Comparative anatomy of the cochlea and auditory nerve in mammals. *Hear. Res.* 34: 253.

Nelkin I., Kim P.J., and Young E.D. 1997. Linear and nonlinear spectral integration in type IV neurons of the dorsal cochlear nucleus. II. Predicting responses with the use of nonlinear models. *J. Neurophysiol.* 78: 800–811.

Nummela S. 1995. Scaling of the mammalian middle ear. *Hear. Res.* 85: 18–30.

Oertel D. and Young E.D. 2004. What's a cerebellar circuit doing in the auditory system? *Trends Neurosci.* 27: 104–110.

Parks T.N., Rubel E.W., Popper A.N., and Fay R.R. (Eds.) 2004. *Plasticity of the Auditory System.* Springer Handbook of Auditory Research, New York: Springer-Verlag, 23: 323.

Parsons J.E., Lim E., and Voigt H.F. 2001. Type III units in the gerbil dorsal cochlear nucleus may be spectral notch detectors. *Ann. Biomed. Eng.* 29: 887–896.

Ravicz M.E. and Rosowski J.J. 1997. Sound-power collection by the auditory periphery of the Mongolian gerbil *Meriones unguiculatus*: III. Effect of variations in middle-ear volume. *J. Acoust. Soc. Am.* 101: 2135–2147.

Razak K.A. and Fuzessery Z.M. 2002. Functional organization of the pallid bat auditory cortex: Emphasis on binaural organization. *J. Neurophysiol.* 87: 72–86.

Recio A., Rhode W.S., Kiefte M., and Kluender K.R. 2002. Responses to cochlear normalized speech stimuli in the auditory nerve of cat. *J. Acoust. Soc. Am.* 111: 2213–2218.

Rhode W.S. 1971. Observations of the vibration of the basilar membrane in squirrel monkeys using the Mössbauer technique. *J. Acoust. Soc. Am.* 49: 1218–1231.

Sachs M.B. and Young E.D. 1979. Encoding of steady-state vowels in the auditory nerve: Representation in terms of discharge rate. *J. Acoust. Soc. Am.* 66: 470.

Spirou G.A., Davis K.A., Nelken I., and Young E.D. 1999. Spectral integration by Type II interneurons in dorsal cochlear nucleus. *J. Neurophysiol.* 82: 48–663.

Spirou G.A. and Young E.D. 1991. Organization of dorsal cochlear nucleus type IV unit response maps and their relationship to activation by band-limited noise. *J. Neurophysiol.* 66: 1750–1768.

Suga N. 1990. Biosonar and neural computation in bats. *Sci. Am.* 262: 60–68.

Tollin D.J. and Yin T.C.T. 2001. Investigation of spatial location coding in the lateral superior olive using virtual space stimulation. In *Physiological and Psychophysical Bases of Auditory Function*. Houtsma A.J.M., Kohlrausch A., Prijs V.F., and Schoonhoven R. (Eds.), Maastricht: Shaker Publishing, pp. 236–243.

Voigt H.F. and Davis K.A. 1996. Computer simulations of neural correlations in the dorsal cochlear nucleus. In: *Cochlear Nucleus: Structure and Function in Relation to Modeling*. Ainsworth W.A. (Ed.), London: JAI Press, pp. 351–375.

Voigt H.F. and Young E.D. 1980. Evidence of inhibitory interactions between neurons in the dorsal cochlear nucleus. *J. Neurophysiol.* 44: 76–96.

Voigt H.F. and Young E.D. 1990. Cross-correlation analysis of inhibitory interactions in dorsal cochlear nucleus. *J. Neurophysiol.* 64: 1590–1610.

von Békésy G. 1960. *Experiments in Hearing*. New York: McGraw-Hill.

Weiner F.M. and Ross D.A. 1946. The pressure distribution in the auditory canal in a progressive sound field. *J. Acoust. Soc. Am.* 18: 401–408.

Wever E.G. and Lawrence M. 1954. *Physiological Acoustics*. Princeton: Princeton University Press.

Wightman F.L. and Kistler D.J. 1989. Headphone simulation of free-field listening. II: Psychophysical validation. *J. Acoust. Soc. Am.* 85: 868–878.

Wilson P.J. 1986. Otoacoustic emissions and tinnitus. *Scand. Audiol. Suppl.* 25: 109–119.

Young E.D. 1984. Response characteristics of neurons of the cochlear nuclei. In: *Hearing Science: Recent Advances*. C.I. Berlin (Ed.), San Diego, California: College-Hill Press.

Young E.D. 1998. The cochlear nucleus. In: *Synaptic Organization of the Brain*. Shepard G.M. (Ed.), New York: Oxford Press, pp. 121–157.

Young E.D. and Brownell W.E. 1976. Responses to tones and noise of single cells in dorsal cochlear nucleus of unanesthetized cats. *J. Neurophysiol.* 39: 282–300.

Young E.D. and Davis K.A. 2002. Circuitry and function of the dorsal cochlear nucleus. In: *Integrative Functions in the Mammalian Auditory Pathway*. Oertel D., Fay R.R., and Popper A.N. (Eds.), New York: Springer-Verlag.

Young E.D. and Voigt H.F. 1981. The internal organization of the dorsal cochlear nucleus. In: *Neuronal Mechanisms in Hearing*, Syka J. and Aitkin L. (Eds.), New York: Plenum Press. pp. 127–133.

6

Gastrointestinal System

6.1	Introduction	6-1
6.2	GI Electrical Oscillations	6-3
	Main Features • Intercellular Communication • Coupled Nonlinear Oscillators	
6.3	A Historical Perspective	6-6
	Minute Rhythms • Hour Rhythms • Terminology	
6.4	The Stomach	6-8
	Anatomical Features • Gastric ECA Slow-Wave Activity • The Electrogastrogram	
6.5	The Small Intestine	6-10
	Anatomical Features • Small Intestinal Slow-Wave Activity • Small Intestinal MMC	
6.6	The Colon	6-11
	Anatomical Features • Colonic Slow-Wave Activity	
6.7	Epilogue	6-12
	Acknowledgments	6-12
	References	6-12

Berj L. Bardakjian
University of Toronto

6.1 Introduction

The primary function of the gastrointestinal (GI) system (Figure 6.1) is to supply the body with nutrients and water. The ingested food is moved along the alimentary canal at an appropriate rate for digestion, absorption, storage, and expulsion. To fulfill the various requirements of the system, each organ has adapted one or more functions. The esophagus acts as a conduit for the passage of food into the stomach for trituration and mixing. The ingested food is then emptied into the small intestine, which plays a major role in the digestion and absorption processes. The chyme is mixed thoroughly with secretions and it is propelled distally (1) to allow further gastric emptying, (2) to allow for uniform exposure to the absorptive mucosal surface of the small intestine, and (3) to empty into the colon. The vigor of mixing and the rate of propulsion depend on the required contact time of chyme with enzymes and the mucosal surface for efficient performance of digestion and absorption. The colon absorbs water and electrolytes from the chyme, concentrating and collecting waste products that are expelled from the system at appropriate times. All of these motor functions are performed by contractions of the muscle layers in the GI wall (Figure 6.2).

The discovery that normal GI motility requires interstitial cells of Cajal (ICC) has altered our understanding of the cellular basis of GI function. It has modified our original concept about the core unit that controls GI motility being made up of nerves and smooth muscle, to one that includes ICC. This core unit fundamentally regulates smooth muscle rhythmic contraction. The ICC provide several important functions in the GI tract: (a) generation of electrical slow-wave activity, (b) coordination of generation and active propagation of slow waves, (c) transduction of motor neural inputs from the

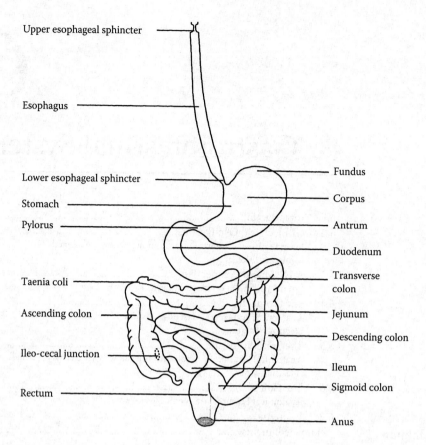

Upper esophageal sphincter

Esophagus

Lower esophageal sphincter

Stomach

Pylorus

Taenia coli

Ascending colon

Ileo-cecal junction

Rectum

Fundus

Corpus

Antrum

Duodenum

Transverse colon

Jejunum

Descending colon

Ileum

Sigmoid colon

Anus

FIGURE 6.1 The GI tract.

enteric nervous system, and (d) mechanosensation to the stretch of GI muscles. These are important functions that contribute to both the regulation of excitation–contraction coupling in the gut and to the connectivity between smooth muscle cells and the motor output of the enteric nervous system. Motility patterns require timed contractions to create ring-like peristaltic and segmental contractions, and slow waves provide oscillations in the open probability of calcium channels of smooth muscle cells that facilitate phasic contractions. It would not be possible to generate the motor programs stored in the enteric nervous system without the patterned electrical activity and synaptic connectivity provided by the ICC (Sanders et al., 2006; Huizinga et al., 2009). The ICC pace GI smooth muscle by initiating slow waves in both the longitudinal and circular muscle layers, and they appear to be preferred sites for the reception of neurotransmitters (Ward and Sanders, 2001; Sanders et al., 2002; Daniel, 2004). The ICC are distributed throughout the GI tract, where the ICC of the myenteric plexus play a crucial role in pacing slow waves and contractions while intramuscular ICC appear to play a role in receiving neural messages (Ward et al., 2001; Sanders et al., 2002). A variety of motility disorders, such as gastroparesis, pseudoobstruction, chronic constipation, and posttraumatic or postinfectious dysfunction, have been associated with either profound or partial loss of ICC. The important physiological roles of ICC also suggest the possibility of a causative role for ICC loss in a variety of motor disorders.

Recently, significant steps forward have been made in our understanding of the physiology of ICC as well as the mechanisms of injury and recovery. These advances have been recently reviewed by Huizinga et al. (2009). A decrease in ICC replenishment from either adult ICC or ICC precursors is associated with several GI motility disorders, an uncontrolled increase may result in GI stromal tumors. Different mechanisms have been proposed for ICC loss. Ultrastructural studies have suggested that in diseased

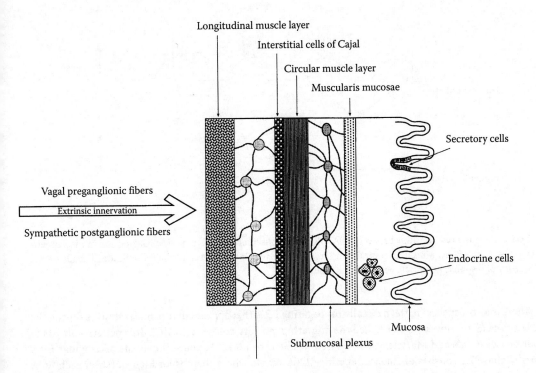

FIGURE 6.2 The layers of the GI wall.

states, ICC might dedifferentiate into an earlier developmental stage, more reminiscent of smooth muscle cells or fibroblasts from an ultrastructural viewpoint. Whether this changed phenotype is reversible into ICC or is destined to be lost is not yet known. ICC can be lost through apoptosis. Apoptotic ICC could be detected in all layers of the human colonic muscle.

6.2 GI Electrical Oscillations

6.2.1 Main Features

GI motility is governed by myogenic, neural, and chemical control systems. The myogenic control system is manifest by rhythmic depolarizations of the ICC and smooth muscle cells, which constitute electrical oscillations called the electrical control activity (ECA) or slow waves (Daniel and Chapman, 1963). The properties of this myogenic system and its electrical oscillations dictate to a large extent the contraction patterns in the stomach, small intestine, and colon (Szurszewski, 1987). The ECA controls the contractile excitability of smooth muscle cells since the cells may contract only when depolarization of the membrane voltage exceeds an excitation threshold. The normal spontaneous amplitude of ECA depolarization does not exceed this excitation threshold except when neural or chemical excitation is present. The myogenic system affects the frequency, direction, and velocity of the contractions. It also affects the coordination or lack of coordination between adjacent segments of the gut wall. Hence, the electrical activities in the gut wall provide an electrical basis for GI motility.

In the distal stomach, small intestine, and colon, there are intermittent bursts of rapid electrical oscillations, called the electrical response activity (ERA) or spike bursts. The ERA occurs during the depolarization plateaus of the ECA if a cholinergic stimulus is present and it is associated with muscular contractions (Figure 6.3). Thus, neural and chemical control systems determine whether contractions will occur or not, but when contractions are occurring, the myogenic control system (Figure 6.4) determines the spatial and temporal patterns of contractions.

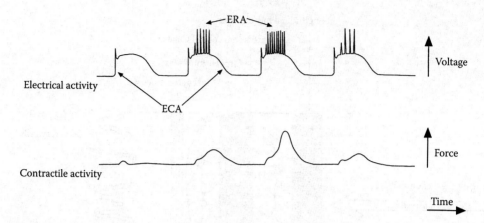

FIGURE 6.3 The relationships between ECA, ERA, and muscular contractions. The ERA occurs in the depolarized phase of the ECA. Muscular contractions are associated with the ERA, and their amplitude depends on the frequency of response potentials within an ERA burst.

There is also a cyclical pattern distally propagating ERA that appears in the small intestine during the fasted state (Szurszewski, 1969), called the migrating motility complex (MMC). This pattern consists of four phases (Code and Marlett, 1975): Phase I has little or no ERA, phase II consists of irregular ERA bursts, phase III consists of intense repetitive ERA bursts where there is an ERA burst on each ECA cycle, and phase IV consists of irregular ERA bursts but is usually much shorter than phase II and may not be always present. The initiation and propagation of the MMC is controlled by enteric cholinergic neurons in the intestinal wall (Figure 6.2). The propagation of the MMC may be modulated by inputs from extrinsic nerves or circulating hormones (Sarna et al., 1981). The MMC keeps the small intestine clean of residual food, debris, and desquamated cells.

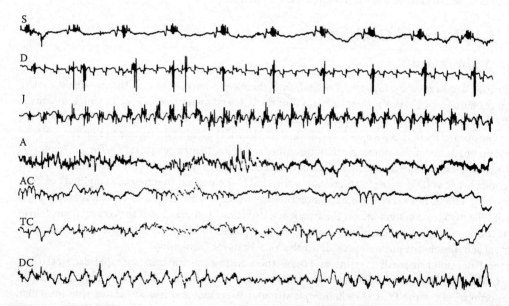

FIGURE 6.4 The GI ECA and ERA, recorded in a conscious dog from electrode sets implanted subserosally on stomach (S), duodenum (D), jejunum (J), proximal ascending colon (A), distal ascending colon (AC), transverse colon (TC), and descending colon (DC), respectively. Each trace is of 2 min duration.

6.2.2 Intercellular Communication

Coupling between ICC and smooth muscle networks is essential for the entrainment of ECA to obtain coordinated muscle contraction. Gap junctions play an important role in intercellular communication since they provide direct electrical and metabolic coupling between the cytoplasm of neighboring cells (Chanson and Spray, 1995), but cells are also coupled by a variety of other structures (Daniel et al., 1976; Huizinga et al., 1992). ICC may be coupled to the smooth muscle by gap junctions as found at the inner border of the circular muscle layer in the canine colon (Berezin et al., 1988), but at other sites, such as between ICC and the muscle layers of the mouse small intestine, gap junctions were not found; however, there was an abundance of close apposition junctions (Thuneberg, 1982). Within certain muscle layers, no gap junctions can be recognized by electron microscopic techniques such as in the longitudinal muscle of the intestine and colon of a variety of species (Zamir and Hanani, 1990; Liu et al., 1998). In such tissues, close apposition junctions are always observed. Such contacts may contain small groups of connexons, which would allow electrical and metabolic communication although it could not be identified as a gap junction; only a large aggregate of connexons can be recognized as a gap junction by electron microscopy. Nevertheless, electrical communication other than purely resistive is likely to occur.

One type of conspicuous contact is the peg-and-socket junction, where an extrusion of one cell forms a peg, which penetrates a neighboring cell and fits into an intrusion that forms a socket with an intracellular gap of 20 nm. This extrusion can be up to 10 μm long, undergo a 90° bend upon entering a cell, and be up to 1.5 μm in diameter (Thuneberg et al., 1998). The abundance of these structures in areas of no demonstrable gap junctions and their absence in areas that have many gap junctions suggest that they may provide an intercellular communication pathway other than a direct low-resistance pathway as provided by a gap junction.

Daniel (2004) reviewed communication between ICC and GI smooth muscle and he considered structural, theoretical, and experimental difficulties with the possible role of gap junctions in pacing and in neurotransmission. Furthermore, he considered the following alternate possibilities for the transmission of ICC pacing and neural messages: (a) The production of an electric field potential in narrow clefts between cells, such as in close apposition junctions, which was shown to be sufficient to allow electrical coupling (Sperelakis and Mann, 1977; Vigmond and Bardakjian, 1995; Sperelakis, 2002; Sperelakis and McConnell, 2002; Sperelakis and Ramasamy, 2002) and (b) potassium accumulation in the narrow clefts, such as in peg-and-socket junctions, which was shown to facilitate electrical coupling without gap junctions (Sperelakis et al., 1984; Vigmond et al., 2000).

6.2.3 Coupled Nonlinear Oscillators

There is an extensive literature on the mathematical modeling of the generation of oscillations, their coupling, their entrainment, and frequency pulling (Fitzhugh, 1961; Pavlidis, 1973; Plant and Kim, 1976; Winfree, 1980; Ermentrout and Kopell, 1984; Grasman, 1984; Rinzel, 1987; Sherman and Rinzel, 1991; Bardakjian and Diamant, 1994; Zarrifa and Bardakjian, 2006; Zalay and Bardakjian, 2008, 2009). The entrainment of coupled oscillators is governed by both intrinsic oscillator properties and coupling mechanisms. The theory of second-order relaxation oscillators, as "traditionally" formulated was qualitative in nature. Two types of oscillators were described: (a) Van der Pol type oscillators (Van der Pol and Van der Mark, 1928), which were generalized (Fitzhugh, 1961) to exhibit neuronal-like features and (b) Winfree-type oscillators (Winfree, 1980, 1989), which focused on rate processes of phase and amplitude of oscillation and they were helpful in elucidating the nature of "phase-resetting" phenomena in biological oscillators. Furthermore, quantitative fourth-order models of the Hodgkin–Huxley type (Hodgkin and Huxley, 1952; Plant and Kim, 1976) have been described that closely reproduce neuronal transmembrane voltages. However, development of these quantitative oscillator models requires a full biophysical description of ionic transport mechanisms through membrane channels, pumps, and exchangers. A simpler alternative is the leaky integrate-and-fire model (Stein, 1967), which can only reproduce basic spiking behavior and it is mostly useful for the investigation of large networks where the focus is not on individual cells.

On the other hand, the mapped clock oscillator (MCO) (Bardakjian and Diamant, 1994) is a multi-portal generalization of the Winfree-type oscillator that is quantitative in nature and exhibits refractory properties. Its parameters are the coefficients of the Fourier series representation of the intrinsic trans-membrane voltage oscillation. Hence, they can be obtained directly from the Fourier analysis of the biologically measured intrinsic waveform of the isolated oscillator (e.g., in experiments where segments of an organ are isolated from each other by transaction). Each oscillator consists of, first, a dynamic nonlinearity represented by two nonlinear simultaneous differential equations that govern the state variables of the system and, second, a static nonlinearity that maps the two state variables onto the observable output. The dynamic nonlinearity represents the clock mechanism of the oscillator. The values of its state variables can be modified by three input "portals," each of which correspond to a different type of coupling pathway (gap junctions, field effects, and membrane receptors). The static nonlinearity represents the cellular membrane. This mapper can be changed to represent the waveform of the specific cell being modeled. The MCO can represent transmembrane voltage oscillations in different systems (e.g., neurons, cardiac cells, GI muscle, and pancreatic beta cells).

6.3 A Historical Perspective

6.3.1 Minute Rhythms

Alvarez and Mahoney (1922) reported the presence of a rhythmic electrical activity (which they called "action currents") in the smooth muscle layers of the stomach, small intestine, and colon. Their data were acquired from cat (stomach and small intestine), dog (stomach, small intestine, and colon), and rabbit (small intestine and colon). They also demonstrated the existence of frequency gradients in excised stomach and bowel. Puestow (1933) confirmed the presence of a rhythmic electrical activity (which he called "waves of altered electrical potential") and a frequency gradient in isolated canine small intestinal segments. He also demonstrated the presence of an electrical spiking activity (associated with muscular contractions) superimposed on the rhythmic electrical activity. He implied that the rhythmic electrical activity persisted at all times, whereas the electrical spike activity was of an intermittent nature. Bozler (1938, 1939, 1941) confirmed the occurrence of an electrical spiking activity associated with muscular contractions both *in vitro* in isolated longitudinal muscle strips from guinea pig (colon and small intestine) and rabbit (small intestine), and *in situ* in exposed loops of the small intestine of anesthetized cat, dog, and rabbit, as well as in cat stomach. He also suggested that the strength of a spontaneous muscular contraction is proportional to the frequency and duration of the spikes associated with it.

The presence of two types of electrical activity in the smooth muscle layers of the GI tract in several species had been established (Milton and Smith, 1956; Bulbring et al., 1958; Gillespie, 1962; Burnstock et al., 1963; Daniel and Chapman, 1963; Bass, 1965; Duthie, 1974; Christensen, 1975; Daniel, 1975; Sarna, 1975a). The autonomous electrical rhythmic activity is an omnipresent myogenic activity (Burnstock et al., 1963) whose function is to control the appearance in time and space of the electrical spiking activity (an intermittent activity associated with muscular contractions) when neural and chemical factors are appropriate (Daniel and Chapman, 1963). Neural and chemical factors determine whether or not contractions will occur, but when contractions are occurring, the myogenic control system determines the spatial and temporal patterns of contractions.

Isolation of a distal segment of canine small intestine from a proximal segment (using surgical tran-section or clamping) had been reported to produce a decrease in the frequency of both the rhythmic muscular contractions (Douglas, 1949; Milton and Smith, 1956) and the electrical rhythmic activity (Milton and Smith, 1956) of the distal segment, suggesting frequency entrainment or pulling of the distal segment by the proximal one. It was demonstrated (Milton and Smith, 1956) that the repetition of the electrical spiking activity changed in the same manner as that of the electrical rhythmic activity, thus confirming a one-to-one temporal relationship between the frequency of the electrical rhythmic activity, the repetition rate of the electrical spiking activity, and the frequency of the muscular contractions (when all are present at any one site). Nelson and Becker (1968) suggested that the electrical rhythmic activity of the small intestine behaves like a system of coupled relaxation oscillators. They used two forward-coupled relaxation oscillators, having different intrinsic frequencies, to demonstrate frequency entrainment of the two coupled oscillators. Uncoupling of the two oscillators caused a decrease in the frequency of the distal oscillator simulating the effect of transection of the canine small intestine.

The electrical rhythmic activity in canine stomach (Sarna et al., 1972), canine small intestine (Nelson and Becker, 1968; Diamant et al., 1970; Sarna et al., 1971), human small intestine (Robertson-Dunn and Linkens, 1974), human colon (Bardakjian and Sarna, 1980), and human rectosigmoid (Linkens et al., 1976) has been modeled by populations of coupled nonlinear oscillators. The interaction between coupled nonlinear oscillators is governed by both intrinsic oscillator properties and coupling mechanisms.

6.3.2 Hour Rhythms

The existence of periodic gastric activity in the fasted state in both dog (Morat, 1882) and man (Morat, 1893) has been reported. The occurrence of a periodic pattern of motor activity, comprising bursts of contractions alternating with "intervals of repose," in the GI tracts of fasted animals was noted early in the twentieth century by Boldireff (1905). He observed that (1) the bursts recurred with a periodicity of about 1.5–2.5 h, (2) the amplitude of the gastric contractions during the bursts were larger than those seen postprandially, (3) the small bowel was also involved, and (4) with longer fasting periods, the bursts occurred less frequently and had a shorter duration. Periodic bursts of activity were also observed in (1) the lower esophageal sphincter (Cannon and Washburn, 1912), and (2) the pylorus (Wheelon and Thomas, 1921). Further investigation of the fasting contractile activity in the upper small intestine was undertaken in the early 1920s with particular emphasis on the coordination between the stomach and duodenum (Wheelon and Thomas, 1922; Alvarez and Mahoney, 1923). More recently, evidence was obtained (Itoh et al., 1978) that the cyclical activity in the lower esophageal sphincter noted by Cannon and Washburn (1912) was also coordinated with that of the stomach and small intestine.

With the use of implanted strain gauges, it was possible to observe contractile activity over long periods of time and it was demonstrated that the cyclical fasting pattern in the duodenum was altered by feeding (Jacoby et al., 1963). The types of contractions observed during fasting and feeding were divided into four groups (Reinke et al., 1967; Carlson et al., 1972). Three types of contractile patterns were observed in fasted animals: (1) quiescent interval, (2) a shorter interval of increasing activity, and (3) an interval of maximal activity. The fourth type was in fed animals and it consisted of randomly occurring contractions of varying amplitudes. With the use of implanted electrodes in the small intestine of fasted dogs, Szurszewski (1969) demonstrated that the cyclical appearance of electrical spiking activity at each electrode site was due to the migration of the cyclical pattern of quiescence, increasing activity, and maximal electrical activity down the small intestine from the duodenum to the terminal ileum. He called this electrical pattern the migrating myoelectric complex (MMC). Grivel and Ruckebusch (1972) demonstrated that the mechanical correlate of this electrical pattern, which they called the migrating motor complex, occurs in other species such as sheep and rabbits. They also observed that the velocity of propagation of the maximal contractile activity was proportional to the length of the small intestine. Code and Marlett (1975) observed the electrical correlate of the cyclical activity in dog stomach that was reported by Morat (1882, 1893) and they demonstrated that the stomach MMC was coordinated with the duodenal MMC.

The MMC pattern has been demonstrated in other mammalian species (Ruckebusch and Fioramonti, 1975; Ruckebusch and Bueno, 1976), including humans. Bursts of distally propagating contractions have been noted in the GI tract of man (Beck et al., 1965), and their cyclical nature was reported by Stanciu and Bennett (1975). The MMC has been described in both normal volunteers (Vantrappen et al., 1977; Fleckenstein, 1978; Thompson et al., 1980; Kerlin and Phillips, 1982; Rees et al., 1982) and in patients (Vantrappen et al., 1977; Thompson et al., 1980; Summers et al., 1982).

6.3.3 Terminology

A nomenclature to describe the GI electrical activities has been proposed to describe the minute rhythm (Sarna, 1975b; Sanders et al., 2006) and the hour rhythm (Carlson et al., 1972; Code and Marlett, 1975).

Control cycle is one depolarization and repolarization of the transmembrane voltage. Control wave (or slow wave) is the continuing rhythmic electrical activity recorded at any one site. It was assumed to be generated by the smooth muscle cells behaving like a relaxation oscillator at that site. However, recent evidence (Hara et al., 1986; Suzuki et al. 1986; Barajas–Lopez et al., 1989; Serio et al., 1991) indicates that it is generated by a system of ICC and smooth muscle cells at that site. ECA or slow-wave activity is the totality of the control waves recorded at one or several sites. Response potentials (or spikes) are the rapid oscillations of transmembrane voltage in the depolarized state of smooth muscle cells. They are associated with muscular contraction and their occurrence is assumed to be in response to a control cycle when acetylcholine is present. ERA is the totality of the groups of response potentials at one or several sites.

Migrating motility complex (MMC) is the entire cycle, which is composed of four phases. Initially, the electrical and mechanical patterns were referred to as the migrating myoelectric complex and the migrating motor complex, respectively. Phase I is the interval during which fewer than 5% of ECA have associated ERA and no or very few contractions are present. Phase II is the interval when 5–95% of the ECA has associated ERA, and intermittent contractions are present. Phase III is the interval when more than 95% of ECA have associated ERA and large cyclical contractions are present. Phase IV is a short and waning interval of intermittent ERA and contractions. Phases II and IV are not always present and are difficult to characterize, whereas phases I and III are always present. MMC cycle time is the interval from the end of one phase III to the end of a subsequent phase III at any one site. Migration time is the time taken for the MMC to migrate from the upper duodenum to the terminal ileum.

6.4 The Stomach

6.4.1 Anatomical Features

The stomach is somewhat pyriform in shape with its large end directed upward at the lower esophageal sphincter and its small end bent to the right at the pylorus. It has two curvatures, the greater curvature which is four to five times as long as the lesser curvature, and it consists of three regions, namely, the fundus, the corpus (or body), and the antrum, respectively. It has three smooth muscle layers. The outermost layer is the longitudinal muscle layer, the middle is the circular muscle layer, and the innermost is the oblique muscle layer. These layers thicken gradually in the distal stomach toward the pylorus, which is consistent with stomach function since trituration occurs in the distal antrum. The size of the stomach varies considerably Famong subjects. In an adult male, its greatest length when distended is about 25–30 cm and its widest diameter is about 10–12 cm (Pick and Howden, 1977).

The structural relationships of nerve, muscle, and ICC in the canine corpus indicated a high density of gap junctions indicating very tight coupling between cells. Nerves in the corpus are not located close to the circular muscle cells but are found exterior to the muscle bundles, whereas ICC have gap junction contact with smooth muscle cells and are closely innervated (Daniel and Sakai, 1984).

6.4.2 Gastric ECA Slow-Wave Activity

In the canine stomach, the fundus does not usually exhibit spontaneous electrical oscillations, but the corpus and antrum do exhibit such oscillations. In the intact stomach, the ECA is entrained to a frequency of about 5 cpm (about 3 cpm in humans) throughout the electrically active region with phase lags in both the longitudinal and circumferential directions (Sarna et al., 1972). The phase lags decrease distally from corpus to antrum.

There is a marked intrinsic frequency gradient along the axis of the stomach and a slight intrinsic frequency gradient along the circumference. The intrinsic frequency of gastric ECA in isolated circular muscle of the orad and midcorpus is the highest (about 5 cpm) compared to about 3.5 cpm in the rest of the corpus, and about 0.5 cpm in the antrum. Also, there is an orad to aboral intrinsic gradient in the resting membrane potential, with the terminal antrum having the most negative resting membrane potential, about 30 mV more negative than the fundal regions (Szurszewski, 1987). The relatively depolarized state of the fundal muscle may explain its electrical inactivity since the voltage-sensitive ionic channels may be kept in a state of inactivation. Hyperpolarization of the fundus to a transmembrane voltage of -60 mV produces fundal control waves similar to those recorded from mid and orad corpus.

The slow-wave activity in canine stomach was modeled (Sarna et al., 1972) using an array of 13 bidirectionally coupled relaxation oscillators. The model featured (1) an intrinsic frequency decline from corpus to the pylorus and from greater curvature to the lesser curvature, (2) entrainment of all coupled oscillators at a frequency close to the highest intrinsic frequency, and (3) distally decreasing phase lags between the entrained oscillators. A simulated circumferential transection caused the formation of another frequency plateau aboral to the transection. The frequency of the orad plateau remained unaffected while that of the aboral plateau was decreased. This is consistent with the observed experimental data.

Recent studies employed high-resolution (HR) mapping to evaluate human gastric slow-wave activity (O'Grady et al., 2010). The application of HR mapping has been constrained by the complex and laborious task of analyzing the large volumes of retrieved data. Recently, a rapid and reliable method for automatically identifying activation times (ATs) of slow waves, whereby automated methods for partitioning identified ATs into their propagation cycles, and for visualizing the HR spatiotemporal maps were described (Erickson et al., 2011). HR mapping performed in 12 patients with normal stomachs undergoing upper abdominal surgery, using up to six flexible printed circuit board arrays (interelectrode distance 7.6 mm, 192 electrodes, area 93 cm^2) was reported (O'Grady et al., 2010). The spatiotemporal characteristics of the human gastric slow-wave activity in terms of regional frequencies, amplitudes, and velocities were described as follows: (i) Slow-wave activity in the mid- to upper corpus on the greater curvature, was of greater amplitude (mean 0.57 mV) and higher velocity (8.0 mm/s) than the corpus (0.25 mV, 3.0 mm/s) and displayed isotropic propagation. (ii) A marked transition to higher amplitude and velocity activity occurred in the antrum (0.52 mV, 5.9 mm/s). (iii) Multiple wavefronts were found to propagate simultaneously in the organoaxial direction. Frequencies were consistent between regions (2.83 ± 0.35 cycles per min). HR mapping has provided (a) more detailed understanding of normal human gastric slow-wave activity, (b) basis for future HR mapping studies in disease states, and (c) basis for investigating noninvasive diagnostic strategies such as the electrogastrogram.

6.4.3 The Electrogastrogram

In a similar manner to other electrophysiological measures such as the electrocardiogram (EKG) and the electroencephalogram (EEG), the electrogastrogram (EGG) was identified (Stern and Koch, 1985; Chen and McCallum, 1994). The EGG is the signal obtained from cutaneous recording of the gastric myoelectrical activity by using surface electrodes placed on the abdomen over the stomach. Although the first EGG was recorded in the early 1920s (Alvarez, 1922), progress *vis-à-vis* clinical applications has been relatively slow, in particular when compared to the progress made in EKG, which also started in the early 1920s. Despite many attempts made over the decades, visual inspection of the EGG signal has not led to the identification of waveform characteristics that would help the clinician to diagnose functional or organic diseases of the stomach. Even the development of techniques such as time–frequency analysis (Qiao et al., 1998) and artificial neural network-based feature extraction (Liang et al., 1997; Wang et al., 1999) for computer analysis of the EGG did not provide clinically relevant information about gastric motility disorders. It has been demonstrated that increased EGG frequencies (1) were seen in perfectly healthy subjects (Pffafenbach et al., 1995) and (2) did not always correspond to serosally recorded tachygastria in dogs (Mintchev and Bowes, 1997). As yet, there is no effective method of detecting a change in the direction or velocity of propagation of gastric ECA from the EGG.

6.5 The Small Intestine

6.5.1 Anatomical Features

The small intestine is a long hollow organ, which consists of the duodenum, jejunum, and ileum, respectively. Its length is about 650 cm in humans and 300 cm in dogs. The duodenum extends from the pylorus to the ligament of Treitz (about 30 cm in humans and dogs). In humans, the duodenum forms a C-shaped pattern, with the ligament of Treitz near the corpus of the stomach. In dogs, the duodenum lies along the right side of the peritoneal cavity, with the ligament of Treitz in the pelvis. The duodenum receives pancreatic exocrine secretions and bile. In both humans and dogs, the jejunum consists of the next one-third whereas the ileum consists of the remaining two-thirds of the intestine. The major differences between the jejunum and ileum are functional in nature, relating to their absorption characteristics and motor control. The majority of sugars, amino acids, lipids, electrolytes, and water are absorbed in the jejunum and proximal ileum, whereas bile acids and vitamin B12 are absorbed in the terminal ileum.

6.5.2 Small Intestinal Slow-Wave Activity

In the canine small intestine, the slow-wave activity is not entrained throughout the entire length (Diamant and Bortoff, 1969a; Sarna et al., 1971). However, the slow-wave activity exhibits a plateau of constant frequency in the proximal region whereby there is a distal increase in phase lag. The frequency plateau (of about 20 cpm) extends over the entire duodenum and part of the jejunum. There is a marked intrinsic frequency gradient in the longitudinal direction with the highest intrinsic frequency being lesser than the plateau frequency. When the small intestine was transected *in vivo* into small segments (15 cm long), the intrinsic frequency of the slow-wave activity in adjacent segments tended to decrease aborally in an exponential manner (Sarna et al., 1971). A single transection of the duodenum caused the formation of another frequency plateau aboral to the transection. The slow-wave frequency in the orad plateau was generally unaffected, while that in the aborad plateau was decreased (Diamant and Bortoff, 1969b; Sarna et al., 1971). The frequency of the aborad plateau was either higher than or equal to the highest intrinsic frequency distal to the transection, depending on whether the transection of the duodenum was either above or below the region of the bile duct (Diamant and Bortoff, 1969b).

The slow-wave activity in canine small intestine was modeled using a chain of 16 bidirectionally coupled relaxation oscillators (Sarna et al., 1971). Coupling was not uniform along the chain, since the proximal oscillators were strongly coupled and the distal oscillators were weakly coupled. The model featured: (1) an exponential intrinsic frequency decline along the chain, (2) a frequency plateau which is higher than the highest intrinsic frequency, and (3) a temporal variation of the frequencies distal to the frequency plateau region. A simulated transection in the frequency plateau region caused the formation of another frequency plateau aboral to the transection, such that the frequency of the orad plateau was unchanged whereas the frequency of the aborad plateau decreased.

The slow-wave activity in human small intestine was modeled using a chain of 100 bidirectionally coupled relaxation oscillators (Robertson-Dunn and Linkens, 1974). Coupling was nonuniform and asymmetrical. The model featured: (1) a piecewise linear decline in intrinsic frequency along the chain, (2) a piecewise linear decline in coupling similar to that of the intrinsic frequency, (3) forward coupling which is stronger than backward coupling, and (4) a frequency plateau in the proximal region, which is higher than the highest intrinsic frequency in the region.

6.5.3 Small Intestinal MMC

The MMCs in canine small intestine have been observed in intrinsically isolated segments (Sarna et al., 1981, 1983), even after the isolated segment has been stripped of all extrinsic innervation (Sarr and Kelly, 1981) or removed in continuity with the remaining gut as a Thiry Vella loop (Itoh et al., 1981). This intrinsic mechanism is able to function independently of extrinsic innervation, since vagotomy (Weisbrodt et al., 1975; Ruckebusch and Bueno, 1977) does not hinder the initiation of the MMC. The initiation of the small intestinal MMC is controlled by integrative networks within the intrinsic plexuses utilizing nicotinic and muscarinic cholinergic receptors (Ormsbee et al., 1979; El-Sharkawy et al., 1982).

When the canine small intestine was transected into four equal strips (Sarna et al., 1981, 1983), it was found that each strip was capable of generating an independent MMC that would appear to propagate from the proximal to the distal part of each segment. This suggested that the MMC could be modeled by a chain of coupled relaxation oscillators. The average intrinsic periods of the MMC for the four segments were reported to be 106.2, 66.8, 83.1, and 94.8 min, respectively. The segment containing the duodenum had the longest period, while the subsequent segment containing the jejunum had the shortest period. However, in the intact small intestine, the MMC starts in the duodenum and not the jejunum. Bardakjian and Sarna (1981) and Bardakjian et al. (1984) have demonstrated that both the intrinsic frequency gradients and resting level gradients have major roles in the entrainment of a chain of coupled oscillators. In modeling the small intestinal MMC with a chain of four coupled oscillators, it was necessary to include a gradient in the intrinsic resting levels of the MMC oscillators (with the proximal oscillator having the lowest resting level) in order to entrain the oscillators and allow the proximal oscillator to behave as the leading oscillator (Bardakjian and Ahmed, 1992).

6.6 The Colon

6.6.1 Anatomical Features

In humans, the colon is about 100 cm in length. The ileum joins the colon approximately 5 cm from its end, forming the cecum, which has a worm-like appendage—the appendix. The colon is sacculated and the longitudinal smooth muscle is concentrated in three bands (the taeniae). It lies in front of the small intestine against the abdominal wall and it consists of the ascending (on the right side), transverse (across the lower stomach), and descending (on the left side) colon. The descending colon becomes the sigmoid colon in the pelvis as it runs down and forward to the rectum. The major functions of the colon are: (1) to absorb water, certain electrolytes, short-chain fatty acids, and bacterial metabolites; (2) to slowly propel its luminal contents in the caudad direction; (3) to store the residual matter in the distal region; and (4) to rapidly move its contents in the caudad direction during mass movements (Sarna, 1991). In dogs, the colon is about 45 cm in length and the cecum has no appendage. The colon is not sacculated, and the longitudinal smooth muscle coat is continuous around the circumference (Miller et al., 1968). It lies posterior to the small intestine and it consists mainly of ascending and descending segments with a small transverse segment. However, functionally it is assumed to consist of three regions, each of about 15 cm in length, representing the ascending, transverse, and descending colon, respectively.

6.6.2 Colonic Slow-Wave Activity

In the human colon, the slow-wave activity is almost completely phase-unlocked between adjacent sites as close as 1–2 cm apart and its frequency (about 3–15 cpm) and amplitude at each site vary with time (Sarna et al., 1980). This results in short duration contractions that are also disorganized in time and space. The disorganization of slow-wave activity and its associated contractions is consistent with the colonic function of extensive mixing, kneading, and slow net distal propulsion (Sarna, 1991). In the canine colon, the reports about the intrinsic frequency gradient were conflicting (Vanasin et al., 1974; Shearin et al., 1978; El-Sharkawy, 1983).

The human colonic slow-wave activity was modeled (Bardakjian and Sarna, 1980) using a tubular structure of 99 bidirectionally coupled nonlinear oscillators arranged in 33 parallel rings where each ring contained three oscillators. Coupling was nonuniform and it increased in the longitudinal direction. The model featured: (1) no phase-locking in the longitudinal or circumferential directions, (2) temporal and spatial variation of the frequency profile with large variations in the proximal and distal regions and small variations in the middle region, and (3) waxing and waning of the amplitudes of the slow-wave activity, which was more pronounced in the proximal and distal regions. The model demonstrated that the "silent periods" occurred because of the interaction between oscillators and they did not occur when the oscillators were uncoupled. The model was further refined (Bardakjian et al., 1990) such that when the slow-wave amplitude exceeded an excitation threshold, a spike burst of ERA was exhibited. The ERA spike bursts occurred in a seemingly random manner in adjacent sites because (1) the slow-wave activity was not phase-locked and (2) the slow-wave amplitudes and wave shapes varied in a seemingly random manner.

6.7 Epilogue

The slow-wave activity in stomach, small intestine, and colon behaves like the outputs of a population of coupled nonlinear oscillators. The populations in the stomach and the proximal small intestine are entrained, whereas those in the distal small intestine and colon are not entrained. There are distinct intrinsic frequency gradients in the stomach and small intestine but their profile in the colon is ambiguous.

The applicability of modeling of GI slow-wave activity by coupled nonlinear oscillators has been reconfirmed (Daniel et al., 1994) and a novel nonlinear oscillator, the mapped clock oscillator, was proposed (Bardakjian and Diamant, 1994; Zarrifa and Bardakjian, 2006; Zalay and Bardakjian, 2008, 2009) for modeling the cellular slow-wave activity. The oscillator consists of two coupled components: a clock, which represents the ICC and a mapper, which represents the smooth muscle transmembrane ionic transport mechanisms (Skinner and Bardakjian, 1991). Such a model accounts for the mounting evidence supporting the role of the ICC as a pacemaker for the smooth muscle transmembrane voltage oscillations (Hara et al., 1986; Suzuki et al., 1986; Barajas–Lopez et al., 1989; Serio et al., 1991; Sanders, 1996; Sanders et al., 2002; Daniel, 2004).

Modeling of the GI slow-wave activity by populations of coupled nonlinear oscillators (Bardakjian, 1987) suggests that the GI motility disorders associated with abnormal ECA can be effectively treated by: (1) electronic pacemakers to coordinate the oscillators, (2) surgical interventions to remove regional ectopic foci, and (3) pharmacotherapy to stimulate the oscillators. Electronic pacing has been demonstrated in the canine stomach (Kelly and LaForce, 1972; Sarna and Daniel, 1973; Bellahsene et al., 1992) and small intestine (Sarna and Daniel, 1975; Becker et al., 1983). Also, pharmacotherapy with prokinetic drugs such as Domperidone and Cisapride has demonstrated improvements in the coordination of the gastric oscillators.

Acknowledgments

The author thanks his colleagues Dr. Sharon Chung and Dr. Karen Hall for providing biological insight.

References

Alvarez, W.C. 1922. The electrogastrogram and what it shows. *J. Am. Med. Assoc.*, 78: 1116–1119.

Alvarez, W.C. and Mahoney, L.J. 1922. Action current in stomach and intestine. *Am. J. Physiol.*, 58: 476–493.

Alvarez, W.C. and Mahoney, L.J. 1923. The relations between gastric and duodenal peristalsis. *Am. J. Physiol.*, 64: 371–386.

Barajas-Lopez, C., Berezin, I., Daniel, E.E., and Huizinga, J.D. 1989. Pacemaker activity recorded in interstitial cells of Cajal of the gastrointestinal tract. *Am. J. Physiol.*, 257: C830–C835.

Bardakjian, B.L. 1987. Computer models of gastrointestinal myoelectric activity. *Automedica*, 7: 261–276.

Bardakjian, B.L. and Ahmed, K. 1992. Is a peripheral pattern generator sufficient to produce both fasting and postprandial patterns of the migrating myoelectric complex (MMC)? *Dig. Dis. Sci.*, 37: 986.

Bardakjian, B.L. and Diamant, N.E. 1994. A mapped clock oscillator model for transmembrane electrical rhythmic activity in excitable cells. *J. Theor. Biol.*, 166: 225–235.

Bardakjian, B.L., El-Sharkawy, T.Y., and Diamant, N.E. 1984. Interaction of coupled nonlinear oscillators having different intrinsic resting levels. *J. Theor. Biol.*, 106: 9–23.

Bardakjian, B.L. and Sarna, S.K. 1980. A computer model of human colonic electrical control activity (ECA). *IEEE Trans. Biomed. Eng.*, 27: 193–202.

Bardakjian, B.L. and Sarna, S.K. 1981. Mathematical investigation of populations of coupled synthesized relaxation oscillators representing biological rhythms. *IEEE Trans. Biomed. Eng.*, 28: 10–15.

Bardakjian, B.L., Sarna, S.K., and Diamant, N.E. 1990. Composite synthesized relaxation oscillators: Application to modeling of colonic ECA and ERA. *Gastrointest. J. Motil.*, 2: 109–116.

Bass, P. 1965. Electric activity of smooth muscle of the gastrointestinal tract. *Gastroenterology*, 49: 391–394.

Beck, I.T., McKenna, R.D., Peterfy, G., Sidorov, J., and Strawczynski, H. 1965. Pressure studies in the normal human jejunum. *Am. J. Dig. Dis.*, 10: 437–448.

Becker, J.M., Sava, P., Kelly, K.A., and Shturman, L. 1983. Intestinal pacing for canine postgastrectomy dumping. *Gastroenterology*, 84: 383–387.

Bellahsene, B.E., Lind, C.D., Schirmer, B.D. et al. 1992. Acceleration of gastric emptying with electrical stimulation in a canine model of gastroparesis. *Am. J. Physiol.*, 262: G826–G834.

Berezin, I., Huizinga, J.D., and Daniel, E.E. 1988. Interstitial cells of Cajal in the canine colon: A special communication network at the inner border of the circular muscle. *J. Comp. Neurol.* 273: 42–51.

Boldireff, W.N. 1905. Le travail periodique de l'appareil digestif en dehors de la digestion. *Arch. Des. Sci. Biol.*, 11: 1–157.

Bozler, E. 1938. Action potentials of visceral smooth muscle. *Am. J. Physiol.*, 124: 502–510.

Bozler, E. 1939. Electrophysiological studies on the motility of the gastrointestinal tract. *Am. J. Physiol.*, 127: 301–307.

Bozler, E. 1941. Action potentials and conduction of excitation in muscle. *Biol. Symposia*, 3: 95–110.

Bulbring, E., Burnstock, G., and Holman, M.E. 1958. Excitation and conduction in the smooth muscle of the isolated taenia coli of the guinea pig. *J. Physiol.*, 142: 420–437.

Burnstock, G., Holman, M.E., and Prosser, C.L. 1963. Electrophysiology of smooth muscle. *Physiol. Rev.*, 43: 482–527.

Cannon, W.B. and Washburn, A.L. 1912. An explanation of hunger. *Am. J. Physiol.*, 29: 441–454.

Carlson, G.M., Bedi, B.S., and Code, C.F. 1972. Mechanism of propagation of intestinal interdigestive myoelectric complex. *Am. J. Physiol.*, 222: 1027–1030.

Chanson, M. and Spray, D.C. 1995. Electrophysiology of gap junctional communication. In: *Pacemaker Activity and Intercellular Communication*. Huizinga, J.D. (Ed.), CRC Press, Baton Rouge, FL.

Chen, J.Z. and McCallum, R.W. 1994. *Electrogastrography: Principles and Applications*. Raven Press, New York.

Christensen, J. 1975. Myoelectric control of the colon. *Gastroenterology*, 68: 601–609.

Code, C.F. and Marlett, J.A. 1975. The interdigestive myoelectric complex of the stomach and small bowel of dogs. *J. Physiol.*, 246: 289–309.

Daniel, E.E. 1975. Electrophysiology of the colon. *Gut*, 16: 298–329.

Daniel, E.E. 2004. Communication between interstitial cells of Cajal and gastrointestinal muscle. *Neurogastroenterol. Motil.*, 16: 118–122.

Daniel, E.E., Bardakjian, B.L., Huizinga, J.D., and Diamant, N.E. 1994. Relaxation oscillators and core conductor models are needed for understanding of GI electrical activities. *Am. J. Physiol.*, 266: G339–G349.

Daniel, E.E. and Chapman, K.M. 1963. Electrical activity of the gastrointestinal tract as an indication of mechanical activity. *Am. J. Dig. Dis.*, 8: 54–102.

Daniel, E.E., Duchon, D.G., Garfield, R.E., Nichols, M., Malhorta, S.K., and Oki, M. 1976. Is the nexus necessary for cell-to-cell coupling of smooth muscle. *Mem. Biol.*, 28: 207–239.

Daniel, E.E. and Sakai, Y. 1984. Structural basis for function of circular muscle of canine corpus. *Can. J. Physiol. Pharmacol.*, 62: 1304–1314.

Diamant, N.E. and Bortoff, A. 1969a. Nature of the intestinal slow wave frequency gradient. *Am. J. Physiol.*, 216: 301–307.

Diamant, N.E. and Bortoff, A. 1969b. Effects of transection on the intestinal slow wave frequency gradient. *Am. J. Physiol.*, 216: 734–743.

Diamant, N.E., Rose, P.K., and Davison, E.J. 1970. Computer simulation of intestinal slow-wave frequency gradient. *Am. J. Physiol.*, 219: 1684–1690.

Douglas, D.M. 1949. The decrease in frequency of contraction of the jejunum after transplantation to the ileum. *J. Physiol.*, 110: 66–75.

Duthie, H.L. 1974. Electrical activity of gastrointestinal smooth muscle. *Gut,* 15: 669–681.

El-Sharkawy, T.Y. 1983. Electrical activity of the muscle layers of the canine colon. *J. Physiol.*, 342: 67–83.

El-Sharkawy, T.Y., Markus, H., and Diamant, N.E. 1982. Neural control of the intestinal migrating myo-electric complex: A pharmacological analysis. *Can. J. Physiol. Pharm.*, 60: 794–804.

Erickson, J.C., O'Grady, G. Du, P., Egbuji, J.U., Pullan, A.J., and Cheng, L.K. 2011. Automated cycle partitioning and visualization of high-resolution activation time maps of gastric slow wave recordings: The region growing using polynomial surface-estimate stabilization (REGROUPS) method. *Ann. Biomed. Eng.*, 39(1): 469–483.

Ermentrout, G.B. and Kopell, N. 1984. Frequency plateaus in a chain of weakly coupled oscillators. *SIAM J. Math. Anal.*, 15: 215–237.

Fitzhugh, R. 1961. Impulses and physiological states in theoretical models of nerve membranes. *Biophys. J.,* 1: 445–466.

Fleckenstein, P. 1978. Migrating electrical spike activity in the fasting human small intestine. *Dig. Dis. Sci.*, 23: 769–775.

Gillespie, J.S. 1962. The electrical and mechanical responses of intestinal smooth muscle cells to stimulation of their extrinsic parasympathetic nerves. *J. Physiol.*, 162: 76–92.

Grasman, J. 1984. The mathematical modeling of entrained biological oscillators. *Bull. Math. Biol.*, 46: 407–422.

Grivel, M.L. and Ruckebusch, Y. 1972. The propagation of segmental contractions along the small intestine. *J. Physiol.*, 277: 611–625.

Hara, Y.M., Kubota, M., and Szurszewski, J.H. 1986. Electrophysiology of smooth muscle of the small intestine of some mammals. *J. Physiol.*, 372: 501–520.

Hodgkin, A.L. and Huxley, A.F.A. 1952. A quantitative description of membrane current and its application to conduction and excitation in nerve. *J. Physiol.*, 117: 500–544.

Huizinga, J.D., Liu, L.W.C., Blennerhassett, M.G., Thuneberg, L., and Molleman, A. 1992. Intercellular communication in smooth muscle. *Experientia,* 48: 932–941.

Huizinga, J.D., Zarate, N., and Farrugia, G. 2009. Physiology, injury, and recovery of interstitial cells of Cajal: Basic and clinical science. *Gastroenterology* 137: 1548–1556.

Itoh, Z., Aizawa, I., and Takeuchi, S. 1981. Neural regulation of interdigestive motor activity in canine jejunum. *Am. J. Physiol.*, 240: G324–G330.

Itoh, Z., Honda, R., Aizawa, I., Takeuchi, S., Hiwatashi, K., and Couch, E.F. 1978. Interdigestive motor activity of the lower esophageal sphincter in the conscious dog. *Dig. Dis. Sci.*, 23: 239–247.

Jacoby, H.I., Bass, P., and Bennett, D.R. 1963. *In vivo* extraluminal contractile force transducer for gastrointestinal muscle. *J. Appl. Physiol.*, 18: 658–665.

Kelly, K.A. and LaForce, R.C. 1972. Pacing the canine stomach with electric stimulation. *Am. J. Physiol.*, 222: 588–594.

Kerlin, P. and Phillips, S. 1982. The variability of motility of the ileum and jejunum in healthy humans. *Gastroenterology,* 82: 694–700.

Liang, J., Cheung, J.Y., and Chen, J.D.Z. 1997. Detection and deletion of motion artifacts in electrogastrogram using feature analysis and neural networks. *Ann. Biomed. Eng.,* 25: 850–857.

Linkens, D.A., Taylor, I., and Duthie, H.L. 1976. Mathematical modeling of the colorectal myoelectrical activity in humans. *IEEE Trans. Biomed. Eng.,* 23: 101–110.

Liu, L.W.C., Farraway, L.A., Berezin, I., and Huizinga, J.D. 1998. Interstitial cells of Cajal: Mediators of communication between longitudinal and circular muscle cells of canine colon. *Cell Tissue Res.,* 294: 69–79.

Miller, M.E., Christensen, G.C., and Evans, H.E. 1968. *Anatomy of the Dog,* W.B. Saunders, Philadelphia.

Milton, G.W. and Smith, A.W.M. 1956. The pacemaking area of the duodenum. *J. Physiol.,* 132: 100–114.

Mintchev, M.P. and Bowes, K.L. 1997. Do increased electrogastrographic frequencies always correspond to internal tachygastria? *Ann. Biomed. Eng.,* 25: 1052–1058.

Morat, J.P. 1882. Sur l'innervation motrice de l'estomac. *Lyon. Med.,* 40: 289–296.

Morat, J.P. 1893. Sur quelques particularites de l'innervation motrice de l'estomac et de l'intestin. *Arch. Physiol. Norm. Path.,* 5: 142–153.

Nelson, T.S. and Becker, J.C. 1968. Simulation of the electrical and mechanical gradient of the small intestine. *Am. J. Physiol.,* 214: 749–757.

O'Grady, G., Du, P., Cheng, L.K., Egbuji, J.U., Lammers, W.J., Windsor, J.A., and Pullan, A.J. 2010. Origin and propagation of human gastric slow-wave activity defined by high-resolution mapping. *Am. J. Physiol. Gastrointest. Liver. Physiol.* 299: G585–G592.

Ormsbee, H.S., Telford, G.L., and Mason, G.R. 1979. Required neural involvement in control of canine migrating motor complex. *Am. J. Physiol.,* 237: E451–E456.

Pavlidis, T. 1973. *Biological Oscillators: Their Mathematical Analysis.* Academic Press, New York.

Pffafenbach, B., Adamek, R.J., Kuhn, K., and Wegener, M. 1995. Electrogastrography in healthy subjects. Evaluation of normal values: Influence of age and gender. *Dig. Dis. Sci.,* 40: 1445–1450.

Pick, T.P. and Howden, R. 1977. *Gray's Anatomy,* Bounty Books, New York.

Plant, R. E. and Kim, M. 1976. Mathematical description of a bursting pacemaker neuron by a modification of the Hodgkin–Huxley equations. *Biophys. J.,* 16: 227–244.

Puestow, C.B. 1933. Studies on the origins of the automaticity of the intestine: The action of certain drugs on isolated intestinal transplants. *Am. J. Physiol.,* 106: 682–688.

Qiao, W., Sun, H.H., Chey, W.Y., and Lee, K.Y. 1998. Continuous wavelet analysis as an aid in the representation and interpretation of electrogastrographic signals. *Ann. Biomed. Eng.,* 26: 1072–1081.

Rees, W.D.W., Malagelada, J.R., Miller, L.J., and Go, V.L.W. 1982. Human interdigestive and postprandial gastrointestinal motor and gastrointestinal hormone patterns. *Dig. Dis. Sci.,* 27: 321–329.

Reinke, D.A., Rosenbaum, A.H., and Bennett, D.R. 1967. Patterns of dog gastrointestinal contractile activity monitored *in vivo* with extraluminal force transducers. *Am. J. Dig. Dis.,* 12: 113–141.

Rinzel, J. 1987. A formal classification of bursting mechanisms in excitable cells. In *Mathematical Topics in Population Biology, Morphogenesis, and Neurosciences,* Teramoto, E. and Yamaguti, M. (Eds.), Lecture Notes in Biomathematics, Vol. 71. Springer-Verlag, Berlin, 267–281.

Robertson-Dunn, B. and Linkens, D.A. 1974. A mathematical model of the slow wave electrical activity of the human small intestine. *Med. Biol. Eng.,* 12: 750–758.

Ruckebusch, Y. and Bueno, L. 1976. The effects of feeding on the motility of the stomach and small intestine in the pig. *Br. J. Nutr.,* 35: 397–405.

Ruckebusch, Y. and Bueno, L. 1977. Migrating myoelectrical complex of the small intestine. *Gastroenterology,* 73: 1309–1314.

Ruckebusch, Y. and Fioramonti, S. 1975. Electrical spiking activity and propulsion in small intestine in fed and fasted states. *Gastroenterology,* 68: 1500–1508.

Sanders, K.M. 1996. A case for interstitial cells of Cajal as pacemakers and mediators of neurotransmission in the gastrointestinal tract. *Gastroenterology,* 111: 492–515.

Sanders, K.M., Koh, S.D., and Ward, S. M. 2006. Interstitial cells of Cajal as pacemakers in the gastrointestinal tract. *Annu. Rev. Physiol.*, 68: 307–343.

Sanders, K.M., Ordog, T., and Ward, S.M. 2002. Physiology and pathophysiology of the interstitial cells of Cajal: From bench to bedside. IV. Genetic and animal models of GI motility disorders caused by loss of interstitial cells of Cajal. *Am. J. Physiol. Gastrointest. Liver Physiol.*, 282: G747–G756.

Sarna, S., Condon, R.E., and Cowles, V. 1983. Enteric mechanisms of initiation of migrating myoelectric complexes in dogs. *Gastroenterology*, 84: 814–822.

Sarna, S.K. 1975a. Models of smooth muscle electrical activity. In: *Methods in Pharmacology*, Daniel, E.E. and Paton, D.M. (Eds.), Plenum Press, New York, pp. 519–540.

Sarna, S.K. 1975b. Gastrointestinal electrical activity: terminology. *Gastroenterology*, 68: 1631–1635.

Sarna, S.K. 1991. Physiology and pathophysiology of colonic motor activity. *Dig. Dis. Sci.*, 6: 827–862.

Sarna, S.K., Bardakjian, B.L., Waterfall, W.E., and Lind, J.F. 1980. Human colonic electrical control activity (ECA). *Gastroenterology*, 78: 1526–1536.

Sarna, S.K. and Daniel, E.E. 1973. Electrical stimulation of gastric electrical control activity. *Am. J. Physiol.*, 225: 125–131.

Sarna, S.K. and Daniel, E.E. 1975. Electrical stimulation of small intestinal electrical control activity. *Gastroenterology*, 69: 660–667.

Sarna, S.K., Daniel, E.E., and Kingma, Y.J. 1971. Simulation of slow wave electrical activity of small intestine. *Am. J. Physiol.*, 221: 166–175.

Sarna, S.K., Daniel, E.E., and Kingma, Y.J. 1972. Simulation of the electrical control activity of the stomach by an array of relaxation oscillators. *Am. J. Dig. Dis.*, 17: 299–310.

Sarna, S.K., Stoddard, C., Belbeck, L., and McWade, D. 1981. Intrinsic nervous control of migrating myoelectric complexes. *Am. J. Physiol.*, 241: G16–G23.

Sarr, M.G. and Kelly, K.A. 1981. Myoelectric activity of the autotransplanted canine jejunoileum. *Gastroenterology*, 81: 303–310.

Serio, R., Barajas-Lopez, C., Daniel, E.E., Berezin, I., and Huizinga, J.D. 1991. Pacemaker activity in the colon: Role of interstitial cells of Cajal and smooth muscle cells. *Am. J. Physiol.*, 260: G636–G645.

Shearin, N.L., Bowes, K.L., and Kingma, Y.J. 1978. *In vitro* electrical activity in canine colon. *Gut*, 20: 780–786.

Sherman, A. and Rinzel, J. 1991. Model for synchronization of pancreatic beta-cells by gap junction coupling. *Biophys. J.*, 59: 547–559.

Skinner, F.K. and Bardakjian, B.L. 1991. A barrier kinetic mapping unit. Application to ionic transport in gastric smooth muscle. *Gastrointest. J. Motil.*, 3: 213–224.

Sperelakis, N. 2002. An electric field mechanism for transmission of excitation between myocardial cells. *Circ. Res.*, 91: 985–987.

Sperelakis, N., LoBrocco, B., Mann, J.E., and Marshall, R. 1984. Potassium accumulation in intercellular junctions combined with electric field interaction for propagation in cardiac muscle. *Innov. Technol. Biol. Med.*, 6: 24–43.

Sperelakis, N. and Mann, J.E. 1977. Evaluation of electric field change in the cleft between excitable cells. *J. Theor. Biol.*, 64: 71–96.

Sperelakis, N. and McConnell, K. 2002. Electric field interactions between closely abutting excitable cells. *IEEE Eng. Med. Biol. Mag.*, 21: 77–89.

Sperelakis, N. and Ramasamy, L. 2002. Propagation in cardiac and smooth muscle based on electric field transmission at cell junctions: An analysis by Pspice. *IEEE Eng. Med. Biol. Mag.*, 21: 177–190.

Stanciu, C. and Bennett, J.R. 1975. The general pattern of gastroduodenal motility: 24 h recordings in normal subjects. *Rev. Med. Chir. Soc. Med. Nat. Iasi.*, 79: 31–36.

Stein, R.B. 1967. Some models of neuronal variability. *Biophys. J.*, 7: 37–68.

Stern, R.M. and Koch, K.L. 1985. *Electrogastrography: Methodology, Validation, and Applications*. Praeger Publishers, New York.

Summers, R.W., Anuras, S., and Green, J. 1982. Jejunal motility patterns in normal subjects and symptomatic patients with partial mechanical obstruction or pseudo-obstruction. In: *Motility of the Digestive Tract,* Weinbeck, M. (Ed.), Raven Press, New York, pp. 467–470.

Suzuki, N., Prosser, C.L., and Dahms, V., 1986. Boundary cells between longitudinal and circular layers: Essential for electrical slow waves in cat intestine. *Am. J. Physiol.,* 280: G287–G294.

Szurszewski, J.H. 1969. A migrating electric complex of the canine small intestine. *Am. J. Physiol.,* 217: 1757–1763.

Szurszewski, J.H. 1987. Electrical basis for gastrointestinal motility. In: *Physiology of the Gastrointestinal Tract,* Johnson, L.R. (Ed.), Raven Press, New York, Chapter 12.

Thompson, D.G., Wingate, D.L., Archer, L., Benson, M.J., Green, W.J., and Hardy, R.J. 1980. Normal patterns of human upper small bowel motor activity recorded by prolonged radiotelemetry. *Gut,* 21: 500–506.

Thuneberg, L. 1982. Interstitial cells of Cajal: Intestinal pacemaker cells. *Adv. Anat. Embryol. Cell. Biol.,* 71: 1–130.

Thuneberg, L., Rahnamai, M.A., and Riazi, H. 1998. The peg-and-socket junction: An alternative to the gap junction in coupling of smooth muscle cells. *Neurogastroenterol. Motil.,* 10: 479–479.

Van der Pol, B. and Van der Mark, J. 1928. The heart considered as a relaxation oscillator and an electrical model of the heart. *Philos. Mag.,* 6: 763–775.

Vanasin, B., Ustach, T.J., and Schuster, M.M. 1974. Electrical and motor activity of human and dog colon in vitro. *Johns Hopkins Med. J.,* 134: 201–210.

Vantrappen, G., Janssens, J.J., Hellemans, J., and Ghoos, Y. 1977. The interdigestive motor complex of normal subjects and patients with bacterial overgrowth of the small intestine. *J. Clin. Invest.,* 59: 1158–1166.

Vigmond, E.J. and Bardakjian, B.L. 1995. The effect of morphological interdigitation on field coupling between smooth muscle cells. *IEEE Trans. Biomed. Eng.,* 42: 162–171.

Vigmond, E.J., Bardakjian, B.L., Thunberg, L., and Huizinga, J.D. 2000. Intercellular coupling mediated by potassium accumulation in peg-and-socket junctions. *IEEE Trans. Biomed. Eng.,* 47: 1576–1583.

Wang, Z., He, Z., and Chen, J.D.Z. 1999. Filter banks and neural network-based feature extraction and automatic classification of electrogastrogram. *Ann. Biomed. Eng.,* 27: 88–95.

Ward, S.M. and Sanders, K.M. 2001. Interstitial cells of Cajal: Primary targets of enteric motor innervation. *Anat. Rec.,* 262: 125–135.

Weisbrodt, N.W., Copeland, E.M., Moore, E.P., Kearly, K.W., and Johnson, L.R. 1975. Effect of vagotomy on electrical activity of the small intestine of the dog. *Am. J. Physiol.,* 228: 650–654.

Wheelon, H. and Thomas, J.E. 1921. Rhythmicity of the pyloric sphincter. *Am. J. Physiol.,* 54: 460–473.

Wheelon, H. and Thomas, J.E. 1922. Observations on the motility of the duodenum and the relation of duodenal activity to that of the pars pylorica. *Am. J. Physiol.,* 59: 72–96.

Winfree, A.T. 1980. *The Geometry of Biological Time.* Springer-Verlag, New York.

Winfree, A.T. 1989. Electrical instability in cardiac muscle: Phase singularities and rotors. *J. Theor. Biol.,* 138: 353–405.

Zalay, O. C. and Bardakjian, B. L. 2008. Mapped clock oscillators as ring devices and their application to neuronal electrical rhythms. *IEEE Trans. Neural Syst. Rehabil. Eng.,* 16(3): 233–244.

Zalay, O.C. and Bardakjian, B.L. 2009. Theta phase precession and phase selectivity: A cognitive device description of neural coding. *J. Neural Eng.,* 6(3): 036002.

Zamir, O. and Hanani, M. 1990. Intercellular dye-coupling in intestinal smooth muscle: Are gap junctions required for intercellular coupling. *Experientia,* 46: 1002–1005.

Zarrifa, J. and Bardakjian B.L. 2006. Neuronal electrical rhythms described by composite mapped clock oscillators. *Ann. Biomed. Eng.,* 34: 128–141.

7

Respiratory System

7.1	Respiration Anatomy	7-1
	Lungs • Conducting Airways • Alveoli • Pulmonary Circulation • Respiratory Muscles	
7.2	Lung Volumes and Gas Exchange	7-5
7.3	Perfusion of the Lung	7-7
7.4	Gas Partial Pressure	7-8
7.5	Pulmonary Mechanics	7-10
7.6	Respiratory Control	7-14
7.7	Pulmonary Function Laboratory	7-16
	Spirometry • Body Plethysmography • Diffusing Capacity	
	Defining Terms	7-20
	References	7-20
	Further Reading	7-21

Arthur T. Johnson
University of Maryland

Christopher G. Lausted
Institute for Systems Biology

Joseph D. Bronzino
Trinity College

As functioning units, the lung and heart are usually considered as a single complex organ, but because these organs contain essentially two compartments—one for blood and one for air—they are usually separated in terms of the tests conducted to evaluate heart or pulmonary function. This chapter focuses on some of the physiologic concepts responsible for the normal function and specific measures of the lung's ability to supply tissue cells with enough oxygen while removing excess carbon dioxide.

7.1 Respiration Anatomy

The respiratory system consists of the lungs, conducting airways, pulmonary vasculature, respiratory muscles, and surrounding tissues and structures (Figure 7.1). Each plays an important role in influencing respiratory responses.

7.1.1 Lungs

There are two lungs in the human chest; the right lung is composed of three incomplete divisions called lobes, and the left lung has two, leaving room for the heart. The right lung accounts for 55% of total gas volume and the left lung for 45%. Lung tissue is spongy because of the very small (200–300 × 10^{-6} m diameter in normal lungs at rest) gas-filled cavities called *alveoli*, which are the ultimate structures for gas exchange. There are 250–350 million alveoli in the adult lung, with a total alveolar surface area of 50–100 m^2 depending on the degree of lung inflation (Johnson, 2009).

7.1.2 Conducting Airways

Air is transported from the atmosphere to the alveoli beginning with the oral and nasal cavities, through the pharynx (in the throat), past the glottal opening, and into the trachea or windpipe. The conduction of air begins at the larynx, or voice box, at the entrance to the trachea, which is a fibromuscular tube

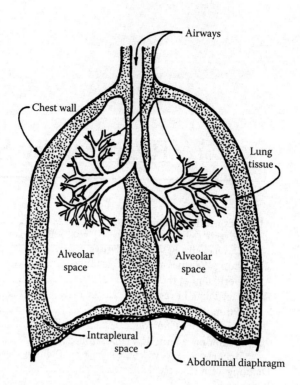

FIGURE 7.1   Schematic representation of the respiratory system.

10–12 cm in length and 1.4–2.0 cm in diameter (Kline, 1976). At a location called the carina, the trachea terminates and divides into the left and right bronchi. Each bronchus has a discontinuous cartilaginous support in its wall. Muscle fibers capable of controlling airway diameter are incorporated into the walls of the bronchi, as well as in those of air passages closer to the alveoli. Smooth muscle is present throughout the respiratory bronchiolus and alveolar ducts but is absent in the last alveolar duct, which terminates in one to several alveoli. The alveolar walls are shared by other alveoli and are composed of highly pliable and collapsible squamous epithelium cells.

The bronchi subdivide into subbronchi, which further subdivide into bronchioli, which further subdivide, and so on, until finally reaching the alveolar level. Table 7.1 provides a description and dimensions of the airways of adult humans. A model of the geometric arrangement of these air passages is presented in Figure 7.2. It will be noted that each airway is considered to branch into two subairways. In the adult human, there are considered to be 23 such branchings, or generations, beginning at the trachea and ending in the alveoli.

Movement of gases in the respiratory airways occurs mainly by bulk flow (convection) throughout the region from the mouth to the nose to the fifteenth generation. Beyond the fifteenth generation, gas diffusion is relatively more important. With the low gas velocities that occur in *diffusion*, dimensions of the space over which diffusion occurs (alveolar space) must be small for adequate oxygen delivery into the walls; smaller alveoli are more efficient in the transfer of gas than are larger ones. Thus, animals with high levels of oxygen consumption are found to have smaller-diameter alveoli compared with animals with low levels of oxygen consumption.

7.1.3 Alveoli

Alveoli are the structures through which gases diffuse to and from the body. To ensure that gas exchange occurs efficiently, alveolar walls are extremely thin. For example, the total tissue thickness between the

TABLE 7.1 Classification and Approximate Dimensions of Airways of Adult Human Lung (Inflated to about 3/4 of TLC)[a]

Common Name	Numerical Order of Generation	Number of Each	Diameter (mm)	Length (mm)	Total Cross-Sectional Area (cm^2)	Description and Comment
Trachea	0	1	18	120	2.5	Main cartilaginous airway; partly in thorax
Main bronchus	1	2	12	47.6	2.3	First branching of airway; one to each lung; in lung root; cartilage
Lobar bronchus	2	4	8	19.0	2.1	Named for each lobe; cartilage
Segmental bronchus	3	8	6	7.6	2.0	Named for radiographical and surgical anatomy; cartilage
Subsegmental bronchus	4	16	4	12.7	2.4	Last generally named bronchi; may be referred to as medium-sized bronchi; cartilage
Small bronchi	5–10	1024[b]	1.3[b]	4.6[b]	13.4[b]	Not generally named; contain decreasing amounts of cartilage. Beyond this level, airways enter the lobules as defined by a strong elastic lobular-limiting membrane
Bronchioles	11–13	8192[b]	0.8[b]	2.7[b]	44.5[b]	Not named; contain no cartilage, mucus-secreting elements, or cilia. Tightly embedded in lung tissue
Terminal bronchioles	14–15	32,768[b]	0.7[b]	2.0[b]	113.0[b]	Generally 2 or 3 orders so designated; morphology not significantly different from orders 11–13
Respiratory bronchioles	16–18	262,144[b]	0.5[b]	1.2[b]	534.0[b]	Definite class; bronchiolar cuboidal epithelium present, but scattered alveoli are present giving these airways a gas exchange function. Order 165 often called first-order respiratory bronchiole; 17, second-order; 18, third-order
Alveolar ducts	19–22	4,194,304[b]	0.4[b]	0.8[b]	5880.0[b]	No bronchial epithelium; have no surface except connective tissue framework; open into alveoli
Alveolar sacs	23	8,388,608	0.4	0.6	11,800.0	No reason to assign a special name; are really short alveolar ducts
Alveoli	24	300,000,000	0.2			Pulmonary capillaries are in the septae that form the alveoli

Source: Used with permission from Suki, B. and Bates, J.H.T. 1991. *J. Appl. Physiol.* 71: 826–833; Weibel, E.R. 1963. *Morphometry of the Human Lung* New York, Academic Press; adapted from Comroe, J.H. 1965. *Physiology of Respiration.* Chicago, IL, Year Book Medical Publishers.

[a] The number of airways in each generation is based on regular dichotomous branching.

[b] Numbers refer to last generation in each group.

inside of the alveolus to pulmonary capillary blood plasma is only about 0.4×10^{-6} m. Consequently, the principal barrier to diffusion occurs at the plasma and red blood cell level, not at the alveolar membrane (Ruch and Patton, 1966). Molecular diffusion within the alveolar volume is responsible for mixing of the enclosed gas. Owing to small alveolar dimensions, complete mixing probably occurs in less than 10 ms, fast enough that alveolar mixing time does not limit gaseous diffusion to or from the blood (Astrand and Rodahl, 1970).

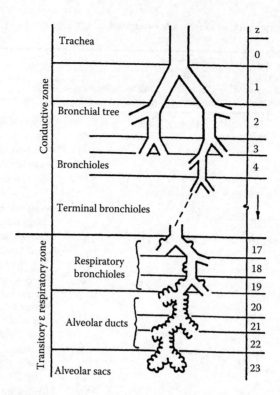

FIGURE 7.2 General architecture of conductive and transitory airways. In the conductive zone, air is conducted to and from the lungs, while in the respiration zone, gas exchange occurs. (Used with permission from Weibel, E.R. 1963. *Morphometry of the Human Lung.* New York, Academic Press.)

Of particular importance to proper alveolar operation is a thin surface coating of surfactant. Without this material, large alveoli would tend to enlarge and small alveoli would collapse. It is the present view that surfactant acts like a detergent, changing the stress–strain relationship of the alveolar wall and thereby stabilizing the lung (Johnson, 2009).

7.1.4 Pulmonary Circulation

There is no true pulmonary analog to the systemic arterioles, since the *pulmonary circulation* occurs under relatively low pressure (West, 1977). Pulmonary blood vessels, especially capillaries and venules, are very thin walled and flexible. Unlike systemic capillaries, pulmonary capillaries increase in diameter, and pulmonary capillaries within alveolar walls separate adjacent alveoli with increases in blood pressure or decreases in alveolar pressure. Flow, therefore, is significantly influenced by elastic deformation. Although pulmonary circulation is largely unaffected by neural and chemical control, it does respond promptly to hypoxia.

There is also a high-pressure systemic blood delivery system to the bronchi that is completely independent of the pulmonary low-pressure ($\sim$3330 N/m^2) circulation in healthy individuals. In diseased states, however, bronchial arteries are reported to enlarge when pulmonary blood flow is reduced, and some arteriovenous shunts become prominent (West, 1977).

Total pulmonary blood volume is approximately 300–500 cm^3 in normal adults, with about 60–100 cm^3 in the pulmonary capillaries (Astrand and Rodahl, 1970). This value, however, is quite variable, depending on such things as posture, position, disease, and chemical composition of the blood (Kline, 1976).

Since pulmonary arterial blood is poor in oxygen and rich in carbon dioxide, it exchanges excess carbon dioxide for oxygen in the pulmonary capillaries, which are in close contact with alveolar walls. At rest, the transit time for blood in the pulmonary capillaries is computed as

$$t = V_c/\dot{V}_c$$

where t is the blood transmit time, s; V_c is the capillary blood volume, m³; and $\dot{V}_c$ is the total capillary blood flow (cardiac output, m³/s), and is somewhat less than 1 s, while during exercise it may be only 500 ms or even less.

7.1.5 Respiratory Muscles

The lungs fill because of a rhythmic expansion of the chest wall. The action is indirect in that no muscle acts directly on the lung. The diaphragm, the muscular mass accounting for 75% of the expansion of the chest cavity, is attached around the bottom of the thoracic cage, arches over the liver, and moves downward like a piston when it contracts. The external intercostal muscles are positioned between the ribs and aid *inspiration* by moving the ribs up and forward. This, then, increases the volume of the thorax. Other muscles are important in the maintenance of thoracic shape during breathing. For details, see Ruch and Patton (1966) and Johnson (2009).

Quiet *expiration* is usually considered to be passive, that is, the pressure to force air from the lungs comes from the elastic expansion of the lungs and chest wall. During moderate to severe exercise, the abdominal and internal intercostal muscles are very important in forcing air from the lungs much more quickly than would otherwise occur. Inspiration requires intimate contact between lung tissues, pleural tissues (the *pleura* is the membrane surrounding the lungs), and chest wall and diaphragm. This is accomplished by reduced intrathoracic pressure (which tends toward negative values) during inspiration.

Viewing the lungs as an entire unit, one can consider the lungs to be elastic sacs within an airtight barrel—the thorax—which is bounded by the ribs and the diaphragm. Any movement of these two boundaries alters the volume of the lungs. The normal breathing cycle in humans is accomplished by the active contraction of the inspiratory muscles, which enlarges the thorax. This enlargement lowers the intrathoracic and interpleural pressure even further, pulls on the lungs, and enlarges the alveoli, alveolar ducts, and bronchioli, expanding the alveolar gas and decreasing its pressure below atmospheric. As a result, air at atmospheric pressure flows easily into the nose, mouth, and trachea.

7.2 Lung Volumes and Gas Exchange

Of primary importance to lung functioning is the movement and mixing of gases within the respiratory system. Depending on the anatomic level under consideration, gas movement is determined mainly by diffusion or convection.

Without the thoracic musculature and rib cage, as mentioned above, the barely inflated lungs would occupy a much smaller space than they occupy *in situ*. However, the thoracic cage holds them open. Conversely, the lungs exert an influence on the thorax, holding it smaller than should be the case without the lungs. Because the lungs and thorax are connected by tissue, the volume occupied by both together is between the extremes represented by relaxed lungs alone and thoracic cavity alone. The resting volume VR, then, is that volume occupied by the lungs with glottis open and muscles relaxed.

Lung volumes greater than resting volume are achieved during inspiration. Maximum inspiration is represented by inspiratory reserve volume (IRV). IRV is the maximum additional volume that can be accommodated by the lung at the end of inspiration. Lung volumes less than resting volume do not normally occur at rest but do occur during exhalation while exercising (when exhalation is active). Maximum additional expiration, as measured from lung volume at the end of expiration, is called expiratory reserve volume (ERV). Residual volume is the amount of gas remaining in the lungs at the end of maximal expiration.

Tidal volume V_T is normally considered to be the volume of air entering the nose and mouth with each breath. Alveolar *ventilation* volume, the volume of fresh air that enters the alveoli during each breath, is always less than tidal volume. The extent of this difference in volume depends primarily on the anatomic *dead space*, the 150- to 160-mL internal volume of the conducting airway passages. The term "dead" is quite appropriate, since it represents wasted respiratory effort; that is, no significant gas exchange occurs across the thick walls of the trachea, bronchi, and bronchiolus. Since normal tidal volume at rest is usually about 500 mL of air per breath, one can easily calculate that because of the presence of this dead space, about 340–350 mL of fresh air actually penetrates the alveoli and becomes involved in the gas exchange process. An additional 150–160 mL of stale air exhaled during the previous breath is also drawn into the alveoli.

The term "volume" is used for elemental differences of lung volume, whereas the term "capacity" is used for a combination of lung volumes. Figure 7.3 illustrates the interrelationship between each of the following lung volumes and capacities:

1. *Total lung capacity (TLC)*: The amount of gas contained in the lung at the end of maximal inspiration.
2. *Forced vital capacity (FVC)*: The maximal volume of gas that can be forcefully expelled after maximal inspiration.
3. *Inspiratory capacity (IC)*: The maximal volume of gas that can be inspired from the resting expiratory level.
4. *Functional residual capacity (FRC)*: The volume of gas remaining after normal expiration. It will be noted that FRC is the same as the resting volume. There is a small difference, however, between resting volume and FRC because FRC is measured while the patient breathes, whereas resting volume is measured with no breathing. FRC is properly defined only at end-expiration at rest and not during exercise.

These volumes and specific capacities, represented in Figure 7.3, have led to the development of specific tests (that will be discussed below) to quantify the status of the pulmonary system. Typical values for these volumes and capacities are provided in Table 7.2.

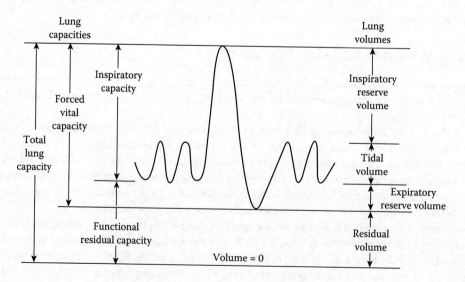

FIGURE 7.3 Lung capacities and lung volumes.

TABLE 7.2 Typical Lung Volumes for Normal, Healthy Males

Lung Volume	Normal Values	
Total lung capacity (TLC)	6.0×10^{-3} m³	(6000 cm³)
Residual volume (RV)	1.2×10^{-3} m³	(1200 cm³)
Vital capacity (VC)	4.8×10^{-3} m³	(4800 cm³)
Inspiratory reserve volume (IRV)	3.6×10^{-3} m³	(3600 cm³)
Expiratory reserve volume (ERV)	1.2×10^{-3} m³	(1200 cm³)
Functional residual capacity (FRC)	2.4×10^{-3} m³	(2400 cm³)
Anatomic dead volume (V_D)	1.5×10^{-4} m³	(150 cm³)
Upper airways volume	8.0×10^{-5} m³	(80 cm³)
Lower airways volume	7.0×10^{-5} m³	(70 cm³)
Physiologic dead volume (V_D)	1.8×10^{-3} m³	(180 cm³)
Minute volume ($\dot{V}_e$) at rest	1.0×10^{-4} m³/s	(6000 cm³/min)
Respiratory period (T) at rest	4 s	
Tidal volume (V_T) at rest	4.0×10^{-4} m³	(400 cm³)
Alveolar ventilation volume (V_A) at rest	2.5×10^{-4} m³	(250 cm³)
Minute volume during heavy exercise	1.7×10^{-3} m³/s	(10,000 cm³/min)
Respiratory period during heavy exercise	1.2 s	
Tidal volume during heavy exercise	2.0×10^{-3} m³	(2000 cm³)
Alveolar ventilation volume during exercise	1.8×10^{-3} m³	(1820 cm³)

Source: Adapted and used with permission from Forster, R.E. et al. 1986. *The Lung*. Chicago, IL, Year Book Medical Publishers, pp. 251–252.

7.3 Perfusion of the Lung

For gas exchange to occur properly in the lung, air must be delivered to the alveoli via the conducting airways, gas must diffuse from the alveoli to the capillaries through extremely thin walls, and the same gas must be removed to the cardiac atrium by blood flow. This three-step process involves (1) alveolar ventilation, (2) the process of diffusion, and (3) ventilatory *perfusion*, which involves pulmonary blood flow. Obviously, an alveolus that is ventilated but not perfused cannot exchange gas. Similarly, a perfused alveolus that is not properly ventilated cannot exchange gas. The most efficient gas exchange occurs when ventilation and perfusion are matched.

There is a wide range of ventilation-to-perfusion ratios that occur naturally in various regions of the lung (Johnson, 2009). Blood flow is somewhat affected by posture because of the effects of gravity. In the upright position, there is a general reduction in the volume of blood in the thorax, allowing for larger lung volume. Gravity also influences the distribution of blood, such that the perfusion of equal lung volumes is about five times greater at the base compared with the top of the lung (Astrand and Rodahl, 1970). There is no corresponding distribution of ventilation; hence the ventilation-to-perfusion ratio is nearly five times smaller at the top of the lung (Table 7.3). A more uniform ventilation-to-perfusion ratio is found in the supine position and during exercise (Jones, 1984).

Blood flow through the capillaries is not steady. Rather, blood flows in a halting manner and may even be stopped if intra-alveolar pressure exceeds intracapillary blood pressure during diastole. Mean blood flow is not affected by heart rate (West, 1977), but the highly distensible pulmonary blood vessels admit more blood when the blood pressure the and cardiac output increase. During exercise, higher pulmonary blood pressures allow more blood to flow through the capillaries. Even mild exercise favors more uniform perfusion of the lungs (Astrand and Rodahl, 1970). Pulmonary artery systolic pressures increases from 2670 N/m² (20 mm Hg) at rest to 4670 N/m² (35 mm Hg) during moderate exercise to 6670 N/m² (50 mm Hg) at maximal work (Astrand and Rodahl, 1970).

TABLE 7.3   Ventilation-to-Perfusion Ratios from the Top to Bottom of the Lung of Normal Man in the Sitting Position

Percent Lung Volume (%)	Alveolar Ventilation Rate (cm³/s)	Perfusion Rate (cm³/s)	Ventilation-to-Perfusion Ratio
		Top	
7	4.0	1.2	3.3
8	5.5	3.2	1.8
10	7.0	5.5	1.3
11	8.7	8.3	1.0
12	9.8	11.0	0.90
13	11.2	13.8	0.80
13	12.0	16.3	0.73
13	13.0	19.2	0.68
		Bottom	
13	13.7	21.5	0.63
100	84.9	100.0	

Source: Used with permission from West, J. 1962. *J. Appl. Physiol.* 17: 893–898.

7.4 Gas Partial Pressure

The primary purpose of the respiratory system is gas exchange. In the gas exchange process, gas must diffuse through the alveolar space, across tissue, and through plasma into the red blood cell, where it finally chemically joins to hemoglobin. A similar process occurs for carbon dioxide elimination.

As long as intermolecular interactions are small, most gases of physiologic significance can be considered to obey the ideal gas law:

$$pV = nRT$$

where p is the pressure; N/m²; V is the volume of the gas, m³; n is the number of moles, mol; R is the gas constant, $(N \times m)/(mol \times K)$; and T is the absolute temperature, K.

The ideal gas law can be applied without error up to atmospheric pressure; it can be applied to a mixture of gases, such as air, or to its constituents, such as oxygen or nitrogen. All individual gases in a mixture are considered to fill the total volume and have the same temperature but reduced pressures. The pressure exerted by each individual gas is called the *partial pressure* of the gas.

Dalton's law states that the total pressure is the sum of the partial pressures of the constituents of a mixture:

$$p = \sum_{i=1}^{N} p_i$$

where p_i is the partial pressure of the ith constituent, N/m², and N is the total number of constituents.

Dividing the ideal gas law for a constituent by that for the mixture gives

$$\frac{P_i V}{PV} = \frac{n_i R_i T}{nRT}$$

so that

$$\frac{p_i}{p} = \frac{n_i R_i}{nR}$$

which states that the partial pressure of a gas may be found if the total pressure, the mole fraction, and the ratio of gas constants are known. For most respiratory calculations, p will be considered to be the pressure of 1 atm, 101 kN/m². Avogadro's principle states that different gases at the same temperature and pressure contain equal numbers of molecules:

$$\frac{V_1}{V_2} = \frac{nR_1}{nR_2} = \frac{R_1}{R_2}$$

Thus

$$\frac{p_i}{p} = \frac{V_i}{V}$$

where V_i/V is the volume fraction of a constituent in air and is therefore dimensionless. Table 7.4 provides individual gas constants, as well as volume fractions, of constituent gases of air.

Gas pressures and volumes can be measured for many different temperature and humidity conditions. Three of these are body temperature and pressure, saturated (*BTPS*); ambient temperature and pressure (ATP); and standard temperature and pressure, dry (*STPD*). To calculate constituent partial pressures at STPD, total pressure is taken as barometric pressure minus vapor pressure of water in the atmosphere:

$$p_i = (V_i/V)(p - pH_2O)$$

where p is the total pressure, kN/m²; pH_2O is the vapor pressure of water in atmosphere, kN/m²; and V_i/V as a ratio does not change in the conversion process.

The gas volume at STPD is converted from ambient condition volume as

$$V_i = V_{amb}[273/(273 + \Theta)][(p - pH_2O)/101.3]$$

TABLE 7.4 Molecular Masses, Gas Constants, and Volume Fractions for Air and Constituents

Constituent	Molecular Mass (kg/mol)	Gas Constant (N·m/(mol·K))	Volume Fraction in Air (m³/m³)
Air	29.0	286.7	1.0000
Ammonia	17.0	489.1	0.0000
Argon	39.9	208.4	0.0093
Carbon dioxide	44.0	189.0	0.0003
Carbon monoxide	28.0	296.9	0.0000
Helium	4.0	2078.6	0.0000
Hydrogen	2.0	4157.2	0.0000
Nitrogen	28.0	296.9	0.7808
Oxygen	32.0	259.8	0.2095

Note: Universal gas constant is 8314.43 N m/kg mol K.

TABLE 7.5 Gas Partial Pressures (kN/m^2) throughout the Respiratory and Circulatory Systems

Gas	Inspired Air[a]	Alveolar Air	Expired Air	Mixed Venous Blood	Arterial Blood	Muscle Tissue
H_2O	—	6.3	6.3	6.3	6.3	6.3
CO_2	0.04	5.3	4.2	6.1	5.3	6.7
O_2	21.2	14.0	15.5	5.3	13.3	4.0
N_2[b]	80.1	75.7	75.3	76.4	76.4	76.4
Total	101.3	101.3	101.3	94.1	101.3	93.4

Source: Used with permission from Astrand, P.O. and Rodahl, K. 1970. *Textbook of Work Physiology.* New York, McGraw-Hill.

[a] Inspired air considered dry for convenience.

[b] Includes all other inert components.

where V_i is the volume of gas i corrected to STPD, m^3; V_{amp} is the volume of gas i at ambient temperature and pressure, m^3; Θ is the ambient temperature, °C; p is the ambient total pressure, kN/m^2; and pH_2O is the vapor pressure of water in the air, kN/m^2.

Partial pressures and gas volumes may be expressed in BTPS conditions. In this case, gas partial pressures are usually known from other measurements. Gas volumes are converted from ambient conditions by

$$V_i = V_{amb}[310/(273 + \Theta)][(p - pH_2O)/p - 6.28]$$

Table 7.5 provides the gas partial pressure throughout the respiratory and circulatory systems.

7.5 Pulmonary Mechanics

The respiratory system exhibits properties of resistance, compliance, and inertance analogous to the electrical properties of resistance, capacitance, and inductance. Of these, inertance is generally considered to be of less importance than the other two properties.

Resistance is the ratio of pressure to flow:

$$R = P/V$$

where R is the resistance, $N \times s/m^5$; P is the pressure, N/m^2; and V is the volume flow rate, m^3/s.

Resistance in the respiratory system appears in several places: in the airways, in the lung tissue, and in the chest wall. Airway resistance occurs due to the movement of air through the conducting air passages; lung tissue and chest wall resistances appear due to viscous dissipation of energy when tissues slide past, or move relative to, one another. Resistance that includes airways and lung tissue components is called *pulmonary resistance*. Resistance that includes all three components is called *respiratory resistance*.

Airways exhalation resistance is usually higher than airways inhalation resistance because the surrounding lung tissue pulls the smaller, more distensible airways open when the lung is being inflated. Thus, airways inhalation resistance is somewhat dependent on lung volume, and airways exhalation resistance can be very lung-volume-dependent (Johnson, 2009). Respiratory tissue resistance varies with frequency, lung volume, and volume history. Tissue resistance is relatively small at high frequencies but increases greatly at low frequencies, nearly proportional to $1/f$. Tissue resistance often exceeds airway resistance below 2 Hz. Lung tissue resistance also increases with decreasing volume amplitude (Stamenovic et al., 1990). One of the first attempts to quantify flow rate dependence was given by Rohrer (1915). Rohrer reasoned that pressure reduction in the airways should be due to laminar flow effects and turbulent effects. To account for these, he postulated

$$R = P/\dot{V} = K_1 + K_2\dot{V}$$

where K_1 is the first Rohrer coefficient, N × s/m⁵; K_2 is the second Rohrer coefficient, N × s²/m⁸; and $\dot{V}$ is the volume flow rate, m³/s.

Rohrer's equation has been applied to tissue as well as airway resistance. In applying it to tissue resistances, airflow rate is still used to obtain the pressure difference despite the fact that air does not flow through the lung tissue and chest wall. There is great variation in Rohrer's coefficients for different individuals, and exhalation coefficients are generally higher than inhalation coefficients. Most pressure–flow nonlinearities are found in the mouth and upper airways. Higher airflow rates occur in these segments compared with those in the lower airways, and therefore turbulence and nonlinearity are more likely to be found in the upper flow segments.

The description of exhalation resistance is complicated by the fact that pressures surrounding the airways tend to close them. It has been known for years that if transpulmonary pressure and expiratory flow rate are plotted along lines of equal lung volume, (1) a point is reached on each of these curves beyond which the flow cannot be increased, (2) sometimes flow rate is actually seen to decrease with increased pressure, and (3) the limiting flow rate decreases as lung volume decreases. Since resistance is the pressure divided by the flow rate, exhalation resistance becomes very high once the flow is limited.

Collapse (or pinching) of the air passages increases the resistance, thus increasing friction and reducing flow rate. Therefore, a dynamic balance is established, whereby flow rate remains constant. An increase in external pressure, which can occur during a particularly forceful exhalation, can actually decrease maximum flow rate because of its adverse effect on airway transmural pressure. Similarly, a decrease in lung volume, which tends to reduce tissue rigidity, would cause tube pinching, or collapse, at a lower flow rate.

Smaller air passages contribute to higher respiratory resistances in children (Figure 7.4). As they grow, their airways become larger and the resistance decreases (Johnson et al., 2005). Adult women normally have higher respiratory resistances than men, presumably also related to differences in body size (Johnson et al., 2005).

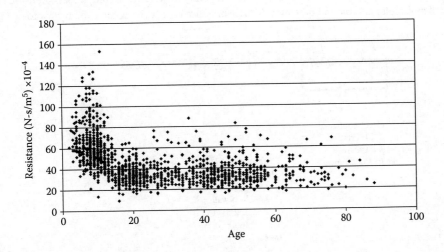

FIGURE 7.4 Respiratory resistance measured on 1400 people aged 2–88. Resistance decreases with age in childhood and appears to be relatively stable during adult years. (From Johnson, A.T. et al. 2005. *Int. J. Med. Dev. Implants.* 1: 137–151.)

Compliance is the ratio of lung volume to lung pressure:

$$C = V/P$$

where C is the compliance, m^5/N; V is the lung volume, m^3; and P is the pressure, N/m^2.

As the lung is stretched, it acts as an expanded balloon that tends to push air out and return to its normal size. The static pressure–volume relationship is nonlinear, exhibiting decreased static compliance at the extremes of lung volume (Johnson, 2009). As with tissue resistance, dynamic tissue compliance does not remain constant during breathing. Dynamic compliance tends to increase with increasing volume and decrease with increasing frequency (Stamenovic et al., 1990).

Two separate approaches can be used to model lung tissue mechanics. The traditional approach places a linear viscoelastic system in parallel with a plastoelastic system. A linear viscoelastic system consists of ideal resistive and compliant elements and can exhibit the frequency dependence of respiratory tissue. A plastoelastic system consists of dry-friction elements and compliant elements and can exhibit the volume dependence of respiratory tissue (Hildebrandt, 1970). An alternate approach is to utilize a nonlinear viscoelastic system that can characterize both the frequency dependence and the volume dependence of respiratory tissue (Suki and Bates, 1991).

Lung tissue hysteresivity relates resistance and compliance:

$$\omega R = \eta/C_{dyn}$$

where ω is the frequency, rad/s; R is the resistance, $N \times s/m^5$; η is the hysteresivity, unitless; and C_{dyn} is the dynamic compliance, m^5/n.

Hysteresivity, analogous to the structural damping coefficient used in solid mechanics, is an empirical parameter arising from the assumption that resistance and compliance are related at the microstructural level. Hysteresivity is independent of frequency and volume. Typical values range from 0.1 to 0.3 (Fredberg and Stamenovic, 1989).

A lumped-parameter, greatly simplified analog model of the respiratory system appears in Figure 7.5. A lumped-parameter respiratory model considers similar properties collected in a small number of elements. Although these properties are really distributed throughout the respiratory system, their lumped-parameter depiction can assist understanding. Three components of airways, lung tissue, and chest wall are shown. Each of these components has elements of resistance (diagrammed as an electrical resistor), compliance (electrical capacitor), and inertances (electrical inductor). Between components there are pressures denoted as alveolar and pleural pressures. Muscle pressure is the driving force for airflow to occur.

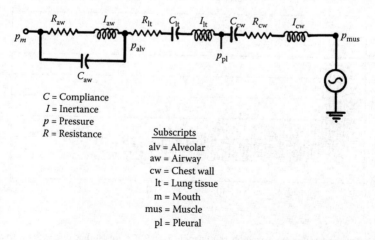

C = Compliance
I = Inertance
p = Pressure
R = Resistance

Subscripts
alv = Alveolar
aw = Airway
cw = Chest wall
lt = Lung tissue
m = Mouth
mus = Muscle
pl = Pleural

FIGURE 7.5 Lumped-parameter model of the respiratory system considered as three compartments comprising airways, lung tissue, and chest wall.

A pressure balance on the components of the model in Figure 7.5 gives

$$(p_m - p_{atm}) + (p_{alv} - p_m) + (p_{pl} - p_{alv}) + (p_{mus} - p_{pl}) + (p_{atm} - p_{mus}) = 0$$

where p_m is the mouth pressure, N/m²; p_{atm} is the atmospheric pressure, N/m²; p_{alv} is the alveolar pressure, N/m²; p_{atm} is the atmospheric pressure, N/m²; p_{pl} is the pleural pressure, N/m²; and p_{mus} is the muscle pressure, N/m².

Each pressure difference can be expressed as

$$\Delta p = R\dot{V} + V/C + \ddot{V}I$$

where R is the resistance, N × s/m⁵; C is the compliance, m⁵/N; I is the inertance, N × s²/m⁵; Δp is the pressure difference, N/m²; V is the lung volume, m³; $\dot{V}$ is the volume flow rate, m³/s; and $\ddot{V}$ is the volume acceleration, m³/s².

The model of Figure 7.5 is actually too complicated for most purposes. A simplified two-parameter respiratory system model comprising one resistance and one compliance component can be used for practical purposes at low frequencies. Lung compliance dominates inertance at frequencies less than the natural frequency of the lung (≈6 cps). At higher frequencies, the two elements appearing in the model would be resistance and inertance.

Table 7.6 gives typical values of mechanical elements appearing in the model of Figure 7.5. To obtain values for resistance R and compliance C appearing in Figure 7.5, use standard methods of combining electrical elements:

$$R = R_{aw} + R_{lt} + R_{cw}$$

$$C \cong \frac{C_{lt}C_{cw}}{C_{lt} + C_{cw}}$$

TABLE 7.6   Mechanical Properties of Lungs and Thorax at Rest

	Resistance
Total	392 kN s/m⁵
Chest wall	196
Total lung	196
Lung tissue	39.2
Total airways	157
Upper airways	39.2
Lower airways	118
	Compliance
Total	1.22×10^{-6} m⁵/N
Chest wall	2.45×10^{-6}
Total lung	2.45×10^{-6}
Airway	0.000
Lung tissue	2.45×10^{-6}
	Inertance
Total	2600 N s²/m⁵
Chest wall	1690
Total lung	911
Airway (gas)	137
Lung tissue	774
Upper airway	519
Lower airway	255

TABLE 7.7 Oxygen Cost of Breathing as Related to Total Oxygen Cost of Exercise

Total Oxygen Cost of Exercise (cm³/s)	Oxygen Cost of Ventilation (cm³/s)	Cost of Breathing Compared of Total (%)
5.0[a]	0.10[a]	2.0[a]
19.5	0.40	2.1
26.7	0.60	2.25
39.7	0.97	2.1
89.5	7.17	8.0

[a] Oxygen cost at rest.

The latter approximation is valid because airway compliance is nearly zero. Airway compliance can be considered to be the compliance of the enclosed air. Some investigators consider airway compliance to be the compliance of the tissue of the lung, the parenchyma.

Drugs, too, can significantly affect mechanical parameter values. A series of bronchoreactive drugs has been developed for use by asthmatics and others to reduce airway resistance. Even as common a drug as aspirin has been found to increase nasal resistance significantly (Jones et al., 1985), and airborne contaminants normally present in the atmosphere can have significant respiratory effects (Love, 1983).

Pulmonary mechanical parameters are especially important in lung pathology. Asthma and chronic obstructive pulmonary disease (COPD) have been increasing until respiratory diseases are some of the leading causes of death in the United States. Asthma, in particular, may be caused by changes in the composition, content, or organization of the cellular and molecular constituents of the airway wall (called *airway remodeling*, McParland et al., 2003). The mechanical properties of the lung depend on the history of the lung and challenges that have been accommodated.

The work of the respiratory muscles consists of two components: the work of breathing and the work of maintaining posture. Although not a great amount of work has been done concerning the latter, it has been stated that a considerable amount of respiratory muscular work is involved in the maintenance of thoracic shape (Grodins and Yamashiro, 1978). For instance, as the diaphragm pulls air into the lungs, the intercostal muscles move the ribs up and out to further increase chest volume. The coordination of this effort requires both positive and negative work. The work of breathing can be expressed as

$$W = p_{pl}V = \int p_{pl}\dot{V}dt$$

where W is the respiratory work, N × m; p_{pl} is the intrapleural pressure, N/m²; V is the lung volume, m³; and t is the time in s.

Because the efficiency of the respiratory muscles has been estimated at 7–11% (mean 8.5%) in normal individuals and at 1–3% (mean 1.8%) for emphysemic individuals (Cherniack, 1959), the amount of oxygen consumption that the body spends on respiration can be considerable (Table 7.7) during exercise.

7.6 Respiratory Control

Control of respiration occurs in many different cerebral structures (Johnson, 2009) and regulates many things (Hornbein, 1981). Respiration must be controlled to produce the respiratory rhythm, ensure adequate gas exchange, protect against inhalation of poisonous substances, assist in the maintenance of body pH, remove irritations, and minimize energy cost. Respiratory control is more complex than cardiac control for at least three reasons:

1. Airways airflow occurs in both directions.
2. The respiratory system interfaces directly with the environment outside the body.
3. Parts of the respiratory system are used for other functions, such as swallowing and speaking.

As a result, respiratory muscular action must be exquisitely coordinated; it must be prepared to protect itself against environmental onslaught, and breathing must be temporarily suspended on demand.

All control systems require sensors, controllers, and effectors. Figure 7.6 presents the general scheme for respiratory control. There are *mechanoreceptors* throughout the respiratory system. For example, nasal receptors are important in sneezing, apnea (cessation of breathing), bronchodilation, bronchoconstriction, and the secretion of mucus. Laryngeal receptors are important in coughing, apnea, swallowing, bronchoconstriction, airway mucus secretion, and laryngeal constriction. Tracheobronchial receptors are important in coughing, pulmonary hypertension, bronchoconstriction, laryngeal constriction, and mucus production. Other mechanoreceptors are important in the generation of the respiratory pattern and are involved with respiratory sensation.

Respiratory *chemoreceptors* exist peripherally in the aortic arch and carotic bodies and centrally in the ventral medulla oblongata of the brain. These receptors are sensitive to partial pressures of CO_2 and O_2 and to blood pH.

The respiratory controller is located in several places in the brain. Each location appears to have its own function. Unlike the heart, the basic respiratory rhythm is not generated within the lungs but rather in the brain and is transmitted to the respiratory muscles by the phrenic nerve.

Effector organs are mainly the respiratory muscles, as described previously. Other effectors are muscles located in the airways and tissues for mucus secretion. Control of respiration appears to be based on two criteria: (1) removal of excess CO_2 and (2) minimization of energy expenditure. It is not the lack of oxygen that stimulates respiration but increased CO_2 partial pressure that acts as a powerful respiratory stimulus. Because of the buffering action of blood bicarbonate, blood pH usually falls as more CO_2 is produced in the working muscles. Lower blood pH also stimulates respiration.

A number of respiratory adjustments are made to reduce energy expenditure during exercise: respiration rate increases, the ratio of inhalation time to exhalation time decreases, respiratory flow wave-shapes become more trapezoidal, and expiratory reserve volume decreases. Other adjustments to reduce energy expenditure have been theorized but not proven (Johnson, 2009).

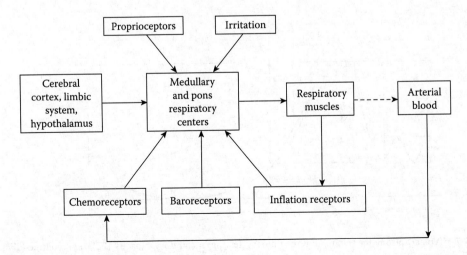

FIGURE 7.6 General scheme of respiratory control.

7.7 Pulmonary Function Laboratory

The purpose of a pulmonary function laboratory is to obtain clinically useful data from patients with respiratory dysfunction. The pulmonary function tests (PFTs) within this laboratory fulfill a variety of functions. They permit (1) quantification of a patient's breathing deficiency, (2) diagnosis of different types of pulmonary diseases, (3) evaluation of a patient's response to therapy, and (4) preoperative screening to determine whether the presence of lung disease increases the risk of surgery.

Although PFTs can provide important information about a patient's condition, the limitations of these tests must be considered. First, they are nonspecific in that they cannot determine which portion of the lungs is diseased, only that the disease is present. Second, PFTs must be considered along with the medical history, physical examination, x-ray examination, and other diagnostic procedures to permit a complete evaluation. Finally, the major drawback of some PFTs is that they require a full patient cooperation and for this reason these tests cannot be conducted on critically ill patients. Consider some of the most widely used PFTs: spirometry, body *plethysmography*, and diffusing capacity.

7.7.1 Spirometry

The simplest PFT is the spirometry maneuver. In this test, the patient inhales to TLC and exhales forcefully to residual volume. The patient exhales into a displacement bell chamber that sits on a water seal. As the bell rises, a pen coupled to the bell chamber inscribes a tracing on a rotating drum. The spirometer offers very little resistance to breathing; therefore, the shape of the spirometry curve (Figure 7.7) is purely a function of the patient's lung compliance, chest compliance, and airway resistance. At high lung volumes, a rise in intrapleural pressure results in greater expiratory flows. However, at intermediate and low lung volumes, the expiratory flow is independent of effort after a certain intrapleural pressure is reached.

Measurements made from the spirometry curve can determine the degree of a patient's ventilatory obstruction. FVC, forced expiratory volumes (FEVs), and forced expiratory flows (FEFs) can be determined. The FEV indicates the volume that has been exhaled from TLC for a particular time interval. For example, FEV0.5 is the volume exhaled during the first half-second of expiration, and FEV1.0 is the volume exhaled during the first second of expiration; these are graphically represented in Figure 7.7. Note that the more severe the ventilatory obstruction, the lower are the timed volumes (FEV0.5 and FEV1.0). The FEF is a measure of the average flow (volume/time) over specified portions of the spirometry curve and is represented by the slope of a straight line drawn between volume levels. The average flow over the

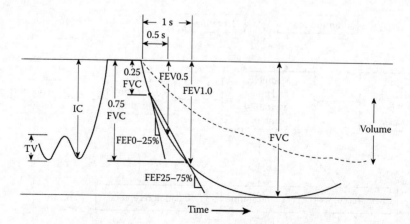

FIGURE 7.7 Typical spirometry tracing obtained during testing; inspiratory capacity (IC), tidal volume (TV), forced vital capacity (FVC), forced expiratory volume (FEV), and forced expiratory flows. Dashed line represents a patient with obstructive lung disease; solid line represents a normal, healthy individual.

first quarter of the forced expiration is the FEF0–25%, whereas the average flow over the middle 50% of the FVC is the FEF25–75%. These values are obtained directly from the spirometry curves. The less steep curves of obstructed patients would result in lower values of FEF0–25% and FEF25–75% compared with normal values, which are predicted on the basis of the patient's sex, age, and height. Equations for normal values are available from statistical analysis of data obtained from a normal population. Test results are then interpreted as a percentage of normal.

Another way of presenting a spirometry curve is as a flow–volume curve. Figure 7.8 represents a typical flow–volume curve. The expiratory flow is plotted against the exhaled volume, indicating the maximum flow that may be reached at each degree of lung inflation. Since there is no time axis, a time must mark the FEV0.5 and FEV1.0 on the tracing. To obtain these flow–volume curves in the laboratory, the patient usually exhales through a *pneumotach*. The most widely used pneumotach measures a pressure drop across a flow-resistive element. The resistance to flow is constant over the measuring range of the device; therefore, the pressure drop is proportional to the flow through the tube. This signal, which is indicative of flow, is then integrated to determine the volume of gas that has passed through the tube.

Another type of pneumotach is the heated-element type. In this device, a small heated mass responds to airflow by cooling. As the element cools, a greater current is necessary to maintain a constant temperature. This current is proportional to the airflow through the tube. Again, to determine the volume that has passed through the tube, the flow signal is integrated.

The flow–volume loop in Figure 7.9 is a dramatic representation displaying inspiratory and expiratory curves for both normal breathing and maximal breathing. The result is a graphic representation of the patient's reserve capacity in relation to normal breathing. For example, the normal patient's tidal breathing loop is small compared with the patient's maximum breathing loop. During these times of stress, this tidal breathing loop can be increased to the boundaries of the outer ventilatory loop. This increase in ventilation provides the greater gas exchange needed during the stressful situation. Compare this condition with that of the patient with obstructive lung disease. Not only is the tidal breathing loop larger than normal, but also the maximal breathing loop is smaller than normal. The result is a decreased ventilatory reserve, limiting the individual's ability to move air in and out of the lungs. As the disease progresses, the outer loop becomes smaller, and the inner loop becomes larger.

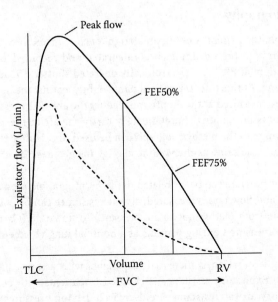

FIGURE 7.8 Flow–volume curve obtained from a spirometry maneuver. Solid line is a normal curve; dashed line represents a patient with obstructive lung disease.

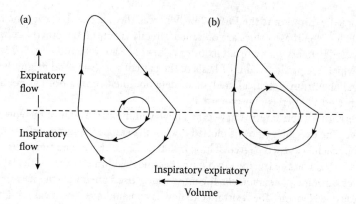

FIGURE 7.9 Typical flow–volume loops. (a) Normal flow–volume loop. (b) Flow–volume loop of patient with obstructive lung disease.

The primary use of spirometry is in the detection of obstructive lung disease that results from increased resistance to flow through the airways. This can occur in several ways:

1. Deterioration of the structure of the smaller airways that results in early airways closure
2. Decreased airway diameters caused by bronchospasm or the presence of secretions increases the airway's resistance to airflow
3. Partial blockage of a large airway by a tumor decreases the airway diameter and causes turbulent flow

Spirometry has its limitations, however. It can measure only ventilated volumes. It cannot measure lung capacities that contain the residual volume. Measurements of TLC, FRC, and RV have a diagnostic value in defining lung overdistension or restrictive pulmonary disease; the body plethysmograph can determine these absolute lung volumes.

7.7.2 Body Plethysmography

In a typical plethysmograph, the patient is put in an airtight enclosure and breathes through a pneumotach. The flow signal through the pneumotach is integrated and recorded as tidal breathing. At the end of a normal expiration (at FRC), an electronically operated shutter occludes the tube through which the patient is breathing. At this time the patient pants lightly against the occluded airway. Since there is no flow, the pressure measured at the mouth must equal the alveolar pressure. But movements of the chest that compress gas in the lung simultaneously rarify the air in the plethysmograph, and vice versa. The pressure change in the plethysmograph can be used to calculate the volume change in the plethysmograph, which is the same as the volume change in the chest. This leads directly to the determination of FRC.

At the same time, alveolar pressure can be correlated to plethysmographic pressure. Therefore, when the shutter is again opened and flow rate is measured, airway resistance can be obtained as the ratio of alveolar pressure (obtainable from plethysmographic pressure) to flow rate (Carr and Brown, 1993). Airway resistance is usually measured during panting, at a nominal lung volume of FRC and flow rate of ±1 L/s.

Airway resistance during inspiration is increased in patients with asthma, bronchitis, and upper respiratory tract infections. Expiratory resistance is elevated in patients with emphysema, since the causes of increased expiratory airway resistance are decreased driving pressures and the airway collapse. Airway resistance also may be used to determine the response of obstructed patients to bronchodilator medications.

7.7.3 Diffusing Capacity

So far the mechanical components of airflow through the lungs have been discussed. Another important parameter is the diffusing capacity of the lung, the rate at which oxygen or carbon dioxide travel from the alveoli to the blood (or vice versa for carbon dioxide) in the pulmonary capillaries. The diffusion of gas across a barrier is directly related to the surface area of the barrier and inversely related to the thickness. Also, diffusion is directly proportional to the solubility of the gas in the barrier material and inversely related to the molecular weight of the gas.

Lung diffusing capacity (Dl) is usually determined for carbon monoxide but can be related to oxygen diffusion. The popular method of measuring carbon monoxide diffusion utilizes a rebreathing technique in which the patient rebreathes rapidly in and out of a bag for approximately 30 s. Figure 7.10 illustrates the test apparatus. The patient begins breathing from a bag containing a known volume of gas consisting of 0.3–0.5% carbon monoxide made with heavy oxygen, 0.3–0.5% acetylene, 5% helium, 21% oxygen, and a balance of nitrogen. As the patient rebreathes the gas mixture in the bag, a modified *mass spectrometer* continuously analyzes it during both inspiration and expiration. During this rebreathing procedure, the carbon monoxide disappears from the patient–bag system; the rate at which this occurs is a function of the lung diffusing capacity.

Helium is inert and insoluble in lung tissue and blood, and equilibrates quickly in unobstructed patients, indicating the dilution level of the test gas. Acetylene, on the other hand, is soluble in blood and is used to determine the blood flow through the pulmonary capillaries. Carbon monoxide is bound very tightly to hemoglobin and is used to obtain diffusing capacity at a constant pressure gradient across the alveolar capillary membrane.

Decreased lung diffusing capacity can occur from the thickening of the alveolar membrane or the capillary membrane as well as the presence of interstitial fluid from edema. All these abnormalities increase the barrier thickness and cause a decrease in diffusing capacity. In addition, a characteristic of specific lung diseases is impaired lung diffusing capacity. For example, fibrotic lung tissue exhibits a decreased permeability to gas transfer, whereas pulmonary emphysema results in the loss of diffusion surface area.

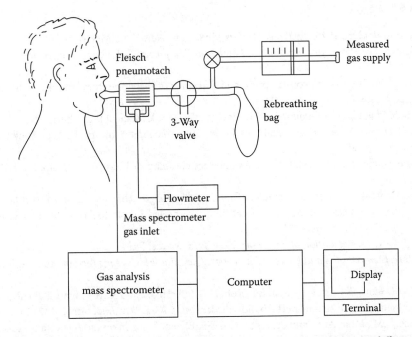

FIGURE 7.10   Typical system configuration for the measurement of rebreathing pulmonary diffusing capacity.

Defining Terms

Alveoli: Respiratory airway terminals where most gas exchange with the pulmonary circulation takes place.

BTPS: Body temperature (37°C) and standard pressure (1 atm), saturated (6.28 kN/m²).

Chemoreceptors: Neural receptors sensitive to chemicals such as gas partial pressures.

Dead space: The portion of the respiratory system that does not take part in gas exchange with the blood.

Diffusion: The process whereby a material moves from a region of higher concentration to a region of lower concentration.

Expiration: The breathing process whereby air is expelled from the mouth and nose. Also called exhalation.

Functional residual capacity: The lung volume at rest without breathing.

Inspiration: The breathing process whereby air is taken into the mouth and noise. Also called inhalation.

Mass spectrometer: A device that identifies relative concentrations of gases by means of mass-to-charge ratios of gas ions.

Mechanoreceptors: Neural receptors sensitive to mechanical inputs such as stretch, pressure, irritants, and so on.

Partial pressure: The pressure that a gas would exert if it were the only constituent.

Perfusion: Blood flow to the lungs.

Plethysmography: Any measuring technique that depends on a volume change.

Pleura: The membrane surrounding the lung.

Pneumotach: A measuring device for airflow.

Pulmonary circulation: Blood flow from the right cardiac ventricle that perfuses the lung and is in intimate contact with alveolar membranes for effective gas exchange.

STPD: Standard temperature (0 °C) and pressure (1 atm), dry (moisture removed).

Ventilation: Airflow to the lungs.

References

Astrand, P.O. and Rodahl, K. 1970. *Textbook of Work Physiology*. New York, McGraw-Hill.

Carr, J.J. and Brown, J.M. 1993. *Introduction to Biomedical Equipment Technology*. Englewood Cliffs, NJ, Prentice-Hall.

Cherniack, R.M. 1959. The oxygen consumption and efficiency of the respiratory muscles in health and emphysema. *J. Clin. Invest.* 38: 494–499.

Comroe, J.H. 1965. *Physiology of Respiration*. Chicago, IL, Year Book Medical Publishers.

Forster, R.E., A. B. Dubois, W. A. Briscoe, and A. B. Fisher. 1986. *The Lung*. Chicago, IL, Year Book Medical Publishers, pp. 251–252.

Fredberg, J.J. and Stamenovic, D. 1989. On the imperfect elasticity of lung tissue. *J. Appl. Physiol.* 67: 2408–2419.

Grodins, F.S., and Yamashiro, S.M. 1978. *Respiratory Function of the Lung and Its Control*. New York, Macmillan.

Hildebrandt, J. 1970. Pressure–volume data of cat lung interpreted by plastoelastic, linear viscoelastic model. *J. Appl. Physiol.* 28: 365–372.

Hornbein, T.F. (Ed.) 1981. *Regulation of Breathing*. New York, Marcel Dekker.

Johnson, A.T. 2009. *Biomechanics and Exercise Physiology: Quantitative Modeling*. Boca Raton, FL, Taylor & Francis.

Johnson, A.T., W.H. Scott, E. Russek-Cohen, F.C. Koh, N.K. Silverman, and K.M. Coyne. 2005. Resistance values obtained with the airflow perturbation device. *Int. J. Med. Dev. Implants.* 1: 137–151.

Jones, A.S., Lancer, J.M., Moir, A.A., and Stevens, J.C. 1985. Effect of aspirin on nasal resistance to airflow. *Br. Med. J.* 290: 1171–1173.

Jones, N.L. 1984. Normal values for pulmonary gas exchange during exercise. *Am. Rev. Respir. Dis.* 129: 544–546.

Kline, J. (Ed.) 1976. *Biologic Foundations of Biomedical Engineering*. Boston, Little, Brown.

Love, R.G. 1983. Lung function studies before and after a work shift. *Br. J. Indus. Med.* 40: 153–159.

McParland, B.E., Macklem, P.T., and Paré, P.D. 2003. Airway wall remodeling: Friend or foe? *J. Appl. Physiol.* 95: 426–434.

Rohrer, F. 1915. Flow resistance in the human air passages and the effect of irregular breathing of the bronchial system on the respiratory process in various regions of the lungs, in *Transitions in Respiratory Physiology*, J. B. West, ed. Stroudsburg, PA, Dowden, Hutchinson, and Ross, pp. 3–66.

Ruch, T.C. and Patton, H.D. (Eds.) 1966. *Physiology Biophysics*. Philadelphia, Saunders.

Stamenovic, D., Glass, G.M., Barnas, G.M., and Fredberg, J.J. 1990. Viscoplasticity of respiratory tissues. *J. Appl. Physiol.* 69: 973–988.

Suki, B. and Bates, J.H.T. 1991. A nonlinear viscoelastic model of lung tissue mechanics. *J. Appl. Physiol.* 71: 826–833.

Weibel, E.R. 1963. *Morphometry of the Human Lung*. New York, Academic Press.

West, J. 1962. Regional differences in gas exchange in the lung of erect man. *J. Appl. Physiol.* 17: 893–898.

West, J.B. (Ed.) 1977. *Bioengineering Aspects of the Lung*. New York, Marcel Dekker.

Further Reading

Fredberg, J.J., Jones, K.A., Nathan, A., Raboudi, S., Prakash, Y.S., Shore, S.A., Butler, J.P., and Sieck, G.C. 1996. Friction in airway smooth muscle: Mechanism, latch, and implications in asthma. *J. Appl. Physiol.* 81: 2703–2712.

Hantos, Z., Daroczy, B., Csendes, T., Suki, B., and Nagy, S. 1990. Modeling of low-frequency pulmonary impedance in dogs. *J. Appl. Physiol.* 68: 849–860.

Hantos, Z., Daroczy, B., Suki, B., and Nagy, S. 1990. Low-frequency respiratory mechanical impedance in rats. *J. Appl. Physiol.* 63: 36–43.

Hantos, Z., Petak, F., Adamicza, A., Asztalos, T., Tolnai, J., and Fredberg, J.J. 1997. Mechanical impedance of the lung periphery. *J. Appl. Physiol.* 83: 1595–1601.

Maksym, G.N. and Bates, J.H.T. 1997. A distributed nonlinear model of lung tissue elasticity. *J. Appl. Physiol.* 82: 32–41.

Parker, J.F. Jr. and West, V.R. (Eds.) 1973. *Bioastronautics Data Book*. Washington, NASA.

Petak, F., Hall, G.L., and Sly, P.D. 1998. Repeated measurements of airway and parenchymal mechanics in rats by using low frequency oscillations. *J. Appl. Physiol.* 84: 1680–1686.

Thorpe, C.W. and Bates, J.H.T. 1997. Effect of stochastic heterogeneity on lung impedance during acute bronchoconstriction: A model analysis. *J. Appl. Physiol.* 82: 1616–1625.

Yuan, H., Ingenito, E.P., and Suki, B. 1997. Dynamic properties of lung parenchyma: Mechanical contributions of fiber network and interstitial cells. *J. Appl. Physiol.* 83: 1420–1431.

II

Biomechanics

Donald R. Peterson
Texas A&M University

8 Mechanics of Hard Tissue *J. Lawrence Katz, Anil Misra, Orestes Marangos, Qiang Ye, and Paulette Spencer* **8**-1
Introduction • Structure of Bone • Composition of Bone • Elastic Properties • Characterizing Elastic Anisotropy • Modeling Elastic Behavior • Viscoelastic Properties • Related Research • Dentin Structure and Composition • Dentin Elasticity • Defining Terms • References • Further Information • Appendix A

9 Musculoskeletal Soft-Tissue Mechanics *Richard L. Lieber, Samuel R. Ward, and Thomas J. Burkholder* **9**-1
Structure of Soft Tissues • References

10 Joint-Articulating Surface Motion *Kenton R. Kaufman and Kai-Nan An* **10**-1
Introduction • Ankle • Knee • Hip • Shoulder • Elbow • Wrist • Hand • Summary • Acknowledgment • References

11 Joint Lubrication *Michael J. Furey* **11**-1
Introduction • Tribology • Lubrication • Synovial Joints • Theories on the Lubrication of Natural and Normal Synovial Joints • *In Vitro* Cartilage Wear Studies • Biotribology and Arthritis: Are There Connections? • Recapitulation and Final Comments • Conclusions • Acknowledgments • Further Information • References

12 Analysis of Gait *Roy B. Davis III, Sylvia Õunpuu, and Peter A. DeLuca* **12**-1
Fundamental Concepts • Measurement Approaches and Systems • Gait Data Reduction: Kinematics and Kinetics • Illustrative Clinical Example • Gait Analysis: Current Status • For Additional Information on Gait Analysis Techniques • For Additional Information on Typically Developing and Pathological Gait • References

13 Mechanics of Head/Neck *Albert I. King and David C. Viano* **13**-1
Mechanisms of Injury • Mechanical Response • Regional Tolerance of the Head and Neck to Blunt Impact • Human Surrogates of the Head and Neck • References

14 Biomechanics of Chest and Abdomen Impact *David C. Viano and Albert I. King* **14**-1
Introduction • Chest and Abdomen Injury Mechanisms • Injury Criteria and Tolerances • Biomechanical Responses during Impact • Injury Risk Assessment • References

15 **Cardiac Biomechanics** *Andrew D. McCulloch and Roy C. P. Kerckhoffs* 15-1
Introduction • Cardiac Geometry and Structure • Cardiac Pump
Function • Myocardial Material Properties • Regional Ventricular Mechanics: Stress and
Strain • Patient-Specific Modeling • Acknowledgments • References

16 **Heart Valve Dynamics** *Choon Hwai Yap, Erin Spinner, Muralidhar Padala,
and Ajit P. Yoganathan*.. 16-1
Introduction • Aortic Valve • Pulmonary Valve • Mitral Valve • Tricuspid
Valve • References

17 **Arterial Macrocirculatory Hemodynamics** *Baruch B. Lieber* 17-1
Blood Vessel Walls • Flow Characteristics • Wave Propagation • Pathology • Defining
Terms • References • Further Information

18 **Mechanics of Blood Vessels** *Thomas R. Canfield and Philip B. Dobrin* 18-1
Assumptions • Vascular Anatomy • Axisymmetric Deformation • Experimental
Measurements • Equilibrium • Strain Energy Density Functions • References

19 **The Venous System** *Artin A. Shoukas and Carl F. Rothe*.. 19-1
Introduction • Definitions • Methods to Measure Venous Characteristics • Typical
Values • Acknowledgments • References

20 **The Microcirculation Physiome** *Aleksander S. Popel and Roland N. Pittman* 20-1
Introduction • Mechanics of Microvascular Blood Flow • Molecular
Transport in the Microcirculation • Regulation of Blood Flow • Defining
Terms • Acknowledgments • References • Further Information

21 **Mechanics and Deformability of Hematocytes** *Richard E. Waugh and
Robert M. Hochmuth*...21-1
Introduction • Fundamentals • Red Cells • Leukocytes • Summary • Definition of
Terms • References • Further Information

22 **Mechanics of Tissue/Lymphatic Transport** *Geert W. Schmid-Schönbein and
Alan R. Hargens*.. 22-1
Introduction • Basic Concepts of Tissue/Lymphatic Transport • Conclusion •
Defining Terms • Acknowledgments • References • Further Reading

23 **Modeling in Cellular Biomechanics** *Alexander A. Spector and
Roger Tran-Son-Tay*..23-1
Introduction • Mechanical Properties of the Cell • Cell Motility • Mechano-,
Mechanoelectrical, and Electromechanical Transduction • Modeling Cells in
Disease • Acknowledgments • References • Further Information

24 **Cochlear Mechanics** *Charles R. Steele and Sunil Puria* 24-1
Anatomy • Passive Models • Active Process • Active Models • Concluding
Comments • References • Further Information

25 **Inner Ear Hair Cell Bundle Mechanics** *Jong-Hoon Nam and Wally Grant*................ 25-1
Introduction • Hair Cell Bundle Structure • Hair Bundle Mechanical
Stiffness • Analytical Models • Computational Model • Mechanical Properties of Hair
Bundle Structures • Hair Bundle Response to Different Types of Stimuli • Effect of
Different Bundle Shapes • Concluding Remarks • References

26 **Exercise Physiology** *Cathryn R. Dooly and Arthur T. Johnson*.................................... 26-1
Introduction • Muscle Energetics • Cardiovascular Adjustments • Maximum
Oxygen Uptake • Respiratory Responses • Optimization • Thermoregulatory
Response • Applications • Defining Terms • References • Further Information

27 **Factors Affecting Mechanical Work in Humans** *Ben F. Hurley and
Arthur T. Johnson*.. 27-1
Exercise Biomechanics • References

Preface

Biomechanics is deeply rooted throughout scientific history and has been influenced by the research work of early mathematicians, engineers, physicists, biologists, and physicians. Not one of these disciplines can claim sole responsibility for maturing biomechanics to its current state; rather, it has been a conglomeration and integration of these disciplines, involving the application of mathematics, physical principles, and engineering methodologies that have been responsible for its advancement. Several examinations exist that offer a historical perspective on biomechanics in dedicated chapters within a variety of biomechanics textbooks. For this reason, a historical perspective is not presented within this brief introduction, and it is left to the reader to discover the material within one of these textbooks. As an example, Y.C. Fung (1993) provides a reasonably detailed synopsis of those who were influential to the progress of biomechanical understanding. A review of this material and similar material from other authors commonly shows that biomechanics has occupied the thoughts of some of the most conscientious minds involved in a variety of the sciences.

The study of biomechanics, or biological mechanics, employs the principles of mechanics, which is a branch of the physical sciences that investigates the effects of energy and forces on matter or material systems. Biomechanics often embraces a broad range of subject matter that may include aspects of classical mechanics, material science, fluid mechanics, heat transfer, and thermodynamics in an attempt to model and predict the mechanical behaviors of living systems.

The contemporary approach to solving problems in biomechanics typically follows a sequence of fundamental steps that are commonly defined as observation, experimentation, theorization, validation, and application. These steps are the basis of the engineering methodologies, and their significance is emphasized within a formal education of the engineering sciences, especially biomedical engineering. Each step is considered to be equally important, and an iterative relationship between steps, with mathematics serving as the common link, is often necessary to converge on a practical understanding of the system in question. An engineering education that ignores these interrelated fundamentals may produce engineers who are ignorant of the ways in which real-world phenomena differs from mathematical models. Since most biomechanical systems are inherently complex and cannot be adequately defined using only theory and mathematics, biomechanics should be considered as a discipline whose progress relies heavily on research and the careful implementation of this approach. When a precise solution is not obtainable, utilizing this approach will assist with identifying critical physical phenomena and obtaining approximate solutions that may provide a deeper understanding as well as improvements to the investigative strategy. Not surprisingly, the need to identify critical phenomena and obtain approximate solutions seems to be more significant in biomedical engineering than any other engineering discipline, which is primarily due to the complex biological processes involved.

Applications of biomechanics have traditionally focused on modeling the system-level aspects of the human body, such as the musculoskeletal system, the respiratory system, and the cardiovascular and cardiopulmonary systems. Technologically, the most progress has been made on system-level device development and implementation, with obvious implications on athletic performance, work environment interaction, clinical rehabilitation, orthotics, prosthetics, and orthopedic surgery. However, more recent biomechanics initiatives are now focusing on the mechanical behaviors of the biological subsystems, such as tissues, cells, and molecules, to relate subsystem functions across all levels by showing how mechanical function is closely associated with certain cellular and molecular processes. These initiatives have a direct impact on the development of biological nano- and micro-technologies involving polymer dynamics, biomembranes, and molecular motors. The integration of system and subsystem models will enhance our overall understanding of human function and performance and advance the principles of biomechanics. Even still, our modern understanding about certain biomechanical processes is limited, but through ongoing biomechanics research, new information that influences the way we think about biomechanics is generated and important applications that are essential to the betterment of human existence are discovered. As a result, our limitations are reduced and our understanding becomes more refined. Recent advances in biomechanics can also be attributed to advances in experimental methods and instrumentation, such as computational and imaging capabilities, which are also subject to constant progress. Therefore, the need to revise and add to the current selections presented within this section becomes obvious, ensuring the presentation of modern viewpoints and developments. The fourth edition of this section presents a total of 20 chapters, 15 of which have been substantially updated and revised to meet this criterion. These 20 selections present material from respected scientists with diverse backgrounds in biomechanics research and application, and the presentation of the chapters has been organized in an attempt to present the material in a systematic manner. The first group of chapters is related to musculoskeletal mechanics and includes hard- and soft-tissue mechanics, joint mechanics, and applications related to human function. The next group of chapters covers several aspects of biofluid mechanics and includes a wide range of circulatory dynamics, such as blood vessel and blood cell mechanics, and transport. It is followed by cellular mechanics, which introduces current methods and strategies for modeling cellular mechanics. The next group consists of two chapters introducing the mechanical functions and significance of the human ear, including a new chapter on the inner ear hair cell mechanics. Finally, the remaining two chapters introduce performance characteristics of the human body system during exercise and exertion.

It is the overall intention of this section to serve as a reference to the skilled professional as well as an introduction to the novice or student of biomechanics. Throughout all the editions of the biomechanics section, an attempt was made to incorporate material that covers a bulk of the biomechanics field; however, as biomechanics continues to grow, some topics may be inadvertently omitted causing a disproportionate presentation of the material. Suggestions and comments from readers are welcomed on the subject matter that may be considered for future editions.

Donald R. Peterson
Section Editor
Texas A&M University
Texarkana, Texas

Reference

Fung, Y.C. 1993. *Biomechanics: Mechanical Properties of Living Tissues* 2nd Edition. New York, Springer-Verlag.

8

Mechanics of Hard Tissue

J. Lawrence Katz
Case Western Reserve University
University of Kansas

Anil Misra
University of Kansas

Orestes Marangos
University of Kansas

Qiang Ye
University of Kansas

Paulette Spencer
University of Kansas

8.1	Introduction	8-1
8.2	Structure of Bone	8-2
8.3	Composition of Bone	8-4
8.4	Elastic Properties	8-4
8.5	Characterizing Elastic Anisotropy	8-10
8.6	Modeling Elastic Behavior	8-12
8.7	Viscoelastic Properties	8-14
8.8	Related Research	8-17
8.9	Dentin Structure and Composition	8-17
8.10	Dentin Elasticity	8-18
Defining Terms		8-20
References		8-20
Further Information		8-24
Appendix A		8-25

8.1 Introduction

Hard tissue, mineralized tissue, and calcified tissue are often used as synonyms for bone when describing the structure and properties of bone or tooth. The hard is self-evident in comparison with all other mammalian tissues, which often are referred to as soft tissues. The use of the terms mineralized and calcified arises from the fact that, in addition to the principle protein, collagen, and other proteins, glycoproteins, and protein-polysaccharides, comprising about 50% of the volume, the major constituent of bone is a calcium phosphate (thus the term calcified). The calcium phosphate occurs in the form of a crystalline carbonate apatite (similar to naturally occurring minerals, thus the term mineralized). Irrespective of its biological function, bone is one of the most interesting materials known in terms of structure–property relationships. Bone is an anisotropic, heterogeneous, inhomogeneous, nonlinear, thermorheologically complex viscoelastic material. It exhibits electromechanical effects, presumed to be due to streaming potentials, both *in vivo* and *in vitro* when wet. In the dry state, bone exhibits piezoelectric properties. Because of the complexity of the structure–property relationships in bone, and the space limitation for this chapter, it is necessary to concentrate on one aspect of the mechanics. Currey (1984, p. 43) states unequivocally that he thinks, "the most important feature of bone material is its stiffness." This is, of course, the premiere consideration for the weight-bearing long bones. Thus, this chapter will concentrate on the elastic and viscoelastic properties of compact cortical bone and the elastic properties of trabecular bone as exemplar of mineralized tissue mechanics.

8.2 Structure of Bone

The complexity of bone's properties arises from the complexity in its structure. Thus it is important to have an understanding of the structure of mammalian bone in order to appreciate the related properties. Figure 8.1 is a diagram showing the structure of a human femur at different levels (Park, 1979). For convenience, the structures shown in Figure 8.1 are grouped into four levels. A further subdivision of structural organization of mammalian bone is shown in Figure 8.2 (Wainwright et al., 1982). The individual figures within this diagram can be sorted into one of the appropriate levels of structure shown in Figure 8.1 and are described as follows in hierarchical order. At the smallest unit of structure we have the tropocollagen molecule and the associated apatite crystallites (abbreviated Ap). The former is approximately 1.5×280 nm, made up of three individual left-handed helical polypeptide (alpha) chains coiled into a right-handed triple helix. Ap crystallites have been found to be carbonate-substituted hydroxyapatite, generally thought to be nonstoichiometric. The crystallites appear to be about $4 \times 20 \times 60$ nm in size. This is denoted at the molecular level. Next is the ultrastructural level. Here, the collagen and Ap are intimately associated and assembled into a microfibrillar composite, several of which are then assembled into fibers from approximately 3 to 5 mm thickness. At the next level, the microstructural, these fibers are either randomly arranged (woven bone) or organized into concentric lamellar groups (osteons) or linear lamellar groups (plexiform bone). This is the level of structure we usually mean when we talk about bone tissue properties. In addition to the differences in lamellar organization at this level, there are also two different types of architectural structure. The dense type of bone found, for example, in the shafts of long bone is known as compact or cortical bone. A more porous or spongy type of bone is found, for example, at the articulating ends of long bones. This is called cancellous bone. It is important to note that the material and structural organization of collagen–Ap making up osteonic or Haversian bone and plexiform bone are the same as the material comprising cancellous bone.

Finally, we have the whole bone itself constructed of osteons and portions of older, partially destroyed osteons (called interstitial lamellae) in the case of humans or of osteons and/or plexiform bone in the case of mammals. This we denote as the macrostructural level. The elastic properties of the whole bone results from the hierarchical contribution of each of these levels.

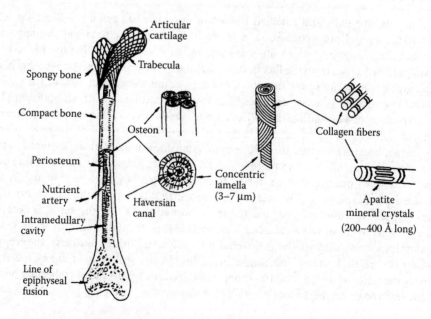

FIGURE 8.1 Hierarchical levels of structure in a human femur. (From Park JB. *Biomaterials: An Introduction.* New York: Plenum, 1979. Courtesy of Plenum Press and Dr. J.B. Park.)

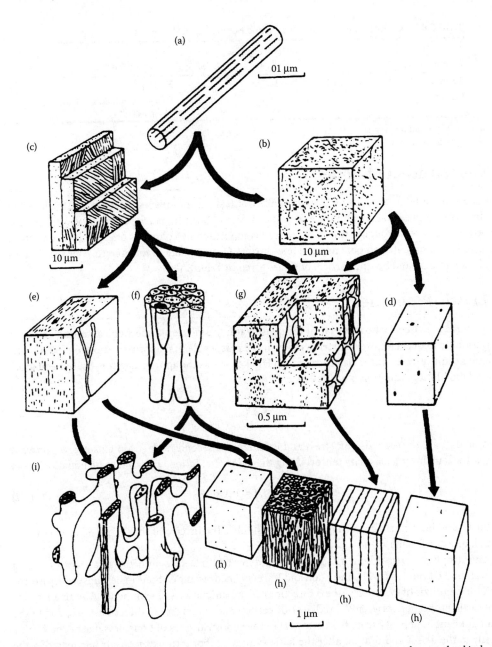

FIGURE 8.2 Diagram showing the structure of mammalian bone at different levels. Bone at the same level is drawn at the same magnification. The arrows show what types may contribute to structures at higher levels. (From Wainwright SA. et al. *Mechanical Design in Organisms*. Princeton, NJ: Princeton University Press, 1982. Courtesy Princeton University Press.) (a) Collagen fibril with associated mineral crystals. (b) Woven bone. The collagen fibrils are arranged more or less randomly. Osteocytes are not shown. (c) Lamellar bone. There are separate lamellae, and the collagen fibrils are arranged in "domains" of preferred fibrillar orientation in each lamella. Osteocytes are not shown. (d) Woven bone. Blood channels are shown as large black spots. At this level woven bone is indicated by light dotting. (e) Primary lamellar bone. At this level lamellar bone is indicated by fine dashes. (f) Haversian bone. A collection of Haversian systems, each with concentric lamellae round a central blood channel. The large black area represents the cavity formed as a cylinder of bone is eroded away. It will be filled in with concentric lamellae and form a new Haversian system. (g) Laminar bone. Two blood channel networks are exposed. Note how layers of woven and lamellar bone alternate. (h) Compact bone of the types shown at the lower levels. (i) Cancellous bone.

TABLE 8.1 Composition of Adult Human and Bovine Cortical Bone

Species	% H$_2$O	Ap	% Dry Weight Collagen	GAG[a]	Reference
Bovine	9.1	76.4	21.5	N.D[b]	Herring (1977)
Human	7.3	67.2	21.2	0.34	Pellegrino and Blitz (1965); Vejlens (1971)

[a] Glycosaminoglycan.
[b] Not determined.

8.3 Composition of Bone

The composition of bone depends on a large number of factors: the species, which bone, the location from which the sample is taken, and the age, sex, and type of bone tissue, for example, woven, cancellous, cortical. However, a rough estimate for overall composition by volume is one-third Ap, one-third collagen and other organic components, and one-third H$_2$O. Some data in the literature for the composition of adult human and bovine cortical bone are given in Table 8.1.

8.4 Elastic Properties

Although bone is a viscoelastic material, at the quasi-static strain rates in mechanical testing and even at the ultrasonic frequencies used experimentally, it is a reasonable first approximation to model cortical bone as an anisotropic, linear elastic solid with Hooke's law as the appropriate constitutive equation. Tensor notation for the equation is written as

$$\sigma_{ij} = C_{ijkl}\varepsilon_{kl} \tag{8.1}$$

where σ_{ij} and ε_{kl} are the second-rank stress and infinitesimal second rank strain tensors, respectively, and C_{ijkl} is the fourth-rank elasticity tensor. Using the reduced notation, we can rewrite Equation 8.1 as

$$\sigma_i = C_{ij}\varepsilon_j \quad i,j = 1 \text{ to } 6 \tag{8.2}$$

where the C_{ij} are the stiffness coefficients (elastic constants). The inverse of the C_{ij}, the S_{ij}, are known as the compliance coefficients.

The anisotropy of cortical bone tissue has been described in two symmetry arrangements. Lang (1969), Katz and Ukraincik (1971), and Yoon and Katz (1976a,b) assumed bone to be transversely isotropic with the bone axis of symmetry (the 3 direction) as the unique axis of symmetry. Any small difference in elastic properties between the radial (1 direction) and transverse (2 direction) axes, due to the apparent gradient in porosity from the periosteal to the endosteal sides of bone, was deemed to be due essentially to the defect and did not alter the basic symmetry. For a transverse isotropic material, the stiffness matrix $[C_{ij}]$ is given by

$$[C_{ij}] = \begin{bmatrix} C_{11} & C_{12} & C_{13} & 0 & 0 & 0 \\ C_{12} & C_{11} & C_{13} & 0 & 0 & 0 \\ C_{13} & C_{13} & C_{33} & 0 & 0 & 0 \\ 0 & 0 & 0 & C_{44} & 0 & 0 \\ 0 & 0 & 0 & 0 & C_{44} & 0 \\ 0 & 0 & 0 & 0 & 0 & C_{66} \end{bmatrix} \tag{8.3}$$

where $C_{66} = 1/2\,(C_{11}-C_{12})$. Of the 12 nonzero coefficients, only 5 are independent.

However, Van Buskirk and Ashman (1981) used the small differences in elastic properties between the radial and tangential directions to postulate that bone is an orthotropic material; this requires that 9 of the 12 nonzero elastic constants be independent, that is,

$$[C_{ij}] = \begin{bmatrix} C_{11} & C_{12} & C_{13} & 0 & 0 & 0 \\ C_{12} & C_{22} & C_{23} & 0 & 0 & 0 \\ C_{13} & C_{23} & C_{33} & 0 & 0 & 0 \\ 0 & 0 & 0 & C_{44} & 0 & 0 \\ 0 & 0 & 0 & 0 & C_{55} & 0 \\ 0 & 0 & 0 & 0 & 0 & C_{66} \end{bmatrix} \tag{8.4}$$

Corresponding matrices can be written for the compliance coefficients, the S_{ij}, based on the inverse equation to Equation 8.2:

$$\varepsilon_i = S_{ij}\sigma_j \quad i, j = 1 \text{ to } 6 \tag{8.5}$$

where the S_{ij}th compliance is obtained by dividing the $[C_{ij}]$ stiffness matrix, minus the ith row and jth column, by the full $[C_{ij}]$ matrix and vice versa to obtain the C_{ij} in terms of the S_{ij}. Thus, although $S_{33} = 1/E_3$, where E_3 is Young's modulus in the bone axis direction, $E_3 \neq C_{33}$, since C_{33} and S_{33}, are not reciprocals of one another even for an isotropic material, let alone for transverse isotropy or orthotropic symmetry.

The relationship between the compliance matrix and the technical constants such as Young's modulus (E_i) shear modulus (G_i), and Poisson's ratio (v_{ij}) measured in mechanical tests such as uniaxial or pure shear is expressed in Equation 8.6.

$$[S_{ij}] = \begin{bmatrix} \dfrac{1}{E_1} & \dfrac{-v_{21}}{E_2} & \dfrac{-v_{31}}{E_3} & 0 & 0 & 0 \\ \dfrac{-v_{12}}{E_1} & \dfrac{1}{E_2} & \dfrac{-v_{32}}{E_3} & 0 & 0 & 0 \\ \dfrac{-v_{13}}{E_1} & \dfrac{-v_{23}}{E_2} & \dfrac{1}{E_3} & 0 & 0 & 0 \\ 0 & 0 & 0 & \dfrac{1}{G_{23}} & 0 & 0 \\ 0 & 0 & 0 & 0 & \dfrac{1}{G_{31}} & 0 \\ 0 & 0 & 0 & 0 & 0 & \dfrac{1}{G_{12}} \end{bmatrix} \tag{8.6}$$

Again, for an orthotropic material, only 9 of the above 12 nonzero terms are independent, due to the symmetry of the S_{ij} tensor:

$$\frac{v_{12}}{E_1} = \frac{v_{21}}{E_2}, \quad \frac{v_{13}}{E_1} = \frac{v_{31}}{E_3}, \quad \frac{v_{23}}{E_2} = \frac{v_{32}}{E_3} \tag{8.7}$$

For the transverse isotropic case, Equation 8.5 reduces to only 5 independent coefficients, since

$$E_1 = E_2, \quad v_{12} = v_{21}, \quad v_{31} = v_{32} = v_{13} = v_{23},$$
$$G_{23} = G_{31}, \quad G_{12} = \frac{E_1}{2(1 + v_{12})} \tag{8.8}$$

In addition to the mechanical tests cited above, ultrasonic wave propagation techniques have been used to measure the anisotropic elastic properties of bone (Lang, 1969; Yoon and Katz, 1976a,b; Van Buskirk and Ashman, 1981). This is possible, since combining Hooke's law with Newton's second law results in a wave equation which yields the following relationship involving the stiffness matrix:

$$\rho V^2 U_m = C_{mrns} N_r N_s U_n \tag{8.9}$$

where ρ is the density of the medium, V is the wave speed, and U and N are unit vectors along the particle displacement and wave propagation directions, respectively, so that U_m, N_r, and others are direction cosines.

Thus to find the five transverse isotropic elastic constants, at least five independent measurements are required, for example, a dilatational longitudinal wave in the 2 and 1(2) directions, a transverse wave in the 13(23) and 12 planes, and so on. The technical moduli must then be calculated from the full set of C_{ij}. For improved statistics, redundant measurements should be made. Correspondingly, for orthotropic symmetry, enough independent measurements must be made to obtain all nine C_{ij}; again, redundancy in measurements is a suggested approach.

One major advantage of the ultrasonic measurements over mechanical testing is that the former can be done with specimens too small for the latter technique. Second, the reproducibility of measurements using the former technique is greater than for the latter. Still a third advantage is that the full set of either five or nine coefficients can be measured on one specimen, a procedure not possible with the latter techniques. Thus, at present, most of the studies of elastic anisotropy in both human and other mammalian bone are done using ultrasonic techniques. In addition to the bulk wave-type measurements described above, it is possible to obtain Young's modulus directly. This is accomplished by using samples of small cross sections with transducers of low frequency so that the wavelength of the sound is much larger than the specimen size. In this case, an extensional longitudinal (bar) wave is propagated (which experimentally is analogous to a uniaxial mechanical test experiment), yielding

$$V^2 = \frac{E}{\rho} \tag{8.10}$$

This technique was used successfully to show that bovine plexiform bone was definitely orthotropic while the bovine Haversian bone could be treated as transversely isotropic (Lipson and Katz, 1984). The results were subsequently confirmed using bulk wave propagation techniques with considerable redundancy (Maharidge, 1984).

Table 8.2 lists the C_{ij} (in GPa) for human (Haversian) bone and bovine (both Haversian and plexiform) bone. With the exception of Knet's (1978) measurements, which were made using quasi-static mechanical testing, all the other measurements were made using bulk ultrasonic wave propagation.

TABLE 8.2 Elastic Stiffness Coefficients for Various Human and Bovine Bones; All Measurements Made with Ultrasound except for Knets (1978) Mechanical Tests

Experiments	C_{11}	C_{22}	C_{33}	C_{44}	C_{55}	C_{66}	C_{12}	C_{13}	C_{23}
(Bone Type)	(GPa)	(GPa)	(GPa)	(GPa)	(GPa)	(GPa)	(GPa)	(GPa)	(GPa)
Van Buskirk and Ashman (1981) (bovine femur)	14.1	18.4	25.0	7.00	6.30	5.28	6.34	4.84	6.94
Knets (1978) (human tibia)	11.6	14.4	22.5	4.91	3.56	2.41	7.95	6.10	6.92
Van Buskirk and Ashman (1981) (human femur)	20.0	21.7	30.0	6.56	5.85	4.74	10.9	11.5	11.5
Maharidge (1984) (bovine femur Haversian)	21.2	21.0	29.0	6.30	6.30	5.40	11.7	12.7	11.1
Maharidge (1984) (bovine femur plexiform)	22.4	25.0	35.0	8.20	7.10	6.10	14.0	15.8	13.6

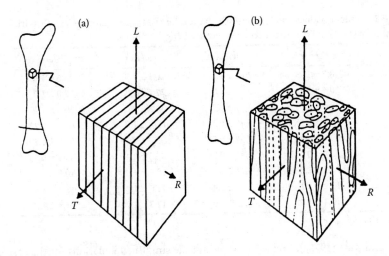

FIGURE 8.3 Diagram showing how laminar (plexiform) bone (a) differs more between radial and tangential directions (R and T) than does Haversian bone (b). The arrows are vectors representing the various directions. (From Wainwright SA et al. *Mechanical Design in Organisms*. Princeton, NJ: Princeton University Press, 1982. Courtesy Princeton University Press.)

In Maharidge's study (1984), both types of tissue specimens, the Haversian and plexiform, were obtained from different aspects of the same level of an adult bovine femur. Thus, the differences in C_{ij} reported between the two types of bone tissue are hypothesized to be due essentially to the differences in microstructural organization (Figure 8.3) (Wainwright et al., 1982). The textural symmetry at this level of structure has dimensions comparable to those of the ultrasound wavelengths used in the experiment, and the molecular and ultrastructural levels of organization in both types of tissues are essentially identical. Note that while C_{11}, almost equals C_{22} and that C_{44} and C_{55} are equal for bovine Haversian bone, C_{11} and C_{22} and C_{44} and C_{55} differ by 11.6% and 13.4%, respectively, for bovine plexiform bone. Similarly, although C_{66} and $\frac{1}{2}(C_{11}-C_{12})$ differ by 12.0% for the Haversian bone, they differ by 31.1% for plexiform bone. Only the differences between C_{13} and C_{23} are somewhat comparable: 12.6% for the Haversian bone and 13.9% for plexiform. These results reinforce the importance of modeling bone as a hierarchical ensemble in order to understand the basis for bone's elastic properties as a composite material–structure system in which the collagen–Ap components define the material composite property. When this material property is entered into calculations based on the microtextural arrangement, the overall anisotropic elastic anisotropy can be modeled.

The human femur data (Van Buskirk and Ashman, 1981) support this description of bone tissue. Although they measured all nine individual C_{ij}, treating the femur as an orthotropic material, their results are consistent with a near transverse isotropic symmetry. However, their nine C_{ij} for bovine femoral bone clearly shows the influence of the orthotropic microtextural symmetry of tissue's plexiform structure.

The data of Knets (1978) on the human tibia are difficult to analyze. This could be due to the possibility of significant systematic errors due to mechanical testing on a large number of small specimens from a multitude of different positions in the tibia.

The variations in bone's elastic properties cited earlier above due to location is appropriately illustrated in Table 8.3, where the mean values and standard deviations (all in GPa) for all g orthotropic C_{ij} are given for bovine cortical bone at each aspect over the entire length of bone.

Since the C_{ij} are simply related to the "technical" elastic moduli, such as Young's modulus (E), shear modulus (G), bulk modulus (K), and others, it is possible to describe the moduli along any given direction. The full equations for the most general anisotropy are too long to present here. However, they can

TABLE 8.3 Mean Values and Standard Deviations for the C_{ij} Measured by Van Buskirk and Ashman (1981) at Each Aspect over the Entire Length of Bone

	Anterior	Medial	Posterior	Lateral
C_{11}	18.7 ± 1.7	20.9 ± 0.8	20.1 ± 1.0	20.6 ± 1.6
C_{22}	20.4 ± 1.2	22.3 ± 1.0	22.2 ± 1.3	22.0 ± 1.0
C_{33}	28.6 ± 1.9	30.1 ± 2.3	30.8 ± 1.0	30.5 ± 1.1
C_{44}	6.73 ± 0.68	6.45 ± 0.35	6.78 ± 1.0	6.27 ± 0.28
C_{55}	5.55 ± 0.41	6.04 ± 0.51	5.93 ± 0.28	5.68 ± 0.29
C_{66}	4.34 ± 0.33	4.87 ± 0.35	5.10 ± 0.45	4.63 ± 0.36
C_{12}	11.2 ± 2.0	11.2 ± 1.1	10.4 ± 1.0	10.8 ± 1.7
C_{13}	11.2 ± 1.1	11.2 ± 2.4	11.6 ± 1.7	11.7 ± 1.8
C_{23}	10.4 ± 1.4	11.5 ± 1.0	12.5 ± 1.7	11.8 ± 1.1

Note: All values in GPa.

be found in Yoon and Katz (1976a). Presented below are the simplified equations for the case of transverse isotropy. Young's modulus is

$$\frac{1}{E(\gamma_3)} = S'_{33} = (1 - \gamma_3^2)2S_{11} + \gamma_3^4 S_{33} + \gamma_3^2(1 - \gamma_3^2)(2S_{13} + S_{44}) \tag{8.11}$$

where $\gamma_3 = \cos\phi$, and ϕ is the angle made with respect to the bone (3) axis.

The shear modulus (rigidity modulus or torsional modulus for a circular cylinder) is

$$\frac{1}{G(\gamma_3)} = \frac{1}{2}(S'_{44} + S'_{55}) = S_{44} + (S_{11} - S_{12}) - \frac{1}{2}S_{44}(1 - \gamma_3^2)$$
$$+ 2(S_{11} + S_{33} - 2S_{13} - S_{44})\gamma_3^2(1 - \gamma_3^2) \tag{8.12}$$

where, again $\gamma_3 = \cos\phi$.

The bulk modulus (reciprocal of the volume compressibility) is

$$\frac{1}{K} = S_{33} + 2(S_{11} + S_{12} + 2S_{13}) = \frac{C_{11} + C_{12} + 2C_{33} - 4C_{13}}{C_{33}(C_{11} + C_{12}) - 2C_{13}^2} \tag{8.13}$$

Conversion of Equations 8.11 and 8.12 from S_{ij} to C_{ij} can be done by using the following transformation equations:

$$S_{11} = \frac{C_{22}C_{33} - C_{23}^2}{\Delta}, \quad S_{22} = \frac{C_{33}C_{11} - C_{13}^2}{\Delta},$$
$$S_{33} = \frac{C_{11}C_{22} - C_{12}^2}{\Delta}, \quad S_{12} = \frac{C_{13}C_{23} - C_{12}C_{33}}{\Delta},$$
$$S_{13} = \frac{C_{12}C_{23} - C_{13}C_{22}}{\Delta}, \quad S_{23} = \frac{C_{12}C_{13} - C_{23}C_{11}}{\Delta}, \tag{8.14}$$
$$S_{44} = \frac{1}{C_{44}}, \quad S_{55} = \frac{1}{C_{55}}, \quad S_{66} = \frac{1}{C_{66}}$$

where

$$\Delta = \begin{vmatrix} C_{11} & C_{12} & C_{13} \\ C_{12} & C_{22} & C_{23} \\ C_{13} & C_{23} & C_{33} \end{vmatrix} = C_{11}C_{22}C_{33} + 2C_{12}C_{23}C_{13} - (C_{11}C_{23}^2 + C_{22}C_{13}^2 + C_{33}C_{12}^2) \tag{8.15}$$

In addition to data on the elastic properties of cortical bone presented above, there is also a considerable set of data available on the mechanical properties of cancellous (trabecullar) bone, including measurements of the elastic properties of single trabeculae. Indeed, as early as 1993, Keaveny and Hayes (1993) presented an analysis of 20 years of studies on the mechanical properties of trabecular bone. Most of the earlier studies used mechanical testing of bulk specimens of a size reflecting a cellular solid, that is, of the order of cubic millimeters or larger. These studies showed that both the modulus and strength of trabecular bone are strongly correlated to the apparent density, where apparent density, ρ_a, is defined as the product of individual trabeculae density, ρ_t, and the volume fraction of bone in the bulk specimen, V_f, and is given by $\rho_a = \rho_t V_f$.

Elastic moduli, E, from these measurements generally ranged from approximately 10 MPa to the order of 1 GPa depending on the apparent density and could be correlated to the apparent density in g/cm^3 by a power-law relationship, $E = 6.13 P_a^{144}$, calculated for 165 specimens with an $r^2 = 0.62$ (Keaveny and Hayes, 1993).

With the introduction of micromechanical modeling of bone, it became apparent that in addition to knowing the bulk properties of trabecular bone it was necessary to determine the elastic properties of the individual trabeculae. Several different experimental techniques have been used for these studies. Individual trabeculae have been machined and measured in buckling, yielding a modulus of 11.4 GPa (wet) and 14.1 GPa (dry) (Townsend et al., 1975), as well as by other mechanical testing methods providing average values of the elastic modulus ranging from less than 1 GPa to about 8 GPa (Table 8.4). Ultrasound measurements (Ashman and Rho, 1988; Rho et al., 1993) have yielded values commensurate with the measurements of Townsend et al. (1975) (Table 8.4). More recently, acoustic microscopy and nanoindentation have been used, yielding values significantly higher than those cited above. Rho et al. (1999) using nanoindentation obtained average values of modulus ranging from 15.0 to 19.4 GPa depending on orientation, as compared to 22.4 GPa for osteons and 25.7 GPa for the interstitial lamellae in cortical bone (Table 8.4). Turner et al. (1999) compared nanoindentation and acoustic microscopy at 50 MHz on the same specimens of trabecular and cortical bone from a common human donor. While the nanoindentation resulted in Young's moduli greater than those measured by acoustic microscopy by 4–14%, the anisotropy ratio of longitudinal modulus to transverse modulus for cortical bone was similar for both modes of measurement; the trabecular values are given in Table 8.4. Acoustic microscopy at 400 MHz has also been used to measure the moduli of both human trabecular and cortical bone (Bumrerraj and Katz, 2001), yielding results comparable with those of Turner et al. (1999) for both types of bone (Table 8.4).

These recent studies provide a framework for micromechanical analyses using material properties measured on the microstructural level. They also point to using nano-scale measurements, such as those

TABLE 8.4 Elastic Moduli of Trabecular Bone Material Measured by Different Experimental Methods

Study	Method	Average Modulus	(GPa)
Townsend et al. (1975)	Buckling	11.4	(Wet)
	Buckling	14.1	(Dry)
Ryan and Williams (1989)	Uniaxial tension	0.760	
Choi and Goldstein (1992)	4-point bending	5.72	
Ashman and Rho (1988)	Ultrasound	13.0	(Human)
	Ultrasound	10.9	(Bovine)
Rho et al. (1993)	Ultrasound	14.8	
	Tensile test	10.4	
Rho et al. (1999)	Nanoindentation	19.4	(Longitudinal)
	Nanoindentation	15.0	(Transverse)
Turner et al. (1999)	Acoustic microscopy	17.5	
	Nanoindentation	18.1	
Bumrerraj and Katz (2001)	Acoustic microscopy	17.4	

provided by atomic force microscopy (AFM), to analyze the mechanics of bone on the smallest unit of structure shown in Figure 8.1.

8.5 Characterizing Elastic Anisotropy

Having a full set of five or nine C_{ij} does permit describing the anisotropy of that particular specimen of bone, but there is no simple way of comparing the relative anisotropy between different specimens of the same bone or between different species or between experimenters' measurements by trying to relate individual C_{ij} between sets of measurements. Adapting a method from crystal physics (Chung and Buessem, 1968), Katz and Meunier (1987) presented a description for obtaining two scalar quantities defining the compressive and shear anisotropy for bone with transverse isotropic symmetry. Later, they developed a similar pair of scalar quantities for bone exhibiting orthotropic symmetry (Katz and Meunier, 1990). For both cases, the percentage compressive (Ac^*) and shear (As^*) elastic anisotropy are given, respectively, by

$$
\begin{aligned}
Ac^* \, (\%) &= 100 \frac{K_V - K_R}{K_V + K_R} \\
As^* \, (\%) &= 100 \frac{G_V - G_R}{G_V + G_R}
\end{aligned}
\tag{8.16}
$$

where K_V and K_R are the Voigt (uniform strain across an interface) and Reuss (uniform stress across an interface) bulk moduli, respectively, and G_V and G_R are the Voigt and Reuss shear moduli, respectively. The equations for K_V, K_R, G_V, and G_R are provided for both transverse isotropy and orthotropic symmetry in Appendix A.

Table 8.5 lists the values of $As^*(\%)$ and $Ac^*(\%)$ for various types of hard tissues and apatites. The graph of $As^*(\%)$ versus $Ac^*(\%)$ is given in Figure 8.4.

$As^*(\%)$ and $Ac^*(\%)$ have been calculated for a human femur, having both transverse isotropic and orthotropic symmetry, from the full set of Van Buskirk and Ashman (1981) C_{ij} data at each of the four aspects around the periphery, anterior, medial, posterior, lateral, as denoted in Table 8.3, at fractional proximal levels along the femur's length, $Z/L = 0.3–0.7$. The graph of $As^*(\%)$ versus Z/L, assuming transverse isotropy, is given in Figure 8.5. Note that the anterior aspect, that is in tension during loading, has values of $As^*(\%)$ in some positions considerably higher than those of the other aspects. Similarly, the graph of $Ac^*(\%)$ versus Z/L is given in Figure 8.6. Note here it is the posterior aspect, that is in compression during loading, that has values of $Ac^*(\%)$ in some positions considerably higher than those of the other aspects. Both graphs are based on the transverse isotropic symmetry calculations, however, the

TABLE 8.5 $As^*(\%)$ versus $Ac^*(\%)$ for Various Types of Hard Tissues and Apatites

Experiments (Specimen Type)	$Ac^*(\%)$	$As^*(\%)$
Van Buskirk et al. (1981) (bovine femur)	1.522	2.075
Katz and Ukraincik (1971) (OHAp)	0.995	0.686
Yoon (redone) in Katz (1984) (FAp)	0.867	0.630
Lang (1969, 1970) (bovine femur dried)	1.391	0.981
Reilly and Burstein (1975) (bovine femur)	2.627	5.554
Yoon and Katz (1976) (human femur dried)	1.036	1.055
Katz et al. (1983) (Haversian)	1.080	0.775
Van Buskirk and Ashman (1981) (human femur)	1.504	1.884
Kinney et al. (2004) (human dentin dry)	0.006	0.011
Kinney et al. (2004) (human dentin wet)	1.305	0.377

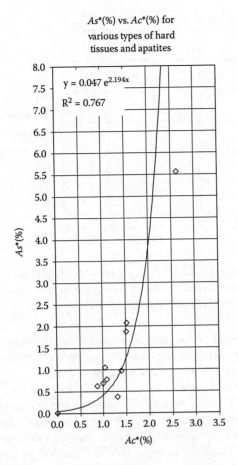

FIGURE 8.4 Values of As^*(%) versus Ac^*(%) from Table 8.5 are plotted for various types of hard tissues and apatites.

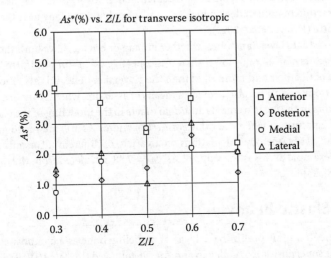

FIGURE 8.5 Values As^*(%) calculated from the data in Table 8.3 for human femoral bone, treated as having transverse isotropic symmetry, is plotted versus Z/L for all four aspects, anterior, medial, posterior, lateral around the bone's periphery; Z/L is the fractional proximal distance along the femur's length.

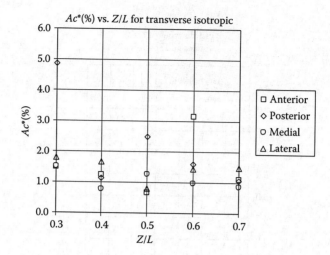

FIGURE 8.6 Values $Ac^*(\%)$ calculated from the data in Table 8.3 for human femoral bone, treated as having transverse isotropic symmetry, is plotted versus Z/L for all four aspects, anterior, medial, posterior, lateral around the bone's periphery; Z/L is the fractional proximal distance along the femur's length.

identical trends were obtained based on the orthotropic symmetry calculations. It is clear that in addition to the moduli varying along the length and over all four aspects of the femur, the anisotropy varies as well, reflecting the response of the femur to the manner of loading.

Recently, Kinney et al. (2004) used the technique of resonant ultrasound spectroscopy (RUS) to measure the elastic constants (C_{ij}) of human dentin from both wet and dry samples. $As^*(\%)$ and $Ac^*(\%)$ calculated from these data are included in both Table 8.5 and Figure 8.4. Their data showed that the samples exhibited transverse isotropic symmetry. However, the C_{ij} for dry dentin implied even higher symmetry. Indeed, the result of using the average value for C_{11} and $C_{12} = 36.6$ GPa and the value for $C_{44} = 14.7$ GP for dry dentin in the calculations suggests that dry human dentin is very nearly elastically isotropic. This isotropic-like behavior of the dry dentin may have clinical significance. There is independent experimental evidence to support this calculation of isotropy based on the ultrasonic data. Small-angle x-ray diffraction of human dentin yielded results implying isotropy near the pulp and mild anisotropy in mid-dentin (Kinney et al. 2001).

It is interesting to note that Haversian bones, whether human or bovine, have both their compressive and shear anisotropy factors considerably lower than the respective values for plexiform bone. Thus, not only is plexiform bone both stiffer and more rigid than the Haversian bone, it is also more anisotropic. These two scalar anisotropy quantities also provide a means of assessing whether there is the possibility either of systematic errors in the measurements and/or artifacts in the modeling of the elastic properties of hard tissues. This is determined when the values of $Ac^*(\%)$ and/or $As^*(\%)$ are much greater than the close range of lower values obtained by calculations on a variety of different ultrasonic measurements (Table 8.5). A possible example of this is the value of $As^*(\%) = 7.88$ calculated from the mechanical testing data of Knets (1978), Table 8.2.

8.6 Modeling Elastic Behavior

Currey (1964) first presented some preliminary ideas of modeling bone as a composite material composed of a simple linear superposition of collagen and Ap. He followed this later (1969) with an attempt to take into account the orientation of the Ap crystallites using a model proposed by Cox (1952) for fiber-reinforced composites. Katz (1971a) and Piekarski (1973) independently showed that the use of Voigt and Reuss or even Hashin and Shtrikman (1963) composite modeling showed the limitations of using linear combinations of either elastic moduli or elastic compliances. The failure of all these early models could be traced to the fact that they were based only on considerations of material properties. This is comparable to trying to determine the properties of an Eiffel Tower built using a composite material by simply modeling the composite material properties without considering void spaces and the interconnectivity of the structure (Lakes, 1993). In neither case is the complexity of the structural organization involved. This consideration of hierarchical organization clearly must be introduced into the modeling.

Katz in a number of papers (1971b, 1976) and meeting presentations put forth the hypothesis that the Haversian bone should be modeled as a hierarchical composite, eventually adapting a hollow fiber composite model by Hashin and Rosen (1964). Bonfield and Grynpas (1977) used extensional (longitudinal) ultrasonic wave propagation in both wet and dry bovine femoral cortical bone specimens oriented at angles of 5°, 10°, 20°, 40°, 50°, 70°, 80°, and 85° with respect to the long bone axis. They compared their experimental results for Young's moduli with the theoretical curve predicted by Currey's model (1969); this is shown in Figure 8.7. The lack of agreement led them to "conclude, therefore that an alternative model is required to account for the dependence of Young's modulus on orientation" (Bonfield and Grynpas, 1977, p. 454). Katz (1980, 1981), applying his hierarchical material–structure composite model, showed that the data in Figure 8.7 could be explained by considering different amounts of Ap crystallites aligned parallel to the long bone axis; this is shown in Figure 8.8. This early attempt at hierarchical micromechanical modeling is now being extended with more sophisticated modeling using either finite-element micromechanical computations (Hogan, 1992) or homogenization theory (Crolet et al., 1993). Further improvements will come by including more definitive information on the structural organization of collagen and Ap at the molecular–ultrastructural level (Wagner and Weiner, 1992; Weiner and Traub, 1989).

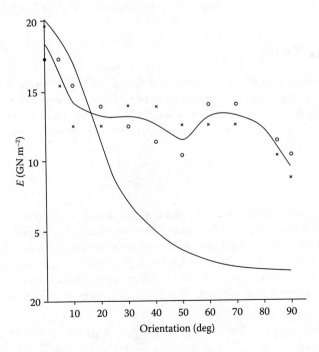

FIGURE 8.7   Variation in Young's modulus of bovine femur specimens (E) with the orientation of specimen axis to the long axis of the bone, for wet (o) and dry (x) conditions compared with the theoretical curve (———) predicted from a fiber-reinforced composite model. (Reprinted by permission from Macmillan Publishers Ltd. *Nature, London*, Bonfield W, Grynpas MD. Anisotropy of Young's modulus of bone. 270:453, Copyright 1977.)

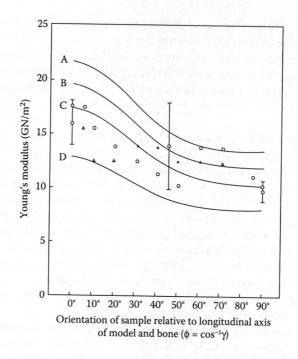

FIGURE 8.8 Comparison of predictions of Katz two-level composite model with the experimental data of Bonfield and Grynpas. Each curve represents a different lamellar configuration within a single osteon, with longitudinal fibers; A, 64%; B, 57%; C, 50%; D, 37%; and the rest of the fibers assumed horizontal. (From Katz JL, *Mechanical Properties of Bone*, AMD, Vol. 45, New York, American Society of Mechanical Engineers, 1981, with permission.)

8.7 Viscoelastic Properties

As stated earlier, bone (along with all other biologic tissues) is a viscoelastic material. Clearly, for such materials, Hooke's law for linear elastic materials must be replaced by a constitutive equation which includes the time dependency of the material properties. The behavior of an anisotropic linear viscoelastic material may be described by using the Boltzmann superposition integral as a constitutive equation:

$$\sigma_{ij}(t) = \int_{-\infty}^{t} C_{ijkl}(t - \tau) \frac{d\epsilon_{kl}(\tau)}{d\tau} d\tau \tag{8.17}$$

where $\sigma_{ij}(t)$ and $\epsilon_{kl}(\tau)$ are the time-dependent second rank stress and strain tensors, respectively, and $C_{ijkl}(t-\tau)$ is the fourth-rank relaxation modulus tensor. This tensor has 36 independent elements for the lowest symmetry case and 12 nonzero independent elements for an orthotropic solid. Again, as for linear elasticity, a reduced notation is used, that is, $11 \rightarrow 1$, $22 \rightarrow 2$, $33 \rightarrow 3$, $23 \rightarrow 4$, $31 \rightarrow 5$, and $12 \rightarrow 6$. If we apply Equation 8.17 to the case of an orthotropic material, for example, plexiform bone, in uniaxial tension (compression) in the 1 direction (Lakes and Katz, 1974), in this case using the reduced notation, we obtain

$$\sigma_1(t) = \int_{-\infty}^{t} \left[C_{11}(t - \tau) \frac{d\epsilon_1(\tau)}{d\tau} + C_{12}(t - \tau) \frac{d\epsilon_2(\tau)}{d\tau} + C_{13}(t - \tau) \frac{d\epsilon_3(\tau)}{d\tau} \right] d\tau \tag{8.18}$$

$$\sigma_2(t) = \int_{-\infty}^{t} \left[C_{21}(t - \tau) \frac{d\epsilon_1(\tau)}{d\tau} + C_{22}(t - \tau) \frac{d\epsilon_2(\tau)}{d\tau} + C_{23}(t - \tau) \frac{d\epsilon_3(\tau)}{d\tau} \right] = 0 \tag{8.19}$$

for all t, and

$$\sigma_3(t) = \int_{-\infty}^{t}\left[C_{31}(t-\tau)\frac{d\epsilon_1(\tau)}{d\tau} + C_{32}(t-\tau)\frac{d\epsilon_2(\tau)}{d\tau} + C_{33}(t-\tau)\frac{d\epsilon_3(\tau)}{d\tau}\right]d\tau = 0 \qquad (8.20)$$

for all t.

Having the integrands vanish provides an obvious solution to Equations 8.19 and 8.20. Solving them simultaneously for $[d\epsilon_2^{(\tau)}]/d\tau$ and $[d\epsilon_3^{(\tau)}]/d\tau$ substituting these values into Equation 8.17 yields

$$\sigma_1(t) = \int_{-\infty}^{t} E_1(t-\tau)\frac{d\epsilon_1(\tau)}{d\tau}d\tau \qquad (8.21)$$

where, if for convenience we adopt the notation C_{ij}; $C_{ij}(t-\tau)$, then Young's modulus is given by

$$E_1(t-\tau) = C_{11} + C_{12}\frac{[C_{31} - (C_{21}C_{33}/C_{23})]}{[(C_{21}C_{33}/C_{23}) - C_{32}]} + C_{13}\frac{[C_{21} - (C_{31}C_{22}/C_{32})]}{[(C_{22}C_{33}/C_{32})/ - C_{23}]} \qquad (8.22)$$

In this case of uniaxial tension (compression), only nine independent orthotropic tensor components are involved, the three shear components being equal to zero. Still, this time-dependent Young's modulus is a rather complex function. As in the linear elastic case, the inverse form of the Boltzmann integral can be used; this would constitute the compliance formulation.

If we consider the bone being driven by a strain at a frequency ω, with a corresponding sinusoidal stress lagging by an angle δ, then the complex Young's modulus $E^*(\omega)$ may be expressed as

$$E^*(\omega) = E'(\omega) + iE''(\omega) \qquad (8.23)$$

where $E'(\omega)$, which represents the stress–strain ratio in phase with the strain, is known as the storage modulus, and $E''(\omega)$, which represents the stress–strain ratio 90° out of phase with the strain, is known as the loss modulus. The ratio of the loss modulus to the storage modulus is then equal to tan d. Usually, data are presented by a graph of the storage modulus along with a graph of tan d, both against frequency. For a more complete development of the values of $E'(\omega)$ and $E''(\omega)$, as well as for the derivation of other viscoelastic technical moduli, see Lakes and Katz (1974); for a similar development of the shear storage and loss moduli, see Cowin (1989).

Thus, for a more complete understanding of bone's response to applied loads, it is important to know its rheologic properties. There have been a number of early studies of the viscoelastic properties of various long bones (Sedlin, 1965; Smith and Keiper, 1965; Lugassy, 1968; Laird and Kingsbury, 1973; Black and Korostoff, 1973). However, none of these was performed over a wide enough range of frequency (or time) to completely define the viscoelastic properties measured, for example, creep or stress relaxation. Thus it is not possible to mathematically transform one property into any other to compare results of three different experiments on different bones (Lakes and Katz, 1974).

In the first experiments over an extended frequency range, the biaxial viscoelastic as well as uniaxial viscoelastic properties of wet cortical human and bovine femoral bone were measured using both dynamic and stress relaxation techniques over eight decades of frequency (time) (Lakes et al., 1979). The results of these experiments showed that bone was both nonlinear and thermorheologically complex, that is, time–temperature superposition could not be used to extend the range of viscoelastic measurements. A nonlinear constitutive equation was developed based on these measurements (Lakes and Katz, 1979a). In addition, relaxation spectrums for both human and bovine cortical bone were obtained; Figure 8.9 shows the former (Lakes and Katz, 1979b). The contributions of several mechanisms to the

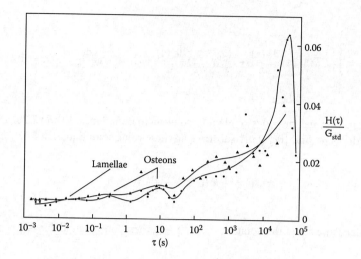

FIGURE 8.9 Comparison of relaxation spectra for wet human bone, specimens 5 and 6 (Lakes et al., 1979) in simple torsion; $T = 37°C$. First approximation from relaxation and dynamic data. • Human tibial bone, specimen 6. Δ Human tibial bone, specimen 5, $G_{std} = G(10\ s)$. $G_{std}(5) = G(10\ s)$. $G_{std}(5) = 0.590 \times 10^6\ lb/in^2$. $G_{std}(6) \times 0.602 \times 10^6$ lb/in^2. (Courtesy *Journal of Biomechanics*, Pergamon Press.)

loss tangent of cortical bone are shown in Figure 8.10 (Lakes and Katz, 1979b). It is interesting to note that almost all the major loss mechanisms occur at frequencies (times) at or close to those in which there are "bumps," indicating possible strain energy dissipation, on the relaxation spectra shown in Figure 8.9. An extensive review of the viscoelastic properties of bone can be found in *Natural and Living Biomaterials*, CRC Press (Lakes and Katz, 1984).

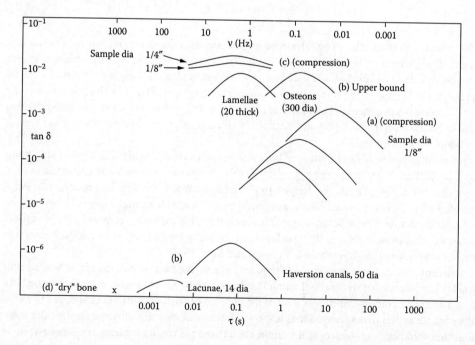

FIGURE 8.10 Contributions of several relaxation mechanisms to the loss tangent of cortical bone. (a) Homogeneous thermoelastic effect. (b) Inhomogeneous thermoelastic effect. (c) Fluid flow effect. (d) Piezoelectric effect. (From Lakes RS, Katz JL. *Natural and Living Tissues*. Boca Raton, FL: CRC Press; 1984. pp. 1–87. Courtesy CRC Press.)

Following on Katz's (1976, 1980) adaptation of the Hashin–Rosen hollow fiber composite model (1964), Gottesman and Hashin (1979) presented a viscoelastic calculation using the same major assumptions.

8.8 Related Research

As stated earlier, this chapter has concentrated on the elastic and viscoelastic properties of compact cortical bone and the elastic properties of trabecular bone. At present there is considerable research activity on the fracture properties of the bone. Professor William Bonfield and his associates at Queen Mary and Westfield College, University of London and Professor Dwight Davy and his colleagues at Case Western Reserve University are among those who publish regularly in this area. Review of the literature is necessary in order to become acquainted with the state of bone fracture mechanics.

An excellent introductory monograph which provides a fascinating insight into the structure–property relationships in bones including aspects of the two areas discussed immediately above is Professor John D. Currey's *Bones Structure and Mechanics* (2002), the 2nd edition of his book, *The Mechanical Adaptations of Bones,* Princeton University Press (1984).

8.9 Dentin Structure and Composition

Dentin is the hydrated composite structure that constitutes the body of each tooth, providing both a protective covering for the pulp and serving as a support for the overlying enamel. Dentin is composed of approximately 45–50% inorganic material, 30–35% organic material, and 20% fluid by volume. Dentin mineral is a carbonate rich, calcium-deficient apatite (Marshall et al. 1997). The organic component is predominantly type I collagen with minor contribution from other proteins (Gage et al. 1989; Linde 1989; Butler 1992). The apatite mineralites are of very small size and are deposited almost exclusively within the collagen fibril (see, e.g., Arsenault 1989). The interactions between collagen and nanocrystalline mineralite gives rise to the stiffness of the dentin structure. The consequent dentin elasticity is an important feature that determines the mechanical behavior of the tooth structure.

The structural characteristics of sound dentin are well known at the micro-scale ($\sim$100 μm). Dentin is described as a system of dentinal tubules surrounded by a collar of highly mineralized peritubular dentin (Wang and Weiner 1998). The tubules traverse the structure from the pulp cavity to the region just below the dentin–enamel junction (DEJ) or the dentin–cementum junction (CEJ). The tubules, which are described as narrow tunnels a few microns or less in diameter as shown in Figure 8.11, represent the tracks taken by the odontoblastic cells from the pulp chamber to the respective junctions. Tubule density, size, and orientation vary from location to location. The density and size are lowest close to the DEJ and highest at the predentin surface at the junction to the pulp chamber. Dentinal tubule diameter measures approximately 2.5 μm near the pulp and 0.9 μm near the DEJ (Ten Cate 1994). The porosity of dentin varies from 0 to 0.25 from the DEJ to the pulp (Manly and Deakins 1940; Koutsi et al. 1994; Sumikawa et al. 1999). The rate of change in porosity with depth depends on the tooth type. In primary tooth dentin, the dentinal tubule density and size is, in general, larger than in permanent dentin (Sumikawa et al. 1999).

The composition of the peritubular dentin is carbonated apatite with very small amounts of organic matrix whereas intertubular dentin, that is, the dentin separating the tubules, is type I collagen matrix reinforced with apatite. Based upon electron microscopic studies, peritubular dentin in primary teeth has been found to be 2–5 times thicker than that of permanent teeth (Hirayama et al. 1986). The composition of intertubular dentin is primarily mineralized collagen fibrils; the fibrils are described as a composite of a collagen framework and thin plate-shaped carbonate apatite crystals whose c-axes are aligned with the collagen fibril axis (Weiner et al. 1999). In sound dentin, the majority of the mineralized collagen fibrils are perpendicular to the tubules (Jones and Boyde 1984). The crystal organization in peritubular and intertubular dentin are similar, but the macromolecular constituents are not. The amino acid compositions of the principal proteins in peritubular dentin are high in

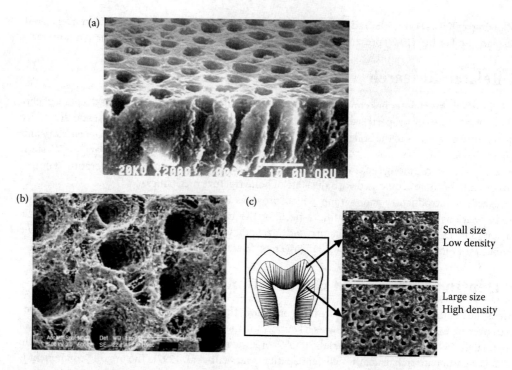

FIGURE 8.11   SEM micrograph showing (a) the spatial distribution of dentin tubules, (b) partially demineralized dentin indicating the orientations of inter-tubular collagen fibrils, and (c) that tubule opening is larger and spacing is denser for deep dentin as opposed to shallow dentin. As shown, the structure and properties of dentin substrate vary with location. (From Marshall GW et al. *J Dent* 1997; 25(6):441–458.)

serine and probably phosphoserine, but they are not similar to the phosphophoryns of intertubular dentin (Weiner et al. 1999). Water in dentin may be classified as either free or bound. Water is present within the dentinal tubules as pulpal fluid and within the interstitial spaces between collagen fibrils. Based upon experimental chemical microanalyses, bound water is likely present as hydroxyl groups bound to the mineral component (Gruner et al. 1937; LeFevre and Hodge 1937; Bird et al. 1940). Mass density measurements were completed more than a century ago. Mass densities of permanent and deciduous dentin were determined by direct measurement of mass and volume of moist dentin slabs (Boyd et al. 1938) and by considering dry powdered fractions of teeth (Manly et al. 1939; Berghash and Hodge 1940). More recently, mineral densities of dentin have been measured using x-ray tomographic microscopy (Kinney et al. 1994) and back scattered scanning electron microscopy (BSEM) (Angker et al. 2004b).

8.10 Dentin Elasticity

Beginning in the 1960s, macro-scale elastic moduli of dentin have been measured by a variety of methods as reviewed by Kinney et al. (2003). Using nanoindentation methods, Kinney et al. (1999), have measured the elastic modulus of peri-tubular dentin and inter-tubular dentin. At somewhat larger, unspecified scales, Katz et al. (2001) measured similar values of dentin elastic modulus using scanning acoustic microscopy (SAM). At even higher scales, Lees and Rollins (1972) used longitudinal and shear wave velocity measurements, Kinney et al. (2004) used resonant ultrasound spectroscopy to determine elastic moduli of millimeter scale samples, and John (2006) used longitudinal velocity measurements on approximately millimeter thick slices to find location-dependent elastic moduli. Primary tooth dentin

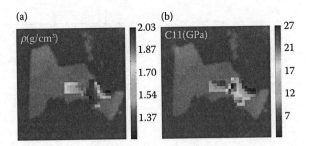

FIGURE 8.12 Micro-scale distribution of (a) density and (b) elastic modulus of carious, caries-affected and sound regions of primary dentin using homotopic measurements from SAM and BSEM. Background image is the SAM C-scan of the tooth sample. (From Marangos, O. et al. *Acta Biomaterial* 2009; 5:1338–1348.)

mechanical properties have been studied at nano-scales using nanoindentation (Hosoya and Marshall 2004; Hosoya and Marshall 2005; Hosoya and Tay 2007). Mechanical properties of primary dentin have also been studied at somewhat higher, unspecified scales (Angker et al. 2003, 2004a).

Recently, Marangos et al. (2009) have performed homotopic (same location) measurements with SAM and BSEM to obtain the micromechanical properties of carious, caries-affected, and sound primary tooth dentin. As a result, the relationships between micro-scale elastic moduli, density and composition of sound, carious, and caries-affected primary dentin were obtained. In Figure 8.12, we show the maps of mass density and the corresponding elastic moduli. In the sound dentin region, the mean and standard deviation of elastic modulus was found to be 10 ± 2 GPa. These values are somewhat lower than Young's moduli reported for inner primary tooth dentin at locations close to the pulp wall (ranging from 2.88 to 19.68 GPa in Angker et al. (2003), and 14.00–22.84 GPa in Hosoya and Marshall (2005)). The low values observed in our measurement were likely caused by resorption prior to natural exfoliation. We further observe that in caries-affected locations, the elastic modulus is higher than the carious or sound dentin regions. Previous studies have indicated the presence of hypermineralized dentin or sclerotic dentin in the vicinity of carious lesions (Driessens and Woltgens 1986; Ten Cate 1994; Nakajima et al. 1999; Marshall et al. 2001). The higher values of elastic modulus could be attributed to a higher level of mineralization in these locations. It is noteworthy however that sclerotic dentin is not always present below carious lesions (Hosoya and Marshall 2004). The conditions under which hypermineralization occurs in proximity of carious dentin remains unclear and needs further investigation. In region 2, that is locations in carious dentin, the elastic modulus varies over a large range. It is well known that carious locations are highly heterogeneous with widely varying degree and extent of demineralization.

Clearly, the mineral content has a significant effect on the elastic modulus. Previous investigators have attempted to correlate the mineral content to elastic modulus in dentin (Angker et al. 2004a; Bembey et al. 2005). Figure 8.13 shows the plot of elastic modulus versus the mineral volume fraction and total porosity for the 89 locations displayed in Figure 8.12. In general, the elastic modulus increases with the mineral content, and it decreases with the porosity. However, a single correlation cannot be used to describe the relationship between the elastic modulus and composition. At certain mineral volume fraction and porosity, the elastic modulus variation is found to be as large as five times. Thus, the mineral content or porosity alone cannot be used to uniquely determine the elastic modulus. Similar observations have been made regarding the elastic properties of bone (Oyen et al. 2008). At the fundamental level, the interactions between collagen and nanocrystalline mineralite gives rise to the stiffness of the dentin structure. Indeed, the various efforts (Hellmich et al. 2004; Nikolov and Raabe 2008) to calculate calcified tissue moduli based upon constituent phases suggest that the mechanical behavior of these tissues at various hierarchical scales may not be determined by simply considering the composition but rather additional interaction at the collagen/mineral interface must be considered.

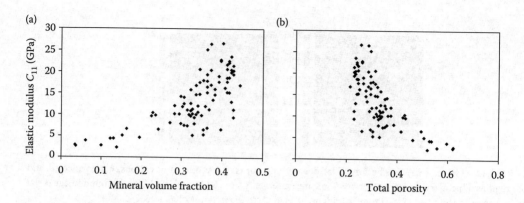

FIGURE 8.13 Elastic modulus plotted against (a) the mass density, and (b) mineral volume fraction. Using data from Figure 8.2. (From Marangos, O. et al. *Acta Biomaterial* 2009; 5:1338–1348.)

Defining Terms

Apatite: Calcium phosphate compound, stoichiometric chemical formula $Ca_5(PO_4)_3 \cdot X$, where X is OH– (hydroxyapatite), F– (fluorapatite), Cl– (chlorapatite), and so on. There are two molecules in the basic crystal unit cell.

Cancellous bone: Also known as porous, spongy, trabecular bone. Found in the regions of the articulating ends of tubular bones, in vertebrae, ribs, and so on.

Cortical bone: The dense compact bone found throughout the shafts of long bones such as the femur, tibia, and so on also found in the outer portions of other bones in the body.

Haversian bone: Also called osteonic. The form of bone found in adult humans and mature mammals, consisting mainly of concentric lamellar structures, surrounding a central canal called the Haversian canal, plus lamellar remnants of older Haversian systems (osteons) called interstitial lamellae.

Interstitial lamellae: See Haversian bone above.

Orthotropic: The symmetrical arrangement of structure in which there are three distinct orthogonal axes of symmetry. In crystals this symmetry is called orthothombic.

Osteons: See Haversian bone above.

Plexiform: Also called laminar. The form of parallel lamellar bone found in younger, immature nonhuman mammals.

Transverse isotropy: The symmetry arrangement of structure in which there is a unique axis perpendicular to a plane in which the other two axes are equivalent. The long bone direction is chosen as the unique axis. In crystals this symmetry is called hexagonal.

References

Angker L, Nijhof N, Swain MV, Kilpatrick NM. Influence of hydration and mechanical characterization of carious primary dentine using an ultra-micro indentation system (UMIS). *Eur J Oral Sci* 2004b; 112(3):231–6.

Angker L, Nockolds C, Swain MV, Kilpatrick N. Correlating the mechanical properties to the mineral content of carious dentine—A comparative study using an ultra-micro indentation system (UMIS) and SEM-BSE signals. *Arch Oral Biol* 2004a; 49(5):369–78.

Angker L, Swain MV, Kilpatrick N. Micro-mechanical characterisation of the properties of primary tooth dentine. *J Dent* 2003; 31(4):261–7.

Arsenault AL. A comparative electron microscopic study of apatite crystals in collagen fibrils of rat bone, dentin and calcified turkey leg tendons. *Bone Miner* 1989; 6(2):165–77.

Ashman RB, Rho JY. Elastic modulus of trabecular bone material. *J Biomech* 1988; 21:177.

Bembey AK, Oyen ML, Ko C-C, Bushby AJ, Boyde A. Elastic modulus and mineral density of dentine and enamel in natural caries lesions. In: Fratzl P, Landis WJ, Wang R, Silver FH (Eds). *Structure and Mechanical Behavior of Biological Materials*. Warrendale: MRS; 2005. pp. 125–130.

Berghash, SR, Hodge HC. Density and refractive index studies of dental hard tissues III: Density distribution of deciduous enamel and dentin. *J Dent Res* 1940; 19(5):487–95.

Bird MJ, French EL, Woodside MR, Morrison MI, Hodge HC. Chemical analyses of deciduous enamel and dentin. *J Dent Res* 1940; 19(4):413–23.

Black J, Korostoff E. Dynamic mechanical properties of viable human cortical bone. *J Biomech* 1973; 6:435.

Bonfield W, Grynpas MD. Anisotropy of Young's modulus of bone. *Nature, London* 1977; 270:453.

Boyd JD, Drain CL, Deakins ML. Method for determining the specific gravity of dentin and its application to permanent and deciduous teeth. *J Dent Res* 1938; 17(6):465–469.

Bumrerraj S, Katz JL. Scanning acoustic microscopy study of human cortical and trabecular bone. *Ann Biomed Eng* 2001; 29:1.

Butler WT. Dentin extracellular matrix and dentinogenesis. *Oper Dent* 1992; Suppl 5:18–23.

Choi K, Goldstein SA. A comparison of the fatigue behavior of human trabecular and cortical bone tissue. *J Biomech* 1992; 25:1371.

Chung DH, Buessem WR. In: Vahldiek FW and Mersol SA (eds), *Anisotropy in Single-Crystal Refractory Compounds*, Vol. 2, New York: Plenum Press; 1968. p. 217.

Cowin SC. *Bone Mechanics*. Boca Raton, FL: CRC Press; 1989

Cowin SC. *Bone Mechanics Handbook*. Boca Raton, FL: CRC Press; 2001.

Cox HL. The elasticity and strength of paper and other fibrous materials. *Br Appl Phys* 1952; 3:72.

Crolet JM, Aoubiza B, Meunier A. Compact bone: Numerical simulation of mechanical characteristics. *J Biomech* 1993; 26(6):677.

Currey JD. *Bone Structure and Mechanics*. New Jersey: Princeton University Press; 2002.

Currey JD. *The Mechanical Adaptations of Bones*. New Jersey: Princeton University Press; 1984.

Currey JD. The relationship between the stiffness and the mineral content of bone. *J Biomech* 1969; (2):477.

Currey JD. Three analogies to explain the mechanical properties of bone. *Biorheology* 1964; (2):1.

Driessens FCM, Woltgens JHM. *Tooth Development and Caries*. Boca Raton, FL: CRC Press; 1986. pp. 132–137.

Gage JP, Francis MJO, Triffitt JT. *Collagen and Dental Matrices*. Boston: Wright; 1989. pp. 21–24.

Gottesman T, Hashin Z. Analysis of viscoelastic behavior of bones on the basis of microstructure. *J Biomech* 1979; 13:89.

Gruner JW, McConnell D, Armstrong WD. The relationship between crystal structure and chemical composition of enamel and dentin. *J Biol Chem* 1937; 121(2):771–781.

Hashin Z, Rosen BW. The elastic moduli of fiber reinforced materials. *J Appl Mech* 1964; (31):223.

Hashin Z, Shtrikman S. A variational approach to the theory of elastic behavior of multiphase materials. *J Mech Phys Solids* 1963; (11):127.

Hastings GW, Ducheyne P (eds). *Natural and Living Biomaterials*, Boca Raton, FL: CRC Press; 1984.

Hellmich C, Ulm FJ, Dormieux L. Can the diverse elastic properties of trabecular and cortical bone be attributed to only a few tissue-independent phase properties and their interactions? *Biomech Model Mechanobiol* 2004; 2(4):219–38.

Herring GM. Methods for the study of the glycoproteins and proteoglycans of bone using bacterial collagenase. Determination of bone sialoprotein and chondroitin sulphate. *Calcif Tiss Res* 1977; (24):29.

Hirayama A, Yamada M, Miake K. An electron microscopic study on dentinal tubules of human deciduous teeth. *Shikwa Gakuho* 1986; 86(6):1021–31.

Hogan HA. Micromechanics modeling of haversian cortical bone properties. *J Biomech* 1992; 25(5):549.

Hosoya Y, Marshall GW. The nano-hardness and elastic modulus of carious and sound primary canine dentin. *Oper Dent* 2004; 29(2):142–9.

Hosoya Y, Marshall GW. The nano-hardness and elastic modulus of sound deciduous canine dentin and young premolar dentin—Preliminary study. *J Mater Sci Mater Med* 2005; 16(1):1–8.

Hosoya Y, Tay FR. Hardness, elasticity, and ultrastructure of bonded sound and caries-affected primary tooth dentin. *J Biomed Mater Res B Appl Biomater* 2007; 81B(1):135–141.

John C. Lateral distribution of ultrasound velocity in horizontal layers of human teeth. *J Acoust Soc Am* 2006; 119(2):1214–1226.

Jones SJ, Boyde A. Ultrastructure of dentine and dentinogenesis. In: Linde A. (ed), *Dentine and Dentinogenesis*. Boca Raton, FL: CRC Press; 1984. pp. 81–134.

Katz JL. Anisotropy of Young's modulus of bone. *Nature* 1980; 283:106.

Katz JL. Composite material models for cortical bone. In: Cowin SC (ed), *Mechanical Properties of Bone*, AMD, Vol. 45, New York: American Society of Mechanical Engineers; 1981. pp. 171–184.

Katz JL. Elastic properties of calcified tissues. *Isr J Med Sci* 1971b; 7:439.

Katz JL. Hard tissue as a composite material: I. Bounds on the elastic behavior. *J Biomech* 1971a; 4:455.

Katz JL. Hierarchical modeling of compact haversian bone as a fiber reinforced material. In: Mates, RE and Smith, CR (eds), *Advances in Bioengineering*. New York: American Society of Mechanical Engineers; 1976. pp. 17–18.

Katz JL, Bumrerraj S, Dreyfuss J, Wang Y, Spencer P. Micromechanics of the dentin/adhesive interface. *J Biomed Mater Res* 2001; 58(4):366.

Katz JL, Meunier A. The elastic anisotropy of bone. *J Biomech* 1987; 20:1063.

Katz JL, Meunier A. A generalized method for characterizing elastic anisotropy in solid living tissues. *J Mat Sci Mater Med* 1990; 1:1.

Katz JL, Ukraincik K. A fiber-reinforced model for compact haversian bone. *Program and Abstracts of the 16th Annual Meeting of the Biophysical Society*, 28a FPM-C15, Toronto, 1972.

Katz JL, Ukraincik K. On the anisotropic elastic properties of hydroxyapatite. *J Biomech* 1971; 4:221.

Keaveny TM, Hayes WC. A 20-year perspective on the mechanical properties of trabecular bone. *J Biomech Eng* 1993; 115:535.

Kinney JH, Balooch M, Marshall GW, Marshall SJ. A micromechanics model of the elastic properties of human dentine. *Arch Oral Biol* 1999; 44(10):813–22.

Kinney JH, Gladden JR, Marshall GW, Marshall SJ, So JH, Maynard JD. Resonant ultrasound spectroscopy measurements of the elastic constants in human dentin. *J Biomech* 2004; 37(4):437–41.

Kinney JH, Marshall GW Jr, Marshall SJ. Three-dimensional mapping of mineral densities in carious dentin: Theory and method. *Scanning Microsc* 1994; 8(2):197–205.

Kinney JH, Marshall SJ, Marshall GW. The mechanical properties of human dentin: A critical review and re-evaluation of the dental literature. *Crit Rev Oral Biol Med* 2003; 14(1):13–29.

Kinney JH, Pople JA, Marshall GW, Marshall SJ. Collagen orientation and crystallite size in human dentin: A small angle x-ray scattering study. *Calcif Tissue Inter* 2001; 69:31.

Knets IV. Mechanics of biological tissues. A review. *Mekhanika Polimerov* 1978; 13:434.

Koutsi V, Noonan RG, Horner JA, Simpson MD, Matthews WG, Pashley DH. The effect of dentin depth on the permeability and ultrastructure of primary molars. *Pediatr Dent* 1994; 16(1):29–35.

Laird GW, Kingsbury HB. Complex viscoelastic moduli of bovine bone. *J Biomech* 1973; 6:59.

Lakes RS. Materials with structural hierarchy. *Nature* 1993; 361:511.

Lakes RS, Katz JL. Interrelationships among the viscoelastic function for anisotropic solids: Application to calcified tissues and related systems. *J Biomech* 1974; 7:259.

Lakes RS, Katz JL. Viscoelastic properties and behavior of cortical bone. Part II. Relaxation mechanisms. *J Biomech* 1979a; 12:679.

Lakes RS, Katz JL. Viscoelastic properties of bone. In: GW Hastings and P Ducheyne (eds), *Natural and Living Tissues*. Boca Raton, FL: CRC Press; 1984. pp. 1–87.

Lakes RS, Katz JL. Viscoelastic properties of wet cortical bone: III. A nonlinear constitutive equation. *J Biomech* 1979b; 12:689.

Lakes RS, Katz JL, Sternstein SS. Viscoelastic properties of wet cortical bone: I. Torsional and biaxial studies. *J Biomech* 1979; 12:657.

Lang SB. Elastic coefficients of animal bone. *Science* 1969; 165:287.

Lees S, Rollins FR. Anisotropy in hard dental tissues. *J Biomech* 1972; 5(6):557–66.

LeFevre ML, Hodge HC. Chemical analysis of tooth samples composed of enamel, dentine and cementum. II. *J Dent Res* 1937; 16(4):279–87.

Linde A. Dentin matrix proteins: Composition and possible functions in calcification. *Anat Record* 1989; 224(2): 154–66.

Lipson SF, Katz JL. The relationship between elastic properties and microstructure of bovine cortical bone. *J Biomech* 1984; 4:231.

Lugassy AA. Mechanical and viscoelastic properties of bone and dentin in compression. Thesis, Metallurgy and Materials Science, University of Pennsylvania, 1968.

Maharidge R. Ultrasonic properties and microstructure of bovine bone and Haversian bovine bone modeling. Thesis, Rensselaer Polytechnic Institute, Troy, NY, 1984.

Manly RS, Deakins ML. Changes in the volume per cent of moisture, organic and inorganic material in dental caries. *J Dent Res* 1940; 19(2):165–70.

Manly RS, Hodge CH, Ange LE. Density and refractive index studies of dental hard tissues II: Density distribution curves. *J Dent Res* 1939; 18(3):203–11.

Marangos O, Misra A, Spencer P, Bohaty B, Katz JL. Physico-mechanical properties determination using microscale homotopic measurement: Application to sound and caries-affected primary tooth dentin. *Acta Biomaterial* 2009; 5:1338–1348.

Marshall GW, Habelitz S, Gallagher R, Balooch M, Balooch G, Marshall SJ. Nanomechanical properties of hydrated carious human dentin. *J Dent Res* 2001; 80(8):1768–1771.

Marshall GW, Marshall SJ, Kinney JH, Balooch M. The dentin substrate: Structure and properties related to bonding. *J Dent* 1997; 25(6):441–458.

Nakajima M, Ogata M, Okuda M, Tagami J, Sano H, Pashley DH. Bonding to caries-affected dentin using self-etching primers. *Am J Dent* 1999; 12(6):309–314.

Nikolov S, Raabe D. Hierarchical modeling of the elastic properties of bone at submicron scales: The role of extrafibrillar mineralization. *Biophys J* 2008; 94(11):4220–4232.

Oyen ML, Ferguson VL, Bembey AK, Bushby AJ, Boyde A. Composite bounds on the elastic modulus of bone. *J Biomech* 2008; 41(11):2585–2588.

Park JB. *Biomaterials: An Introduction*. New York: Plenum, 1979.

Pellegrino ED, Biltz RM. The composition of human bone in uremia. *Medicine* 1965; 44:397.

Piekarski K. Analysis of bone as a composite material. *Int J Eng Sci* 1973; 10:557.

Reuss A. Berechnung der fliessgrenze von mischkristallen auf grund der plastizitatsbedingung fur einkristalle, A. *Zeits Angew Math Mech* 1929; 9:49–58.

Rho JY, Ashman RB, Turner CH. Young's modulus of trabecular and cortical bone material; ultrasonic and microtensile measurements. *J Biomech* 1993; 26:111.

Rho JY, Roy ME, Tsui TY, Pharr GM. Elastic properties of microstructural components of human bone tissue as measured by indentation. *J Biomed Mat Res* 1999; 45:48.

Ryan SD, Williams JL. Tensile testing of rodlike trabeculae excised from bovine femoral bone. *J Biomech* 1989; 22:351.

Sedlin E. A rheological model for cortical bone. *Acta Orthop Scand* 1965; 36 (suppl 83).

Smith R, Keiper D. Dynamic measurement of viscoelastic properties of bone. *Am J Med Elec* 1965; 4:156.

Sumikawa DA, Marshall GW, Gee L, Marshall SJ. Microstructure of primary tooth dentin. *Pediatr Dent* 1999; 21(7): 439–44.

Ten Cate AR. Repair and regeneration of dental tissue. In: Ten Cate AR (ed), *Oral Histology. Development, Structure, and Function*. St. Louis: Mosby; 1994. pp. 456–468.

Townsend PR, Rose RM, Radin EL. Buckling studies of single human trabeculae. *J Biomech* 1975; 8:199.

Turner CH, Rho JY, Takano Y, Tsui TY, Pharr GM. The elastic properties of trabecular and cortical bone tissues are similar: Results from two microscopic measurement techniques. *J Biomech* 1999; 32:437.

Van Buskirk WC, Ashman RB. The elastic moduli of bone. In: Cowin SC (ed), *Mechanical Properties of Bone AMD*, Vol. 45, New York: American Society of Mechanical Engineers; 1981. pp. 131–143.

Vejlens L. Glycosaminoglycans of human bone tissue: I. Pattern of compact bone in relation to age. *Calcif Tiss Res* 1971; 7:175.

Voigt W. Lehrbuch der Kristallphysik Teubner, Leipzig 1910; *Reprinted (1928) with an additional appendix.* Leipzig, Teubner, New York: Johnson Reprint; 1966.

Wagner HD, Weiner S. On the relationship between the microstructure of bone and its mechanical stiffness. *J Biomech* 1992; 25:1311.

Wainwright SA, Briggs WD, Currey JD, Gosline JM. *Mechanical Design in Organisms.* Princeton, NJ: Princeton University Press, 1982.

Wang R, Weiner S. Human root dentin: Structure anisotropy and Vickers microhardness isotropy. *Connect Tissue Res* 1998;39(4):269–279.

Weiner S, Traub W. Crystal size and organization in bone. *Conn Tissue Res* 1989; 21:259.

Weiner S, Veis A, Beniash E, Arad T, Dillon JW, Sabsay B, Siddiqui F. Peritubular dentin formation: Crystal organization and the macromolecular constituents in human teeth. *J Struct Biol* 1999; 126(1):27–41.

Yoon HS, Katz JL. Ultrasonic wave propagation in human cortical bone: I. Theoretical considerations of hexagonal symmetry. *J Biomech* 1976a; 9:407.

Yoon HS, Katz JL. Ultrasonic wave propagation in human cortical bone: II. Measurements of elastic properties and microhardness. *J Biomech* 1976b; 9:459.

Zheng, L, Hilton JF, Habelitz S, Marshall SJ, Marshall GW. Dentin caries activity status related to hardness and elasticity. *Eur J Oral Sci* 2003; 111(3):243–252.

Further Information

Several societies both in the United States and abroad hold annual meetings during which many presentations, both oral and poster, deal with hard tissue biomechanics. In the United States these societies include the Orthopaedic Research Society, the American Society of Mechanical Engineers, the Biomaterials Society, the American Society of Biomechanics, the Biomedical Engineering Society, and the Society for Bone and Mineral Research. In Europe there are alternate year meetings of the European Society of Biomechanics and the European Society of Biomaterials. Every four years there is a World Congress of Biomechanics; every three years there is a World Congress of Biomaterials. All of these meetings result in documented proceedings; some with extended papers in book form.

The two principal journals in which bone mechanics papers appear frequently are the *Journal of Biomechanics* published by Elsevier and the *Journal of Biomechanical Engineering* published by the American Society of Mechanical Engineers. Other society journals which periodically publish papers in the field are the *Journal of Orthopaedic Research* published for the Orthopaedic Research Society, the *Annals of Biomedical Engineering* published for the Biomedical Engineering Society, and the *Journal of Bone and Joint Surgery* (both American and English issues) for the American Academy of Orthopaedic Surgeons and the British Organization, respectively. Additional papers in the field may be found in the journal *Bone and Calcified Tissue International*.

The 1984 CRC volume, *Natural and Living Biomaterials* (Hastings GW and Ducheyne P, Eds.) provides a good historical introduction to the field. A recent more advanced book is *Bone Mechanics Handbook* (Cowin SC, Ed. 2001) the 2nd edition of *Bone Mechanics* (Cowin SC, Ed. 1989).

Many of the biomaterials journals and society meetings will have occasional papers dealing with hard tissue mechanics, especially those dealing with implant–bone interactions.

Appendix A

The Voigt and Reuss moduli for both transverse isotropic and orthotropic symmetry are given below:

Voigt Transverse Isotropic

$$K^V = \frac{2(C_{11} + C_{12}) + 4(C_{13} + C_{33})}{9}$$
$$G^V = \frac{(C_{11} + C_{12}) - 4C_{13} + 2C_{33} + 12(C_{44} + C_{66})}{30}$$
(A.1)

Reuss Transverse Isotropic

$$K_R = \frac{C_{33}(C_{11} + C_{12}) - 2C_{13}^2}{(C_{11} + C_{12} - 4C_{13} + 2C_{33})}$$
$$G_R = \frac{5[C_{33}(C_{11} + C_{12}) - 2C_{13}^2]C_{44}C_{66}}{2\{[C_{33}(C_{11} + C_{12}) - 2C_{13}^2](C_{44} + C_{66}) + [C_{44}C_{66}(2C_{11} + C_{12}) + 4C_{13} + C_{33}]/3\}}$$
(A.2)

Voigt Orthotropic

$$K^V = C_{11} + C_{22} + C_{33} + 2(C_{12} + C_{13} + C_{23})$$
$$G^V = \frac{[C_{11} + C_{22} + C_{33} + 3(C_{44} + C_{55} + C_{66}) - (C_{12} + C_{13} + C_{23})]}{15}$$
(A.3)

Reuss Orthotropic

$$K_R = \frac{\Delta}{\begin{array}{l} C_{11}C_{22} + C_{22}C_{33} + C_{33}C_{11} - 2(C_{11}C_{23} + C_{22}C_{13} + C_{33}C_{12}) \\ + 2(C_{12}C_{23} + C_{23}C_{13} + C_{13}C_{12}) - (C_{12}^2 + C_{13}^2 + C_{23}^2) \end{array}}$$
$$\begin{aligned} G_R = 15/(4\{&(C_{11}C_{22} + C_{22}C_{33} + C_{33}C_{11} + C_{11}C_{23} + C_{22}C_{13} + C_{33}C_{22}) \\ &- [C_{12}(C_{12} + C_{23}) + C_{23}(C_{23} + C_{13}) + C_{13}(C_{13} + C_{12})]\}/\Delta \\ &+ 3(1/C_{44} + 1/C_{55} + 1/C_{66})) \end{aligned}$$
(A.4)

where D is given in Equation 8.15.

9

Richard L. Lieber
*University of California,
San Diego*

*Veterans Administration
Medical Centers*

Samuel R. Ward
*University of California,
San Diego*

*Veterans Administration
Medical Centers*

Thomas J.
Burkholder
*Georgia Institute of
Technology*

Musculoskeletal Soft-Tissue Mechanics

9.1   Structure of Soft Tissues 9-1
      Cartilage • Tendon and Ligament • Muscle • Material
      Properties • Modeling
References.. 9-13

9.1 Structure of Soft Tissues

9.1.1 Cartilage

Articular cartilage is found at the ends of bones, where it serves as a shock absorber and reduces friction between articulating bones. It is best described as a hydrated proteoglycan (PG) gel supported by a sparse population of chondrocytes, and its composition and properties vary dramatically over its 1–2 mm thickness. The bulk composition of articular cartilage consists of approximately 20% collagen, 5% PG, primarily aggrecan bound to hyaluronic acid, with most of the remaining 75% water (Ker, 1999). At the articular surface, collagen fibrils are most dense, and arranged primarily in parallel with the surface. PG content is very low and chondrocytes are rare in this region. At the bony interface, collagen fibrils are oriented perpendicular to the articular surface, chondrocytes are more abundant, but PG content is low. PGs are most abundant in the middle zone, where collagen fibrils lack obvious orientation in association with the transition from parallel to perpendicular alignment.

Collagen itself is a fibrous protein composed of tropocollagen molecules. Tropocollagen is a triple-helical protein, which self-assembles into the long collagen fibrils observable at the ultrastructural level. These fibrils, in turn, aggregate and intertwine to form the ground substance of articular cartilage. When crosslinked into a dense network, as in the superficial zone of articular cartilage, collagen has a low permeability to water and helps to maintain the water cushion of the middle and deep zones. Collagen fibrils arranged in a random network, as in the middle zone, structurally immobilize the large PG aggregates, creating the solid phase of the composite material.

PGs consist of a number of negatively charged glycosaminoglycan chains bound to an aggrecan protein core. Aggrecan molecules, in turn, bind to a hyaluronic acid backbone, forming a PG of 50–100 MDa which carries a dense negative charge. This negative charge attracts positively charged ions (Na^+) from the extracellular fluid, and the resulting Donnan equilibrium results in rich hydration of the tissue creating an osmotic pressure that enables the tissue to function well as a shock absorber.

The overall structure of articular cartilage is analogous to a jelly-filled balloon. The PG-rich middle zone is osmotically pressurized, with fluid restrained from exiting the tissue by the dense collagen network of the superficial zone and the calcified structure of the deep bone. The interaction between the mechanical loading forces and osmotic forces yields the complex material properties of articular cartilage.

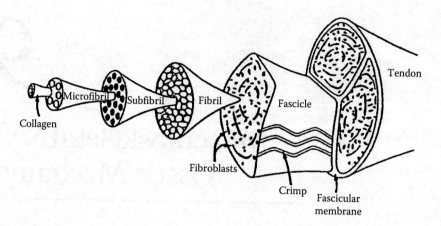

FIGURE 9.1 Tendons are organized in progressively larger filaments, beginning with molecular tropocollagen, and building to a complete tendon encased in a reticular sheath.

9.1.2 Tendon and Ligament

The passive tensile tissues, tendon and ligament, are also composed largely of water and collagen, but contain very little of the PGs that give cartilage its unique mechanical properties. In keeping with the functional role of these tissues, the collagen fibrils are organized primarily in long strands parallel to the axis of loading (Figure 9.1; Kastelic et al., 1978). The collagen fibrils, which may be hollow tubes (Gutsmann et al., 2003), combine in a hierarchical structure, with the 20–40 nm fibrils being bundled into 0.2–12 μm fibers. These fibers are birefringent under polarized light, reflecting an underlying wave or crimp structure with a periodicity between 20 and 100 μm. The fibers are bundled into fascicles, supported by fibroblasts or tenocytes, and surrounded by a fascicular membrane. Finally, multiple fascicles are bundled into a complete tendon or ligament encased in a reticular membrane.

As the tendon is loaded, the bending angle of the crimp structure of the collagen fibers can be seen to reversibly decrease, indicating that deformation of this structure is one source of elasticity. Individual collagen fibrils also display some inherent elasticity, and these two features are believed to determine the bulk properties of passive tensile tissues.

9.1.3 Muscle

9.1.3.1 Gross Morphology

Muscles are described as running from a proximal origin to a distal insertion. While these attachments are frequently discrete, distributed attachments, or even distinctly bifurcated attachments, are also common. The main mass of muscle fibers can be referred to as the belly. In a muscle with distinctly divided origins, the separate origins are often referred to as heads, and in a muscle with distinctly divided insertions, each mass of fibers terminating on distinct tendons is often referred to as a separate belly.

A muscle generally receives its blood supply from one main artery, which enters the muscle in a single, or sometimes two branches. Likewise, the major innervation is generally by a single nerve, which carries both motor efferents and sensory afferents.

Some muscles are functionally and structurally subdivided into compartments. A separate branch of the principle nerve generally innervates each compartment, and motor units of the compartments do not overlap. Generally, a dense connective tissue, or fascial, plane separates the compartments.

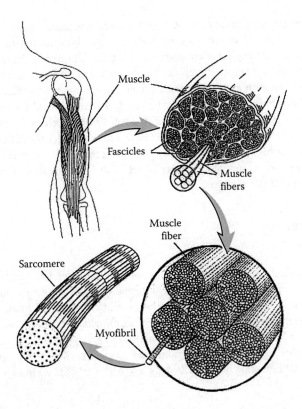

FIGURE 9.2 Skeletal muscle is organized in progressively larger filaments, beginning with molecular actin and myosin, arranged as myofibrils. Myofibrils assemble into sarcomeres and myofilaments. Myofilaments are assembled into myofibers, which are organized into the fascicles that form a whole muscle.

9.1.3.2 Fiber Architecture

Architecture, the arrangement of fibers within a muscle, determines the relationship between whole muscle length changes and force generation. The stereotypical muscle architecture is fusiform, with the muscle originating from a small tendonous attachment, inserting into a discrete tendon, and having fibers running generally parallel to the muscle axis (Figure 9.2). Fibers of unipennate muscles run parallel to each other but at an angle (pennation angle) to the muscle axis. Bipennate muscle fibers run in two distinct directions. Multipennate or fan-like muscles have one distinct attachment and one broad attachment, and pennation angle is different for every fiber. Strap-like muscles have parallel fibers that run from a broad bony origin to a broad insertion. As the length of each of these muscles is changed, the change in length of its fibers depends on fiber architecture. For example, fibers of a strap-like muscle undergo essentially the same length change as the muscle, where the length change of highly pennate fibers is reduced by their angle.

9.1.3.3 Sarcomere

Force generation in skeletal muscle results from the interaction between myosin and actin proteins. These molecules are arranged in antiparallel filaments, a 2–3 nm diameter thin filament composed mainly of actin, and a 20 nm diameter thick filament composed mainly of myosin. Myosin filaments are arranged in a hexagonal array, rigidly fixed at the M-line, and are the principal constituent of the A-band (anisotropic, light bending). Actin filaments are arranged in a complimentary hexagonal array and rigidly fixed at the Z-line, comprising the I-band (isotropic, light transmitting). The sarcomere is a nearly crystalline structure, composed of an A-band and two adjacent I-bands, and is the fundamental unit of muscle force generation. Sarcomeres are arranged into arrays of myofibrils, and one muscle cell or myofiber contains many myofibrils. Myofibers themselves are multinucleated syncitia, hundreds of microns in diameter and may be tens of millimeters in length that are derived during development by the fusion of myoblasts.

The myosin protein occurs in several different isoforms, each with different force generating characteristics, and each associated with expression of characteristic metabolic and calcium-handling proteins. Broadly, fibers can be characterized as either fast or slow, with slow fibers having a lower rate of actomyosin ATPase activity, slower velocity of shortening, slower calcium dynamics, and greater activity of oxidative metabolic enzymes. The lower ATPase activity makes these fibers more efficient for generating force, while the high oxidative capacity provides a plentiful energy source, making slow fibers ideal for extended periods of activity. Their relatively slow speed of shortening results in poor performance during fast or ballistic motions.

9.1.4 Material Properties

9.1.4.1 Cartilage

The behavior of cartilage is highly viscoelastic. A compressive load applied to articular cartilage drives the positively charged fluid phase through the densely intermeshed and negatively charged solid phase while deforming the elastic PG–collagen structure. The mobility of the fluid phase is relatively low, and, for rapid changes in load, cartilage responds nearly as a uniform linear elastic solid with a Young's modulus of approximately 6 MPa (Carter and Wong, 2003).

At lower loading rates, cartilage displays more nonlinear properties. Ker (1999) reports that human limb articular cartilage stiffness can be described as $E = E_0(1 + \sigma^{0.366})$, with $E_0 = 3.0$ MPa and σ expressed in MPa.

9.1.4.2 Tendon and Ligament

At rest, collagen fibrils are significantly crimped or wavy so that initial loading acts primarily to straighten these fibrils. At higher strains, the straightened collagen fibrils must be lengthened. Thus, tendons are more compliant at low loads and less compliant at high loads. The highly nonlinear low load region has been referred to as the "toe" region and occurs up to approximately 3% strain and 5 MPa (Butler et al. 1978; Zajac, 1989). Typically, tendons have nearly linear properties from about 3% strain until ultimate strain, which ranges from 9% to 10% (Table 9.1). The tangent modulus in this linear region is approximately 1.5 GPa. Ultimate tensile stress reported for tendons is approximately 100 MPa (McElhaney et al., 1976). However, under physiological conditions, tendons operate at stresses of only 5–10 MPa (Table 9.1) yielding a typical safety factor of 10.

9.1.4.3 Muscle

Tension generated by skeletal muscle depends on length, velocity, level of activation, and history. Performance characteristics of a muscle depend on both its intrinsic properties and the extrinsic organization of that tissue. Whole muscle maximum shortening velocity depends both upon the sliding velocity of its component sarcomeres and on the number of those sarcomeres arranged in series. Likewise, maximum isometric tension depends on both the intrinsic tension generating capacity of the actomyosin cross-bridges and on the number of sarcomeres arranged in parallel. The relationship between intrinsic properties and extrinsic function is further complicated by pennation of the fibers. Given the orthotropic nature of the muscle fiber, material properties should be considered relative to the fiber axis. That is, the relevant area for stress determination is not the geometric cross section, but the physiological cross section, perpendicular to the fiber axis. The common form for estimation of the physiological cross-sectional area (PCSA) is

$$PCSA = \frac{M\cos\theta}{\rho FL}$$

TABLE 9.1 Tendon Biomechanical Properties

Tendon	Ultimate Stress (MPa)	Ultimate Strain (%)	Stress under Normal Loads (MPa)	Strain under Normal Loads (%)	Tangent Modulus (GPa)	Reference
	40	9				Woo et al. (1980)
Wallaby			15–40		1.56	Bennett et al. (1986)
Porpoise					1.53	Bennett et al. (1986)
Dolphin					1.43	Bennett et al. (1986)
Deer			28–74		1.59	Bennett et al. (1986)
Sheep					1.65	Bennett et al. (1986)
Donkey			22–44		1.25	Bennett et al. (1986)
Human leg			53		1.0–1.2	Bennett et al. (1986)
Cat leg					1.21	Bennett et al. (1986)
Pig tail					0.9	Bennett et al. (1986)
Rat tail					0.8–1.5	Bennett et al. (1986)
Horse				4–10		Ker et al. (1988)
Dog leg			84			Ker et al. (1988)
Camel ankle			18			Ker et al. (1988)
Human limb (various)	60–120					McElhaney et al. (1976)
Human calcaneal	55	9.5				McElhaney et al. (1976)
Human wrist	52–74	11–17	3.2–3.3	1.5–3.5		Loren and Lieber (1994)

where M is muscle mass, θ is pennation angle, ρ is muscle density (1.06 g/cm^3), and FL is fiber length. Likewise, the relevant gage length for strain determination is not muscle length, but fiber length, or fascicle length in muscles composed of serial fibers.

Maximum muscle stress: Maximum active stress, or specific tension, varies somewhat among fiber types and species (Table 9.2) around a generally accepted average of 250 kPa. This specific tension can be determined in any system in which it is possible to measure force and estimate the area of contractile material. Given muscle PCSA, maximum force produced by a muscle can be predicted by multiplying this PCSA by specific tension (Table 9.2). Specific tension can also be calculated for isolated muscle fibers or motor units in which estimates of cross-sectional area have been made.

Maximum muscle contraction velocity: Muscle maximum contraction velocity is primarily dependent on the type and number of sarcomeres in series along the muscle fiber length (Gans, 1982). The intrinsic velocity of shortening has been experimentally determined for a number of muscle types (Table 9.3). Maximum contraction velocity of a given muscle can thus be calculated based on knowledge of the number of serial sarcomeres within the muscle multiplied by the maximum contraction velocity of an individual sarcomere (Tables 9.4 through 9.6). Sarcomere shortening velocity varies widely among species and fiber types (Table 9.3).

Muscle force–length relationship: Under conditions of constant length, muscle force generated is proportional to the magnitude of the interaction between the actin and myosin contractile filaments. Myosin filament length in most species is approximately 1.6 μm, but actin filament length varies (Table 9.7). Optimal sarcomere length and maximum sarcomere length can be calculated using these filament lengths. For optimal force generation, each half myosin filament must completely overlap an actin filament, without opposing actin filaments overlapping, so peak force generation occurs at a sarcomere length of twice the thin filament length. No active force is produced at sarcomere spacings shorter than 1.3 μm or longer than the sum of the myosin and the pair of actin filament lengths. The range of operating sarcomere lengths varies among muscles, but generally covers a range of ±15% of optimal length (Burkholder and Lieber, 2003). At submaximal activation, the peak of the force–length relationship shifts to longer lengths (Rack and Westbury, 1969; Balnave and Allen, 1996).

TABLE 9.2 Skeletal Muscle-Specific Tension

Species	Muscle Type	Preparation	Specific Tension (kPa)	Reference
		Synthesis	300	Josephson (1989)
Rat	SO	Single fiber	134	Fitts et al. (1991)
Human	Slow	Single fiber	133	Fitts et al. (1991)
Rat	FOG	Single fiber	108	Fitts et al. (1991)
Rat	FG	Single fiber	108	Fitts et al. (1991)
Human	Fast	Single fiber	166	Fitts et al. (1991)
Cat	1	Motor unit	59	Dum et al. (1982)
Cat	S	Motor unit	172	Bodine et al. (1987)
Cat	2A	Motor unit	284	Dum et al. (1982)
Cat	FR	Motor unit	211	Bodine et al. (1987)
Cat	2B + 2AB	Motor unit	343	Dum et al. (1982)
Cat	FF/FI	Motor unit	249	Bodine et al. (1987)
Human	Elbow	Whole muscle	230–420	Edgerton et al. (1990)
Human	Ankle	Whole muscle	45–250	Fukunaga et al. (1996)
Rat	TA	Whole muscle	272	Wells (1965)
Rat	Soleus	Whole muscle	319	Wells (1965)
Guinea pig	Hindlimb	Whole muscle	225	Powell et al. (1984)
Guinea pig	Soleus	Whole muscle	154	Powell et al. (1984)

TABLE 9.3 Muscle Dynamic Properties

Species	Muscle Type	Preparation	V_{max}^a	a/P_o	b/V_{max}	Reference
Rat	SO	Single fiber	1.49 L/s			Fitts et al. (1991)
Human	Slow	Single fiber	0.86 L/s			Fitts et al. (1991)
Rat	FOG	Single fiber	4.91 L/s			Fitts et al. (1991)
Rat	FG	Single fiber	8.05 L/s			Fitts et al. (1991)
Human	Fast	Single fiber	4.85 L/s			Fitts et al. (1991)
Mouse	Soleus	Whole muscle	31.7 μm/s			Close (1972)
Rat	Soleus	Whole muscle	18.2 μm/s			Close (1972)
Rat	Soleus	Whole muscle	5.4 cm/s	0.214	0.23	Wells (1965)
Cat	Soleus	Whole muscle	13 μm/s			Close (1972)
Mouse	EDL	Whole muscle	60.5 μm/s			Close (1972)
Rat	EDL	Whole muscle	42.7 μm/s			Close (1972)
Cat	EDL	Whole muscle	31 μm/s			Close (1972)
Rat	TA	Whole muscle	14.4 cm/s	0.356	0.38	Wells (1965)

[a] L/s fiber or sarcomere lengths per second, μm/s sarcomere velocity; cm/s whole muscle velocity.

Muscle force–velocity relationship: Under conditions of constant load the relationship between force and velocity is nearly hyperbolic during shortening (Hill, 1938, Figure 9.5). The normalized shortening force–velocity relation can be described by

$$(F + a)v = b(1 - F)$$

TABLE 9.4 Architectural Properties of the Human Arm and Forearm[a]

Muscle	Muscle Mass (g)	Muscle Length (mm)	Fiber Length (mm)	Pennation Angle (deg.)	Cross-Sectional Area (cm²)	FL/ML Ratio
BR ($n = 8$)	16.6 ± 2.8	175 ± 8.3	121 ± 8.3	2.4 ± .6	1.33 ± .22	.69 ± .062
PT ($n = 8$)	15.9 ± 1.7	130 ± 4.7	36.4 ± 1.3	9.6 ± .8	4.13 ± .52	.28 ± .012
PQ ($n = 8$)	5.21 ± 1.0	39.3 ± 2.3	23.3 ± 2.0	9.9 ± .3	2.07 ± .33	.58 ± .021
EDC I ($n = 8$)	3.05 ± .45	114 ± 3.4	56.9 ± 3.6	3.1 ± .5	.52 ± .08	.49 ± .024
EDC M ($n = 5$)	6.13 ± 1.2	112 ± 4.7	58.8 ± 3.5	3.2 ± 1.0	1.02 ± .20	.50 ± .014
EDC R ($n = 7$)	4.70 ± .75	125 ± 10.7	51.2 ± 1.8	3.2 ± .54	.86 ± .13	.42 ± .023
EDC S ($n = 6$)	2.23 ± .32	121 ± 8.0	52.9 ± 5.2	2.4 ± .7	.40 ± .06	.43 ± .029
EDQ ($n = 7$)	3.81 ± .70	152 ± 9.2	55.3 ± 3.7	2.6 ± .6	.64 ± .10	.36 ± .012
FPLEIP ($n = 6$)	2.86 ± .61	105 ± 6.6	48.4 ± 2.3	6.3 ± .8	.56 ± .11	.46 ± .023
EPL ($n = 7$)	4.54 ± .68	138 ± 7.2	43.6 ± 2.6	5.6 ± 1.3	.98 ± .13	.31 ± .020
PL ($n = 6$)	3.78 ± .82	134 ± 11.5	52.3 ± 3.1	3.5 ± 1.2	.69 ± .17	.40 ± .032
FDS I(P) ($n = 6$)	6.0 ± 1.1	92.5 ± 8.4	31.6 ± 3.0	5.1 ± 0.2	1.81 ± .83	.34 ± .022
FDS I(D) ($n = 9$)	6.6 ± 0.8	119 ± 6.1	37.9 ± 3.0	6.7 ± 0.3	1.63 ± .22	.32 ± .013
FDS I(C) ($n = 6$)	12.4 ± 2.1	207 ± 10.7	67.6 ± 2.8	5.7 ± 0.2	1.71 ± .28	.33 ± .025
FDS M ($n = 9$)	16.3 ± 2.2	183 ± 11.5	60.8 ± 3.9	6.9 ± 0.7	2.53 ± .34	.34 ± .014
FDS R ($n = 9$)	10.2 ± 1.1	155 ± 7.7	60.1 ± 2.7	4.3 ± 0.6	1.61 ± .18	.39 ± .023
FDS S ($n = 9$)	1.8 ± 0.3	103 ± 6.3	42.4 ± 2.2	4.9 ± 0.7	0.40 ± .05	.42 ± .014
FDP I ($n = 9$)	11.7 ± 1.2	149 ± 3.8	61.4 ± 2.4	7.2 ± 0.7	1.77 ± .16	.41 ± .018
FDP M ($n = 9$)	16.3 ± 1.7	200 ± 8.2	68.4 ± 2.7	5.7 ± 0.3	2.23 ± .22	.34 ± .011
FDP R ($n = 9$)	11.9 ± 1.4	194 ± 7.0	64.6 ± 2.6	6.8 ± 0.5	1.72 ± .18	.33 ± .009
FDP S ($n = 9$)	13.7 ± 1.5	150 ± 4.7	60.7 ± 3.9	7.8 ± 0.9	2.20 ± .30	.40 ± .015
FPL ($n = 9$)	10.0 ± 1.1	168 ± 10.0	45.1 ± 2.1	6.9 ± 0.2	2.08 ± .22	.24 ± .010

Source: Data from Lieber, R.L. et al. 1990. *J. Hand Surg.* 15:244–250; Lieber, R.L. et al. 1992. *J. Hand Surg.* 17:787–798.

[a] BR, brachioradialis; EDC I, EDC M, EDC R, and EDC S, extensor digitorum communis to the index, middle, ring, and small fingers, respectively; EDQ, extensor digiti quinti; EIP, extensor indicis proprious; EPL, extensor pollicis longus; FDP I, FDP M, FDP R, and FDP S, flexor digitorum profundus muscles; FDS I, FDS M, FDS R, and FDS S, flexor digitorum superficialis muscles; FDS I (P) and FDS I (D), proximal and distal bellies of the FDS I; FDS I (C), the combined properties of the two bellies as if they were a single muscle; FPL, flexor pollicis longus; PQ, pronator quadratus; PS, palmaris longus; PT, pronator teres.

while the lengthening relation can be described by

$$F = 1.8 - 0.8 \frac{V_{max} + v}{V_{max} - 7.6\, v}$$

The dynamic parameters (a, b, and V_{max}) vary across species and fiber types (Table 9.3).

9.1.5 Modeling

9.1.5.1 Cartilage

Although cartilage can be modeled as a simple elastic element, more accurate results are obtained using a biphasic model (Mow et al., 1980), which describes the motion of the hydrating fluid relative to the charged organic matrix. The total stress acting on the cartilage is separated into independent solid and fluid phases:

$$\sigma^T = \sigma^s + \sigma^f$$

TABLE 9.5 Architectural Properties of Human Lower Limb[a]

Muscle	Muscle Mass (g)	Muscle Length (cm)	Fiber Length (cm)	Pennation Angle (deg.)	Cross-Sectional Area (cm²)	FL/ML Ratio
Psoas	97.69 ± 33.58	24.25 ± 4.75	11.69 ± 1.66	10.66 ± 3.20	7.73 ± 2.31	0.50 ± 0.14
Iliacus	113.74 ± 37.01	20.61 ± 4.02	10.66 ± 1.86	14.29 ± 5.32	9.88 ± 3.40	0.56 ± 0.26
Gluteus maximus	547.24 ± 162.17	26.95 ± 6.42	15.69 ± 2.57	21.94 ± 26.24	28.17 ± 11.05	0.62 ± 0.22
Glut. medius	273.45 ± 76.86	19.99 ± 2.86	7.33 ± 1.57	20.47 ± 17.34	33.78 ± 14.39	0.37 ± 0.08
Sartorius	78.45 ± 31.13	44.81 ± 4.19	40.30 ± 4.63	1.33 ± 1.76	1.86 ± 0.74	0.90 ± 0.04
Rectus femoris	110.55 ± 43.33	36.28 ± 4.73	7.59 ± 1.28	13.93 ± 3.49	13.51 ± 4.97	0.21 ± 0.03
Vastus lateralis	375.85 ± 137.18	27.34 ± 4.62	9.94 ± 1.76	18.38 ± 6.78	35.09 ± 16.14	0.38 ± 0.11
Vastus intermedius	171.86 ± 72.89	41.20 ± 8.17	9.93 ± 2.03	4.54 ± 4.45	16.74 ± 6.91	0.24 ± 0.04
Vastus medialis	239.44 ± 94.83	43.90 ± 9.85	9.68 ± 2.30	29.61 ± 6.89	20.58 ± 7.17	0.22 ± 0.04
Gracilis	52.53 ± 16.72	28.69 ± 3.29	22.78 ± 4.38	8.16 ± 2.51	2.23 ± 0.81	0.79 ± 0.08
Adductor longus	74.67 ± 28.42	21.84 ± 4.46	10.82 ± 2.02	7.08 ± 3.43	6.50 ± 2.17	0.50 ± 0.07
Adductor brevis	54.56 ± 24.83	15.39 ± 2.46	10.31 ± 1.42	6.10 ± 3.14	4.95 ± 2.11	0.68 ± 0.06
Adductor magnus	324.72 ± 127.82	37.90 ± 7.36	14.44 ± 2.74	15.54 ± 7.27	20.48 ± 7.82	0.39 ± 0.07
Biceps femoris LH	113.37 ± 48.53	34.73 ± 3.65	9.76 ± 2.62	11.58 ± 5.50	11.33 ± 4.75	0.28 ± 0.08
Biceps femoris SH	59.79 ± 22.62	22.39 ± 2.50	11.03 ± 2.06	12.33 ± 3.61	5.06 ± 1.69	0.49 ± 0.07
Semitendinosus	99.74 ± 37.81	29.67 ± 3.86	19.30 ± 4.12	12.86 ± 4.94	4.82 ± 2.01	0.65 ± 0.11
Semimembranosus	134.31 ± 57.56	29.34 ± 3.42	6.90 ± 1.83	15.09 ± 3.43	18.40 ± 7.53	0.24 ± 0.06
Tibialis anterior	80.13 ± 26.63	25.98 ± 3.25	6.83 ± 0.79	9.56 ± 3.11	10.89 ± 3.01	0.27 ± 0.05
Extensor hallucis longus	20.93 ± 9.86	24.25 ± 3.27	7.48 ± 1.13	9.44 ± 2.15	2.67 ± 1.52	0.31 ± 0.06
Extensor digitorum longus	40.98 ± 12.62	29.00 ± 2.33	6.93 ± 1.14	10.83 ± 2.75	5.55 ± 1.68	0.24 ± 0.04
Peroneus longus	57.74 ± 22.64	27.08 ± 3.02	5.08 ± 0.63	14.08 ± 5.14	10.39 ± 3.75	0.19 ± 0.03
Peroneus brevis	24.15 ± 10.59	23.75 ± 3.11	4.54 ± 0.65	11.46 ± 2.96	4.91 ± 2.01	0.19 ± 0.03
GastrocnemiusMH	113.46 ± 31.97	26.94 ± 4.65	5.10 ± 0.98	9.88 ± 4.39	21.12 ± 5.66	0.19 ± 0.03
Gastrocnemius	62.24 ± 24.56	22.35 ± 3.70	5.88 ± 0.95	12.04 ± 3.11	9.72 ± 3.26	0.27 ± 0.03
Soleus	275.77 ± 98.50	40.54 ± 8.32	4.40 ± 0.99	28.25 ± 10.05	51.79 ± 14.91	0.11 ± 0.02
Flexor hallucis longus	38.89 ± 17.09	26.88 ± 3.55	5.27 ± 1.29	16.89 ± 4.62	6.85 ± 2.72	0.20 ± 0.05
Flexor digitorum longus	20.27 ± 10.75	27.33 ± 5.62	4.46 ± 1.06	13.64 ± 4.73	4.37 ± 2.02	0.16 ± 0.09
Tibialis posterior	58.44 ± 19.20	31.03 ± 4.68	3.78 ± 0.49	13.71 ± 4.11	14.42 ± 4.94	0.12 ± 0.02

[a] Data from Ward, J.S. et al. 2009. *Clin Orthop Relat Res.* 467:1074–82.

where s denotes the solid phase and f the fluid phase. The relative motion of the phases defines the equilibrium equations

$$\nabla \cdot \sigma^s = \frac{(v^s - v^f)}{k(1 + \alpha)^2} = -\nabla \cdot \sigma^f$$

where α is tissue solid content and k the tissue permeability coefficient. In addition to the equilibrium equations, each phase is subject to separate constitutive relations:

$$\sigma^f = -p_a \underline{I} \quad \text{and} \quad \sigma^s = -\alpha p_a \underline{I} + \underline{D}e$$

where p_a is the apparent tissue stress, $\underline{D}$ is the material property tensor and $\underline{e}$ is the strain tensor. For a hyperelastic solid phase

TABLE 9.6　Architectural Properties of Human Foot[a]

Muscle	Muscle Volume (cm³)	Muscle Length (mm)	Fiber Length (mm)	Cross-Sectional Area (cm²)
ABDH	15.2 ± 5.3	115.8 ± 4.9	23.0 ± 5.5	6.68 ± 2.07
ABDM	8.8 ± 4.7	112.8 ± 19.0	23.9 ± 7.4	3.79 ± 1.83
ADHT	1.1 ± 0.6	24.8 ± 4.2	18.7 ± 5.2	0.62 ± 0.26
ADHO	9.1 ± 3.1	67.4 ± 4.6	18.6 ± 5.3	4.94 ± 1.36
EDB2	2.1 ± 1.2	69.8 ± 16.8	28.0 ± 6.5	0.79 ± 0.43
EDB3	1.3 ± 0.7	82.2 ± 20.7	26.4 ± 5.1	0.51 ± 0.30
EDB4	1.0 ± 0.7	70.4 ± 21.1	23.1 ± 3.8	0.44 ± 0.29
EHB	3.6 ± 1.5	65.7 ± 8.5	27.9 ± 5.7	1.34 ± 0.66
FDB2	4.5 ± 2.3	92.9 ± 15.0	25.4 ± 4.5	1.78 ± 0.79
FDB3	3.2 ± 1.5	98.8 ± 18.1	22.8 ± 4.0	1.49 ± 0.71
FDB4	2.6 ± 1.0	103.0 ± 9.2	20.8 ± 4.5	1.26 ± 0.47
FDB5	0.7 ± 0.3	83.2 ± 3.0	18.2 ± 2.2	0.35 ± 0.16
FDMB	3.4 ± 1.7	51.0 ± 5.3	17.7 ± 3.8	2.00 ± 1.02
FHBM	3.1 ± 1.3	76.0 ± 19.8	17.5 ± 4.8	1.80 ± 0.75
FHBL	3.4 ± 1.4	65.3 ± 7.1	16.5 ± 3.4	2.12 ± 0.84
DI1	2.7 ± 1.4	51.0 ± 4.9	16.1 ± 4.4	1.70 ± 0.64
DI2	2.5 ± 1.4	49.9 ± 5.1	15.3 ± 4.0	1.68 ± 0.80
DI3	2.5 ± 1.2	44.3 ± 5.6	15.6 ± 5.4	1.64 ± 0.58
DI4	4.2 ± 2.0	61.4 ± 4.5	16.0 ± 4.8	2.72 ± 1.33
LB2	0.6 ± 0.4	53.9 ± 11.8	22.4 ± 6.5	0.28 ± 0.17
LB3	0.5 ± 0.4	45.2 ± 8.7	22.3 ± 6.7	0.28 ± 0.09
LB4	0.6 ± 0.4	37.3 ± 19.9	21.1 ± 9.3	0.30 ± 0.32
LB5	0.4 ± 0.4	41.0 ± 12.1	16.2 ± 7.0	0.18 ± 0.13
PI1	1.5 ± 0.5	46.2 ± 4.0	13.6 ± 3.7	1.23 ± 0.65
PI2	1.9 ± 0.7	56.6 ± 6.6	13.9 ± 3.5	1.41 ± 0.48
PI3	1.8 ± 0.6	48.8 ± 9.9	14.2 ± 5.9	1.38 ± 0.55
QPM	5.6 ± 3.4	81.3 ± 20.1	27.5 ± 7.0	1.96 ± 0.94
QPL	2.4 ± 1.2	55.3 ± 3.9	23.4 ± 7.1	1.00 ± 0.41

Source:　Data from Kura, H. et al. 1997. *Anat. Rec.* 249:143–151.

[a] ABDH, abductor hallucis; FHBM flexor hallucis brevis medialis; FHBL, flexor hallucis brevis lateralis; ADHT, adductor hallucis transverse; ADHO, adductor hallucis oblique; ABDM, abductor digiti minimi; FDMB, flexor digiti minimi brevis; DI, dorsal interosseous; PI, plantar interosseous; FDB, flexor digitorum brevis; LB, lumbrical; QPM, quadratus plantaris medialis; QPL, quadratus plantaris lateralis; EHB, extensor hallucis brevis; EDB, extensor digitorum brevis.

$$\underline{D}\underline{e} = \lambda Tr(\underline{e})\underline{I} + 2\mu\underline{e}$$

where λ and μ are the Lamé constants.

These equations can be solved analytically for the special case of confined compression against a porous platen (Mow et al., 1980). The surface displacement during creep under an applied load f_0 is

$$\frac{u}{h} = \frac{f_0}{H_A}\left(1 - \frac{2}{\pi^2}\sum_{n=0}^{\infty}(n+12)^{-2}\exp\left\{-\pi^2(n+12)^2\frac{H_A k f}{(1+2a_0)h^2}\right\}\right)$$

where h is the tissue thickness, and H_A is the aggregate modulus ($\lambda + 2\mu$). Those authors estimate k as $7.6 \pm 3.0 \times 10^{-13}\,\mathrm{m^4/Ns}$ and H_A as 0.70 ± 0.09 MPa for bovine articular cartilage. Chen et al. (2001) report

TABLE 9.7 Actin Filament Lengths

Species	Actin Filament Length (μm)	Optimal Length (μm)	Reference
Cat	1.12	2.24	Herzog et al. (1992)
Rat	1.09	2.18	Herzog et al. (1992)
Rabbit	1.09	2.18	Herzog et al. (1992)
Frog	0.98	1.96	Page and Huxley (1963)
Monkey	1.16	2.32	Walker and Schrodt (1973)
Human	1.27	2.54	Walker and Schrodt (1973)
Hummingbird	1.75	3.50	Mathieu-Costello et al. (1992)
Chicken	0.95	1.90	Page (1969)
Wild rabbit	1.12	2.24	Dimery (1985)
Carp	0.98	1.92	Sosnicki et al. (1991)

strongly depth-dependent values for H_A ranging between 1.16 ± 0.20 MPa in the superficial zone to 7.75 ± 1.45 MPa in the deep zone in human articular cartilage. The biphasic approach has been extended to finite element modeling, resulting in the u–p class of models (Wayne et al., 1991).

9.1.5.2 Tendon and Ligament

The composition and structure of the tensile soft tissues is quite similar to that of cartilage, and the biphasic theory can be applied to them as well (Yin and Elliott, 1983). Fluid pressure serves a smaller role in tissues loaded in tension, and the complication of the biphasic model is generally unnecessary. For modeling of segmental mechanics, it is frequently sufficient to treat these structures according to a one-dimensional approximation.

While considering tendons and ligaments as simple nonlinear elastic elements (Table 9.6) is often sufficient, additional accuracy can be obtained by incorporating viscous damping. The quasi-linear viscoelastic approach (Fung, 1967) introduces a stress relaxation function, $G(t)$, that depends only on time, is convoluted with the elastic response, $T^e(\lambda)$, that depends only on the stretch ratio, to yield the complete stress response, $K(\lambda,t)$. To obtain the stress at any point in time requires that the contribution of all preceding deformations be assessed:

$$T(t) = \int G(t - \tau) \frac{\partial T^e(\lambda)}{\partial \lambda} \frac{\partial \lambda}{\partial \tau} d\tau$$

Both the elastic response and the relaxation function are empirically determined. The common form for the relaxation function is a sum of exponentials

$$G(t) = A + \sum_i B_i e^{-t/\tau_i}$$

The form of the elastic response varies, but usually includes a power or exponential term to accommodate the toe region.

9.1.5.3 Muscle

9.1.5.3.1 Types of Muscle Models

There are three general classes of models for predicting muscle force: biochemical, or crossbridge, models, constitutive models, and phenomenological, or Hill, models. Cross-bridge models (Huxley, 1957;

Huxley and Simmons, 1971) attempt to determine force from the chemical reactions of the cross-bridge cycle. Though accurate at the cross-bridge level, it is generally computationally prohibitive to model a whole muscle in this manner. Constitutive models, such as that described by Zahalak and Ma (1990), generally attempt to determine muscle behavior by describing populations of cross-bridges. A potentially powerful approach, this technique has not yet been widely adopted. In the context of whole-body biomechanics, the primary modeling approach uses the phenomenological model first described by Hill (1939), which incorporates the steady-state force–length and force–velocity properties into a contractile element, which is dynamically isolated by a series elastic element (Figure 9.3). The parallel elastic element represents the passive properties of the muscle, which reflect the properties of titin and extracellular connective tissue. The series elastic element provides the dynamic response during time-varying force and velocity conditions. Some of this elasticity resides in extracellular connective tissue, including tendon and aponeurosis, but series elasticity of 5–10% Lo/Po is found even in muscles lacking any external tendon or in segments of single fibers. The contractile component is described by independent isometric force–length (Figure 9.4) and isotonic force–velocity relations (Figure 9.5) and an activation function (Zajac, 1989).

Force production by the contractile component can be calculated as the product of three independent functions, each bounded by 0 and 1, and the maximal isometric tension, F_0: $F = a * afl * afv * F_0$. The activation function (a) depends only on an input representing neural drive or a descending command if excitation–contraction coupling is intact. Often, it is a first-order transformation intended to represent calcium and troponin dynamics, but activation dynamics and series elasticity are both first-order processes, so the extent to which the activation function improves model results depends strongly on the extent to which modeled series elasticity accurately represents muscle mechanics. The active force–length function (afl) depends only on muscle fiber or sarcomere length. The active force–velocity function (afv) depends only on fiber velocity.

In forward simulation, initial conditions are known and an activation function is given or derived from a control model. The muscle model is coupled with a physical model, and the physical model provides a muscle–tendon unit (MTU) length. The muscle model must calculate force

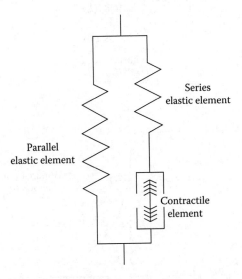

Series
elastic element

Parallel
elastic element

Contractile
element

FIGURE 9.3 The Hill model of muscle separates the active properties of muscle into a contractile element, in series with a purely elastic element. The properties of the passive muscle are represented by the parallel elastic element.

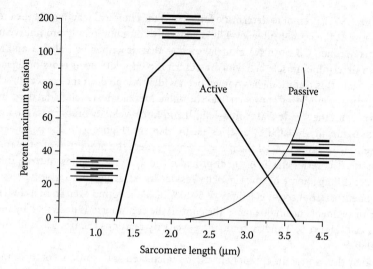

FIGURE 9.4 The force generating capacity of a sarcomere depends strongly on the degree of overlap of myosin and actin filaments.

production in order to update the physical model. Mathematically, this reduces to solving the following equations:

$$\frac{dx}{dt} = f(F)$$

$$\frac{dF}{dt} = k\left(\frac{dx}{dt} - \frac{dL}{dt}\right)$$

$$\frac{dL}{dt} = afv^{-1}\left(\frac{F}{F_0 a(t) afl(L)}\right)$$

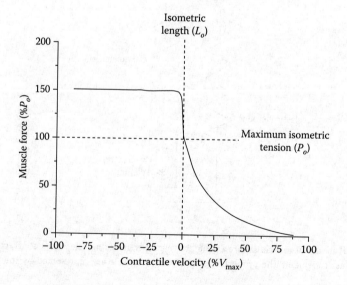

FIGURE 9.5 Active force generation depends strongly on shortening velocity.

where x is MTU length, calculated from the physical model; F is the force in the series elastic and contractile elements, calculated from the elasticity of the SEE; L is the length of the contractile element, calculated from the applied force and inversion of the force–velocity relationship.

It should be noted that this formulation omits several potentially important force-generating phenomena. Notable among these are the persistent extra tension obtained following stretch (Edman et al., 1982) and changes in the force–length relation associated with activation level (Rack and Westbury, 1969). Some of these features can be accommodated by considering series elasticity and sarcomere length inhomogeneity (Morgan, 1990), and each represents a nonlinearity that substantially complicates modeling and may not be necessary for first approximations of muscle function.

Common applications of muscle modeling include forward simulation to predict output forces or motions, as for control of functional electrical stimulation (Park and Durand 2008), and inverse analysis to estimate the muscle forces that produced an observed motion (Thelen and Anderson 2006). In neither of these cases is it necessarily practical to determine muscle contractile properties empirically, and it is frequently necessary to resort to estimation of the force–length and force–velocity relations from muscle structure. If a muscle is considered to be a composition of uniform sarcomeres in series and in parallel, then the deformation of single sarcomeres can be estimated from whole muscle length changes. A simplified view of a muscle is an array of identical fibers of uniform length arranged at a common pennation angle to the line of force. Peak isometric tension can be estimated from PCSA. Pennation angle determines the relationship between muscle and fiber length changes:

$$\frac{\Delta L_m}{L_m} = \frac{\Delta L_f}{L_f} \cos\theta$$

If sarcomere length is known at any muscle length, it is then possible to scale the sarcomere length–tension and velocity–tension relations to the whole muscle. When reporting architectural data (tables), muscle and fiber lengths should be normalized to optimal sarcomere length. Even with direct measurements of the steady-state afl and afv, errors in force estimates during dynamic, submaximal activations can be substantial (Perreault and Heckman, 2003).

References

Balnave, C.D. and Allen, D.G. 1996. The effect of muscle length on intracellular calcium and force in single fibres from mouse skeletal muscle. *J Physiol.* 492(Pt 3):705–713.

Bennett, M.B., Ker, R.F., Dimery, N.J., and Alexander, R. M. 1986. Mechanical properties of various mammalian tendons. *J Zoology* 209, 537–548.

Bodine, S.C., Roy, R.R., Eldred, E., and Edgerton, V.R. 1987. Maximal force as a function of anatomical features of motor units in the cat tibialis anterior. *J Neurophysiol.* 57, 1730–45.

Burkholder, T.J. and Lieber, R.L. Sarcomere length operating range of vertebrate muscles during movement. *J Exp Biol.* 204:1529–36.

Butler, D.L., Grood, E.S., Noyes, F.R., and Zernicke, R.F. 1978. Biomechanics of ligaments and tendons. *Exerc. Sport Sci. Rev.* Vol. 6: 125–181, Hutton, R.S. (Ed.). The Franklin Institute Press.

Carter, D.R. and Wong, M. 2003. Modeling Cartilage mechanobiology. *Philos Trans R Soc Lond B Biol Sci.* 29; 358(1437): 1461–1471.

Close, R.I. 1972. Dynamic properties of mammalian skeletal muscles. *Physiological Reviews* 52, 129–97.

Chen, A.C., Bae, W.C., Schinagl, R.M., and Sah, R.L. 2001. Depth- and strain-dependent mechanical and electromechanical properties of full-thickness bovine articular cartilage in confined compression. *J Biomech.* 34(1):1–12.

Dimery, N.J. 1985. Muscle and sarcomere lengths in the hind limb of the rabbit (Oryctolagus cuniculus) during a galloping stride. *J Zoology* 205, 373–383.

Dum, R.P., Burke, R.E., O'Donovan, M.J., Toop, J., and Hodgson, J.A. 1982. Motor-unit organization in flexor digitorum longus muscle of the cat. *J Neurophysiol.* 47(6):1108–25.

Edgerton, V.R., Apor, P., and Roy, R.R. 1990. Specific tension of human elbow flexor muscles. *Acta Physiologica Hungarica.* 75, 205–16.

Edman, K.A., Elzinga, G., and Noble, M.I. 1982. Residual force enhancement after stretch of contracting frog single muscle fibers. *J Gen Physiol.* 80(5):769–784.

Fitts, R.H., McDonald, K.S., and Schluter, J.M. 1991. The determinants of skeletal muscle force and power: their adaptability with changes in activity pattern. *J Biomech.* 24 Suppl 1, 111–22.

Fukunaga, T., Roy, R.R., Shellock, F.G., Hodgson, J.A., and Edgerton, V.R. 1996. Specific tension of human plantar flexors and dorsiflexors. *J Appl Physiol.* 80(1):158–65.

Fung, Y.C. 1967. Elasticity of soft tissues in simple elongation. *Am. J. Physiol.* 213(6):1532–1544.

Gans, C. 1982. Fiber architecture and muscle function. *Exerc. Sport Sci. Rev.* 10:160–207.

Gordon, A.M., Huxley, A.F., and Julian, F.J. 1966. The variation in isometric tension with sarcomere length in vertebrate muscle fibres. *J. Physiol.* 184:170–192.

Gutsmann, T., Fantner, G.E., Venturoni, M., Ekani-Nkodo, A., Thompson, J.B., Kindt, J.H., Morse, D.E., Fygenson, D.K., and Hansma, P.K. 2003. Evidence that collagen fibrils in tendons are inhomogeneously structured in a tubelike manner. *Biophys. J.* 84(4):2593–2598.

Herzog, W., Leonard, T.R., Renaud, J.M., Wallace, J., Chaki, G., and Bornemisza, S. 1992. Force-length properties and functional demands of cat gastrocnemius, soleus and plantaris muscles. *J Biomech.* 25(11):1329–35.

Hill, A.V. 1938. The heat of shortening and the dynamic constants of muscle. *Proc. R. Soc. Lond. Series B: Biol. Sci.* 126:136–195.

Huxley, A.F. 1957. Muscle structure and theories of contraction. *Prog. Biophys. Mol. Biol.* 7:255–318.

Huxley, A.F. and Simmons, R.M. 1971. Proposed mechanism of force generation in striated muscle. *Nature* 233:533–538.

Josephson, R.K. 1989. Power output from skeletal muscle during linear and sinusoidal shortening. *J Exp Biol.* 147:533–37.

Kastelic, J., Galeski, A., and Baer, E. 1978. The multicomposite structure of tendon. *Connect. Tissue Res.* 6:11–23.

Ker, R.F. 1999. The design of soft collagenous load-bearing tissues. *J. Exp. Biol.* 202(Pt 23):3315–3324.

Ker, R.F., Alexander, R.M. and Bennett, M.B. 1988. Why are mammalian tendons so thick. *J Zoolog.* 216:309–24.

Kura, H., Luo, Z., Kitaoka, H.B., and An, K. 1997. Quantitative analysis of the intrinsic muscles of the foot. *Anat. Rec.* 249:143–151.

Lieber, R.L., Fazeli, B.M., and Botte, M.J. 1990. Architecture of selected wrist flexor and extensor muscles. *J. Hand Surg.* 15:244–250.

Lieber, R.L., Jacobson, M.D., Fazeli, B.M., Abrams, R.A., and Botte, M.J. 1992. Architecture of selected muscles of the arm and forearm: Anatomy and implications for tendon transfer. *J. Hand Surg.* 17:787–798.

Loren, G.J. and Lieber, R.L. 1995. Tendon biomechanical properties enhance human wrist muscle specialization. *J Biomech.* 28:791–9.

Mathieu-Costello, O., Suarez, R.K., and Hochachka, P.W. 1992. Capillary-to-fiber geometry and mitochondrial density in hummingbird flight muscle. *Respir Physiol.* 89(1):113–32.

McElhaney, J.H., Roberts, V.L., and Hilyard, J.F. 1976. *Handbook of Human Tolerance.* Japan Automobile Research Institute, Inc. (JARI), Tokyo, Japan.

Morgan, D.L. 1990. New insights into the behavior of muscle during active lengthening. *Biophys J.* 57(2):209–221.

Mow, V.C., Kuei, S.C., Lai, W.M., and Armstrong, C.G. 1980. Biphasic creep and stress relaxation of articular cartilage in compression: Theory and experiments. *J Biomech. Eng.* 102:73–84.

Page, S.G. 1969. Structure and some contractile properties of fast and slow muscles of the chicken. *J Physiol.* 205(1):131–45.

Page, S.G. and Huxley, H.E. 1996. Filament lengths in striated muscle. *J Cell Biol.* 19:369–90.

Park, H. and Durand, D.M. 2008. Motion control of musculoskeletal systems with redundancy. *Biol. Cybern.* 99(6):503–516.

Perreault, E.J., Heckman, C.J., and Sandercock, T.G. 2003. Hill muscle model errors during movement are greatest within the physiologically relevant range of motor unit firing rates. *J. Biomech.* 36(2):211–218.

Powell, P.L., Roy, R.R., Kanim, P., Bello, M.A., and Edgerton, V.R. 1984. Predictability of skeletal muscle tension from architectural determinations in guinea pig hindlimbs. *J. Appl. Physiol.* 57:1715–1721.

Rack, P.M. and Westbury, D.R. 1969. The effects of length and stimulus rate on tension on the isometric cat soleus muscle. *J. Physiol.* 204(2): 443–460.

Sosnicki, A.A., Loesser, K.E., and Rome, L.C. 1991. Myofilament overlap in swimming carp. I. Myofilament lengths of red and white muscle. *Am J Physiol.* 260(2 Pt1):C283–8.

Thelen, D.G. and Anderson, F.C. 2006. Using computed muscle control to generate forward dynamic simulations of human walking from experimental data. *J. Biomech.* 39(6):1107–1115.

Walker, S.M. and Schrodt, G.R. 1974. I segment lengths and thin filament periods in skeletal muscle fibers of the Rhesus monkey and the human. *Anatomical Record* 178, 63–81.

Ward, S.R., Eng, C.M., Smallwood, L.H. and Lieber, R.L. 2009. Are current measurements of lower extremity muscle architecture accurate? *Clin Orthop Relat Res.* 467:1074–82.

Wayne, J.S., Woo, S.L., and Kwan, M.K. 1991. Application of the u-p finite element method to the study of articular cartilage. *J. Biomech. Eng.* 113:397–403.

Weiss, J.A. and Gardiner, J.C. 2001. Computational modeling of ligament mechanics. *Crit. Rev. Biomed. Eng.* 29:303–371.

Wells, J.B. 1965. Comparison of Mechanical Properties between Slow and Fast Mammalian Muscles. *J Physiol.* 178, 252–69.

Wickiewicz, T.L., Roy, R.R., Powell, P.L., and Edgerton, V.R. 1983. Muscle architecture of the human lower limb. *Clin. Orthop. Rel. Res.* 179:275–283.

Woo, S.L., Ritter, M.A., Amiel, D., Sanders, T.M., Gomez, M.A., Kuei, S.C., Garfin, S.R., and Akeson, W.H. 1980. The biomechanical and biochemical properties of swine tendons—long term effects of exercise on the digital extensors. *Connect Tissue Res.* 7(3):177–183.

Yin, Y. and Elliott, D.M. 2003. A biphasic and transversely isotropic mechanical model for tendon: Application to mouse tail fascicles in uniaxial tension. *J. Biomech.* 37(6):907–914.

Zahalak, G.I. and Ma S.P. 1990. Muscle activation and contraction: Constitutive relations based directly on cross-bridge kinetics. *J. Biomech. Eng.* 112:52–62.

Zajac, F.E. 1989. Muscle, and tendon: Properties, models, scaling and application to biomechanics and motor control. *CRC Crit. Rev. Biomed. Eng.* CRC Press, Inc. 17:359–411.

10

Joint-Articulating Surface Motion

10.1 Introduction **10**-1
10.2 Ankle **10**-2
  Geometry of the Articulating Surfaces • Joint Contact • Axes of
  Rotation
10.3 Knee **10**-5
  Geometry of the Articulating Surfaces • Joint Contact • Axes of
  Rotation
10.4 Hip **10**-13
  Geometry of the Articulating Surfaces • Joint Contact • Axes of
  Rotation
10.5 Shoulder **10**-18
  Geometry of the Articulating Surfaces • Joint Contact • Axes of
  Rotation
10.6 Elbow **10**-21
  Geometry of the Articulating Surfaces • Joint Contact • Axes of
  Rotation
10.7 Wrist **10**-28
  Geometry of the Articulating Surfaces • Joint Contact • Axes of
  Rotation
10.8 Hand **10**-32
  Geometry of the Articulating Surfaces • Joint Contact • Axes of
  Rotation
10.9 Summary **10**-38
Acknowledgment **10**-40
References **10**-40

Kenton R. Kaufman
Mayo Clinic

Kai-Nan An
Mayo Clinic

10.1 Introduction

Knowledge of joint-articulating surface motion is essential for design of prosthetic devices to restore function; assessment of joint wear, stability, and degeneration; and determination of proper diagnosis and surgical treatment of joint disease. In general, kinematic analysis of human movement can be arranged into two separate categories, (1) gross movement of the limb segments interconnected by joints, or (2) detailed analysis of joint articulating surface motion which is described in this chapter. Gross movement is the relative three-dimensional joint rotation as described by adopting the Eulerian angle system. Movement of this type is described in Chapter 5: Analysis of Gait. In general, the three-dimensional unconstrained rotation and translation of an articulating joint can be described utilizing the concept of the screw displacement axis. The most commonly used analytic method for the description

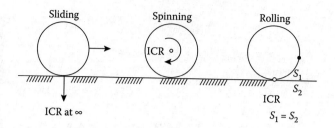

FIGURE 10.1 Three types of articulating surface motion in human joints.

of 6-degree-of-freedom displacement of a rigid body is the screw displacement axis (Kinzel et al., 1972; Spoor and Veldpaus, 1980; Woltring et al., 1985).

Various degrees of simplification have been used for kinematic modeling of joints. A hinged joint is the simplest and most common model used to simulate an anatomic joint in planar motion about a single axis embedded in the fixed segment. Experimental methods have been developed for determination of the instantaneous center of rotation for planar motion. The *instantaneous center of rotation* is defined as the point of zero velocity. For a true hinged motion, the instantaneous center of rotation will be a fixed point throughout the movement. Otherwise, loci of the instantaneous center of rotation or centrodes will exist. The center of curvature has also been used to define joint anatomy. The *center of curvature* is defined as the geometric center of coordinates of the articulating surface.

For more general planar motion of an articulating surface, the term *sliding, rolling,* and *spinning* are commonly used (Figure 10.1). Sliding (gliding) motion is defined as the pure translation of a moving segment against the surface of a fixed segment. The contact point of the moving segment does not change, while the contact point of the fixed segment has a constantly changing contact point. If the surface of the fixed segment is flat, the instantaneous center of rotation is located at infinity. Otherwise, it is located at the center of curvature of the fixed surface. Spinning motion (rotation) is the exact opposite of sliding motion. In this case, the moving segment rotates, and the contact points on the fixed surface does not change. The instantaneous center of rotation is located at the center of curvature of the spinning body that is undergoing pure rotation. Rolling motion occurs between moving and fixed segments where the contact points in each surface are constantly changing and the arc lengths of contact are equal on each segment. The instantaneous center of rolling motion is located at the contact point. Most planar motion of anatomic joints can be described by using any two of these three basic descriptions.

In this chapter, various aspects of joint-articulating motion are covered. Topics include the anatomical characteristics, joint contact, and axes of rotation. Joints of both the upper and lower extremity are discussed.

10.2 Ankle

The ankle joint is composed of two joints: the talocrural (ankle) joint and the talocalcaneal (subtalar joint). The talocrural joint is formed by the articulation of the distal tibia and fibula with the trochlea of the talus. The talocalcaneal joint is formed by the articulation of the talus with the calcaneus.

10.2.1 Geometry of the Articulating Surfaces

Morphological measurements of the ankle joint were collected in 36 normal subjects using a radiographic measurement method (Stagni et al., 2005). Three-dimensional characteristics of this articulation were collected (Figure 10.2, Table 10.1). A significant correlation was found among some of the measures but none of the measures correlated with malleolar width. Most measurements were larger in the male group than in the female group but these differences were not significantly different.

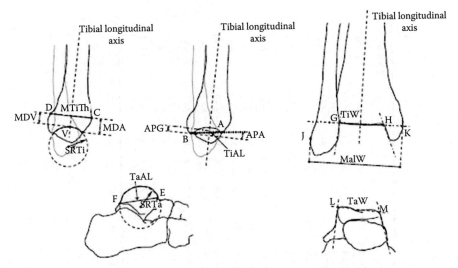

FIGURE 10.2   Sketch of the sagittal (a) and frontal (b) profiles of the tibio-fibular and talar segments. The relevant measurements taken in this work are schematically illustrated. (From Stagni R. et al., 2005. *Clin Biomech*, 20, 307–311. With permission.)

The upper articular surface of the talus is wedge-shaped, its width diminishing from front to back. The talus can be represented by a conical surface. The superior talar dome surface has an average anterior width of 29.9 ± 2.6 mm, a middle width of 27.9 ± 3.0 mm, and a posterior width of 25.2 ± 3.7 mm. Thus, the wedge shape of the talus is about 20% wider in front than behind. The talar dome radius is 20.7 ± 2.6 mm (Hayes et al., 2006). The wedge shape of the talus is about 25% wider in front than behind with an average difference of 2.4 ± 1.3 mm and a maximal difference of 6 mm (Inman, 1976).

10.2.2 Joint Contact

The talocrural joint contact area varies with flexion of the ankle (Table 10.2). During plantarflexion, such as would occur during the early stance phase of gait, the contact area is limited and the joint is incongruous. As the position of the joint progresses from neutral to dorsiflexion, as would occur during the midstance of gait, the contact area increases and the joint becomes more stable. The area of the subtalar articulation is smaller than that of the talocrural joint. The contact area of the subtalar joint is 0.89 ± 0.21 cm² for the posterior facet and 0.28 ± 15 cm² for the anterior and middle facets (Wang et al., 1994). The total contact area (1.18 ± 0.35 cm²) is only 12.7% of the whole subtalar articulation area (9.31 ± 0.66 cm²) (Wang et al., 1994). The contact area/joint area ratio increases with increases in applied load (Figure 10.3).

10.2.3 Axes of Rotation

Joint motion of the talocrural joint has been studied to define the axes of rotation and their location with respect to specific anatomic landmarks (Table 10.3). The axis of motion of the talocrural joint essentially passes through the inferior tibia at the fibular and tibial malleoli (Figure 10.4). Three types of motion have been used to describe the axes of rotation: fixed, quasi-instantaneous, and instantaneous axes. The motion that occurs in the ankle joints consists of dorsiflexion and plantarflexion. Minimal or no transverse rotation takes place within the talocrural joint. The motion in the talocrural joint is intimately related to the motion in the talocalcaneal joint which is described next.

The motion axes of the talocalcaneal joint have been described by several authors (Table 10.4). The axis of motion in the talocalcaneal joint passes from the anterior medial superior aspect of the navicular bone to the posterior lateral inferior aspect of the calcaneus (Figure 10.5). The motion that occurs in the talocalcaneal joint consists of inversion and eversion.

TABLE 10.1 Morphometry of the Ankle Joint

Measurement	Abbreviation Used in Figure 10.2	All (n = 36)					Male (n = 23)					Female (n = 13)					Male > Female
		Mean	SD	Max	Min	Median	Mean	SD	Max	Min	Median	Mean	SD	Max	Min	Median	P Value
Tibial arc length	TiAL	31.4	3.5	39.8	24.3	31.5	33.1	2.7	39.8	28.8	33.3	28.1	2.5	34.6	24.3	27.8	0.99
Sagittal radius of the tibial mortise	SRTi	27.8	4.4	34.9	21.2	26.8	29.3	4.2	41.5	23.1	27.9	24.7	4.4	32.4	21.2	24.1	0.97
Anteroposterior gap	APG	2.7	1.8	6.8	0.0	2.5	2.6	1.6	5.5	0.1	2.6	2.7	2.3	6.8	0.0	2.4	0.01
Anteroposterior inclination angle of the tibial mortise	APA	5.0	3.4	12.4	0.0	5.1	4.7	2.9	10.1	0.2	4.8	5.5	4.3	12.4	0.0	5.4	0.03
Tibial width	TiW	31.9	3.5	40.4	25.9	32.1	33.6	2.8	40.4	27.0	33.6	28.6	2.1	31.9	25.9	29.1	0.99
Malleolar width	MalW	69.0	7.6	79.6	54.0	69.9	71.0	7.4	79.6	54.0	71.9	63.5	5.1	70.3	55.1	63.4	0.91
Trochlea tali length	TaAL	41.7	4.4	49.6	34.2	41.5	43.6	3.9	49.6	35.1	44.2	37.9	2.4	41.6	34.2	37.6	0.99
Sagittal radius of the trochlea tali arc	SRTa	23.4	3.1	32.5	19.1	23.3	24.5	3.0	32.5	19.9	24.5	21.1	1.9	26.4	19.1	20.9	0.98
Tarsal width	TaW	30.4	3.3	40.2	24.2	30.1	31.5	3.5	40.2	24.2	31.9	28.3	1.4	31.0	26.2	28.1	0.97
Maximal tibial thickness	MTiTh	41.4	3.9	48.9	33.7	41.2	42.2	3.6	48.9	33.7	43.2	38.3	2.2	41.2	33.7	38.7	0.99
Distance of level of MTiTh from the vertex of the mortise	MDV	8.7	3.5	18.0	3.2	8.0	9.3	2.9	16.5	5.6	8.1	7.7	4.2	18.0	3.2	7.3	0.29
Distance of level of MTiTh from the anterior limit of the mortise	MDA	11.5	3.5	21.4	6.7	10.7	12.2	3.2	20.4	8.0	11.2	10.4	3.9	21.4	6.7	9.6	0.14

Source: Stagni R et al., 2005. *Clin. Biomech.,* 20: 307–311.

Note: All measurements in mm but APA in degrees.

TABLE 10.2   Talocalcaneal (Ankle) Joint Contact Area

Investigators	Plantarflexion	Neutral	Dorsiflexion
Ramsey and Hamilton (1976)		4.40 ± 1.21	
Kimizuka et al. (1980)		4.83	
Libotte et al. (1982)	5.01 (30°)	5.41	3.60 (30°)
Paar et al. (1983)	4.15 (10°)	4.15	3.63 (10°)
Macko et al. (1991)	3.81 ± 0.93 (15°)	5.2 ± 0.94	5.40 ± 0.74 (10°)
Driscoll et al. (1994)	2.70 ± 0.41 (20°)	3.27 ± 0.32	2.84 ± 0.43 (20°)
Hartford et al. (1995)		3.37 ± 0.52	
Pereira et al. (1996)	1.49 (20°)	1.67	1.47 (10°)
Rosenbaum et al. (2003)		2.11 ± 0.72	

Note: The contact area is expressed in square centimeters.

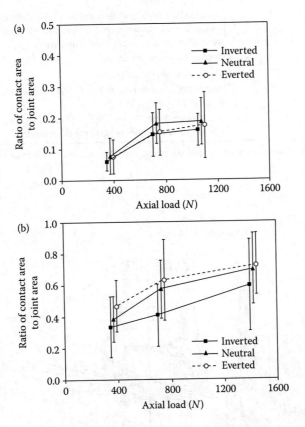

FIGURE 10.3   Ratio of total contact area to joint area in the (a) anterior/middle facet and (b) posterior facet of the subtalar joint as a function of applied axial load for three different positions of the foot. (From Wagner U.A. et al. 1992. *J. Orthop. Res.* 10: 535. With permission.)

10.3 Knee

The knee is the intermediate joint of the lower limb. It is composed of the distal femur and proximal tibia. It is the largest and most complex joint in the body. The knee joint is composed of the tibiofemoral articulation and the patellofemoral articulation.

TABLE 10.3   Axis of Rotation for the Ankle

Investigators	Axis[a]	Position
Elftman (1945)	Fix.	67.6 ± 7.4° with respect to sagittal plane
Isman and Inman (1969)	Fix.	8 mm anterior, 3 mm inferior to the distal tip of the lateral malleolus; 1 mm posterior, 5 mm inferior to the distal tip of the medial malleolus
Inman and Mann (1979)	Fix.	79° (68–88°) with respect to the sagittal plane
Allard et al. (1987)	Fix.	95.4 ± 6.6° with respect to the frontal plane, 77.7 ± 12.3° with respect to the sagittal plane, and 17.9 ± 4.5° with respect to the transverse plane
Singh et al. (1992)	Fix.	3.0 mm anterior, 2.5 mm inferior to distal tip of lateral malleolus; 2.2 mm posterior, 10 mm inferior to distal tip of medial malleolus
Sammarco et al. (1973)	Ins.	Inside and outside the body of the talus
D'Ambrosia et al. (1976)	Ins.	No consistent pattern
Parlasca et al. (1979)	Ins.	96% within 12 mm of a point 20 mm below the articular surface of the tibia along the long axis
Van Langelaan (1983)	Ins.	At an approximate right angle to the longitudinal direction of the foot, passing through the corpus tali, with a direction from anterolaterosuperior to posteromedioinferior
Barnett and Napier	Q-I	Dorsiflexion: down and lateral
		Plantarflexion: down and medial
Hicks (1953)	Q-I	Dorsiflexion: 5 mm inferior to tip of lateral malleolus to 15 mm anterior to tip of medial malleolus
		Plantarflexion: 5 mm superior to tip of lateral malleolus to 15 mm anterior, 10 mm inferior to tip of medial malleolus

[a] Fix. = fixed axis of rotation; Ins. = instantaneous axis of rotation; Q-I = quasi-instantaneous axis of rotation.

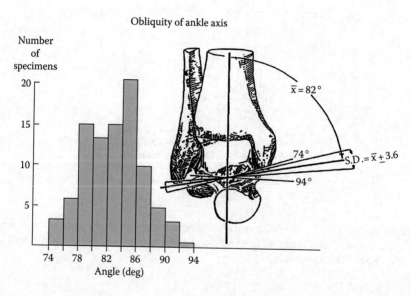

FIGURE 10.4   Variations in angle between middle of tibia and empirical axis of ankle. The histogram reveals a considerable spread of individual values. (From Inman V.T. 1976. *The Joints of the Ankle*, Baltimore, Williams and Wilkins. With permission.)

TABLE 10.4 Axis of Rotation for the Talocalcaneal (Subtalar) Joint

Investigators	Axis[a]	Position
Manter (1941)	Fix.	16° (8–24°) with respect to sagittal plane, and 42° (29–47°) with respect to transverse plane
Shephard (1951)	Fix.	Tuberosity of the calcaneus to the neck of the talus
Hicks (1953)	Fix.	Posterolateral corner of the heel to superomedial aspect of the neck of the talus
Root et al. (1966)	Fix.	17° (8–29°) with respect to sagittal plane, and 41° (22–55°) with respect to transverse plane
Isman and Inman (1969)	Fix.	23° ± 11° with respect to sagittal plane, and 41° ± 9° with respect to transverse plane
Kirby (1947)	Fix.	Extends from the posterolateral heel, posteriorly, to the first intermetatarsal space, anteriorly
Rastegar et al. (1980)	Ins.	Instant centers of rotation pathways in posterolateral quadrant of the distal articulating tibial surface, varying with applied load
Van Langelaan (1983)	Ins.	A bundle of axes that make an acute angle with the longitudinal direction of the foot passing through the tarsal canal having a direction from anteromediosuperior to posterolateroinferior
Engsberg (1987)	Ins.	A bundle of axes with a direction from anteromediosuperior to posterolateroinferior

[a] Fix. = fixed axis of rotation; Ins. = instantaneous axis of rotation.

10.3.1 Geometry of the Articulating Surfaces

The shape of the articular surfaces of the proximal tibia and distal femur must fulfill the requirement that they move in contact with one another. The profile of the femoral condyles varies with the condyle examined (Figure 10.6 and Table 10.5). The tibial plateau widths are greater than the corresponding widths of the femoral condyles (Figure 10.7 and Table 10.6). However, the tibial plateau depths are less than those of the femoral condyle distances. The medial and lateral tibial plateaus have a posterior slope in the sagittal plane (Table 10.7). The medial and lateral tibial slopes are greater in female subjects than in male subjects ($p < 0.05$) (Hashemi et al., 2008). There is also a slope in the coronal plane with the lateral point of the tibial plateau located proximal to the medial point (Table 10.7). The medial condyle of the tibia is concave superiorly (the center of curvature lies above the tibial surface) with a radius of curvature of 80 mm (Kapandji, 1987). The lateral condyle is convex superiorly (the center of curvature lies below the tibial surface) with a radius of curvature of 70 mm (Kapandji, 1987). The shape of the femoral surfaces is complementary to the shape of the tibial plateaus. The shape of the posterior femoral condyles may be approximated by spherical surfaces (Table 10.8).

The geometry of the patellofemoral articular surfaces remains relatively constant as the knee flexes. The knee sulcus angle changes only ±3.4° from 15° to 75° of knee flexion (Figure 10.8). The mean depth index varies by only ±4% over the same flexion range (Figure 10.8). Similarly, the medial and lateral patellar facet angles (Figure 10.9) change by less than a degree throughout the entire knee flexion range (Table 10.9). However, there is a significant difference between the magnitude of the medial and lateral patellar facet angles.

10.3.2 Joint Contact

The mechanism for movement between the femur and tibia is a combination of rolling and gliding. Backward movement of the femur on the tibia during flexion has long been observed in the human knee. The magnitude of the rolling and gliding changes through the range of flexion. The tibiofemoral contact area decreases as the knee flexion increases (Table 10.10). The tibial–femoral contact point has been shown to move posteriorly as the knee is flexed, reflecting the coupling of posterior motion with

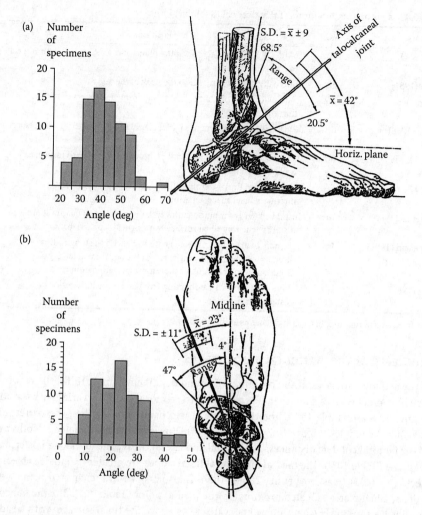

FIGURE 10.5 (a) Variations in inclination of axis of subtalar joint as projected upon the sagittal plane. The distribution of the measurements on the individual specimens is shown in the histogram. The single observation of an angle of almost 70° was present in a markedly cavus foot. (b) Variations in position of subtalar axis as projected onto the transverse plane. The angle was measured between the axis and the midline of the foot. The extent of individual variation is shown on the sketch and revealed in the histogram. (From Inman V.T. 1976. *The Joints of the Ankle*, Baltimore, Williams and Wilkins. With permission.)

flexion (Figure 10.10). In the intact knee at full extension, the center of pressure is approximately 25 mm from the anterior edge of the tibial plateau (Andriacchi et al., 1986). The medial femoral condyle rests further anteriorly on the tibial plateau than the lateral plateau. The medial femoral condyle is positioned 35 ± 4 mm from the posterior edge while the lateral femoral condyle is positioned 25 ± 4 mm from the posterior edge (Figure 10.10). During knee flexion to 90°, the medial femoral condyle moves back by 15 ± 2 mm and the lateral femoral condyle moves back by 12 ± 2 mm. Thus, during flexion, the femur moves posteriorly on the tibia (Table 10.11).

The patellofemoral contact area is smaller than the tibiofemoral contact area (Table 10.12). As the knee joint moves from extension to flexion, a band of contact moves upward over the patellar surface (Figure 10.11). As knee flexion increases, not only does the contact area move superiorly, but it also becomes larger. At 90° of knee flexion, the contact area has reached the upper level of the patella. As the knee

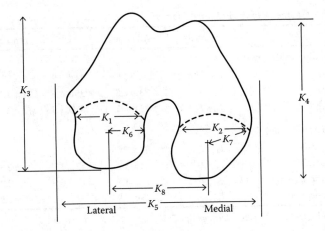

FIGURE 10.6 Geometry of the distal femur. The distances are defined in Table 10.5.

TABLE 10.5 Geometry of the Distal Femur

	Condyle					
	Lateral		Medial		Overall	
Parameter	Symbol	Distance (mm)	Symbol	Distance (mm)	Symbol	Distance (mm)
Medial/lateral distance	K_1	31 ± 2.3 (male)	K_2	32 ± 31 (male)		
		28 ± 1.8 (female)		27 ± 3.1 (female)		
Anterior/posterior distance	K_3	72 ± 4.0 (male)	K_4	70 ± 4.3 (male)		
		65 ± 3.7 (female)		63 ± 4.5 (female)		
Posterior femoral condyle spherical radii	K_6	19.2 ± 1.7	K_7	20.8 ± 2.4		
Epicondylar width					K_5	90 ± 6 (male)
						80 ± 6 (female)
Medial/lateral spacing of center of spherical surfaces					K_8	45.9 ± 3.4

Source: Yoshioka Y., Siu D., and Cooke T.D.V. 1987. *J. Bone Joint Surg.* 69A: 873–880; Kurosawa H. et al. 1985. *J. Biomech.* 18: 487.

Note: See Figure 10.6 for location of measurements.

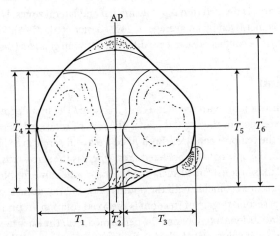

FIGURE 10.7 Contour of the tibial plateau (transverse plane). The distances are defined in Table 10.6.

TABLE 10.6   Geometry of the Proximal Tibia

Parameter	Symbols	All Limbs	Male	Female
Tibial plateau with widths (mm)				
Medial plateau	T_1	32 ± 3.8	34 ± 3.9	30 ± 22
Lateral plateau	T_3	33 ± 2.6	35 ± 1.9	31 ± 1.7
Overall width	$T_1 + T_2 + T_3$	76 ± 6.2	81 ± 4.5	73 ± 4.5
Tibial plateau depths (mm)				
AP depth, medial	T_4	48 ± 5.0	52 ± 3.4	45 ± 4.1
AP depth, lateral	T_5	42 ± 3.7	45 ± 3.1	40 ± 2.3
Interspinous width (mm)	T_2	12 ± 1.7	12 ± 0.9	12 ± 2.2
Intercondylar depth (mm)	T_6	48 ± 5.9	52 ± 5.7	45 ± 3.9

Source: Yoshioka Y. et al. 1989. *J. Orthop. Res.* 7: 132.

TABLE 10.7   Tibial Plateau Slope (deg)

	Sagittal Plane		
Gender	Medial Plateau	Lateral Plateau	Coronal Plane
Female ($n = 33$)	5.9 ± 3.0	7.0 ± 3.1	2.5 ± 1.9
Male ($n = 22$)	3.7 ± 3.1	5.4 ± 2.8	3.5 ± 1.9
P Value	0.01	0.02	0.03

Source: Hashemi J et al. 2008. *J. Bone Joint Surg.—Am.* Vol. 90: 2724–2734.

TABLE 10.8   Posterior Femoral Condyle Spherical Radius

	Normal Knee	Varus Knees	Valgus Knees
Medial condyle	20.3 ± 3.4 (16.1–28.0)	21.2 ± 2.1 (18.0–24.5)	21.1 ± 2.0 (17.84–24.1)
Lateral condyle	19.0 ± 3.0 (14.7–25.0)	20.8 ± 2.1 (17.5–30.0)	$21.1^{a} \pm 2.1$ (18.4–25.5)

Source: Matsuda S. et al. 2004. *J. Ortho. Res.* 22: 104–109.

[a] Significantly different from normal knees ($p < 0.05$).

continues to flex, the contact area is divided into separate medial and lateral zones. Under weight-bearing conditions, the contact area is increased by an average of 24% (Besier et al., 2005). When normalized by patellar dimensions ($Ht \times Wt$), the contact areas are no different between genders (Besier et al., 2005).

10.3.3 Axes of Rotation

The tibiofemoral joint is mainly a joint with two degrees of freedom. The first degree of freedom allows movements of flexion and extension in the sagittal plane. The axis of rotation lies perpendicular to the sagittal plane and intersects the femoral condyles. Both fixed axes and screw axes have been calculated (Figure 10.12). In Figure 10.12, the optimal axes are fixed axes, whereas the screw axis is an instantaneous axis. The symmetric optimal axis is constrained such that the axis is the same for both the right and left knee. The screw axis may sometimes coincide with the optimal axis but not always, depending upon the motions of the knee joint. The second degree of freedom is the axial rotation around the long axis of the tibia. Rotation of the leg around its long axis can only be performed with the knee flexed. There is also an automatic axial rotation which is involuntarily linked to flexion and extension. When the knee is flexed, the tibia internally rotates. Conversely, when the knee is extended, the tibia externally rotates.

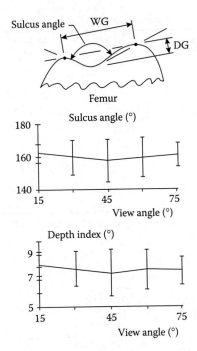

FIGURE 10.8 The trochlear geometry indices. The sulcus angle is the angle formed by the lines drawn from the top of the medial and lateral condyles to the deepest point of the sulcus. The depth index is the ratio of the width of the groove (WG) to the depth (DG). Mean and SD; $n = 12$. (From Farahmand et al. 1988. *J. Orthop. Res.* 16: 1, 136.)

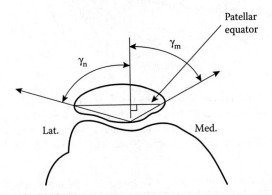

FIGURE 10.9 Medial (γ_m) and lateral (γ_n) patellar facet angles. (From Ahmed A.M., Burke D.L., and Hyder A. 1987. *J. Orthop. Res.* 5: 69–85.)

TABLE 10.9 Patellar Facet Angles

Facet angle (deg)	Knee Flexion Angle				
	0	30	60	90	120
γ_m (deg)	60.88	60.96	61.43	61.30	60.34
	3.89[a]	4.70	4.12	4.18	4.51
γ_n (deg)	67.76	68.05	68.36	68.39	68.20
	4.15	3.97	3.63	4.01	3.67

Source: Ahmed A.M., Burke D.L., and Hyder A. 1987. *J. Orthop. Res.* 5: 69–85.
[a] SD.

TABLE 10.10 Tibiofemoral Contact Area

Knee Flexion (deg)	Contact Area (cm²)
−5	20.2
5	19.8
15	19.2
25	18.2
35	14.0
45	13.4
55	11.8
65	13.6
75	11.4
85	12.1

Source: Maquet P.G., Vandberg A.J., and Simonet J.C. 1975. *J. Bone Joint Surg.* 57A: 766–771.

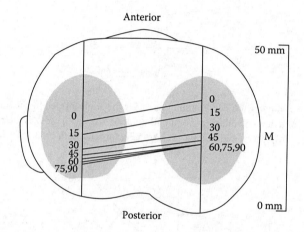

FIGURE 10.10 Diagram of the tibial plateau, showing the tibiofemoral contact pattern from 0° to 90° of knee flexion, in the loaded knee. In both medial and lateral compartments, the femoral condyle rolls back along the tibial plateau from 0° to 30°. Between 30° and 90° the lateral condyle continues to move posteriorly, while the medial condyle moves back little. (From Scarvell, J.M. et al. 2004. *J. Orthop. Res.* 22: 788–793.)

TABLE 10.11 Posterior Displacement of the Femur Relative to the Tibia

Authors	Condition	A/P Displacement (mm)
Kurosawa (1985)	*In vitro*	14.8
Andriacchi (1986)	*In vitro*	13.5
Draganich et al. (1987)	*In vitro*	13.5
Nahass et al. (1991)	*In vivo* (walking)	12.5
	In vivo (stairs)	13.9

During knee flexion, the patella makes a rolling/gliding motion along the femoral articulating surface. Throughout the entire flexion range, the gliding motion is clockwise (Figure 10.13). In contrast, the direction of the rolling motion is counter-clockwise between 0° and 90° and clockwise between 90° and 120° (Figure 10.13). The mean amount of patellar gliding for all knees is approximately 6.5 mm per 10° of flexion between 0° and 80° and 4.5 mm per 10° of flexion between 80° and 120°. The relationship

TABLE 10.12 Patellofemoral Contact Area

Knee Flexion (deg)	Contact Area (cm^2)
20	2.6 ± 0.4
30	3.1 ± 0.3
60	3.9 ± 0.6
90	4.1 ± 1.2
120	4.6 ± 0.7

Source: Huberti H.H. and Hayes W.C. 1984. *J. Bone Joint Surg.* 66A: 715–725.

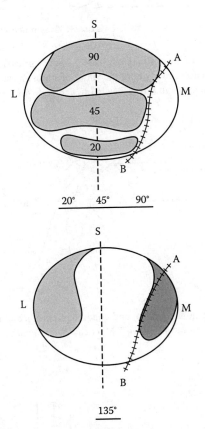

FIGURE 10.11 Diagrammatic representation of patella contact areas for varying degrees of knee flexion. (From Goodfellow J., Hungerford D.S., and Zindel M., 1976. *J. Bone Joint Surg.* 58-B: 3, 288. With permission.)

between the angle of flexion and the mean rolling/gliding ratio for all knees is shown in Figure 10.14. Between 80° and 90° of knee flexion, the rolling motion of the articulating surface comes to a standstill and then changes direction. The reversal in movement occurs at the flexion angle where the quadriceps tendon first contacts the femoral groove.

10.4 Hip

The hip joint is composed of the head of the femur and the acetabulum of the pelvis. The hip joint is one of the most stable joints in the body. The stability is provided by the rigid ball-and-socket configuration.

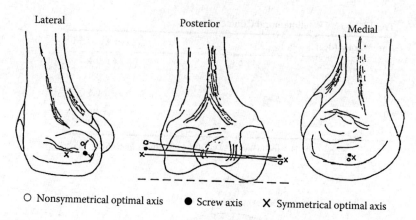

O Nonsymmetrical optimal axis   ● Screw axis   X Symmetrical optimal axis

FIGURE 10.12   Approximate location of the optimal axis (case 1—nonsymmetric, case 3—symmetric), and the screw axis (case 2) on the medial and lateral condyles of the femur of a human subject for the range of motion of 0–90° flexion (standing to sitting, respectively). (From Lewis J.L. and Lew W.D. 1978. *J. Biomech. Eng.* 100: 187. With permission.)

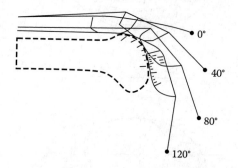

FIGURE 10.13   Position of patellar ligament, patella, and quadriceps tendon and location of the contact points as a function of the knee flexion angle. (From van Eijden T.M. et al. 1986. *J Biomech.* 19: 227. With permission.)

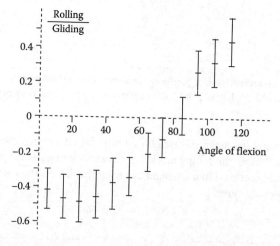

FIGURE 10.14   Calculated rolling/gliding ratio for the patellofemoral joint as a function of the knee flexion angle. (From van Eijden T.M. et al. 1986. *J Biomech.* 19: 226. With permission.)

10.4.1 Geometry of the Articulating Surfaces

The femoral head is spherical in its articular portion which forms two-thirds of a sphere. The diameter of the femoral head is smaller for female than for male individuals (Table 10.13). In the normal hip, the center of the femoral head coincides exactly with the center of the acetabulum. The rounded part of the femoral head is spheroidal rather than spherical because the uppermost part is flattened slightly. This causes the load to be distributed in a ringlike pattern around the superior pole. The geometrical center of the femoral head is traversed by the three axes of the joint, the horizontal axis, the vertical axis, and the anterior/posterior axis. The head is supported by the neck of the femur, which joins the shaft. The axis of the femoral neck is obliquely set and runs superiorly, medially, and anteriorly. The angle of inclination of the femoral neck to the shaft in the frontal plane is the neck–shaft angle (Figure 10.15). In most adults, this angle is about 130° (Table 10.13). An angle exceeding 130° is known as *coxa valga*; an angle less than 130° is known as *coxa vara*. The femoral neck forms an acute angle with the transverse axis of the femoral condyles. This angle faces medially and anteriorly and is called the *angle of anteversion* (Figure 10.16). In the adult, this angle averages about 7.5° (Table 10.13).

The acetabulum receives the femoral head and lies on the lateral aspect of the hip. The acetabulum of the adult is a hemispherical socket. Its cartilage area is approximately 16 cm² [(Von Lanz and Wauchsmuth, 1938). Together with the labrum, the acetabulum covers slightly more than 50% of the femoral head (Tönnis, 1987). Only the sides of the acetabulum are lined by articular cartilage, which is interrupted inferiorly by the deep acetabular notch. The central part of the cavity is deeper than the articular cartilage and is nonarticular. This part is called the *acetabular fossae* and is separated from the interface of the pelvic bone by a thin plate of bone.

TABLE 10.13 Geometry of the Proximal Femur

Parameter	Females	Males
Femoral head diameter (mm)	45.0 ± 3.0	52.0 ± 3.3
Neck shaft angle (deg)	133 ± 6.6	129 ± 7.3
Anteversion (deg)	8 ± 10	7.0 ± 6.8

Source: Yoshioka Y., Siu D., and Cooke T.D.V. 1987. *J. Bone Joint Surg.* 69A: 873.

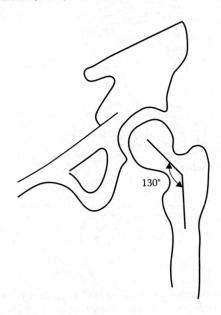

FIGURE 10.15 The neck–shaft angle.

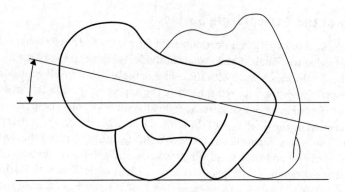

FIGURE 10.16 The normal anteversion angle formed by a line tangent to the femoral condyles and the femoral neck axis, as displayed in the superior view.

10.4.2 Joint Contact

Miyanaga et al. (1984) studied the deformation of the hip joint under loading, the contact area between the articular surfaces, and the contact pressures. They found that at loads up to 1000 N, pressure was distributed largely to the anterior and posterior parts of the lunate surface with very little pressure applied to the central portion of the roof itself. As the load increased, the contact area enlarged to include the outer and inner edges of the lunate surface (Figure 10.17). However, the highest pressures

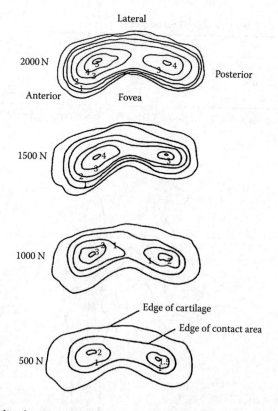

FIGURE 10.17 Pressure distribution and contact area of hip joint. The pressure is distributed largely to the anterior and posterior parts of the lunate surface. As the load increased, the contact area increased. (From Miyanaga Y., Fukubayashi T., and Kurosawa H. 1984. *Arch. Orth. Trauma Surg.* 103: 13–17. With permission.)

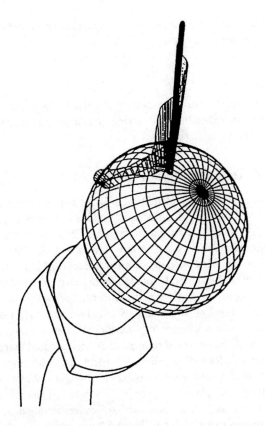

FIGURE 10.18 Scaled three-dimensional plot of resultant force during the gait cycle with crutches. The lengths of the lines indicate the magnitude of force. Radial line segments are drawn at equal increments of time, so the distance between the segments indicates the rate at which the orientation of the force was changing. For higher amplitudes of force during stance phase, line segments in close proximity indicate that the orientation of the force was changing relatively little with the cone angle between 30° and 40° and the polar angle between −25° and −15°. (From Davy D.T. et al. 1989. *J. Bone Joint Surg.* 70A: 45. With permission.)

were still measured anteriorly and posteriorly. Of five hip joints studied, only one had a pressure maximum at the zenith or central part of the acetabulum.

Davy et al. (1989) utilized a telemetered total hip prosthesis to measure forces across the hip after total hip arthroplasty. The orientation of the resultant joint contact force varies over a relatively limited range during the weight-load-bearing portions of gait. Generally, the joint contact force on the ball of the hip prosthesis is located in the anterior/superior region. A three-dimensional plot of the resultant joint force during the gait cycle, with crutches, is shown in Figure 10.18.

10.4.3 Axes of Rotation

The human hip is a modified spherical (ball-and-socket) joint. Thus, the hip possesses three degrees of freedom of motion with three correspondingly arranged, mutually perpendicular axes that intersect at the geometric center of rotation of the spherical head. The transverse axis lies in the frontal plane and controls movements of flexion and extension. An anterior/posterior axis lies in the sagittal plane and controls movements of adduction and abduction. A vertical axis which coincides with the long axis of the limb when the hip joint is in the neutral position controls movements of internal and external rotation. Surface motion in the hip joint can be considered as spinning of the femoral head on the acetabulum. The pivoting of the bone socket in three planes around the center of rotation in the femoral head produces the spinning of the joint surfaces.

10.5 Shoulder

The shoulder represents the group of structures connecting the arm to the thorax. The combined movements of four distinct articulations—glenohumeral, acromioclavicular, sternoclavicular, and scapulothoracic—allow the arm to be positioned in space.

10.5.1 Geometry of the Articulating Surfaces

The articular surface of the humerus is approximately one-third of a sphere (Figure 10.19). The articular surface is oriented with an upward tilt of approximately 45° and is retroverted approximately 30° with respect to the condylar line of the distal humerus (Morrey and An, 1990). The average radius of curvature of the humeral head in the coronal plane is 24.0 ± 2.1 mm (Iannotti et al., 1992). The radius of curvature in the anteroposterior and axillary-lateral view is similar, measuring 13.1 ± 1.3 and 22.9 ± 2.9 mm, respectively (McPherson et al., 1997). The humeral articulating surface is spherical in the center. However, the peripheral radius is 2 mm less in the axial plane than in the coronal plane. Thus, the peripheral contour of the articular surface is elliptical with a ratio of 0.92 (Iannotti et al., 1992). The major axis is superior to inferior and the minor axis is anterior to posterior (McPherson et al., 1997). More recently, the three-dimensional geometry of the proximal humerus has been studied extensively. The articular surface, which is part of a sphere, varies individually in its orientation with respect to inclination and retroversion, and it has variable medial and posterior offsets (Boileau and Walch, 1997). These findings have great impact in implant design and placement in order to restore soft-tissue function.

The glenoid fossa consists of a small, pear-shaped, cartilage-covered bony depression that measures 39.0 ± 3.5 mm in the superior/inferior direction and 29.0 ± 3.2 mm in the anterior/posterior direction (Iannotti et al., 1992). The anterior/posterior dimension of the glenoid is pear-shaped with the lower half being larger than the top half. The ratio of the lower half to the top half is 1:0.80 ± 0.01 (Iannotti et al., 1992). The glenoid radius of curvature is 32.2 ± 7.6 mm in the anteroposterior view and 40.6 ± 14.0 mm in the axillary–lateral view (McPherson et al., 1997). The glenoid is therefore more curved superior to inferior (coronal plane) and relatively flatter in an anterior to posterior direction (sagittal plane). Glenoid

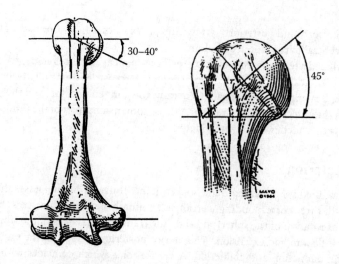

FIGURE 10.19 The two-dimensional orientation of the articular surface of the humerus with respect to the bicondylar axis. (With permission of the Mayo Foundation.)

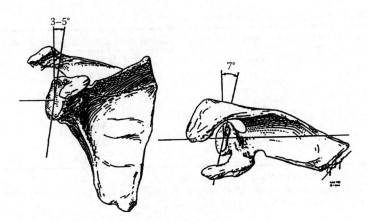

FIGURE 10.20 The glenoid faces slightly superior and posterior (retroverted) with respect to the body of the scapula. (With permission of the Mayo Foundation.)

depth is 5.0 ± 1.1 mm in the anteroposterior view and 2.9 ± 1.0 mm in the axillary–lateral (McPherson et al., 1997), again confirming that the glenoid is more curved superior to inferior. In the coronal plane the articular surface of the glenoid comprises an arc of approximately 75° and in the transverse plane the arc of curvature of the glenoid is about 50° (Morrey and An, 1990). The glenoid has a slight upward tilt of about 5° (Basmajian and Bazant, 1959) with respect to the medial border of the scapula (Figure 10.20) and is retroverted a mean of approximately 7° (Saha, 1971). The relationship of the dimension of the humeral head to the glenoid head is approximately 0.8 in the coronal plane and 0.6 in the horizontal or transverse plane (Saha, 1971). The surface area of the glenoid fossa is only one-third to one-fourth that of the humeral head (Kent, 1971). The arcs of articular cartilage on the humeral head and glenoid in the frontal and axial planes were measured (Jobe and Iannotti, 1995). In the coronal plane, the humeral heads had an arc of 159° covered by 96° of glenoid, leaving 63° of cartilage uncovered. In the transverse plane, the humeral arc of 160° is opposed by 74° of glenoid, leaving 86° uncovered.

10.5.2 Joint Contact

The degree of conformity and constraint between the humeral head and glenoid has been represented by conformity index (radius of head/radius of glenoid) and constraint index (arc of enclosure/360) (McPherson et al., 1997). Based on the study of 93 cadaveric specimens, the mean conformity index was 0.72 in the coronal and 0.63 in the sagittal plane. There was more constraint to the glenoid in the coronal versus sagittal plane (0.18 versus 0.13). These anatomic features help prevent superior–inferior translation of the humeral head but allow translation in the sagittal plane. Joint contact areas of the glenohumeral joint tend to be greater at mid-elevation positions than at either of the extremes of joint position (Table 10.14). These results suggest that the glenohumeral surface is maximum at these more functional positions, thus distributing joint load over a larger region in a more stable configuration. In general, the contact area between the glenohumeral joint over the glenolabral complex was between 49.0% and 61.5% of the calculated surface area for the intact specimens (Greis et al., 2002). The contact point moves forward and inferior during internal rotation (Figure 10.21). With external rotation, the contact is posterior/inferior. With elevation, the contact area moves superiorly. Lippitt and associates (1993) calculated the stability ratio, which is defined as a force necessary to translate the humeral head from the glenoid fossa divided by the compressive load times 100. The stability ratios were in the range of 50–60% in the superior–inferior direction and 30–40% in the anterior–posterior direction. After the labrum was removed, the ratio decreased by approximately 20%. Joint conformity was found to have significant influence on translations of humeral head during active positioning by muscles (Karduna et al., 1996).

TABLE 10.14 Glenohumeral Contact Areas

Elevation Angle (deg)	Contact Areas at SR (cm²)	Contact Areas at 20° Internal to SR (cm²)
0	0.87 ± 1.01	1.70 ± 1.68
30	2.09 ± 1.54	2.44 ± 2.15
60	3.48 ± 1.69	4.56 ± 1.84
90	4.95 ± 2.15	3.92 ± 2.10
120	5.07 ± 2.35	4.84 ± 1.84
150	3.52 ± 2.29	2.33 ± 1.47
180	2.59 ± 2.90	2.51 ± NA

Source: Soslowsky L.J. et al. 1992. *J. Orthop. Res.* 10: 524.

Note: SR, starting external rotation which allowed the shoulder to reach maximal elevation in the scapular plane (≈40° ± 8°); NA, not applicable.

The glenohumeral articular contact kinematics of normal healthy subjects and patients after total shoulder arthroplasty was assessed by using dual-plane fluoroscopic images and computer-aided design models (Boyer et al., 2008, Massimini et al., 2010). In all positions studied at 0°, 45°, and 90° of abduction, and maximal internal and external rotation, the centroid of contact on the glenoid surface for each individual, on average, was more than 5 mm away from the geometric center of the glenoid articular surface and on the humeral head surface, the centroids of contact were located at the superomedial quarter (Boyer et al., 2008). For patients with joint replacement, the superior–posterior quadrant seems to experience the most articular contact in all the shoulder positions tested. In a cadaveric experiment using Fiji film, the posterior edge loading was also consistently observed in the total shoulder specimens in positions of increased horizontal adduction and variably in positions of less adduction (Schamblin et al., 2009).

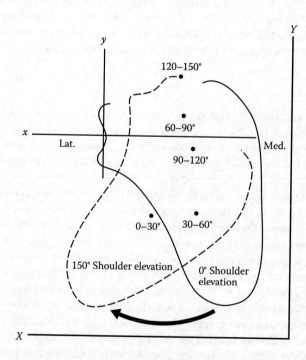

FIGURE 10.21 Humeral contact positions as a function of glenohumeral motion and positions. (From Morrey B.F. and An K.N. 1990. *The Shoulder*, pp. 208–245, Philadelphia, Saunders. With permission.)

TABLE 10.15   Arm Elevation: Glenohumeral–Scapulothoracic Rotation

Investigator	Glenohumeral/Scapulothoracic Motion Ratio
Inman et al. (1944)	2:1
Freedman and Munro (1966)	1.35:1
Doody et al. (1970)	1.74:1
Poppen and Walker (1976)	4.3:1 (<24° elevation)
	1.25:1 (>24° elevation)
Saha (1971)	2.3:1 (30–135° elevation)
Sugamoto (2002)	2.4 (Low speed)
	2.9 (High speed, 60° elevation)
	1.7 (High speed, 150° elevation)

10.5.3 Axes of Rotation

The shoulder complex consists of four distinct articulations: the glenohumeral joint, the acromioclavicular joint, the sternoclavicular joint, and the scapulothoracic articulation. The wide range of motion of the shoulder (exceeding a hemisphere) is the result of synchronous, simultaneous contributions from each joint. The most important function of the shoulder is arm elevation. Several investigators have attempted to relate glenohumeral and scapulothoracic motion during arm elevation in various planes (Table 10.15). About two-thirds of the motion takes place in the glenohumeral joint and about one-third in the scapulothoracic articulation, resulting in a 2:1 ratio. By using image intensifier combined with a video system, Sugamoto et al. (2002) found that the ratio can be influenced by the speed of rotation (Table 10.15).

Surface motion at the glenohumeral joint is primarily rotational. The center of rotation of the glenohumeral joint has been defined as a locus of points situated within 6.0 ± 1.8 mm of the geometric center of the humeral head (Poppen and Walker, 1976). However, the motion is not purely rotational. The humeral head displaces, with respect to the glenoid. From 0° to 30°, and often from 30° to 60°, the humeral head moves upward in the glenoid fossa by about 3 mm, indicating that rolling and/or gliding has taken place. Thereafter, the humeral head has only about 1 mm of additional excursion. During arm elevation in the scapular plane, the scapula moves in relation to the thorax (Poppen and Walker, 1976). From 0° to 30° the scapula rotates about its lower mid-portion, and then from 60° onward the center of rotation shifts toward the glenoid, resulting in a large lateral displacement of the inferior tip of the scapula (Figure 10.22). The center of rotation of the scapula for arm elevation is situated at the tip of the acromion as viewed from the edge on (Figure 10.23). The mean amount of scapular twisting at maximum arm elevation is 40°. The superior tip of the scapula moves away from the thorax, and the inferior tip moves toward it.

Recently, relative motion of the scapula with respect to the clavicle or the acromioclavicular joint motion was studied *in vivo* using 3D MR images obtained by a vertically open MRI (Sahara et al., 2006). They found that the scapula rotated about the clavicle at a specific screw axis passing through the insertions of both the acromioclavicular and the coracoclavicular ligaments on the coracoid process and the average rotation was 35° (Figure 10.24).

10.6 Elbow

The bony structures of the elbow are the distal end of the humerus and the proximal ends of the radius and ulna. The elbow joint complex allows two degrees of freedom in motion: flexion/extension and pronation/supination. The elbow joint complex is three separate synovial articulations. The humeral–ulnar joint is the articulation between the trochlea of the distal radius and the trochlear fossa of the proximal ulna. The humero–radial joint is formed by the articulation between the capitulum of the distal humerus and the head of the radius. The proximal radioulnar joint is formed by the head of the radius and the radial notch of the proximal ulna.

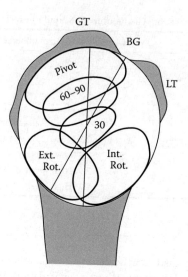

FIGURE 10.22 Rotation of the scapula on the thorax in the scapular plane. Instant centers of rotation (solid dots) are shown for each 30° interval of motion during shoulder elevation in the scapular plane from 0 to 150°. The x and y axes are fixed in the scapula, whereas the X and Y axes are fixed in the thorax. From 0 to 30° in the scapula rotated about its lower midportion; from 60° onward, rotation took place about the glenoid area, resulting in a medial and upward displacement of the glenoid face and a large lateral displacement of the inferior tip of the scapula. (From Poppen N.K. and Walker P.S. 1976. *J. Bone Joint Surg.* 58A: 195. With permission.)

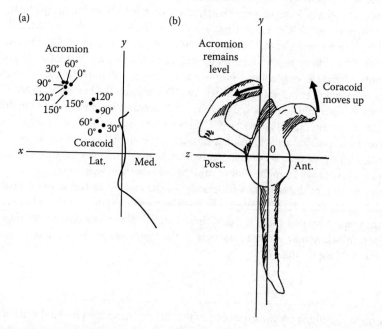

FIGURE 10.23 (a) A plot of the tips of the acromion and coracoid process on roentgenograms taken at successive intervals of arm elevation in the scapular plane shows upward movement of the coracoid and only a slight shift in the acromion relative to the glenoid face. This finding demonstrates twisting, or external rotation, of the scapula about the x-axis. (b) A lateral view of the scapula during this motion would show the coracoid process moving upward while the acromion remains on the same horizontal plane as the glenoid. (From Poppen N.K. and Walker P.S. 1976. *J. Bone Joint Surg.* 58A: 195. With permission.)

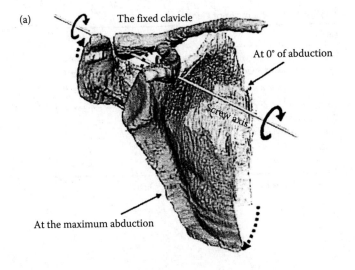

(a) The fixed clavicle

At 0° of abduction

Screw axis

At the maximum abduction

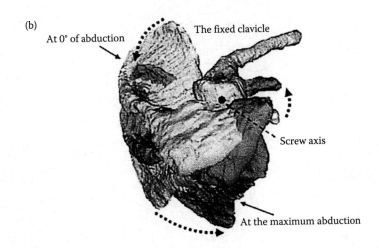

(b)

At 0° of abduction

The fixed clavicle

Screw axis

At the maximum abduction

FIGURE 10.24 These figures show the motion of a representative case. The models of the scapula at both 0° (white) and the maximum abduction (gray) are shown when the clavicular motion is fixed. (a) Is in the anterior view. The white pole is the screw axis. (b) Is in the superolateral view of the acromion parallel to the screw axis. The black dot is the screw axis. The scapula relative to the clavicle was rotated counterclockwise on the screw axis in this view, and the average rotation around this axis was approximately 35°. (From Sahara W. et al. 2006. *J. Orthop. Res.*, 24, 1823–1831. With permission.)

10.6.1 Geometry of the Articulating Surfaces

The curved, articulating portions of the trochlea and capitulum are approximately circular in a cross-section. The radius of the capitulum is larger than the central trochlear groove (Table 10.16). The centers of curvature of the trochlea and capitulum lie in a straight line located on a plane that slopes at 45°–50° anterior and distal to the transepicondylar line and is inclined at 2.5° from the horizontal transverse plane (Shiba et al., 1988). The curves of the ulnar articulations form two surfaces (coronoid and olecranon) with centers on a line parallel to the transepicondylar line but are distinct from it (Shiba et al., 1988). The carrying angle is an angle made by the intersection of the longitudinal axis of the humerus and the forearm in the frontal plane with the elbow in an extended position. The carrying angle is contributed to, in part, by the oblique axis of the distal humerus and, in part, by the shape of the proximal ulna (Figure 10.25).

TABLE 10.16 Elbow Joint Geometry

Parameter	Size (mm)
Capitulum radius	10.6 ± 1.1
Lateral trochlear flange radius	10.8 ± 1.0
Central trochlear groove radius	8.8 ± 0.4
Medial trochlear groove radius	13.2 ± 1.4
Distal location of flexion/extension axis from transepicondylar line:	
Lateral	6.8 ± 0.2
Medial	8.7 ± 0.6

Source: Shiba R. et al. 1988. *J. Orthop. Res.* 6: 897.

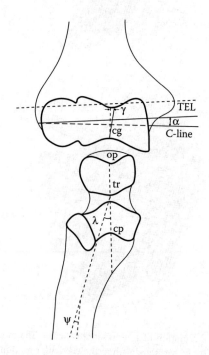

FIGURE 10.25 Components contributing to the carrying angles: $\alpha + \lambda + \psi$. α, angle between C-line and TEL; γ, inclination of central groove (cg); λ, angle between trochlear notch (tn); ψ, reverse angulation of shaft of ulna; TLE, transepicondylar line; C-line, line joining centers of curvature of the trochlea and capitellum; cg, central groove; op, olecranon process; tr, trochlear ridge; cp, coronoid process. $\alpha = 2.5 \pm 0.0$; $\lambda = 17.5 \pm 5.0$ (females) and 12.0 ± 7.0 (males); $\psi = -6.5 \pm 0.7$ (females) and -9.5 ± 3.5 (males). (From Shiba R. 1988. *J. Orthop. Res.* 6: 897. With permission.)

10.6.2 Joint Contact

The contact area on the articular surfaces of the elbow joint depends on the joint position and the loading conditions. Increasing the magnitude of the load not only increases the size of the contact area but shifts the locations as well (Figure 10.26). As the axial loading is increased, there is an increased lateralization of the articular contact (Stormont et al., 1985). The area of contact, expressed as a percentage of the total articulating surface area, is given in Table 10.17. Based on a finite element model of the humero–ulnar joint, Merz et al. (1997) demonstrated that the humero–ulnar joint incongruity brings about a bicentric distribution of contact pressure, a tensile stress exists in the notch that is the same order of magnitude as the compressive stress (Merz et al., 1997).

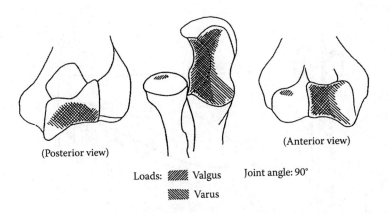

(Posterior view)

(Anterior view)

Loads: ░░ Valgus   Joint angle: 90°
       ▓▓ Varus

FIGURE 10.26 Contact of the ulnohumeral joint with varus and valgus loads and the elbow at 90°. Notice only minimal radiohumeral contact in this loading condition. (Reprinted from *J. Biomech.*, 18, Stormont T.J. et al. Elbow joint contact study: Comparison of technique, 329, Copyright 1985, with permission of Elsevier.)

TABLE 10.17   Elbow Joint Contact Area

Position	Total Articulating Surface Area of Ulna and Radial Head (mm²)	Contact Area (%)
Full extension	1598 ± 103	8.1 ± 2.7
90° flexion	1750 ± 123	10.8 ± 2.0
Full flexion	1594 ± 120	9.5 ± 2.1

Source: Goel V.K., Singh D., and Bijlani V. 1982. *J. Biomech. Eng.* 104: 169–175.

By using pressure-sensitive film, Ahmad et al. (2004) found that release of the medial ulnar collateral ligament condition and valgus load had significant effects on contact area and pressure. For a given load and flexion angle, in general, the contact area in the posteromedial olecranon decreased and the pressure increased with increasing medial ulnar collateral ligament insufficiency, especially when the elbow was at 30° of flexion.

Using magnetic resonance images and 3D registration, the *in vivo* three-dimensional kinematics of the elbow joint during elbow flexion was carried out by Goto et al. (2004). The inferred contact areas based on the proximity on the ulna against the trochlea tended to occur only on the medial facet of the trochlear notch in all of the elbow positions, and those on the radial head against the capitellum occurred on the central depression of the radial head (Goto et al., 2004).

10.6.3 Axes of Rotation

The axes of flexion and extension can be approximated by a line passing through the center of the trochlea, bisecting the angle formed by the longitudinal axes of the humerus and the ulna (Morrey and Chao, 1976). The instant centers of flexion and extension vary within 2–3 mm of this axis (Figures 10.27 through 10.29). With the elbow fully extended and the forearm fully supinated, the longitudinal axes of humerus and ulna normally intersect at a valgus angle referred to as the *carrying angle*. In adults, this angle is usually 10–15° and normally is greater on average in women (Zuckerman and Matsen, 1989). As the elbow flexes, the carrying angle varies as a function of flexion (Figures 10.30 through 10.32). In extension there is a valgus angulation of 10°; at full flexion there is a varus angulation of 8° (Morrey and Chao, 1976). More recently, the three-dimensional kinematics of the ulno–humeral joint under simulated active elbow joint flexion–extension was obtained by using an electromagnetic tracking device (Tanaka et al., 1998). The optimal axis to best represent flexion–extension motion was found to be close to the line joining the centers of the capitellum and the trochlear groove. Furthermore, the joint laxity

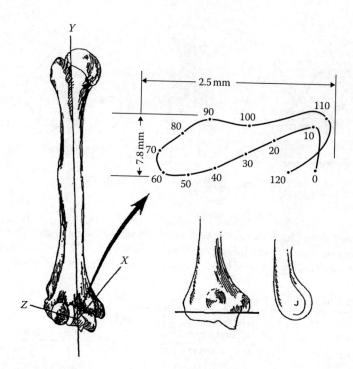

FIGURE 10.27 Very small locus of instant center of rotation for the elbow joint demonstrates that the axis may be replicated by a single line drawn from the inferior aspect of the medial epicondyle through the center of the lateral epicondyle, which is in the center of the lateral projected curvature of the trochlea and capitellum. (From Morrey B.F. and Chao E.Y.S. 1976. *J. Bone Joint Surg.* 58A: 501. With permission.)

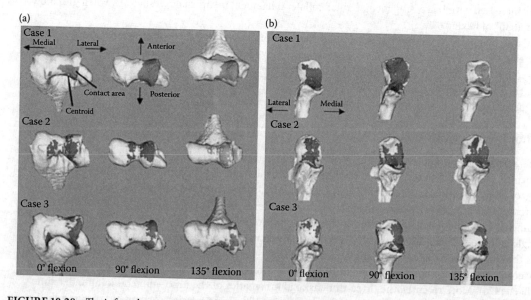

FIGURE 10.28 The inferred contact areas of articular surfaces and their centroids of the ulnohumeral joint in 0°, 90°, and 135° flexion. (a) Contact areas on the humerus. (b) Contact areas on the ulna. (From Goto A. et al. 2004. *J. Shoulder Elbow Surg.* 13, 441–447. With permission.)

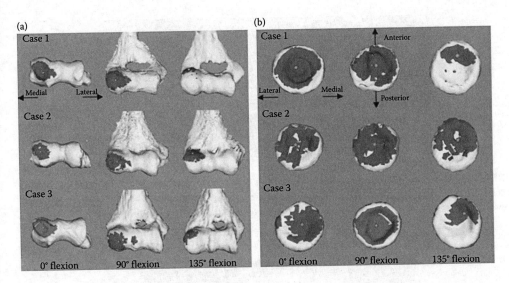

FIGURE 10.29 The inferred contact areas of articular surfaces and their centroids of the ulnohumeral joint in 0°, 90°, and 135° flexion. (a) Contact areas on the humerus. (b) Contact areas on the radius. (From Goto A. et al. 2004. *J. Shoulder Elbow Surg.* 13, 441–447. With permission.)

under valgus–varus stress was also examined. With the weight of the forearm as the stress, a maximum of 7.6° valgus–varus and 5.3° of axial rotation laxity were observed.

The screw axes of rotation of the elbow joint were evaluated *in vivo* using magnetic resonance images and 3D registration (Goto et al., 2004). They found that the pathway of the axis exhibits a roller configuration tracing the surface of a double conic shape, with the frustum waist being located in the medial portion of the trochlea (Figure 10.27). The locus of the axis of rotation traced on the surface of the condyles tended to be larger on the lateral side than on the medial side and that the locus of the averaged axis of rotation on the lateral condyle showed a counterclockwise circular pattern (Goto et al., 2004).

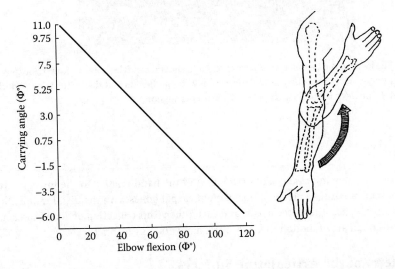

FIGURE 10.30 During elbow flexion and extension, a linear change in the carrying angle is demonstrated, typically going from the valgus in extension to the varus in flexion. (From Morrey B.F. and Chao E.Y.S. 1976. *J. Bone Joint Surg.* 58A: 501. With permission.)

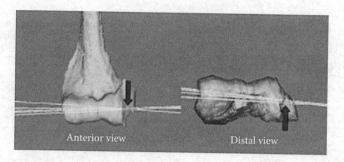

FIGURE 10.31 Superimposed images of the instantaneous axes of rotation of the ulnohumeral joint showing roller configuration tracing the surface of a double conic shape, with the frustum waist being located in the medial portion of the trochlea (arrows). (From Goto A. et al. 2004. *J. Shoulder Elbow Surg.* 13, 441–447. With permission.)

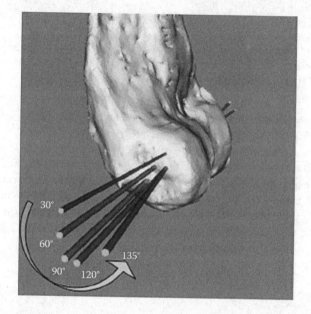

FIGURE 10.32 The locus of the averaged axis of rotation on the lateral condyle shows a counterclockwise circular pattern, where it initially moves anteriorly in the range from 0° to 60° flexion and then returns posteriorly. (From Goto A. et al. 2004. *J. Shoulder Elbow Surg.* 13, 441–447. With permission.)

10.7 Wrist

The wrist functions by allowing changes of orientation of the hand relative to the forearm. The wrist joint complex consists of multiple articulations of eight carpal bones with the distal radius, the structures of the ulnocarpal space, the metacarpals, and each other. This collection of bones and soft tissues is capable of a substantial arc of motion that augments hand and finger function.

10.7.1 Geometry of the Articulating Surfaces

The global geometry of the carpal bones has been quantified for grasp and active isometric contraction of the elbow flexors (Schuind et al., 1992). During grasping there is a significant proximal migration of the

TABLE 10.18 Changes of Wrist Geometry with Grasp

	Resting	Grasp	Analysis of Variance (p = Level)
Distal radioulnar joint space (mm)	1.6 ± 0.3	1.8 ± 0.6	0.06
Ulnar variance (mm)	-0.2 ± 1.6	0.7 ± 1.8	0.003
Lunate, uncovered length (mm)	6.0 ± 1.9	7.6 ± 2.6	0.0008
Capitate length (mm)	21.5 ± 2.2	20.8 ± 2.3	0.0002
Carpal height (mm)	33.4 ± 3.4	31.7 ± 3.4	0.0001
Carpal ulnar distance (mm)	15.8 ± 4.0	15.8 ± 3.0	NS
Carpal radial distance (mm)	19.4 ± 1.8	19.7 ± 1.8	NS
Third metacarpal length (mm)	63.8 ± 5.8	62.6 ± 5.5	NS
Carpal height ratio	52.4 ± 3.3	50.6 ± 4.1	0.02
Carpal ulnar ratio	24.9 ± 5.9	25.4 ± 5.3	NS
Lunate uncovering index	36.7 ± 12.1	45.3 ± 14.2	0.002
Carpal radial ratio	30.6 ± 2.4	31.6 ± 2.3	NS
Radius—third metacarpal angle (deg)	-0.3 ± 9.2	-3.1 ± 12.8	NS
Radius—capitate angle (deg)	0.4 ± 15.4	-3.8 ± 22.2	NS

Source: Schuind F.A. et al. 1992. *J. Hand Surg.* 17A: 698.
Note: 15 normal subjects with forearm in neutral position and elbow at 90° flexion.

radius of 0.9 mm, apparent shortening of the capitate, a decrease in the carpal height ratio, and an increase in the lunate uncovering index (Table 10.18). There is also a trend toward increase of the distal radioulnar joint with grasping. The addition of elbow flexion with concomitant grasping did not significantly change the global geometry, except for a significant decrease in the forearm interosseous space (Schuind et al., 1992).

10.7.2 Joint Contact

Studies of the normal biomechanics of the proximal wrist joint have determined that the scaphoid and lunate bones have separate, distinct areas of contact on the distal radius/triangular fibrocartilage complex surface (Viegas et al., 1987) so that the contact areas were localized and accounted for a relatively small fraction of the joint surface, regardless of wrist position (average of 20.6%). The contact areas shift from a more volar location to a more dorsal location as the wrist moves from flexion to extension. Overall, the scaphoid contact area is 1.47 times greater than that of the lunate. The scapho-lunate contact area ratio generally increases as the wrist position is changed from radial to ulnar deviation and/or from flexion to extension. Palmer and Werner (1984) also studied pressures in the proximal wrist joint and found that there are three distinct areas of contact: the ulno-lunate, radio-lunate, and radio-scaphoid. They determined that the peak articular pressure in the ulno-lunate fossa is 1.4 N/mm^2, in the radio-ulnate fossa is 3.0 N/mm^2, and in the radio-scaphoid fossa is 3.3 N/mm^2. Viegas et al. (1989) found a nonlinear relationship between increasing load and the joint contact area (Figure 10.33). In general, the distribution of load between the scaphoid and lunate was consistent with all loads tested, with 60% of the total contact area involving the scaphoid and 40% involving the lunate. Loads greater than 46 lbs were found to not significantly increase the overall contact area. The overall contact area, even at the highest loads tested, was not more than 40% of the available joint surface.

Horii et al. (1990) calculated the total amount of force borne by each joint with the intact wrist in the neutral position in the coronal plane and subjected to a total load of 143 N (Table 10.19). They found that 22% of the total force in the radio-ulno–carpal joint is dissipated through the ulna (14% through the ulno-lunate joint, and 18% through the ulno–triquetral joint) and 78% through the radius (46% through the scaphoid fossa and 32% through the lunate fossa). At the midcarpal joint, the scapho–trapezial joint transmits 31% of the total applied force, the scapho–capitate joint transmits 19%, the luno-capitate joint transmits 29%, and the triquetral-hamate joints transmits 21% of the load.

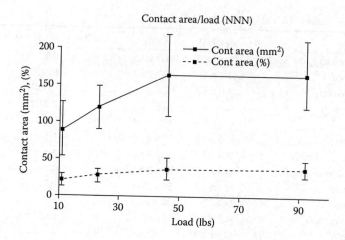

FIGURE 10.33 The nonlinear relation between the contact area and the load at the proximal wrist joint. The contact area was normalized as a percentage of the available joint surface. The load of 11, 23, 46, and 92 lbs was applied at the position of neutral pronation/supination, neutral radioulnar deviation, and neutral flexion/extension. (From Viegas S.F. et al. 1989. *J. Hand Surg.* 14A: 458. With permission.)

A limited amount of studies have been done to determine the contact areas in the midcarpal joint. Viegas et al. (1990) have found four general areas of contact: the scapho-trapezial-trapezoid (STT), the scapho-capitate (SC), the capito-lunate (CL), and the triquetral-hamate (TH). The high-pressure contact area accounted for only 8% of the available joint surface with a load of 32 lbs and increased to a maximum of only 15% with a load of 118 lbs. The total contact area, expressed as a percentage of the total available joint area for each fossa was: STT = 1.3%, SC = 1.8%, CL = 3.1%, and TH = 1.8%.

The correlation between the pressure loading in the wrist and the progress of degenerative osteoarthritis associated with pathological conditions of the forearm was studied in a cadaveric model (Sato, 1995). Malunion after distal radius fracture, tear of triangular fibrocartilage, and scapholunate dissociation were all responsible for the alteration of the articulating pressure across the wrist joint. Residual articular incongruity of the distal radius following intra-articular fracture has been correlated with early osteoarthritis. In an *in vitro* model, step-offs of the distal radius articular incongruity were created. Mean contact stress was significantly greater than the anatomically reduced case at only 3 mm of step-off (Anderson et al., 1996).

TABLE 10.19 Force Transmission at the Intercarpal Joints

Joint	Force (N)
Radio-ulno-carpal	
Ulno-triquetral	12 ± 3
Ulno-lunate	23 ± 8
Radio-lunate	52 ± 8
Radio-scaphoid	74 ± 13
Midcarpal	
Triquetral-hamate	36 ± 6
Luno-capitate	51 ± 6
Scapho-capitate	32 ± 4
Scapho-trapezial	51 ± 8

Source: Horii E. et al. 1990. *J. Bone Joint Surg.* 15A: 393.
Note: A total of 143 N axial force applied across the wrist.

10.7.3 Axes of Rotation

The complexity of joint motion at the wrist makes it difficult to calculate the instant center of motion. However, the trajectories of the hand during radioulnar deviation and flexion/extension, when they occur in a fixed plane, are circular, and the rotation in each plane takes place about a fixed axis. These axes are located within the head of the capitate and are not altered by the position of the hand in the plane of rotation (Youm et al., 1978). During radioulnar deviation, the instant center of rotation lies at a point in the capitate situated distal to the proximal end of this bone by a distance equivalent to approximately one-quarter of its total length (Figure 10.34). During flexion/extension, the instant center is close to the proximal cortex of the capitate, which is somewhat more proximal than the location for the instant center of radioulnar deviation.

Recently, an in vivo kinematic study of normal forearm rotation used computed tomographic (CT) images in five positions: neutral, 60° pronation, maximal pronation, 60° supination, and maximal supination. Surface registration of the image with the neutral position was performed, and the kinematics were expressed as motion of the radius relative to the ulna (Tay et al., 2008). The axes of the forearm rotation passed through the volar region of the radial head at the proximal radioulnar joint extending toward the dorsal region of the ulnar head at the distal radioulnar joint (Tay et al., 2008) (Figure 10.35).

Normal carpal kinematics was studied in 22 cadaver specimens using a biplanar radiography method. The kinematics of the trapezium, capitate, hamate, scaphoid, lunate, and triquetrum were determined during wrist rotation in the sagittal and coronal plane (Kobayashi et al., 1997). The results were expressed using the concept of the screw displacement axis and covered to describe the magnitude of rotation about and translation along three orthogonal axes. The orientation of these axes is expressed relative to the radius during sagittal plane motion of the wrist (Table 10.20). The scaphoid exhibited the greatest magnitude of rotation and the lunate displayed the least rotation. The proximal carpal bones exhibited some ulnar deviation in 60° of wrist flexion. During coronal plane motion (Table 10.21), the magnitude of radial–ulnar deviation of the distal carpal bones was mutually similar and generally of a greater magnitude than that of the proximal carpal bones. The proximal carpal bones experienced some flexion during radial deviation of the wrist and extension during ulnar deviation of the wrist.

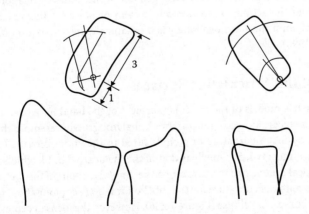

FIGURE 10.34 The location of the center of rotation during ulnar deviation (a) and extension (b), determined graphically using two metal markers embedded in the capitate. Note that during radial–ulnar deviation the center lies at a point in the capitate situated distal to the proximal end of this bone by a distance equivalent to approximately one-quarter of its total longitudinal length. During flexion–extension, the center of rotation is close to the proximal cortex of the capitate. (From Youm Y. et al. 1978. *J. Bone Joint Surg.* 60A: 423. With permission.)

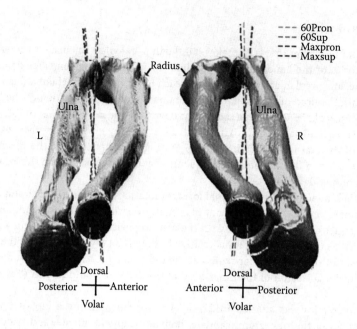

FIGURE 10.35 Distal view of three-dimensional reconstructions of the subject's left and right forearms in neutral rotation. The FHA of the four forearm positions (60° pronation, 60° supination, maximal pronation, and maximal supination), are distinctly shown. They all pass through the colar region of the proximal radial head and dorsal region of the distal ulnar head. The axis of forearm rotation appears to move largely in a linear manner during pronation and supination. (From Tay S.C. et al. 2008. *J. Biomech.* 41, 56–62. With permission.)

10.8 Hand

The hand is an extremely mobile organ that is capable of conforming to a large variety of object shapes and coordinating an infinite variety of movements in relation to each of its components. The mobility of this structure is possible through the unique arrangement of the bones in relation to one another, the articular contours, and the actions of an intricate system of muscles. Theoretical and empirical evidence suggest that limb joint surface morphology is mechanically related to joint mobility, stability, and strength (Hamrick, 1996).

10.8.1 Geometry of the Articulating Surfaces

Three-dimensional geometric models of the articular surfaces of the hand have been constructed. The sagittal contours of the metacarpal head and proximal phalanx grossly resemble the arc of a circle (Tamai et al., 1988). The radius of curvature of a circle fitted to the entire proximal phalanx surface ranges from 11 to 13 mm, almost twice as much as that of the metacarpal head, which ranges from 6 to 7 mm (Table 10.22). The local centers of curvature along the sagittal contour of the metacarpal heads are not fixed. The locus of the center of curvature for the subchondral bony contour approximates the locus of the center for the acute curve of an ellipse (Figure 10.36). However, the locus of center of curvature for the articular cartilage contour approximates the locus of the obtuse curve of an ellipse.

The surface geometry of the thumb carpometacarpal (CMC) joint has also been quantified (Athesian et al., 1992). The surface area of the CMC joint is significantly greater for male than for female individuals (Table 10.23). The minimum, maximum, and mean square curvature of these joints is reported in Table 10.23. The curvature of the surface is denoted by κ and the radius of curvature is $\rho = 1/\kappa$. The curvature is negative when the surface is concave and positive when the surface is convex.

TABLE 10.20 Individual Carpal Rotation Relative to the Radius (Deg) (Sagittal Plane Motion of the Wrist)

Wrist Motion[a] Carpal Bone	X (+) Pronation; (−) Supination				Y (+) Flexion; (−) Extension				Z (+) Ulnar Deviation; (−) Radial Deviation			
	N-E60	N-E30	N-F30	N-F60	N-E60	N-E30	N-F30	N-F60	N-E60	N-E30	N-F30	N-F60
Trapezium (N = 13)	−0.9	−1.3	0.9	−1.4	−59.4	−29.3	28.7	54.2	1.2	0.3	−0.4	2.5
SD	2.8	2.2	2.6	2.7	2.3	1	1.8	3	4	2.7	1.3	2.8
Capitate (N = 22)	0.9	−1	1.3	−1.6	60.3	−30.2	21.5	63.5	0	0	0.6	3.2
SD	2.7	1.8	2.5	3.5	2.5	1.1	1.2	2.8	2	1.4	1.6	3.6
Hamate (N = 9)	0.4	−1	1.3	−0.3	−59.5	−29	28.8	62.6	2.1	0.7	0.1	1.8
SD	3.4	1.7	2.5	2.4	1.4	0.8	10.2	3.6	4.4	1.8	1.2	4.1
Scaphoid (N = 22)	−2.5	−0.7	1.6	2	−52.3	−26	20.6	39.7	4.5	0.8	2.1	7.8
SD	3.4	2.6	2.2	3.1	3	3.2	2.8	4.3	3.7	2.1	2.2	4.5
Lunate (N = 22)	1.2	0.5	0.3	−2.2	−29.7	−15.4	11.5	23	4.3	0.9	3.3	11.1
SD	2.8	1.8	1.7	2.8	6.6	3.9	3.9	5.9	2.6	1.5	1.9	3.4
Triquetrum (N = 22)	−3.5	−2.5	2.5	−0.7	−39.3	−20.1	15.5	30.6	0	−0.3	2.4	9.8
SD	3.5	2	2.2	3.7	4.8	2.7	3.8	5.1	2.8	1.4	2.6	4.3

Source: Kobayashi M. et al. 1997. *J. Biomech.* 30: 787.

Note: SD, standard deviation.

[a] N-E60: neutral to 60° of extension; N-E30: neutral to 30° of extension; N-F30: neutral to 30° of flexion; N-F60: neutral to 60° of flexion.

TABLE 10.21   Individual Carpal Rotation to the Radius (Deg) (Coronal Plane Motion of the Wrist)

Wrist Motion[a] Carpal Bone	X (+) Pronation; (−) Supination			Y (+) Flexion; (−) Extension			Z (+) Ulnar Deviation; (−) Radial Deviation		
	N-RD15	N-UD15	N-UD30	N-RD15	N-UD15	N-UD30	N-RD15	N-UD15	N-UD30
Trapezium (N = 13)	−4.8	9.1	16.3	0	4.9	9.9	−14.3	16.4	32.5
SD	2.4	3.6	3.6	1.5	1.3	2.1	2.3	2.8	2.6
Capitate (N = 22)	−3.9	6.8	11.8	1.3	2.7	6.5	−14.6	15.9	30.7
SD	2.6	2.6	2.5	1.5	1.1	1.7	2.1	1.4	1.7
Hamate (N = 9)	−4.8	6.3	10.6	1.1	3.5	6.6	−15.5	15.4	30.2
SD	1.8	2.4	3.1	1.1	3.2	4.1	2.4	2.6	3.6
Scaphoid (N = 22)	0.8	2.2	6.6	8.5	−12.5	−17.1	−4.2	4.3	13.6
SD	1.8	2.4	3.1	3	3.2	4.1	2.4	2.6	3.6
Lunate (N = 22)	−1.2	1.4	3.9	7	−13.9	−22.5	−1.7	5.7	15
SD	1.6	0	3.3	3.1	4.3	6.9	1.7	2.8	4.3
Triquetrum (N = 22)	−1.1	−1	0.8	4.1	−10.5	−17.3	−5.1	7.7	18.4
SD	1.4	2.6	4	3	3.8	6	2.4	2.2	4

Source: Kobayashi M. et al. 1997. *J. Biomech.* 30: 787.

Note: SD, standard deviation.

[a] N-RD15: neutral to 15° of radial deviation; N-UD30: neutral to 30° of ulnar deviation; N-UD15: neutral to 15° of ulnar deviation.

TABLE 10.22 Radius of Curvature of the Middle Sections of the
Metacarpal Head and Proximal Phalanx Base

	Radius (mm)	
	Bony Contour	Cartilage Contour
MCH index	6.42 ± 1.23	6.91 ± 1.03
Long	6.44 ± 1.08	6.66 ± 1.18
PPB index	13.01 ± 4.09	12.07 ± 3.29
Long	11.46 ± 2.30	11.02 ± 2.48

Source: Tamai K. et al. 1988. *J. Hand Surg.* 13A: 521.

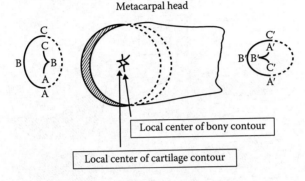

Metacarpal head

Local center of bony contour

Local center of cartilage contour

FIGURE 10.36 The loci of the local centers of curvature for subchondral bony contour of the metacarpal head approximates the loci of the center for the acute curve of an ellipse. The loci of the local center of curvature for articular cartilage contour of the metacarpal head approximates the loci of the bony center of the obtuse curve of an ellipse. (From Tamai K. et al. 1988. *J. Hand Surg.* 13A: 521. Reprinted with permission of Churchill Livingstone.)

TABLE 10.23 Curvature of Carpometacarpal Joint Articular Surfaces

	n	Area (cm²)	$\bar{\kappa}_{min}$ (m⁻¹)	$\bar{\kappa}_{max}$ (m⁻¹)	$\bar{\kappa}_{rms}$ (m⁻¹)
Trapezium					
Female	8	1.05 ± 0.21	− 61 ± 22	190 ± 36	165 ± 32
Male	5	1.63 ± 0.18	− 87 ± 17	114 ± 19	118 ± 6
Total	13	1.27 ± 0.35	− 71 ± 24	161 ± 48	147 ± 34
Female versus male		$p \le 0.01$	$p \le 0.05$	$p \le 0.01$	$p \le 0.01$
Metacarpal					
Female	8	1.22 ± 0.36	− 49 ± 10	175 ± 25	154 ± 20
Male	5	1.74 ± 0.21	− 37 ± 11	131 ± 17	116 ± 8
Total	13	1.42 ± 0.40	− 44 ± 12	158 ± 31	140 ± 25
Female versus male		$p \le 0.01$	$p \le 0.05$	$p \le 0.01$	$p \le 0.01$

Source: Athesian J.A., Rosenwasser M.P., and Mow V.C. 1992. *J. Biomech.* 25: 591.
Note: Radius of curvature: $\rho = 1/\kappa$.

10.8.2 Joint Contact

The size and location of joint contact areas of the metacarpophalangeal (MCP) joint changes as a function of the joint flexion angle (Figure 10.37). The radioulnar width of the contact area becomes narrow in the neutral position and expands in both the hyperextended and fully flexed positions (An and Cooney, 1991). In the neutral position, the contact area occurs in the center of the phalangeal base, this area being slightly larger on the ulnar than on the radial side.

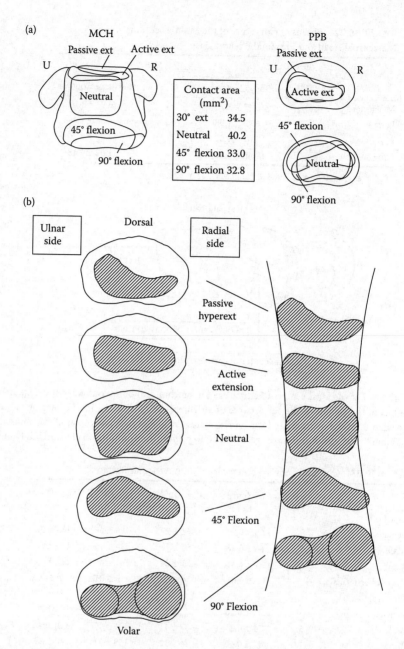

Contact area (mm²)	
30° ext	34.5
Neutral	40.2
45° flexion	33.0
90° flexion	32.8

FIGURE 10.37 (a) Contact area of the MCP joint in five joint positions. (b) End on view of the contact area on each of the proximal phalanx bases. The radioulnar width of the contact area becomes narrow in the neutral position and expands in both the hyperextended and fully flexed positions. (From An K.N. and Cooney W.P. 1991. *Joint Replacement Arthroplasty*, pp. 137–146, New York, Churchill Livingstone. By permission of Mayo Foundation.)

The contact areas of the thumb carpometacarpal joint under the functional position of lateral key pinch and in the extremes of range of motion were studied using a stereophotogrammetric technique (Ateshian et al., 1995). The lateral pinch position produced contact predominately on the central, volar, and volar–ulnar regions of the trapezium and the metacarpals (Figure 10.38). Pellegrini et al. (1993) noted that the palmar compartment of the trapeziometacarpal joint was the primary contact area during

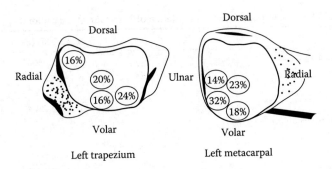

FIGURE 10.38 Summary of the contact areas for all specimens, in lateral pinch with a 25 N load. All results from the right hand are transposed onto the schema of a carpometacarpal joint from the left thumb. (From Ateshian G.A. et al. 1995. *J. Orthop. Res.* 13: 450.)

flexion adduction of the thumb in lateral pinch. Detachment of the palmar beak ligament resulted in dorsal translation of the contact area producing a pattern similar to that of cartilage degeneration seen in the osteoarthritic joint.

10.8.3 Axes of Rotation

Rolling and sliding actions of articulating surfaces exist during finger joint motion. The geometric shapes of the articular surfaces of the metacarpal head and proximal phalanx, as well as the insertion location of the collateral ligaments, significantly govern the articulating kinematics, and the center of rotation is not fixed but rather moves as a function of the angle of flexion (Pagowski and Piekarski, 1977). The instant centers of rotation are within 3 mm of the center of the metacarpal head (Walker and Erhman, 1975). Recently the axis of rotation of the MCP joint has been evaluated *in vivo* by Fioretti (1994). The instantaneous helical axis of the MCP joint tends to be more palmar and tends to be displaced distally as flexion increases (Figure 10.39).

The axes of rotation of the CMC joint have been described as being fixed (Hollister et al., 1992), but others believe that a polycentric center of rotation exists (Imaeda et al., 1994). Hollister et al. (1992) found

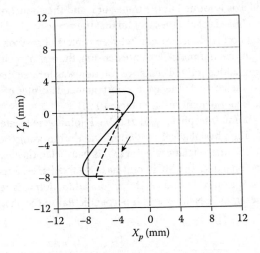

FIGURE 10.39 Intersections of the instantaneous helical angles with the metacarpal sagittal plane. They are relative to one subject tested twice in different days. The origin of the graph is coincident with the calibrated center of the metacarpal head. The arrow indicates the direction of flexion. (From Fioretti S. 1994. *Advances in the Biomechanics of the Hand and Wrist*, pp. 363–375, New York, Plenum Press. With permission.)

TABLE 10.24 Location of Center of Rotation of Trapeziometacarpal Joint

	Mean ± SD (mm)
Circumduction	
X	0.1 ± 1.3
Y	−0.6 ± 1.3
Z	−0.5 ± 1.4
Flexion/extension (in x–y plane)	
X	
Centroid	−4.2 ± 1.0
Radius	2.0 ± 0.5
Y	
Centroid	−0.4 ± 0.9
Radius	1.6 ± 0.5
Abduction/adduction (in x–z plane)	
X	
Centroid	6.7 ± 1.7
Radius	4.6 ± 3.1
Z	
Centroid	−0.2 ± 0.7
Radius	1.7 ± 0.5

Source: Imaeda T. et al. 1994. *J. Orthop. Res.* 12: 197.

Note: The coordinate system is defined with the x-axis corresponding to internal/external rotation, the y-axis corresponding to abduction/adduction, and the z-axis corresponding to flexion/extension. The x-axis is positive in the distal direction, the y-axis is positive in the dorsal direction for the left hand and in the palmar direction for the right hand, and the z-axis is positive in the radial direction. The origin of the coordinate system was at the intersection of a line connecting the radial and ulnar prominences and a line connecting the volar and dorsal tubercles.

that axes of the CMC joint are fixed and are not perpendicular to each other, or to the bones, and do not intersect. The flexion/extension axis is located in the trapezium, and the abduction/adduction axis is on the first metacarpal. In contrast, Imaeda et al. (1994) found that there was no single center of rotation, but rather the instantaneous motion occurred reciprocally between centers of rotations within the trapezium and the metacarpal base of the normal thumb. In flexion/extension, the axis of rotation was located within the trapezium, but for abduction/adduction the center of rotation was located distally to the trapezium and within the base of the first metacarpal. The average instantaneous center of circumduction was at approximately the center of the trapezial joint surface (Table 10.24).

The axes of rotation of the thumb interphalangeal and MCP joint were located using a mechanical device (Hollister et al., 1995). The physiological motion of the thumb joints occur about these axes (Figure 10.40 and Table 10.25). The interphalangeal joint axis is parallel to the flexion crease of the joint and is not perpendicular to the phalanx. The MCP joint has two fixed axes: a fixed flexion–extension axis just distal and volar to the epicondyles, and an abduction–adduction axis related to the proximal phalanx passing between the sesamoids. Neither axis is perpendicular to the phalanges.

10.9 Summary

It is important to understand the biomechanics of joint-articulating surface motion. The specific characteristics of the joint will determine the musculoskeletal function of that joint. The unique geometry of the joint surfaces and the surrounding capsule ligamentous constraints will guide the unique characteristics of the articulating surface motion. The range of joint motion, the stability of

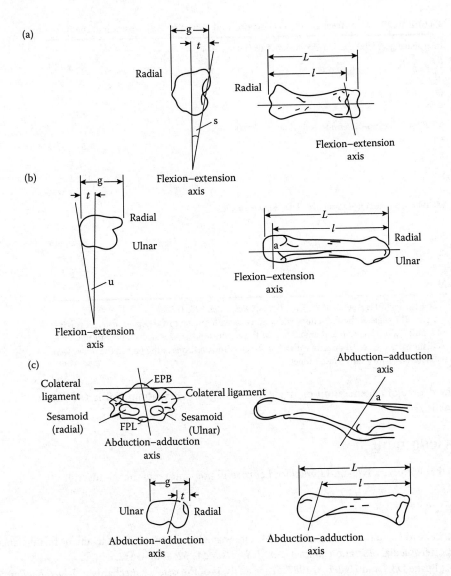

FIGURE 10.40   (a) The angles and length and breadth measurements defining the axis of rotation of the interphalangeal joint of the right thumb. (t/T = ratio of anatomic plane diameter; l/L = ratio of length). (b) The angles and
length and breadth measurements of the MCP flexion–extension axis' position in the metacarpal. (c) The angles and
length and breadth measurements that locate the MCP abduction–adduction axis. The measurements are made in
the metacarpal when the metacarpophalangeal joint is at neutral flexion extension. The measurements are made
relative to the metacarpal because the axis passes through this bone, not the proximal phalanx with which it moves.
This method of recording the abduction–adduction measurements allows the measurements of the axes to each
other at a neutral position to be made. The MCP abduction–adduction axis passes through the volar plate of the
proximal phalanx. (From Hollister A. et al. 1995. *Clin. Orthop. Relat. Res.* 320: 188.)

the joint, and the ultimate functional strength of the joint will depend on these specific characteristics. A congruent joint usually has a relatively limited range of motion but a high degree of stability,
whereas a less congruent joint will have a relatively larger range of motion but less degree of stability.
The characteristics of the joint-articulating surface will determine the pattern of joint contact and
the axes of rotation. These characteristics will regulate the stresses on the joint surface which will

TABLE 10.25 Measurement of Axis Location and Values for Axis Position in the Bone

Interphalangeal Joint Flexion–Extension Axis (Figure 10.40a)	
t/T	$44 \pm 17\%$
l/L	$90 \pm 5\%$
Θ	$5 \pm 2°$
β	$83 \pm 4°$
MCP Joint Flexion–Extension Axis (Figure 10.40b)	
t/T	$57 \pm 17\%$
l/L	$87 \pm 5\%$
α	$101 \pm 6°$
β	$5 \pm 2°$
MCP Joint Abduction–Adduction Axis (Figure 10.40c)	
t/T	$45 \pm 8\%$
l/L	$83 \pm 13\%$
α	$80 \pm 9°$
β	$74 \pm 8°$
M	

Source: Hollister A. et al. 1995. *Clin. Orthop. Relat. Res.* 320: 188.

Note: The angle of the abduction–adduction axis with respect to the flexion–extension axis is $84.8 \pm 12.2°$. The location and angulation of the K-wires of the axes with respect to the bones were measured (Θ, α, β) directly with a goniometer. The positions of the pins in the bones were measured (T, L) with a Vernier caliper.

influence the degree of degeneration of articular cartilage in an anatomic joint and the amount of wear of an artificial joint.

Acknowledgment

The authors thank Barbara Iverson-Literski for her careful preparation of the manuscript.

References

Ahmad C.S., Park M.C., and Elattrache N.S. 2004. Elbow medial ulnar collateral ligament insufficiency alters posteromedial olecranon contact. *Am. J. Sports Med.*, 32: 1607–1612.

Ahmed A.M., Burke D.L., and Hyder A. 1987. Force analysis of the patellar mechanism. *J. Orthop. Res.* 5: 69–85.

Allard P., Duhaime M., Labelle H. et al. 1987. Spatial reconstruction technique and kinematic modeling of the ankle. *IEEE Eng. Med. Biol.* 6: 31.

An K.N. and Cooney W.P. 1991. Biomechanics, Section II. The hand and wrist. In B.F. Morrey (Ed.), *Joint Replacement Arthroplasty*, pp. 137–146, New York, Churchill Livingstone.

Anderson D.D., Bell A.L., Gaffney M.B. et al. 1996. Contact stress distributions in malreduced intra-articular distal radius fractures. *J. Orthop. Trauma* 10: 331.

Andriacchi T.P., Stanwyck T.S., and Galante J.O. 1986. Knee biomechanics in total knee replacement. *J. Arthroplasty* 1: 211.

Ateshian G.A., Ark J.W., Rosenwasser M.D. et al. 1995. Contact areas in the thumb carpometacarpal joint. *J. Orthop. Res.* 13: 450.

Athesian J.A., Rosenwasser M.P., and Mow V.C. 1992. Curvature characteristics and congruence of the thumb carpometacarpal joint: Differences between female and male joints. *J. Biomech.* 25: 591.

Barnett C.H. and Napier J.R. 1952. The axis of rotation at the ankle joint in man. Its influence upon the form of the talus and the mobility of the fibula. *J. Anat.* 86: 1.

Basmajian J.V. and Bazant F.J. 1959. Factors preventing downward dislocation of the adducted shoulder joint. An electromyographic and morphological study. *J. Bone Joint Surg.* 41A: 1182.

Besier T.F., Draper C.E., Gold G.E., Beaupre G.S., and Delp S.L. 2005. Patellofemoral joint contact area increases with knee flexion and weight-bearing. *J. Orthop. Res.* 23: 345–350.

Boileau P. and Walch G. 1997. The three-dimensional geometry of the proximal humerus. *J. Bone Joint Surg.* 79B: 857.

Boyer P.J., Massimini D.F., Gill T.J., Papannagari R., Stewart S.L., Warner J.P., and Li G. 2008. *In vivo* articular cartilage contact at the glenohumeral joint: Preliminary report. *J. Orthop. Sci.* 13: 359–365.

D'Ambrosia R.D., Shoji H., and Van Meter J. 1976. Rotational axis of the ankle joint: Comparison of normal and pathological states. *Surg. Forum* 27: 507.

Davy D.T., Kotzar D.M., Brown R.H. et al. 1989. Telemetric force measurements across the hip after total arthroplasty. *J. Bone Joint Surg.* 70A: 45.

Doody S.G., Freedman L., and Waterland J.C. 1970. Shoulder movements during abduction in the scapular plane. *Arch. Phys. Med. Rehabil.* 51: 595.

Draganich L.F., Andriacchi T.P., and Andersson G.B.J. 1987. Interaction between intrinsic knee mechanics and the knee extensor mechanism. *J. Orthop. Res.* 5: 539.

Driscoll H.L., Christensen J.C., and Tencer A.F. 1994. Contact characteristics of the ankle joint. *J. Am. Pediatr. Med. Assoc.* 84: 491.

Elftman H. 1945. The orientation of the joints of the lower extremity. *Bull. Hosp. Joint Dis.* 6: 139.

Engsberg J.R. 1987. A biomechanical analysis of the talocalcaneal joint *in vitro*. *J. Biomech.* 20: 429.

Farahmand F., Senavongse W., and Amis A.A. 1998. Quantitative study of the quadriceps muscles and trochlear groove geometry related to instability of the patellofemoral joint. *J. Orthop. Res.* 16: 136.

Fioretti S. 1994. Three-dimensional *in-vivo* kinematic analysis of finger movement. In F. Schuind et al. (Eds.), *Advances in the Biomechanics of the Hand and Wrist*, pp. 363–375, New York, Plenum.

Freedman L. and Munro R.R. 1966. Abduction of the arm in the scapular plane: Scapular and glenohumeral movements. A roentgenographic study. *J. Bone Joint Surg.* 48A: 1503.

Goel V.K., Singh D., and Bijlani V. 1982. Contact areas in human elbow joints. *J. Biomech. Eng.* 104: 169–175.

Goodfellow J., Hungerford D.S., and Zindel M. 1976. Patellofemoral joint mechanics and pathology. *J. Bone Joint Surg.* 58B: 287.

Goto A., Moritomo H., Murase T., Oka K., Sugamoto K., Arimura T., Nakajima Y. et al. 2004. *In vivo* elbow biomechanical analysis during flexion: Three-dimensional motion analysis using magnetic resonance imaging. *J. Shoulder Elbow Surg.* 13: 441–447.

Greis P.E., Scuderi M.G., Mohr A., Bachus K.N., and Burks R.T. 2002. Glenohumeral articular contact areas and pressures following labral and osseous injury to the anteroinferior quadrant of the glenoid. *J. Shoulder Elbow Surg.* 11: 442–451.

Hamrick M.W. 1996. Articular size and curvature as detriments of carpal joint mobility and stability in strepsirhine primates. *J. Morphol.* 230: 113.

Hartford J.M., Gorczyca J.T., McNamara J.L. et al. 1985. Tibiotalar contact area. *Clin. Orthop.* 320: 82.

Hashemi J., Chandrashekar N., Gill B., Beynnon B.D., Slauterbeck J.R., Schutt R.C., Jr., Mansouri H., and Dabezies E. 2008. The geometry of the tibial plateau and its influence on the biomechanics of the tibiofemoral joint. *J. Bone Joint Surg.—Am. Vol.* 90: 2724–2734.

Hayes A., Tochigi Y., and Saltzman C.L. 2006. Ankle morphometry on 3D-CT images. *Iowa Orthop. J.* 26: 1–4.

Hicks J.H. 1953. The mechanics of the foot. The joints. *J. Anat.* 87: 345–357.

Hollister A., Buford W.L., Myers L.M. et al. 1992. The axes of rotation of the thumb carpometacarpal joint. *J. Orthop. Res.* 10: 454.

Hollister A., Guirintano D.J., Bulford W.L. et al. 1995. The axes of rotation of the thumb interphalangeal and metacarpophalangeal joints. *Clin. Orthop. Relat. Res.* 320: 188.

Horii E., Garcia-Elias M., An K.N. et al. 1990. Effect of force transmission across the carpus in procedures used to treat Kienböck's disease. *J. Bone Joint Surg.* 15A: 393.

Huberti H.H. and Hayes W.C. 1984. Patellofemoral contact pressures: The influence of Q-angle and tendo-femoral contact. *J. Bone Joint Surg.* 66A: 715–725.

Iannotti J.P., Gabriel J.P., Schneck S.L. et al. 1992. The normal glenohumeral relationships: An anatomical study of 140 shoulders. *J. Bone Joint Surg.* 74A: 491.

Imaeda T., Niebur G., Cooney W.P. et al. 1994. Kinematics of the normal trapeziometacarpal joint. *J. Orthop. Res.* 12: 197.

Inman V.T. 1976. *The Joints of the Ankle*, Baltimore, MD. Williams and Wilkins.

Inman V.T. and Mann R.A. 1979. Biomechanics of the foot and ankle. In V.T. Inman (Ed.), *DuVrie's Surgery of the Foot*. St Louis, Mosby.

Inman V.T., Saunders J.B. deCM, and Abbott L.C. 1944. Observations on the function of the shoulder joint. *J. Bone Joint Surg.* 26A: 1.

Iseki F. and Tomatsu T. 1976. The biomechanics of the knee joint with special reference to the contact area. *Keio. J. Med.* 25: 37.

Isman R.E. and Inman V.T. 1969. Anthropometric studies of the human foot and ankle. *Pros. Res.* 10–11: 97.

Jobe C.M. and Iannotti J.P. 1995. Limits imposed on glenohumeral motion by joint geometry. *J. Shoulder Elbow Surg.* 4: 281.

Kapandji I.A. 1987. *The Physiology of the Joints*, Vol. 2, *Lower Limb*. Edinburgh, Churchill-Livingstone.

Karduna A.R., Williams G.R., Williams J.I. et al. 1996. Kinematics of the glenohumeral joint: Influences of muscle forces, ligamentous constraints, and articular geometry. *J. Orthop. Res.* 14: 986.

Kent B.E. 1971. Functional anatomy of the shoulder complex. A review. *Phys. Ther.* 51: 867.

Kimizuka M., Kurosawa H., and Fukubayashi T. 1980. Load-bearing pattern of the ankle joint. Contact area and pressure distribution. *Arch. Orthop. Trauma Surg.* 96: 45–49.

Kinzel G.L., Hall A.L., and Hillberry B.M. 1972. Measurement of the total motion between two body segments: Part I. Analytic development. *J. Biomech.* 5: 93.

Kirby K.A. 1947. Methods for determination of positional variations in the subtalar and transverse tarsal joints. *Anat. Rec.* 80: 397.

Kobayashi M., Berger R.A., Nagy L. et al. 1997. Normal kinematics of carpal bones: A three-dimensional analysis of carpal bone motion relative to the radius. *J. Biomech.* 30: 787.

Kurosawa H., Walker P.S., Abe S. et al. 1985. Geometry and motion of the knee for implant and orthotic design. *J. Biomech.* 18: 487.

Lewis J.L. and Lew W.D. 1978. A method for locating an optimal "fixed" axis of rotation for the human knee joint. *J. Biomech. Eng.* 100: 187.

Libotte M., Klein P., Colpaert H. et al. 1982. Contribution à l'étude biomécanique de la pince malléolaire. *Rev. Chir. Orthop.* 68: 299.

Lippitt B., Vanderhooft J.E., Harris S.L. et al. 1993. Glenohumeral stability from concavity-compression: A quantitative analysis. *J. Shoulder Elbow Surg.* 2: 27–35.

Macko V.W., Matthews L.S., Zwirkoski P. et al. 1991. The joint contract area of the ankle: The contribution of the posterior malleoli. *J. Bone Joint Surg.* 73A: 347.

Manter J.T. 1941. Movements of the subtalar and transverse tarsal joints. *Anat. Rec.* 80: 397–402.

Maquet P.G., Vandberg A.J., and Simonet J.C. 1975. Femorotibial weight bearing areas: Experimental determination. *J. Bone Joint Surg.* 57A: 766–771.

Massimini D.F., Li G., and Warner J.P. 2010. Glenohumeral contact kinematics in patients after total shoulder arthroplasty. *J. Bone Joint Surg.* 92: 916–926.

Matsuda S., Miura H., Nagamine R., Mawatari T., Tokunaga M., Nabeyama R., and Iwamoto Y. 2004. Anatomical analysis of the femoral condyle in normal and osteoarthritic knees. *J. Orthop. Res.* 22: 104–109.

McPherson E.J., Friedman R.J., An Y.H. et al. 1997. Anthropometric study of normal glenohumeral relationships. *J. Shoulder Elbow Surg.* 6: 105.

Merz B., Eckstein F., Hillebrand S. et al. 1997. Mechanical implication of humero-ulnar incongruity-finite element analysis and experiment. *J. Biomech.* 30: 713.

Miyanaga Y., Fukubayashi T., and Kurosawa H. 1984. Contact study of the hip joint: Load deformation pattern, contact area, and contact pressure. *Arch. Orth. Trauma Surg.* 103: 13–17.

Morrey B.F. and An K.N. 1990. Biomechanics of the shoulder. In C.A. Rockwood and F.A. Matsen (Eds.), *The Shoulder*, pp. 208–245, Philadelphia, Saunders.

Morrey B.F. and Chao E.Y.S. 1976. Passive motion of the elbow joint: A biomechanical analysis. *J. Bone Joint Surg.* 58A: 501.

Nahass B.E., Madson M.M., and Walker P.S. 1991. Motion of the knee after condylar resurfacing—An in vivo study. *J. Biomech.* 24: 1107.

Paar O., Rieck B., and Bernett P. 1983. Experimentelle untersuchungen über belastungsabhängige Drukund Kontaktflächenverläufe an den Fussgelenken. *Unfallheilkunde* 85: 531.

Pagowski S. and Piekarski K. 1977. Biomechanics of metacarpophalangeal joint. *J. Biomech.* 10: 205.

Palmer A.K. and Werner F.W. 1984. Biomechanics of the distal radio–ulnar joint. *Clin. Orthop.* 187: 26.

Parlasca R., Shoji H., and D'Ambrosia R.D. 1979. Effects of ligamentous injury on ankle and subtalar joints. A kinematic study. *Clin. Orthop.* 140: 266.

Pellegrini V.S., Olcott V.W., and Hollenberg C. 1993. Contact patterns in the trapeziometacarpal joint: The role of the palmar beak ligament. *J. Hand Surg.* 18A: 238.

Pereira D.S., Koval K.J., Resnick R.B. et al. 1996. Tibiotalar contact area and pressure distribution: The effect of mortise widening and syndesmosis fixation. *Foot Ankle* 17: 269.

Poppen N.K. and Walker P.S. 1976. Normal and abnormal motion of the shoulder. *J. Bone Joint Surg.* 58A: 195.

Ramsey P.L. and Hamilton W. 1976. Changes in tibiotalar area of contact caused by lateral talar shift. *J. Bone Joint Surg.* 58A: 356.

Rastegar J., Miller N., and Barmada R. 1980. An apparatus for measuring the load-displacement and load-dependent kinematic characteristics of articulating joints—Application to the human ankle. *J. Biomech. Eng.* 102: 208.

Root M.L., Weed J.H., Sgarlato T.E., and Bluth D.R. 1966. Axis of motion of the subtalar joint. *J. Am. Pediatry Assoc.* 56: 149.

Rosenbaum D., Eils E., and Hillmann A. 2003. Changes in talocrural joint contact stress characteristics after simulated rotationplasty. *J. Biomech.* 36: 81–86.

Saha A.K. 1971. Dynamic stability of the glenohumeral joint. *Acta Orthop. Scand.* 42: 491.

Sahara W., Sugamoto K., Murai M., Tanaka H., and Toshikawa H. 2006. 3D kinematic analysis of the acromioclavicular joint during arm abduction using vertically open MRI. *J. Orthop. Res.* 24: 1823–1831.

Sammarco G.J., Burstein A.J., and Frankel V.H. 1973. Biomechanics of the ankle: A kinematic study. *Orthop. Clin. North Am.* 4: 75–96.

Sato S. 1995. Load transmission through the wrist joint: A biomechanical study comparing the normal and pathological wrist. *Nippon Seikeigeka Gakkai Zasshi-Journal of the Japanese Orthopaedic Association* 69: 470–483.

Scarvell J.M., Smith P.N., Refshauge K.M., Galloway H.R., and Woods K.R. 2004. Evaluation of a method to map tibiofemoral contact points in the normal knee using MRI. *J. Orthop. Res.* 22: 788–793.

Schamblin M., Gupta R., Yang B.Y., Mcgarry M.H., Mcmaster W.C., and Lee T.Q. 2009. In vitro quantitative assessment of total and bipolar shoulder arthroplasties: A biomechanical study using human cadaver shoulders. *Clin Biomech (Bristol, Avon)*, 24: 626–631.

Schuind F.A., Linscheid R.L., An K.N. et al. 1992. Changes in wrist and forearm configuration with grasp and isometric contraction of elbow flexors. *J. Hand Surg.* 17A: 698.

Shephard E. 1951. Tarsal movements. *J. Bone Joint Surg.* 33B: 258.

Shiba R., Sorbie C., Siu D.W. et al. 1988. Geometry of the humeral–ulnar joint. *J. Orthop. Res.* 6: 897.

Singh A.K., Starkweather K.D., Hollister A.M. et al. 1992. Kinematics of the ankle: A hinge axis model. *Foot Ankle* 13: 439.

Soslowsky L.J., Flatow E.L., Bigliani L.U. et al. 1992. Quantitation of *in situ* contact areas at the glenohumeral joint: A biomechanical study. *J. Orthop. Res.* 10: 524.

Spoor C.W. and Veldpaus F.E. 1980. Rigid body motion calculated from spatial coordinates of markers. *J. Biomech.* 13: 391.

Stagni R., Leardini A., Ensini A., and Cappello A. 2005. Ankle morphometry evaluated using a new semi-automated technique based on X-ray pictures. *Clin. Biomech.*, 20: 307–311.

Stormont T.J., An K.A., Morrey B.F. et al. 1985. Elbow joint contact study: Comparison of techniques. *J. Biomech.* 18: 329.

Sugamoto K., Harada T., Machida A., Inui H., Miyamoto T., Takeuchi E., Yoshikawa H., and Ochi T. 2002. Scapulohumeral rhythm: Relationship between motion velocity and rhythm. *Clin. Orthop. Relat. Res.* 401: 119–124.

Tamai K., Ryu J., An K.N. et al. 1988. Three-dimensional geometric analysis of the metacarpophalangeal joint. *J. Hand Surg.* 13A: 521.

Tanaka S., An K.N., and Morrey B.F. 1998. Kinematics and laxity of ulnohumeral joint under valgus–varus stress. *J. Musculoskeletal Res.* 2: 45.

Tay S.C., Van Riet R., Kazunari T., Koff M.F., Amrami K.K., An K.N., and Berger R.A. 2008. A method for in-vivo kinematic analysis of the forearm. *J. Biomech.* 41: 56–62.

Tönnis D. 1987. *Congenital Dysplasia and Dislocation of the Hip and Shoulder in Adults*, pp. 1–12. Berlin, Springer-Verlag.

Van Eijden T.M.G.J., Kouwenhoven E., Verburg J. et al. 1986. A mathematical model of the patellofemoral joint. *J. Biomech.* 19: 219.

Van Langelaan E.J. 1983. A kinematical analysis of the tarsal joints. An x-ray photogrammetric study. *Acta Orthop. Scand.* 204: 211.

Viegas S.F., Patterson R.M., Peterson P.D. et al. 1989. The effects of various load paths and different loads on the load transfer characteristics of the wrist. *J. Hand Surg.* 14A: 458.

Viegas S.F., Patterson R.M., Todd P. et al. 1990. Load transfer characteristics of the midcarpal joint. *Wrist Biomechanics Symposium, Wrist Biomechanics Workshop*, Mayo Clinic, Rochester, MN.

Viegas S.F., Tencer A.F., Cantrell J. et al. 1987. Load transfer characteristics of the wrist: Part I. The normal joint. *J. Hand Surg.* 12A: 971.

Von Lanz D. and Wauchsmuth W. 1938. *Das Hüftgelenk, Praktische Anatomie* I Bd, pp. 138–175, Teil 4: *Bein und Statik*, Berlin, Springer-Verlag.

Wagner U.A., Sangeorzan B.J., Harrington R.M. et al. 1992. Contact characteristics of the subtalar joint: Load distribution between the anterior and posterior facets. *J. Orthop. Res.* 10: 535.

Walker P.S. and Erhman M.J. 1975. Laboratory evaluation of a metaplastic type of metacarpophalangeal joint prosthesis. *Clin. Orthop.* 112: 349.

Wang C.-L., Cheng C.-K., Chen C.-W. et al. 1994. Contact areas and pressure distributions in the subtalar joint. *J. Biomech.* 28: 269.

Woltring H.J., Huiskes R., deLange A., and Veldpaus F.E. 1985. Finite centroid and helical axis estimation from noisy landmark measurements in the study of human joint kinematics. *J. Biomech.* 18: 379.

Yoshioka Y., Siu D., and Cooke T.D.V. 1987. The anatomy and functional axes of the femur. *J. Bone Joint Surg.* 69A: 873.

Yoshioka Y., Siu D., Scudamore R.A. et al. 1989. Tibial anatomy in functional axes. *J. Orthop. Res.* 7: 132.

Youm Y., McMurty R.Y., Flatt A.E. et al. 1978. Kinematics of the wrist: An experimental study of radioulnar deviation and flexion/extension. *J. Bone Joint Surg.* 60A: 423.

Zuckerman J.D. and Matsen F.A. 1989. Biomechanics of the elbow. In M. Nordine and V.H. Frankel (Eds.), *Basic Biomechanics of the Musculoskeletal System*, pp. 249–260. Philadelphia, Lea & Febiger.

11

Joint Lubrication

11.1   Introduction 11-1
11.2   Tribology 11-2
       Friction • Wear and Surface Damage
11.3   Lubrication 11-3
       Hydrodynamic Lubrication Theories • Transition from
       Hydrodynamic to Boundary Lubrication
11.4   Synovial Joints 11-7
11.5   Theories on the Lubrication of Natural and Normal
       Synovial Joints 11-8
11.6   *In Vitro* Cartilage Wear Studies 11-11
11.7   Biotribology and Arthritis: Are There Connections? 11-15
11.8   Recapitulation and Final Comments 11-18
       Terms and Definitions • Experimental Contact Systems • Fluids
       and Materials Used as Lubricants in *In Vitro* Biotribology
       Studies • The Preoccupation with Rheology and Friction • The
       Probable Existence of Various Lubrication Regimes • Recent
       Developments
11.9   Conclusions 11-21
       Acknowledgments 11-22
       Further Information 11-23
       References 11-23

Michael J. Furey
*Virginia Polytechnic
Institute and State
University*

The Fabric of the Joints in the Human Body is a subject so much the more entertaining, as it must strike every one that considers it attentively with an Idea of fine Mechanical Composition. Wherever the Motion of one Bone upon another is requisite, there we find an excellent Apparatus for rendering that Motion safe and free: We see, for Instance, the Extremity of one Bone molded into an orbicular Cavity, to receive the Head of another, in order to afford it an extensive Play. Both are covered with a smooth elastic Crust, to prevent mutual Abrasion; connected with strong Ligaments, to prevent Dislocation; and inclosed in a Bag that contains a proper Fluid Deposited there, for lubricating the Two contiguous Surfaces. So much in general.

The above is the opening paragraph of the classic paragraph of the classic paper by the surgeon, Sir William Hunter, "Of the Structure and Diseases of Articulating Cartilages" which he read at a meeting of the Royal Society, June 2, 1743 [1]. Since then, a great deal of research has been carried out on the subject of synovial joint lubrication. However, the mechanisms involved are still unknown.

11.1 Introduction

The purpose of this chapter is twofold: (1) to introduce the reader to the subject of tribology—the study of friction, wear, and lubrication; and (2) to extend this to the topic of *biotribology*, which includes the lubrication of natural synovial joints. It is not meant to be an exhaustive review of joint lubrication theories; space does not permit this. Instead, major concepts or principles will be discussed not only in the light of what is known about synovial joint lubrication but perhaps more importantly what is not known. Several references are given for those who wish to learn more about the topic. It is clear that synovial joints are by far the most complex and sophisticated tribological systems that exist. We shall see that although numerous theories have been put forth to attempt to explain joint lubrication, the mechanisms involved are still far from being understood. And when one begins to examine possible connections between tribology and degenerative joint disease or osteoarthritis (OA), the picture is even more complex and controversial. Finally, this chapter does not treat (1) the tribological behavior of artificial joints or partial joint replacements, (2) the possible use of elastic or poroplastic materials as artificial cartilage, and (3) new developments in cartilage repair using transplanted chondrocytes. These are separate topics, which would require detailed discussion and additional space.

11.2 Tribology

The word tribology, derived from the Greek "to rub," covers all frictional processes between solid bodies moving relative to one another that are in contact [2]. Thus, tribology may be defined as the study of friction, wear, and lubrication.

Tribological processes are involved whenever one solid slides or rolls against another, as in bearings, cams, gears, piston rings and cylinders, machining and metalworking, grinding, rock drilling, sliding electrical contacts, frictional welding, brakes, the striking of a match, music from a cello, articulation of human synovial joints (e.g., hip joints), machinery, and in numerous less obvious processes (e.g., walking, holding, stopping, writing, and the use of fasteners such as nails, screws, and bolts).

Tribology is a multidisciplinary subject involving at least the areas of materials science, solid and surface mechanics, surface science and chemistry, rheology, engineering, mathematics, and even biology and biochemistry. Although tribology is still an emerging science, interest in the phenomena of friction, wear, and lubrication is an ancient one. Unlike thermodynamics, there are no generally accepted laws in tribology. But there are some important basic principles that are needed to understand any study of lubrication and wear and even more so in a study of biotribology or biological lubrication phenomena. These basic principles follow.

11.2.1 Friction

Much of the early work in tribology was in the area of friction—possibly because frictional effects are more readily demonstrated and measured. Generally, early theories of friction dealt with dry or unlubricated systems. The problem was often treated strictly from a mechanical viewpoint, with little or no regard for the environment, surface films, or chemistry.

In the first place, *friction may be defined as the tangential resistance that is offered to the sliding of one solid body over another.* Friction is the result of many factors and cannot be treated as something as singular as density or even viscosity. Postulated sources of friction have included (1) the lifting of one asperity over another (increase in potential energy), (2) the interlocking of asperities followed by shear, (3) interlocking followed by plastic deformation or plowing, (4) adhesion followed by shear, (5) elastic hysteresis and waves of deformation, (6) adhesion or interlocking followed by tensile failure, (7) intermolecular attraction, (8) electrostatic effects, and (9) viscous drag. The coefficient of friction, indicated in the literature by μ or f, is defined as the ratio F/W where F = friction force and W = the normal load. It is emphasized that friction is a force and not a property of a solid material or lubricant.

11.2.2 Wear and Surface Damage

One definition of wear in a tribological sense is that it is the *progressive loss of substance from the operating surface of a body as a result of relative motion at the surface.* In comparison with friction, very little theoretical work has been done on the extremely important area of wear and surface damage. This is not too surprising in view of the complexity of wear and how little is known of the mechanisms by which it can occur. Variations in wear can be, and often are, enormous compared with variations in friction. For example, practically all the coefficients of sliding friction for diverse dry or lubricated systems fall within a relatively narrow range of 0.1–1. In some cases (e.g., certain regimes of hydrodynamic or "boundary" lubrication), the coefficient of friction may be <0.1 and as low as 0.001. In other cases (e.g., very clean unlubricated metals in vacuum), friction coefficients may exceed 1. Reduction of friction by a factor of 2 through changes in design, materials, or lubricant would be a reasonable, although not always attainable, goal. On the other hand, it is not uncommon for wear rates to vary by a factor of 100, 1000, or even more.

For systems consisting of common materials (e.g., metals, polymers, ceramics), there are at least four main mechanisms by which wear and surface damage can occur between solids in relative motion: (1) abrasive wear, (2) adhesive wear, (3) fatigue wear, and (4) chemical or corrosive wear. A fifth, fretting wear and fretting corrosion, combines elements of more than one mechanism. For complex biological materials such as articular cartilage, most likely other mechanisms are involved.

Again, wear is the removal of material. The idea that friction causes wear and therefore, low friction means low wear, is a common mistake. Brief descriptions of five types of wear; abrasive, adhesive, fatigue, chemical or corrosive, and fretting—may be found in Reference 2 as well as in other references in this chapter. Next, it may be useful to consider some of the major concepts of lubrication.

11.3 Lubrication

Lubrication is a process of reducing friction *and/or* wear (or other forms of surface damage) between relatively moving surfaces by the application of a solid, liquid, or gaseous substance (i.e., a lubricant). Since friction and wear do not necessarily correlate with each other, the use of the word *and* in place of *and/or* in the above definition is a common mistake to be avoided. The primary function of a lubricant is to reduce friction or wear or both between moving surfaces in contact with each other.

Examples of lubricants are wide and varied. They include automotive engine oils, wheel bearing greases, transmission fluids, electrical contact lubricants, rolling oils, cutting fluids, preservative oils, gear oils, jet fuels, instrument oils, turbine oils, textile lubricants, machine oils, jet engine lubricants, air, water, molten glass, liquid metals, oxide films, talcum powder, graphite, molybdenum disulfide, waxes, soaps, polymers, and the synovial fluid in human joints.

A few general principles of lubrication may be mentioned here:

1. The lubricant must be present at the place where it can function.
2. Almost any substance under carefully selected or special conditions can be shown to reduce friction or wear in a particular test, but that does not mean these substances are lubricants.
3. Friction and wear do not necessarily go together. This is an extremely important principle which applies to nonlubricated (dry) as well as lubricated systems. It is particularly true under conditions of "boundary lubrication," to be discussed later. An additive may reduce friction and increase wear, reduce wear and increase friction, reduce both or increase both. Although the reasons are not fully understood, this is an experimental observation. Thus, friction and wear should be thought of as separate phenomena—an important point when we discuss theories of synovial joint lubrication.
4. The effective or active lubricating film in a particular system may or may not consist of the original or bulk lubricant phase.

In a broad sense, it may be considered that the main function of a lubricant is to keep the surfaces apart so that interaction (e.g., adhesion, plowing, and shear) between the solids cannot occur; thus friction and wear can be reduced or controlled.

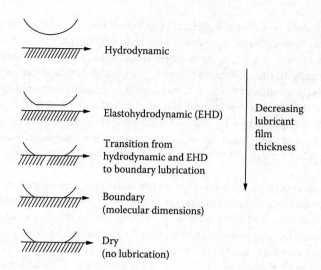

FIGURE 11.1 Regimes of lubrication.

The following regimes or types of lubrication may be considered in the order of increasing severity or decreasing lubricant film thickness (Figure 11.1):

1. Hydrodynamic lubrication
2. Elastohydrodynamic lubrication (EHL)
3. Transition from hydrodynamic and EHL to boundary lubrication
4. Boundary lubrication

A fifth regime, sometimes referred to as *dry* or *unlubricated*, may also be considered as an extreme or limit. In addition, there is another form of lubrication that does not require relative movement of the bodies either parallel or perpendicular to the surface, that is, as in externally pressurized hydrostatic or aerostatic bearings.

11.3.1 Hydrodynamic Lubrication Theories

In hydrodynamic lubrication, the load is supported by the pressure developed due to relative motion and the geometry of the system. In the regime of hydrodynamic or fluid film lubrication, there is no contact between the solids. The film thickness is governed by the bulk physical properties of the lubricants, the most important being viscosity; friction arises purely from shearing of viscous lubricant.

Contributions to our knowledge of hydrodynamic lubrication, with special focus on journal bearings, have been made by numerous investigators including Reynolds. The classic Reynolds treatment considered the equilibrium of a fluid element and the pressure and shear forces on this element. In this treatment, eight assumptions were made (e.g., surface curvature is large compared to lubricant film thickness, fluid is Newtonian, flow is laminar, viscosity is constant through film thickness). Velocity distributions due to relative motion and pressure buildup were developed and added together. The solution of the basic Reynolds equation for a particular bearing configuration results in a pressure distribution throughout the film as a function of viscosity, film shape, and velocity.

The total load W and frictional (viscous) drag F can be calculated from this information. For rotating disks with parallel axes, the "simple" Reynolds equation yields

$$\frac{h_o}{R} = 4.9\left(\frac{\eta U}{W}\right) \tag{11.1}$$

where h_o is the minimum lubricant film thickness, η is the absolute viscosity, U is the average velocity $(U_1 + U_2)/2$, W is the applied normal load per unit width of disk, and R is the reduced radius of curvature $(1/R = 1/R_1 + 1/R_2)$.

The dimensionless term $(\eta U/W)$ is sometimes referred to as the hydrodynamic factor. It can be seen that doubling either the viscosity or velocity doubles the film thickness, and that doubling the applied load halves the film thickness. This regime of lubrication is sometimes referred to as the *rigid isoviscous or classical Martin condition*, since the solid bodies are assumed to be perfectly rigid (nondeformable), and the fluid is assumed to have a constant viscosity.

At high loads with systems such as gears, ball bearings, and other high-contact-stress geometries, two additional factors have been considered in further developments of the hydrodynamic theory of lubrication. One of these is that the surfaces deform elastically; this leads to a localized change in geometry more favorable to lubrication. The second is that the lubricant becomes more viscous under the high pressure existing in the contact zone, according to relationships such as

$$\eta/\eta_o = \exp\alpha(p - p_o) \tag{11.2}$$

where η is the viscosity at pressure p, η_o is the viscosity at atmospheric pressure p_o, and α is the pressure–viscosity coefficient (e.g., in Pa^{-1}). In this concept, the lubricant pressures existing in the contact zone approximate those of dry contact Hertzian stress. This is the regime of elastohydrodynamic lubrication, sometimes abbreviated as EHL or EHD. It may also be described as the elastic–viscous type or mode of lubrication, since elastic deformation exists and the fluid viscosity is considerably greater due to the pressure effect.

The comparable Dowson–Higginson expression for minimum film thickness between cylinders or disks in contact with parallel axes is

$$\frac{h_o}{R} = 2.6\left(\frac{\eta U}{W}\right)^{0.7}\left(\frac{\alpha W}{R}\right)^{0.54}\left(\frac{W}{RE'}\right)^{0.03} \tag{11.3}$$

The term E' represents the reduced modulus of elasticity:

$$\frac{1}{E'} = \frac{(1 - v_1^2)}{E_1} + \frac{(1 - v_2^2)}{E_2} \tag{11.4}$$

where E is the modulus, v is Poisson's ratio, and the subscripts 1 and 2 refer to the two solids in contact. All the other terms are the same as previously stated. In addition to the hydrodynamic factor $(\eta U/W)$, a pressure–viscosity factor $(\alpha W/R)$, and an elastic deformation factor (W/RE') can be considered. Thus, properties of both the lubricant and the solids as materials are included. In examining the elastohydrodynamic film thickness equations, it can be seen that the velocity U is an important factor ($h_o \propto U^{0.7}$) but the load W is rather unimportant ($h_o \propto W^{-0.13}$).

Experimental confirmation of the EHL theory has been obtained in certain selected systems using electrical capacitance, x-ray transmission, and optical interference techniques to determine film thickness and shape under dynamic conditions. Research is continuing in this area, including studies on micro-EHL or asperity lubrication mechanisms, since surfaces are never perfectly smooth. These studies may lead to a better understanding of not only lubricant film formation in high-contact-stress systems but lubricant film failure as well.

Two other possible types of hydrodynamic lubrication, rigid–viscous and elastic–isoviscous, complete the matrix of four, considering the two factors of elastic deformation and pressure–viscosity effects. In addition, *squeeze film* lubrication can occur when surfaces approach one another. For more information on hydrodynamic and EHL, see Cameron [3] and Dowson and Higginson [4].

11.3.2 Transition from Hydrodynamic to Boundary Lubrication

Although prevention of contact is probably the most important function of a lubricant, there is still much to be learned about the transition from hydrodynamic and EHL to boundary lubrication. This is the region in which lubrication goes from the desirable hydrodynamic condition of no contact to the less acceptable "boundary" condition, where increased contact usually leads to higher friction and wear. This regime is sometimes referred to as a condition of *mixed lubrication*.

Several examples of experimental approaches to thin-film lubrication have been reported [3]. It is important in examining these techniques to make the distinction between methods that are used to determine lubricant film thickness under hydrodynamic or elastohydrodynamic conditions (e.g., optical interference, electrical capacitance, or x-ray transmission), and methods that are used to determine the occurrence or frequency of contact. As we will see later, most experimental studies of synovial joint lubrication have focused on friction measurements, using the information to determine the lubrication regime involved; this approach can be misleading.

11.3.2.1 Boundary Lubrication

Although there is no generally accepted definition of boundary lubrication, it is often described as a condition of lubrication in which the friction and wear between two surfaces in relative motion are determined by the surface properties of the solids and the chemical nature of the lubricant rather than its viscosity. An example of the difficulty in defining boundary lubrication can be seen if the term *bulk viscosity* is used in place of viscosity in the preceding sentence—another frequent form. This opens the door to the inclusion of elastohydrodynamic effects which depend in part on the influence of pressure on viscosity. Increased friction under these circumstances could be attributed to increased viscous drag rather than solid–solid contact. According to another common definition, boundary lubrication occurs or exists when the surfaces of the bearing solids are separated by films of molecular thickness. That may be true, but it ignores the possibility that "boundary" layer surface films may indeed be very thick (i.e., 10, 20, or 100 molecular layers). The difficulty is that boundary lubrication is complex.

Although a considerable amount of research has been done on this topic, an understanding of the basic mechanisms and processes involved is by no means complete. Therefore, definitions of boundary lubrication tend to be nonoperational. This is an extremely important regime of lubrication because it involves more extensive solid–solid contact and interaction as well as generally greater friction, wear, and surface damage. In many practical systems, the occurrence of the boundary lubrication regime is unavoidable or at least quite common. The condition can be brought about by high loads, low relative sliding speeds (including zero for stop-and-go, motion reversal, or reciprocating elements) and low lubricant viscosity—factors that are important in the transition from hydrodynamic to boundary lubrication.

The most important factor in boundary lubrication is the chemistry of the tribological system—the contacting solids and total environment including lubricants. More particularly, the surface chemistry and interactions occurring with and on the solid surfaces are important. This includes factors such as physisorption, chemisorption, intermolecular forces, surface chemical reactions, and the nature, structure, and properties of thin films on solid surfaces. It also includes many other effects brought on by the process of moving one solid over another, such as (1) changes in topography and the area of contact, (2) high surface temperatures, (3) the generation of fresh reactive metal surfaces by the removal of oxide and other layers, (4) catalysis, (5) the generation of electrical charges, and (6) the emission of charged particles such as electrons.

In examining the action of boundary lubricant compounds in reducing friction or wear or both between solids in sliding contact, it may be helpful to consider at least the following five modes of film formation on or protection of surfaces: (1) physisorption, (2) chemisorption, (3) chemical reactions with the solid surface, (4) chemical reactions on the solid surface, and (5) mere interposition of a solid or other material. These modes of surface protection are discussed in more detail in Reference 2.

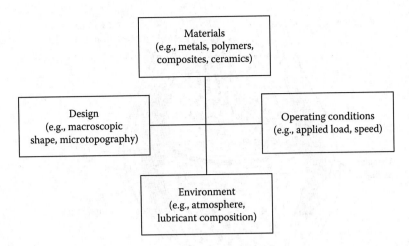

FIGURE 11.2 In any tribological system, friction, wear, and surface damage depend on four interrelated factors.

The beneficial and harmful effects of minor changes in chemistry of the environment (e.g., the lubricant) are often enormous in comparison with hydrodynamic and elastohydrodynamic effects. Thus, the surface and chemical properties of the solid materials used in tribological applications become especially important. One might expect that this would also be the case in biological (e.g., human joint) lubrication where biochemistry is very likely an important factor.

11.3.2.2 General Comments on Tribological Processes

It is important to recognize that friction and wear depend upon four major factors, that is, materials, design, operating conditions, and total environment (Figure 11.2). This four-block figure may be useful as a guide in thinking about synovial joint lubrication either from a theoretical or experimental viewpoint—the topic discussed in the next section.

Readers are cautioned against the use of various terms in tribology which are either vaguely defined or not defined at all. These would include such terms as "lubricating ability," "lubricity," and even "boundary lubrication." For example, do "boundary lubricating properties" refer to effects on friction or effects on wear and damage? It makes a difference. It is emphasized once again that friction and wear are different phenomena. Low friction does not necessarily mean low wear. We will see several examples of this common error in the discussion of joint lubrication research.

11.4 Synovial Joints

Examples of natural synovial or movable joints include the human hip, knee, elbow, ankle, finger, and shoulder. A simplified representation of a synovial joint is shown in Figure 11.3. The bones are covered by a thin layer of articular cartilage bathed in synovial fluid confined by synovial membrane. Synovial joints are truly remarkable systems—providing the basis of movement by allowing bones to articulate on one another with minimal friction and wear. Unfortunately, various joint diseases occur even among the young—causing pain, loss of freedom of movement, or instability.

Synovial joints are complex, sophisticated systems not yet fully understood. The loads are surprisingly high and the relative motion is complex. Articular cartilage has the deceptive appearance of simplicity and uniformity. But it is an extremely complex material with unusual properties. Basically, it consists of water (~75%) enmeshed in a network of collagen fibers and proteoglycans with high molecular weight. In a way, cartilage could be considered as one of nature's composite materials. Articular cartilage also has no blood supply, no nerves, and very few cells (chondrocytes).

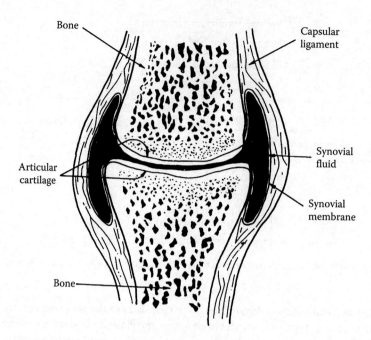

FIGURE 11.3   Representation of a synovial joint.

The other major component of an articular joint is *synovial fluid*, named by Paracelsus after "synovia" (egg-white). It is essentially a dialysate of blood plasma with added hyaluronic acid. Synovial fluid contains complex proteins, polysaccharides, and other compounds. Its chief constituent is water (~85%). Synovial fluid functions as a joint lubricant, nutrient for cartilage, and carrier for waste products.

For more information on the biochemistry, structure, and properties of articular cartilage, Freeman [5], Sokoloff [6], Stockwell [7], and articles referenced in these works are suggested.

11.5 Theories on the Lubrication of Natural and Normal Synovial Joints

As stated, the word *tribology* means the study of friction, wear, and lubrication. Therefore, *biotribology* may be thought of as the study of biological lubrication processes, for example, as in synovial joints. A surprisingly large number of concepts and theories of synovial joint lubrication have been proposed [8–10] (as shown in Table 11.1). And even if similar ideas are grouped together, there are still well over a dozen fundamentally different theories. These have included a wide range of lubrication concepts, for example, hydrodynamic, hydrostatic, elasto-hydrodynamic, squeeze-film, "boundary," mixed-regime, "weeping," osmotic, synovial mucin gel, "boosted," lipid, electrostatic, porous layers, and special forms of boundary lubrication (e.g., "lubricating glycoproteins," structuring of boundary water "surface-active" phospholipids). This chapter will not review these numerous theories, but excellent reviews on the lubrication of synovial joints have been written by McCutchen [11], Swanson [12], and Higginsworth and Unsworth [13]. The book edited by Dumbleton is also recommended [14]. In addition, theses by Droogendijk [15] and Burkhardt [16] contain extensive and detailed reviews of theories of joint lubrication.

McCutchen was the first to propose an entirely new concept of lubrication, "weeping lubrication," applied to synovial joint action [17,18]. He considered unique and special properties of cartilage and how this could affect flow and lubrication. The work of Mow et al. continued along a more complex and sophisticated approach in which a biomechanical model is proposed for the study of the dynamic

TABLE 11.1 Examples of Proposed Mechanisms and Studies of Synovial Joint Lubrication

Mechanism	Authors	Date
1. Hydrodynamic	MacConnail	1932
2. Boundary	Jones	1934
3. Hydrodynamic	Jones	1936
4. Boundary	Charnley	1959
5. Weeping	McCutchen	1959
6. Floating	Barnett and Cobbold	1962
7. Elastohydrodynamic	Tanner	1966
	Dowson	1967
8. Thixotropic/elastic fluid	Dintenfass	1963
9. Osmotic (boundary)	McCutchen	1966
10. Squeeze-film	Fein	1966
	Higginson et al.	1974
11. Synovial gel	Maroudas	1967
12. Thin-film	Faber et al.	1967
13. Combinations of hydrostatic, boundary, and EHL	Linn	1968
14. Boosted	Walker et al.	1968
15. Lipid	Little et al.	1969
16. Weeping + boundary	McCutchen and Wilkins	1969
	McCutchen	1969
17. Boundary	Caygill and West	1969
18. Fat (or mucin)	Freeman et al.	1970
19. Electrostatic	Roberts	1971
20. Boundary + fluid squeeze-film	Radin and Paul	1972
21. Mixed	Unsworth et al.	1974
22. Imbibe/exudate composite model	Ling	1974
23. Complex biomechanical model	Mow et al.	1974
	Mansour and Mow	1977
24. Two porous layer model	Dinnar	1974
25. Boundary	Reimann et al.	1975
26. Squeeze-film + fluid film + boundary	Unsworth, Dowson et al.	1975
27. Compliant bearing model	Rybicki	1977
28. Lubricating glycoproteins	Swann et al.	1977
29. Structuring of boundary water	Sokoloff et al.	1979
30. Surface flow	Kenyon	1980
31. Lubricin	Swann et al.	1985
32. Micro-EHL	Dowson and Jin	1986
33. Lubricating factor	Jay	1992
34. Lipidic component	LaBerge et al.	1993
35. Constitutive modeling of cartilage	Lai et al.	1993
36. Asperity model	Yao et al.	1993
37. Bingham fluid	Tandon et al.	1994
38. Filtration/gel/squeeze film	Hlavacek et al.	1995
39. Surface-active phospholipid	Schwarz and Hills	1998
40. Interstitial fluid pressurization	Ateshian et al.	1998

interaction between synovial fluid and articular cartilage [19,20]. These ideas are combined in the more recent work of Ateshian [21] which uses a framework of the biphasic theory of articular cartilage to model interstitial fluid pressurization. Several additional studies have also been made of effects of porosity and compliance, including the behavior of elastic layers, in producing hydrodynamic and squeeze-film lubrication. A good review in this area was given by Unsworth who discussed both human and artificial joints [22].

The following general observations are offered on the theories of synovial joint lubrication that have been proposed:

1. Most of the theories are strictly mechanical or rheological—involving such factors as deformation, pressure, and fluid flow.
2. There is a preoccupation with *friction*, which of course is very low for articular cartilage systems.
3. None of the theories consider *wear*—which is neither the same as friction nor related to it.
4. The detailed structure, biochemistry, complexity, and living nature of the total articular cartilage–synovial fluid system are generally ignored.

These are only general impressions. And although mechanical/rheological concepts seem dominant (with a focus on friction), wear and biochemistry are not completely ignored. For example, Simon [23] abraded articular cartilage from human patellae and canine femoral heads with a stainless-steel rotary file, measuring the depth of penetration with time and the amount of wear debris generated. Cartilage wear was also studied experimentally by Bloebaum and Wilson [24], Radin and Paul [25], and Lipshitz et al. [26–28]. The latter researchers carried out several *in vitro* studies of wear of articular cartilage using bovine cartilage plugs or specimens in sliding contact against stainless-steel plates. They developed a means of measuring cartilage wear by determining the hydroxyproline content of both the lubricant and solid wear debris. Using this system and technique, effects of variables such as time, applied load, and chemical modification of articular cartilage on wear and profile changes were determined. This work is of particular importance in that they addressed the question of *cartilage wear and damage* rather than friction, recognizing that wear and friction are different phenomena.

Special note is also made of two researchers, Swann and Sokoloff, who considered biochemistry as an important factor in synovial joint lubrication. Swann et al. very carefully isolated fractions of bovine synovial fluid using sequential sedimentation techniques and gel permeation chromatography. They found a high molecular weight glycoprotein to be the major constituent in the articular lubrication fraction from bovine synovial fluid and called this LGP-I (from lubricating glycoprotein). This was based on friction measurements using cartilage in sliding contact against a glass disc. An excellent summary of this work with additional references is presented in a chapter by Swann in *The Joints and Synovial Fluid: I* [6].

Sokoloff et al. [29] examined the "boundary lubricating ability" of several synovial fluids using a latex-glass test system and cartilage specimens obtained at necropsy from knees. Measurements were made of friction. The research was extended to other *in vitro* friction tests using cartilage obtained from the nasal septum of cows and widely differing artificial surfaces [30]. As a result of this work, a new model of boundary lubrication by synovial fluid was proposed—the structuring of boundary water. The postulate involves adsorption of one part of a glycoprotein on a surface followed by the formation of hydration shells around the polar portions of the adsorbed glycoprotein; the net result is a thin layer of viscous "structured" water at the surface. This work is of particular interest in that it involves not only a specific and more detailed mechanism of boundary lubrication in synovial joints but also takes into account the possible importance of water in this system.

In more recent research by Jay, an interaction between hyaluronic acid and a "purified synovial lubricating factor" (PSLF) was observed, suggesting a possible synergistic action in the boundary lubrication of synovial joints [31]. The definition of "lubricating ability" was based on friction measurements made with a latex-covered stainless-steel stud in oscillating contact against polished glass.

The above summary of major synovial joint lubrication theories is taken from References 10 and 31 as well as the thesis by Burkhardt [32].

Two more recent studies are of interest since cartilage wear was considered although not as a part of a theory of joint lubrication. Stachowiak et al. [33] investigated the friction and wear characteristics of adult rat femur cartilage against a stainless-steel plate using an environmental scanning microscope (ESM) to examine damaged cartilage. One finding was evidence of a load limit to lubrication of cartilage, beyond which high friction and damage occurred. Another study, by Hayes et al. [34] on the influence of crystals on cartilage wear, is particularly interesting not only in the findings reported (e.g., certain crystals can increase cartilage wear), but also in the full description of the biochemical techniques used.

A special note should be made concerning the doctoral thesis by Lawrence Malcom in 1976 [35]. This is an excellent study of cartilage friction and deformation, in which a device resembling a rotary plate rheometer was used to investigate the effects of static and dynamic loading on the frictional behavior of bovine cartilage. The contact geometry consisted of a circular cylindrical annulus in contact with a concave hemispherical section. It was found that dynamically loaded specimens in bovine synovial fluid yielded the more efficient lubrication based on friction measurements. The Malcom study is thorough and excellent in its attention to detail (e.g., specimen preparation) in examining the influence of type of loading and time effects on cartilage friction. It does not, however, consider cartilage wear and damage except in a very preliminary way. And it does not consider the influence of fluid biochemistry on cartilage friction, wear, and damage. In short, the Malcom work represents a superb piece of systematic research along the lines of mechanical, dynamic, rheological, and viscoelastic behavior—one important dimension of synovial joint lubrication.

11.6 *In Vitro* Cartilage Wear Studies

Over the last 15 years, studies aimed at exploring possible connections between tribology and mechanisms of synovial joint lubrication and degeneration (e.g., OA) have been conducted by the author and his graduate and undergraduate students in the Department of Mechanical Engineering at Virginia Polytechnic Institute and State University. The basic approach used involved *in vitro* tribological experiments using bovine articular cartilage, with an emphasis on the effects of fluid composition and biochemistry on cartilage wear and damage. This research is an outgrowth of earlier work carried out during a sabbatical study in the Laboratory for the Study of Skeletal Disorders, The Children's Hospital Medical Center, Harvard Medical School in Boston. In that study, bovine cartilage test specimens were loaded against a polished steel plate and subjected to reciprocating sliding for several hours in the presence of a fluid (e.g., bovine synovial fluid or a buffered saline reference fluid containing biochemical constituents kindly provided by Dr. David Swann). Cartilage wear was determined by sampling the test fluid and determining the concentration of 4-hydroxyproline—a constituent of collagen. The results of that earlier study have been reported and summarized elsewhere [36–39]. Figure 11.4 shows the average hydroxyproline contents of wear debris obtained from these *in vitro* experiments. These numbers are related to the cartilage wear which occurred. However, since the total quantities of collected fluids varied somewhat, the values shown in the bar graph should not be taken as exact or precise measures of fluid effects on cartilage wear.

The main conclusions of that study were as follows:

1. Normal bovine synovial fluid is very effective in reducing cartilage wear under these *in vitro* conditions as compared to the buffered saline reference fluid.
2. There is no significant difference in wear between the saline reference and distilled water.
3. The addition of hyaluronic acid to the reference fluid significantly reduces wear; but its effect depends on the source.
4. Under these test conditions, Swann's LGP-I, known to be extremely effective in reducing friction in cartilage-on-glass tests, does not reduce cartilage wear.
5. However, a protein complex isolated by Swann is extremely effective in reducing wear—producing results similar to those obtained with synovial fluid. The detailed structure of this constituent is complex and has not yet been fully determined.

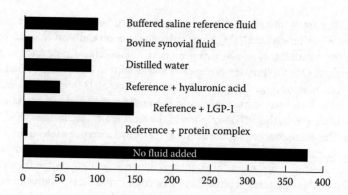

FIGURE 11.4 Relative cartilage wear based on hydroxyproline content of debris (*in vitro* tests with cartilage on stainless steel).

6. Last, the lack of an added fluid in these experiments leads to extremely high wear and damage of the articular cartilage.

In discussing the possible significance of these findings from a tribological point of view, it may be helpful first of all to emphasize once again that friction and wear are different phenomena. Furthermore, as suggested by Figure 11.5, certain constituents of synovial fluid (e.g., Swann's LGP) may act to reduce friction in synovial joints while other constituents (e.g., Swann's protein complex or hyaluronic acid) may act to reduce cartilage *wear*. Therefore, it is necessary to distinguish between biochemical antifriction and antiwear compounds present in synovial fluid.

In more recent years, this study has been greatly enhanced by the participation of interested faculty and students from the Virginia-Maryland College of Veterinary Medicine and Department of Biochemistry and Animal Science at Virginia Tech. One major hypothesis tested is a continuation of previous work showing that the detailed biochemistry of the fluid–cartilage system has a pronounced and possibly controlling influence on cartilage wear. A consequence of the above hypothesis is that a lack or deficiency of certain biochemical constituents in the synovial joint may be one factor contributing to the initiation and progression of cartilage damage, wear, and possibly OA. A related but somewhat different hypothesis concerns synovial fluid constituents which may act to increase the wear and further damage of articular cartilage under tribological contact.

To carry out continued research on biotribology, a new device for studies of cartilage deformation, wear, damage, and friction under conditions of tribological contact was designed by Burkhardt [32] and later modified, constructed, and instrumented. A simplified sketch is shown in Figure 11.6. The key features of this test device are shown in Table 11.2. The apparatus is designed to accommodate cartilage-on-cartilage specimens. Motion of the lower specimen is controlled by a computer-driven *x–y* table, allowing simple oscillating motion or complex motion patterns. An octagonal strain ring with two full semi-conductor bridges is used to measure the normal load as well as the tangential load (friction). An

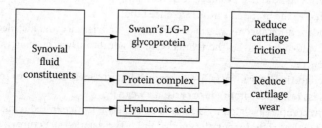

FIGURE 11.5 Friction and wear are different phenomena.

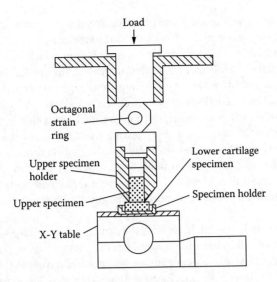

FIGURE 11.6   Device for *in vitro* cartilage-on-cartilage wear studies.

LVDT, not shown in the figure, is used to measure cartilage deformation and linear wear during a test. However, hydroxyproline analysis of the wear debris and washings is used for the actual determination of total cartilage wear on a mass basis.

In one study by Schroeder [40], two types of experiments were carried out, that is, cartilage-on-stainless steel and cartilage-on-cartilage at applied loads up to 70 N—yielding an average pressure of 2.2 MPa in the contact area. Reciprocating motion (40 cps) was used. The fluids tested included (1) a buffered saline solution, (2) saline plus hyaluronic acid, and (3) bovine synovial fluid. In cartilage-on-stainless-steel tests, scanning electron microscopy, and histological staining showed distinct effects of the lubricants on surface and subsurface damage. Tests with the buffered saline fluid resulted in the most damage, with large wear tracks visible on the surface of the cartilage plug, as well as subsurface voids and cracks. When hyaluronic acid, a constituent of the natural synovial joint lubricant, was added

TABLE 11.2   Key Features of Test Device Designed for Cartilage Wear Studies

Contact System	Cartilage-on-Cartilage
Contact geometry	Flat-on-flat, convex-on-flat, irregular-on-irregular
Cartilage type	Articular, any source (e.g., bovine)
Specimen size	Upper specimen, 4–6 mm diam., lower specimen, ca. 15–25 mm diam.
Applied load	50–660 N
Average pressure	0.44–4.4 MPa
Type of motion	Linear, oscillating; circular, constant velocity; more complex patterns
Sliding velocity	0–20 mm/s
Fluid temperature	Ambient (20°C); or controlled humidity
Environment	Ambient or controlled humidity
Measurements	Normal load, cartilage deformation, friction; cartilage wear and damage, biochemical analysis of cartilage specimens, synovial fluid, and wear debris; sub-surface changes

Source: Burkhardt, B.M. Development and design of a test device for cartilage wear studies, MS thesis, Mechanical Engineering, Virginia Polytechnic Institute and State University, Blacksburg, VA, December 1988.

to the saline reference fluid, less severe damage was observed. Little or no cartilage damage was evident in tests in which the natural synovial joint fluid was used as the lubricant.

These results were confirmed in a later study by Owellen [41] in which hydroxyproline analysis was used to determine cartilage wear. It was found that increasing the applied load from 20 to 65 N increased cartilage wear by eightfold for the saline solution and approximately threefold for synovial fluid. Furthermore, the coefficient of friction increased from an initial low value of 0.01–0.02 to a much higher value, for example, 0.20–0.30 and higher, during a normal test which lasted 3 h; the greatest change occurred during the first 20 min. Another interesting result was that a thin film of transferred or altered material was observed on the stainless-steel disks—being most pronounced with the buffered saline lubricant and not observed with synovial fluid. Examination of the film with Fourier transfer infrared microspectrometry shows distinctive bio-organic spectra which differs from that of the original bovine cartilage. We believe this to be an important finding since it suggests a possible bio-tribo-chemical effect [42].

In another phase of this research, the emphasis is on the cartilage-on-cartilage system and the influence of potentially beneficial as well as harmful constituents of synovial fluid on wear and damage. In cartilage-on-cartilage tests, the most severe wear and damage occurred during tests with buffered saline as the lubricant. The damage was less severe than in the stainless-steel tests, but some visible wear tracks were detectable with scanning electron microscopy. Histological sectioning and staining of both the upper and lower cartilage samples show evidence of elongated lacunae and coalesced voids that could lead to wear by delamination. An example is shown in Figure 11.7 (original magnification of 500 × on 35 mm slide). The proteoglycan content of the subsurface cartilage under the region of contact was also reduced. When synovial fluid was used as the lubricant, no visible wear or damage was detected [43]. These results demonstrate that even in *in vitro* tests with bovine articular cartilage, the nature of the fluid environment can have a dramatic effect on the severity of wear and subsurface damage.

In a more recent study carried out by Berrien in the biotribology program at Virginia Tech, a different approach was taken to examine the role of joint lubrication in joint disease, particularly OA. A degradative biological enzyme, collagenase-3, suspected of playing a role in a cartilage degeneration was used to create a physiologically adverse biochemical fluid environment. Tribological tests were performed with the same device and procedures described previously. The stainless-steel disk was replaced with a 1 in. diameter plug of bovine cartilage to create a cartilage sliding on cartilage configuration more closely related to the *in vivo* condition. Normal load was increased to 78.6 N and synovial fluid and buffered saline were used as lubricants. Prior to testing, cartilage plugs were exposed to a fluid medium containing three concentrations of collagenase-3 for 24 h. The major discovery of this work was that exposure to the collagenase-3 enzyme had a substantial adverse effect on cartilage wear *in vitro*, increasing average

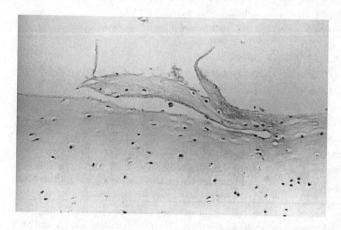

FIGURE 11.7 Cartilage damage produced by sliding contact.

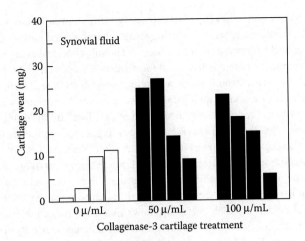

FIGURE 11.8 Effect of collagenase-3 on cartilage wear.

wear values by three and one-half times those of the unexposed cases. Figure 11.8 shows an example of the effect of enzyme treatment when bovine synovial fluid was used as the lubricant. Scanning electron microscopy showed disruption of the superficial layer and collagen matrix with exposure to collagenase-3, where unexposed cartilage showed none. Histological sections showed a substantial loss of the superficial layer of cartilage and a distinct and abnormal loss of proteoglycans in the middle layer of collagenase-treated cartilage. Unexposed cartilage showed only minor disruption of the superficial layer [44].

This study indicates that some of the biochemical constituents that gain access to the joint space, during normal and pathological functions, can have a significant adverse effect on the wear and damage of the articular cartilage. Future studies will include determination of additional constituents that have harmful effects on cartilage wear and damage. This research, using bovine articular cartilage in *in vitro* sliding contact tests, raises a number of interesting questions:

1. Has "Nature" designed a special biochemical compound which has as its function the protection of articular cartilage?
2. What is the mechanism (or mechanisms) by which biochemical constituents of synovial fluid can act to reduce wear of articular cartilage?
3. Could a lack of this biochemical constituent lead to increased cartilage wear and damage?
4. Does articular cartilage from osteoarthritic patients have reduced wear resistance?
5. Do any of the findings on the importance of synovial fluid biochemistry on cartilage wear in our *in vitro* studies apply to living or *in vitro* systems as well?
6. How does collagenase-3 treatment of cartilage lead to increased wear and does this finding have any significance in the *in vivo* situation? This question is addressed in the next section.

11.7 Biotribology and Arthritis: Are There Connections?

Arthritis is an umbrella term for more than 100 rheumatic diseases affecting joints and connective tissue. The two most common forms are OA and rheumatoid arthritis (RA). Osteoarthritis—also referred to as *osteoarthrosis or degenerative joint disease*—is the most common form of arthritis. It is sometimes simplistically described as the "wear and tear" form of arthritis. The causes and progression of degenerative joint disease are still not understood. RA is a chronic and often progressive disease of the synovial membrane leading to release of enzymes which attack, erode, and destroy articular cartilage. It is an inflammatory response involving the immune system and is more prevalent in female individuals. RA is extremely complex. Its causes are still unknown.

Sokoloff defines degenerative joint disease as "an extremely common, noninflammatory, progressive disorder of movable joints, particularly weight-bearing joints, characterized pathologically by deterioration of articular cartilage and by formation of new bone in the sub-chondral areas and at the margins of the 'joint'" [45]. As mentioned, osteoarthritis or osteoarthrosis is sometimes referred to as the "wear and tear" form of arthritis; but, wear itself is rarely a simple process even in well-defined systems.

It has been noted by the author that tribological terms occasionally appear in hypotheses which describe the etiology of OA (e.g., "reduced wear resistance of cartilage" or "poor lubricity of synovial fluid"). It has also been noted that there is a general absence of hypotheses connecting normal synovial joint *lubrication* (or lack thereof) and synovial joint *degeneration*. Perhaps it is natural (and unhelpful) for a tribologist to imagine such a connection and that, for example, cartilage wear under certain circumstances might be due to or influenced by a lack of proper "boundary lubrication" by the synovial fluid. In this regard, it may be of interest to quote Swanson [12] who said in 1979 that "there exists at present no experimental evidence which certainly shows that a failure of lubrication is or is not a causative factor in the first stages of cartilage degeneration." A statement made by Professor Glimcher (discussions with M.J. Glimcher, The Children's Hospital Medical Center) may also be appropriate here. Glimcher fully recognized the fundamental difference between friction and wear as well as the difference between joint lubrication (one area of study) and joint degeneration (another area of study). Glimcher said that wearing or abrading cartilage with a steel file is not OA; and neither is digesting cartilage in a test tube with an enzyme. But both forms of cartilage deterioration can occur in a living joint and in a way which is still not understood. It is interesting that essentially none of the many synovial joint lubrication theories consider enzymatic degradation of cartilage as a factor whereas practically all the models of the etiology of degenerative joint disease include this as an important factor.

It was stated earlier that there are at least two main areas to consider, that is, (1) mechanisms of synovial joint lubrication and (2) the etiology of synovial joint degeneration (e.g., as in osteoarthrosis). Both areas are extremely complex. And the key questions as to what actually happens in each have yet to be answered (and perhaps asked). It may therefore be presumptuous of the present author to suggest possible connections between two areas which in themselves are still not fully understood.

Tribological processes in a movable joint involve not only the contacting surfaces (articular cartilage), but the surrounding medium (synovial fluid) as well. Each of these depends on the synthesis and transport of necessary biochemical constituents to the contact region or interface. As a result of relative motion (sliding, rubbing, rolling, and impact) between the joint elements, friction and wear can occur.

It has already been shown and discussed—at least in *in vitro* tests with articular cartilage—that compounds which reduce friction do not necessarily reduce wear; the latter was suggested as being more important [10]. It may be helpful first of all to emphasize once again that friction and wear are different phenomena. Furthermore, certain constituents of synovial fluid (e.g., Swann's LGP) may act to reduce *friction* in synovial joints while other constituents (e.g., Swann's protein complex or hyaluronic acid) may act to reduce cartilage *wear*.

A significant increase in joint friction could lead to a slight increase in local temperatures or possibly to reduce mobility. But the effects of cartilage wear would be expected to be more serious. When cartilage wear occurs, a very special material is lost and the body is neither capable of regenerating cartilage of the same quality nor at the desired rate. Thus, there are at least two major tribological dimensions involved—one concerning the nature of the synovial fluid and the other having to do with the properties of articular cartilage itself. Changes in *either* the synovial fluid or cartilage could conceivably lead to increased wear or damage (or friction) as shown in Figure 11.9.

A simplified model or illustration of possible connections between OA and tribology is offered in Figure 11.10 taken from Furey [46]. Its purpose is to stimulate discussion. There are other pathways to the disease, pathways which may include genetic factors.

In some cases, the body makes an unsuccessful attempt at repair, and bone growth may occur at the periphery of contact. As suggested by Figure 11.10, this process and the generation of wear particles could lead to joint inflammation and the release of enzymes which further soften and degrade the

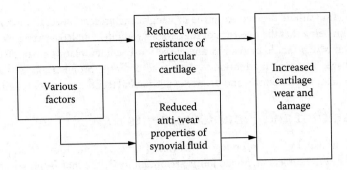

FIGURE 11.9   Two tribological aspects of synovial joint lubrication.

articular cartilage. This softer, degraded cartilage does not possess the wear-resistance of the original. It has been shown previously that treatment of cartilage with collagenase-3 increases wear significantly, thus supporting the idea of enzyme release as a factor in OA. Thus, there exists a feedback process in which the occurrence of cartilage wear can lead to even more damage. Degradative enzymes can also be released by trauma, shock, or injury to the joint. Ultimately, as the cartilage is progressively thinned and bony growth occurs, a condition of OA or degenerative joint disease may exist. There are other pathways to the disease, pathways which may include genetic factors. It is not argued that arthritis is a tribological problem. However, the inclusion of tribological processes in one set of pathways to osteoarthrosis would not seem strange or unusual.

A specific example of a different tribological dimension to the problem of synovial joint lubrication (i.e., third-body abrasion), was shown by the work of Hayes et al. [47]. In an excellent study of the effect of crystals on the wear of articular cartilage, they carried out *in vitro* tests using cylindrical cartilage sub-chondral bone plugs obtained from equine fetlock joints in sliding contact against a stainless-steel plate. They examined the effects of three types of crystals (orthorhombic calcium pyrophosphate tetra-hydrate, monoclinic calcium pyrophosphate dehydrate, and calcium hydroxyapatite) on wear using a Ringer's solution as the carrier fluid. Concentration of cartilage wear debris in the fluid was determined

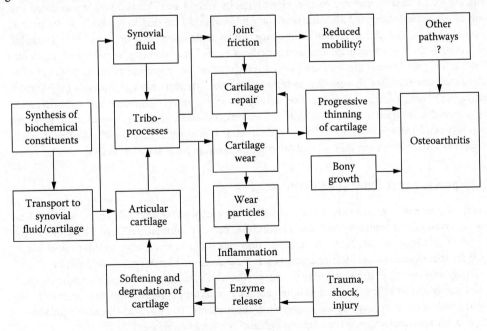

FIGURE 11.10   Osteoarthritis–tribology connections?

by analyzing for inorganic sulfate derived from the proteoglycans present. Several interesting findings were made, one of them being that the presence of the crystals roughly doubled cartilage wear. This is an important contribution which should be read by anyone seriously contemplating research on the tribology of articular cartilage. The careful attention to detail and potential problems, as well as the precise description of the biochemical procedures and diverse experimental techniques used, set a high standard.

11.8 Recapitulation and Final Comments

It is obvious from the unusually large number of theories of synovial joint lubrication proposed, that very little is known about the subject. Synovial joints are undoubtedly the most sophisticated and complex tribological systems that exist or will ever exist. It will require a great deal more research—possibly very different approaches—before we even begin to understand the processes involved.

Some general comments and specific suggestions are offered—not for the purpose of criticizing any particular study but hopefully to provide ideas which may be helpful in further research as well as in the re-interpretation of some past research.

11.8.1 Terms and Definitions

First of all, as mentioned earlier in this chapter, part of the problem has to do with the use and misuse of various terms in tribology—the study of friction, wear, and lubrication. A glance at any number of the published papers on synovial joint lubrication will reveal such terms and phrases as "lubricating ability," "lubricity," "lubricating properties," "lubricating component," and many others, all undefined. We also see terms such as "boundary lubricant," "lubricating glycoprotein," or "lubricin." There is nothing inherently wrong with this but one should remember that lubrication is a process of reducing friction and/or wear between rubbing surfaces. Saying that a fluid is a "good" lubricant does not distinguish between friction and wear. And assuming that friction and wear are correlated and go together is the first pitfall in any tribological study. It cannot be overemphasized that friction and wear are different, though sometimes related, phenomena. Low friction does not mean low wear. The terms and phrases used are therefore extremely important. For example, in a brief and early review article by Wright and Dowson [48], it was stated that "Digestion of hyaluronate does not alter the boundary lubrication," referring to the work of Radin et al. [49]. In another article, McCutchen re-states this conclusion in another way, saying "... the lubricating ability did not reside in the hyaluronic acid" and later asks the question "Why do the glycoprotein molecules (of Swann) lubricate?" [50] These statements are based on effects of various constituents on friction, not wear. The work of the present author showed that in tests with bovine articular cartilage, Swann's LGP-I which was effective in reducing friction did not reduce cartilage wear. However, hyaluronic acid—shown earlier not to be responsible for friction-reduction—did reduce cartilage wear. Thus, it is important to make the distinction between friction-reduction and wear-reduction. It is suggested that operational definitions be used in place of vague "lubricating ability," and other terms in future papers on the subject.

11.8.2 Experimental Contact Systems

Second, some comments are made on the experimental approaches that have been reported in the literature on synovial joint lubrication mechanisms. Sliding contact combinations in *in vitro* studies have consisted of (1) cartilage-on-cartilage, (2) cartilage-on-some other surface (e.g., stainless steel, glass), and (3) solids other than cartilage sliding against each other in X-on-X or X-on-Y combinations.

The cartilage-on-cartilage combination is of course the most realistic and yet most complex contact system. But variations in shape or macroscopic geometry, microtopography, and the nature of contact present problems in carrying out well-controlled experiments. There is also the added problem of acquiring suitable specimens which are large enough and reasonably uniform.

The next combination—cartilage-on-another material—allows for better control of contact, with the more elastic, deformable cartilage loaded against a well-defined hard surface (e.g., a polished, flat solid made of glass or stainless steel). This contact configuration can provide useful tribological information on effects of changes in biochemical environment (e.g., fluids), on friction, wear, and sub-surface damage. It also could parallel the situation in a partial joint replacement in which healthy cartilage is in contact with a metal alloy.

The third combination, which appears in some of the literature on synovial joint lubrication, does not involve any articular cartilage at all. For example, Jay made friction measurements using a latex-covered stainless-steel stud in oscillating contact against polished glass [31]. Williams et al., in a study of a lipid component of synovial fluid, used reciprocating contact of borosilicate glass-on-glass [51]. And in a recent paper on the action of a surface-active phospholipid as the "lubricating component of lubricin," Schwarz and Hills carried out friction measurements using two optically flat quartz plates in sliding contact [52]. In another study, a standard four-ball machine using alloy steel balls was used to examine the "lubricating ability" of synovial fluid constituents. Such tests, in the absence of cartilage, are easiest to control and carry out. However, they are not relevant to the study of synovial joint lubrication. With a glass sphere sliding against a glass flat, almost anything will reduce friction—including a wide variety of chemicals, biochemicals, semi-solids, and fluids. This has little if anything to do with the lubrication of synovial joints.

11.8.3 Fluids and Materials Used as Lubricants in *In Vitro* Biotribology Studies

Fluids used as lubricants in synovial joint lubrication studies have consisted of (1) "normal" synovial fluid (e.g., bovine), (2) buffered saline solution containing synovial fluid constituents (e.g., hyaluronic acid), and (3) various aqueous solutions of surface-active compounds neither derived from nor present in synovial fluid. In addition, a few studies used synovial fluids from patients suffering from either OA or RA.

The general comment made here is that the use of synovial fluids—whether derived from human or animal sources and whether "healthy" or "abnormal"—is important in *in vitro* studies of synovial joint lubrication. The documented behavior of synovial fluid in producing low friction and wear with articular cartilage sets a reference standard and demonstrates that useful information can indeed come from *in vitro* tests.

Studies that are based on adding synovial fluid constituents to a reference fluid (e.g., a buffered saline solution) can also be useful in attempting to identify which biochemical compound or compounds are responsible for reductions in frictions or wear. But if significant interactions between compounds exist, then such an approach may require an extensive program of tests. It should also be mentioned that in the view of the present author, the use of a pure undissolved constituent of synovial fluid, either derived or synthetic, in a sliding contact test is not only irrelevant but may be misleading. An example would be the use of a pure lipid (e.g., phospholipid) at the interface rather than in the concentration and solution form in which this compound would normally exist in synovial fluid. This is basic in any study of lubrication and particularly in the case of boundary lubrication where major effects on wear or friction can be brought on by minor, seemingly trivial, changes in chemistry.

11.8.4 The Preoccupation with Rheology and Friction

The synovial joint as a system—the articular cartilage and underlying bone structure as well as the synovial fluid as important elements—is extremely complex and far from being understood. It is noted that there is a proliferation of mathematical modeling papers stressing rheology and the mechanics of deformation, flow, and fluid pressures developed in the cartilage model. One recent example is the paper "The Role of Interstitial Fluid Pressurization and Surface Properties on the Boundary Friction of Articular Cartilage" by Ateshian et al. [21]. This study, a genuine contribution, grew out of the early work by Mow and connects also with the "weeping lubrication" model of McCutchen. Both McCutchen and

Mow have made significant contributions to our understanding of synovial joint lubrication, although each approach is predominantly rheological and friction-oriented with little regard for biochemistry and wear. This is not to say that rheology is unimportant. It could well be that, as suggested by Ateshian, the mechanism of interstitial fluid pressurization that leads to low friction in cartilage could also lead to low wear rates (private communication, letter to Michael J. Furey from Gerard A. Ateshian, July 1998).

11.8.5 The Probable Existence of Various Lubrication Regimes

In an article by Wright and Dowson, it is suggested that a variety of types of lubrication operate in human synovial joints at different parts of a walking cycle stating that, "At heel-strike a squeeze-film situation may develop, leading to elastohydrodynamic lubrication and possibly both squeeze-film and boundary lubrication, while hydrodynamic lubrication may operate during the free-swing phase of walking" [48].

In a simplified approach to examining the various regimes of lubrication that could exist in a human joint, it may be useful to look at Figure 11.11a which shows the variation in force (load) and velocity for a human hip joint at different parts of the walking cycle (taken from Graham and Walker [53]). As discussed earlier in this chapter, theories of hydrodynamic and EHL all include the hydrodynamic factor $(\eta U/W)$ as the key variable, where η = fluid viscosity, U = the relative sliding velocity, and W = the normal load. High values of $(\eta U/W)$ lead to thicker hydrodynamic films—a more desirable condition

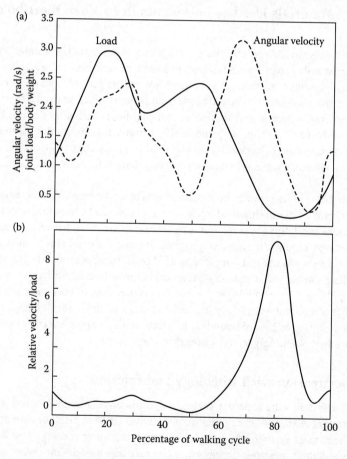

FIGURE 11.11 (a) Hip joint forces and angular velocities at different parts of the walking cycle. (After Graham, J.D. and Walker, T.W. *Perspectives in Biomedical Engineering*, University Park Press, Baltimore, MD, pp. 161–164, 1973.) (b) Calculated ratio of velocity to force for the hip joint (from (a)).

if one wants to keep surfaces apart. It can be seen from Figure 11.11a that there is considerable variation in load and velocity, with peaks and valleys occurring at different parts of the cycle. Note also that in this example, the loads can be quite high (e.g., up to three times body weight). The maximum load occurs at 20% of the walking cycle illustrated in Figure 11.11a, with a secondary maximum occurring at a little over the 50% point. The maximum angular velocity occurs at approximately 67% of the cycle. If one now creates a new curve of relative velocity/load or (U/W) from Figure 11.11a, the result obtained is shown in Figure 11.11b. We now see a very different and somewhat simplified picture. There is a clear and distinct maximum in the ratio of velocity to load (U/W) at 80% of walking cycle, favoring the formation of a hydrodynamic film of maximum thickness. However, for most of the cycle (e.g., from 0 to 60%), the velocity/load ratio is significantly lower, thus favoring a condition of minimum film thickness and "boundary lubrication." However, we also know that synovial fluid is non-Newtonian; at higher rates of shear, its viscosity decreases sharply, approaching that of water. The shear rate is equal to the relative velocity divided by fluid film thickness (U/h) and is expressed in per second. This means that at the regions of low (U/W) ratios or thinner hydrodynamic films, the viscosity term in $(\eta U/W)$ is even lower, thus pushing the minima to lower values favoring a condition of boundary lubrication. This is only a simplified view and does not consider those periods in which the relative sliding velocity is zero at motion reversal and where squeeze-film lubrication may come into play. A good example of the complexity of load and velocity variation in a human knee joint—including several zero-velocity periods—may be found in the chapter by Higginson and Unsworth [54] citing the work of Seedhom et al., which deals with biomechanics in the design of a total knee replacement [55].

The major point made here is that (1) there are parts of a walking cycle that would be expected to approach a condition of minimum fluid film thickness and boundary lubrication and (2) it is during these parts of the cycle that cartilage wear and damage resulting from contact is more likely to occur. Thus, approaches to reducing cartilage wear in a synovial joint could be broken down into two categories (i.e., promoting thicker hydrodynamic films and providing special forms of "boundary lubrication").

11.8.6 Recent Developments

Recent developments in addressing some of the problems that involve cartilage damage and existing joint replacements include (1) progress in promoting cartilage repair [56], (2) possible use of artificial cartilage materials (e.g., synthetic hydrogels) [57,58], and (3) the development and application of more compliant joint replacement materials to promote a more favorable formation of an elastohydrodynamic film [59]. Although these are not strictly "lubricant-oriented" developments, they do and will involve important tribological aspects discussed in this chapter. For example, if new cartilage growth can be promoted by transplanting healthy chondrocytes to a platform in a damaged region of a synovial joint, how long will this cartilage last? If a hydrogel is used as an artificial cartilage, how long will it last? And if softer, elastomeric materials are used as partial joint replacements or coatings, how long will they last? These are questions of wear, not friction. And although the early fundamental studies of hydrogels as artificial cartilage measured only friction, and often only after a few moments of sliding, we know from recent work that even for hydrogels, low friction does not mean low wear [60].

11.9 Conclusions

The following main conclusions relating to the tribological behavior of natural, "normal" synovial joints are presented:

1. An unusually large number of theories and studies of joint lubrication have been proposed over the years. All of the theories focus on friction, none address wear, many do not involve experimental studies with cartilage, and very few consider the complexity and detailed biochemistry of the synovial-fluid articular-cartilage system.

2. It was shown by *in vitro* tests with bovine articular cartilage that the detailed biochemistry of synovial fluid has a significant effect on cartilage wear and damage. "Normal" bovine synovial fluid was found to provide excellent protection against wear. Various biochemical constituents isolated from bovine synovial fluid by Dr. David Swann, of the Shriners Burns Institute in Boston, showed varying effects on cartilage wear when added back to a buffered saline reference fluid. This research demonstrates once again the importance of distinguishing between friction and wear.

3. In a collaborative study of biotribology involving researchers and students in Mechanical Engineering, the Virginia-Maryland College of Veterinary Medicine, and Biochemistry, *in vitro* tribological tests using bovine articular cartilage demonstrated among other things that (1) normal synovial fluid provides better protection than a buffered saline solution in a cartilage-on-cartilage system, (2) tribological contact in cartilage systems can cause subsurface damage, delamination, changes in proteoglycan content, and in chemistry via a "biotribochemical" process not understood, and (3) pretreatment of articular cartilage with the enzyme collagenase-3—suspected as a factor in OA—significantly increases cartilage wear.

4. It is suggested that these results could change significantly the way mechanisms of synovial joint lubrication are examined. Effects of biochemistry of the system on wear of articular cartilage are likely to be important; such effects may not be related to physical/rheological models of joint lubrication.

5. It is also suggested that connections between tribology/normal synovial joint lubrication and degenerative joint disease are not only possible but likely; however, such connections are undoubtedly complex. It is *not* argued that OA is a tribological problem or that it is necessarily the result of a tribological deficiency. Ultimately, a better understanding of how normal synovial joints function from a tribological point of view could conceivably lead to advances in the prevention and treatment of OA.

6. Several problems exist that make it difficult to understand and interpret many of the published works on synovial joint lubrication. One example is the widespread use of nonoperational and vague terms such as "lubricating activity," "lubricating factor," "boundary lubricating ability," and similar undefined terms which not only fail to distinguish between friction (which is usually measured) and cartilage wear (which is rarely measured), but tend to lump these phenomena together—a common error. Another problem is that a significant number of the published experimental studies of biotribology do not involve cartilage at all—relying on the use of glass-on-glass, rubber-on-glass, and even steel-on-steel. Such approaches may be a reflection of the incorrect view that "lubricating activity" is a property of a fluid and can be measured independently. Some suggestions are offered.

7. Last, the topic of synovial joint lubrication is far from being understood. It is a complex subject involving at least biophysics, biomechanics, biochemistry, and tribology. For a physical scientist or engineer, carrying out research in this area is a humbling experience.

Acknowledgments

The author acknowledges the support of the Edward H. Lane, G. Harold, and Leila Y. Mathers Foundations for their support during the sabbatical study at The Children's Hospital Medical Center. He also thanks Dr. David Swann for his invaluable help in providing the test fluids and carrying out the biochemical analyses as well as Ms Karen Hodgens for conducting the early scanning electron microscopy studies of worn cartilage specimens.

The author is also indebted to the following researchers for their encouraging and stimulating discussions of this topic over the years and for teaching a tribologist something of the complexity of synovial joints, articular cartilage, and arthritis: Drs. Leon Sokoloff, Charles McCutchen, Melvin Glimcher, David Swann, Henry Mankin, Clement Sledge, Helen Muir, Paul Dieppe, Heikki Helminen, as well as his colleagues at Virginia Tech—Hugo Veit, E. T. Kornegay, and E. M. Gregory.

Last, the author expresses his appreciation for and recognition of the valuable contributions made by students interested in biotribology over the years. These include graduate students Bettina Burkhardt, Michael Owellen, Matt Schroeder, Mark Freeman, and especially La Shaun Berrien, who contributed to this chapter, as well as the following summer undergraduate research students: Jean Yates, Elaine Ashby, Anne Newell, T. J. Hayes, Bethany Revak, Carolina Reyes, Amy Diegelman, and Heather Hughes.

Further Information

For more information on synovial joints and arthritis, the following books are suggested: *The Biology of Degenerative Joint Disease* [45], *Adult Articular Cartilage* [5], *The Joints and Synovial Fluid: I* [6], *Textbook of Rheumatology* [61], *Osteoarthritis: Diagnosis and Management* [62], Degenerative joints: Test tubes, tissues, models, and man [63], Biology of the articular cartilage in health and disease [64], and *Crystals and Joint Disease* [65].

References

1. Hunter, W. Of the structure and diseases of articulating cartilages, *Philos. Trans.*, 42, 514–521, 1742–1743.
2. Furey, M.J. Tribology, In: *Encyclopedia of Materials Science and Engineering*, Pergamon Press, Oxford, 1986, pp. 5145–5158.
3. Cameron, A. *The Principles of Lubrication*, Longmans Green & Co. Ltd, London, 1966.
4. Dowson, D. and Higginson, G.R. *Elastohydrodynamic Lubrication*, SI Edition, Pergamon Press, Oxford, 1977.
5. Freeman, M.A.R. *Adult Articular Cartilage*, 2nd ed., Pitman Medical Publishing Co., Ltd., Tunbridge Wells, Kent, England, 1979.
6. Sokoloff, L., Ed. *The Joints and Synovial Fluid*, Vol. I, Academic Press, New York, 1978.
7. Stockwell, R.A. *Biology of Cartilage Cells*, Cambridge University Press, Cambridge, 1979.
8. Furey, M.J. Biochemical aspects of synovial joint lubrication and cartilage wear, European Society of Osteoarthrology. *Symposium on Joint Destruction in Arthritis and Osteoarthritis*, Noordwijkerhout, the Netherlands, May 24–27, 1992.
9. Furey, M.J. Biotribology: Cartilage lubrication and wear, *6th International Congress on Tribology, EUROTRIB '93*, Budapest, Hungary, August 30–September 2, 1993.
10. Furey, M.J. and Burkhardt, B.M. Biotribology: Friction, wear, and lubrication of natural synovial joints, *Lubrication Sci.*, 255–271, 3–9, 1997.
11. McCutchen, C.W. Lubrication of joints. In: *The Joints and Synovial Fluid*, Vol. I, Academic Press, New York, 1978, pp. 437–483.
12. Swanson, S.A.V. Friction, wear and lubrication. In *Adult Articular Cartilage*, M.A.R. Freeman, Ed., Pitman Medical Publishing Co., Ltd., Tunbridge Wells, Kent, England, 2nd ed., 1979, pp. 415–460.
13. Higginson, G.R. and Unsworth, T. The lubrication of natural joints. In *Tribology of Natural and Artificial Joints*, J. H. Dumbleton, Ed. Elsevier Scientific Publishing Co., Amsterdam, 1981, pp. 47–73.
14. Dumbleton, J.H. *Tribology of Natural and Artificial Joints*, Elsevier Scientific Publishing Co., Amsterdam, the Netherlands, 1981.
15. Droogendijk, L. *On the Lubrication of Synovial Joints*, PhD Thesis, Twente University of Technology, the Netherlands, 1984.
16. Burkhardt, B.M. *Development and Design of a Test Device for Cartilage Wear Studies*, MS thesis, Mechanical Engineering, Virginia Polytechnic Institute & State University, Blacksburg, VA, December 1988.
17. McCutchen, C.W. Mechanisms of animal joints: Sponge-hydrostatic and weeping bearings, *Nature (Lond.)*, 184, 1284–1285, 1959.

18. McCutchen, C.W. The frictional properties of animal joints, *Wear*, 5, 1–17, 1962.

19. Torzilli, P.A. and Mow, V.C. On the fundamental fluid transport mechanisms through normal and pathological articular cartilage during friction-1. The formulation. *J. Biomech.*, 9, 541–552, 1976.

20. Mansour, J.M. and Mow, V.C. On the natural lubrication of synovial joints: Normal and degenerated. *J. Lubrication Technol.*, 163–173, 1977.

21. Ateshian, G. A., Wang, H., and Lai, W. M. The role of interstitial fluid pressurization and surface porosities on the boundary friction of articular cartilage, *ASMS J. Biomed. Eng.*, 120, 241–251, 1998.

22. Unsworth, A. Tribology of human and artificial joints. *Proc. I. Mech. E., Part II: J. Eng. Med.*, 205, 1991.

23. Simon, W.H. Wear properties of articular cartilage. *In vitro*, Section on Rheumatic Diseases, Laboratory of Experimental Pathology, National Institute of Arthritis and Metabolic Diseases, National Institutes of Health, February 1971.

24. Bloebaum, R.D. and Wilson, A.S. The morphology of the surface of articular cartilage in adult rats, *J. Anatomy*, 131, 333–346, 1980.

25. Radin, E.L. and Paul, I.L. Response of joints to impact loading I. *In vitro* wear tests, *Arthritis Rheumatism*, 14, 1971.

26. Lipshitz, H. and Glimcher, M.J. A technique for the preparation of plugs of articular cartilage and subchondral bone, *J. Biomech.*, 7, 293–298.

27. Lipshitz, H. and Etheredge, III, R. *In vitro* wear of articular cartilage. *J. Bone Joint Surg.*, 57-A, 527–534, 1975.

28. Lipshitz, H. and Glimcher, M.J. *In vitro* studies of wear of articular cartilage, II. Characteristics of the wear of articular cartilage when worn against stainless steel plates having characterized surfaces. *Wear*, 52, 297–337, 1979.

29. Sokoloff, L., Davis, W.H., and Lee, S.L. Boundary lubricating ability of synovial fluid in degenerative joint disease, *Arthritis Rheum.*, 21, 754–760, 1978.

30. Sokoloff, L., Davis, W.H., and Lee, S.L. A proposed model of boundary lubrication by synovial fluid: Structuring of boundary water, *J. Biomech. Eng.*, 101, 185–192, 1979.

31. Jay, D.J. Characterization of bovine synovial fluid lubricating factor, I. Chemical surface activity and lubrication properties, *Connective Tissue Res.*, 28, 71–88, 1992.

32. Burkhardt, B.M. *Development and Design of a Test Device for Cartilage Wear Studies*, MS thesis, Mechanical Engineering, Virginia Polytechnic Institute and State University, Blacksburg, VA, December 1988.

33. Stachowiak, G.W., Batchelor, A.W., and Griffiths, L.J. Friction and wear changes in synovial joints, *Wear*, 171, 135–142, 1994.

34. Hayes, A., Harris, B., Dieppe, P.A., and Clift, S.E. Wear of articular cartilage: The effect of crystals, *IMechE*, 41–58, 1993.

35. Malcolm, L.L. *An Experimental Investigation of the Frictional and Deformational Responses of Articular Cartilage Interfaces to Static and Dynamic Loading*, PhD thesis, University of California, San Diego, 1976.

36. Furey, M.J. Biotribology: An *in vitro* study of the effects of synovial fluid constituents on cartilage wear. *Proc., XVth Symposium of the European Society of Osteoarthrology*, Kuopio, Finland, June 25–27, 1986, abstract in *Scandanavian Journal of Rheumatology*, Supplement.

37. Furey, M.J. The influence of synovial fluid constituents on cartilage wear: A scanning electron microscope study. *Conference on Joint Destruction, XVth Symposium on the European Society of Osteoarthrology*, Sochi, USSR, September 28–October 3, 1987.

39. Furey, M.J. Biotribology: Cartilage lubrication and wear. *Proceedings of the 6th International Congress on Tribology EUROTRIB; '93*, Vol. 2, pp. 464–470, Budapest, Hungary, August 30–September 2, 1993.

40. Schroeder, M.O. *Biotribology: Articular Cartilage Friction, Wear, and Lubrication*, MS thesis, Mechanical Engineering, Virginia Polytechnic Institute and State University, Blacksburg, VA, July 1995.

41. Owellen, M.C. *Biotribology: The Effect of Lubricant and Load on Articular Cartilage Wear and Friction*, MS thesis, Mechanical Engineering, Virginia Polytechnic Institute and State University, Blacksburg, VA, July 1997.

42. Furey, M.J., Schroeder, M.O., Hughes, H.L., Owellen, M.C., Berrien, L.S., Veit, H., Gregory, E.M., and Kornegay, E.T. Observations of subsurface damage and cartilage degradation in *in vitro* tribological tests using bovine articular cartilage, *21st Symposium of the European Society for Osteoarthrology*, Vol. 15, Gent, Belgium, September 1996, 5, 3.2.

43. Furey, M.J., Schroeder, M.O., Hughes, H.L., Owellen, M.C., Berrien, L.S., Veit, H., Gregory, E.M., and Kornegay, E.T. *Biotribology, Synovial Joint Lubrication and Osteoarthritis*, Paper in Session W5 on Biotribology, *World Tribology Congress*, London, September 8–12, 1997.

44. Berrien, L.S., Furey, M.J., Veit, H.P., and Gregory, E.M. The Effect of collagenase-3 on the *in vitro* wear of bovine articular cartilage, paper, Biotribology Session, *Fifth International Tribology Conference*, Brisbane, Australia, December 6–9, 1998.

45. Sokoloff, L. *The Biology of Degenerative Joint Disease*, University of Chicago Press, Chicago, IL, 1969. Boston, MA, Fall 1983.

46. Furey, M.J. Exploring possible connections between tribology and osteoarthritis, *Lubricat. Sci.*, 273, May 1997.

47. Hayes, A., Harris, B., Dieppe, P.A., and Clift, S.E. Wear of articular cartilage: The effect of crystals, *Proc. I.Mech.E.*, 207, 41–58, 1993.

48. Wright, V. and Dowson, D. Lubrication and cartilage, *J. Anat.*, 121, 107–118, 1976.

49. Radin, E.L., Swann, D.A., and Weisser, P.A. Separation of a hyaluronate-free lubricating fraction from synovial fluid, *Nature*, 228, 377–378, 1970.

50. McCutchen, C.W. Joint lubrication, *Bull. Hosp. Joint Dis. Orthop. Inst.* XLIII, 118–129, 1983.

51. Williams, III, P.F., Powell, G.L., and LaBerge, M. Sliding friction analysis of phosphatidylcholine as a boundary lubricant for articular cartilage, *Proc. I. Mech. E.*, 207, 41–166, 1993.

52. Schwarz, I. M. and Hills, B. A. Surface-active phospholipid as the lubricating component of lubrician, *Br. J. Rheumatol.*, 37, 21–26, 1998.

53. Graham, J.D. and Walker, T.W. Motion in the hip: The relationship of split line patterns to surface velocities, a paper in *Perspectives in Biomedical Engineering*, R.M. Kenedi, Ed., University Park Press, Baltimore, MD, pp. 161–164, 1973.

54. Higginson, G.R. and Unsworth, T. The lubrication of natural joints. In *Tribology by Natural and Artificial Joints*, J.H. Dumbleton, Ed., Elsevier Scientific Publishing Co., Amsterdam, pp. 47–73, 1981.

55. Seedhom, B.B., Longton, E.B., Dowson, D., and Wright, V. Biomechanics background in the design of total replacement knee prosthesis. *Acta Orthop. Belgica*, 39(1), 164–180, 1973.

56. Brittberg, M. Cartilage repair, *A Collection of Five Articles on Cartilaginous Tissue Engineering with an Emphasis on Chondrocyte Transplantation*, 2nd ed., Institute of Surgical Sciences and Department of Clinical Chemistry and Institute of Laboratory Medicine, Goteborg University, Sweden, 1996.

57. Corkhill, P.H., Trevett, A.S., and Tighe, B.J. The potential of hydrogels as synthetic articular cartilage. *Proc. Inst. Mech. Eng.*, 204, 147–155, 1990.

58. Caravia, L., Dowson, D., Fisher, J., Corkhill, P.H., and Tighe, B.J. A comparison of friction in hydrogel and polyurethane materials for cushion form joints. *J. Mater. Sci.: Mater. Med.*, 4, 515–520, 1993.

59. Caravia, L., Dowson, D., Fisher, J., Corkhill, P.H., and Tighe, B.J. Friction of hydrogel and polyurethane elastic layers when sliding against each other under a mixed lubrication regime. *Wear*, 181–183, 236–240, 1995.

60. Freeman, M.E., Furey, M.J., Love, B.J., and Hampton, J.M. Friction, wear, and lubrication of hydrogels as synthetic articular cartilage, paper, Biotribology Session, *Fifth International Tribology Conference*, AUSTRIB '98, Brisbane, Australia, December 6–9, 1998.

61. Kelley, W.N., Harris, Jr., E.D., Ruddy, S., and Sledge, C.B. *Textbook of Rheumatology*, W.B. Saunders Co., Philadelphia, 1981.

62. Moskowitz, R.W., Howell, D.S., Goldberg, V.M., and Mankin, H.J. *Osteoarthritis: Diagnosis and Management*, W.B. Saunders Co., Philadelphia, 1984.

63. Verbruggen, G. and Veyes, E.M. Degenerative joints: Test tubes, tissues, models, and man. *Proceedings of the First Conference on Degenerative Joint Diseases*, Excerpta Medica, Amsterdam, 1982.

64. Gastpar, H. Biology of the articular cartilage in health and disease. *Proceedings of the Second Munich Symposium on Biology of Connective Tissue*, Munich, July 23–24, 1979; F.K. Schattauer Verlag, Stuttgart, 1980.

65. Dieppe, P. and Calvert, P. *Crystals and Joint Disease*, Chapman & Hall, London, 1983.

12

Analysis of Gait

12.1 Fundamental Concepts.. 12-2
    Clinical Gait Analysis Components • Gait Data Reference
    System • Motion Data Collection Protocol
12.2 Measurement Approaches and Systems...................... 12-3
    Stride and Temporal Parameters • Motion Measurement • Ground
    Reaction Measurement • Dynamic EMG
12.3 Gait Data Reduction: Kinematics and Kinetics......................... 12-6
12.4 Illustrative Clinical Example 12-8
12.5 Gait Analysis: Current Status 12-11
For Additional Information on Gait Analysis Techniques 12-12
For Additional Information on Typically Developing
    and Pathological Gait.. 12-12
References.. 12-12

Roy B. Davis III
*Shriners Hospitals for
Children*

Sylvia Õunpuu
*Connecticut Children's
Medical Center*

Peter A. DeLuca
*Connecticut Orthopaedic
Specialists*

The analysis of gait is the quantitative measurement and assessment of human locomotion which may include walking, running, and stair assent and descent. A number of different disciplines use gait or movement analysis techniques. Basic scientists seek a better understanding of how typically developing ambulators use muscle contractions about articulating joints to accomplish functional tasks, such as level walking [1] and stair climbing [2]. Physicians seek a better understanding of atypical movement patterns to assist in treatment decision making. Sports biomechanists, athletes, and their coaches use movement analysis techniques to investigate performance improvement [3–5] and injury mechanisms [6]. Sports equipment manufacturers seek to quantify the perceived advantages of their products relative to a competitor's offering.

With respect to the analysis of gait in the clinical setting, medical professionals measure and analyze the walking patterns of patients with locomotor impairment in the planning of treatment protocols, for example, orthotic prescription and surgical intervention. Clinical gait analysis is an evaluation tool that may determine the extent to which an individual's gait has been affected by an already diagnosed disorder [7] or provide a baseline for gait disorders that are progressive. Examples of clinical pathologies currently served by gait analysis include

- Amputation [8]
- Cerebral palsy [9,10]
- Degenerative joint disease [11,12]
- Joint pain [13]
- Joint replacement [14]
- Poliomyelitis [15]
- Multiple sclerosis [16]
- Muscular dystrophy [17]
- Myelodysplasia [18,19]

- Rheumatoid arthritis [20]
- Spinal cord injury [21]
- Stroke [22]
- Traumatic brain injury [23]

Generally, gait analysis data collection protocols and data reduction models have been developed to meet the requirements specific to the research, sport or clinical setting. For example, gait measurement protocols in a research setting might include an extensive physical examination to detail the anthropometrics of each subject. This time expenditure may not be possible in a clinical setting. This chapter focuses on the methods to assess the walking patterns of persons with locomotor impairment, that is, clinical gait analysis. The discussion will include a description of the available measurement technology, the components of data collection and reduction, the type of gait information produced for clinical interpretation, and the strengths and limitations of clinical gait analysis.

12.1 Fundamental Concepts

12.1.1 Clinical Gait Analysis Components

A comprehensive clinical gait analysis consists of a variety of components, the final combination of which is predicated on the individual patient's movement-related pathology and ability. Data that are currently provided for the assessment of gait in a clinical setting may include

- A video recording of the individual's gait (before instrumentation) for qualitative review and quality control purposes.
- Static physical examination measures, such as passive joint range of motion, muscle strength, ability to isolate movement, muscle tone, and the presence and degree of bony deformity.
- Segment and joint angular positions associated with standing posture.
- Stride and temporal parameters, such as step length and walking velocity.
- Segment and joint angular displacements during gait (level walking), commonly referred to as *kinematics*.
- The forces and torque applied to the patient's foot by the ground, or ground reaction loads during gait.
- The reactive intersegmental moments produced about the lower extremity joints by active and passive soft-tissue forces as well as the associated mechanical power of the intersegmental moment during gait, collectively referred to as *kinetics*.
- Indications of muscle activity, that is, voltage potentials produced by contracting muscles, during gait, relaxed standing and muscle tone assessment, known as dynamic *electromyography* (EMG).
- The dynamic pressure distributions on the plantar surface of the foot during standing and gait, referred to as *pedobarography*.
- A measure of metabolic energy expenditure during rest (sitting) and gait, for example, oxygen consumption, energy cost.
- The time to complete these steps can range from 1 to 3 h (Table 12.1).

12.1.2 Gait Data Reference System

Gait is a cyclic activity for which certain discrete events have been defined as significant. Typically, the *gait cycle* is defined as a period of time from the point of *initial contact* (also referred to as *foot contact*) of the patient's foot with the ground to the next point of initial contact for that same limb. Dividing the gait cycle into stance and swing phases is the point in the cycle where the stance limb leaves the ground, called *toe off* or *foot off*. Gait variables that change over time such as the patient's joint angular displacements are normally presented for clinical analysis as a function of the individual's gait cycle. This is

TABLE 12.1 A Typical Gait Data Collection Protocol

Test Component	Approximate Time (min)
Pretest tasks: test explanation to the adult patient or the pediatric patient and parent, system calibration	10
Video taping: brace, barefoot, close-up, standing	5–10
Clinical examination: range of motion, muscle strength, etc.	15–30
Motion marker placement	15–20
Motion data collection: subject calibration and multiple walks, per test condition (barefoot and orthosis)	10–60
EMG (surface electrodes and fine wire electrodes)	20–60
Data reduction of all trials	15–90
Data interpretation	20–30
Report dictation, generation, and distribution	120–180

done to facilitate the comparison of different walking trials and the use of a reference database from a matched, typical population [24].

12.1.3 Motion Data Collection Protocol

Motion data collection is typically the longest component of a comprehensive clinical gait assessment. After anatomical measures are acquired from the patient, such as leg length and joint widths, the patient is equipped with external markers (see Section 12.2.2.3). A static calibration of the "instrumented" patient is then completed followed by multiple walks along a pathway that is commonly both level and smooth. While the baseline for analysis is typically barefoot gait, patients are tested in other conditions as well, for example, while using lower extremity orthoses and walking aids such as crutches or a walker. Requirements and constraints associated with clinical gait data collection include the following:

- The patient should not be intimidated or distracted by the testing environment.
- The measurement equipment and protocols should not alter the patient's gait.
- Patient preparation and testing time must be minimized, and rest (or play) intervals must be included in the process as needed.
- Data collection techniques must be repeatable.
- Methodology must be sufficiently robust and flexible to allow the evaluation of a variety of gait abnormalities where the patient's dynamic range of motion and anatomy may be significantly different from typically developing persons of a similar age.
- The quality of the collected data must be assured before the patient leaves the facility.

12.2 Measurement Approaches and Systems

The purpose of this section is to provide an overview of the several technologies that are available to measure the dynamic gait variables listed earlier, including stride and temporal parameters, kinematics, kinetics, and dynamic EMG. Methods of data reduction will be described in a following section.

12.2.1 Stride and Temporal Parameters

The gait cycle events of first and second initial contact and toe off must be identified for the computation of the stride and temporal parameters. These measures may be obtained through a wide variety of approaches ranging from the use of simple tools such as a stopwatch and tape measure to sophisticated arrays of photoelectric monitors. Foot switches may be applied to the plantar surface of the patient's foot, for example, under the heel, first and fifth metatarsal heads and great toe. In clinical populations, foot switch placement is challenging because of the variability of foot deformities and the associated foot-ground contact patterns. This foot switch placement difficulty is avoided through the use of either shoe insoles instrumented with one or two large foot switches or entire contact-sensitive walkways. These gait events may also be quantified using simultaneous synchronized video recordings, the camera-based motion measurement or the force platform technology described below.

12.2.2 Motion Measurement

A number of alternative technologies are available for the measurement of body segment spatial position and orientation. These include the use of electrogoniometry, accelerometry, and video-based digitizers. These approaches are described below.

12.2.2.1 Electrogoniometry

A simple electrogoniometer consists of a rotary potentiometer with arms fixed to the shaft and base for attachment to the body segments juxtaposed to the joint of interest. Multi-axial goniometers extend this capability by providing additional, simultaneous, orthogonal measures of rotational displacement, more appropriate for human joint motion measurement. Electrogoniometers offer the advantages of real-time display and the rapid collection of single joint information. These devices are, however, limited to the measurement of relative angles and may be cumbersome in typical clinical applications such as the simultaneous, bilateral assessment of hip, knee, and ankle motion during gait.

12.2.2.2 Accelerometry

Multi-axis accelerometers can be employed to measure both linear and angular accelerations (if multiple transducers are properly configured). Velocity and position data may then be derived through numerical integration although care must be taken with respect to the selection of initial conditions and the handling of gravitational effects.

12.2.2.3 Video Camera–Based Systems

This approach to human motion measurement involves the use of external markers that are placed on the patient's body segments and aligned with specific anatomical landmarks. Marker trajectories are then monitored by a system of motion capture cameras (generally from 6 to 12) placed around a measurement volume (Figure 12.1). In a frame-by-frame analysis, stereophotogrammetric techniques are then used to produce the instantaneous three-dimensional (3-D) coordinates of each marker (relative to a fixed laboratory coordinate system) from the set of two-dimensional camera images. The processing of the 3-D marker coordinate data is described in a later section.

The video camera-based systems employ either passive (retroreflective) or active (light-emitting diodes [LEDs]) markers. Passive marker camera systems incorporate strobe light sources (LED rings around the camera lens). The cameras then capture the light returned from the highly reflective markers (usually small spheres). Active marker camera systems record the light that is produced by small LED markers that are placed directly on the patient. Advantages and disadvantages are associated with each approach. For example, the anatomical location (or identity) of each marker used in an active marker system is immediately known because the markers are sequentially pulsed by a controlling computer. Active markers and the associated electronics worn by the patients are heavier and more cumbersome than comparable passive markers. Passive marker systems require user interaction for marker identification although algorithms have been developed to expedite this process through semi-automated tracking.

12.2.3 Ground Reaction Measurement

12.2.3.1 Force Platforms

The 3-D ground reaction force vector, the vertical ground reaction torque and the point of application of the ground reaction force vector (referred to as the center of pressure) are measured with force platforms

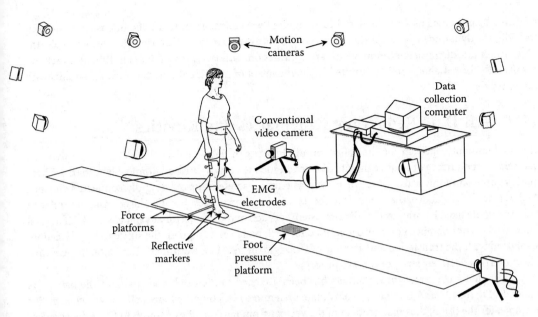

FIGURE 12.1 An "instrumented" patient with reflective spheres or markers and EMG electrodes. She walks along a level pathway while being monitored by 6–12 motion cameras (that monitor the displacement of the reflective markers) and 2–4 force platforms (that measure ground reaction loads). She might also walk over a foot pressure platform that measures the plantar pressure distribution. Her walk is also videotaped with 1 or 2 conventional video cameras. All of these signals (from the motion cameras, force platforms, EMG electrodes, foot pressure platform) are sent to the central data collection computer in the lab. These signals are then processed by the operator to produce the information used, along with the video recordings and other clinical examination data, to identify gait abnormalities and guide treatment planning.

embedded in the walkway. Force platforms with typical measurement surface dimensions of 0.5×0.5 m are comprised of several strain gauge or piezoelectric sensor arrays rigidly mounted together.

12.2.3.2 Pedobarography

The dynamic distributed load that corresponds to the vertical ground reaction force can be evaluated with the use of a flat, two-dimensional array of small piezoresistive force sensors. Overall resolution of the pedobarograph is dictated by the size of the individual sensor "cell." Sensor arrays configured as shoe insole inserts or flat plates offer the clinical user two measurement alternatives. Although this technology does afford the clinical practitioner better insight into the interaction between the plantar surface of the patient's foot and the ground, careful data interpretation is essential in patients with both foot deformity and altered gait patterns.

12.2.4 Dynamic EMG

Electrodes placed on the skin's surface and fine wires inserted into muscle are used to measure the voltage potentials produced by contracting muscles. The activity of the lower limb musculature is evaluated in this way with respect to the timing and the intensity of the contraction. Data collection variables that affect the quality of the EMG signal include the placement and distance between recording electrodes, skin surface conditions, distance between electrode and target muscle, signal amplification and filtering, and the rate of data acquisition. The quality of the EMG signal needs to be evaluated in all EMG data collection using the raw (unprocessed) signal. The phasic characteristics of the muscle activity may then be estimated from the raw EMG signal when referenced to the phases of the gait cycle. The EMG data may also be presented as a rectified and/or integrated waveform. To evaluate the intensity of the contraction, the dynamic EMG amplitudes are typically normalized by a reference value, for example, the EMG amplitude during a maximum voluntary contraction. This latter requirement is difficult to achieve consistently for patients who have limited isolated control of individual muscles, such as patients with cerebral palsy.

12.3 Gait Data Reduction: Kinematics and Kinetics

The predominant approach for the collection of clinical gait data involves the placement of external markers on the surface of body segments that are aligned with particular anatomical landmarks. These markers are commonly attached to the patient as either discrete units or in rigidly connected clusters. As described briefly above, the products of the data-acquisition process are the 3-D coordinates (relative to an inertially fixed laboratory coordinate system) of each marker trajectory over a gait cycle. If at least three markers or reference points are identified for each body segment, then the six degrees-of-freedom associated with the translation and attitude of the segment may be determined. The following example illustrates this relatively straightforward process.

Assume that a cluster of three markers has been attached to the thigh and shank of the patient as shown in Figure 12.2a. A body-fixed coordinate system may be computed for each marker cluster. For example, for the thigh, the cross product of the vectors from markers B to A and B to C produces a vector that is perpendicular to the cluster plane. From these vectors, the unit vectors $\mathbf{T}_{TX}$ and $\mathbf{T}_{TY}$ may be determined and used to compute the third orthogonal coordinate direction $\mathbf{T}_{TZ}$. In a similar manner, the marker-based, or technical, coordinate system may be calculated for the shank, that is, $\mathbf{S}_{TX}$, $\mathbf{S}_{TY}$, and $\mathbf{S}_{TZ}$. At this point, one might use these two technical coordinate systems to provide an estimate of

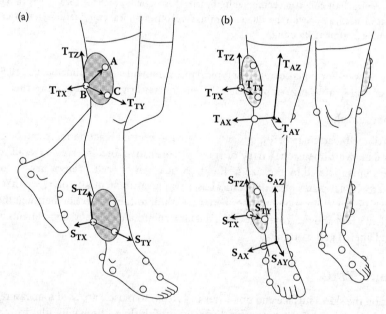

FIGURE 12.2 (a) Technical or marker-based coordinate systems "fixed" to the thigh and shank. A body fixed coordinate system may be computed for each cluster of three or more markers. On the thigh, for example, the vector cross product of the vectors from markers B to A and B to C produces a vector that is perpendicular to the cluster plane. From these vectors, the unit vectors $\mathbf{T}_{TX}$ and $\mathbf{T}_{TY}$ may be determined and used to compute the third orthogonal coordinate direction $\mathbf{T}_{TZ}$. (b) A subject calibration relates technical coordinate systems with anatomical coordinate systems, for example, $\{\mathbf{T}_T\}$ with $\{\mathbf{T}_A\}$, through the identification of anatomical landmarks, for example, the medial and lateral femoral condyles and medial and lateral malleoli.

the absolute orientation of the thigh or shank or the relative angles between the thigh and shank. This assumes that the technical coordinate systems reasonably approximate the anatomical axes of the body segments, for example, that T_{TZ} approximates the long axis of the thigh. A more rigorous approach incorporates the use of a subject calibration procedure to relate technical coordinate systems with relevant anatomical axes [25].

In a subject calibration, usually performed with the patient in a relaxed standing position, additional data are collected by the motion measurement system that relates the technical coordinate systems to the underlying anatomical structure. For example, as shown in Figure 12.2b, the medial and lateral femoral condyles and the medial and lateral malleoli may be used as anatomical references with the application of additional markers. With the hip center location estimated from markers placed on the pelvis [26,27] and knee and ankle center locations based on the additional markers, anatomical coordinate systems may be computed, for example, $\{T_A\}$ and $\{S_A\}$. The relationship between the respective anatomical and technical coordinate system pairs as well as the location of the joint centers in terms of the appropriate technical coordinate system may be stored, to be recalled in the reduction of each frame of the walking data. In this way, the technical coordinate systems (shown in Figure 12.2b) are transformed into alignment with the anatomical coordinate systems.

Once anatomically aligned coordinate systems have been computed for each body segment under investigation, one may compute relative joint angles and absolute segment attitudes in a number of ways. The classical approach of Euler, or more specifically, Cardan angles is commonly used in clinical gait analysis to describe the motion of the thigh relative to the pelvis (or hip angles), the motion of the shank relative to the thigh (or knee angles), the motion of the foot relative to the shank (or ankle angles), as well as the absolute attitudes of the pelvis and foot in space. The joint rotation sequence commonly used for the Cardan angle computation is flexion–extension, adduction–abduction, and transverse plane rotation [28]. Alternatively, joint motion has been described through the use of helical axes [29].

The intersegmental moments that soft tissue (e.g., muscle, ligaments, joint capsule) forces produce about approximate joint centers may be computed using Newtonian mechanics. For example, the free body diagram of the foot shown in Figure 12.3 depicts the various external loads to the foot as well as the intersegmental reactions produced at the ankle. The mass, mass moments of inertia, and location of the center of mass may be estimated from regression-based anthropometric relationships [30–32], and linear and angular velocity and acceleration may be determined by numerical differentiation. If the ground reaction loads, F_G and T, are measured by a force platform, then the unknown ankle intersegmental force, F_A, may be solved for with Newton's translational equation of motion. Note that intersegmental force values underestimate the magnitude of the actual joint contact forces. Newton's rotational equation of motion may then be applied to compute the net ankle intersegmental moment, M_A. This

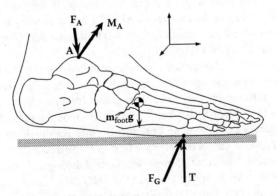

FIGURE 12.3 A free body diagram of the foot that illustrates the external loads to the foot, for example, the ground reaction loads, F_G and T, and the weight of the foot, $m_{foot}g$, as well as the unknown intersegmental reactions produced at the ankle, F_A and M_A, which may be solved for through the application of Newtonian mechanics.

process may then be repeated for the shank and thigh by using computed (distal) intersegmental force and moment values to solve for the unknown (proximal) intersegmental reactions. The mechanical power associated with an intersegmental moment and the corresponding joint angular velocity may be computed from the vector dot product of the two vectors, for example, ankle intersegmental power is computed through $\mathbf{M}_A \cdot \omega_A$ where ω_A is the angular velocity of the foot relative to the shank. Readers are referred to descriptions by Õunpuu et al. [33] and Palladino and Davis [34] for more details associated with this process.

Although sometimes referred to as "muscle moments," these net intersegmental moments reflect the moments produced by several mechanisms, for example, bony restrictions to motion, ligamentous forces, passive muscle and tendon force, and active muscle contractile force, in response to external loads. Currently, the evaluation of individual muscle forces in a patient population is not feasible because optimization strategies that may be successful for typically developing ambulation [35,36] may not be appropriate for pathological muscle behavior, for example, spasticity, overactivity, hyper- or hypotonicity [37].

With respect to assumptions associated with these gait models, the body segments are assumed to be rigid, for example, soft-tissue movement relative to underlying bone is small. The external markers are assumed to move with the underlying anatomical references. In this way, estimated joint center locations are assumed to remain fixed relative to the respective segmental coordinate systems, for example, the knee center is fixed relative to the thigh coordinate system. Moreover, the mass distribution changes during motion are assumed to be negligible. Consequently, the marker or instrumentation attachment sites must be selected carefully, for example, over tendinous structures of the distal shank as opposed to the more proximal muscle masses of the gastrocnemius and soleus.

12.4 Illustrative Clinical Example

As indicated above, the information available for clinical gait interpretation may include static physical examination measures, stride and temporal data, segment and joint kinematics, joint kinetics, electromyograms, and a video record. With this information, the clinical team can assess the patient's gait deviations, attempt to identify the etiology of the abnormalities and recommend treatment alternatives. In this way, clinicians are able to isolate the biomechanical insufficiency that may produce a locomotor impairment and require a compensatory response from the patient. For example, a patient may excessively elevate a pelvis (compensatory) in order to gain additional foot clearance in swing which may be inadequate due to a weak ankle dorsiflexor muscle (primary problem).

The following example illustrates how gait analysis data are used in the treatment decision-making process for a six-year-old child with cerebral palsy, left spastic hemiplegia. All gait video records, clinical examination data, and quantitative gait data are reviewed and a list of primary problems and possible causes is generated. The reviewed gait data would include 3-D kinematic data (Figure 12.4) and kinetic data (Figure 12.5) and dynamic EMG data (Figure 12.6).

In the sagittal plane, increased left plantar flexion in stance and swing (Figure 12.4, Point **A**) is secondary to spasticity of the ankle plantar flexor muscles as the patient has a passive range of motion of the ankle that is within normal limits and can stand plantigrade. Premature plantar flexion of the right ankle in mid stance (Figure 12.4, Point **B**) is a vault compensation as the patient can isolate motion about the right ankle on clinical examination and produce an internal dorsiflexor moment following initial contact (Figure 12.5, Point **A**). Increased left knee flexion at initial contact (Figure 12.4, Point **C**) is secondary to hamstring muscle spasticity/tightness (appreciated during the clinical examination and evidenced by hamstring over-activity during gait, seen in the EMG data, Figure 12.6, Point **A**). Reduced left knee flexion in swing (Figure 12.4, Point **D**) is secondary to rectus femoris muscle over-activity in mid swing (Figure 12.6, Point **B**), an absence of ankle power generation in terminal stance (Figure 12.5, Point **B**), reduced hip power generation in pre-swing (Figure 12.5, Point **C**), and out-of-plane positioning of the lower extremity due to internal hip rotation (Figure 12.4, Point **E**). Increasing anterior pelvic

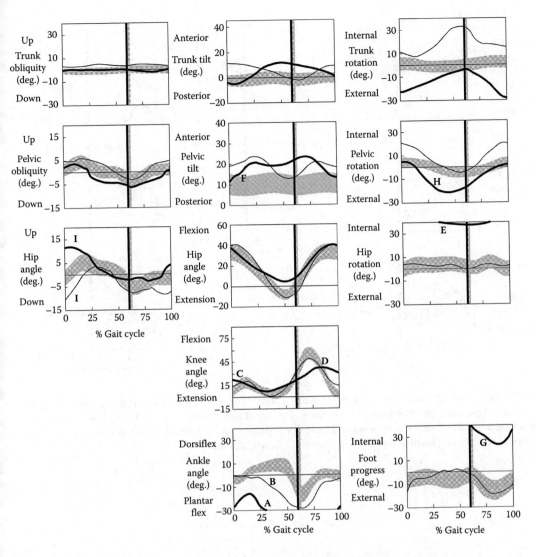

FIGURE 12.4 The left (thick lines) and right (thin lines) trunk, pelvic, and lower extremity kinematics for a six-year-old child with cerebral palsy, left spastic hemiplegia. Also shown are shaded bands that indicate one standard deviation about mean values associated with the reference (typically developing children) database used in the Motion Analysis Laboratory at Shriners Hospitals for Children, Greenville, South Carolina.

tilt during left-side stance (Figure 12.4, Point **F**) is related to the patient's limited ability to isolate movement between the pelvis and femur on the left side (determined from the clinical examination). In the transverse plane, increased left internal hip rotation (Figure 12.4, Point **E**), increased left internal foot progression (Figure 12.4, Point **G**), and asymmetric pelvic rotation with the left side externally rotated (Figure 12.4, Point **H**) are all secondary to increased internal femoral torsion (noted during the clinical examination). In the coronal plane, asymmetrical hip rotations (Figure 12.4, Point **I**) are secondary to pelvic transverse plane asymmetry.

After all of the primary gait issues are identified and possible causes are determined, treatment options for each primary issue are proposed. For the child presented above, treatment options include a left femoral derotation osteotomy to correct for internal femoral torsion and associated internal hip rotation (primary problem). Expected secondary outcomes of this intervention include improved foot

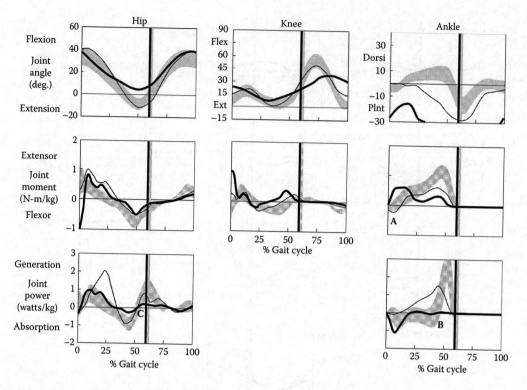

FIGURE 12.5 The left (thick lines) and right (thin lines) sagittal lower extremity kinetics for a six-year-old child with cerebral palsy, left spastic hemiplegia. Also shown are shaded bands that indicate one standard deviation about mean values associated with the reference (typically developing children) database used in the Motion Analysis Laboratory at Shriners Hospitals for Children, Greenville, South Carolina.

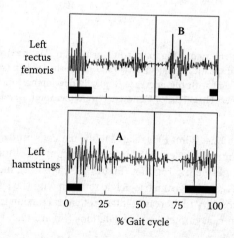

FIGURE 12.6 EMG tracing for the left rectus femoris and hamstring muscles for a six-year-old child with cerebral palsy, left spastic hemiplegia. The horizontal bars on the graphs indicate the approximate typical activity of these muscles during walking associated with the reference database used in the Motion Analysis Laboratory at Shriners Hospitals for Children, Greenville, South Carolina.

progression and symmetrical pelvic position in the transverse plane. A left intramuscular plantar flexor muscle lengthening is recommended to provide more length to the ankle plantar flexor muscles and reduce the impact of muscle stretch on the spastic plantar flexor muscles, thereby reducing (or resolving) the excessive ankle equinus and provide improved stability in stance and foot clearance in swing. A left hamstring muscle lengthening is also recommended to reduce the impact of muscle stretch on hamstring muscle spasticity, thereby improving knee extension at initial contact and overall knee motion in stance. A rectus femoris muscle transfer is recommended to reduce the impact of inappropriate activity of the rectus femoris muscle in mid swing and therefore improve peak knee flexion in swing and the associated clearance in swing. The premature plantar flexion of the right ankle in stance is secondary to a vault compensation and therefore, is predicted to resolve secondary to the surgery on the left side, that is, does not require any treatment. A standard protocol in most clinical gait laboratories is to repeat the gait analysis at about one year post surgery. At this time, surgical hypotheses and progress with respect to resolution of pretreatment gait abnormalities can be evaluated objectively.

12.5 Gait Analysis: Current Status

Comprehensive gait analysis techniques as described above have had a profound impact on the understanding of gait pathology, defining indications for specific treatments and ultimately, improving treatment outcomes. As with any kind of measurement, the utility of gait analysis information may be limited by sources of error, for example, soft-tissue displacement relative to the underlying bone. However, gains continue to be made with respect to analytical techniques to address this potential artifact [38–41]. The estimation of the location of the hip joint center is required in the determination of both hip kinematics and kinetics. Recent improvements in technology and computational techniques [42–44] have made the dynamic estimation of the instantaneous joint center locations, suggested by Cappozzo [25] in 1984, more viable clinically. Functional joint centering of the hip and all motion measurement using external markers, however, is challenged by excessive pelvic adipose tissue in patients who are overweight or obese. The evaluation of small patients weakens the quality of the data because inter-marker distances are reduced, thereby reducing the precision of angular computations, although recent improvements in camera resolution and camera image processing have addressed this limitation to a degree. Other errors associated with data collection alter the results as well, such as, a marker improperly placed or a force platform inadvertently contacted by the swing limb. To minimize the impact of these issues on motion data and its utility, it is essential that the potential adverse effects of these errors on the gait information be understood and appreciated by the clinical team in the interpretation process.

In addition to the kinematic (segment and joint angles), kinetic, and dynamic EMG data, estimations of musculo-tendon length are coming into use in clinical assessment and research [45,46]. This alternative expression of gait kinematics is also subject to the measurement and modeling issues associated with soft-tissue artifact and joint center determination with the additional challenge of approximating muscle origin and insertion anatomical locations. However, the assessment of musculo-tendon lengths in combination with other motion measurement and clinical data may assist in our understanding of the complex relationships between adjacent joints during gait. Gait forward simulation models are proving increasingly useful as exploratory tools in the investigation of the mechanisms associated with pathological gait [47,48]. These simulations will be strengthened when more is understood about the pathomechanics of impaired muscle and tendon and when they can be applied on an individual patient basis in the clinical setting.

Carefully performed gait analysis facilitates the systematic, quantitative documentation of walking patterns in comparison to qualitative observational techniques which represent the standard of care for the assessment of complex gait disorders in many medical facilities. With the various gait data, the clinician has the opportunity to separate the primary causes of a gait abnormality from the secondary deviations and compensatory gait mechanisms. Apparent contradictions between the different types of gait information, specifically visual impression versus joint angles (kinematics), can result in a more carefully developed understanding of the gait deviations and an appreciation for the additional knowledge and understanding gained through gait analysis data interpretation. Gait analysis provides the clinical user the ability to more precisely (than observational gait analysis alone) understand the gait pathomechanics; therefore, plan complex multi-level surgeries and ultimately objectively evaluate the efficacy of different interventions, for example, surgical approaches and orthotic designs. Through gait analysis, movement in planes of motion not easily observed, such as about the long axes of the lower limb segments, may be quantified. Finally, quantities that cannot be observed may be assessed, for example, muscular activity and joint kinetics. In the future, it is anticipated that our understanding of gait will be enhanced through the application of pattern recognition strategies, and coupled dynamics. The systematic and objective evaluation of gait both before and after intervention will continue to lead to improved treatment outcomes.

For Additional Information on Gait Analysis Techniques

Allard, P., Stokes, I.A.F., and Blanchi, J.P. (Eds.), *Three-Dimensional Analysis of Human Movement*, Human Kinetics, Champaign, Illinois, 1995.

Berme, N. and Cappozzo, A. (Eds.), *Biomechanics of Human Movement: Applications in Rehabilitation, Sports and Ergonomics*, Bertec Corporation, Worthington, Ohio, 1990.

Harris, G.F. and Smith, P.A., (Eds.), *Human Motion Analysis*, IEEE Press, Piscataway, New Jersey, 1996.

Rose, J. and Gamble, J.G. (Eds), *Human Walking*, 3rd Edition, Lippincott Williams & Wilkins, Philadelphia, 2006.

Winter, D.A., *Biomechanics and Motor Control of Human Movement*, John Wiley and Sons, New Jersey, 2009.

For Additional Information on Typically Developing and Pathological Gait

Gage, J.R., Koop, S.E., Schwartz, M.H., Novacheck, T.F. (Eds.), *The Treatment of Gait Problems in Cerebral Palsy*, 2nd Edition, Mac Keith Press, London, 2009.

Perry, J. and Burnfield, J.M., *Gait Analysis: Normal and Pathological Function*, 2nd Edition, Slack, New Jersey, 2010.

Rose, J. and Gamble, J.G. (Eds.), *Human Walking*, 3rd Edition, Lippincott Williams & Wilkins, Philadelphia, 2006.

Sutherland, D.H. et al., *The Development of Mature Walking*, Mac Keith Press, London, 1988.

References

1. Neptune, R.R., Zajac, F.E., and Kautz, S.A., Muscle force redistributes segmental power for body progression during walking, *Gait Posture*, 19, 194, 2004.
2. Heller, M.O. et al., Musculo-skeletal loading conditions at the hip during walking and stair climbing, *J. Biomech.*, 34, 883, 2001.
3. Ferber, R., Davis, I.M., and Williams, D.S. 3rd, Gender differences in lower extremity mechanics during running, *Clin. Biomech.*, 18, 350, 2003.
4. Kerrigan D.C. et al., The effect of running shoes on lower extremity joint torques, *Arch. Phys. Med. Rehabil.*, 1, 1058, 2009.
5. Kautz, S.A. and Hull, M.L., Dynamic optimization analysis for equipment setup problems in endurance cycling, *J. Biomech.*, 28, 1391, 1995.
6. Tashman, S. et al., Abnormal rotational knee motion during running after anterior cruciate ligament reconstruction, *Am. J. Sports Med.*, 32, 975, 2004.

7. Brand, R.A. and Crowninshield, R.D., Comment on criteria for patient evaluation tools, *J. Biomech.*, 14, 655, 1981.

8. Mâaref, K. et al., Kinematics in the terminal swing phase of unilateral transfemoral amputees: Microprocessor-controlled versus swing-phase control prosthetic knees, *Arch. Phys. Med. Rehabil.*, 91, 919, 2010.

9. Stebbins, J. et al., Gait compensations caused by foot deformity in cerebral palsy, *Gait Posture*, 32, 226, 2010.

10. Adolfsen, S.E. et al., Kinematic and kinetic outcomes after identical multilevel soft tissue surgery in children with cerebral palsy, *J. Pediatr. Orthop.*, 27, 658, 2007.

11. Kaufman, K.R. et al., Gait characteristics of patients with knee osteoarthritis, *J. Biomech.*, 34, 907, 2001.

12. Vanwanseele, B. et al., The relationship between knee adduction moment and cartilage and meniscus morphology in women with osteoarthritis, *Osteoarthritis Cartilage*, 18, 894, 2010.

13. Koutakis, P. et al., Abnormal joint powers before and after the onset of claudication symptoms, *J. Vasc. Surg.*, 52, 340, 2010.

14. Pospischill, M. et al., Minimally invasive compared with traditional transgluteal approach for total hip arthroplasty: A comparative gait analysis, *J. Bone Joint Surg. Am.*, 92, 328, 2010.

15. Perry, J., Mulroy, S.J., and Renwick, S.E., The relationship of lower extremity strength and gait parameters in patients with post-polio syndrome, *Arch. Phys. Med. Rehabil.*, 74, 165, 1993.

16. Kelleher, K.J. et al., The characterisation of gait patterns of people with multiple sclerosis, *Disabil. Rehabil.*, 32, 1242, 2010.

17. D'Angelo, M.G. et al., Gait pattern in Duchenne muscular dystrophy, *Gait Posture*, 29, 36, 2009.

18. Õunpuu, S. et al., An examination of knee function during gait in children with myelomeningocele, *J. Pediatr. Orthop.*, 20, 629, 2000.

19. Bartonek, A., Eriksson, M., and Gutierrez-Farewik, E.M., Effects of carbon fibre spring orthoses on gait in ambulatory children with motor disorders and plantarflexor weakness, *Dev. Med. Child. Neurol.*, 49, 615, 2007.

20. Weiss, R.J. et al., Gait pattern in rheumatoid arthritis, *Gait Posture*, 28, 229, 2008.

21. Gordon, K.E. et al., Ankle load modulates hip kinetics and EMG during human locomotion, *J. Neurophysiol.*, 101, 2062, 2009.

22. Mulroy, S. et al., Use of cluster analysis for gait pattern classification of patients in the early and late recovery phases following stroke, *Gait Posture*, 18, 114, 2003.

23. Perry, J., The use of gait analysis for surgical recommendations in traumatic brain injury, *J. Head Trauma Rehabil.*, 14, 116, 1999.

24. Õunpuu, S., Gage, J.R., and Davis, R.B., Three-dimensional lower extremity joint kinetics in normal pediatric gait, *J. Pediatr. Orthop.*, 11, 341, 1991.

25. Cappozzo, A., Gait analysis methodology, *Hum. Move. Sci.*, 3, 27, 1984.

26. Davis, R.B. et al., A gait analysis data collection and reduction technique, *Hum. Move. Sci.*, 10, 575, 1991.

27. Bell, A.L., Pederson, D.R., and Brand, R.A., Prediction of hip joint center location from external landmarks, *Hum. Move. Sci.*, 8, 3, 1989.

28. Grood, E.S. and Suntay, W.J., A joint coordinate system for the clinical description of three-dimensional motions: Application to the knee, *J. Biomech. Eng.*, 105, 136, 1983.

29. Woltring, H.J., Huskies, R., and DeLange, A., Finite centroid and helical axis estimation from noisy landmark measurement in the study of human joint kinematics, *J. Biomech.*, 18, 379, 1985.

30. Dempster, W.T., Space requirements of the seated operator: Geometrical, kinematic, and mechanical aspects of the body with special reference to the limbs, WADC-55-159, AD-087-892, Wright Air Development Center, Wright-Patterson Air Force Base, Ohio, 1955.

31. McConville, J.T. et al., Anthropometric relationships of body and body segment moments of inertia, Technical report AFAMRL-TR-80-119, Air Force Aerospace Medical Research Laboratory,

Aerospace Medical Division, Air Force Systems Command, Wright-Patterson Air Force Base, Ohio, 1980.

32. Jenson, R.K., Body segment mass, radius and radius of gyration proportions of children, *J. Biomech.*, 19, 359, 1986.

33. Õunpuu, S., Davis, R.B., and DeLuca, P.A., Joint kinetics: Methods, interpretation and treatment decision-making in children with cerebral palsy and myelomeningocele, *Gait Posture*, 4, 62, 1996.

34. Palladino, J. and Davis, R.B., Biomechanics, in *Introduction to Biomedical Engineering*, Enderle, J., Blanchard, S., and Bronzino, J., Eds., Elsevier Academic Press, Amsterdam, 133, 2012.

35. Chao, E.Y. and Rim, K., Application of optimization principles in determining the applied moments in human leg joints during gait, *J. Biomech.*, 6, 497, 1973.

36. Anderson, F.C. and Pandy, M.G., Static and dynamic optimization solutions for gait are practically equivalent, *J. Biomech.*, 34, 153, 2001.

37. Bleck, E.E., *Orthopaedic Management in Cerebral Palsy*, Mac Keith Press, Philadelphia, 1987, 87.

38. Stagni R., Fantozzi S., and Cappello A., Double calibration vs. global optimization: Performance and effectiveness for clinical application, *Gait Posture*, 1, 119, 2009.

39. Peters A. et al., Determination of the optimal locations of surface-mounted markers on the tibial segment, *Gait Posture*, 1, 42, 2009.

40. De Groote F. et al., Kalman smoothing improves the estimation of joint kinematics and kinetics in marker-based human gait analysis, *J. Biomech.*, 41, 3390, 2008.

41. Cappello A. et al., Soft tissue artifact compensation in knee kinematics by double anatomical land-mark calibration: Performance of a novel method during selected motor tasks, *IEEE Trans Biomed Eng.*, 52, 992, 2005.

42. Leardini, A. et al., Validation of a functional method for the estimation of hip joint centre location, *J. Biomech.*, 32, 99, 1999.

43. Piazza, S.J. et al., Assessment of the functional method of hip joint center location subject to reduced range of hip motion, *J. Biomech.*, 37, 349, 2004.

44. Schwartz, M.H. and Rozumalskia, A., A new method for estimating joint parameters from motion data, *J. Biomech.*, 38, 107, 2005.

45. Jahn, J., Vasavada, A.N., and McMulkin, M.L., Calf muscle-tendon lengths before and after tendo-Achilles lengthenings and gastrocnemius lengthenings for equinus in cerebral palsy and idiopathic toe walking, *Gait Posture*, 29, 612, 2009.

46. van der Krogt, M.M. et al., Walking speed modifies spasticity effects in gastrocnemius and soleus in cerebral palsy gait, *Clin. Biomech.*, 24, 422, 2009.

47. Damiano, D.L. et al., Can strength training predictably improve gait kinematics? A pilot study on the effects of hip and knee extensor strengthening on lower-extremity alignment in cerebral palsy, *Phys. Ther.*, 90, 269, 2010.

48. Fox, M.D. et al., Mechanisms of improved knee flexion after rectus femoris transfer surgery, *J. Biomech.*, 42, 614, 2009.

13

Mechanics of Head/Neck

13.1 Mechanisms of Injury... 13-1
    Head Injury Mechanisms • Neck Injury Mechanisms
13.2 Mechanical Response... 13-3
    Mechanical Response of the Brain • Mechanical Response of the Neck
13.3 Regional Tolerance of the Head and Neck to Blunt Impact..... 13-7
    Regional Tolerance of the Head • Regional Tolerance of the Neck
13.4 Human Surrogates of the Head and Neck.............................. 13-10
    The Experimental Surrogate • The Injury-Assessment
    Tool • Computer Models
References.. 13-11

Albert I. King
Wayne State University

David C. Viano
Wayne State University

Injury is a major societal problem in the United States. Approximately 140,000 fatalities occur each year due to both intentional and unintentional injuries. Two-thirds of these are unintentional, and of these, about one-half are attributable to automotive-related injuries. In 1993, the estimated number of automotive-related fatalities dipped under 40,000 for the first time in the last three decades due to a continuing effort by both the industry and the government to render vehicles safer in crash situations. However, for people under 40 years of age, automotive crashes, falls, and other unintentional injuries are the highest risks of fatality in the United States in comparison with all other causes.

The principal aim of impact biomechanics is the prevention of injury through environmental modification, such as the provision of an airbag for automotive occupants to protect them during a frontal crash. To achieve this aim effectively, it is necessary that workers in the field have a clear understanding of the *mechanisms of injury*, be able to describe the *mechanical response* of the tissues involved, have some basic information on *human tolerance* to impact, and be in possession of tools that can be used as *human surrogates* to assess a particular injury (Viano et al., 1989). This chapter deals with the biomechanics of blunt impact injury to the head and neck.

13.1 Mechanisms of Injury

13.1.1 Head Injury Mechanisms

Among the more popular theories of brain injury due to blunt impact are changes in intracranial pressure and the development of shear strains in the brain. Positive pressure increases are found in the brain behind the site of impact on the skull. Rapid acceleration of the head, in-bending of the skull, and the propagation of a compressive pressure wave are proposed as mechanisms for the generation of intracranial compression that causes local contusion of brain tissue. At the contrecoup site, there is an opposite response in the form of a negative-pressure pulse that also causes bruising. It is not clear as to whether the injury is due to the negative pressure itself (tensile loading) or to a cavitation phenomenon similar to that seen on the surfaces of propellers of ships (compression loading). The pressure differential across the brain necessarily results in a pressure gradient that can give rise to shear strains developing within the deep structures of the brain. Furthermore, when the head is impacted, it not only translates but also rotates about the neck, causing relative motion of the brain with respect to the skull. Gennarelli (1983) has found that rotational acceleration of the head can cause a diffuse injury to the white matter of the brain in animal models, as evidenced by retraction balls developing along the axons of injured nerves. This injury was described by Strich (1961) as diffuse axonal injury (DAI) that she found in the white matter of autopsied human brains. Other researchers, including Lighthall et al. (1990), have been able to cause the development of DAI in the brain of an animal model (ferrets) by the application of direct impact to the brain without the associated head angular acceleration. Adams et al. (1986) indicated that DAI is the most important factor in severe head injury because it is irreversible and leads to incapacitation and dementia. It is postulated that DAI occurs as a result of the mechanical insult but cannot be detected by staining techniques at autopsy unless the patient survives the injury for at least several hours.

13.1.2 Neck Injury Mechanisms

The neck or the cervical spine is subjected to several forms of unique injuries that are not seen in the thoracolumbar spine. Injuries to the upper cervical spine, particularly at the atlanto-occipital joint, are considered to be more serious and life threatening than those at the lower level. The atlanto-occipital joint can be dislocated either by an axial torsional load or a shear force applied in the anteroposterior direction, or vice versa. A large compression force can cause the arches of Cl to fracture, breaking it up into two or four sections. The odontoid process of C2 is also a vulnerable area. Extreme flexion of the neck is a common cause of odontoid fractures, and a large percentage of these injuries are related to automotive accidents (Pierce and Barr, 1983). Fractures through the pars interarticularis of C2, commonly known as "hangman's fractures" in automotive collisions, are the result of a combined axial compression and extension (rearward bending) of the cervical spine. Impact of the forehead and face of unrestrained occupants with the windshield can result in this injury. Garfin and Rothman (1983) discussed this injury in relation to hanging and traced the history of this mode of execution. It was estimated by a British judiciary committee that the energy required to cause a hangman's fracture was 1708 N m (1260 ft lb).

In automotive-type accidents, the loading on the neck due to head contact forces is usually a combination of an axial or shear load with bending. Bending loads are almost always present, and the degree of axial or shear force depends on the location and direction of the contact force. For impacts near the crown of the head, compressive forces predominate. If the impact is principally in the transverse plane, there is less compression and more shear. Bending modes are infinite in number because the impact can come from any angle around the head. To limit the scope of the discussion, the following injury modes are considered: tension–flexion, tension–extension, compression–flexion, and compression–extension in the midsagittal plane and lateral bending.

13.1.2.1 Tension–Flexion Injuries

Forces resulting from inertial loading of the head–neck system can result in flexion of the cervical spine while it is being subjected to a tensile force. In experimental impacts of restrained subjects undergoing forward deceleration, Thomas and Jessop (1983) reported atlanto-occipital separation and C1–C2 separation occurring in subhuman primates at 120 g. Similar injuries in human cadavers were found at 34–38 g by Cheng et al. (1982), who used a preinflated driver airbag system that restrained the thorax but allowed the head and neck to rotate over the bag.

13.1.2.2 Tension–Extension Injuries

The most common type of injury due to combined tension and extension of the cervical spine is the "whiplash" syndrome. However, a large majority of such injuries involve the soft tissues of the neck, and the pain is believed to reside in the joint capsules of the articular facets of the cervical vertebrae (Wallis et al., 1997).

In severe cases, teardrop fractures of the anterosuperior aspect of the vertebral body can occur. Alternately, separation of the anterior aspect of the disk from the vertebral endplate is known to occur. More severe injuries occur when the chin impacts the instrument panel or when the forehead impacts the windshield. In both cases, the head rotates rearward and applies a tensile and bending load on the neck. In the case of windshield impact by the forehead, hangman's fracture of C2 can occur. Garfin and Rothman (1983) suggested that it is caused by spinal extension combined with compression on the lamina of C2, causing the pars to fracture.

13.1.2.3 Compression–Flexion Injuries

When a force is applied to the posterosuperior quadrant of the head or when a crown impact is administered while the head is in flexion, the neck is subjected to a combined load of axial compression and forward bending. Anterior wedge fractures of vertebral bodies are commonly seen, but with increased load, burst fractures, and fracture-dislocations of the facets can result. The latter two conditions are unstable and tend to disrupt or injure the spinal cord, and the extent of the injury depends on the penetration of the vertebral body or its fragments into the spinal canal. Recent experiments by Pintar et al. (1989, 1990) indicate that burst fractures of lower cervical vertebrae can be reproduced in cadaveric specimens by a crown impact to a flexed cervical spine. A study by Nightingale et al. (1993) showed that fracture dislocations of the cervical spine occur very early in the impact event (within the first 10 ms) and that the subsequent motion of the head or bending of the cervical spine cannot be used as a reliable indicator of the mechanism of injury.

13.1.2.4 Compression–Extension Injuries

Frontal impacts to the head with the neck in extension will cause compression–extension injuries. These involve the fracture of one or more spinous processes and, possibly, symmetrical lesions of the pedicles, facets, and laminae. If there is a fracture dislocation, the inferior facet of the upper vertebra is displaced posteriorly and upward and appears to be more horizontal than normal on x-ray.

13.1.2.5 Injuries Involving Lateral Bending

If the applied force or inertial load on the head has a significant component out of the midsagittal plane, the neck will be subjected to lateral or oblique along with axial and shear loading. The injuries characteristic of lateral bending are lateral wedge fractures of the vertebral body and fractures to the posterior elements on one side of the vertebral column.

Whenever there is lateral or oblique bending, there is the possibility of twisting the neck. The associated torsional loads may be responsible for unilateral facet dislocations or unilateral locked facets (Moffat et al., 1978). However, the authors postulated that pure torsional loads on the neck are rarely encountered in automotive accidents.

13.2 Mechanical Response

13.2.1 Mechanical Response of the Brain

Skull impact response was presented in the previous edition in which remarks were made regarding the unavailability of data on the response of the brain during an injury-producing impact. Such data are now available. For intact heads, the motion of the brain inside the skull has been recently studied by Hardy et al. (2001). Isolated cadaveric heads were subjected to a combined linear and angular acceleration and exposed to a biplanar high-speed x-ray system. Neutral density targets made of tin or tungsten were preinserted into the brain. Video data collected from such impacts showed that most of the motion was in the center of the brain and that target motion was in the form of a figure 8, as shown in Figure 13.1. This motion was limited to ±5 mm regardless of the severity of the impact. Angular acceleration levels in excess of 10,000 rad/s² were reached.

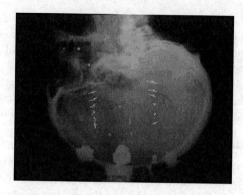

FIGURE 13.1 Brain response to blunt impact.

In another experiment, a Hybrid III dummy head and neck system was accelerated into a variety of plastic foams to assess head response with and without the use of a helmet used in American football. It was found that the helmet reduced the linear acceleration of the head substantially but did not change its angular acceleration significantly. However, it is believed by many that angular acceleration is the cause of brain injury. So if angular acceleration is the culprit, then how does the helmet protect the brain? In an attempt to answer this question, video data from NFL helmet impacts were analyzed and the helmet velocities were computed using stereophotogrammetric methods. The helmet impacts were reproduced in the laboratory by Newman et al. (1999) to yield head angular and linear accelerations, using helmeted Hybrid III dummies. These head accelerations were fed into a brain injury computer model developed by Zhang et al. (2001) to compute brain responses, such as strain (ε), strain rate ($d\varepsilon/dt$), and pressure. A total of 58 cases were studied, involving 25 cases of concussion or mild traumatic brain injury (MTBI), as reported by Pellman et al. (2003). The results of the model were analyzed statistically to determine the best predictors of MTBI, using the logist analysis. It was found brain response parameters such as the product of strain and strain rate, were good predictors whereas angular acceleration was a poor predictor, as shown in Table 13.1. The chi square value is a measure of the ability of the parameter to predict injury and in this analysis, its ability to predict injury is high if the chi square value is high. These results are consistent with the findings of Viano and Lövsund (1999) who used animal data to determine the parameter most likely to cause DAI in a living brain. It was the product of the velocity (V) of the impactor and depth of penetration of the impactor as percentage of the brain depth (C). For the brain, the product, $V \cdot C$, is analogous to $\varepsilon \cdot d\varepsilon/dt$. Note that head injury criterion (HIC) is the current criterion used in Federal Motor Vehicle Safety Standard (FMVSS) 208 to assess head injury and GSI (Gadd Severity Index) is the previous head injury criterion, now referred to as the Gadd Severity Index. The cumulative strain

TABLE 13.1 List of Best Predictors of MTBI

Rank Order	Predictor Variable	Chi Square	*p*-value
1	$\varepsilon \cdot d\varepsilon/dt$	41.0	0.0000
2	$d\varepsilon/dt$	33.1	0.0000
3	HIC	31.5	0.0000
4	SI	31.2	0.0000
5	Linear acceleration	28.3	0.0000
6	ε_{max}	28.0	0.0000
7	Max. principal stress	27.3	0.0000
8	Cumulative strain at 15%	26.0	0.0000
9	Angular acceleration	24.9	0.0000

at 15% is a measure of the volume of brain that experienced a strain of 15% or higher throughout the impact. It is concluded that response variable of the brain are better predictors of injury than input variables.

13.2.2 Mechanical Response of the Neck

The mechanical response of the cervical spine was studied by Mertz and Patrick (1967, 1971), Patrick and Chou (1976), Schneider et al. (1975), and Ewing et al. (1978). Mertz et al. (1973) quantified the response in terms of rotation of the head relative to the torso as a function of bending moment at the occipital condyles. Loading corridors were obtained for flexion and extension, as shown in Figures 13.2 and 13.3. An exacting definition of the impact environments to be used in evaluating dummy necks relative to the loading corridors illustrated in these figures is included in SAE J1460 (1985). It should be noted that the primary basis for these curves is volunteer data and that the extension of these corridors to dummy tests in the injury-producing range is somewhat surprising.

The issue of whiplash is a controversial one principally because researchers in the field cannot agree on an injury mechanism. Currently, five such mechanisms have been proposed. It began with the hyperextension theory, which was discarded when the automotive headrest did not reduce the incidence of injury. The flexion theory is also considered untenable because head and neck flexion after the rear end collision is much less severe than that resulting from a frontal impact and the whiplash syndrome is not frequently seen in frontal impacts. The theory that a momentary increase in pressure in the cerebrospinal fluid during whiplash could induce neck pain was also considered invalid because injury to the nerve roots require prolonged pressure and root compression leads to radiculopathy and not direct neck pain. The fourth theory of impingement of the facet joint surfaces was proposed but has not been demonstrated. It claims that the synovial lining can be trapped between the facets resulting in pain. Finally, the shear theory appears to be the most promising. A shear force is developed at every level of the cervical spine before the head and can be brought forward along with the torso, which is pushed forward by the seat back. This shear force causes relative motion between adjacent cervical vertebrae in the form of relative translation and rotation. Deng et al. (2000) performed a series of cadaveric tests and measured this relative displacement and also estimated the amount of stretch the facet capsules would undergo. Wallis et al. (1997) have shown that removal of nerve endings in the cervical facet capsules can relieve neck pain for an average of about nine months.

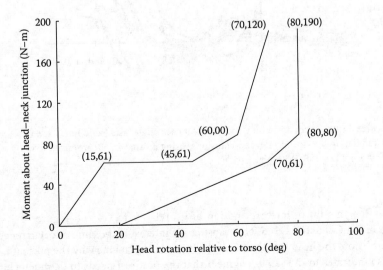

FIGURE 13.2 Loading corridor for neck flexion.

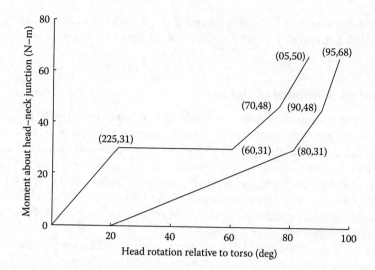

FIGURE 13.3 Loading corridor for neck extension.

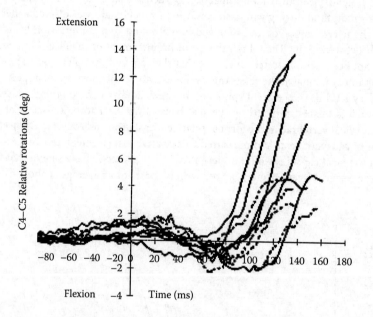

FIGURE 13.4 Relative displacement of C4 on C5 for 20° seat back angle tests (solid lines) and 0° seat back angle tests (dotted lines) simulating low-speed rear-end collisions, using a cadaver. (Reproduced from Deng, B. et al. 2000. *Stapp Car Crash J.* 44: 171–188. With permission.)

Figure 13.4 shows the amount of forward motion of C5 relative to C4 and Figure 13.5 shows the estimated stretch of the C4–5 and C5–6 facet capsule. Of interest is the time of occurrence of these events. They occur before the head hits the headrest. It not only explains why the present headrest is ineffective but also indicates to the safety engineer that the headrest needs to be much closer to the head if it is to be effective.

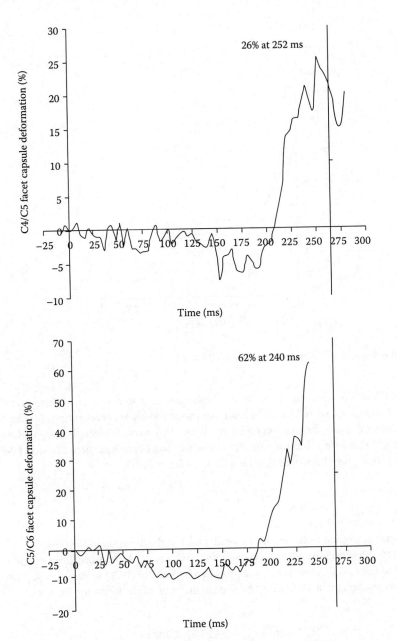

FIGURE 13.5 Estimated cervical facet capsule stretch during the simulated test described in Figure 13.4. (Reproduced from Deng, B. et al. 2000. *Stapp Car Crash J.* 44: 171–188. With permission.)

13.3 Regional Tolerance of the Head and Neck to Blunt Impact

13.3.1 Regional Tolerance of the Head

The most commonly measured parameter for head injury is acceleration. It is therefore natural to express human tolerance to injury in terms of head acceleration. The first known tolerance criterion is the Wayne State Tolerance Curve, proposed by Lissner et al. (1960) and subsequently modified by

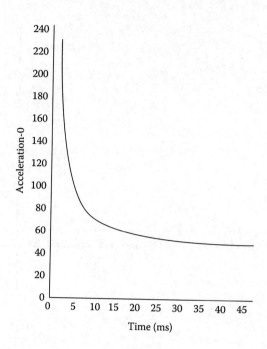

Time (ms)

FIGURE 13.6 The Wayne State Tolerance Curve for head injury.

Patrick et al. (1965) by the addition of animal and volunteer data to the original cadaveric data. The modified curve is shown in Figure 13.13. The head can withstand higher accelerations for shorter durations and any exposure above the curve is injurious. When this curve is plotted on logarithmic paper, it becomes a straight line with a slope of −2.5. This slope was used as an exponent by Gadd (1961) in his proposed severity index, now known as the *Gadd Severity Index* (GSI):

$$\text{GSI} = \int_0^T a^{2.5} \, dt \tag{13.1}$$

where a is the instantaneous acceleration of the head, and T is the duration of the pulse.

If the integrated value exceeds 1000, a severe injury will result. A modified form of the GSI, now known as the *Head Injury Criterion* (HIC), was proposed by Versace (1970) to identify the most damaging part of the acceleration pulse by finding the maximum value of the following integral:

$$\text{HIC} = (t_2 - t_1) \left[(t_2 - t_1)^{-1} \int_{t_1}^{t_2} a(t) \, dt \right]^{2.5} \Bigg|_{\text{max}} \tag{13.2}$$

where $a(t)$ is the resultant instantaneous acceleration of the head, and $t_2 - t_1$ is the time interval over which HIC is a maximum.

A severe but not life-threatening injury would have occurred if the HIC reached or exceeded 1000. Subsequently, Prasad and Mertz (1985) proposed a probabilistic method of assessing head injury and developed the curve shown in Figure 13.7. At an HIC of 1000, approximately 16% of the population would sustain a severe-to-fatal injury. It is apparent that this criterion is useful in automotive safety design and in the design of protective equipment for the head, such as football and bicycle helmets. However, there is another school of thought that believes in the injurious potential of angular acceleration in its ability to cause DAI and rupture of the parasagittal bridging veins between the brain and

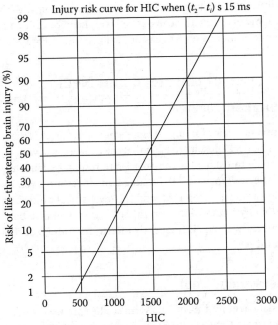

FIGURE 13.7 Head injury risk curve based on HIC.

TABLE 13.2 Tolerance Estimates for MTBI

Variable	Tolerance Estimate (Probability of Injury)		
	25%	50%	75%
HIC	136	235	333
Linear acceleration (m/s²)	559	778	965
Angular acceleration (rad/s²)	4384	5757	7130
Max. principal strain, ε (%)	25	37	49
Max. principal strain rate, $d\varepsilon/dt$ (s⁻¹)	46	60	79
$\varepsilon \cdot d\varepsilon/dt$ (s⁻¹)	14	20	25

Source: King, A.I. et al. 2003. *Bertil Aldman Lecture, Proceedings of the 2003 International IRCOBI Conference on the Biomechanics of Impact,* pp. 1–12.

dura mater. The MTBI data referred to above show that this may not be case and that a strain-related parameter should be designated as a brain injury criterion, regardless of the input. However, for the moment, HIC remains as the head injury criterion in FMVSS 208 and attempts to replace it have so far been unsuccessful.

As a matter of interest, tolerance data for MTBI, data obtained from the National Football League (NFL) data are presented in Table 13.2, taken from King et al. (2003).

13.3.2 Regional Tolerance of the Neck

Currently there are no universally accepted tolerance values for the neck for the various injury modes. This is not due to a lack of data but rather to the many injury mechanisms and several levels of injury severity, ranging from life-threatening injuries to the spinal cord to minor soft-tissue injuries that cannot be identified on radiographic or magnetic scans. It is likely that a combined criterion of axial load and bending moment about one or more axes will be adopted as a future FMVSS.

13.4 Human Surrogates of the Head and Neck

13.4.1 The Experimental Surrogate

The most effective experimental surrogate for impact biomechanics research is the unembalmed cadaver. This is also true for the head and neck, despite the fact that the cadaver is devoid of muscle tone because the duration of impact is usually too short for the muscles to respond adequately. It is true, however, that muscle pretensioning in the neck may have to be added under certain circumstances. Similarly, for the brain, the cadaveric brain cannot develop DAI, and the mechanical properties of the brain change rapidly after death. If the pathophysiology of the central nervous system is to be studied, the ideal surrogate is an animal brain. Currently, the rat is frequently used as the animal of choice and there is some work in progress using the mini-pig.

13.4.2 The Injury-Assessment Tool

The response and tolerance data acquired from cadaveric studies are used to design human-like surrogates, known as *anthropomorphic test devices* (ATD). These surrogates are required not only to have biofidelity and the ability to simulate human response but also need to provide physical measurements that are representative of human injury. In addition, they are designed to be repeatable and reproducible. The current frontal impact dummy is the Hybrid III family of dummies ranging from the 95th percentile male to the 3-year-old infant. The 50th percentile male dummy is human like in many of its responses, including that of the head and neck. The head consists of an aluminum headform covered by an appropriately designed vinyl "skin" to yield human-like acceleration responses for frontal and lateral impacts against a flat, rigid surface. Two-dimensional physical models of the brain were proposed by Margulies et al. (1990) using a silicone gel in which preinscribed grid lines would deform under angular acceleration. No injury criterion is associated with this gel model.

The dummy neck was designed to yield responses in flexion and extension that would fit within the corridors shown in Figures 13.2 and 13.3. The principal function of the dummy neck is to place the head in the approximate position of a human head in the same impact involving a human occupant.

13.4.3 Computer Models

Models of head impact first appeared over 50 years ago (Holbourn, 1943). Extensive reviews of such models were made by King and Chou (1977) and Hardy et al. (1994). The use of the finite-element method (FEM) to simulate the various components of the head appears to be the most effective and popular means of modeling brain response. A recent model by Zhang et al. (2001) is extremely detailed, with over 300,000 elements. It simulates the brain, the meninges, the cerebrospinal fluid and ventricles, the skull, scalp, and most of the facial bones and soft tissues. Validation was attempted against all available experimental data. It has been used in many applications, including the prediction of MTBI for helmeted football players described earlier. Other less detailed models include those by Kleiven and Hardy (2002), Willinger et al. (1999), and Takhounts et al. (2003).

A large number of neck and spinal models also have been developed over the past four decades. A paper by Kleinberger (1993) provides a brief and incomplete review of these models. However, the method of choice for modeling the response of the neck is the finite-element method, principally because of the complex geometry of the vertebral components and the interaction of several different materials.

A partially validated model for impact response was developed by Yang et al. (1998) to simulate both crown impact as well as the whiplash phenomenon due to a rear-end impact.

References

Adams, J.H., Doyle, D., Graham, D.I. et al. 1986. Gliding contusions in nonmissile head injury in humans. *Arch. Pathol. Lab. Med.* 110: 485.

Cheng, R., Yang, K.H., Levine, R.S. et al. 1982. Injuries to the cervical spine caused by a distributed frontal load to the chest. In *Proceedings of the 26th Stapp Car Crash Conference*, pp. 1–40.

Deng, B., Begeman, P.C., Yang, K.H. et al. 2000. Kinematics of human cadaver cervical spine during low speed rear-end impacts. *Stapp Car Crash J.* 44: 171–188.

Ewing, C.L., Thomas, D.J., Lustick, L. et al. 1978. Effect of initial position on the human head and neck response to + Y impact acceleration. In *Proceedings of the 22nd Stapp Car Crash Conference*, pp. 101–138.

Gadd, C.W. 1961. Criteria for injury potential. In *Impact Acceleration Stress Symposium, National Research Council Publication No. 977*, pp. 141–144. Washington, National Academy of Sciences.

Garfin, S.R. and Rothman, R.H. 1983. Traumatic spondylolisthesis of the axis (Hangman's fracture). In R.W. Baily (Ed.), *The Cervical Spine*, pp. 223–232. Philadelphia, PA, Lippincott.

Gennarelli, T.A. 1983. Head injuries in man and experimental animals: Clinical aspects. *Acta Neurochir. Suppl.* 32: 1.

Hardy, W.N., Foster, C.D., Mason, M.J. et al. 2001. Investigation of head injury mechanisms using neutral density technology and high-speed biplanar x-ray. *Stapp Car Crash J.* 45: 337–368.

Hardy, W.N., Khalil, T.B., and King, A.I. 1994. Literature review of head injury biomechanics. *Int. J. Impact Eng.* 15: 561–586.

Holbourn, A.H.S. 1943. Mechanics of head injury. *Lancet* 2: 438.

King, A.I. and Chou, C. 1977. Mathematical modelling, simulation and experimental testing of biomechanical system crash response. *J. Biomech.* 9: 3–10.

King, A.I., Yang, K.H., Zhang, L. et al. 2003. Is head injury caused by linear or angular acceleration? In *Bertil Aldman Lecture, Proceedings of the 2003 International IRCOBI Conference on the Biomechanics of Impact*, pp. 1–12.

Kleinberger, M. 1993. Application of finite element techniques to the study of cervical spine mechanics. In *Proceedings of the 37th Stapp Car Crash Conference*, pp. 261–272.

Kleiven, S. and Hardy, W.N. 2002. Correlation of an FE model of the human head with experiments on localized motion of the brain—Consequences for injury prediction. *Stapp Car Crash J.* 46: 123–144.

Lighthall, J.W., Goshgarian, H.G., and Pinderski, C.R. 1990. Characterization of axonal injury produced by controlled cortical impact. *J. Neurotrauma* 7(2): 65.

Lissner, H.R., Lebow, M., and Evans, F.G. 1960. Experimental studies on the relation between acceleration and intracranial pressure changes in man. *Surg. Gynecol. Obstet.* 111: 329.

Margulies, S.S., Thibault, L.E., and Gennarelli, T.A. 1990. Physical model simulation of brain injury in the primate. *J. Biomech.* 23: 823.

Mertz, H.J., Neathery, R.F., and Culver, C.C. 1973. Performance requirements and characteristics of mechanical necks. In W.F. King and H.I. Mertz (Eds.), *Human Impact Response: Measurement and Simulations*, pp. 263–288. New York, Plenum Press.

Mertz, H.J. and Patrick, L.M. 1967. Investigation of the kinematics and kinetics of whiplash. In *Proceedings of the 11th Stapp Car Crash Conference*, pp. 267–317.

Mertz, H.J. and Patrick, L.M. 1971. Strength and response of the human neck. In *Proceedings of the 15th Stapp Car Crash Conference*, pp. 207–255.

Moffat, E.A., Siegel, A.W., and Huelke, D.F. 1978. The biomechanics of automotive cervical fractures. In *Proceedings of the 22nd Conference of American Association for Automotive Medicine*, pp. 151–168.

Newman, J., Beusenberg, M., Fournier, E. et al. 1999. A new biomechanical assessment of mild traumatic brain injury—Part I: methodology. In *Proceedings of the 1999 International IRCOBI Conference on the Biomechanics of Impact*, pp. 17–36.

Nightingale, R.W., McElhaney, J.H., Best, T.M. et al. 1993. The relationship between observed head motion and cervical spine injury mechanism. In *Proceedings of the 39th Meeting of the Orthopedic Research Society*, p. 233.

Patrick, L.M. and Chou, C. 1976. Response of the human neck in flexion, extension, and lateral flexion, Vehicle Research Institute Report No. VRI-7-3. Warrendale, PA, Society of Automotive Engineers.

Patrick, L.M., Lissner, H.R., and Gurdjian, E.S. 1965. Survival by design: Head protection. In *Proceedings of the 7th Stapp Car Crash Conference*, pp. 483–499.

Pellman, E.J., Viano D.C., Tucker, A.M. et al. 2003. Concussion in professional football: Reconstruction of game impacts and injuries. *Neurosurgery*, 53: 799–814.

Pierce, D.A. and Barr, J.S. 1983. Fractures and dislocations at the base of the skull and upper spine. In R.W. Baily (Ed.), *The Cervical Spine*, pp. 196–206. Philadelphia, PA, Lippincott.

Pintar, F.A., Sances, A. Jr, Yoganandan, N. et al. 1990. Biodynamics of the total human cadaveric spine. In *Proceedings of the 34th Stapp Car Crash Conference*, pp. 55–72.

Pintar, F.A., Yoganandan, N., Sances, A. Jr et al. 1989. Kinematic and anatomical analysis of the human cervical spinal column under axial loading. In *Proceedings of the 33rd Stapp Car Crash Conference*, pp. 191–214.

Prasad, P. and Mertz, H.J. 1985. The Position of the United States Delegation to the ISO Working Group 6 on the Use of HIC in the Automotive Environment, SAE Paper No. 851246. Warrendale, PA, Society of Automotive Engineers.

Schneider, L.W., Foust, D.R., Bowman, B.M. et al. 1975. Biomechanical properties of the human neck in lateral flexion. In *Proceedings of the 19th Stapp Car Crash Conference*, pp. 455–486.

Society of Automotive Engineers, Human Mechanical Response Task Force. 1985. *Human Mechanical Response Characteristics, SAE J1460*. Warrendale, PA, Society of Automotive Engineers.

Strich, S.J. 1961. Shearing of nerve fibres as a cause of brain damage due to head injury. *Lancet* 2: 443.

Takhounts, E.G., Eppinger, R.H., Campbell, J.Q. et al. 2003. On the development of the SIMon finite element head model. *Stapp Car Crash J.* 47: 107–134.

Thomas, D.J. and Jessop, M.E. 1983. Experimental head and neck injury. In C.L. Ewing et al. (Eds.), *Impact Injury of the Head and Spine*, pp. 177–217. Springfield, IL, Charles C. Thomas.

Versace, J. 1970. A review of the severity index. In *Proceedings of the 15th Stapp Car Crash Conference*, pp. 771–796.

Viano, D.C., King, A.I., Melvin, J.W., and Weber, K. 1989. Injury biomechanics research: An essential element in the prevention of trauma. *J. Biomech.* 21: 403.

Viano, D.C. and Lövsund, P. 1999. Biomechanics of brain and spinal cord injury: Analysis of neurophysiological experiments. *Crash Prevention and Injury Control* 1: 35–43.

Wallis, B.J., Lord, S.M., and Bogduk, N. 1997. Resolution of psychological distress of whiplash patients following treatment by radiofrequency neurotomy: A randomized, double-blind, placebo controlled trial. *Pain* 73: 15–22.

Willinger, R., Kang, H.S., and Diaw, B. 1999. Three-dimensional human head finite-element model validation against two experimental impacts. *Ann. Biomed. Eng.* 27(3): 403–410.

Yang, K.H., Zhu, F., Luan, F. et al. 1998. Development of a finite element model of the human neck. In *Proceedings of the 42nd Stapp Car Crash Conference*, pp. 195–205.

Zhang, L., Yang, K.H., Dwarampudi, R. et al. 2001. Recent advances in brain injury research: A new human head model, development and validation. *Stapp Car Crash J.* 45: 369–394.

14

Biomechanics of Chest and Abdomen Impact

David C. Viano
Wayne State University

Albert I. King
Wayne State University

14.1 Introduction 14-1
14.2 Chest and Abdomen Injury Mechanics 14-1
14.3 Injury Criteria and Tolerances... 14-2
　　　Acceleration Injury • Force Injury • Compression Injury • Viscous Injury
14.4 Biomechanical Responses during Impact............................. 14-6
14.5 Injury Risk Assessment.. 14-8
References... 14-11

14.1 Introduction

Injury is caused by energy transfer to the body by an impacting object. It occurs when sufficient force is concentrated on the chest or abdomen by striking a blunt object, such as a vehicle instrument panel or side interior, or being struck by a baseball or blunt ballistic mass. The risk of injury is influenced by the object's shape, stiffness, point of contact, and orientation. It can be reduced by energy-absorbing padding or crushable materials, which allow the surfaces in contact to deform, extend the duration of impact, and reduce loads. The torso is viscoelastic, so reaction force increases with the speed of body deformation.

The biomechanical response of the body has three components, (1) inertial resistance by acceleration of body masses, (2) elastic resistance by compression of stiff structures and tissues, and (3) viscous resistance by rate-dependent properties of tissue. For low-impact speeds, the elastic stiffness protects from crush injuries; whereas, for high rates of body deformation, the inertial and viscous properties determine the force developed and limit deformation. The risk of skeletal and internal organ injury relates to energy stored or absorbed by the elastic and viscous properties. The reaction load is related to these responses and inertial resistance of body masses, which combine to resist deformation and prevent injury. When tissues are deformed beyond their recoverable limit, injuries occur.

14.2 Chest and Abdomen Injury Mechanisms

The primary mechanism of chest and abdomen injury is compression of the body at high rates of loading. This causes deformation and stretching of internal organs and vessels. When torso compression exceeds the rib-cage tolerance, fractures occur and internal organs and vessels can be contused or ruptured. In some chest impacts, internal injury occurs without skeletal damage. This can happen during high-speed loading, such as with a baseball impact causing ventricular fibrillation in a child without rib fractures. Injury is due to the viscous or rate-sensitive nature of human tissue as biomechanical responses differ for low- and high-speed impact.

When organs or vessels are loaded slowly, the input energy is absorbed gradually through deformation, which is resisted by elastic properties and pressure buildup in tissue. This is the situation when the shoulder belt loads the upper body in a frontal crash. When loaded rapidly, reaction force is proportional to the speed of tissue deformation as the viscous properties of the body resist deformation and provide a natural protection from impact. However, there is also a considerable inertial component to the reaction force. In this case, the body develops high internal pressure and injuries can occur before the ribs deflect much. The ability of an organ or other biological system to absorb impact energy without failure is called tolerance.

If an artery is stretched beyond its tensile strength, the tissue will tear. Organs and vessels can be stretched in different ways, which result in different types of injury. Motion of the heart during chest compression stretches the aorta along its axis from points of tethering in the body. This elongation generally leads to a transverse laceration when the strain limit is exceeded. In contrast, an increase in vascular pressure dilates the vessel and produces biaxial strain, which is larger in the transverse than axial direction. If pressure rises beyond the vessel's limit, it will burst. For severe impacts, intra-aortic pressure exceeds 500–1000 mm Hg, which is a significant, nonphysiological level, but is tolerable for short durations. When laceration occurs, the predominant mode of aortic failure is axial so the combined effects of stretch and internal pressure contribute to injury. Chest impact also compresses the rib cage causing tensile strain on the outer surface of the ribs. As compression increases, the risk of rib fracture increases. In both cases, the mechanism of injury is tissue deformation. Shah et al. (2001) found right-side impacts caused a higher risk of aortic injury than other impact directions.

The abdomen is more vulnerable to injury than the chest, because there is little bony structure below the ribcage to protect internal organs in front and lateral impact. Blunt impact of the upper abdomen can compress and injure the liver and spleen, before significant whole-body motion occurs. In the liver, compression increases intrahepatic pressure and generates tensile or shear strains. If the tissue is sufficiently deformed, laceration of the major hepatic vessels can result in hemoperitoneum. The injury tolerance of the solid organs in the abdomen is rate sensitive. Abdominal deformation also causes lobes of the liver to move relative to each other, stretching and shearing the vascular attachment at the hilar region.

Effective occupant restraints, safety systems, and protective equipment not only spread impact energy over the strongest body structures but also reduce contact velocity between the body and the impacted surface or striking object. The design of protective systems is aided by an understanding of injury mechanisms, quantification of human tolerance levels and development of numerical relationships between measurable engineering parameter, such as force, acceleration or deformation, and human injury. These relationships are called injury criteria.

14.3 Injury Criteria and Tolerances

14.3.1 Acceleration Injury

Stapp (1970) conducted rocket-sled experiments in the 1940s on belt-restraint systems and achieved a substantial human tolerance to long-duration, whole-body acceleration. Safety belts protected military personnel exposed to rapid but sustained acceleration. The experiments enabled Eiband (1959) to show in Figure 14.1 that the tolerance to whole-body acceleration increased as the exposure duration decreased. This linked human tolerance and acceleration for exposures of 2–1000 ms duration. The tolerance data are based on average sled acceleration rather than the acceleration of the volunteer subject, which would be higher due to compliance of the restraint system. Even with this limitation, the data provide useful early guidelines for the development of military and civilian restraint systems.

More recent side impact tests have led to other tolerance formulas for chest injury. Morgan et al. (1986) evaluated rigid, side-wall cadaver tests and developed TTI, a thoracic trauma index, which is the average rib and spine acceleration. TTI limits human tolerance to 85–90 g in vehicle crash tests. Better

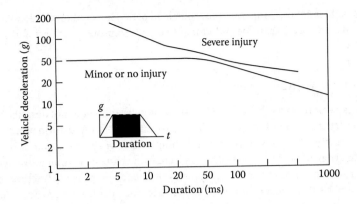

FIGURE 14.1 Whole-body human tolerance to vehicle acceleration based on impact duration. (Redrawn from Eiband A.M. Human tolerance to rapidly applied acceleration. A survey of the literature. National Aeronautics and Space Administration, Washington, DC, NASA Memo No. 5-19-59E, 1959; Viano D.C., *Bull. NY Acad. Med.*, 2nd Series, 64: 376–421, 1988. With permission.)

injury assessment was achieved by Cavanaugh et al. (1993) using average spinal acceleration (ASA), which is the average slope of the integral of spinal acceleration. ASA is the rate of momentum transfer during side impact, and a value of 30 g is proposed. In most cases, the torso can withstand 60–80 g peak, whole-body acceleration by a well-distributed load.

14.3.2 Force Injury

Whole-body tolerance is related to Newton's second law of motion, where acceleration of a rigid mass is proportional to the force acting on it, or $F = ma$. While the human body is not a rigid mass, a well-distributed restraint system allows the torso to respond as though it were fairly rigid when load is applied through the shoulder and pelvis. The greater the acceleration, the greater the force and risk of injury. For a high-speed frontal crash, a restrained occupant can experience 60 g acceleration. For a body mass of 76 kg, the inertial load is 44.7 kN (10,000 lb) and is tolerable if distributed over strong skeletal elements for a short period of time.

The ability to withstand high acceleration for short durations implies that tolerance is related to momentum transfer, because an equivalent change in velocity can be achieved by increasing the acceleration and decreasing its duration, as $\Delta V = a\Delta t$. The implication for occupant-protection systems is that the risk of injury can be decreased if the crash deceleration is extended over a greater period of time. For occupant restraint in 25 ms, a velocity change of 14.7 m/s (32.7 mph) occurs with 60 g whole-body acceleration. This duration can be achieved by crushable vehicle structures and occupant restraints (Mertz and Gadd, 1971).

Prior to the widespread use of safety belts, safety engineers needed information on the tolerance of the chest to design energy-absorbing instrument panels and steering systems. The concept was to limit impact force below human tolerance by crushable materials and structures. Using the highest practical crush force, safety was extended to the greatest severity of vehicle crashes. GM Research and Wayne State University collaborated on the development of the first crash sled, which was used to simulate progressively more severe frontal impacts. Embalmed human cadavers were exposed to head, chest, and knee impact on 15 cm (6″) diameter load cells until bone fracture was observed on x-ray. Patrick et al. (1965, 1967) demonstrated that blunt chest loading of 3.3 kN (740 lb) could be tolerated with minimal risk of serious injury. This is a pressure of 187 kPa. Gadd and Patrick (1968) later found a tolerance of 8.0 kN (1800 lb) if the load was distributed over the shoulders and chest by a properly designed steering wheel and column. Cavanaugh et al. (1993) found that side-impact tolerance is similar to frontal tolerance, and that shoulder contact is also an important load path. However, for the abdomen, side padding needs to crush at lower force than the abdominal tolerance to protect the liver and spleen (Viano and Andrzejak, 1993).

14.3.3 Compression Injury

High-speed films of cadaver impacts show that whole-body acceleration does not describe torso impact biomechanics. Tolerance of the chest and abdomen must consider body deformation. Force acting on the body causes two simultaneous responses, (1) compression of the compliant structures of the torso, and (2) acceleration of body masses. The neglected mechanism of injury was compression, which causes the sternum to displace toward the spine as ribs bend and possibly fracture. Acceleration and force, *per se*, are not sufficient indicators of impact tolerance because they cannot discriminate between the two responses. Numerous studies have shown that acceleration is less related to injury than compression.

The importance of chest deformation was confirmed by Kroell et al. (1971, 1974) in blunt thoracic impacts of unembalmed cadavers. Peak spinal acceleration and impact force were poorer injury predictors than the maximum compression of the chest, as measured by the percent change in the anteroposterior thickness of the body. A relationship was found between injury risk and compression and that it involves energy stored by elastic deformation of the body for moderate rates of chest compression. The stored energy (E_s) by a spring representing the ribcage and soft tissues is related to the displacement integral of force: $E_s = \int F dx$. Force in a spring is proportional to deformation: $F = kx$, where k is a spring constant representing the stiffness of the chest and is in the range of 26 kN/m. Stored energy is $E_s = k \int x dx = 0.5\ kx^2$. Over a compression range of 20–40%, stored energy is proportional to deformation or compression, so $E_s \approx C$.

Tests with human volunteers showed that compression up to 20% during moderate-duration loading was fully reversible. Cadaver impacts with compression greater than 20% showed (Figure 14.2a) an increase in rib fractures and internal organ injury as the compression increased to 40%. The deflection tolerance was originally set at 8.8 cm (3.5″) for moderate but recoverable injury. This represents 39% compression. However, at this level of compression, multiple rib fractures and serious injury can occur, so a more conservative tolerance of 32% has been used to avert the possibility of flail chest (Figure 14.2b).

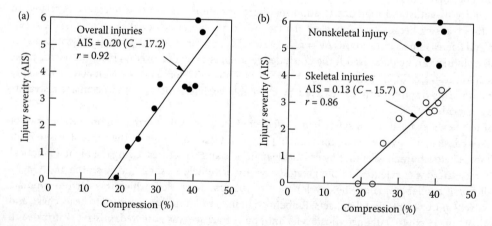

FIGURE 14.2 (a) Injury severity from blunt impact of human cadavers as a function of the maximum chest compression. (From Viano, D.C., *Bull. NY Acad. Med.*, 2nd Series, 64: 376–421, 1988. With permission.) (b) Severity of skeletal injury and incidence of internal organ injury as a function of maximum chest compression for blunt impacts of human cadavers. (From Viano D.C., *Bull. NY Acad. Med.*, 2nd Series, 64: 376–421, 1988. With permission.)

This reduces the risk of direct loading on the heart, lungs, and internal organs by a loss of the protective function of the ribcage.

14.3.4 Viscous Injury

The velocity of body deformation is an important factor in impact injury. For example, when a fluid-filled organ is compressed slowly, energy can be absorbed by tissue deformation without damage. When loaded rapidly, the organ cannot deform fast enough and rupture may occur without significant change in shape, even though the load is substantially higher than for the slow-loading condition. This situation depends on the viscous and inertial characteristics of the tissues.

The viscoelastic behavior of soft tissues becomes progressively more important as the velocity of body deformation exceeds 3 m/s. For lower speeds, such as in slow-crushing loads or for a belt-restrained occupant in a frontal crash, tissue compression is limited by elastic properties resisting skeletal and internal organ injury. For higher speeds of deformation, such as occupant loading by the door in a side impact, an unrestrained occupant or pedestrian impact, or chest impact by a nonpenetrating bullet, maximum compression does not adequately address the viscous and inertial properties of the torso, nor the time of greatest injury risk. In these conditions, the tolerance to compression is progressively lower as the speed of deformation increases, and the velocity of deformation becomes a dominant factor in injury.

Insight on a rate-dependent injury mechanism came from over 20 years of research by Jonsson et al. (1979) on high-speed impact and blast-wave exposures. The studies confirmed that tolerable compression inversely varied with the velocity of impact. The concept was further studied in relation to the abdomen by Lau and Viano (1981) for frontal impacts in the range of 5–20 m/s (10–45 mph). The liver was the target organ. Using a maximum compression of 16%, the severity of injury increased with the speed of loading, including serious mutilation of the lobes and major vessels in the highest-speed impacts. While the compression was within limits of volunteer loading at low speeds, the exposure produced critical injury at higher speeds. Subsequent tests on other animals and target organs verified an interrelationship between body compression, deformation velocity, and injury.

The previous observations led Viano and Lau (1988) to propose a viscous injury mechanism for soft biological tissues. The viscous response (*VC*) is defined as the product of velocity of deformation (*V*) and compression (*C*), which is a time-varying function in an impact. The parameter has physical meaning to absorbed energy (E_a) by a viscous dashpot under impact loading. Absorbed energy is related to the displacement integral of force: $E_a = \int F dx$, and force in a dashpot representing the viscous characteristics of the body is proportional to the velocity of deformation: $F = cV$, where *c* is a dashpot parameter in the range of 0.5 kN/m/s for the chest. Absorbed energy is $E_a = c \int V dx$, or a time integral by substitution: $E_a = c \int V^2 dt$. The integrand is composed of two responses, so: $E_a = c(\int d(Vx) - \int ax \, dt)$, where *a* is acceleration across the dashpot. The first term is the viscous response and the second an inertial term related to the deceleration of fluid set in motion. Absorbed energy is given by: $E_a = c(Vx - \int ax \, dt)$. The viscous response is proportional to absorbed energy, or $E_a \approx VC$, during the rapid phase of impact loading prior to peak compression.

Subsequent tests by Lau and Viano (1986, 1988) verified that serious injury occurred at the time of peak *VC*, much earlier than peak compression. For blunt chest impact, peak *VC* occurs in about half the time for maximum compression. Rib fractures also occur progressively with chest compression, as early as 9–14 ms—at peak *VC*—in a cadaver impact requiring 30 ms to reach peak compression. Upper-abdominal injury by steering wheel contact also relates to viscous loading. Lau et al. (1987) showed that limiting the viscous response by a self-aligning steering wheel reduced the risk of liver injury, as does force limiting an armrest in side impacts. Animal tests have also shown that *VC* is a good predictor of functional injury to heart and respiratory systems. In these experiments, Stein et al. (1982) found that the severity of cardiac arrhythmia and traumatic apnea was related to *VC*. This situation is important to baseball impact protection of children, Viano et al. (1992), and in the definition of human biomechanical responses used in the assessment of bullet-proof protective vests and blunt ballistics (Bir et al., 2004).

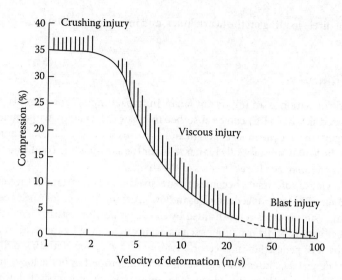

FIGURE 14.3 Biomechanics of chest injury by a crushing injury mechanism limited by tolerable compression at $C_{max} = 35\%$, a viscous injury mechanism limited by the product of velocity and extent of deformation at $VC_{max} = 1.0$ m/s, and a blast injury mechanism for shock wave loading.

With the increasing use of bullet-proof vests and nonpenetrating munitions by the police and military, blunt, high-velocity impacts are occurring to the chest. Although rarely lethal, there has been a concern for improving the understanding of injury mechanisms and means to establish standards for the technology. Behind-body-armor standards use the depth of the cavity created in clay after a bullet is stopped by the vest. The roots of this approach involve military research. However, the clay may not adequately simulate the human viscoelastic properties and biomechanical responses. Recent research has defined the blunt ballistic characteristics of the chest and the mechanisms for ventricular fibrillation (Bir and Viano, 1999; Bir et al., 2004).

Sturdivan et al. (2004) developed the blunt criterion (BC) in the 1970s. It is energy based and assesses vulnerability to blunt weapons, projectile impacts, and behind-body-armor exposures. $BC = \ln[E/(W^{0.33}TD)]$, where $E = 1\,2\,MV^2$ is the kinetic energy of the projectile at impact in Joules, M is the projectile mass in kg, V is projectile velocity in m/s, D is the projectile diameter in cm, W is the mass of the individual in kg, and T is body-wall thickness in cm. BC is an energy ratio. The numerator is the striking kinetic energy of the blunt projectile, the energy available to cause injury. The denominator is a semiempirical expression of the capacity of the body to absorb the impact energy without lethal damage to the vulnerable organs, scaled by the mass of the individual. The viscous and blunt criteria are both energy-based and have been correlated for chest and abdominal impacts.

Figure 14.3 summarizes injury mechanisms associated with torso impact deformation. For low speeds of deformation, the limiting factor is crush injury from compression of the body (C). This occurs at $C = 35–40\%$ depending on the contact area and orientation of loading. For deformation speeds above 3 m/s, injury is related to a peak viscous response of $VC = 1.0$ m/s. In a particular situation, injury can occur by a compression or viscous responses, or both, as these responses occur at different times in an impact. At extreme rates of loading, such as in a blast-wave exposure, injury occurs with less than 10–15% compression by high-energy transfer to viscous elements of the body.

14.4 Biomechanical Responses during Impact

The reaction force developed by the chest varies with the velocity of deformation, and biomechanics is best characterized by a family of force–deflection responses. Figure 14.4 summarizes frontal and lateral

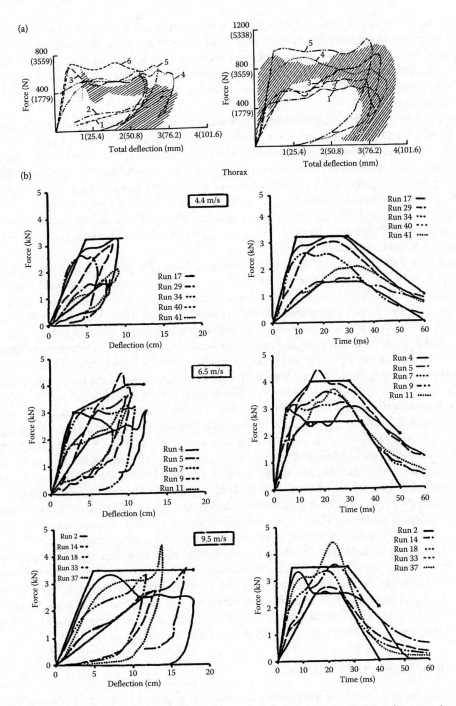

FIGURE 14.4 Frontal (a) and lateral (b) force–deflection response of the human cadaver chest at various speeds of blunt pendulum impact. The initial stiffness is followed by a plateau force until unloading. (From Kroell et al., *Proceedings of the 18th Stapp Car Crash Conference*, pp. 383–457, SAE Paper No. 741187, Society of Automotive Engineers, Warrendale, PA, 1974; Viano, D.C., *Proceedings of the 33rd Stapp Car Crash Conference*, pp. 113–142, SAE Paper No. 892432, Society of Automotive Engineers, Warrendale, PA, 1989; with kind permission from Springer Science+Business Media: *Accidental Injury: Biomechanics and Prevention*, The biomechanics of thoracic trauma, 1993, pp. 362–391, Cavanaugh, J.M.)

chest biomechanics for various impact speeds. The dynamic compliance is related to viscous, inertial, and elastic properties of the body. The initial rise in force is due to inertia as the sternal mass, which is rapidly accelerated to the impact speed as the chest begins to deform. The plateau force is related to the viscous component, which is rate-dependent, and a superimposed elastic stiffness, which increases force with chest compression. Unloading provides a hysteresis loop representing the energy absorbed by body deformation.

Melvin et al. (1988) analyzed frontal biomechanics of the chest. The dynamic compliance is related to viscous, inertial, and elastic properties of the body. There is an initial rise in force, which is related to the inertia of the sternal mass, which is rapidly accelerated to the impact speed. This is followed by a plateau in force, which is related to the viscous properties and is rate dependent. There is also an elastic stiffness component from chest compression that adds to the force. The force–deflection response can be modeled as an initial stiffness $k = 0.26 + 0.60(V − 1.3)$ and a plateau force $F = 1.0 + 0.75(V − 3.7)$, where k is in kN/cm, F is in kN, and the velocity of impact V is in m/s. The force F reasonably approximates the plateau level for lateral chest and abdominal impact, but the initial stiffness is lower at $F = 0.12(V − 1.2)$ for side loading (Melvin and Weber, 1988).

The reaction force developed by the chest varies with the velocity of impact, so biomechanics is best characterized by the force–deflection response of the torso (25.6). The dynamic compliance is related to viscous, inertial, and elastic properties of the body. There is an initial rise in force, which is related to inertial responses as the sternal mass is rapidly accelerated to the impact speed. This is followed by a plateau in force, which is related to the viscous response and is rate dependent, and a superimposed stiffness component related to chest compression. By analyzing frontal biomechanics, the chest response can be modeled as an initial stiffness $k = 0.26 + 0.60(V − 1.3)$ and a plateau force $F = 1.0 + 0.75(V − 3.7)$, where k is in kN/cm, F is in kN, and the velocity of impact V is in m/s. The force F reasonably approximates the plateau level for lateral chest and abdominal impact, but the initial stiffness is lower at $F = 0.12(V − 1.2)$ for side loading.

A simple, but relevant, lumped-mass model of the chest was developed by Lobdell et al. (1973) and is shown in Figure 14.5. The impacting mass is m_1 and skin compliance is represented by k_{12}. An energy-absorbing interface was added by Viano (1987) to evaluate protective padding. Chest structure is represented by a parallel Voigt and Maxwell spring–dashpot system, which couples the sternal m_2 and spinal m_3 masses. When subjected to a blunt sternal impact, the model follows established force–deflection corridors. The biomechanical model is effective in studying compression and viscous responses. It also simulates military exposures to high-speed, nonpenetrating projectiles (Figure 14.6), even though the loading conditions are quite different from the cadaver database used to develop the model. This mechanical system characterizes the elastic, viscous, and inertial components of the torso.

The Hybrid III dummy was the first to demonstrate humanlike chest responses typical of the biomechanical data for frontal impacts (Foster et al., 1977). Rouhana (1989) developed a frangible abdomen, useful in predicting injury for lap-belt submarining. More recent work by Schneider et al. (1992) led to a new prototype frontal dummy. Lateral impact tests of cadavers against a rigid wall and blunt pendulum led to side-impact dummies, such as the Eurosid and Biosid (Mertz, 1993). Even more recently, a small female-sized side-impact dummy has been developed (Scherer et al., 1998).

14.5 Injury Risk Assessment

Over years of study, tolerances have been established for most responses of the chest and abdomen. Table 14.1 provides tolerance levels from reviews by Cavanaugh (1993), Rouhana (1993), and Viano et al. (1989). While these are single thresholds, they are commonly used to evaluate safety systems. The implication is that for biomechanical responses below tolerance, there is no injury, and for responses above tolerance, there is injury. An additional factor is biomechanical response scaling for individuals of different size and weight. The commonly accepted procedure involves equal stress and velocity, which enabled Mertz et al. (1989) to predict injury tolerances and biomechanical responses for different size adult dummies.

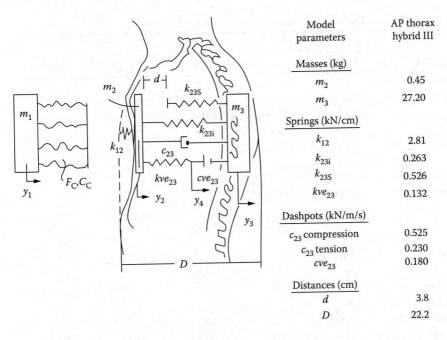

Model parameters	AP thorax hybrid III
Masses (kg)	
m_2	0.45
m_3	27.20
Springs (kN/cm)	
k_{12}	2.81
k_{23i}	0.263
k_{23S}	0.526
kve_{23}	0.132
Dashpots (kN/m/s)	
c_{23} compression	0.525
c_{23} tension	0.230
cve_{23}	0.180
Distances (cm)	
d	3.8
D	22.2

FIGURE 14.5 Lumped-mass model of the human thorax with impacting mass and energy-absorbing material interface. The biomechanical parameters are given for mass, spring, and damping characteristics of the chest in blunt frontal impact. (Modified from Lobdell T.E. et al., In *Human Impact Response Measurement and Simulation*, Plenum Press, New York, pp. 201–245, 1973; Viano, D.C., *Proceedings of the 31st Stapp Car Crash Conference*, pp. 185–224, SAE Paper No. 872213, Society of Automotive Engineers, Warrendale, PA, 1987. With permission.)

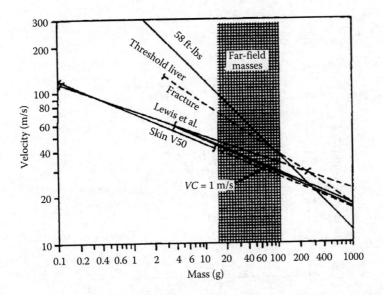

FIGURE 14.6 Tolerance levels for blunt loading as a function of impact mass and velocity. The plot includes information from automotive impact situations and from high-speed military projectile impacts. The Lobdell model is effective over the entire range of impact conditions. (Modified from Quatros J.H., *Proceedings of the 14th International Symposium on Ballistics*, Quebec, Canada, September 26–29, 1993. With permission.)

TABLE 14.1 Human Tolerance for Chest and Abdomen Impact

Criteria	Chest		Abdomen		Criteria
	Frontal	Lateral	Frontal	Lateral	
Acceleration					*Acceleration*
3 ms limit	60 g				
TTI		85–90 g			
ASA		30 g			
AIS 4+		45 g		39 g	AIS 4+
Force					*Force*
Sternum	3.3 kN				
Chest + shoulder	8.8 kN	10.2 kN			
AIS 3+			2.9 kN	3.1 kN	AIS 3+
AIS 4+		5.5 kN	3.8 kN	6.7 kN	AIS 4+
Pressure					*Pressure*
	187 kPa		166 kPa		AIS 3+
			216 kPa		AIS 4+
Compression					*Compression*
Rib fracture	20%				
Stable ribcage	32%		38%		AIS 3+
Flail chest	40%	38%	48%	44%	AIS 4+
Viscous					*Viscous*
AIS 3+	1.0 m/s				AIS 3+
AIS 4+	1.3 m/s	1.47 m/s	1.4 m/s	1.98 m/s	AIS 4+

Source: With kind permission from Springer Science+Business Media: *Accidental Injury: Biomechanics and Prevention*, The biomechanics of thoracic trauma, 1993, pp. 362–391, Cavanaugh, J.M.; *Accidental Injury: Biomechanics and Prevention*, Biomechanics of abdominal trauma, 1993, pp. 391–428, Rouhana, S.W.

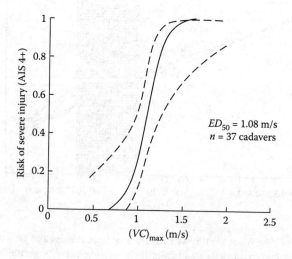

FIGURE 14.7 Typical logist injury probability function relating the risk of serious injury to the viscous response of the chest. (From Viano D.C., *Bull. NY Acad. Med.*, 2nd Series, 64: 376–421, 1988. With permission.)

TABLE 14.2 Injury Probability Functions for Blunt Impact

Body Region	$ED_{25\%}$	α	β	X^2	p	R
		Frontal Impact				
Chest (AIS 4+)						
VC	1.0 m/s	11.42	11.56	25.6	0.000	0.68
C	34%	10.49	0.277	15.9	0.000	0.52
		Lateral Impact				
Chest (AIS 4+)						
VC	1.5 m/s	10.02	6.08	13.7	0.000	0.77
C	38%	31.22	0.79	13.5	0.000	0.76
Abdomen (AIS 4+)						
VC	2.0 m/s	8.64	3.81	6.1	0.013	0.60
C	47%	16.29	0.35	4.6	0.032	0.48
Pelvis (pubic ramus facture)						
C	27%	84.02	3.07	11.5	0.001	0.91

Source: Modified from Viano, D.C. et al., *J. Biomech.*, 22: 403–417, 1989.

Injury risk assessment is frequently used. It evaluates the probability of injury as a continuous function of a biomechanical response. A logist function relates injury probability p to a biomechanical response x by $p(x) = [1 + \exp(\alpha - \beta x)]^{-1}$ where α and β are parameters derived from statistical analysis of biomechanical data. This function provides a sigmoidal relationship with three distinct regions in Figure 14.7. For low biomechanical response levels, there is a low probability of injury. Similarly, for very high levels, the risk asymptotes to 100%. The transition region between the two extremes involves risk, which is proportional to the biomechanical response. A sigmoidal function is typical of human tolerance because it represents the distribution in weak through strong subjects in a population exposed to impact. Table 14.2 summarizes available parameters for chest and abdominal injury risk assessment.

References

Bir, C. and Viano, D.C., Biomechanics of commotio cordis. *J. Trauma*, 47(3): 468–473, 1999.

Bir, C., Viano, D.C., and King, A.I., Human response of the thorax to blunt ballistic impacts. *J. Biomech.*, 37(1): 73–79, 2004.

Cavanaugh, J.M., The biomechanics of thoracic trauma, In *Accidental Injury: Biomechanics and Prevention*, Nahum A.M. and Melvin J.W. (Eds.), pp. 362–391, Springer-Verlag, New York, 1993.

Cavanaugh, J.M. et al., Injury and response of the thorax in side impact cadaveric tests, *Proceedings of the 37th Stapp Car Crash Conference*, pp. 199–222, SAE Paper No. 933127, Society of Automotive Engineers, Warrendale, PA, 1993.

Eiband, A.M., Human Tolerance to Rapidly Applied Acceleration. A Survey of the Literature. National Aeronautics and Space Administration, Washington DC, NASA Memo No. 5-19-59E, 1959.

Foster, J.K., Kortge, J.O., and Wolanin, M.J., Hybrid III—A biomechanically-based crash test dummy, *Stapp Car Crash Conference*, pp. 975–1014, SAE Paper No. 770938, Society of Automotive Engineers, Warrendale, PA, 1977.

Gadd, C.W. and Patrick, L.M., Systems versus laboratory impact tests for estimating injury hazards, SAE Paper No. 680053, Society of Automotive Engineers, Warrendale, PA, 1968.

Jonsson, A., Clemedson, C.J. et al., Dynamic factors influencing the production of lung injury in rabbits subjected to blunt chest wall impact, *Aviation, Space Environ. Med.*, 50: 325–337, 1979.

King, A.I., Regional tolerance to impact acceleration, In SP-622, SAE 850852, Society of Automotive Engineers, Warrendale, PA, 1985.

Kroell, C.K., Schneider, D.C., and Nahum, A.M., Impact tolerance and response to the human thorax, *Proceedings of the 15th Stapp Car Crash Conference*, pp. 84–134, SAE Paper No. 710851, Society of Automotive Engineers, Warrendale, PA, 1971.

Kroell, C.K., Schneider, D.C., and Nahum, A.M., Impact tolerance and response to the human thorax II, *Proceedings of the 18th Stapp Car Crash Conference*, pp. 383–457, SAE Paper No. 741187, Society of Automotive Engineers, Warrendale, PA, 1974.

Lau, I.V., Horsch, J.D. et al., Biomechanics of liver injury by steering wheel loading, *J. Trauma*, 27: 225–237, 1987.

Lau, I.V. and Viano, D.C., How and when blunt injury occurs: Implications to frontal and side impact protection. *Proceedings of the 32nd Stapp Car Crash Conference*, pp. 81–100, SAE Paper No. 881714, Society of Automotive Engineers, Warrendale, PA, 1988.

Lau, I.V. and Viano, D.C., Influence of impact velocity on the severity of nonpenetrating hepatic injury, *J. Trauma*, 21(2): 115–123, 1981.

Lau, I.V. and Viano, D.C., The viscous criterion—Bases and application of an injury severity index for soft tissue, *Proceedings of the 30th Stapp Car Crash Conference*, pp. 123–142, SAE Paper No. 861882, Society of Automotive Engineers, Warrendale, PA, 1986.

Lobdell, T.E., Kroell, C.K., Schneider, D.C., Hering, W.E., and Nahum, A.M., Impact response of the human thorax, In *Human Impact Response Measurement and Simulation*, King W.F. and Mertz H.J. (Eds.), Plenum Press, New York, pp. 201–245, 1973.

Melvin, J.W., King, A.I., and Alem, N.M., AATD system technical characteristics, design concepts, and trauma assessment criteria, AATD task E-F Final Report, DOT-HS-807-224, US Department of Transportation, National Highway Traffic Safety Administration, Washington, DC, 1988.

Melvin, J.W. and Weber, K. (Eds.), Review of biomechanical response and injury in the automotive environment, AATD Task B Final Report, DOT-HS-807-224, US Department of Transportation, National Highway Traffic Safety Administration, Washington, DC, 1988.

Mertz, H.J., Anthropomorphic test devices, In *Accidental Injury: Biomechanics and Prevention*, Nahum, A.M. and Melvin, J.W. (Eds.), pp. 66–84, Springer-Verlag, New York, 1993.

Mertz, H.J. and Gadd, C.W., Thoracic tolerance to whole-body deceleration, *Proceedings of the 15th Stapp Car Crash Conference*, pp. 135–157, SAE Paper No. 710852, Society of Automotive Engineers, Warrendale, PA, 1971.

Mertz, H.J., Irwin, A. et al., Size, weight and biomechanical impact response requirements for adult size small female and large male dummies, SAE Paper No. 890756, Society of Automotive Engineers, Warrendale, PA, 1989.

Morgan, R.M., Marcus, J.H., and Eppinger, R.H., Side impact—The biofidelity of NHTSA's proposed ATD and efficacy of TTI, *Proceedings of the 30th Stapp Car Crash Conference*, pp. 27–40, SAE Paper No. 861877, Society of Automotive Engineers, Warrendale, PA, 1986.

Patrick, L.M., Kroell, C.K., and Mertz, H.J., Forces on the human body in simulated crashes, *Proceedings of the 9th Stapp Car Crash Conference*, SAE, pp. 237–260, Society of Automotive Engineers, Warrendale, PA, 1965.

Patrick, L.M., Mertz, H.J., and Kroell, C.K., Cadaver knee, chest, and head impact loads, *Proceedings of the 11th Stapp Car Crash Conference*, pp. 168–182, SAE Paper No. 670913, Society of Automotive Engineers, Warrendale, PA, 1967.

Quatros, J.H., Terminal ballistics of non-lethal projectiles, *Proceedings of the 14th International Symposium on Ballistics*, Quebec, Canada, September 26–29, 1993.

Rouhana, S.W., Biomechanics of abdominal trauma, In *Accidental Injury: Biomechanics and Prevention*, Nahum A.M. and Melvin J.W. (Eds.), pp. 391–428, Springer-Verlag, New York, 1993.

Rouhana, S.W. et al., Assessing submarining and abdominal injury risk in the Hybrid III family of dummies, *Proceedings of the 33rd Stapp Car Crash Conference*, pp. 257–279, SAE Paper No. 892440, Society of Automotive Engineers, Warrendale, PA, 1989.

Scherer, R.D., Kirkish, S.L., McCleary, J.P., Rouhana, S.W. et al., SIDS-IIs Beta\u+- prototype dummy biomechanical responses. SAE 983151, *Proceedings of the 42nd Stapp Car Crash Conference*, Society of Automotive Engineers, Warrendale, PA, 1998.

Schneider, L.W., Haffner, M.P. et al., Development of an advanced ATD thorax for improved injury assessment in frontal crash environments, *Proceedings of the 36th Stapp Car Crash Conference*, pp. 129–156, SAE Paper No. 922520, Society of Automotive Engineers, Warrendale, PA, 1992.

Shah, C.S., Yang, K.H., Hardy, W.N., Wang, H.K., and King, A.I., Development of a computer model to predict aortic rupture due to impact loading. SAE 2001-22-0007, Society of Automotive Engineers, Warrendale, PA, *Stapp Car Crash J.*, 45: 161–182, 2001.

Society of Automotive Engineers, *Human Tolerance to Impact Conditions as Related to Motor Vehicle Design*, SAE J885, Society of Automotive Engineers, Warrendale, PA, 1986.

Stapp, J.P., Voluntary human tolerance levels, In *Impact Injury and Crash Protection*, Gurdjian, E.S., Lange, W.A., Patrick, L.M., and Thomas, L.M. (Eds.), pp. 308–349, Charles C. Thomas, Springfield, IL, 1970.

Stein, P.D., Sabbah, H.N. et al., Response of the heart to nonpenetrating cardiac trauma. *J. Trauma*, 22(5): 364–373, 1982.

Sturdivan, L.M., Viano, D.C., and Champion, H., Analysis of injury criteria to assess chest and abdominal injury risks in blunt and ballistic impacts. *J. Trauma*, 56: 651–663, 2004.

Viano, D.C., Biomechanical responses and injuries in blunt lateral impact, *Proceedings of the 33rd Stapp Car Crash Conference*, pp. 113–142, SAE Paper No. 892432, Society of Automotive Engineers, Warrendale, PA, 1989.

Viano, D.C., Cause and control of automotive trauma, *Bull. NY Acad. Med.*, 2nd Series, 64: 376–421, 1988.

Viano, D.C., Evaluation of the benefit of energy-absorbing materials for side impact protection, *Proceedings of the 31st Stapp Car Crash Conference*, pp. 185–224, SAE Paper No. 872213, Society of Automotive Engineers, Warrendale, PA, 1987.

Viano, D.C. and Andrzejak, D.V., Biomechanics of abdominal injury by armrest loading. *J. Trauma*, 34(1): 105–115, 1993.

Viano, D.C., Andrzejak, D.V., Polley, T.Z., and King, A.I., Mechanism of fatal chest injury by baseball impact: Development of an experimental model, *Clin. J. Sport Med.*, 2: 166–171, 1992.

Viano, D.C., King, A.I. et al., Injury biomechanics research: An essential element in the prevention of trauma, *J. Biomech.*, 22: 403–417, 1989.

Viano, D.C. and Lau, I.V., A viscous tolerance criterion for soft tissue injury assessment, *J. Biomech.*, 21: 387–399, 1988.

15

Cardiac Biomechanics

15.1 Introduction 15-1
15.2 Cardiac Geometry and Structure.. 15-1
    Ventricular Geometry • Myofiber Architecture • Extracellular
    Matrix Organization
15.3 Cardiac Pump Function 15-9
    Ventricular Hemodynamics • Ventricular Pressure–Volume
    Relations and Energetics
15.4 Myocardial Material Properties 15-13
    Muscle Contractile Properties • Resting Myocardial Properties
15.5 Regional Ventricular Mechanics: Stress and Strain 15-20
15.6 Patient-Specific Modeling 15-22
Acknowledgments 15-22
References... 15-22

Andrew D.
McCulloch
University of California,
San Diego

Roy C. P. Kerckhoffs
University of California,
San Diego

15.1 Introduction

The primary function of the heart, to pump blood through the circulatory system, is fundamentally mechanical. In this chapter, cardiac function is discussed in the context of the mechanics of the ventricular walls from the perspective of the determinants of myocardial stresses and strains (Table 15.1). Many physiological, pathophysiological, and clinical factors are directly or indirectly affected by myocardial stress and strain (Table 15.2). Of course, the factors in Tables 15.1 and 15.2 are closely interrelated—most of the factors affected by myocardial stress and strain in turn affect the stress and strain in the ventricular wall. For example, changes in wall stress due to altered hemodynamic load may cause ventricular remodeling, which in turn alters the geometry, structure, and material properties. This chapter is organized around the governing determinants in Table 15.1, but mention is made where appropriate of some of the factors in Table 15.2.

15.2 Cardiac Geometry and Structure

The mammalian heart consists of four pumping chambers, the left and right atria and ventricles communicating through the atrioventricular (mitral and tricuspid) valves, which are structurally connected by chordae tendineae to papillary muscles that extend from the anterior and posterior aspects of the right and left ventricular lumens. The muscular cardiac wall is perfused via the coronary vessels that originate at the left and right coronary ostia located in the sinuses of Valsalva immediately distal to the aortic valve leaflets. Surrounding the whole heart is the collagenous parietal pericardium that fuses with the diaphragm and great vessels. These are the anatomical structures that are most commonly studied in the field of cardiac mechanics. Particular emphasis is given in this chapter to the ventricular walls, which are the most important for the pumping function of the heart. Most studies of cardiac mechanics have focused on the left ventricle, but many of the important conclusions apply equally to the right ventricle.

TABLE 15.1   Basic Determinants of Myocardial Stress and Strain

Geometry and Structure	
3D shape	Wall thickness
	Curvature
	Stress-free and unloaded reference configurations
Tissue structure	Muscle fiber architecture
	Connective tissue organization
	Pericardium, epicardium, and endocardium
	Coronary vascular anatomy
Boundary/Initial Conditions	
Pressure	Filling pressure (preload)
	Arterial pressure (afterload)
	Direct and indirect ventricular interactions
	Thoracic and pericardial pressure
Constraints	Effects of inspiration and expiration
	Constraints due to the pericardium and its attachments
	Valves and fibrous valve annuli, chordae tendineae
	Great vessels, lungs
Material Properties	
Resting or passive	Nonlinear finite elasticity
	Quasilinear viscoelasticity
	Anisotropy
	Biphasic poroelasticity
Active dynamic	Activation sequence
	Myofiber isometric and isotonic contractile dynamics
	Sarcomere length and length history
	Cellular calcium kinetics and metabolic energy supply

15.2.1 Ventricular Geometry

From the perspective of engineering mechanics, the ventricles are three-dimensional thick-walled pressure vessels with substantial variations in wall thickness and principal curvatures both regionally and temporally through the cardiac cycle. The ventricular walls in the normal heart are thickest at the equator and base of the left ventricle and thinnest at the left ventricular apex and right ventricular free wall. There are also variations in the principal dimensions of the left ventricle with species, age, phase of the cardiac cycle, and disease (Table 15.3). But, in general, the ratio of wall thickness to radius is too high to be treated accurately by all but the most sophisticated thick-wall shell theories [1].

Ventricular geometry has been studied in most quantitative detail in the dog heart [2,3]. Geometric models have been very useful in the analysis, especially the use of confocal and nonconfocal ellipses of revolution to describe the epicardial and endocardial surfaces of the left and right ventricular walls (Figure 15.1). The canine left ventricle is reasonably modeled by a thick ellipsoid of revolution truncated at the base. The crescentic right ventricle wraps about 180° around the heart wall circumferentially and extends longitudinally about two-thirds of the distance from the base to the apex. Using a truncated ellipsoidal model, the left ventricular geometry in the dog can be defined by the major and minor radii of two surfaces, the left ventricular endocardium, and a surface defining the free wall epicardium and the septal endocardium of the right ventricle. Streeter and Hanna [2] described the position of the basal plane using a truncation factor f_b defined as the ratio between the longitudinal distances from equator-to-base and equator-to-apex. Hence, the overall longitudinal distance from base to apex is $(1 + f_b)$ times

TABLE 15.2 Factors Affected by Myocardial Stress and Strain

Direct factors	Regional muscle work
	Myocardial oxygen demand and energetics
	Coronary blood flow
Electrophysiological responses	Action potential duration (QT interval)
	Repolarization (T wave morphology)
	Excitability
	Risk of arrhythmia
Development and morphogenesis	Growth rate
	Cardiac looping and septation
	Valve formation
Vulnerability to injury	Ischemia
	Arrhythmia
	Cell dropout
	Aneurysm rupture
Remodeling, repair, and adaptation	Eccentric and concentric hypertrophy
	Fibrosis
	Scar formation
Progression of disease	Transition from hypertrophy to failure
	Ventricular dilation
	Infarct expansion
	Response to reperfusion
	Aneurysm formation

TABLE 15.3 Representative Left Ventricular Minor-Axis Dimensions

Species	Comments	Inner Radius (mm)	Outer Radius (mm)	Wall Thickness: Inner Radius
Dog (21 kg)	Unloaded diastole (0 mm Hg)	16	26	0.62
Dog	Normal diastole (2–12 mm Hg)	19	28	0.47
Dog	Dilated diastole (24–40 mm Hg)	22	30	0.36
Dog	Normal systole (1–9 mm Hg EDP)	14	26	0.86
Dog	Long axis, apex-equator (normal diastole)	42	47	0.12
Young rats	Unloaded diastole (0 mm Hg)	1.4	3.5	1.50
Mature rats	Unloaded diastole (0 mm Hg)	3.2	5.8	0.81
Human	Normal	24	32	0.34
Human	Compensated pressure overload	27	42	0.56
Human	Compensated volume overload	32	42	0.33

Note: Dog data from Ross et al. [177] and Streeter and Hanna [2]. Human data from Grossman et al. [178,179]. Rat data are from unpublished observations in the author's laboratory.

the major radius of the ellipse. Since variations in f_b between diastole and systole are relatively small (0.45–0.51), they suggested a constant value of 0.5.

The focal length d of an ellipsoid is defined from the major and minor radii (a and b) by $d^2 = a^2 - b^2$, and varies only slightly in the dog from endocardium to epicardium between end-diastole (37.3–37.9 mm) and end-systole (37.7–37.1 mm) [2]. Hence, within the accuracy that the boundaries of the left ventricular wall can be treated as ellipsoids of revolution, the assumption that the ellipsoids are confocal appears to be a good one. This has motivated the choice of prolate spheroidal (elliptic–hyperbolic–polar) coordinates (λ, μ, θ) as a system for economically representing ventricular geometries obtained post mortem or by noninvasive tomography [3,4]. The Cartesian coordinates of a point are given in terms of its prolate spheroidal coordinates by

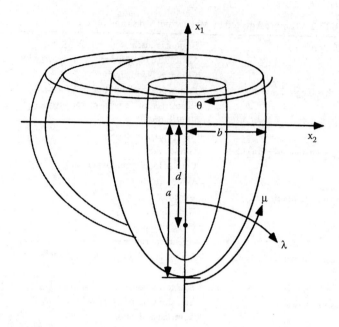

FIGURE 15.1 Truncated ellipsoid representation of ventricular geometry, showing major left ventricular radius (*a*), minor radius (*b*), focal length (*d*), and prolate spheroidal coordinates (λ, μ, θ).

$$x_1 = d \cosh \lambda \cos \mu,$$

$$x_2 = d \sinh \lambda \sin \mu \cos \theta, \tag{15.1}$$

$$x_3 = d \sinh \lambda \sin \mu \sin \theta.$$

Here, the focal length *d* defines a family of coordinate systems that vary from spherical polar when $d = 0$ to cylindrical polar in the limit when $d \to \infty$. A surface of constant transmural coordinate λ (Figure 15.1) is an ellipse of revolution with major radius $a = d \cosh \lambda$ and minor radius $b = d \sinh \lambda$. In an ellipsoidal model with a truncation factor of 0.5, the longitudinal coordinate μ varies from zero at the apex to 120° at the base. Integrating the Jacobian in prolate spheroidal coordinates gives the volume of the wall or cavity:

$$d^3 \int_0^{2\pi} \int_0^{\mu_2} \int_{\lambda_1}^{\lambda_2} ((\sinh^2 \lambda + \sin^2 \mu) \sinh \lambda \sin \mu) d\lambda \, d\mu \, d\theta = \frac{2\pi d^3}{3} \left| (1 - \cos \mu_2) \cosh^3 \lambda - (1 - \cos^3 \mu_2) \cosh \lambda \right|_{\lambda_1}^{\lambda_2}$$

$$\tag{15.2}$$

The scaling between heart mass M_H and body mass M within or between species is commonly described by the allometric formula

$$M_H = kM^\alpha. \tag{15.3}$$

Using combined measurements from a variety of mammalian species with *M* expressed in kilograms, the coefficient *k* is 5.8 g and the power α is close to unity (0.98) [5]. Within individual species, the ratio of heart weight to body weight is somewhat lower in mature rabbits and rats (about 2 g kg^{-1}) than in humans (5 g kg^{-1}), and higher in horses and dogs (8 g kg^{-1}) [6]. The rate α of heart growth with body weight decreases with age in most species but not humans. At birth, left and right ventricular weights are similar, but the left ventricle is substantially more massive than the right by adulthood.

15.2.2 Myofiber Architecture

The cardiac ventricles have a complex three-dimensional muscle fiber architecture (for a comprehensive review, see Reference 7). Although the myocytes are relatively short, they are connected such that at any point in the normal heart wall there is a clear predominant fiber axis that is approximately tangent to the wall (within 3–5° in most regions, except near the apex and papillary muscle insertions). Each ventricular myocyte is connected via gap junctions at intercalated disks to an average of 11.3 neighbors, 5.3 on the sides and 6.0 at the ends [8]. The classical anatomists dissected discrete bundles of fibrous swirls, though later investigations showed that the ventricular myocardium could be unwrapped by blunt dissection into a single continuous muscle "band" [9]. However, more modern histological techniques have shown that in the plane of the wall, the mean muscle fiber angle makes a smooth transmural transition from epicardium to endocardium (Figure 15.2). About the mean, myofiber angle dispersion is typically 10–15° [10] except in certain pathologies. Similar patterns have been described for humans, dogs, baboons, macaques, pigs, guinea pigs, and rats. In the human or dog left ventricle, the muscle fiber angle typically varies continuously from about −60° (i.e., 60° clockwise from the circumferential axis) at the epicardium to about +70° at the endocardium. The rate of change of fiber angle is usually greatest at the epicardium, so that circumferential (0°) fibers are found in the outer half of the wall, and begins to slow down on approaching the inner third near the trabeculata–compacta interface. There are also small increases in fiber orientation from end-diastole to systole (7–19°), with greatest changes at the epicardium and apex [11].

Regional variations in ventricular myofiber orientations are generally smooth except at the junction between the right ventricular free wall and septum. A detailed study in the dog that mapped fiber angles throughout the entire right and left ventricles described the same general transmural pattern in all regions, including the septum and right ventricular free wall, but with definite regional variations [3]. Transmural differences in the fiber angle were about 120–140° in the left ventricular free wall, larger in the septum (160–180°), and smaller in the right ventricular free wall (100–120°). A similar study of fiber angle distributions in the rabbit left and right ventricles has recently been reported [12]. For the most part, fiber angles in the rabbit heart were very similar to those in the dog, except for on the anterior wall, where average fiber orientations were 20–30° counterclockwise of those in the dog. While the most reliable reconstructions of ventricular myofiber architecture have been made using quantitative histological techniques, diffusion tensor magnetic resonance imaging (DTI) has proven to be a reliable technique for estimating fiber orientation nondestructively in fixed [13,14] and even intact beating human hearts [15].

The locus of fiber orientations at a given depth in the ventricular wall has a spiral geometry that may be modeled as a general helix by simple differential geometry. The position vector $\mathbf{x}$ of a point on a helix inscribed on an ellipsoidal surface that is symmetric about the x_1 axis and has major and minor radii, a and b, is given by the parametric equation

$$\mathbf{x} = a \sin t \, \mathbf{e}_1 + b \cos t \sin wt \, \mathbf{e}_2 + b \cos t \cos wt \, \mathbf{e}_3, \tag{15.4}$$

where the parameter is t and the helix makes $w/4$ full turns between the apex and the equator. A positive w defines a left-handed helix with a positive pitch. The fiber angle or helix pitch angle η varies along the arc length:

$$\sin \eta = \sqrt{\frac{a^2 \cos^2 t + b^2 \sin^2 t}{(a^2 + b^2 w^2)\cos^2 t + b^2 \sin^2 t}}. \tag{15.5}$$

If another deformed configuration $\hat{\mathbf{x}}$ is defined in the same way as Equation 15.4, the fiber segment extension ratio $d\hat{s}/ds$ associated with a change in the ellipsoid geometry [16] can be derived from

$$\frac{d\hat{s}}{ds} = \frac{\dfrac{d\hat{s}}{dt}}{\dfrac{ds}{dt}} = \frac{\left|\dfrac{d\hat{\mathbf{x}}}{dt}\right|}{\left|\dfrac{d\mathbf{x}}{dt}\right|}. \tag{15.6}$$

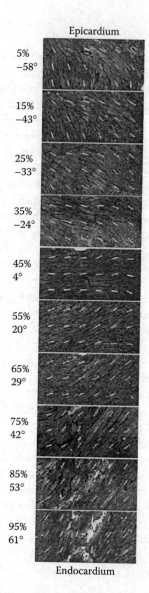

Epicardium

5%
−58°

15%
−43°

25%
−33°

35%
−24°

45%
4°

55%
20°

65%
29°

75%
42°

85%
53°

95%
61°

Endocardium

FIGURE 15.2 Cardiac muscle fiber orientations vary continuously through the left ventricular wall from a negative angle at the epicardium (0%) to near zero (circumferential) at the midwall (50%) and to increasing positive values toward the endocardium (100%). (Micrographs of murine myocardium from the author's laboratory, courtesy of Jyoti Rao.)

Although the traditional notion of discrete myofiber bundles has been revised in view of the continuous transmural variation of muscle fiber angle in the plane of the wall, there is a transverse laminar structure in the myocardium that groups fibers together in sheets at an average of 4 ± 2 myocytes thick (48 ± 20 μm) separated by histologically distinct cleavage planes [17–19]. LeGrice and colleagues investigated these structures in a detailed morphometric study of four dog hearts [19]. They describe an ordered laminar arrangement of myocytes with extensive cleavage planes running approximately radially from the endocardium toward the epicardium in transmural section. Like the fibers, the sheets also have a branching pattern with the number of branches varying considerably through the wall thickness. Recent reports suggest that, in addition to fiber orientations, DTI may be able to detect laminar sheet orientations [20]. The tensor of diffusion coefficients in the myocardium detected by DTI has been shown to be orthotropic, and the principal axis of slowest diffusion was seen to coincide with the direction normal to the sheet planes.

The fibrous architecture of the myocardium has motivated models of myocardial material symmetry as transversely isotropic. The transverse laminae are the first structural evidence for material orthotropy and have motivated the development of models describing the variation of fiber, sheet, and sheet-normal axes throughout the ventricular wall [21]. This has led to the idea that the laminar architecture of the ventricular myocardium affects the significant transverse shears [22] and myofiber rearrangement [18] described in the intact heart during systole. By measuring three-dimensional distributions of strain across the wall thickness using biplane radiography of radiopaque markers, LeGrice and colleagues [23] found that the cleavage planes coincide closely with the planes of maximum shearing during ejection, and that the consequent reorientation of the myocytes may contribute 50% or more of normal systolic wall thickening. Arts et al. [24] showed that the distributions of sheet orientations measured within the left ventricular wall of the dog heart coincided closely with those predicted from observed three-dimensional wall strains using the assumption that laminae are oriented in planes that contain the muscle fibers and maximize interlaminar shearing. This assumption also leads to the conclusion that two families of sheet orientations may be expected. Indeed, a retrospective analysis of the histology supported this prediction and more recent observations confirm the presence of two distinct populations of sheet plane in the inner half of the ventricular wall.

A detailed description of the morphogenesis of the muscle fiber system in the developing heart is not available but there is evidence of an organized myofiber pattern by day 12 in the fetal mouse heart that is similar to that seen at birth (day 20) [25]. Abnormalities of cardiac muscle fiber patterns have been described in some disease conditions. In hypertrophic cardiomyopathy, which is often familial, there is substantial myofiber disarray, typically in the interventricular septum [10,26].

15.2.3 Extracellular Matrix Organization

The cardiac extracellular matrix primarily consists of the fibrillar collagens, type I (85%) and III (11%), synthesized by the cardiac fibroblasts, the most abundant cell type in the heart. Collagen is the major structural protein in connective tissues, but only comprises 2–5% of the myocardium by weight, compared with the myocytes, which make up 90% [27]. The collagen matrix has a hierarchical organization (Figure 15.3), and has been classified according to conventions established for skeletal muscle into endomysium, perimysium, and epimysium [28,29]. The endomysium is associated with individual cells and includes a fine weave surrounding the cell and transverse structural connections 120–150 nm long connecting adjacent myocytes, with attachments localized near the z-line of the sarcomere. The primary purpose of the endomysium is probably to maintain registration between adjacent cells. The perimysium groups cells together and includes the collagen fibers that wrap bundles of cells into the laminar sheets described above as well as large coiled fibers typically 1–3 μm in diameter composed of smaller collagen fibrils (40–50 nm) [30]. The helix period of the coiled perimysial fibers is about 20 μm and the convolution index (ratio of fiber arc length to midline length) is approximately 1.3 in the unloaded state of the ventricle [31,32]. These perimysial fibers are most likely to be the major structural elements of the collagen extracellular matrix though they probably contribute to myocardial strain energy by uncoiling rather than stretching [31]. Finally, a thick epimysial collagen sheath surrounds the entire myocardium forming the protective epicardium (visceral pericardium) and endocardium.

Collagen content, organization, cross-linking, and ratio of types I to III change with age and in various disease conditions, including myocardial ischemia and infarction, hypertension, and hypertrophy (Table 15.4). Changes in myocardial collagen content and organization coincide with alterations in diastolic myocardial stiffness [33]. Collagen intermolecular cross-linking is mediated by two separate mechanisms. The formation of enzymatic hydroxylysyl pyridinoline cross-links is catalyzed by lysyl oxidase, which requires copper as a cofactor. Nonenzymatic collagen cross-links known as advanced

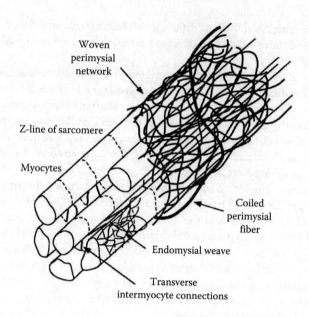

Woven perimysial network

Z-line of sarcomere

Myocytes

Coiled perimysial fiber

Endomysial weave

Transverse intermyocyte connections

FIGURE 15.3 Schematic representation of cardiac tissue structure showing the association of endomysial and perimysial collagen fibers with cardiac myocytes. (Courtesy of Dr. Deidre MacKenna.)

TABLE 15.4 Changes in Ventricular Collagen Structure and Mechanics with Age and Disease

Condition	Collagen Morphology	Types and Cross-Linking	Passive Stiffness	Others
Pressure overload hypertrophy	[Hydroxyproline]: ⇑-⇑⇑⇑ [147,148] Area fraction: ⇑⇑⇑⇑ [148,149]	Type III: ⇑[150] Cross-links: No change [151]	Chamber: ⇑-⇑⇑ [148,149] Tissue: ⇑⇑⇑ [152]	Perivascular fibrosis: ⇑⇑⇑ [148] Focal scarring: [153,154]
Volume overload hypertrophy	[Hydroxyproline]: No change-⇓: [155,156] Area fraction: No change [147,157]	Cross-links: ⇑ [151,156] Type III/I: ⇑ [156]	Chamber: ⇓[158] Tissue: No change/⇑ [158]	Parallel changes
Acute ischemia/ stunning	[Hydroxyproline]: ⇓ [180] Light microscopy: No change/⇓ [159] ⇓⇓ endomysial fibers [160]		⇓ early [161] ⇑ late [162]	Collagenase activity: ⇑ [163,164]
Chronic myocardial infarction	[Hydroxyproline]: ⇑⇑⇑ [165,166] Loss of birefringence [167]	Type III: ⇑[168]	Chamber: ⇑ early [169] Chamber: ⇓ late [169]	Organization: ⇑-⇑⇑⇑ [170,171]
Age	[Hydroxyproline]: ⇑-⇑⇑⇑ [163,172] Collagen fiber diameter ⇑⇑[172]	Type III/I: ⇓[173] Cross-links: ⇑[173]	Chamber: ⇑ [174] Papillary muscle: ⇑[175]	Light microscopy: fibril diameter ⇑ [172]

glycation end products can be formed in the presence of reducing sugars. This mechanism has been seen to significantly increase ventricular wall stiffness independent of changes in tissue collagen content, not only in diabetics but also in an animal model of volume overload hypertrophy [34]. Hence, the collagen matrix plays an important role in determining the elastic material properties of the ventricular myocardium.

15.3 Cardiac Pump Function

15.3.1 Ventricular Hemodynamics

The most basic mechanical parameters of the cardiac pump are blood pressure and volume flow rate, especially in the major pumping chambers, the ventricles. From the point of view of wall mechanics, the ventricular pressure is the most important boundary condition. Schematic representations of the time courses of pressure and volume in the left ventricle are shown in Figure 15.4. Ventricular filling immediately following mitral valve opening (MVO) is initially rapid because the ventricle produces a diastolic suction as the relaxing myocardium recoils elastically from its compressed systolic configuration below the resting chamber volume. The later slow phase of ventricular filling (diastasis) is followed finally by atrial contraction. The deceleration of the inflowing blood reverses the pressure gradient across the mitral valve leaflets and causes them to close (MVC). Valve closure may not, however, be completely passive because the atrial side of the mitral valve leaflets, which, unlike the pulmonic and aortic valves, are cardiac in embryological origin, have muscle [35] and nerve cells, and are electrically coupled to atrial conduction [36].

Ventricular contraction is initiated by excitation, which is almost synchronous (the duration of the QRS complex of the ECG is only about 60 ms in the normal adult) and begins about 0.1–0.2 s after atrial depolarization. Pressure rises rapidly during the isovolumic contraction phase (about 50 ms in adult humans), and the aortic valve opens (AVO) when the developed pressure exceeds the aortic pressure (afterload). Most of the cardiac output is ejected within the first quarter of the ejection phase before the pressure has peaked. The aortic valve closes (AVC) 200–300 ms after AVO when the ventricular pressure falls below the aortic pressure owing to the deceleration of the ejecting blood. The dichrotic notch, a characteristic feature of the aortic pressure waveform and a useful marker of aortic valve closure, is caused by pulse wave reflections in the aorta. Since the pulmonary artery pressure against which the

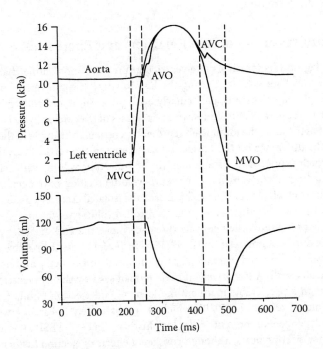

FIGURE 15.4 Left ventricular pressure, aortic pressure, and left ventricular volume during a single cardiac cycle showing the times of mitral valve closure (MVC), aortic valve opening (AVO), aortic valve closure (AVC), and mitral valve opening (MVO).

right ventricle pumps is much lower than the aortic pressure, the pulmonic valve opens before and closes after the aortic valve. The ventricular pressure falls during isovolumic relaxation, and the cycle continues. The rate of pressure decay from the value P_0 at the time of the peak rate of pressure fall until MVO is commonly characterized by a single exponential time constant, that is

$$P(t) = P_0\, e^{-t/\tau} + P_\infty, \tag{15.7}$$

where P_∞ is the (negative) baseline pressure to which the ventricle would eventually relax if MVO were prevented [37]. In dogs and humans, τ is normally about 40 ms, but it is increased by various factors, including elevated afterload, asynchronous contraction associated with abnormal activation sequence or regional dysfunction, and slowed cytosolic calcium reuptake to the sarcoplasmic reticulum associated with cardiac hypertrophy and failure. The pressure and volume curves for the right ventricle look essentially the same; however, the right ventricular and pulmonary artery pressures are only about a fifth of the corresponding pressures on the left side of the heart. The intraventricular septum separates the right and left ventricles and can transmit forces from one to the other. An increase in right ventricular volume may increase the left ventricular pressure by deformation of the septum. This direct interaction is most significant during filling [38].

The phases of the cardiac cycle are customarily divided into systole and diastole. The end of diastole—the start of systole—is generally defined as the time of mitral valve closure. Mechanical end-systole is usually defined as the end of ejection, but Brutsaert and colleagues proposed extending systole until the onset of diastasis (see the review by Brutsaert and Sys [39]) since there remains considerable myofilament interaction and active tension during relaxation. The distinction is important from the point of view of cardiac muscle mechanics: the myocardium is still active for much of diastole and may never be fully relaxed at sufficiently high heart rates (over 150 beats per minute). Here, we will retain the traditional definition of diastole, but consider the ventricular myocardium to be "passive" or "resting" only in the final slow-filling stage of diastole.

15.3.2 Ventricular Pressure–Volume Relations and Energetics

A useful alternative to Figure 15.4 for displaying ventricular pressure and volume changes is the pressure–volume loop shown in Figure 15.5a. During the last 20 years, the ventricular pressure–volume relationship has been explored extensively, particularly by Sagawa, Suga, and colleagues, who wrote a comprehensive book on the approach [40]. The isovolumic phases of the cardiac cycle can be recognized as the vertical segments of the loop, the lower limb represents ventricular filling, and the upper segment is the ejection phase. The difference on the horizontal axis between the vertical isovolumic segments is the stroke volume, which expressed as a fraction of the end-diastolic volume is the ejection fraction. The effects of altered loading on the ventricular pressure–volume relation have been studied in many preparations, but the best controlled experiments have used the isolated cross-circulated canine heart in which the ventricle fills and ejects against a computer-controlled volume servo-pump.

Changes in the filling pressure of the ventricle (preload) move the end-diastolic point along the unique end-diastolic pressure–volume relation (EDPVR), which represents the passive filling mechanics of the chamber that are determined primarily by the thick-walled geometry and nonlinear elasticity of the resting ventricular wall. Alternatively, if the afterload seen by the left ventricle is increased, stroke volume decreases in a predictable manner. The locus of end-ejection points (AVC) forms the end-systolic pressure–volume relation (ESPVR), which is approximately linear in a variety of conditions and also largely independent of the ventricular load history. Hence, the ESPVR is almost the same for isovolumic beats as for ejecting beats, although consistent effects of ejection history have been well characterized [41]. Connecting pressure–volume points at corresponding times in the cardiac cycle also results in a relatively linear relationship throughout systole with the intercept on the volume axis V_0 remaining nearly constant (Figure 15.5b). This leads to the valuable approximation that the ventricular

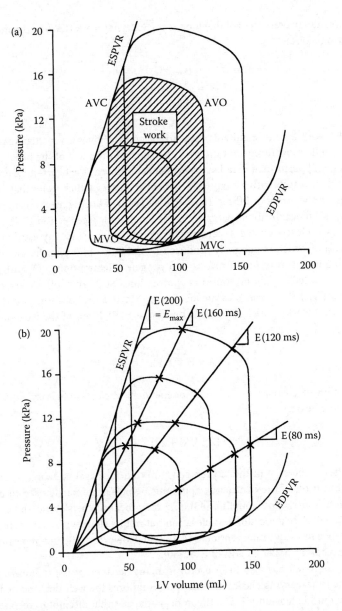

FIGURE 15.5 Schematic diagram of left ventricular pressure–volume loops: (a) end-systolic pressure–volume relation (ESPVR), end-diastolic pressure–volume relation (EDPVR), and stroke work. The three P–V loops show the effects of changes in preload and afterload. (b) Time-varying elastance approximation of ventricular pump function (see text).

volume $V(t)$ at any instance during systole is simply proportional to the instantaneous pressure $P(t)$ through a time-varying elastance $E(t)$:

$$P(t) = E(t)\{V(t) - V_0\}. \tag{15.8}$$

The maximum elastance E_{max}, the slope of the ESPVR, has acquired considerable significance as an index of cardiac contractility that is independent of ventricular loading conditions. As the inotropic state of the myocardium increases, for example, with catecholamine infusion, E_{max} increases, and with a negative inotropic effect such as a reduction in coronary artery pressure, it decreases.

The area of the ventricular pressure–volume loop is the external work (EW) performed by the myocardium on the ejecting blood:

$$EW = \int_{EDV}^{ESV} P(t)dV \qquad (15.9)$$

Plotting this stroke work against a suitable measure of preload gives a ventricular function curve, which illustrates the single most important intrinsic mechanical property of the heart pump. In 1914, Patterson and Starling [42] performed detailed experiments on the canine heart–lung preparation, and Starling summarized their results with his famous "Law of the Heart," which states that the work output of the heart increases with ventricular filling. The so-called Frank–Starling mechanism is now well recognized to be an intrinsic mechanical property of the cardiac muscle (see Section 15.4).

External stroke work is closely related to cardiac energy utilization. Since myocardial contraction is fueled by ATP, 90–95% of which is normally produced by oxidative phosphorylation, cardiac energy consumption is often studied in terms of myocardial oxygen consumption, VO_2 (mL O_2 g^{-1} beat^{-1}). Since energy is also expended during nonworking contractions, Suga and colleagues [43] defined the pressure–volume area (PVA) (J g^{-1} beat^{-1}) as the loop area (external stroke work) plus the end-systolic potential energy (internal work), which is the area under the ESPVR left of the isovolumic relaxation line (Figure 15.5a)

$$PVA = EW + PE. \qquad (15.10)$$

The PVA has strong linear correlation with VO_2 independent of ejection history. Equation 15.11 has typical values for the dog heart:

$$VO_2 = 0.12(PVA) + 2.0 \times 10^{-4}. \qquad (15.11)$$

The intercept represents the sum of the oxygen consumption for basal metabolism and the energy associated with the activation of the contractile apparatus, which is primarily used to cycle intracellular Ca^{2+} for excitation–contraction coupling [43]. The reciprocal of the slope is the contractile efficiency [44,45]. The VO_2–PVA relation shifts its elevation but not its slope with increments in E_{max} with most positive and negative inotropic interventions [44,46–49]. However, ischemic–reperfused viable but "stunned" myocardium has a smaller O_2 cost of PVA [50].

Although the PVA approach has also been useful in many settings, it is fundamentally phenomenological. Because the time-varying elastance assumptions ignores the well-documented load-history dependence of cardiac muscle tension [51–53], theoretical analyses that attempt to reconcile PVA with cross-bridge mechanoenergetics [54] are usually based on isometric or isotonic contractions. So that regional oxygen consumption in the intact heart can be related to myofiber biophysics, regional variations on the PVA have been proposed, such as the tension–area area [55], normalization of E_{max} [56], and the fiber stress–strain area [57].

In mammals, there are characteristic variations in cardiac function with heart size. In the power law relation for heart rate as a function of body mass (analogous to Equation 15.3), the coefficient k is 241 beats min^{-1} and the power α is −0.25 [5]. In the smallest mammals, like soricine shrews that weigh only a few grams, maximum heart rates exceeding 1000 beats min^{-1} have been measured [58]. Ventricular cavity volume scales linearly with heart weight, and ejection fraction and blood pressure are reasonably invariant from rats to horses. Hence, stroke work also scales directly with heart size [59], and thus work rate and energy consumption would be expected to increase with decreased body size in the same manner as heart rate. However, careful studies have demonstrated only a twofold increase in myocardial heat production as body mass decreases in mammals ranging from humans to rats, despite a 4.6-fold increase in heart rate [60]. This suggests that cardiac energy expenditure does not scale in proportion to heart rate and that cardiac metabolism is a lower proportion of total body metabolism in the smaller species.

The primary determinants of the EDPVR are the material properties of resting myocardium, the chamber dimensions and wall thickness, and the boundary conditions at the epicardium, endocardium, and valve annulus [61]. The EDPVR has been approximated by an exponential function of volume (see, e.g., Chapter 9 in Reference 62), though a cubic polynomial also works well. Therefore, the passive chamber stiffness dP/dV is approximately proportional to the filling pressure. Important influences on the EDPVR include the extent of relaxation, ventricular interaction and pericardial constraints, and coronary vascular engorgement. The material properties and boundary conditions in the septum are important since they determine how the septum deforms [63,64]. Through septal interaction, the end-diastolic pressure–volume relationship of the left ventricle may be directly affected by changes in the hemodynamic loading conditions of the right ventricle. The ventricles also interact indirectly since the output of the right ventricle is returned as the input to the left ventricle via the pulmonary circulation. Slinker and Glantz [65], using pulmonary artery and venae caval occlusions to produce direct (immediate) and indirect (delayed) interaction transients, concluded that the direct interaction is about half as significant as the indirect coupling. The pericardium provides a low friction mechanical enclosure for the beating heart that constrains ventricular overextension [66]. Since the pericardium has stiffer elastic properties than the ventricles [67], it contributes to direct ventricular interactions. The pericardium also augments the mechanical coupling between the atria and ventricles [68]. Increasing coronary perfusion pressure has been seen to increase the slope of the diastolic pressure–volume relation (an "erectile" effect) [69,70].

15.4 Myocardial Material Properties

15.4.1 Muscle Contractile Properties

Cardiac muscle mechanics testing is far more difficult than skeletal muscle testing mainly owing to the lack of ideal test specimens like the long single fiber preparations that have been so valuable for studying the mechanisms of skeletal muscle mechanics. Moreover, under physiological conditions, cardiac muscle cannot be stimulated to produce sustained tetanic contractions due to the absolute refractory period of the myocyte cell membrane. Cardiac muscle also exhibits a mechanical property analogous to the relative refractory period of excitation. After a single isometric contraction, some recovery time is required before another contraction of equal amplitude can be activated. The time constant for this mechanical restitution property of cardiac muscle is about 1 s [71].

Unlike skeletal muscle, in which maximal active force generation occurs at a sarcomere length that optimizes myofilament overlap (~2.1 μm), the isometric twitch tension developed by isolated cardiac muscle continues to rise with increased sarcomere length in the physiological range (1.6–2.4 μm). Early evidence for a descending limb of the cardiac muscle isometric length–tension curve was found to be caused by shortening in the central region of the isolated muscle at the expense of stretching at the damaged ends where specimen was tethered to the test apparatus. If muscle length is controlled so that sarcomere length in the undamaged part of the muscle is indeed constant, or if the developed tension is plotted against the instantaneous sarcomere length rather than the muscle length, the descending limb is eliminated [72]. Thus, the increase with chamber volume of end-systolic pressure and stroke work is reflected in isolated muscle as a monotonic increase in peak isometric tension with sarcomere length. Unlike in skeletal muscle, resting tension becomes very significant at sarcomere lengths over 2.3 μm. The increase in slope of the ESPVR associated with increased contractility is mirrored by the effects of increased calcium concentration in the length–tension relation. The duration as well as the tension developed in the active cardiac twitch also increases substantially with sarcomere length.

The relationship between cytosolic calcium concentration and isometric muscle tension has mostly been investigated in muscle preparations in which the sarcolemma has been chemically permeabilized.

Because there is evidence that this chemical "skinning" alters the calcium sensitivity of myofilament interaction, recent studies have also investigated myofilament calcium sensitivity in intact muscles tetanized by high-frequency stimulation in the presence of a compound such as ryanodine that open calcium release sites in the sarcoplasmic reticulum. Intracellular calcium concentration was estimated using calcium-sensitive optical indicators such as Fura. The myofilaments are activated in a graded manner by micromolar concentrations of calcium, which binds to troponin-C according to a sigmoidal relation [73]. Half-maximal tension in cardiac muscle is developed at intracellular calcium concentrations of 10^{-6} to 10^{-5} M (the C_{50}) depending on factors such as species and temperature [71]. Hence, relative isometric tension T_0/T_{max} may be modeled using [74,75].

$$\frac{T_0}{T_{max}} = \frac{[Ca]^n}{[Ca]^n + C_{50}^n}.$$
(15.12)

The Hill coefficient (n) governs the steepness of the sigmoidal curve. A wide variety of values have been reported but most have been in the range 3–6 [76–79]. The steepness of the isometric length–tension relation, compared with that of skeletal muscle is due to length-dependent calcium sensitivity. That is, the C_{50} (M) changes with sarcomere length, L (μm). Kentish et al. [77] also reported a dependence of the Hill coefficient n on sarcomere length, but this was probably due to shortening during contraction of their specimens. In experiments in which sarcomere length was tightly controlled, no length dependence of n was found [80]. Niederer et al. [181] used a Hill coefficient of 5 for intact rat preparations at room temperature and the following approximation for C_{50} to fit the data of skinned rat cardiac muscle:

$$C_{50} = 4.72\left(1 - 4.0\left(\frac{L}{L_{ref} - 1}\right)\right),$$
(15.13)

where the reference sarcomere length L_{ref} was taken to be 2.0 μm.

The isotonic force–velocity relation of cardiac muscle is similar to that of skeletal muscle, and A. V. Hill's well-known hyperbolic relation is a good approximation except at larger forces greater than about 85% of the isometric value. The maximal (unloaded) velocity of shortening is essentially independent of preload, but does change with time during the cardiac twitch and is affected by factors that affect contractile ATPase activity and hence cross-bridge cycling rates. De Tombe and colleagues [81], using sarcomere length-controlled isovelocity release experiments, found that viscous forces impose a significant internal load opposing sarcomere shortening. If the isotonic shortening response is adjusted for the confounding effects of passive viscoelasticity, the underlying cross-bridge force–velocity relation is found to be linear.

Cardiac muscle contraction also exhibits other significant length-history-dependent properties. An important example is "deactivation" associated with length transients. Following a brief length transient that dissociates cross-bridges, the tension that is redeveloped reaches the original isometric value when the transient is imposed early in the twitch before peak tension is reached. But, following transients applied at times after the peak twitch tension has occurred, the fraction of tension redeveloped declines progressively since the activator calcium has fallen to levels below that necessary for all cross-bridges to reattach [82].

There have been many model formulations of cardiac muscle contractile mechanics, too numerous to summarize here. In essence, they may be grouped into three categories. Time-varying elastance models include the essential dependence of cardiac active force development on muscle length and time. These models would seem to be well suited to create EDPVR and ESPVR curves in the continuum analysis of whole heart mechanics [1,83,84] by virtue of the success of the time-varying elastance concept of ventricular function (see Section 15.3.2 above). However, to obtain more realistic flow and pressure waveforms when a whole-heart model is coupled to an afterload, or in the presence of an asynchronous ventricular activation pattern, contractile models that incorporate a force–velocity relation are more appropriate. In

"Hill" models, the active fiber stress development is modified by shortening or lengthening according to the force–velocity relation, so that fiber tension is reduced by increased shortening velocity [85,86]. Fully history-dependent models are more complex and are generally based on A. F. Huxley's cross-bridge theory [53,87–89]. A statistical approach known as the distribution moment model has also been shown to provide an excellent approximation to cross-bridge theory [90]. Alternative, more phenomenological approaches are Hunter's fading memory theory [75]—which captures the complete length-history dependence of cardiac muscle contraction—and Markov models of myofilament activation [91–93] without requiring all the biophysical complexity of cross-bridge models.

Recently, Campbell et al. proposed a mechanistic Markov model of cardiac thin filament activation in which emphasis was put on interactions among nearest-neighbor regulatory units (RUs) [94]. In the model, RUs are composed of seven actin monomers, troponin C, troponin I, and tropomyosin, together with the S1 region of myosin (Figure 15.6) [95]. Interactions were assumed to arise from structural coupling of adjacent tropomyosins, such that tropomyosin shifting within each RU was influenced by the tropomyosin status of its neighbors. Model results suggested that this single mechanism was capable of producing cooperative activation of force-Ca^{2+} dynamics in intact cardiac muscle (Figure 15.7).

The appropriate choice of model will depend on the purpose of the analysis. For many models of global ventricular function, a time-varying elastance or Hill-type model will suffice, but for an analysis of sarcomere dynamics in isolated muscle or the ejecting heart, a history-dependent analysis is more appropriate.

Although Hill's basic assumption that resting and active muscle fiber tensions are additive is axiomatic in one-dimensional tests of isolated cardiac mechanics, there remains little experimental information on how the passive and active material properties of myocardium superpose in two dimensions or three. The simplest and commonest assumption is that active stress is strictly one-dimensional and adds to the fiber component of the three-dimensional passive stress. However, even this addition will indirectly affect all the other components of the stress response, since myocardial elastic deformations are finite, nonlinear, and approximately isochoric (volume conserving). In an interesting and important new development, biaxial testing of tetanized and barium-contracted ventricular myocardium has shown that the developed systolic stress also has a large component in directions transverse to the mean myofiber axis that can exceed 50% of the axial fiber component [96]. The magnitude of this transverse active stress depended significantly on the biaxial loading conditions. Moreover, evidence from osmotic swelling and other studies suggests that transverse strain can affect contractile tension development along the fiber axis by altering myofibril lattice spacing [97,98]. The mechanisms of transverse active stress development

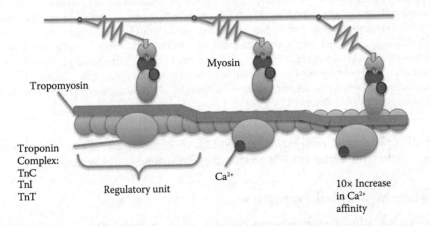

FIGURE 15.6 Diagram of myofilament Ca^{2+} activation. This depiction is based on concepts reviewed in Reference 95. (Reproduced with permission from S. G. Campbell, *The Role of Regulatory Light Chain Phosphorylation in Left Ventricular Function*, La Jolla: University of California, San Diego, 2010, p. 215.)

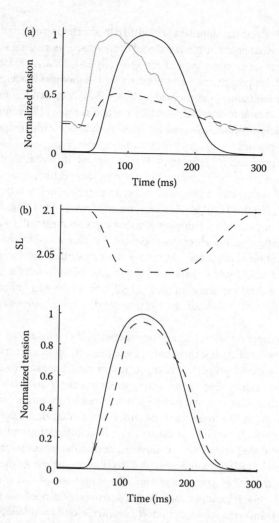

FIGURE 15.7 Twitches simulated with a Markov model of myofilament activation that properly accounts for structural interactions among regulatory proteins [176]. (a) Twitch tension was simulated in response to an intracellular Ca^{2+} transient measured in mouse papillary muscle (gray trace in background). In the absence of cooperative interactions between neighboring tropomyosin molecules along the length of actin filaments, diastolic tension is high, and the time course of twitch very nearly follows that of the driving Ca^{2+} transient (dashed trace). When neighboring tropomyosin molecules interact (solid trace), the cooperative effects can be seen as low diastolic tension (cooperative inhibition) as well as enhanced peak tension (cooperative activation). (b) An illustration of length and velocity dependence in the same model, responding to isometric (solid traces) and nonisometric (dashed traces) conditions. (Courtesy of Dr. Stuart Campbell.)

remain unclear but two possible contributors are the geometry of the cross-bridge head itself, which is oriented oblique to the myofilament axis [99], and the dispersion of myofiber orientation [10].

15.4.2 Resting Myocardial Properties

Since, by the Frank–Starling mechanism, end-diastolic volume directly affects systolic ventricular work, the mechanics of resting myocardium also have fundamental physiological significance. Most biomechanics studies of passive myocardial properties have been conducted in isolated, arrested whole-heart or tissue preparations. Passive cardiac muscle exhibits most of the mechanical properties characteristic of soft tissues in general [100]. In cyclic uniaxial loading and unloading, the stress–strain relationship is nonlinear with small but significant hysteresis. Depending on the preparation used, resting cardiac muscle typically requires 2–10 repeated loading cycles to achieve a reproducible (preconditioned) response. Intact cardiac muscle experiences finite deformations during the normal cardiac cycle, with maximum Lagrangian strains (which are generally radial and endocardial) that may easily exceed 0.5 in magnitude. Hence, the classical linear theory of elasticity is quite inappropriate for resting myocardial mechanics. The hysteresis of the tissue is consistent with a viscoelastic response, which is undoubtedly related to the substantial water content of the myocardium (about 80% by mass). Changes in water content, such as edema, can cause substantial alterations in the passive stiffness and viscoelastic properties of myocardium. The viscoelasticity of passive cardiac muscle has been characterized in creep and relaxation studies of papillary muscle from cat and rabbit. In both species, the tensile stress in response to a step in strain relaxes 30–40% in the first 10 s [101,102]. The relaxation curves exhibit a short exponential time constant (<0.02 s) and a long one (about 1000 s), and are largely independent of the strain magnitude, which supports the approximation that myocardial viscoelasticity is quasilinear. Myocardial creep under isotonic loading is 2–3% of the original length after 100 s of isotonic loading and is also quasilinear with an exponential time course. There is also evidence that passive ventricular muscle exhibits other anelastic properties such as maximum-strain-dependent "strain softening" [103,104], a well-known property in elastomers first described by Mullins [105].

Since the hysteresis of passive cardiac muscle is small and only weakly affected by changes in strain rate, the assumption of pseudoelasticity [100] is often appropriate. That is, the resting myocardium is considered to be a finite elastic material with different elastic properties in loading versus unloading. Although various preparations have been used to study resting myocardial elasticity, the most detailed and complete information has come from biaxial and multiaxial tests of isolated sheets of cardiac tissue, mainly from the dog [106–108]. These experiments have shown that the arrested myocardium exhibits significant anisotropy with substantially greater stiffness in the muscle fiber direction than transversely. In equibiaxial tests of muscle sheets cut from planes parallel to the ventricular wall, fiber stress was greater than the transverse stress (Figure 15.8) by an average factor of close to 2.0 [109]. Moreover, because of the structural organization of the myocardium described in Section 15.2, there is also significant anisotropy

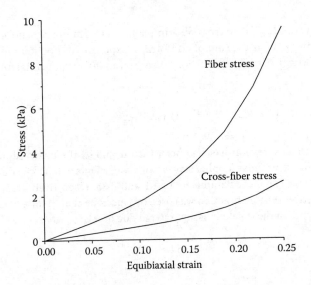

FIGURE 15.8 Representative stress–strain curves for passive rat myocardium computed using Equations 15.17 and 15.19. Fiber and cross-fiber stresses are shown for equibiaxial strain. (Courtesy of Dr. Jeffrey Omens.)

in the plane of the tissue transverse to the fiber axis, with the fiber direction being the stiffest, followed by the cross-fiber direction within a sheet, with the direction normal to a sheet being the softest [110]. Dokos and coworkers [110] have demonstrated that myocardial shear properties are also anisotropic.

The biaxial stress–strain properties of passive myocardium display some heterogeneity. Recently, Novak et al. [111] measured regional variations of biaxial mechanics in the canine left ventricle. Specimens from the inner and outer thirds of the left ventricular free wall were stiffer than those from the midwall and interventricular septum, but the degree of anisotropy was similar in each region. Significant species variations in myocardial stiffness have also been described. Using measurements of two-dimensional regional strain during left ventricular inflation in the isolated whole heart, a parameter optimization approach showed that canine cardiac tissue was several times stiffer than that of the rat, though the nonlinearity and anisotropy were similar [112]. Biaxial testing of the collagenous parietal pericardium and epicardium has shown that these tissues have distinctly different properties than the myocardium being very compliant and isotropic at low biaxial strains (<0.1–0.15) but rapidly becoming very stiff and anisotropic as the strain is increased [67,107].

Various constitutive models have been proposed for the elasticity of passive cardiac tissues. Because of the large deformations and nonlinearity of these materials, the most useful framework has been provided by the pseudostrain-energy formulation for hyperelasticity. For a detailed review of the material properties of passive myocardium and approaches to constitutive modeling, the reader is referred to Chapters 1 through 6 of Reference 113. In hyperelasticity, the components of the stress* are obtained from the strain energy W as a function of the Lagrangian (Green's) strain E_{RS}.

The myocardium is generally assumed to be an incompressible material, which is a good approximation in the isolated tissue, although in the intact heart there can be significant redistribution of tissue volume associated with phasic changes in regional coronary blood volume. Incompressibility is included as a kinematic constraint in the finite elasticity analysis, which introduces a new pressure variable that is added as a Lagrange multiplier in the strain energy. The examples that follow are various strain-energy functions, with representative parameter values (for W in kPa, i.e., mJ mL⁻¹), that have been suggested for cardiac tissues. For the two-dimensional properties of canine myocardium, Yin and colleagues [109] obtained reasonable fits to experimental data with an exponential function

$$W = 0.47e^{(35E_{11}^{1.2} + 20E_{22}^{1.2})}, \tag{15.14}$$

where E_{11} is the fiber strain and E_{22} is the cross-fiber in-plane strain. Humphrey and Yin [114] proposed a three-dimensional form for W as the sum of an isotropic exponential function of the first principal invariant I_1 of the right Cauchy–Green deformation tensor and another exponential function of the fiber stretch ratio λ_F:

$$W = 0.21(e^{9.4(I_1-3)} - 1) + 0.35(e^{66(\lambda_F-1)^2} - 1), \tag{15.15}$$

The isotropic part of this expression has also been used to model the myocardium of the embryonic chick heart during the ventricular looping stages, with coefficients of 0.02 kPa during diastole and 0.78 kPa at end-systole, and exponent parameters of 1.1 and 0.85, respectively [115]. Another transversely related isotropic strain-energy function was used by Guccione et al. [116] and Omens et al. [117] to model material properties in the isolated mature rat and dog hearts:

$$W = 0.6\,(e^Q - 1), \tag{15.16}$$

---

* In a hyperelastic material, the *second Piola Kirchhoff* stress tensor is given by $P_{RS} = \dfrac{1}{2}\left(\dfrac{\partial W}{\partial E_{RS}} + \dfrac{\partial W}{\partial E_{SR}} \right)$.

where, in the dog

$$Q = 26.7E_{11}^2 + 2.0(E_{22}^2 + E_{33}^2 + E_{23}^2 + E_{32}^2) + 14.7(E_{12}^2 + E_{21}^2 + E_{13}^2 + E_{31}^2), \tag{15.17}$$

and, in the rat

$$Q = 9.2E_{11}^2 + 2.0(E_{22}^2 + E_{33}^2 + E_{23}^2 + E_{32}^2) + 3.7(E_{12}^2 + E_{21}^2 + E_{13}^2 + E_{31}^2). \tag{15.18}$$

In Equations 15.17 and 15.18, normal and shear strain components involving the radial (x_3) axis are included. Humphrey and colleagues [118] determined a new polynomial form directly from biaxial tests. Novak et al. [111] gave representative coefficients for canine myocardium from three layers of the left ventricular free wall. For the outer third, they obtained

$$W = 4.8(\lambda_F - 1)^2 + 3.4(\lambda_F - 1)^3 + 0.77(I_1 - 3) - 6.1(I_1 - 3)(\lambda_F - 1) + 6.2(I_1 - 3)^2, \tag{15.19}$$

for the midwall region

$$W = 5.3(\lambda_F - 1)^2 + 7.5(\lambda_F - 1)^3 + 0.43(I_1 - 3) - 7.7(I_1 - 3)(\lambda_F - 1) + 5.6(I_1 - 3)^2, \tag{15.20}$$

and for the inner layer of the wall

$$W = 0.51(\lambda_F - 1)^2 + 27.6(\lambda_F - 1)^3 + 0.74(I_1 - 3) - 7.3(I_1 - 3)(\lambda_F - 1) + 7.0(I_1 - 3)^2. \tag{15.21}$$

A power law strain-energy function expressed in terms of circumferential, longitudinal, and transmural extension ratios (λ_1, λ_2, and λ_3) was used [119] to describe the biaxial properties of sheep myocardium 2 weeks after experimental myocardial infarction, in the scarred infarct region:

$$W = 0.36\left(\frac{\lambda_1^{32}}{32} + \frac{\lambda_2^{30}}{30} + \frac{\lambda_3^{31}}{31} - 3\right), \tag{15.22}$$

and in the remote, noninfarcted tissue:

$$W = 0.11\left(\frac{\lambda_1^{22}}{22} + \frac{\lambda_2^{26}}{26} + \frac{\lambda_3^{24}}{24} - 3\right), \tag{15.23}$$

Based on the observation that resting stiffness rises steeply at strains that extend coiled collagen fibers to the limit of uncoiling, Hunter and colleagues have proposed a pole-zero constitutive relation in which the stresses rise asymptotically as the strain approaches a limiting elastic strain [75].

Recently, Holzapfel and Ogden [120] proposed a convex, strong elliptic and stable orthotropic strain-energy law for the myocardium:

$$W = \frac{a}{2b}\exp[b(I_1 - 3)] + \sum_{i=f,s}\frac{a_i}{2b_i}(\exp[b_i(I_{4i} - 1)^2 - 1) + \frac{a_{fs}}{2b_{fs}}(\exp[b_{fs}I_{8fs}^2] - 1) \tag{15.24}$$

consisting of an isotropic term in I_1, transversely isotropic terms in I_{4f} and I_{4s} and an orthotropic term in I_{8fs}. Here, f, s, and n refer to fiber, cross-fiber within the sheet, and sheet-normal directions. The a parameters have unit of stress, whereas the b parameters are dimensionless. The quasi-invariant I_4 is a right Cauchy–Green strain in a preferred direction and I_{8fs} is the right Cauchy–Green fiber-sheet shear strain. Special care was taken to fit this model with data from Yin et al. [109] and Dokos et al. [110].

The strain in the constitutive equation must generally be referred to the stress-free state of the tissue. However, the unloaded state of the passive left ventricle is not stress-free; residual stress exists in the intact, unloaded myocardium, as shown by Omens and Fung [121]. Cross-sectional equatorial rings from potassium-arrested rat hearts spring open elastically when the left ventricular wall is resected radially. The average opening angle of the resulting curved arc is $45 \pm 10°$ in the rat. Subsequent radial cuts produce no further change. Hence, a slice with one radial cut is considered to be stress-free, and there is a nonuniform distribution of residual strain across the intact wall, being compressive at the endocardium and tensile at the epicardium, with some regional differences. Stress analyses of the diastolic left ventricle have shown that residual stress acts to minimize the endocardial stress concentrations that would otherwise be associated with diastolic loading [116]. An important physiological consequence of residual stress is that the sarcomere length is nonuniform in the unloaded resting heart. Rodriguez et al. [122] showed that sarcomere length is about 0.13 μm greater at the epicardium than the endocardium in the unloaded rat heart, and this gradient vanishes when residual stress is relieved. Three-dimensional studies have also revealed the presence of substantial transverse residual shear strains [123]. Residual stress and strain may have an important relationship to cardiac growth and remodeling. Theoretical studies have shown that residual stress in tissues can arise from growth fields that are kinematically incompatible [124,125].

15.5 Regional Ventricular Mechanics: Stress and Strain

Although ventricular pressures and volumes are valuable for assessing the global pumping performance of the heart, myocardial stress and strain distributions are needed to characterize regional ventricular function, especially in pathological conditions, such as myocardial ischemia and infarction, where profound localized changes may occur. The measurement of stress in the intact myocardium involves resolving the local forces acting on defined planes in the heart wall. Attempts to measure local forces [126,127] have had limited success because of the large deformations of the myocardium and the uncertain nature of the mechanical coupling between the transducer elements and the tissue. Efforts to measure intramyocardial pressures using miniature implanted transducers have been more successful but have also raised a controversy over the extent to which they accurately represent changes in interstitial fluid pressure. In all cases, these methods provide an incomplete description of three-dimensional wall stress distributions. Therefore, the most common approach for estimating myocardial stress distributions is the use of mathematical models based on the laws of continuum mechanics. Although there is no room to review these analyses here, the important elements of such models are the geometry and structure, boundary conditions, and material properties, described in the foregoing sections. An excellent review of ventricular wall stress analysis is given by Yin [128]. The most versatile and powerful method for ventricular stress analysis is the finite element method, which has been used in cardiac mechanics for over 20 years [129]. However, models must also be validated with experimental measurements. Since the measurement of myocardial stresses is not yet reliable, the best experimental data for model validation are measurements of strains in the ventricular wall.

The earliest myocardial strain gauges were mercury-in-rubber transducers sutured to the epicardium. These days, local segment length changes are routinely measured with various forms of the piezoelectric crystal sonomicrometer. However, since the ventricular myocardium is a three-dimensional continuum, the local strain is only fully defined by all the normal and shear components of the myocardial strain tensor. Villarreal et al. [130] measured two-dimensional midwall strain components by arranging three piezoelectric crystals in a small triangle so that three segment lengths could be measured simultaneously. They showed that the principal axis of greatest shortening is not aligned with circumferential midwall fibers, and that this axis changes with altered ventricular loading and contractility. Therefore, uniaxial segment measurements do not reveal the full extent of alterations in regional function caused by an experimental intervention. Another approach to measuring regional myocardial strains is the use of clinical imaging techniques, such as magnetic resonance imaging tagging [4] with sophisticated strain analyses like HARP [131] and two- and three-dimensional speckle tracking echocardiography [132]. In unusual circumstances, radiopaque markers are implanted in the myocardium during cardiac surgery or transplantation [133].

In experimental research, implantable radiopaque markers are used for tracking myocardial motions with high spatial and temporal resolution. Meier et al. [134,135] placed triplets of metal markers 10–15 mm apart near the epicardium of the canine right ventricle and reconstructed their positions from biplane cinéradiographic recordings. By polar decomposition, they obtained the two principal epicardial strains, the principal angle, and the local rotation in the region. The use of radiopaque markers was extended to three dimensions by Waldman and colleagues [22], who implanted three closely separated columns of 5–6 metal beads in the ventricular wall. With this technique, it is possible to find all six components of strain and all three rigid-body rotation angles at sites through the wall. For details of this method, see the review by Waldman in Chapter 7 of Glass et al. [113]. An enhancement to this method uses high-order finite element interpolation of the marker positions to compute continuous transmural distributions of myocardial deformation [136].

Studies and models like these are producing an increasingly detailed picture of regional myocardial stress and strain distributions. Of the many interesting observations, there are some useful generalizations, particularly regarding the strain. Myocardial deformations are large and three-dimensional, and hence the nonlinear finite strain tensors are more appropriate measures than the linear infinitesimal Cauchy strain. During filling in the normal heart, the wall stretches biaxially but nonuniformly in the plane of the wall, and thins in the transmural direction. During systole, shortening is also two-dimensional and the wall thickens. There are substantial regional differences in the time course, magnitude, and pattern of myocardial deformations. In humans and dogs, in-plane systolic myocardial shortening and diastolic lengthening vary with longitudinal position on the left and right ventricular free walls generally increasing in magnitude from base to apex.

During both systole and diastole, there are significant shear strains in the wall. In-plane (torsional) shears are negative during diastole, consistent with a small left-handed torsion of the left ventricle during filling, and positive as the ventricular twist reverses during ejection. Consequently, the principal axes of the greatest diastolic segment lengthening and systolic shortening are not circumferential or longitudinal but at oblique axes, that are typically rotated 10–60° clockwise from circumferential. There are circumferential variations in regional left ventricular strain. The principal axes of greatest diastolic lengthening and systolic shortening tend to be more longitudinal on the posterior wall and more circumferentially oriented on the anterior wall. Perhaps the most significant regional variations are transmural. In-plane and transmural, normal or principal strains, are usually significantly greater in magnitude at the endocardium than at the epicardium, both in filling and ejection. However, when the strain is resolved in the local muscle fiber direction, the transmural variation of fiber strain becomes insignificant. The combination of torsional deformation and the transmural variation in fiber direction means that systolic shortening and diastolic lengthening tend to be maximized in the fiber direction at the epicardium and minimized at the endocardium. Hence, whereas maximum shortening and lengthening are closely aligned with muscle fibers at the subepicardium, they are almost perpendicular to the fibers at the subendocardium. In the left ventricular wall, there are also substantial transverse shear strains (i.e., in the circumferential-radial and longitudinal-radial planes) during systole, though during filling they are smaller. Their functional significance remains unclear, though they change substantially during acute myocardial ischemia or ventricular pacing and are apparently associated with the transverse laminae described earlier [23].

Sophisticated continuum mechanics models are needed to determine the stress distributions associated with these complex myocardial deformations. With modern finite element methods, it is now possible to include in the analysis the three-dimensional geometry and fiber architecture, finite deformations, nonlinear material properties, and muscle contraction of the ventricular myocardium. Some models have included other factors such as viscoelasticity, poroelasticity, coronary perfusion, growth and remodeling, regional ischemia, residual stress, and electrical activation. To date, continuum models have provided some valuable insight into regional cardiac mechanics. These include the importance of muscle fiber orientation, torsional deformations and residual stress, and the substantial inhomogeneities associated with regional variations in geometry and fiber angle or myocardial ischemia and infarction. A new arena in which models promise to make important contributions is the rapidly growing field of cardiac resynchronization therapy [137–139]. The use of biventricular pacing in cases of congestive heart failure that are accompanied by electrical conduction asynchrony has been seen to significantly improve ventricular pump function. However, the improvement in mechanical function is not well predicted by the improvement in electrical synchrony. New electromechanical models promise to provide insights into the mechanisms of cardiac resynchronization therapy and potentially to optimize the pacing protocols used [140–142].

15.6 Patient-Specific Modeling

The maturation of computational biology may lead to a new approach to medicine. During the last decade, there have been many improvements in diagnostic medical technologies such as multislice cardiac CT imaging, three-dimensional electroanatomic mapping, and many types of applications of magnetic resonance imaging (i.e., tagging and DTI). Combined with more powerful computing resources and more accurate predictive computational models, it is feasible to begin developing mechanistic patient-specific models that may help diagnosis, guide therapy or surgery, and predict outcomes of the latter. Indeed, in recent years, there have been successes in patient-specific modeling in various clinical domains such as cardiology, orthopedics, brain surgery, cancer, and periodontia [143]. Of these disciplines, the cardiovascular system is an excellent candidate for patient-specific modeling [144], since cardiac models represent one of the most advanced areas of computational biology, bridging the subcellular level to the circulatory level [145]. Despite the advances in medical technology, patient-specific modeling has not yet become a standard of care in clinical practice because the evaluation of the predictive capability of these models has not yet been performed on a large scale [143,146].

Acknowledgments

We are indebted to many colleagues and students, past and present, for their input and perspective of cardiac biomechanics. Owing to space constraints, we have relied on much of their work without adequate citation, especially in the final section. Special thanks to Drs. Jeffrey Omens, Deidre MacKenna, Stuart Campbell, and Jyoti Rao, who provided illustrations used in this chapter.

References

1. L. A. Taber, On a nonlinear theory for muscle shells. Part II—Application to the beating left ventricle, *ASME J Biomech Eng,* 113, 63–71, 1991.
2. D. D. Streeter, Jr and W. T. Hanna, Engineering mechanics for successive states in canine left ventricular myocardium: I. Cavity and wall geometry, *Circ Res,* 33, 639–655, 1973.
3. P. M. F. Nielsen, I. J. Le Grice, B. H. Smaill, and P. J. Hunter, Mathematical model of geometry and fibrous structure of the heart, *Am J Physiol,* 260, H1365–H1378, 1991.
4. A. A. Young and L. Axel, Three-dimensional motion and deformation in the heart wall: Estimation from spatial modulation of magnetization—A model-based approach, *Radiology,* 185, 241–247, 1992.
5. W. R. Stahl, Scaling of respiratory variable in mammals, *J Appl Physiol,* 22, 453–460, 1967.
6. K. Rakusan, Cardiac growth, maturation and aging, in *Growth of the Heart in Health and Disease,* R. Zak, Ed. New York: Raven Press, 1984, 131–164.
7. D. D. Streeter, Jr, Gross morphology and fiber geometry of the heart, in *Handbook of Physiology, Section 2: The Cardiovascular System, Chapter 4.* vol. I, B. R. M, Ed. Bethesda, MD: American Physiological Society, 1979, pp. 61–112.

8. J. E. Saffitz, H. L. Kanter, K. G. Green, T. K. Tolley, and E. C. Beyer, Tissue-specific determinants of anisotropic conduction velocity in canine atrial and ventricular myocardium, *Circ Res*, 74, 1065–1070, 1994.

9. F. Torrent-Guasp, *The Cardiac Muscle*. Madrid: Juan March Foundation, 1973.

10. W. J. Karlon, J. W. Covell, A. D. McCulloch, J. J. Hunter, and J. H. Omens, Automated measurement of myofiber disarray in transgenic mice with ventricular expression of ras, *Anat Rec*, 252, 612–625, 1998.

11. D. D. Streeter, Jr, H. M. Spotnitz, D. P. Patel, J. Ross, Jr, and E. H. Sonnenblick, Fiber orientation in the canine left ventricle during diastole and systole, *Circ Res*, 24, 339–347, 1969.

12. F. J. Vetter and A. D. McCulloch, Three-dimensional analysis of regional cardiac function: A model of rabbit ventricular anatomy, *Prog Biophys Mol Biol*, 69, 157–183, 1998.

13. E. W. Hsu, A. L. Muzikant, S. A. Matulevicius, R. C. Penland, and C. S. Henriquez, Magnetic resonance myocardial fiber-orientation mapping with direct histological correlation, *Am J Physiol*, 274, H1627–H1634, 1998.

14. D. F. Scollan, A. Holmes, R. Winslow, and J. Forder, Histological validation of myocardial microstructure obtained from diffusion tensor magnetic resonance imaging, *Am J Physiol*, 275, H2308–H2318, 1998.

15. J. Dou, W. Y. Tseng, T. G. Reese, and V. J. Wedeen, Combined diffusion and strain MRI reveals structure and function of human myocardial laminar sheets in vivo, *Magn Reson Med*, 50, 107–113, 2003.

16. A. D. McCulloch, B. H. Smaill, and P. J. Hunter, Regional left ventricular epicardial deformation in the passive dog heart, *Circ Res*, 64, 721–733, 1989.

17. B. H. Smaill and P. J. Hunter, Structure and function of the diastolic heart, in *Theory of Heart*, L. Glass, P. J. Hunter, and A. D. McCulloch, Eds. New York: Springer-Verlag, 1991, pp. 1–29.

18. H. M. Spotnitz, W. D. Spotnitz, T. S. Cottrell, D. Spiro, and E. H. Sonnenblick, Cellular basis for volume related wall thickness changes in the rat left ventricle, *J Mol Cell Cardiol*, 6, 317–331, 1974.

19. I. J. LeGrice, B. H. Smaill, L. Z. Chai, S. G. Edgar, J. B. Gavin, and P. J. Hunter, Laminar structure of the heart: Ventricular myocyte arrangement and connective tissue architecture in the dog, *Am J Physiol*, 269, H571–H582, 1995.

20. W. Y. Tseng, V. J. Wedeen, T. G. Reese, R. N. Smith, and E. F. Halpern, Diffusion tensor MRI of myocardial fibers and sheets: Correspondence with visible cut-face texture, *J Magn Reson Imaging*, 17, 31–42, 2003.

21. I. J. Legrice, P. J. Hunter, and B. H. Smaill, Laminar structure of the heart: A mathematical model, *Am J Physiol*, 272, H2466–H2476, 1997.

22. L. K. Waldman, Y. C. Fung, and J. W. Covell, Transmural myocardial deformation in the canine left ventricle: Normal *in vivo* three-dimensional finite strains, *Circ Res*, 57, 152–163, 1985.

23. I. J. LeGrice, Y. Takayama, and J. W. Covell, Transverse shear along myocardial cleavage planes provides a mechanism for normal systolic wall thickening, *Circ Res*, 77, 182–193, 1995.

24. T. Arts, K. D. Costa, J. W. Covell, and A. D. McCulloch, Relating myocardial laminar architecture to shear strain and muscle fiber orientation, *Am J Physiol Heart Circ Physiol*, 280, H2222–H2229, 2001.

25. M. McLean, M. A. Ross, and J. Prothero, Three-dimensional reconstruction of the myofiber pattern in the fetal and neonatal mouse heart, *Anat Rec*, 224, 392–406, 1989.

26. B. J. Maron, R. O. Bonow, R. O. D. Cannon, M. B. Leon, and S. E. Epstein, Hypertrophic cardiomyopathy. Interrelations of clinical manifestations, pathophysiology, and therapy (1), *N Engl J Med*, 316, 780–789, 1987.

27. K. T. Weber, Cardiac interstituim in health and disease: The fibrillar collagen network, *J Am Coll Cardiol*, 13, 1637–165, 1989.

28. T. F. Robinson, L. Cohen-Gould, and S. M. Factor, Skeletal framework of mammalian heart muscle: Arrangement of inter- and pericellular connective tissue structures, *Lab Invest*, 49, 482–498, 1983.

29. J. B. Caulfield and T. K. Borg, The collagen network of the heart, *Lab Invest*, 40, 364–371, 1979.

30. T. F. Robinson, M. A. Geraci, E. H. Sonnenblick, and S. M. Factor, Coiled perimysial fibers of papillary muscle in rat heart: Morphology, distribution, and changes in configuration, *Circ Res*, 63, 577–592, 1988.

31. D. A. MacKenna, J. H. Omens, and J. W. Covell, Left ventricular perimysial collagen fibers uncoil rather than stretch during diastolic filling, *Basic Res Cardiol*, 91, 111–122, 1996.

32. D. A. MacKenna, S. M. Vaplon, and A. D. McCulloch, Microstructural model of perimysial collagen fibers for resting myocardial mechanics during ventricular filling, *Am J Physiol*, 273, H1576– H1586, 1997.

33. D. A. MacKenna and A. D. McCulloch, Contribution of the collagen extracellular matrix to ventricular mechanics, in *Systolic and Diastolic Function of the Heart*, N. B. Ingels, G. T. Daughters, J. Baan, J. W. Covell, R. S. Reneman, and F. C.-P. Yin, Eds. Amsterdam: IOS Press, 1996, pp. 35–46.

34. K. L. Herrmann, A. D. McCulloch, and J. H. Omens, Glycated collagen cross-linking alters cardiac mechanics in volume-overload hypertrophy, *Am J Physiol Heart Circ Physiol*, 284, H1277–H1284, 2003.

35. A. Itoh, G. Krishnamurthy, J. C. Swanson, D. B. Ennis, W. Bothe, E. Kuhl, M. Karlsson, L. R. Davis, D. C. Miller, and N. B. Ingels, Jr., Active stiffening of mitral valve leaflets in the beating heart, *Am J Physiol Heart Circ Physiol*, 296, H1766–H1773, 2009.

36. E. H. Sonnenblick, L. M. Napolitano, W. M. Daggett, and T. Cooper, An intrinsic neuromuscular basis for mitral valve motion in the dog, *Circ Res*, 21, 9–15, 1967.

37. E. L. Yellin, M. Hori, C. Yoran, E. H. Sonnenblick, S. Gabbay, and R. W. M. Frater, Left ventricular relaxation in the filling and nonfilling intact canine heart, *Am J Physiol*, 250, H620–H629, 1986.

38. J. S. Janicki and K. T. Weber, The pericardium and ventricular interaction, distensibility and function, *Am J Physiol*, 238, H494–H503, 1980.

39. D. L. Brutsaert and S. U. Sys, Relaxation and diastole of the heart, *Physiol Rev*, 69, 1228, 1989.

40. K. Sagawa, L. Maughan, H. Suga, and K. Sunagawa, *Cardiac Contraction and the Pressure-Volume Relationship*. New York: Oxford University Press, 1988.

41. W. C. Hunter, End-systolic pressure as a balance between opposing effects of ejection, *Circ Res*, 64, 265–275, 1989.

42. S. W. Patterson and E. H. Starling, On the mechanical factors which determine the output of the ventricles, *J Physiol*, 48, 357–379, 1914.

43. H. Suga, T. Hayashi, and M. Shirahata, Ventricular systolic pressure-volume area as predictor of cardiac oxygen consumption, *Am J Physiol*, 240, H39–H44, 1981.

44. H. Suga and Y. Goto, Cardiac oxygen costs of contractility (Emax) and mechanical energy (PVA): New key concepts in cardiac energetics, in *Recent Progress in Failing Heart Syndrome*, S. Sasayama and H. Suga, Eds. Tokyo: Springer-Verlag, 1991, pp. 61–115.

45. H. Suga, Y. Goto, O. Kawaguchi, K. Hata, T. Takasago, A. Saeki, and T. W. Taylor, Ventricular perspective on efficiency, *Basic Res Cardiol*, 88 Suppl 2, 43–65, 1993.

46. H. Suga, Ventricular energetics, *Physiol Rev*, 70, 247–277, 1990.

47. H. Suga, Y. Goto, Y. Yasumura, T. Nozawa, S. Futaki, N. Tanaka, and M. Uenishi, O_2 consumption of dog heart under decreased coronary perfusion and propranolol, *Am J Physiol*, 254, H292–H303, 1988.

48. D. D. Zhao, T. Namba, J. Araki, K. Ishioka, M. Takaki, and H. Suga, Nipradilol depresses cardiac contractility and O_2 consumption without decreasing coronary resistance in dogs, *Acta Med Okayama*, 47, 29–33, 1993.

49. T. Namba, M. Takaki, J. Araki, K. Ishioka, and H. Suga, Energetics of the negative and positive inotropism of pentobarbitone sodium in the canine left ventricle, *Cardiovasc Res*, 28, 557–564, 1994.

50. Y. Ohgoshi, Y. Goto, S. Futaki, H. Taku, O. Kawaguchi, and H. Suga, Increased oxygen cost of contractility in stunned myocardium of dog, *Circ Res*, 69, 975–988, 1991.

51. D. Burkhoff, M. Schnellbacher, R. A. Stennett, D. Zwas, K. Ogino, and J. P. Morgan, Explaining load-dependent ventricular performance and energetics based on a model of E-C coupling, in *Cardiac Energetics: From Emax to Pressure-Volume Area*, M. M. LeWinter, H. Suga, and M. W. Watkins, Eds. Boston: Kluwer Academic Publishers, 1995.

52. H. E. ter Keurs and P. P. de Tombe, Determinants of velocity of sarcomere shortening in mammalian myocardium, *Adv Exp Med Biol*, 332, 649–664; discussion 664–665, 1993.

53. J. M. Guccione and A. D. McCulloch, Mechanics of active contraction in cardiac muscle: Part I—Constitutive relations for fiber stress that describe deactivation, *J Biomech Eng*, 115, 72–81, 1993.

54. T. W. Taylor, Y. Goto, and H. Suga, Variable cross-bridge cycling-ATP coupling accounts for cardiac mechanoenergetics, *Am J Physiol*, 264, H994–H1004, 1993.

55. Y. Goto, S. Futaki, O. Kawaguchi, K. Hata, T. Takasago, A. Saeki, T. Nishioka, T. W. Taylor, and H. Suga, Coupling between regional myocardial oxygen consumption and contraction under altered preload and afterload, *J Am Coll Cardiol*, 21, 1522–1531, 1993.

56. M. Sugawara, Y. Kondoh, and K. Nakano, Normalization of Emax and PVA, in *Cardiac Energetics: From Emax to Pressure-Volume Area*, M. M. LeWinter, H. Suga, and M. W. Watkins, Eds. Boston: Kluwer Academic Publishers, 1995, pp. 65–78.

57. T. Delhaas, T. Arts, F. W. Prinzen, and R. S. Reneman, Regional fibre stress-fibre strain area as an estimate of regional blood flow and oxygen demand in the canine heart, *J Physiol (Lond)*, 477, 481–496, 1994.

58. M. Vornanen, Maximum heart rate of sorcine shrews: Correlation with contractile properties and myosin composition, *Am J Physiol*, 31, R842–RR851, 1992.

59. J. P. Holt, E. A. Rhode, S. A. Peoples, and H. Kines, Left ventricular function in mammals of greatly different size, *Circ Res*, 10, 798–806, 1962.

60. D. S. Loiselle and C. L. Gibbs, Species differences in cardiac energetics, *Am J Physiol*, 237(1), H90–H98, 1979.

61. J. C. Gilbert and S. A. Glantz, Determinants of left ventricular filling and of the diastolic pressure-volume relation, *Circ Res*, 64, 827–852, 1989.

62. W. H. Gaasch and M. M. LeWinter, *Left Ventricular Diastolic Dysfunction and Heart Failure*. Philadelphia: Lea & Febiger, 1994.

63. S. A. Glantz, G. A. Misbach, W. Y. Moores, D. G. Mathey, J. Lekuen, D. F. Stowe, W. W. Parmley, and J. V. Tyberg, The pericardium substantially affects the left ventricular diastolic pressure-volume relationship in the dog, *Circ Res*, 42, 433–441, 1978.

64. S. A. Glantz and W. W. Parmley, Factors which affect the diastolic pressure-volume curve, *Circ Res*, 42, 171–180, 1978.

65. B. K. Slinker and S. A. Glantz, End-systolic and end-diastolic ventricular interaction, *Am J Physiol*, 251, H1062–H1075, 1986.

66. I. Mirsky and J. S. Rankin, The effects of geometry, elasticity, and external pressures on the diastolic pressure-volume and stiffness-stress relations: How important is the pericardium?, *Circ Res*, 44, 601–611, 1979.

67. M. C. Lee, Y. C. Fung, R. Shabetai, and M. M. LeWinter, Biaxial mechanical properties of human pericardium and canine comparisons, *Am J Physiol*, 253, H75–H82, 1987.

68. C. A. Gibbons-Kroeker, N. G. Shrive, I. Belenkie, and J. V. Tyberg, Pericardium modulates left and right ventricular stroke volumes to compensate for sudden changes in atrial volume, *Am J Physiol Heart Circ Physiol*, 284, H2247–H2254, 2003.

69. K. May-Newman, J. H. Omens, R. S. Pavelec, and A. D. McCulloch, Three-dimensional transmural mechanical interaction between the coronary vasculature and passive myocardium in the dog, *Circ Res*, 74, 1166–1178, 1994.

70. P. F. Salisbury, C. E. Cross, and P. A. Rieben, Influence of coronary artery pressure upon myocardial elasticity, *Circ Res*, 8, 794–800, 1960.

71. D. M. Bers, *Excitation-Contraction Coupling and Cardiac Contractile Force*. Dordrecht: Kluwer, 1991.

72. H. E. D. J. ter Keurs, W. H. Rijnsburger, R. van Heuningen, and M. J. Nagelsmit, Tension development and sarcomere length in rat cardiac trabeculae: Evidence of length-dependent activation, *Circ Res*, 46, 703–713, 1980.

73. J. C. Rüegg, *Calcium in Muscle Activation: A Comparative Approach*, 2nd ed. vol. 19. Berlin: Springer-Verlag, 1988.

74. A. Tözeren, Continuum rheology of muscle contraction and its application to cardiac contractility, *Biophys J*, 47, 303–309, 1985.

75. P. J. Hunter, A. D. McCulloch, and H. E. ter Keurs, Modelling the mechanical properties of cardiac muscle, *Prog Biophys Mol Biol*, 69, 289–331, 1998.

76. P. H. Backx, W. D. Gao, M. D. Azan-Backx, and E. Marban, The relationship between contractile force and intracellular [Ca^{2+}] in intact rat cardiac trabeculae, *J Gen Physiol*, 105, 1–19, 1995.

77. J. C. Kentish, H. E. D. J. Ter Keurs, L. Ricciari, J. J. J. Bucx, and M. I. M. Noble, Comparisons between the sarcomere length-force relations of intact and skinned trabeculae from rat right ventricle, *Circ Res*, 58, 755–768, 1986.

78. D. T. Yue, E. Marban, and W. G. Wier, Relationship between force and intracellular [Ca^{2+}] in tetanized mammalian heart muscle, *J Gen Physiol*, 87, 223–242, 1986.

79. W. D. Gao, P. H. Backx, M. Azan-Backx, and E. Marban, Myofilament Ca^{2+} sensitivity in intact versus skinned rat ventricular muscle, *Circ Res*, 74, 408–415, 1994.

80. D. P. Dobesh, J. P. Konhilas, and P. P. de Tombe, Cooperative activation in cardiac muscle: Impact of sarcomere length, *Am J Physiol Heart Circ Physiol*, 282, H1055–H1062, 2002.

81. P. P. de Tombe and H. E. ter Keurs, An internal viscous element limits unloaded velocity of sarcomere shortening in rat myocardium, *J Physiol (Lond)*, 454, 619–642, 1992.

82. H. E. D. J. ter Keurs, W. H. Rijnsburger, and R. van Heuningen, Restoring forces and relaxation of rat cardiac muscle, *Eur Heart J*, 1, 67–80, 1980.

83. T. Arts, R. S. Reneman, and P. C. Veenstra, A model of the mechanics of the left ventricle, *Ann Biomed Eng*, 7, 299–318, 1979.

84. R. S. Chadwick, Mechanics of the left ventricle, *Biophys J*, 39, 279–288, 1982.

85. E. Nevo and Y. Lanir, Structural finite deformation model of the left ventricle during diastole and systole, *J Biomech Eng*, 111, 342–349, 1989.

86. T. Arts, P. C. Veenstra, and R. S. Reneman, Epicardial deformation and left ventricular wall mechanics during ejection in the dog, *Am J Physiol*, 243, H379–H390, 1982.

87. R. B. Panerai, A model of cardiac muscle mechanics and energetics, *J Biomech*, 13, 929–940, 1980.

88. A. Landesberg, V. S. Markhasin, R. Beyar, and S. Sideman, Effect of cellular inhomogeneity on cardiac tissue mechanics based on intracellular control mechanisms, *Am J Physiol*, 270, H1101–H1114, 1996.

89. A. Landesberg and S. Sideman, Coupling calcium binding to troponin C and cross-bridge cycling in skinned cardiac cells, *Am J Physiol*, 266, H1260–H1271, 1994.

90. S. P. Ma and G. I. Zahalak, A distribution-moment model of energetics in skeletal muscle [see comments], *J Biomech*, 24, 21–35, 1991.

91. F. B. Sachse, G. Seemann, K. Chaisaowong, and D. Weiss, Quantitative reconstruction of cardiac electromechanics in human myocardium: Assembly of electrophysiologic and tension generation models, *J Cardiovasc Electrophysiol*, 14, S210–S218, 2003.

92. J. J. Rice, F. Wang, D. M. Bers, and P. P. de Tombe, Approximate model of cooperative activation and crossbridge cycling in cardiac muscle using ordinary differential equations, *Biophys J*, 95, 2368–2390, 2008.

93. A. Landesberg, L. Livshitz, and H. E. Ter Keurs, The effect of sarcomere shortening velocity on force generation, analysis, and verification of models for crossbridge dynamics, *Ann Biomed Eng*, 28, 968–978, 2000.

94. S. G. Campbell, F. V. Lionetti, K. S. Campbell, and A. D. McCulloch, Coupling of adjacent tropomyosins enhances cross-bridge-mediated cooperative activation in a Markov model of the cardiac thin filament, *Biophys J*, 98, 2254–2264, 2010.

95. A. M. Gordon, E. Homsher, and M. Regnier, Regulation of contraction in striated muscle, *Physiol Rev*, 80, 853–924, 2000.

96. D. H. S. Lin and F. C. P. Yin, A multiaxial constitutive law for mammalian left ventricular myocardium in steady-state barium contracture or tetanus, *J Biomech Eng*, 120, 504–517, 1998.

97. M. Schoenberg, Geometrical factors influencing muscle force development. I. The effect of filament spacing upon axial forces, *Biophys J*, 30, 51–67, 1980.
98. G. I. Zahalak, Non-axial muscle stress and stiffness, *J Theor Biol*, 182, 59–84, 1996.
99. M. Schoenberg, Geometrical factors influencing muscle force development. II. Radial forces, *Biophys J*, 30, 69–77, 1980.
100. Y. C. Fung, *Biomechanics: Mechanical Properties of Living Tissues*, 2nd ed. New York: Springer-Verlag Inc., 1993.
101. J. G. Pinto and P. J. Patitucci, Creep in cardiac muscle, *Am J Physiol*, 232, H553–H563, 1977.
102. J. G. Pinto and P. J. Patitucci, Visco-elasticity of passive cardiac muscle, *J Biomech Eng*, 102, 57–61, 1980.
103. J. L. Emery, J. H. Omens, and A. D. McCulloch, Strain softening in rat left ventricular myocardium, *J Biomech Eng*, 119, 6–12, 1997.
104. J. L. Emery, J. H. Omens, and A. D. McCulloch, Biaxial mechanics of the passively overstretched left ventricle, *Am J Physiol*, 272, H2299–H2305, 1997.
105. L. Mullins, Effect of stretching on the properties of rubber, *J Rubber Res*, 16, 275–289, 1947.
106. H. R. Halperin, P. H. Chew, M. L. Weisfeldt, K. Sagawa, J. D. Humphrey, and F. C. P. Yin, Transverse stiffness: A method for estimation of myocardial wall stress, *Circ Res*, 61, 695–703, 1987.
107. J. D. Humphrey, R. K. Strumpf, and F. C. P. Yin, Biaxial mechanical behavior of excised ventricular epicardium, *Am J Physiol*, 259, H101–H108, 1990.
108. L. L. Demer and F. C. P. Yin, Passive biaxial mechanical properties of isolated canine myocardium, *J Physiol*, 339, 615–630, 1983.
109. F. C. P. Yin, R. K. Strumpf, P. H. Chew, and S. L. Zeger, Quantification of the mechanical properties of noncontracting canine myocardium under simultaneous biaxial loading, *J Biomech*, 20, 577–589, 1987.
110. S. Dokos, B. H. Smaill, A. A. Young, and I. J. LeGrice, Shear properties of passive ventricular myocardium, *Am J Physiol Heart Circ Physiol*, 283, H2650–H2659, 2002.
111. V. P. Novak, F. C. P. Yin, and J. D. Humphrey, Regional mechanical properties of passive myocardium, *J Biomech*, 27, 403–412, 1994.
112. J. H. Omens, D. A. MacKenna, and A. D. McCulloch, Measurement of strain and analysis of stress in resting rat left ventricular myocardium, *J Biomech*, 26, 665–676, 1993.
113. L. Glass, P. Hunter, and A. D. McCulloch, Theory of heart: Biomechanics, biophysics and nonlinear dynamics of cardiac function, in *Institute for Nonlinear Science*, H. Abarbanel, Ed. New York: Springer-Verlag, 1991.
114. J. D. Humphrey and F. C. P. Yin, A new constitutive formulation for characterizing the mechanical behavior of soft tissues, *Biophys J*, 52, 563–570, 1987.
115. I.-E. Lin and L. A. Taber, Mechanical effects of looping in the embryonic chick heart, *J Biomech*, 27, 311–321, 1994.
116. J. M. Guccione, A. D. McCulloch, and L. K. Waldman, Passive material properties of intact ventricular myocardium determined from a cylindrical model, *J Biomech Eng*, 113, 42–55, 1991.
117. J. H. Omens, D. A. MacKenna, and A. D. McCulloch, Measurement of two-dimensional strain and analysis of stress in the arrested rat left ventricle, *Adv Bioeng*, BED-20, 635–638, 1991.
118. J. D. Humphrey, R. K. Strumpf, and F. C. P. Yin, Determination of a constitutive relation for passive myocardium: I. A New functional form, *J Biomech Eng*, 112, 333–339, 1990.
119. K. B. Gupta, M. B. Ratcliff, M. A. Fallert, L. H. Edmunds, Jr, and D. K. Bogen, Changes in passive mechanical stiffness of myocardial tissue with aneurysm formation, *Circulation*, 89, 2315–2326, 1994.
120. G. A. Holzapfel and R. W. Ogden, Constitutive modelling of passive myocardium: A structurally based framework for material characterization, *Philos Transact A Math Phys Eng Sci*, 367, 3445–3475, 2009.
121. J. H. Omens and Y. C. Fung, Residual strain in rat left ventricle, *Circ Res*, 66, 37–45, 1990.

122. E. K. Rodriguez, J. H. Omens, L. K. Waldman, and A. D. McCulloch, Effect of residual stress on transmural sarcomere length distribution in rat left ventricle, *Am J Physiol,* 264, H1048–H1056, 1993.

123. K. Costa, K. May-Newman, D. Farr, W. O'Dell, A. McCulloch, and J. Omens, Three-dimensional residual strain in canine mid-anterior left ventricle, *Am J Physiol,* 273, H1968–H1976, 1997.

124. R. Skalak, G. Dasgupta, M. Moss, E. Otten, P. Dullemeijer, and H. Vilmann, Analytical description of growth, *J Theor Biol,* 94, 555–577, 1982.

125. E. K. Rodriguez, A. Hoger, and A. D. McCulloch, Stress-dependent finite growth in soft elastic tissues, *J Biomech,* 27, 455–467, 1994.

126. E. O. Feigl, G. A. Simon, and D. L. Fry, Auxotonic and isometric cardiac force transducers, *J Appl Physiol,* 23, 597–600, 1967.

127. R. M. Huisman, G. Elzinga, N. Westerhof, and P. Sipkema, Measurement of left ventricular wall stress, *Cardiovasc Res,* 14, 142–153, 1980.

128. F. C. P. Yin, Ventricular wall stress, *Circ Res,* 49, 829–842, 1981.

129. F. C. P. Yin, Applications of the finite-element method to ventricular mechanics, *CRC Crit Rev Biomed Eng,* 12, 311–342, 1985.

130. F. J. Villarreal, L. K. Waldman, and W. Y. W. Lew, Technique for measuring regional two-dimensional finite strains in canine left ventricle, *Circ Res,* 62, 711–721, 1988.

131. N. F. Osman and J. L. Prince, Visualizing myocardial function using HARP MRI, *Phys Med Biol,* 45, 1665, 2000.

132. T. Kawagishi, Speckle tracking for assessment of cardiac motion and dyssynchrony, *Echocardiography,* 25, 1167–1171, 2008.

133. N. B. Ingels, Jr, G. T. Daughters, II, E. B. Stinson, and E. L. Alderman, Measurement of midwall myocardial dynamics in intact man by radiography of surgically implanted markers, *Circulation,* 52, 859–867, 1975.

134. G. D. Meier, A. A. Bove, W. P. Santamore, and P. R. Lynch, Contractile function in canine right ventricle, *Am J Physiol,* 239, H794–H804, 1980.

135. G. D. Meier, M. C. Ziskin, W. P. Santamore, and A. A. Bove, Kinematics of the beating heart, *IEEE Trans Biomed Eng,* 27, 319–329, 1980.

136. A. D. McCulloch and J. H. Omens, Non-homogeneous analysis of three-dimensional transmural finite deformations in canine ventricular myocardium, *J Biomech,* 24, 539–548, 1991.

137. C. Leclercq, O. Faris, R. Tunin, J. Johnson, R. Kato, F. Evans, J. Spinelli, H. Halperin, E. McVeigh, and D. A. Kass, Systolic improvement and mechanical resynchronization does not require electrical synchrony in the dilated failing heart with left bundle-branch block, *Circulation,* 106, 1760–1763, 2002.

138. R. C. P. Kerckhoffs, J. Lumens, K. Vernooy, J. H. Omens, L. J. Mulligan, T. Delhaas, T. Arts, A. D. McCulloch, and F. W. Prinzen, Cardiac Resynchronization: Insight from experimental and computational models, *Progr Biophys Mol Biol,* 97, 543–561, 2008.

139. R. C. P. Kerckhoffs, J. H. Omens, A. D. McCulloch, and L. J. Mulligan, Ventricular dilation and electrical dyssynchrony synergistically increase regional mechanical non-uniformity but not mechanical dyssynchrony: A computational model, *Circulation: Heart Fail,* 3, 528–536, 2010.

140. T. P. Usyk and A. D. McCulloch, Electromechanical model of cardiac resynchronization in the dilated failing heart with left bundle branch block, *J Electrocardiol,* 36, 57–61, 2003.

141. R. C. Kerckhoffs, A. D. McCulloch, J. H. Omens, and L. J. Mulligan, Effects of biventricular pacing and scar size in a computational model of the failing heart with left bundle branch block, *Med Image Anal,* 13, 362–369, 2009.

142. V. Gurev, J. Constantino, J. J. Rice, and N. A. Trayanova, Distribution of electromechanical delay in the heart: Insights from a three-dimensional electromechanical model, 99, 745–754, 2010.

143. M. L. Neal and R. Kerckhoffs, Current progress in patient-specific modeling, *Brief Bioinform,* 11, 111–126, 2010.

144. R. C. P. Kerckhoffs, *Patient Specific Modeling of the Cardiovascular System: Technology-Driven Personalized Medicine,* New York, NY: Springer, 2010, p. 265.

145. J. Southern, J. Pitt-Francis, J. Whiteley, D. Stokeley, H. Kobashi, R. Nobes, Y. Kadooka, and D. Gavaghan, Multi-scale computational modelling in biology and physiology, *Prog Biophys Mol Biol,* 96, 60–89, 2008.

146. L. Antiga, M. Piccinelli, L. Botti, B. Ene-Iordache, A. Remuzzi, and D. Steinman, An image-based modeling framework for patient-specific computational hemodynamics, *Med Biol Eng Comput,* 46, 1097–1112, 2008.

147. I. Medugorac, Myocardial collagen in different forms of hypertrophy in the rat, *Res Exp Med (Berl),* 177, 201–211, 1980.

148. K. T. Weber, J. S. Janicki, S. G. Shroff, R. Pick, R. M. Chen, and R. I. Bashey, Collagen remodeling of the pressure-overloaded, hypertrophied nonhuman primate myocardium, *Circ Res,* 62, 757–765, 1988.

149. J. E. Jalil, C. W. Doering, J. S. Janicki, R. Pick, W. A. Clark, C. Abrahams, and K. T. Weber, Structural vs. contractile protein remodeling and myocardial stiffness in hypertrophied rat left ventricle, *J Mol Cell Cardiol,* 20, 1179–1187, 1988.

150. D. Mukherjee and S. Sen, Collagen phenotypes during development and regression of myocardial hypertrophy in spontaneously hypertensive rats, *Circ Res,* 67, 1474–1480, 1990.

151. J. Harper, E. Harper, and J. W. Covell, Collagen characterization in volume-overload- and pressure-overload-induced cardiac hypertrophy in minipigs, *Am J Physiol,* 265, H434–H438, 1993.

152. J. H. Omens, D. E. Milkes, and J. W. Covell, Effects of pressure overload on the passive mechanics of the rat left ventricle, *Ann Biomed Eng,* 23, 152–163, 1995.

153. F. Contard, V. Koteliansky, F. Marotte, I. Dubus, L. Rappaport, and J. L. Samuel, Specific alterations in the distribution of extracellular matrix components within rat myocardium during the development of pressure overload, *Lab Invest,* 64, 65–75, 1991.

154. M. A. Silver, R. Pick, C. G. Brilla, J. E. Jalil, J. S. Janicki, and K. T. Weber, Reactive and reparative fibrillar collagen remodelling in the hypertrophied rat left ventricle: Two experimental models of myocardial fibrosis, *Cardiovasc Res,* 24, 741–747, 1990.

155. J. B. Michel, J. L. Salzmann, M. Ossondo Nlom, P. Bruneval, D. Barres, and J. P. Camilleri, Morphometric analysis of collagen network and plasma perfused capillary bed in the myocardium of rats during evolution of cardiac hypertrophy, *Basic Res Cardiol,* 81, 142–154, 1986.

156. D. S. Iimoto, J. W. Covell, and E. Harper, Increase in crosslinking of type I and type III collagens associated with volume overload hypertrophy, *Circ Res,* 63, 399–408, 1988.

157. K. T. Weber, R. Pick, M. A. Silver, G. W. Moe, J. S. Janicki, I. H. Zucker, and P. W. Armstrong, Fibrillar collagen and remodeling of dilated canine left ventricle, *Circulation,* 82, 1387–401, 1990.

158. W. J. Corin, T. Murakami, E. S. Monrad, O. M. Hess, and H. P. Krayenbuehl, Left ventricular passive diastolic properties in chronic mitral regurgitation, *Circulation,* 83, 97–807, 1991.

159. P. Whittaker, D. R. Boughner, R. A. Kloner, and K. Przyklenk, Stunned myocardium and myocardial collagen damage: Differential effects of single and repeated occlusions, *Am Heart J,* 121, 434–441, 1991.

160. M. Zhao, H. Zhang, T. F. Robinson, S. M. Factor, E. H. Sonnenblick, and C. Eng, Profound structural alterations of the extracellular collagen matrix in postischemic dysfunctional (stunned) but viable myocardium, *J Am Coll Cardiol,* 10, 1322–1334, 1987.

161. J. S. Forrester, G. Diamond, W. W. Parmley, and H. J. C. Swan, Early increase in left ventricular compliance after myocardial infarction, *J Clin Invest,* 51, 598–603, 1972.

162. F. A. Pirzada, E. A. Ekong, P. S. Vokonas, C. S. Apstein, and W. B. Hood, Jr, Experimental myocardial infarction XIII. Sequential changes in left ventricular pressure-length relationships in the acute phase, *Circulation,* 53, 970–975, 1976.

163. S. Takahashi, A. C. Barry, and S. M. Factor, Collagen degradation in ischaemic rat hearts, *Biochem J,* 265, 233–241, 1990.

164. R. H. Charney, S. Takahashi, M. Zhao, E. H. Sonnenblick, and C. Eng, Collagen loss in the stunned myocardium, *Circulation*, 85, 1483–1490, 1992.

165. C. M. Connelly, W. M. Vogel, A. W. Wiegner, E. L. Osmers, O. H. Bing, R. A. Kloner, D. M. Dunn-Lanchantin, C. Franzblau, and C. S. Apstein, Effects of reperfusion after coronary artery occlusion on post-infarction scar tissue, *Circ Res*, 57, 562–77, 1985.

166. B. I. Jugdutt and R. W. Amy, Healing after myocardial infarction in the dog: Changes in infarct hydroxyproline and topography, *J Am Coll Cardiol*, 7, 91–102, 1986.

167. P. Whittaker, D. R. Boughner, and R. A. Kloner, Analysis of healing after myocardial infarction using polarized light microscopy, *Am J Pathol*, 134, 879–893, 1989.

168. L. T. Jensen, K. Hørslev-Petersen, P. Toft, K. D. Bentsen, P. Grande, E. E. Simonsen, and I. Lorenzen, Serum aminoterminal type III procollagen peptide reflects repair after acute myocardial infarction, *Circulation*, 81, 52–57, 1990.

169. J. M. Pfeffer, M. A. Pfeffer, P. J. Fletcher, and E. Braunwald, Progressive ventricular remodeling in rat with myocardial infarction, *Am J Physiol*, 260, H1406–H1414, 1991.

170. P. Whittaker, D. R. Boughner, and R. A. Kloner, Role of collagen in acute myocardial infarct expansion, *Circulation*, 84, 2123–2134, 1991.

171. J. W. Holmes, H. Yamashita, L. K. Waldman, and J. W. Covell, Scar remodeling and transmural deformation after infarction in the pig, *Circulation*, 90, 411–420, 1994.

172. M. Eghbali, T. F. Robinson, S. Seifter, and O. O. Blumenfeld, Collagen accumulation in heart ventricles as a function of growth and aging, *Cardiovasc Res*, 23, 723–729, 1989.

173. I. Medugorac and R. Jacob, Characterisation of left ventricular collagen in the rat, *Cardiovasc Res*, 17, 15–21, 1983.

174. T. K. Borg, W. F. Ranson, F. A. Moslehy, and J. B. Caulfield, Structural basis of ventricular stiffness, *Lab Invest*, 44, 49–54, 1981.

175. P. Anversa, E. Puntillo, P. Nikitin, G. Olivetti, J. M. Capasso, and E. H. Sonnenblick, Effects of age on mechanical and structural properties of myocardium of Fischer 344 rats, *Am J Physiol*, 256, H1440–H1449, 1989.

176. S. G. Campbell, *The Role of Regulatory Light Chain Phosphorylation in Left Ventricular Function*, La Jolla, CA: University of California San Diego, 2010, p. 215.

177. J. Ross Jr, E. H. Sonnenblick, J. W. Covell, G. A. Kaiser, and D. Spiro, The architecture of the heart in systole and diastole: Technique of rapid fixation and analysis of left ventricular geometry, *Circ Res*, 21, 409–421, 1967.

178. W. Grossman, Cardiac hypertrophy: Useful adaptation or pathologic process? *Am J Med*, 69, 576–583, 1980.

179. W. Grossman, D. Jones, and L. P. McLaurin, Wall stress and patterns of hypertrophy in the human left ventricle, *J Clin Invest*, 56, 56–64, 1975.

180. R. H. Charney, S. Takahashi, M. Zhao, E. H. Sonnenblick, and C. Eng, Collagen loss in the stunned myocardium, *Circulation*, 85, 1483–1490, 1992.

181. S. A. Niederer, P. J. Hunter, and N. P. Smith, A quantitative analysis of cardiac myocyte relaxation: A simulation study, *Biophys J* 90, 1697–722, 2000.

16

Heart Valve Dynamics

Choon Hwai Yap
*Georgia Institute of
Technology*

Erin Spinner
*Georgia Institute of
Technology*

Muralidhar Padala
*Emory University School of
Medicine*

Ajit P. Yoganathan
*Georgia Institute of
Technology*

16.1   Introduction 16-1
16.2   Aortic Valve 16-3
        Valve Structure • Valve Function • Valve Disease and Treatment
16.3   Pulmonary Valve 16-10
        Valve Structure • Valve Function
16.4   Mitral Valve 16-12
        Valve Structure • Valve Function • Disease of the Mitral Valve and
        Treatment
16.5   Tricuspid Valve... 16-21
        Valve Structure • Valve Function • Disease of the Tricuspid Valve
        and Treatment
References.. 16-24

16.1 Introduction

The heart has four valves (Figure 16.1), which maintain unidirectional blood flow through the heart. They are classified as atrioventricular valves or semilunar valves, depending on their location. The atrioventricular valves are the tricuspid and mitral valves, and the semilunar valves are the pulmonary and aortic valves. The atrioventricular valves control the blood flow entering the ventricles from the atria, and the semilunar valves maintain forward flow from the ventricles to the lungs or distal organs. On the right side of the heart, the tricuspid valve (TV) controls the flow of deoxygenated blood from the right atrium into the right ventricle, and the pulmonary valve maintains forward flow from the right ventricle into the lungs. On the left side, the mitral valve (MV) controls the flow of oxygenated blood from the left atrium into the left ventricle, and the aortic valve maintains forward flow from the left ventricle to the distal organs.

Heart valve function is primarily governed by the pressure gradients across the valves during different cardiac phases, although other active mechanisms have been implicated. During diastole, the ventricular filling phase, the mitral and tricuspid valves open due to higher atrial pressure than the pressure in the relaxed ventricle, thus allowing diastolic filling of both the ventricles. The aortic and pulmonary valves are closed in this phase due to higher pressure in the aorta and pulmonary artery, respectively. Next, as the ventricles contract, ventricular pressure builds up, reaching first the pressure required for closing the atrioventricular valves, and then the pressure required to open the semilunar valves. The period of build up between these two pressures is the isovolumetric contraction phase, where all four valves are closed. During systole, high pressures in the ventricles open the aortic and pulmonary valves, allowing ejection of blood into the arterial tree and the lungs, respectively. Following this, the ventricles relax, reducing pressures, first, to that slightly lower than in the arteries, when the semilunar valves close, and then second, to that slightly lower than that in the atria, when the atrioventricular valves open. The period of reduction of pressures between these two points is known as the isovolumetric

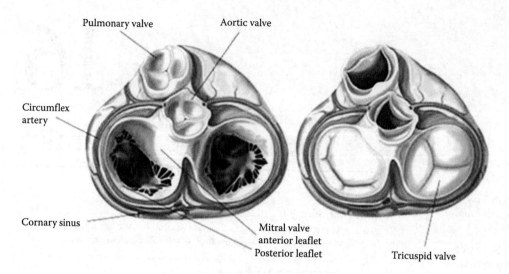

FIGURE 16.1 Superior, short-axis view of the heart showing the heart valves and their anatomies.

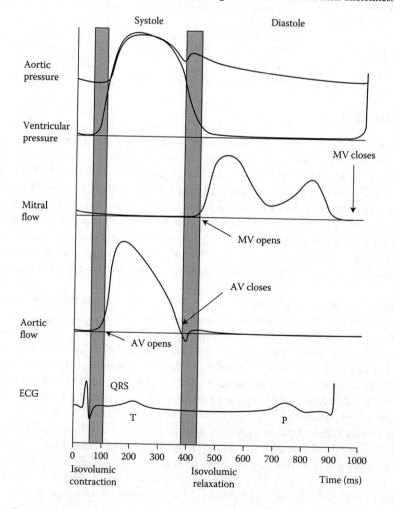

FIGURE 16.2 Typical pressure and flow curve for aortic and mitral valve.

relaxation, when, again, all four valves are closed. The typical pressure and flow curves and the relative durations of all the phases in the cardiac cycle for the aortic and mitral valves are shown in Figure 16.2.

When closed, the pulmonic and tricuspid valves withstand a pressure of approximately 30 mmHg. The closing pressures on the left side of the heart are much higher. The aortic valve withstands pressures of approximately 100 mmHg, while the MV closes against pressures up to 150 mmHg. Diseases of the valves are more prevalent on the left side of the heart than the right side (Lloyd-Jones et al., 2010).

16.2 Aortic Valve

16.2.1 Valve Structure

16.2.1.1 Anatomy

The aortic valve is composed of three semilunar cusps, or leaflets, within the aortic root, which is the base of the aorta abutting the heart. The inferior base of the leaflet is connected to the annulus, which is a fibrous ring embedded in the fibers of the ventricular septum and the anterior leaflet of the MV. The superior base of the leaflet is connected to the valve commissure. The annulus of the aortic valve separates the aorta from the left ventricle, and superior to this ring are bulges in the wall known as the sinuses of Valsalva, or aortic sinuses. Each bulge is aligned with the center of a specific valve leaflet, and the valve leaflets and corresponding sinuses are named according to their anatomical location. The top of the sinus, where it transitions to the tube-like ascending aorta, is termed the sino-tubular junction, and the portion of the aorta between the aortic valve annulus and the sino-tubular junction is known as the aortic root. Two of the aortic sinuses give rise to coronary arteries that branch off the aorta, providing blood flow to the heart itself. The right coronary artery is based at the right or right anterior sinus, the left coronary artery exits the left or left posterior sinus, and the third sinus is called the noncoronary or right posterior sinus. The coronary orifice on the walls of the aortic root has been reported to exhibit variability in location, with a substantial proportion of people having the orifice at or above the sino-tubular junction instead of within the sinus (Muriago et al., 1997). The three valve leaflets are named left coronary leaflet, right coronary leaflet, and noncoronary leaflet due to their anatomical association with the left sinus, the right sinus, and the posterior sinus, and according to the presence or absence of coronaries ostia behind them. Figure 16.3 also shows the configuration of the normal aortic sinuses and valve in the closed position, as well as the average dimensions of various structures in the aortic root, measured from molds of human samples.

The leaflets of the aortic valve show variable dimensions. The posterior leaflet tends to be thicker, have a larger surface area, and weigh more than the right or left coronary leaflets (Silver and Roberts, 1985, Sahasakul et al., 1988), and the average width of the right coronary leaflet is greater than that of the other two (Vollebergh and Becker, 1977). Because the lengths of the aortic valve leaflets are greater than the annular radius, a small overlap of tissue from each leaflet protrudes and forms a coaptation surface within the aorta when the valve is closed (Emery and Arom, 1991). This overlapped tissue, called the lunula, helps to ensure that the valve is sealed.

Each of the aortic valve leaflets is lined with endothelial cells and is composed of collagen, elastin, proteoglycans, protein, polysaccharides, and interstitial cells in a three-layered structure (Figure 16.4). The layer facing the aorta is termed the fibrosa and is the major fibrous layer within the leaflet, and consists mainly of trunk collagen bundle chords in the circumferential direction, interlaced with radially aligned elastin fibers (Vesely and Lozon, 1993). The layer covering the ventricular side of the valve is a thin layer called the ventricularis and is composed of elastin fibers interspersed with some collagen. The ventricularis presents a very smooth surface to the flow of blood (Christie, 1992), while the fibrosa surface is visibly undulating under the microscope. The central portion of the valve, called the spongiosa, contains variable loose connective tissue and proteins, has reduced amount of protein fibers, and is normally not vascularized. It is thought that the semifluid nature of the spongiosa provides the valve leaflet with deformability, allowing the exterior layers of fibers to slide over each other during bending and stretching. Further, the spongiosa layer provides damping to the leaflets to avoid

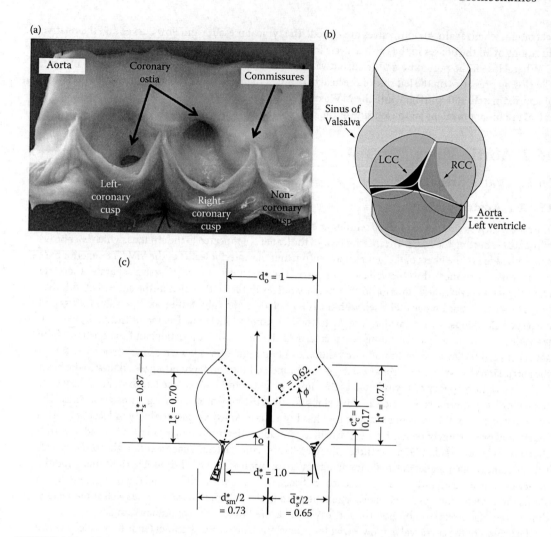

FIGURE 16.3 (a) An excised porcine aortic valve showing (from left to right) the left coronary, right coronary, and noncoronary cusps. The sinuses of Valsalva and the ostia leading to the coronary arteries are also visible. (b) The aortic sinus and valve in the closed position. (c) Dimensions of the aortic valve measured from mold of human samples, expressed as ratios of the outflow tract annulus diameter. (Adapted from Swanson, M. and Clark, R. E. 1974. *Circ Res*, 35, 871–882.)

deformation oscillations (Grande-Allen et al., 2001, 2003, 2007). The collagen fibers within the fibrosa and ventricularis are unorganized in the unstressed state, but when a stress is applied, they become oriented primarily in the circumferential (or width) direction (Christie, 1992, Thubrikar, 1990). The amount of transvalvular pressure required to align the collagen fibers from the relaxed state has been reported to be as low as 1 mmHg (Sacks et al., 1998).

16.2.1.2 Mechanical Properties

Like most biological tissues, the aortic valve leaflets are anisotropic, inhomogeneous, and viscoelastic. The collagen fibers within each leaflet are mostly aligned along the circumferential direction. Vesely and Noseworthy found that both the ventricularis and fibrosa were stiffer in the circumferential direction than in the radial direction (Vesely and Noseworthy, 1992). However, the ventricularis was more extensible radially than circumferentially while the fibrosa had uniform extensibility

(a)   (b)

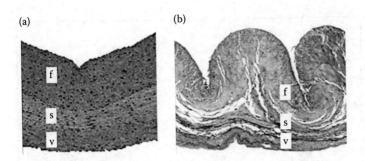

FIGURE 16.4 (a) H&E stain of a cross section of the aortic valve. (Adapted from Hilbert, S. L. et al. 1999. *J Thorac Cardiovasc Surg*, 117, 454–462.) (b) Movat Pentachrome stain of a cross section of the aortic valve showing the three distinct layers with different composition. "f," "s," and "v" indicate fibrosa, spongiosa, and ventricularis, respectively. (Adapted from Schenke-Layland, K. et al. 2009. *Eur Heart J*, 30, 2254–2265.)

in both directions. Elastin fibers are present at a lesser concentration than collagen and are mostly oriented radially. This fiber structure accounts for the anisotropic properties of the valve. The variation in thickness and composition across the leaflets is responsible for their inhomogeneous material properties. Although the aortic valve leaflet as a whole is asymmetric in its distensibility, the basal region tends to be relatively isotropic while the central region shows the greatest degree of anisotropy (Lo and Vesely, 1995). Scott and Vesely (1996) have shown that the elastin in the ventricularis consists of continuous amorphous sheets or compact meshes while elastin in the fibrosa consists of complex arrays of large tubes that extend circumferentially across the leaflet. These tubes may surround the large circumferential collagen bundles in the fibrosa. Mechanical testing of elastin structures from the fibrosa and ventricularis separately have shown that the purpose of elastin in the aortic valve leaflet is to maintain a specific collagen fiber configuration and return the fibers to that state during cyclic loading (Vesely, 1998).

Billiar et al. tested porcine aortic valve leaflets and found that their response curve was similar to those of collagen fibers, with an exponential increase in stress with strain (Billiar and Sacks, 2000). With increasing stress, the leaflets exhibit three distinct responses consecutively, starting a low-stiffness "toe" region, moving on to a transitional "heel" region, and a high-stiffness "linear" region (Figure 16.5). This is in accordance to the fiber architecture of the valve leaflet: the "toe" region represents the uncrimping of the collagen fiber curls and the elastic response of elastins, while the "linear" region represents the stretching of already straightened collagen fibers (Sacks et al., 1998). As expected, the leaflet as a whole was found to have higher stiffness in the circumferential direction than in the radial direction. Further, dynamic testing has revealed that at physiological loading rates, the leaflet material behaves elastically although the leaflets are viscoelastic in nature (Doehring et al., 2004, Stella et al., 2007). The leaflet is capable of undergoing large, rapid anisotropic strains in response to transvalvular pressures and return to its original configuration when unloaded with little hysteresis and creep, leading to its association with the term "quasi-elastic." Performing engineering analysis of the valve structures, Christie et al. concluded that stress in the leaflets in the circumferential direction is the primary load-bearing element, which is in line with the presence of collagen fiber bundles oriented circumferentially (Christie, 1992). Radial stress was found to be small compared to circumferential stress in the closed valve.

In addition to the collagen and elastin, clusters of lipids have been observed in the central spongiosa of porcine aortic valves. Vesely et al. (1994) have shown that the lipids tend to be concentrated at the base of the valve leaflets while the coaptation regions and free edges of the leaflets tend to be devoid of these lipids. In addition, the spatial distribution of the lipids within the spongiosa layer of the aortic leaflets corresponds to areas in which calcification is commonly observed on bioprosthetic valves, suggesting

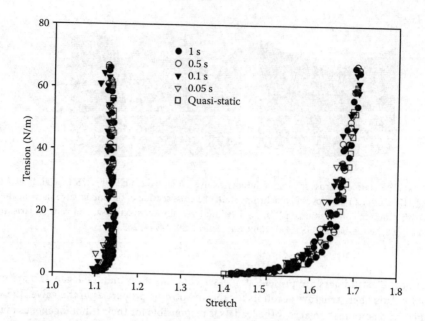

FIGURE 16.5 Mechanical response of fresh aortic valve leaflet to equi-biaxial stress at different loading rates, demonstrating the anisotropy of the tissue as well as the insensitivity of the tissue to loading rates. (Adapted from Stella, J. A., Liao, J., and Sacks, M. S. 2007. *J Biomech*, 40, 3169–3177.)

that these lipid clusters may be potential nucleation sites for calcification. In contrast, pulmonic leaflets showed a substantially lower incidence of lipids (Dunmore-Buyze et al., 1995).

16.2.2 Valve Function

16.2.2.1 Aortic Root Dynamics

During the cardiac cycle, the heart undergoes translation and rotation due to its own contraction pattern. As a result, the base of the aortic valve varies in size and also translates and twists. The dynamics of the aortic root are a result of the combination of passive response to pressures on both sides of the valve as well as active contractions of the muscular shelf on the anterio-medial segment of the annulus. Using marker fluoroscopy in sheeps, Dagum et al. (1999) characterized the aortic root motion. During isovolumetric contraction, the annulus and sino-tubular junction undergo rapid circumferential expansion and the aortic root increases in longitudinal length without shear or torsion. During the ejection phase, the annulus undergoes circumferential contraction whereas the sino-tubular junction continues to expand, and the aortic root undergoes nonuniform shearing, which results in torsional deformation. During the isovolumetric contraction, the aortic root undergoes further circumferential contraction at both the annulus and the sino-tubular junction, and experiences further shearing and torsional deformation, as well as longitudinal compression. During early diastole, the annulus and sino-tubular junction recoils from its dynamically loaded configuration by expanding, and the root is elongated and untwisted from its motion during the other phases. Torsional deformation has been described to be nonuniform over the three sinus segments.

16.2.2.2 Valve Leaflet Dynamics

The systolic motion of the aortic valve can be described in three phases: the rapid opening phase, the slow closing phase, and the rapid closing phase. The rapid opening phase lasts for about 60 ms, when leaflets rapidly open at an average speed of 20 cm/s, the valve opens to the fullest extent, and blood accelerates through the valve. The slow closing phase, which lasts for 330 ms, is when the bulk of ejection occurs, and valve leaflets move approximately 13 mm. The rapid closing phase occurs during late systole, lasts for 40 ms, and witnesses leaflet speed of 26 cm/s (Leyh et al., 1999).

Earlier experiments in measuring the physiologic deformations of the aortic valve leaflets involve using marker fluoroscopy, in which the aortic valve leaflets were surgically tagged with radio-opaque markers and imaged with high-speed x-rays (Thubrikar, 1990). The leaflets were found to be longer during diastole than systole in both the radial and circumferential direction, as is expected due to the high transvalvular pressure across the closed aortic valve stretching the leaflets. Yap et al. (2010) characterized the deformational dynamics of the aortic valve leaflets *in vitro* at high spatial and temporal resolution, and showed the average diastolic stretch ratio of the valve to be 15–18% in the circumferential direction and 45–54% in the radial direction at the base and belly regions of the valve. It was found during diastole that the leaflets rapidly load up to the peak stretch ratios, and plateau at approximately the same stretch ratio until the rapid unloading phase at the end of diastole. During systole, however, the valve stretches slightly in the radial direction (to a lesser extent than during diastole) due to drag forces induced by forward flow, and it compresses slightly in the circumferential direction due to Poisson's effect of radial stretch. It has been reasoned that the stretching of the valve leaflets during diastole is useful in allowing leaflets to come together and achieving proper coaptation, and that the shortening of the leaflets during systole reduces obstruction of the aorta during the ejection of blood (Christie, 1992).

Drastic changes in the valve area described above are results of the valve reacting to the stresses in a passive manner. It is currently unclear if active contractions of aortic valve cells play a role in the deformation dynamics of the leaflets. Active contractions of aortic valve cells have been studied and were found to be able to impart very small forces at physiological biochemical stimulations (Kershaw et al., 2004). On the other hand, stimulants such as serotonin and endothelin were found to alter the stiffness of valve leaflets at the posttransitional zone of the response curve (high-stiffness zone) significantly (El-Hamamsy et al., 2009). It is unclear if the stiffness of the pretransitional zone (low-stiffness zone) is altered, which is the main determinant of the amount of stretch suffered by the leaflets under physiologic loads. Active cell contraction has also been observed to impart additional bending stiffness to the valve leaflet (Merryman et al., 2006). This is an important consideration because the aortic valve leaflet experiences substantial bending during the cardiac cycle: valve leaflet is convex curved toward the ventricle during diastole and curved toward the sinus when open, with the base of the valve leaflet bent to allow the opening. It is hypothesized that leaflet cell contractions is a regulatory mechanism of leaflet kinematics, and biochemical cues are used to control leaflet stiffness tone to influence function.

16.2.2.3 Valve Fluid Dynamics

During the fast opening phase of the valve leaflet, blood is rapidly accelerating through the valve, and peak velocity is reached during the first third of systole. Thereafter, flow begins to decelerate to zero at the end of systole under adverse pressure gradient. The adverse pressure gradient that is developed affects the low momentum fluid near the wall of the aorta more than that at the center; this causes reverse flow into the sinus region (Reul and Talukdar, 1979). The systolic pressure gradient required to accelerate blood through the aortic valve is on the order of a few millimeters of mercury. However, the diastolic pressure difference reaches 80 mmHg across the closed valve in normal individuals.

The aortic valve closes during the end of systole with very little reverse flow through the valve, estimated to be about 2.6 mL per beat (Erasmi et al., 2005). This is often attributed to the influence of the vortical flow in the sinuses behind the leaflets, which is induced by forward flow through the valve during systole. The function of these vortices was first described by Leonardo da Vinci in 1513, and they have been extensively investigated primarily through the use of *in vitro* models (Bellhouse and Reid, 1969, Reul and Talukdar, 1979). More recently, phase contrast magnetic resonance imaging velocity measurements have provided evidence of their presence in humans, as shown in Figure 16.6 (Kvitting et al., 2004, Markl et al., 2005). It has been hypothesized that these vortices create a transverse pressure

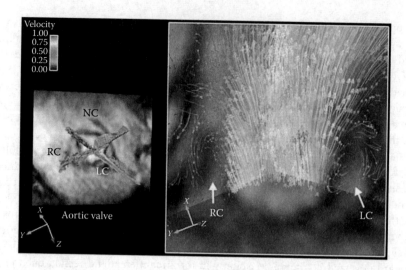

FIGURE 16.6 Three-directional velocity vectors along two-dimensional planes, showing the vortices in the right and left coronary sinuses, obtained through phase contrast magnetic resonance imaging of a healthy subject. (From Markl, M. et al. 2005. *J Thorac Cardiovasc Surg,* 130, 456–463.)

difference that pushes the leaflets toward the center of the aorta and each other at the end of systole, thereby helping with the valve closing process and minimizing regurgitation of blood. However, *in vitro* work showed that the axial pressure difference alone is enough to close the valve (Reul and Talukdar, 1979). Without the sinus vortices, the valve still closes, but the closure is not as quick as when the vortices are present, and the velocity of the leaflet closure motion is not as rapid (Leyh et al., 1999).

The parameters that describe the normal blood flow through the aortic valve are the velocity profile, time course of the blood velocity or flow, and magnitude of the peak velocity. These are influenced in part by the pressure difference between the ventricle and aorta and by the geometry of the aortic valve complex. As seen in Figure 16.7, the velocity profile at the level of the aortic valve annulus is relatively flat. However, there is usually a slight skew toward the septal wall (less than 10% of the center-line velocity), which is caused by the orientation of the aortic valve relative to the long axis of the left ventricle. This skew in the velocity profile has been shown by many experimental techniques, including hot film anemometry, Doppler ultrasound and magnetic resonance imaging (MRI) (Paulsen and Hasenkam, 1983, Rossvoll et al., 1991, Kilner et al., 1993, Sloth et al., 1994). In healthy individuals, blood flows through the aortic valve at the beginning of systole and then rapidly accelerates to its peak value of 1.35 ± 0.35 m/s. For children, this value is slightly higher at 1.5 ± 0.3 m/s (Hatle and Angelsen, 1985). Highly skewed velocity profiles and corresponding helical flow patterns have been observed in the human aortic arch using magnetic resonance phase velocity mapping (Kilner et al., 1993, Markl et al., 2005). The flow patterns just downstream of the aortic valve are of particular interest because of their complexity and relation to valvular and arterial disease. *In vitro* laser Doppler anemometry experiments have shown that these flow patterns are dependent on the valve geometry and thus can be used to evaluate function and performance of the heart valve (Sung and Yoganathan, 1990a).

16.2.3 Valve Disease and Treatment

Diseases of the aortic valve include stenosis, where the valve orifice is narrowed to obstruct blood ejection, and regurgitation, where blood leaks back into the ventricle after valve closure. The leading cause of aortic valve stenosis is the degenerative calcification of the valve leaflets, characterized by lipid accumulation, inflammation, and mineralization. The morphology of such lesions are mostly similar to

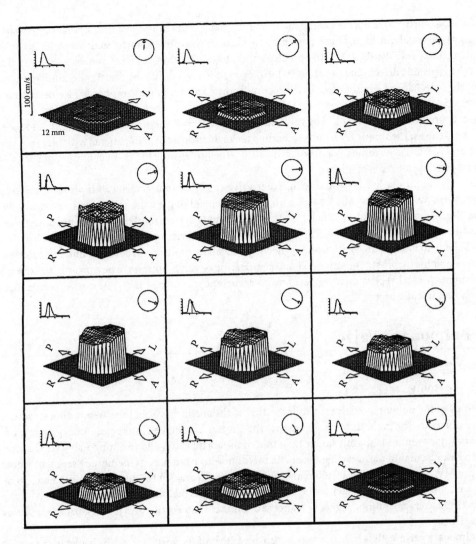

FIGURE 16.7 Velocity profiles measured 2 cm downstream of the aortic valve with hot film anemometry in dogs. The marker on the aortic flow curve shows the timing of the measurements during the cardiac cycle. (From Paulsen, P.K. and Hansenkam, J.M. 1983. *J Biomech*. 16:201–210. With permission.)

that of atherosclerosis, and the two diseases share several common risk factors (Freeman and Otto, 2005), including age, gender, diabetes, hypercholesterolemia, hypertension, rheumatic fever, and congenital malformations such as bicuspid or unicuspid aortic valve (Stewart et al., 1997, Ward, 2000). Rheumatic fever causes scar formation on the valve leaflets, which can independently lead to stenosis, and the scarred surface serves as a calcification site, leading to worsening stenosis. Rheumatic fever is the leading cause of calcific aortic stenosis. Fortunately, in developed countries, the incidences of rheumatic fever have decreased tremendously, and its prevalence is limited to undeveloped countries (Sliwa and Mocumbi, 2010, Lloyd-Jones et al., 2010). Recent studies have shown that the valve responds to mechanical forces and that certain mechanical environment can elicit pathological expressions consistent with native valve degeneration (Butcher et al., 2008). Calcification on the valve leaflet demonstrates specific patterns in most cases. These patterns include calcification only on the aortic surface, along the coaptation line, and at the base of the leaflet (Thubrikar et al., 1986). These patterns have led authors to hypothesize that tissue stress fatigue, such as bending, plays a role in the development of the disease.

The bicuspid aortic valve is a congenital malformation that occurs in 1–2% of the population (Roberts, 1970). This type of valve is highly predisposed to calcification with 50% of aortic stenosis patients having bicuspid aortic valves (Ward, 2000). The predisposition to calcification has been shown to be related to an underlying genetic defect (Garg et al., 2005). However, it is argued that the drastic alteration of geometry and thus mechanical environment in the bicuspid aortic valve is in part responsible for calcification (Robicsek et al., 2004).

Aortic regurgitation may be caused by valve disease or aortic root anomaly. It is commonly associated with aortic stenosis, rheumatic fever, and ascending aorta dilation as seen in patients with bicuspid aortic valve and Marfan syndrome (Tsifansky et al., 2010). The prolapse or the mal-coaptation of the valve is often responsible for regurgitation.

Aortic valve regurgitation is treated with either valve repair or replacement with prosthetic valves, but aortic valve stenosis is typically treated with the replacement of the valve with prosthetic valves due to tissue degeneration. Several prosthetic aortic valve designs are currently available, including fixed xenograft bioprosthetics and mechanical heart valves. These valves however are prone to failure over time, either due to blood damage induced by mechanical valves, or due to structural failure or calcification of xenographic bioprosthetic valves. Tissue engineering of valves appears to be a promising strategy to developing an ideal replacement valves; however, current technology needs to evolve before these valves can be clinically used.

16.3 Pulmonary Valve

16.3.1 Valve Structure

16.3.1.1 Anatomy

The anatomy of the pulmonary valve is similar to that of the aortic valve but the surrounding structure is slightly different. The main differences are that the sinuses are smaller in the pulmonary artery, the pulmonary valve annulus is slightly larger than that of the aortic valve, and the pulmonary valve annulus is entirely muscular in nature while the aortic valve annulus has a fibrous membrane segment where it abuts the MV. An examination of 160 pathologic specimens revealed the aortic valve diameter to be 23.2 ± 3.3 mm, whereas the diameter of the pulmonary valve was measured at 24.3 ± 3.0 mm (Westaby et al., 1984). On average, pulmonary valve leaflets are thinner than aortic valve leaflets: 0.49 mm versus 0.67 mm (Davies, 1980).

The pulmonary valve leaflets have the same structure as that of the aortic valve. The leaflet is composed of three layers, the fibrosa, spongiosa, and ventricularis, with similar composition in each layer (Rabkin-Aikawa et al., 2004), as shown in Figure 16.8. The pulmonary valve has been used as an autograft replacement

(a)   (b)

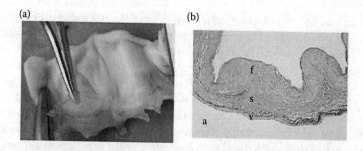

FIGURE 16.8 (a) The fixed pulmonary valve demonstrating the similar valve anatomy to that of the aortic valve. (Adapted from Godart, F. et al. 2009. *J Thorac Cardiovasc Surg*, 137, 1141–1145.) (b) Movat Pentachrom stain of the pulmonary valve leaflet, showing that the three-layered microstructure of the valve similar to that of the aortic valve. (Adapted from Rabkin-Aikawa, E. et al. 2004. *J Thorac Cardiovasc Surg*, 128, 552–561.)

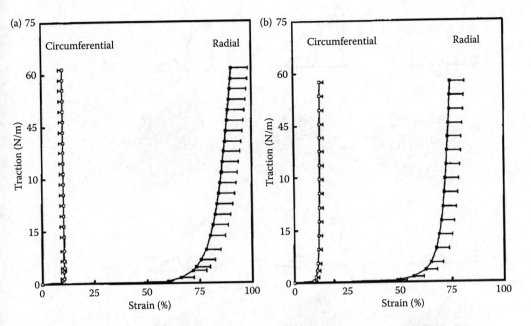

FIGURE 16.9   The mechanical properties of fresh pulmonic valve leaflet (a) versus the aortic valve leaflet (b), from equi-biaxial stress mechanical tests. (Adapted from Christie, G. W. and Barratt-Boyes, B. G. 1995. *Ann Thorac Surg*, 60, S195–S199.)

valve for diseased aortic valve, especially in children, since the valve will remain alive and grows with the patient (Takkenberg et al., 2009). This procedure is commonly known as the Ross procedure after its inventor, and studies on the pulmonary valve is often motivated by this potential use of the valve.

16.3.1.2 Valve Mechanical Properties

The pulmonic valve leaflet has similar mechanical properties as the aortic valve, as shown in Figure 16.9. While the pulmonic valve leaflet is less stiff than the aortic valve in the radial direction, its circumferential direction stiffness is similar to that of the aortic valve, indicating a more pronounced anisotropy (Christie and Barratt-Boyes, 1995). However, the pulmonic valve leaflet has similar extensibilities as the aortic valve leaflet, as well as similar viscoelastic material parameters (Leeson-Dietrich et al., 1995).

16.3.2 Valve Function

16.3.2.1 Valve Dynamics

The pulmonary valve flow behaves similarly to that of the aortic valve but the magnitude of the velocity is smaller. Typical peak velocities for healthy adults are 0.75 ± 0.15 m/s and for children are 0.9 ± 0.2 m/s (Weyman, 1994). As seen in Figure 16.10, a rotation of the peak velocity can be observed in the pulmonary artery velocity profile. During acceleration, the peak velocity is observed inferiorly with the peak rotating counterclockwise throughout the remainder of the ejection phase (Sloth et al., 1994). The mean spatial profile is relatively flat, although there is a region of reverse flow that occurs in late systole, which may be representative of flow separation. Typically, there is only a slight skew in the profile. The peak velocity is generally within 20% of the spatial mean throughout the cardiac cycle. The pulmonary valve is also distinct from the aortic valve in terms of its downstream geometry. The main pulmonary artery splits into the left and right pulmonary artery approximately 5 cm from the pulmonary aortic root, and secondary flow patterns can also be observed in the pulmonary artery and its bifurcation (Sung and Yoganathan, 1990b).

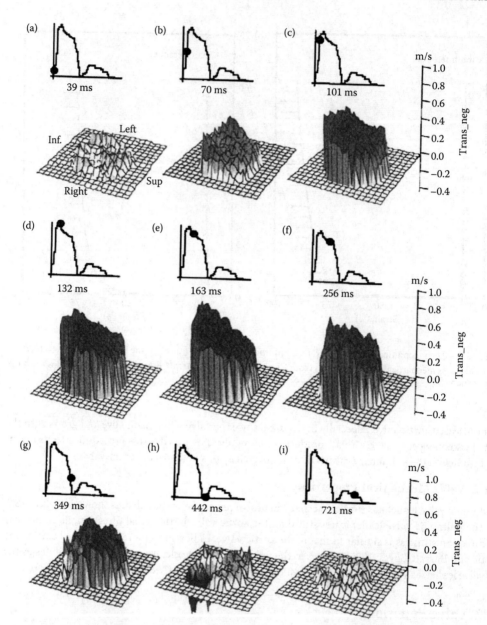

FIGURE 16.10 Velocity profiles downstream of the human pulmonary valve obtained with magnetic resonance phase velocity mapping. The timing of the measurements is shown by the marker on the flow curve. (From Sloth, E. et al. 1994. *Am Heart J.* 128:1130–1138. With permission.)

16.4 Mitral Valve

16.4.1 Valve Structure

16.4.1.1 Anatomy

The MV has a complex geometric structure, with a fibromuscular mitral annulus at the base of the left atrium, two collagenous leaflets, several chordae tendineae, and two papillary muscles (PMs) that emerge from the left ventricular myocardium. Normal MV function requires interplay between the valve's four main components, shown in Figure 16.11. A fibromuscular atrioventricular ring forms the base of the MV at the junction of the left atrium and the left ventricle, with a veil of tissue attached to it along its circumference, which form the mitral leaflets. Fibrous chordae tendineae extend from the ventricular surface of the two leaflets, and extend apically toward the PMs in the left ventricle. These chordae follow a pattern of insertion, such that the leaflets assume an optimal systolic configuration that

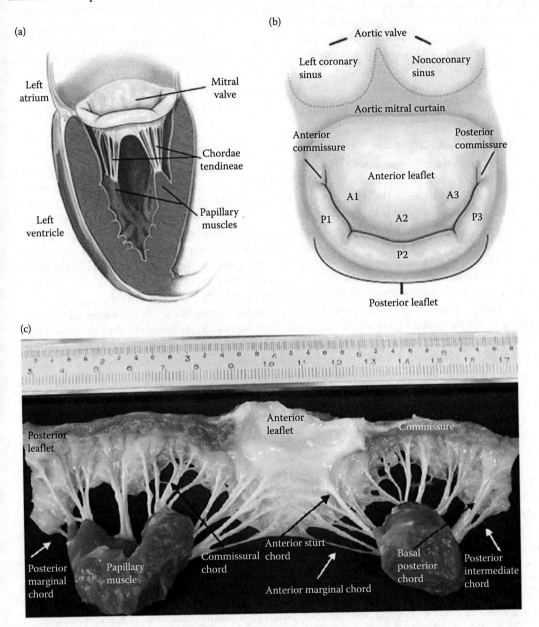

FIGURE 16.11 (a) Schematic of mitral valve structure with different components that constitute the valve. (b) The mitral valve leaflets as located in reference to the aortic valve leaflets with specific distinction between the leaflet cusps. (c) Chordal insertion pattern in an excised porcine mitral valve, depicting the segregation of chordae into primary chordae (inserting into the free edge), secondary (inserting into the base of the leaflet), and tertiary (inserting into the annulus at the commissures).

ensures complete valve competence. Two PMs, antero-lateral and postero-medial, are myocardial structures that extend into the left ventricular cavity (Kalmanson, 1976). Vasculature from the ventricular muscle richly perfuses the PMs, and ensures their contractility during systole.

16.4.1.1.1 Mitral Annulus

The mitral annulus is the anatomical junction between the left atrium and the left ventricle, and serves as the basal insertion site for the MV leaflets. It is an elliptical ring composed of dense collagenous tissue surrounded by muscle. The anterior portion of the annulus is continuous with the base of the noncoronary and left coronary leaflets of the aortic valve. The extremities of this anterior annular section are clearly demarcated by two fibrous protrusions called trigones, from which tendon-like structures extend dorsally along half of the mitral annular ring. The posterior part of the annulus is a nebulous fibrous ring that is not as visually distinct as the anterior annulus. The MV annulus has a three-dimensional saddle shape and is not planar, and dynamically changes its shape over the cardiac cycle (Levine et al., 1987, Glasson et al., 1996).

16.4.1.1.2 Mitral Valve Leaflets

The MV consists of a continuous veil of tissue inserted around the entire circumference of the mitral orifice, which is distinguished into the anterior leaflet and the posterior leaflet. The anterior leaflet has a triangular structure and attaches to the mitral annulus between the trigones, with the greatest leaflet height at the free edge as shown in Figure 16.11. The basal portion of the leaflet is continuous with the aorto-mitral curtain along the noncoronary and left coronary aortic leaflets, while the apical portion of the leaflet forms the free edge of the leaflet that aids coaptation. The posterior leaflet on the other hand covers the entire circumference from one commissure to the other, covering three-fifths of the entire mitral annulus. The leaflet is divided into three individual scallops identified as the P1 (anterior or medial scallop), P2 (the middle scallop), and P3 (posterior or lateral scallop). The height of the posterior leaflet varies from the P1 cusp to the P3 cusp, with P2 cusp having the greatest height from the base to the free edge. The combined area of both leaflets is about twice the size of the mitral orifice; this extra surface area permits a large line of coaptation and ample coverage of the mitral orifice during normal function, and provides compensation during disease (He et al., 1997). The width and height of the anterior leaflet are about 3.3 and 2.3 cm, respectively, and the height of the posterior leaflet is about 1.3 cm, while that of the commissure is about 1.0 cm. The MV tissue can be divided into the rough and smooth zones. The rough zone is defined from the free edge of the valve to the valve's line of closure, and the term rough is used to denote the texture of the leaflet due to the insertion of the chordae tendinae in this area. The smooth zone is thinner and translucent and extends from the line of closure to the annulus in the anterior leaflet and to the basal zone in the posterior leaflet.

Fenoglio and colleagues (Fenoglio et al., 1972) reported that MV leaflets have distinct layers divided by differences in cellularity and collagen density (Figure 16.12). Kunzelman et al. (1993) described the leaflet as consisting of a thick central fibrosa layer, the atrialis or spongiosa layer on the atrial side, and the ventricularis on the ventricular side. The fibrosa has dense collagen fibrils spread in a fan-like arrangement (Figure 16.12), and is thickest near the annulus and thins toward the free edge. The spongiosa has loose collagen with interstitial cells sparsely distributed, extends throughout the entire leaflet, and is the main component of the free edge. Trace randomly oriented collagen and elastin fibers are spread out in the proteoglycan gel in this layer, but elastin and cells diminish toward the free edge. The ventricularis is similar to the spongiosa, but is thinner, rich in elastin, and is continuous with the thin elastin rich layer covering the outer portion of chordae tendinae. This abundance of proteoglycan near the free edge helps sustain the compressive loads during systolic closure, while the abundance of collagen in the other areas helps to sustain tensile load within the leaflet. The atrial and ventricular surfaces of the leaflets are lined with endothelial cells, though of a different morphology on both sides.

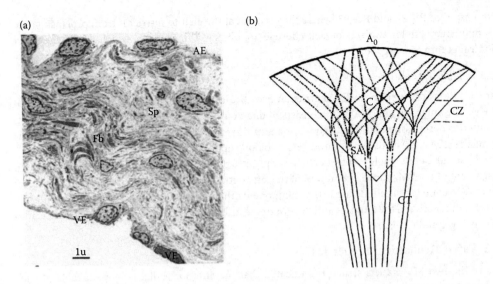

FIGURE 16.12 (a) Histological cross-sectional image of the mitral leaflet showing the atrial and ventricular layers populated with endothelial cells, the fibrosa with collagen fibrils, and spongiosa with interstitial cells. (b) Fan-like arrangement of the collagen fibrils from the region of chordal insertion to the mitral annulus. (From Fenoglio, J. J. et al. 1972. *Circ Res*, 31, 417–430.)

16.4.1.1.3 *Chordae Tendineae*

The mitral chordae are tendinous structure that arise from the PM tips and insert into the ventricular surface of the anterior and posterior leaflets. They differ in number from valve to valve. However, the chordae can be broadly classified into three classes based on the region of their insertion into the leaflet: Primary or marginal chordae tendineae, secondary or strut chordae tendineae, and tertiary or basal or commissural chordae tendineae. The MV typically consists of 8–12 chordae tendineae, 15–20 mm long, and approximately 0.45 mm in diameter before branching, either at the tip of the PM or at their insertion into the leaflet. The chordae inserting into the anterior leaflet are obliquely aligned along their longitudinal axis, while those on the posterior leaflet insert parallel to each other.

On the anterior leaflet, the marginal chordae that insert into the free edge, the secondary that insert into the belly of the leaflet, and the basal that insert closer to the mitral annulus. The marginal chordae split into three branches soon after their origin from the PM, with one branch inserting into the free margin of the leaflet, one into the intermediate area in the rough zone, and one slightly beyond the line of coaptation. These chords are responsible for the proper coaptation of the MV, since severing them will result in prolapsed leaflet and regurgitation (Obadia et al., 1997). The secondary chordae, which are the thickest chordae, originate from the tips of both the anterior lateral and the posterior medial PMs and insert at the transition from the rough to the smooth zones of the leaflets, where dense collagen networks provides continuity to the fibrous trigones, completed a load-bearing loop between the ventricle and the valve (Cochran et al., 1991). Secondary chordae are the thickest and carry the largest load during systolic loading on the valve and are under continuous tension. It has been speculated that they hold the function of maintaining the normal ventricular size and geometry by pulling the annulus and the PMs toward each other (Silbiger and Bazaz, 2009). The basal chordae insert into the anterior leaflet close to the annulus and toward the commissural sections. Their exact function in the global MV hemodynamic or mechanical function is currently unknown. On the posterior leaflet, the chordal distribution is similar to the anterior with a few exceptions. Posterior basal chordae, which are unique to this leaflet, are a set of chordae that extend directly from the PM to the insertion of the leaflet and do not divide along their entire stem. Additionally, cleft chordae are also seen at the regions dividing the posterior cusp into P1–P2 and P2–P3, where they fan out at the cleft to restrict it from prolapsing into the atrium during systole. Two sets of cleft chordae are observed in humans, which divide the entire posterior leaflet into three scallops.

16.4.1.1.4 Papillary Muscles

There are two PMs arising from the left ventricular myocardium: the antero-lateral PM and the postero-medial PM. The antero-lateral PM often consists of one body or tip and obtains its blood supply from the left anterior descending and the diagonal or a marginal branch of the circumflex artery, while the postero-medial PM consists of two tips and gets its blood supply from the left circumflex or right coronary artery. Because of its single system of blood supply, it is prone to injury from myocardial infarction. The attachment of the PMs to the lateral wall of the left ventricle makes the ventricular wall an integral part of the MV complex. The PMs are active components that contract during systole and maintain a constant distance between the annulus and the PM tip, restricting the prolapse of the mitral leaflets into the atria during systolic closure.

16.4.1.2 Valve Mechanical Properties

Analysis of the two MV leaflets structure indicated that the anterior leaflet is more capable of supporting large tensile loads than the posterior leaflet, since the anterior leaflet has thicker collagen-rich fibrosa layer. This is confirmed by uniaxial tensile testing (Kunzelman and Cochran, 1992). Grashow et al. (2006) performed equi-biaxial mechanical testing of the anterior leaflet. The leaflet was found to exhibit a mechanical response curve similar to that of collagen, with a very long toe region of large strain and slow loading followed by a region of small strain and rapid loading (Figure 16.13). The leaflet exhibits no hysteresis in the circumferential direction, and a very small amount in the radial direction. The valve leaflet was found to be strain rate insensitive over a range of loading rates from 0.07 to 20 Hz, maintaining the same mechanical response and hysteresis.

The mechanical properties of chordae tendineae vary with their type and size. Liao and colleagues reported that chordal grouping based on cross-sectional area demonstrates a stark correlation between the chordal size, type, and mechanical properties (Liao and Vesely, 2003, 2004a, 2004b, 2007, Liao et al., 2009). They reported that the thicker strut chordae are more extensible and less stiff than the thinner marginal chordae. The marginal chordae that are the thinnest had smaller fibril diameters and a greater

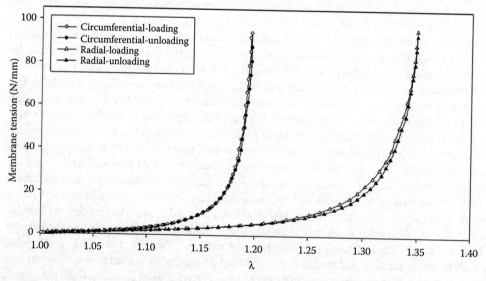

FIGURE 16.13 Mechancial response of the mitral valve anterior leaflet to equibiaxial tensile testing. (Adapted from Grashow, J. S., Yoganathan, A. P., and Sacks, M. S. 2006. *Ann Biomed Eng*, 34, 315–325.)

average fibril density than the other chordae, thus contributing to their stiffness. On the other hand, the extensibility of the chordae seems to increase with increasing chordal diameter or with a reduction in the tensile modulus. In the thicker chordae, the collagen fibrils are extensively crimped and thus allow better elongation than their thinner counterparts.

16.4.2 Valve Function

16.4.2.1 Valve Dynamics

The primary function of the MV is to allow blood flow from the left atrium to the left ventricle during diastole, and prevent the backflow of blood from the left ventricle to the atrium during systole. To perform this physiological function synchronously with the cardiac phase, the MV components works in tandem with one another to ensure proper closure of the leaflets. At the beginning of systole, higher pressure in the left ventricle and lower pressure in the left atrium accelerates the valve leaflets basally toward the mitral annulus. As the leaflets move closer to the mitral annulus, the limited extensibility of the chordae tendineae restricts the leaflets from prolapsing into the atrium. The chordae tendineae are inserted along the leaflet surface such that they not only restrict leaflet prolapse but also impart a curvature to the leaflets that results in good anterior and posterior leaflet overlap and good coaptation. Typically, in humans, the coaptation height measured along the A2–P2 ranges between 5 and 8 mm and varies with the valve size and body surface area. At peak systole, the PMs also contract and transfer an apically directed force to the annulus. This force has been speculated to change the shape of the mitral annulus from a flat diastolic configuration to a three-dimensional systolic saddle shape. Though the exact dynamics and interaction between each MV component are currently unknown, it has been demonstrated to some extent that the transfer of forces from the subannular components to the annular plane plays a critical role in optimizing leaflet coaptation (Nolan et al., 1969). As the ventricular pressure falls during late systole, rapid left atrial filling increases the chamber pressure until an inflection point is reached when the MV opens. The positive pressure gradient between the left atrium and the ventricle displaces the mitral leaflets apically to their completely open position. The strut chordae on the anterior leaflet ensure that the open mitral leaflets do not obstruct the left ventricular outflow tract, and unobstructed left ventricular filling occurs. Figure 16.14a and b depicts the different forces acting on the MV during the systolic and diastolic phase of the cardiac cycle, and

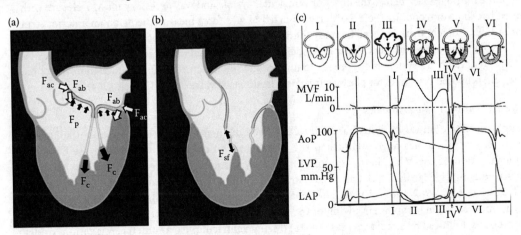

FIGURE 16.14 Forces acting on the mitral valve structure during systolic (a) and diastole (b). F_p: ventricular pressure exerted on the leaflets; F_c: force of systolic papillary muscle contraction; F_{ac}: the annular contraction force; F_{ab}: the annular bending force components; F_{sf}: tension in the strut chordae during diastole preventing systolic anterior motion of the leaflet. (c) Chamber pressures and mitral valve flow recorded during different phases on the cardiac cycle in calves. (Adapted from Nolan, S. P. et al. 1969. *Am Heart J*, 77, 784–791.)

illustrates the structure-to-function relationship between the chamber pressures and the kinematics of the MV components.

Figure 16.14c presents the synchronous recording of the MV flow, and ventricular and atrial chamber pressures in a calf. The duration of the total cardiac cycle is divided into six cardiac phases. Phase I is the period of low flow rate and volume at pre-diastole, when the MV is just about to open. Phase II begins at the time point when the atrioventricular pressure gradient is positive and during this period the flow from the left atrium rapidly accelerates into the left ventricle and slowly declines. Phase III commences at atrial systole, when the left atrium contracts and pushes the fluid volume remaining in the chamber into the left ventricle, creating a second peak in the transmitral flow curve. Phase IV is the only period of flow reversal, occurring during the isovolumetric contraction. This volume could either be slight regurgitation or can be the volume of the fluid displaced by the valve leaflets into the left atrium, termed as the closing volume. Phase V varied between 15 and 40 ms and consisted of minor flow rates related to outflow from the ventricle and motion of the MV. Phase VI extended throughout systole when no MV flow will be detectable for a healthy valve.

16.4.2.1.1 Valve Leaflet Dynamics

The first studies on understanding MV function focused on understanding the opening and closure dynamics of the valve in relevance to the atrial and ventricular hemodynamics. Henderson and Johnson (1912) demonstrated that atrial contraction begins the basal motion of the mitral leaflets toward leaflet closure, with subsequent increase in left ventricular pressure inducing complete valve closure (Henderson and Johnson, 1912). In 1916, Dean repeated the experiments in a perfused cat heart model with a constant atrial pressure head and measured the anterior leaflet mobility using a sensitive lever mechanism with changing left ventricular pressures (Dean, 1916). He observed that with the complete absence of left atrial contraction/systole, the leaflets closed only upon the onset of ventricular contraction and such passive left ventricular pressure-driven closure was associated with large backward flow of blood through the MV into the left atrium. Between 1916 and 1970, a few investigators used large animals to study the role of atrial and ventricular contraction to MV closure, by ablating the left atrial fibers or by inducing a left atrioventricular block (Paravisini, 1953, Brockman, 1962, Sarnoff et al., 1962, Meadows et al., 1963, Braunwald et al., 1966, Williams et al., 1967, 1968, Vandenberg et al., 1969, Zaky et al., 1969, Shah et al., 1970, Bellhouse, 1970b). The conclusion from these studies was that atrial systole contributed to the closure of the mitral leaflets, before the onset of ventricular systole and was necessary for MV closure with limited backflow of blood. In 1962, Salisbury reported *in vivo* force measurements on an anterior strut chord under different drug-induced hemodynamic conditions in anesthetized Mongrel dogs (Salisbury et al., 1963). In the same decade, Frater et al. defined the functional anatomy of the mammalian MV (1961), and developed a systematic approach to understand the structure-to-function relationship of the valve, and proposed principles for plastic surgery of the diseased valve (1964) (Frater, 1964).

16.4.2.1.2 Valve Annulus Dynamics

Though the entire mitral annulus has historically been defined as an incomplete and diaphanous structure, several studies have established the importance of the mitral annulus in the hemodynamic function of the MV. The mitral annulus is a dynamic structure, which changes its shape and size during the cardiac cycle, as demonstrated in animal and human studies (Tsakiris et al., 1971, Levine et al., 1987, 1989). The size of the annulus increased in late diastole until it reached its maximum area. Then, a rapid narrowing of the ring was observed during the atrial and ventricular contractions, followed by a rapid increase in size during ventricular isovolumetric relaxation. Under control conditions in dogs, a decrease in annular area of 19–34% was observed during systole as compared to the diastolic ring size (Tsakiris et al., 1975). The most striking observation was that nearly two-thirds of the annular size reduction occurred during atrial contraction, and the valve annulus was significantly reduced before the onset of ventricular systole as shown in Figure 16.15. A substantial amount of this reduction in annular size is attributable to atrial systole because it is

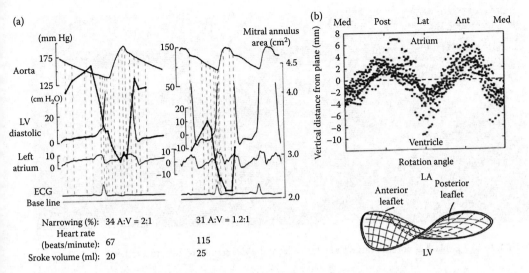

FIGURE 16.15 (a) Temporal contraction of the mitral annulus through the cardiac cycle as measured from fluo-roscopic images in anesthetized dogs, with maximal contraction occurring before onset of systole. (Adapted from Tsakiris, A. G. et al. 1971. *J Appl Physiol*, 30, 611–618.) (b) 3D saddle-shaped structure of the mitral annulus as measured from echocardiographic images in normal subjects. (Adapted from Levine, R. A. et al. 1989. *Circulation*, 80, 589–598.)

not seen when atrial activity is absent, such as in the instance of atrial fibrillation (Pai et al., 2003). Further, Tsakiris et al. demonstrated that the mitral annulus moves apically during systole, and toward the left atrium during diastole, with the magnitude and frequency of motion correlating with the left atrial size (Tsakiris et al., 1971).

The mitral annulus in addition also undergoes an apical-basal flexing, imparting it a saddle shape during systole from its flat diastolic configuration, first reported by Levine et al. as shown in Figure 16.15 (Levine et al., 1987, 1988, 1989). When studied *in vitro*, it was found that this saddle shape of the annulus minimizes the stretch of the MV as well as the forces experienced by the chordae as opposed to the flat planar annulus shape (Jimenez et al., 2003, 2007, Padala et al., 2009a).

16.4.2.2 Chordae Tendineae Dynamics

The locations of the chordae tendineae relative to the valve leaflets and papillary muscles are shown in Figure 16.16. Studies on the chordae tendineae mechanics focused on force measurements in the chor-dae under physiological loading conditions. Chordae forces are elevated during systole but are reduced during diastole. *In vitro* studies using a flexible saddle-shaped annulus revealed that the marginal, sec-ondary, and basal chordae experiences peak systolic forces of approximately 0.2, 1.0, and 0.1 N, respec-tively (Jimenez et al., 2005b). With the displacement of the PMs, such as in the case of hypertrophy of the ventricle secondary to diseases, it was found that forces in the basal chordae increased significantly while those in the marginal and secondary chordae were unaffected (Jimenez et al., 2005a).

16.4.2.3 Papillary Muscle Dynamics

The locations of the papillary muscles relative to the valve leaflets and chordae tendineae are shown in Figure 16.16. The contraction of the left ventricle is torsional in nature, given that ventricular muscle fibers are arranged helically. This results in the PMs experiencing rotational motion about the long axis of the left ventricle (Gorman et al., 1996). The PMs experiences contractions as well, being muscular in compo-sition. Their shortening coincides with ventricular contraction durations and serves to maintain the dis-tance between the mitral annulus and the tips of the PMs constant (Sanfilippo et al., 1992). The dynamics

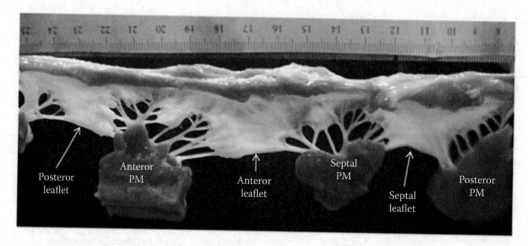

FIGURE 16.16 Explanted porcine valve, showing leaflet and PM locations relative to another.

of the PM aid the formation of ventricular inflow. During diastole, they protrude only minimally into the submitral space, providing room for mitral inflow with reduced resistance. During systole, they bulge into the ventricular cavity, directing flow toward the outflow tract (Armour and Randall, 1970).

16.4.2.4 Valve Fluid Dynamics

In 1971, Bellhouse attempted to explain the movements of the mitral cusps by flow patterns within the left ventricle, and by acceleration and deceleration of blood flow through the MV (Bellhouse, 1970a, 1970b, 1972). He reported stable vortex formation behind the anterior leaflet, which corroborated with previous observations reported in animals by Taylor and Wade, and speculated their role in early diastolic closure of the mitral leaflets (Taylor and Wade, 1969). Even though his model MV did not have chordae tendineae, the diastolic motion of the mitral leaflets matched that measured in animals, challenging existing hypothesis that PM traction governs diastolic opening of valve leaflets (Rushmer et al., 1956). At the same time, using electromagnetic flow probes, Taylor et al. measured the impedance of the MV to transmitral flow, and reported that the MV adapts to changing cardiac output so as to optimize the increase in energy loss (Rushmer et al., 1956, Taylor and Wade, 1969, Taylor, 1972, 1976). At the level of the mitral annulus, the velocity profile was flat and consistent with a plug flow, analogous to the entrance of a pipe. At the free cusp margin, the velocity profile becomes more skewed with higher velocities along the anterior leaflet, with a skewed profile at the free margin outlet; yet the overall profile did not seem to change significantly at higher heart rates.

16.4.3 Disease of the Mitral Valve and Treatment

MV pathologies encompass a spectrum of lesions, which include congenital defects, degeneration of valve tissue, and geometric distortions to the valve secondary to other diseases. Congenital lesions of the MV include annular calcification leading to mitral stenosis, leaflet prolapse due to Marfan syndrome, isolated cleft valve, undivided atrioventricular valve in ostium primum or septum secondum defects, and mitral regurgitation due to congestive heart failure caused by severe stenosis of the left main coronary artery. Though the underlying etiology of each congenital lesion is different, the common manifestations between all the lesions are leaflet and subannular malformations that reduce valve competence. Degenerative MV lesions occur in both children and adults due to genetic mutations such as Marfan syndrome, acquired diseases such as rheumatic heart disease in developing countries, fibroelastic deficiency in adult life due to collagen deficiencies, or Barlow's syndrome speculated to be caused due to genetic and mechanical factors. The last classification of MV lesions, termed as the functional

MV defects, are caused due to perturbations to the MV geometry secondary to other lesions such as ischemic dilated cardiomyopathy or hypertrophic dilated cardiomyopathy.

MV pathologies can be treated with either valve replacement with a prosthetic valve, or surgical repair. The latter is currently the accepted standard of care over valve replacement due to risks associated with anticoagulation therapy, growth of cardiac structure in pediatric patients, and lack of durability of the artificial valves. Surgical therapy for valvular heart disease has seen tremendous progress in the last two decades. In the current era of cardiothoracic surgery, surgical repair of a diseased MV has become a routine procedure that is associated with low mortality rates and excellent acute outcomes. With better understanding of pathological anatomy of MV lesions and increasing surgical experience, several innovative methods for MV repair have been established. However, the long-term durability and chronic outcomes of these techniques are not optimal, with failure rates range from 5% to 40% for the repair of different MV lesions. These disconcerting statistics indicate that MV repair for acute correction of regurgitation or stenosis is achieved, but chronic failure of these repairs is inevitable. The mechanisms of this long-term failure are currently poorly understood. Engineering studies to understand the structural and functional mechanisms of MV dysfunction and recurrent failure of surgical repairs are thus necessary to enable the development of novel MV therapies and devices.

A very common repair technique for mitral regurgitation is the surgical installation of a mitral annuloplasty ring to correct annular dilation. Since its conception in the 1960s (Tsakiris et al., 1967), and made famous by Carpentier in 1983 (Carpentier, 1983), several types of mitral annuloplasty rings have since been developed, and there is a lack of consensus on which ring performs better. Mitral annuloplasty inevitably reduced native annular dynamics, flattened the mitral annular shape, restricted the posterior leaflet mobility (He et al., 1997, Green et al., 1999), and adversely affected ventricular motion (Cheng et al., 2006), although they improve valve coaptation.

In vitro studies have been useful for the evaluation of different surgical repair techniques for prolapsed MV. Padala et al. demonstrated that both resective and nonresective MV repair techniques are effective at acutely eliminating regurgitation, but resective techniques significantly reduce the motion of the resected leaflet and may impact chronic outcomes (Padala et al., 2009a, 2009b). Studies from the same group also demonstrated that the success of percutaneous edge-to-edge repair also largely depends on the size of the mitral annulus and the extent of leaflet distension, and thus indicate proper patient selection for use of this repair (Croft et al., 2007).

16.5 Tricuspid Valve

16.5.1 Valve Structure

16.5.1.1 Anatomy

The TV is located on the right side of the heart between the right atrium and right ventricle. Its perimeter is lined with the septal wall and the right free wall of the heart. The valve consists of an annulus, three leaflets, chordae tendineae, and three PMs. The three leaflets are named according to their position in the heart: anterior, posterior, and septal leaflet. The septal leaflet is located along the septal wall and is attached to the wall with short chordae (Silver et al., 1971). The anterior and posterior leaflets are located along the free wall with the anterior leaflet reported to be the largest (Skwarek et al., 2006, Anwar et al., 2007a, Shah and Raney, 2008). While it is typically accepted that the TV has three main leaflets, numerous studies have reported there to be a variable number of leaflets ranging from 2 up to 7 leaflets (Joudinaud, 2006, Victor and Nayak, 2000). The septal leaflet is always present but the number of leaflets along the free wall can vary.

The annulus is a fibrous ring located on the perimeter of the valve and connects the leaflets to the myocardial wall. The annulus has a complex 3D geometry as seen in Figure 16.17 (Silver et al., 1971, Hiro et al., 2004, Fukuda et al., 2006b, Jouan et al., 2007, Kwan et al., 2007, Anwar et al., 2007b). While some studies have reported the annulus to be oval (Anwar et al., 2007a, 2007b), others report that it

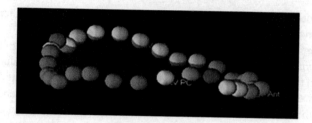

FIGURE 16.17 3D representation of the complex shape of the tricuspid annulus using 3D echocardiography and 3D in house software. (Adapted from Kwan, J. et al. 2007. *Eur J Echocardiogr,* 8, 375–383.)

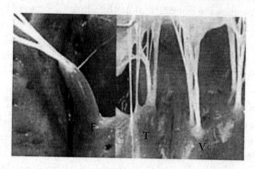

FIGURE 16.18 Classification of the three groups of papillary muscles: F—finger-like, T—tethered, and V—vestigial. Classified using excised porcine hearts by Joudinaud in 2006. (Adapted from Joudinaud, T. M., Flecher, E. M., and Duran, C. M. G. 2006. *J Heart Valve Dis,* 15, 382–388.)

is triangular (Silver et al., 1971). Annulus areas range from 7.6 to 11.2 cm^2 during systole and 11.3 to 18.35 cm^2 during diastole (Tei et al., 1982, Anwar et al., 2007a, Kwan et al., 2007).

There are three PMs located in the right ventricle, which connect to the leaflets via chordae tendineae. The PMs on the right side of the hearts are not as well defined as those seen on the left side of the heart as with the MV (Joudinaud et al., 2006). The PMs are named according to their location in the ventricle: septal, anterior, and posterior. The septal PM is located on the anterior side of the septum between the septal and anterior leaflets, while the posterior PM is located on the posterior side between the septal and posterior leaflets. The anterior PM is located on the free wall between the anterior and posterior leaflets. The PMs are classified into three groups based upon structure: finger-like, with the muscle protruding, tethered, with the muscle imbedded in the wall, and vestigial with the chords attaching directly to the well (Joudinaud et al., 2006) (Figure 16.18). Each PM has several chords that attach to the two corresponding leaflets, for example, the anterior PM has chords that insert into the anterior and posterior leaflets. The chords insert into different locations on the leaflet, including the free-edge, base, and belly of the leaflet, and are classified as marginal/primary, inserting into the free edge of the leaflet, rough zone/supplemental, inserting between the marginal and intermediate chords, and deep/intermediate, inserting into the belly of the leaflet, respectively. Silver et al. report the deep/strut chordae to be the longest (1.7 ± 0.4 cm). All chords have similar thickness ranging from 0.8 ± 0.3 to 1.1 ± 0.4 cm (Silver et al., 1971).

16.5.2 Valve Function

16.5.2.1 Valve Dynamics

The main function of the TV is to prevent the backflow of blood from the ventricle to the atrium during systole, when blood is being pumped from the right ventricle to the pulmonary artery. The typical pressures on the right side of the heart range from 0 to 5 mmHg for the atrium and from 5 to 40 mmHg for the ventricle as reported using catheter measurements (Hurst and O'Rourke, 2004). The TV closes with

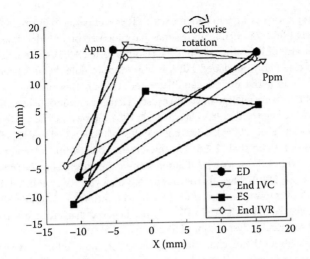

FIGURE 16.19 Results from an *in vivo* sonomicrometry study on sheep show the clockwise rotation motion of the papillary muscles over the cardiac cycle. (Adapted from Jouan, J. et al. 2007. *J Heart Valve Dis*, 16, 511–518.)

the initiation of isovolumetric contraction, and remains closed throughout the systole and isovolumetric relaxation. Once the pressure in the right ventricle is lower than that in the atrium, the valve opens. The valve remains closed for approximately one-third of the cardiac cycle.

The TV annulus area significantly increases from early to late systole in healthy subjects by 5.4 ± 1.6% (Kwan et al., 2007) and experiences differences ranging from 28 to 48% from its minimum to maximum area throughput the cardiac cycle (Tei et al., 1982, Fukuda et al., 2006b, Jouan et al., 2007). The area of the TV annulus is at its maximum during diastole, increasing the efficiency of filling by providing a larger orifice (Jouan et al., 2007) and minimum during systole aiding coaptation of the leaflets. In addition to changes in area throughout the cardiac cycle, the annulus changes its shape as well. The annulus of the TV has a three-dimensional saddle (Hiro et al., 2004, Fukuda et al., 2006b, Kwan et al., 2007), as seen in Figure 16.17, with the annulus becoming more planar during diastole (Hiro et al., 2004).

Juaon et al. (2007) studied the dynamics of the three PMs of the right side of heart during the cardiac cycle and found that the PMs move in a clockwise manner during systole as shown in Figure 16.19. The anterior PM experiences the greatest movement during the cardiac cycle due to the contraction of the myocardium since the PM is located on the free wall. The motion of the PMs has been observed to twist, shift, and bend in relation to the annulus plane, while the distance from the PMs to the annulus plane remains relatively constant (Jouan et al., 2007).

16.5.3 Disease of the Tricuspid Valve and Treatment

Tricuspid regurgitation (TR) is defined as the backflow of blood from the right ventricle to the right atrium through the TV and occurs in 8–35% of the population (Antunes and Barlow, 2007). Commonly, TR occurs in conjunction with MV regurgitation (Antunes and Barlow, 2007). Clinically, small levels of TR are detected by color Doppler imaging in many normal persons (Bonow et al., 1998) and is left untreated as it is not seen as life threatening. TR is commonly secondary to another disease and not due to changes in the natural structure of the valve and its leaflets (King et al., 1984, Matsuyama et al., 2003). Mechanisms of TR include, but are not limited to, changes in preload, afterload, such as in the case of pulmonary hypertension (Abe et al., 1996, Matsuyama et al., 2003), and right ventricular function (Sadeghi et al., 2004, Dreyfus et al., 2005).

Alterations in right ventricular function have detrimental effects on the mechanics of the TV, including less-than-normal systolic reduction in annulus (Tei et al., 1982). Human clinical studies have reported that the tricuspid annulus is twice as large in patients with TR as compared to normal subjects, measuring 35 and 70 mm, respectively (Tei et al., 1982). Studies may have focused on annular dilatation because it is believed to be a better indicator of TV pathology than TR (Dreyfus et al., 2005), since patients with no initial TR and a dilated annulus eventually developed TR. It is important to note that it is believed that only the anterior and posterior segments of the annulus can dilate, since they are the only segments on the free wall (Dreyfus et al., 2005). Right ventricle enlargement also causes tricuspid annulus deformations and displacement of PMs (Tei et al., 1982, Ubago et al., 1983, Gibson et al., 1984, Come and Riley, 1985, Sagie et al., 1994, Hinderliter et al., 2003, Fukuda et al., 2006a), which contributes to TR. It is believed that RV dilatation may affect the anterior PM position (Kim et al., 2006, Anyanwu et al., 2008), while interventricular mechanics have been shown to affect PM positions, with LV dilation significantly displacing the septal PM toward the center of the RV (Spinner et al., 2010). It has also been reported that with RV systolic failure, diastolic pressure rises and the septum moves toward the left side of the heart (Antunes and Barlow, 2007), thus increasing pulmonary pressure, believed to be a factor in TR. It is also believed that TR occurs in conjunction with left-side heart disease and ventricular dysfunction (Fukuda et al., 2006a).

Although little is known about the mechanisms that cause TR, many efforts have been made to correct it. Most recent efforts at correcting TR have been focused on repairing the annulus and reconstructing to its native structure and size, with the use of annuloplasty. Another option for treatment is valve replacement although it is uncommon because functional TR can be repaired with annuloplasty (Chang et al., 2006). It is believed that a complete understanding of valvular and subvalvular mechanics will significantly aid in better treatment options.

References

Abe, T., Tukamoto, M., Yanagiya, M., Morikawa, M., Watanabe, N., and Komatsu, S. 1996. De Vega's annuloplasty for acquired tricuspid disease: Early and late results in 110 patients. *Ann Thorac Surg*, 62, 1876–1877.

Antunes, M. J. and Barlow, J. B. 2007. Management of tricuspid valve regurgitation. *Heart*, 93, 271–276.

Anwar, A. M., Geleijnse, M. L., Soliman, O. I. I., Mcghie, J. S., Frowijn, R., Nemes, A., Van den Bosch, A. E., Galema, T. W., and Ten Cate, F. J. 2007a. Assessment of normal tricuspid valve anatomy in adults by real-time three-dimensional echocardiography. *Int J Cardiovasc Imaging*, 23, 717–724.

Anwar, A. M., Soliman, O. I. I., Nemes, A., Van Geuns, R. J. M., Geleijnse, M. L., and Ten Cate, F. J. 2007b. Value of assessment of tricuspid annulus: Real-time three-dimensional echocardiography and magnetic resonance imaging. *Int J Cardiovasc Imaging*, 23, 701–705.

Anyanwu, A. C., Chikwe, J., and Adams, D. H. 2008. Tricuspid valve repair for treatment and prevention of secondary tricuspid regurgitation in patients undergoing mitral valve surgery. *Curr Cardiol Rep*, 10, 110–117.

Armour, J. A. and Randall, W. C. 1970. Structural basis for cardiac function. *Am J Physiol*, 218, 1517–1523.

Bellhouse, B. J. 1970a. Fluid mechanics of a model mitral valve. *J Physiol*, 207, 72P–73P.

Bellhouse, B. J. 1970b. Mechanism of closure of the mitral valve. *Clin Sci*, 39, 13P–14P.

Bellhouse, B. J. 1972. Fluid mechanics of a model mitral valve and left ventricle. *Cardiovasc Res*, 6, 199–210.

Bellhouse, B. J. and Reid, K. G. 1969. Fluid mechanics of the aortic valve. *Br Heart J*, 31, 391.

Billiar, K. L. and Sacks, M. S. 2000. Biaxial mechanical properties of the natural and glutaraldehyde treated aortic valve cusp—Part I: Experimental results. *J Biomech Eng*, 122, 23–30.

Bonow, R. O., Carabello, B., De Leon, A. C., Edmunds, L. H., Fedderly, B. J., Freed, M. D., Gaasch, W. H. et al. 1998. Acc/Aha guidelines for the management of patients with valvular heart disease—A report of the American College of Cardiology American Heart Association Task Force on practice guidelines (Committee on Management of Patients with Valvular Heart Disease). *J Am Coll Cardiol*, 32, 1486–1582.

Braunwald, E., Rockoff, S. D., Oldham, H. N., Jr., and Ross, J., Jr. 1966. Effective closure of the mitral valve without atrial systole. *Circulation*, 33, 404–409.

Brockman, S. K. 1962. The physiology of closure of the mitral valve. *Surg Forum*, 13, 206–207.

Butcher, J. T., Simmons, C. A., and Warnock, J. N. 2008. Mechanobiology of the aortic heart valve. *J Heart Valve Dis*, 17, 62–73.

Carpentier, A. 1983. Cardiac valve surgery—The "French correction". *J Thorac Cardiovasc Surg*, 86, 323–337.

Chang, B. C., Lim, S. H., Yi, G. Y., Hong, Y. S., Lee, S., Yoo, K. J., Kang, M. S., and Cho, B. K. 2006. Long-term clinical results of tricuspid valve replacement. *Ann Thorac Surg*, 81, 1317–1324.

Cheng, A., Nguyen, T. C., Malinowski, M., Liang, D., Daughters, G. T., Ingels, N. B., Jr., and Miller, D. C. 2006. Effects of undersized mitral annuloplasty on regional transmural left ventricular wall strains and wall thickening mechanisms. *Circulation*, 114, I600–I609.

Christie, G. W. 1992. Anatomy of aortic heart valve leaflets: The influence of glutaraldehyde fixation on function. *Eur J Cardiothorac Surg*, 6 Suppl 1, S25–S32; discussion S33.

Christie, G. W. and Barratt-Boyes, B. G. 1995. Mechanical properties of porcine pulmonary valve leaflets: How do they differ from aortic leaflets? *Ann Thorac Surg*, 60, S195–S199.

Cochran, R. P., Kunzelman, K. S., Chuong, C. J., Sacks, M. S., and Eberhart, R. C. 1991. Nondestructive analysis of mitral valve collagen fiber orientation. *ASAIO Trans*, 37, M447–M448.

Come, P. C. and Riley, M. F. 1985. Tricuspid anular dilatation and failure of tricuspid leaflet coaptation in tricuspid regurgitation. *Am J Cardiol*, 55, 599–601.

Croft, L. R., Jimenez, J. H., Gorman, R. C., Gorman, J. H. 3rd, and Yoganathan, A. P. 2007. Efficacy of the edge-to-edge repair in the setting of a dilated ventricle: An *in vitro* study. *Ann Thorac Surg*, 84, 1578–1584.

Dagum, P., Green, G. R., Nistal, F. J., Daughters, G. T., Timek, T. A., Foppiano, L. E., Bolger, A. F., Ingels, N. B., Jr., and Miller, D. C. 1999. Deformational dynamics of the aortic root: Modes and physiologic determinants. *Circulation*, 100, II54–II62.

Davies, M. J. 1980. *Pathology of Cardiac Valves*, London, Butterworths.

Dean, A. L. 1916. The movements of the mitral cusps in relation to the cardiac cycle. *Am J Physiol*, 40, 206–217.

Doehring, T. C., Carew, E. O., and Vesely, I. 2004. The effect of strain rate on the viscoelastic response of aortic valve tissue: A direct-fit approach. *Ann Biomed Eng*, 32, 223–232.

Dreyfus, G. D., Corbi, P. J., Chan, J., and Bahrami, T. 2005. Secondary tricuspid regurgitation or dilatation: Which should be the criteria for surgical repair? *Ann Thorac Surg*, 79, 127–132.

Dunmore-Buyze, J., Boughner, D. R., Macris, N., and Vesely, I. 1995. A comparison of macroscopic lipid content within porcine pulmonary and aortic valves. Implications for bioprosthetic valves. *J Thorac Cardiovasc Surg*, 110, 1756–1761.

El-Hamamsy, I., Balachandran, K., Yacoub, M. H., Stevens, L. M., Sarathchandra, P., Taylor, P. M., Yoganathan, A. P., and Chester, A. H. 2009. Endothelium-dependent regulation of the mechanical properties of aortic valve cusps. *J Am Coll Cardiol*, 53, 1448–1455.

Emery, R. W. and Arom, K. V. 1991. *The Aortic Valve*, Philadelphia, Henry & Belfus.

Erasmi, A., Sievers, H. H., Scharfschwerdt, M., Eckel, T., and Misfeld, M. 2005. *In vitro* hydrodynamics, cusp-bending deformation, and root distensibility for different types of aortic valve-sparing operations: Remodeling, sinus prosthesis, and reimplantation. *J Thorac Cardiovasc Surg*, 130, 1044–1049.

Fenoglio, J. J., Jr., Tuan Duc, P., Wit, A. L., Bassett, A. L., and Wagner, B. M. 1972. Canine mitral complex. Ultrastructure and electromechanical properties. *Circ Res*, 31, 417–430.

Frater, R. W. 1964. Anatomical rules for the plastic repair of a diseased mitral valve. *Thorax*, 19, 458–464.

Freeman, R. V. and Otto, C. M. 2005. Spectrum of calcific aortic valve disease: Pathogenesis, disease progression, and treatment strategies. *Circulation*, 111, 3316–3326.

Fukuda, S., Gillinov, A. M., Mccarthy, P. M., Stewart, W. J., Song, J. M., Kihara, T., Daimon, M., Shin, M. S., Thomas, J. D., and Shiota, T. 2006a. Determinants of recurrent or residual functional tricuspid regurgitation after tricuspid annuloplasty. *Circulation*, 114, I582–I587.

Fukuda, S., Saracino, G., Matsumura, Y., Daimon, M., Tran, H., Greenberg, N. L., Hozumi, T., Yoshikawa, J., Thomas, J. D., and Shiota, T. 2006b. Three-dimensional geometry of the tricuspid annulus in healthy subjects and in patients with functional tricuspid regurgitation—A real-time, 3-dimensional echocardiographic study. *Circulation,* 114, 1492–1498.

Garg, V., Muth, A. N., Ransom, J. F., Schluterman, M. K., Barnes, R., King, I. N., Grossfeld, P. D., and Srivastava, D. 2005. Mutations in NOTCH1 cause aortic valve disease. *Nature,* 437, 270–274.

Gibson, T. C., Foale, R. A., Guyer, D. E., and Weyman, A. E. 1984. Clinical-significance of incomplete tri-cuspid-valve closure seen on two-dimensional echocardiography. *J Am Coll Cardiol,* 4, 1052–1057.

Glasson, J. R., Komeda, M. K., Daughters, G. T., Niczyporuk, M. A., Bolger, A. F., Ingels, N. B., and Miller, D. C. 1996. Three-dimensional regional dynamics of the normal mitral anulus during left ventricu-lar ejection. *J Thorac Cardiovasc Surg,* 111, 574–585.

Godart, F., Bouzguenda, I., Juthier, F., Wautot, F., Prat, A., Rey, C., Corseaux, D., Ung, A., Jude, B., and Vincentelli, A. 2009. Experimental off-pump transventricular pulmonary valve replacement using a self-expandable valved stent: A new approach for pulmonary incompetence after repaired tetralogy of Fallot? *J Thorac Cardiovasc Surg,* 137, 1141–1145.

Gorman, J. H., 3rd, Gupta, K. B., Streicher, J. T., Gorman, R. C., Jackson, B. M., Ratcliffe, M. B., Bogen, D. K., and Edmunds, L. H., Jr. 1996. Dynamic three-dimensional imaging of the mitral valve and left ventricle by rapid sonomicrometry array localization. *J Thorac Cardiovasc Surg,* 112, 712–726.

Grande-Allen, K. J., Cochran, R. P., Reinhall, P. G., and Kunzelman, K. S. 2001. Mechanisms of aortic valve incompetence: Finite-element modeling of Marfan syndrome. *J Thorac Cardiovasc Surg,* 122, 946–954.

Grande-Allen, K. J., Griffin, B. P., Ratliff, N. B., Cosgrove, D. M., and Vesely, I. 2003. Glycosaminoglycan profiles of myxomatous mitral leaflets and chordae parallel the severity of mechanical alterations. *J Am Coll Cardiol,* 42, 271–277.

Grande-Allen, K. J., Osman, N., Ballinger, M. L., Dadlani, H., Marasco, S., and Little, P. J. 2007. Glycosaminoglycan synthesis and structure as targets for the prevention of calcific aortic valve dis-ease. *Cardiovasc Res,* 76, 19–28.

Grashow, J. S., Yoganathan, A. P., and Sacks, M. S. 2006. Biaixal stress-stretch behavior of the mitral valve anterior leaflet at physiologic strain rates. *Ann Biomed Eng,* 34, 315–325.

Green, G. R., Dagum, P., Glasson, J. R., Nistal, J. F., Daughters, G. T., 2nd, Ingels, N. B., Jr., and Miller, D. C. 1999. Restricted posterior leaflet motion after mitral ring annuloplasty. *Ann Thorac Surg,* 68, 2100–2106.

Hatle, L. and Angelsen, B. 1985. *Doppler Ultrasound in Cardiology Physical Principals and Clinical Applications,* Philadelphia, Lea and Febiger.

He, S., Fontaine, A. A., Schwammenthal, E., Yoganathan, A. P., and Levine, R. A. 1997. Integrated mecha-nism for functional mitral regurgitation: Leaflet restriction versus coapting force: *In vitro* studies. *Circulation,* 96, 1826–1834.

Henderson, Y. and Johnson, F.E. 1912. Two modes of closure of the heart valves. *Heart,* 4, 69–82.

Hilbert, S. L., Luna, R. E., Zhang, J., Wang, Y., Hopkins, R. A., Yu, Z. X., and Ferrans, V. J. 1999. Allograft heart valves: The role of apoptosis-mediated cell loss. *J Thorac Cardiovasc Surg,* 117, 454–462.

Hinderliter, A. L., Willis, P. W., Long, W. A., Clarke, W. R., Ralph, D., Caldwell, E. J., Williams, W. et al. 2003. Frequency and severity of tricuspid regurgitation determined by Doppler echocardiography in primary pulmonary hypertension. *Am J Cardiol,* 91, 1033–1037.

Hiro, M. E., Jouan, J., Pagel, M. R., Lansac, E., Lim, K. H., Lim, H. S., and Duran, C. M. G. 2004. Sonometric study of the normal tricuspid valve annulus in sheep. *J Heart Valve Dis,* 13, 452–460.

Hurst, J. W. and O'Rourke, R. A. 2004. *The Heart,* McGraw-Hill Professional.

Jimenez, J. H., Liou, S. W., Padala, M., He, Z., Sacks, M., Gorman, R. C., Gorman, J. H. 3rd, and Yoganathan, A. P. 2007. A saddle-shaped annulus reduces systolic strain on the central region of the mitral valve anterior leaflet. *J Thorac Cardiovasc Surg,* 134, 1562–1568.

Jimenez, J. H., Soerensen, D. D., He, Z., He, S., and Yoganathan, A. P. 2003. Effects of a saddle shaped annulus on mitral valve function and chordal force distribution: An *in vitro* study. *Ann Biomed Eng,* 31, 1171–1181.

Jimenez, J. H., Soerensen, D. D., He, Z., Ritchie, J., and Yoganathan, A. P. 2005a. Effects of papillary muscle position on chordal force distribution: An *in vitro* study. *J Heart Valve Dis*, 14, 295–302.

Jimenez, J. H., Soerensen, D. D., He, Z., Ritchie, J., and Yoganathan, A. P. 2005b. Mitral valve function and chordal force distribution using a flexible annulus model: An *in vitro* study. *Ann Biomed Eng*, 33, 557–566.

Jouan, J., Pagel, M. R., Hiro, M. E., Lim, K. H., Lansac, E., and Duran, C. M. G. 2007. Further information from a sonometric study of the normal tricuspid valve annulus in sheep: Geometric changes during the cardiac cycle. *J Heart Valve Dis*, 16, 511–518.

Joudinaud, T. M., Flecher, E. M., and Duran, C. M. G. 2006. Functional terminology for the tricuspid valve. *J Heart Valve Dis*, 15, 382–388.

Kalmanson, D. (ed.) 1976. *The Mitral Valve: A Pluridisciplinary Approach*, Acton, MA, Publishing Sciences Group Inc.

Kershaw, J. D., Misfeld, M., Sievers, H. H., Yacoub, M. H., and Chester, A. H. 2004. Specific regional and directional contractile responses of aortic cusp tissue. *J Heart Valve Dis*, 13, 798–803.

Kilner, P. J., Yang, G. Z., Mohiaddin, R. H., Firmin, D. N., and Longmore, D. B. 1993. Helical and retrograde secondary flow patterns in the aortic arch studied by three-directional magnetic resonance velocity mapping. *Circulation*, 88, 2235–2247.

Kim, H. K., Kim, Y. J., Park, J. S., Kim, K. H., Kim, K. B., Ahn, H., Sohn, D. W., Oh, B. H., Park, Y. B., and Choi, Y. S. 2006. Determinants of the severity of functional tricuspid regurgitation. *Am J Cardiol*, 98, 236–242.

King, R. M., Schaff, H. V., Danielson, G. K., Gersh, B. J., Orszulak, T. A., Piehler, J. M., Puga, F. J., and Pluth, J. R. 1984. Surgery for tricuspid regurgitation late after mitral-valve replacement. *Circulation*, 70, 193–197.

Kunzelman, K. S. and Cochran, R. P. 1992. Stress/strain characteristics of porcine mitral valve tissue: Parallel versus perpendicular collagen orientation. *J Card Surg*, 7, 71–78.

Kunzelman, K. S., Cochran, R. P., Murphree, S. S., Ring, W. S., Verrier, E. D., and Eberhart, R. C. 1993. Differential collagen distribution in the mitral valve and its influence on biomechanical behaviour. *J Heart Valve Dis*, 2, 236–244.

Kvitting, J. P., Ebbers, T., Wigstrom, L., Engvall, J., Olin, C. L., and Bolger, A. F. 2004. Flow patterns in the aortic root and the aorta studied with time-resolved, 3-dimensional, phase-contrast magnetic resonance imaging: Implications for aortic valve-sparing surgery. *J Thorac Cardiovasc Surg*, 127, 1602–1607.

Kwan, J., Kim, G. C., Jeon, M. J., Kim, D. H., Shiota, T., Thomas, J. D., Park, K. S., and Lee, W. H. 2007. 3D geometry of a normal tricuspid annulus during systole: A comparison study with the mitral annulus using real-time 3D echocardiography. *Eur J Echocardiogr*, 8, 375–383.

Leeson-Dietrich, J., Boughner, D., and Vesely, I. 1995. Porcine pulmonary and aortic valves: A comparison of their tensile viscoelastic properties at physiological strain rates. *J Heart Valve Dis*, 4, 88–94.

Levine, R. A., Handschumacher, M. D., Sanfilippo, A. J., Hagege, A. A., Harrigan, P., Marshall, J. E., and Weyman, A. E. 1989. Three-dimensional echocardiographic reconstruction of the mitral valve, with implications for the diagnosis of mitral valve prolapse. *Circulation*, 80, 589–598.

Levine, R. A., Stathogiannis, E., Newell, J. B., Harrigan, P., and Weyman, A. E. 1988. Reconsideration of echocardiographic standards for mitral valve prolapse: Lack of association between leaflet displacement isolated to the apical four chamber view and independent echocardiographic evidence of abnormality. *J Am Coll Cardiol*, 11, 1010–1019.

Levine, R. A., Triulzi, M. O., Harrigan, P., and Weyman, A. E. 1987. The relationship of mitral annular shape to the diagnosis of mitral valve prolapse. *Circulation*, 75, 756–767.

Leyh, R. G., Schmidtke, C., Sievers, H. H., and Yacoub, M. H. 1999. Opening and closing characteristics of the aortic valve after different types of valve-preserving surgery. *Circulation*, 100, 2153–2160.

Liao, J., Priddy, L. B., Wang, B., Chen, J., and Vesely, I. 2009. Ultrastructure of porcine mitral valve chordae tendineae. *J Heart Valve Dis*, 18, 292–299.

Liao, J. and Vesely, I. 2003. A structural basis for the size-related mechanical properties of mitral valve chordae tendineae. *J Biomech,* 36, 1125–1133.

Liao, J. and Vesely, I. 2004a. Relationship between collagen fibrils, glycosaminoglycans, and stress relaxation in mitral valve chordae tendineae. *Ann Biomed Eng,* 32, 977–983.

Liao, J. and Vesely, I. 2004b. Skewness angle of interfibrillar proteoglycan increases with applied load on chordae tendineae. *Conf Proc IEEE Eng Med Biol Soc,* 5, 3741–3744.

Liao, J. and Vesely, I. 2007. Skewness angle of interfibrillar proteoglycans increases with applied load on mitral valve chordae tendineae. *J Biomech,* 40, 390–398.

Lloyd-Jones, D., Adams, R. J., Brown, T. M., Carnethon, M., Dai, S., De Simone, G., Ferguson, T. B. et al. 2010. Heart disease and stroke statistics—2010 update: A report from the American Heart Association. *Circulation,* 121, e46–e215.

Lo, D. and Vesely, I. 1995. Biaxial strain analysis of the porcine aortic valve. *Ann Thorac Surg,* 60, S374–S378.

Markl, M., Draney, M. T., Miller, D. C., Levin, J. M., Williamson, E. E., Pelc, N. J., Liang, D. H., and Herfkens, R. J. 2005. Time-resolved three-dimensional magnetic resonance velocity mapping of aortic flow in healthy volunteers and patients after valve-sparing aortic root replacement. *J Thorac Cardiovasc Surg,* 130, 456–463.

Matsuyama, K., Matsumoto, M., Sugita, T., Nishizawa, J., Tokuda, Y., and Matsuo, T. 2003. Predictors of residual tricuspid regurgitation after mitral valve surgery. *Ann Thorac Surg,* 75, 1826–1828.

Meadows, W. R., Vanpraagh, S., Indreika, M., and Sharp, J. T. 1963. Premature mitral valve closure: A hemodynamic explanation for absence of the first sound in aortic insufficiency. *Circulation,* 28, 251–258.

Merryman, W. D., Huang, H. Y., Schoen, F. J., and Sacks, M. S. 2006. The effects of cellular contraction on aortic valve leaflet flexural stiffness. *J Biomech,* 39, 88–96.

Muriago, M., Sheppard, M. N., Ho, S. Y., and Anderson, R. H. 1997. Location of the coronary arterial orifices in the normal heart. *Clin Anat,* 10, 297–302.

Nolan, S. P., Dixon, S. H., Jr., Fisher, R. D., and Morrow, A. G. 1969. The influence of atrial contraction and mitral valve mechanics on ventricular filing. A study of instantaneous mitral valve flow *in vivo. Am Heart J,* 77, 784–791.

Obadia, J. F., Casali, C., Chassignolle, J. F., and Janier, M. 1997. Mitral subvalvular apparatus: Different functions of primary and secondary chordae. *Circulation,* 96, 3124–3128.

Padala, M., Hutchison, R. A., Croft, L. R., Jimenez, J. H., Gorman, R. C., Gorman, J. H., 3rd, Sacks, M. S., and Yoganathan, A. P. 2009a. Saddle shape of the mitral annulus reduces systolic strains on the P2 segment of the posterior mitral leaflet. *Ann Thorac Surg,* 88, 1499–1504.

Padala, M., Powell, S. N., Croft, L. R., Thourani, V. H., Yoganathan, A. P., and Adams, D. H. 2009b. Mitral valve hemodynamics after repair of acute posterior leaflet prolapse: Quadrangular resection versus triangular resection versus neochordoplasty. *J Thorac Cardiovasc Surg,* 138, 309–315.

Pai, R. G., Varadarajan, P., and Tanimoto, M. 2003. Effect of atrial fibrillation on the dynamics of mitral annular area. *J Heart Valve Dis,* 12, 31–37.

Paravisini, J. 1953. [On the mechanism of the closure of the mitral valve.]. *Rev Esp Fisiol,* 9, 9–13.

Paulsen, P. K. and Hasenkam, J. M. 1983. Three-dimensional visualization of velocity profiles in the ascending aorta in dogs, measured with a hot-film anemometer. *J Biomech,* 16, 201–210.

Rabkin-Aikawa, E., Aikawa, M., Farber, M., Kratz, J. R., Garcia-Cardena, G., Kouchoukos, N. T., Mitchell, M. B., Jonas, R. A., and Schoen, F. J. 2004. Clinical pulmonary autograft valves: Pathologic evidence of adaptive remodeling in the aortic site. *J Thorac Cardiovasc Surg,* 128, 552–561.

Reul, H. and Talukdar, N. 1979. Heart valve mechanics. In: Hwang N. H. C., G. D. R., and Patel D. J. (ed.) *Quantitative Cardiovascular Studies Clinical and Research Applications of Engineering Principles.* Baltimore, University Park Press.

Roberts, W. C. 1970. The congenitally bicuspid aortic valve. A study of 85 autopsy cases. *Am J Cardiol,* 26, 72–83.

Robicsek, F., Thubrikar, M. J., Cook, J. W., and Fowler, B. 2004. The congenitally bicuspid aortic valve: How does it function? Why does it fail? *Ann Thorac Surg*, 77, 177–185.

Rossvoll, O., Samstad, S., Torp, H. G., Linker, D. T., Skjaerpe, T., Angelsen, B. A., and Hatle, L. 1991. The velocity distribution in the aortic annulus in normal subjects: A quantitative analysis of two-dimensional Doppler flow maps. *J Am Soc Echocardiogr*, 4, 367–378.

Rushmer, R. F., Finlayson, B. L., and Nash, A. A. 1956. Movements of the mitral valve. *Circ Res*, 4, 337–342.

Sacks, M. S., Smith, D. B., and Hiester, E. D. 1998. The aortic valve microstructure: Effects of transvalvular pressure. *J Biomed Mater Res*, 41, 131–141.

Sadeghi, H. M., Kimura, B. J., Raisinghani, A., Blanchard, D. G., Mahmud, E., Fedullo, P. F., Jamieson, S. W., and Demaria, A. N. 2004. Does lowering pulmonary arterial pressure eliminate severe functional tricuspid regurgitation? *J Am Coll Cardiol*, 44, 126–132.

Sagie, A., Schwammenthal, E., Padial, L. R., Vazquez, J. A., Weyman, A. E., and Levine, R. A. 1994. Determinants of functional tricuspid regurgitation in incomplete tricuspid-valve closure—Doppler color-flow study of 109 patients. *J Am Coll Cardiol*, 24, 446–453.

Sahasakul, Y., Edwards, W. D., Naessens, J. M., and Tajik, A. J. 1988. Age-related changes in aortic and mitral valve thickness: Implications for two-dimensional echocardiography based on an autopsy study of 200 normal human hearts. *Am J Cardiol*, 62, 424–430.

Salisbury, P. F., Cross, C. E., and Rieben, P. A. 1963. Chorda tendinea tension. *Am J Physiol*, 205, 385–392.

Sanfilippo, A. J., Harrigan, P., Popovic, A. D., Weyman, A. E., and Levine, R. A. 1992. Papillary muscle traction in mitral valve prolapse: Quantitation by two-dimensional echocardiography. *J Am Coll Cardiol*, 19, 564–571.

Sarnoff, S. J., Gilmore, J. P., and Mitchell, J. H. 1962. Influence of atrial contraction and relaxation on closure of mitral valve. Observations on effects of autonomic nerve activity. *Circ Res*, 11, 26–35.

Schenke-Layland, K., Stock, U. A., Nsair, A., Xie, J., Angelis, E., Fonseca, C. G., Larbig, R. et al. 2009. Cardiomyopathy is associated with structural remodelling of heart valve extracellular matrix. *Eur Heart J*, 30, 2254–2265.

Scott, M. J. and Vesely, I. 1996. Morphology of porcine aortic valve cusp elastin. *J Heart Valve Dis*, 5, 464–471.

Shah, P. M., Kramer, D. H., and Gramiak, R. 1970. Influence of the timing of atrial systole on mitral valve closure and on the first heart sound in man. *Am J Cardiol*, 26, 231–237.

Shah, P. M. and Raney, A. A. 2008. Tricuspid valve disease. *Curr Probl Cardiol*, 33, 47–84.

Silbiger, J. J. and Bazaz, R. 2009. Contemporary insights into the functional anatomy of the mitral valve. *Am Heart J*, 158, 887–895.

Silver, M. A. and Roberts, W. C. 1985. Detailed anatomy of the normally functioning aortic valve in hearts of normal and increased weight. *Am J Cardiol*, 55, 454–461.

Silver, M. D., Lam, J. H. C., Ranganat, N., and Wigle, E. D. 1971. Morphology of human tricuspid valve. *Circulation*, 43, 333–334.

Skwarek, M., Hreczecha, J., Dudziak, M., and Grzybiak M. 2006. The morphology of the right atrioventricular valve in the adult human heart. *Folia Morphol*, 65, 200–208.

Sliwa, K. and Mocumbi, A. O. 2010. Forgotten cardiovascular diseases in Africa. *Clin Res Cardiol*, 99, 65–74.

Sloth, E., Houlind, K. C., Oyre, S., Kim, W. Y., Pedersen, E. M., Jorgensen, H. S., and Hasenkam, J. M. 1994. Three-dimensional visualization of velocity profiles in the human main pulmonary artery with magnetic resonance phase-velocity mapping. *Am Heart J*, 128, 1130–1138.

Spinner, E. M., Sundareswaran, K., Dasi, L. P., Thourani, V. H., Oshinski, J., and Yoganathan, A. P. 2010. Altered right ventricular papillary muscle position and orientation in patients with a dilated left ventricle. *J Thorac Cardiovasc Surg*, 744–749.

Stella, J. A., Liao, J., and Sacks, M. S. 2007. Time-dependent biaxial mechanical behavior of the aortic heart valve leaflet. *J Biomech*, 40, 3169–3177.

Stewart, B. F., Siscovick, D., Lind, B. K., Gardin, J. M., Gottdiener, J. S., Smith, V. E., Kitzman, D. W., and Otto, C. M. 1997. Clinical factors associated with calcific aortic valve disease. Cardiovascular Health Study. *J Am Coll Cardiol,* 29, 630–634.

Sung, H. W. and Yoganathan, A. P. 1990a. Axial flow velocity patterns in a normal human pulmonary artery model: Pulsatile *in vitro* studies. *J Biomech,* 23, 201–214.

Sung, H. W. and Yoganathan, A. P. 1990b. Secondary flow velocity patterns in a pulmonary artery model with varying degrees of valvular pulmonic stenosis: Pulsatile *in vitro* studies. *J Biomech Eng,* 112, 88–92.

Swanson, M. and Clark, R. E. 1974. Dimensions and geometric relationships of the human aortic valve as a function of pressure. *Circ Res,* 35, 871–882.

Takkenberg, J. J., Klieverik, L. M., Schoof, P. H., Van Suylen, R. J., Van Herwerden, L. A., Zondervan, P. E., Roos-Hesselink, J. W., Eijkemans, M. J., Yacoub, M. H., and Bogers, A. J. 2009. The Ross procedure: A systematic review and meta-analysis. *Circulation,* 119, 222–228.

Taylor, D. E. 1972. Mitral valve geometry and flow dynamics at varying heart rates in the dog. *J Physiol,* 227, 37P–38P.

Taylor, D. E. 1976. International symposium on the mitral valve. *Biomed Eng,* 11, 59.

Taylor, D. E. and Wade, J. D. 1969. Flow through the mitral valve during diastolic filling of the left ventricle. *J Physiol,* 200, 73P–74P.

Tei, C., Pilgrim, J. P., Shah, P. M., Ormiston, J. A., and Wong, M. 1982. The tricuspid-valve annulus—Study of size and motion in normal subjects and in patients with tricuspid regurgitation. *Circulation,* 66, 665–671.

Thubrikar, M. 1990. *The Aortic Valve,* Boca Raton, FL, CRC Press.

Thubrikar, M. J., Aouad, J., and Nolan, S. P. 1986. Patterns of calcific deposits in operatively excised stenotic or purely regurgitant aortic valves and their relation to mechanical stress. *Am J Cardiol,* 58, 304–308.

Tsakiris, A. G., Gordon, D. A., Mathieu, Y., and Irving, L. 1975. Motion of both mitral valve leaflets: A cineroentgenographic study in intact dogs. *J Appl Physiol,* 39, 359–366.

Tsakiris, A. G., Rastelli, G. C., Banchero, N., Wood, E. H., and Kirklin, J. W. 1967. Fixation of the annulus of the mitral valve with a rigid ring. Hemodynamic studies. *Am J Cardiol,* 20, 812–819.

Tsakiris, A. G., Von Bernuth, G., Rastelli, G. C., Bourgeois, M. J., Titus, J. L., and Wood, E. H. 1971. Size and motion of the mitral valve annulus in anesthetized intact dogs. *J Appl Physiol,* 30, 611–618.

Tsifansky, M., Morell, V. O., and Muñoz, R. 2010. Aortic valve regurgitation. In: Munoz, R., Morell, V., Cruz, E., and Vetterly, C. (eds.) *Critical Care of Children with Heart Disease.* London, Springer.

Ubago, J. L., Figueroa, A., Ochoteco, A., Colman, T., Duran, R. M., and Duran, C. G. 1983. Analysis of the amount of tricuspid-valve anular dilatation required to produce functional tricuspid regurgitation. *Am J Cardiol,* 52, 155–158.

Vandenberg, R. A., Williams, J. C., Sturm, R. E., and Wood, E. H. 1969. Effect of ventricular extrasystoles on closure of mitral valve. *Circulation,* 39, 197–204.

Vesely, I. 1998. The role of elastin in aortic valve mechanics. *J Biomech,* 31, 115–123.

Vesely, I. and Lozon, A. 1993. Natural preload of aortic valve leaflet components during glutaraldehyde fixation: Effects on tissue mechanics. *J Biomech,* 26, 121–131.

Vesely, I., Macris, N., Dunmore, P. J., and Boughner, D. 1994. The distribution and morphology of aortic valve cusp lipids. *J Heart Valve Dis,* 3, 451–456.

Vesely, I. and Noseworthy, R. 1992. Micromechanics of the fibrosa and the ventricularis in aortic valve leaflets. *J Biomech,* 25, 101–113.

Victor, S. and Nayak, V. M. 2000. Tricuspid valve is bicuspid. *Ann Thorac Surg,* 69, 1989–1990.

Volebergh, F. E. and Becker, A. E. 1977. Minor congenital variations of cusp size in tricuspid aortic valves. Possible link with isolated aortic stenosis. *Br Heart J,* 39, 1006–1011.

Ward, C. 2000. Clinical significance of the bicuspid aortic valve. *Heart,* 83, 81–85.

Westaby, S., Karp, R. B., Blackstone, E. H., and Bishop, S. P. 1984. Adult human valve dimensions and their surgical significance. *Am J Cardiol,* 53, 552–556.

Weyman, A. E. 1994. *Principles and Practices of Echocardiography,* Philadelphia, Lea & Febiger.

Williams, J. C., O'Donovan, T. P., Cronin, L., and Wood, E. H. 1967. Influence of sequence of atrial and ventricular systoles on closure of mitral valve. *J Appl Physiol,* 22, 786–792.

Williams, J. C., Vandenberg, R. A., O'Donovan, T. P., Sturm, R. E., and Wood, E. H. 1968. Roentgen video densitometer study of mitral valve closure during atrial fibrillation. *J Appl Physiol,* 24, 217–224.

Yap, C. H., Kim, H. S., Balachandran, K., Weiler, M., Haj-Ali, R., and Yoganathan, A. P. 2010. Dynamic deformation characteristics of porcine aortic valve leaflet under normal and hypertensive conditions. *Am J Physiol Heart Circ Physiol,* 298, H395–H405.

Zaky, A., Steinmetz, E., and Feigenbaum, H. 1969. Role of atrium in closure of mitral valve in man. *Am J Physiol,* 217, 1652–1659.

17

Arterial Macrocirculatory Hemodynamics

17.1 Blood Vessel Walls 17-1
17.2 Flow Characteristics 17-2
17.3 Wave Propagation 17-4
17.4 Pathology 17-9
Defining Terms 17-9
References 17-10
Further Information 17-10

Baruch B. Lieber
State University of
New York, Stony Brook

The arterial circulation is a multiply branched network of compliant tubes. The geometry of the network is complex, and the vessels exhibit nonlinear *viscoelastic* behavior. Flow is pulsatile, and the blood flowing through the network is a suspension of red cells and other particles in plasma, which exhibits complex *non-Newtonian* properties. Whereas the development of an exact biomechanical description of arterial hemodynamics is a formidable task, surprisingly useful results can be obtained with greatly simplified models.

The geometrical parameters of the canine *systemic* and *pulmonary* circulations are summarized in Table 17.1. Vessel diameters vary from a maximum of 19 mm in the proximal aorta to 0.008 mm (8 μm) in the capillaries. Because of the multiple branching, the total cross-sectional area increases from 2.8 cm² in the proximal aorta to 1357 cm² in the capillaries. Of the total blood volume, approximately 83% is in the systemic circulation, 12% is in the pulmonary circulation, and the remaining 5% is in the heart. Most of the systemic blood is in the venous circulation, where changes in compliance are used to control mean circulatory blood pressure. This chapter will be concerned with flow in the larger arteries, classes 1–5 in the systemic circulation and 1–3 in the pulmonary circulation in Table 17.1.

17.1 Blood Vessel Walls

The detailed properties of blood vessels were described earlier in this section, but a few general observations are made here to facilitate the following discussion. Blood vessels are composed of three layers, the intima, media, and adventitia. The inner layer, or intima, is composed primarily of *endothelial* cells, which line the vessel and are involved in control of vessel diameter. The media, composed of *elastin*, *collagen*, and smooth muscle, largely determines the elastic properties of the vessel. The outer layer, or adventitia, is composed mainly of connective tissue. Unlike in structures composed of passive elastic materials, vessel diameter and elastic modulus vary with smooth-muscle tone. Dilation in response to increases in flow and *myogenic* constriction in response to increases in pressure have been observed in some arteries. Smooth-muscle tone is also affected by circulating vasoconstrictors such as norepinephrine and vasodilators such as nitroprusside. Blood vessels, like other soft biological tissues, generally do

TABLE 17.1   Model of Vascular Dimensions in a Dog Weighing 20 kg

Class	Vessels	Mean Diam. (mm)	Number of Vessels	Mean Length (mm)	Total Cross-Section (cm²)	Total Blood Volume (mL)	Percentage of Total Volume
			Systemic				
1	Aorta	(19–4.5)	1		(2.8–0.2)	60	
2	Arteries	4.000	40	150.0	5.0	75	
3	Arteries	1.300	500	45.0	6.6	30	
4	Arteries	0.450	6000	13.5	9.5	13	11
5	Arteries	0.150	110,000	4.0	19.4	8	
6	Arterioles	0.050	2.8×10^6	1.2	55.0	7	
7	Capillaries	0.008	2.7×10^9	0.65	1357.9	88	5
8	Venules	0.100	1.0×10^7	1.6	785.4	126	
9	Veins	0.280	660,000	4.8	406.4	196	
10	Veins	0.700	40,000	13.5	154.0	208	
11	Veins	1.800	2100	45.0	53.4	240	
12	Veins	4.500	110	150.0	17.5	263	67
13	Venae cavae	(5–14)	2		(0.2–1.5)	92	
Total						1406	
			Pulmonary				
1	Main artery	1.600	1	28.0	2.0	6	
2	Arteries	4.000	20	10.0	2.5	25	3
3	Arteries	1.000	1550	14.0	12.2	17	
4	Arterioles	0.100	1.5×10^6	0.7	120.0	8	
5	Capillaries	0.008	2.7×10^9	0.5	1357.0	68	4
6	Venules	0.110	2.0×10^6	0.7	190.0	13	
7	Veins	1.100	1650	14.0	15.7	22	
8	Veins	4.200	25	100.0		35	5
9	Main veins	8.000	4	30.0		6	
Total						200	
			Heart				
	Atria		2			30	
	Ventricles	2			54	54	
Total						84	
Total circulation						1690	100

Source: Milnor WR. 1989. *Hemodynamics*, 2nd ed., p. 45. Baltimore, Williams and Wilkins. With permission.

not obey Hooke's law, becoming stiffer as pressure is increased. They also exhibit viscoelastic character-istics such as hysteresis and creep. Fortunately, for many purposes a linear elastic model of blood vessel behavior provides adequate results.

17.2 Flow Characteristics

Blood is a complex substance containing water, inorganic ions, proteins, and cells. Approximately 50% is plasma, a nearly Newtonian fluid consisting of water, ions, and proteins. The balance contains erythrocytes (red blood cells), leukocytes (white blood cells), and platelets. Whereas the behavior of blood in vessels smaller than approximately 100 H exhibits significant non-Newtonian effects, flow in larger vessels can be described reasonably accurately using the Newtonian assumption. There is some evidence suggesting that in blood analog fluids wall shear stress distributions may differ somewhat from Newtonian values (Liepsch et al. 1991).

Flow in the arterial circulation is predominantly laminar with the possible exception of the proximal aorta and main pulmonary artery. In steady flow, transition to turbulence occurs at Reynolds numbers (N_R) above approximately 2300.

$$N_R = \frac{2rV}{\nu}$$

where r = vessel radius, V = velocity, ν = kinematic viscosity/density. Peak-to-mean flow amplitudes

Flow in the major systemic and pulmonary arteries is highly pulsatile. Peak-to-mean flow amplitudes as high as 6 to 1 have been reported in both human and dog (Milnor, 1989, p. 149). Womersley's analysis of incompressible flow in rigid and elastic tubes (Womersley 1957) showed that the importance of pulsatility in the velocity distributions depended on the parameter

$$N_W = r\sqrt{\frac{\omega}{\nu}}$$

where ω = frequency.

This is usually referred to as the Womersley number (N_W) or α-parameter. Womersley's original report is not readily available; however, Milnor provides a reasonably complete account (Milnor, 1989, pp. 106–121).

Mean and peak Reynolds numbers in human and dog are given in Table 17.2, which also includes mean, peak, and minimum velocities as well as the Womersley number. Mean Reynolds numbers in the entire systemic and pulmonary circulations are below 2300. Peak systolic Reynolds numbers exceed 2300 in the aorta and pulmonary artery, and some evidence of transition to turbulence has been reported. In dogs, distributed flow occurs at Reynolds numbers as low as 1000, with higher Womersley numbers increasing the transition Reynolds number (Nerem and Seed, 1972). The values in Table 17.2 are typical for individuals at rest. During exercise, cardiac output and hence Reynolds numbers can increase several fold. The Womersley number also affects the shape of the instantaneous velocity profiles as discussed in Table 17.3.

TABLE 17.2 Normal Average Hemodynamics Values in Man and Dog

	Dog (20 kg)			Man (70 kg, 1.8 m²)		
	N_W	Velocity (cm/s)	N_R	N_W	Velocity (cm/s)	N_R
Systemic vessels						
Ascending aorta	16	15.8(89/0)[a]	870(4900)[b]	21	18(112/0)[a]	1500(9400)[a]
Abdominal aorta	9	12(60.0)	370(1870)	12	14(75/0)	640(3600)
Renal artery	3	41(74/26)	440(800)	4	40(73/26)	700(1300)
Femoral artery	4	10(42/1)	130(580)	4	12(52/2)	200(860)
Femoral vein	5	5	92	7	4	104
Superior vena cava	10	8(20/0)	320(790)	15	9(23/0)	550(1400)
Inferior vena cava	11	19(40/0)	800(1800)	17	21(46/0)	1400(3000)
Pulmonary vessels						
Main artery	14	18(72/0)	900(3700)	20	19(96/0)	1600(7800)
Main vein[c]	7	18(30/9)	270(800)	10	19(38/10)	800(2200)

Source: Milnor WR. 1989. *Hemodynamics*, 2nd ed., p. 148, Baltimore, Williams and Wilkins. With permission.

[a] Mean (systolic/diastolic).

[b] Mean (peak).

[c] One of the usually four terminal pulmonary veins.

TABLE 17.3 Pressure Wave Velocities in Arteries

Artery	Species	Wave Velocity (cm/s)
Ascending aorta	Man	440–520
	Dog	350–472
Thoracic aorta	Man	400–650
	Dog	400–700
Abdominal aorta	Man	500–620
	Dog	550–960
Iliac	Man	700–880
	Dog	700–800
Femoral	Man	800–1800
	Dog	800–1300
Popliteal	Dog	1220–1310
Tibial	Dog	1040–1430
Carotid	Man	680–830
	Dog	610–1240
Pulmonary	Man	168–182
	Dog	255–275
	Rabbit	100
	Pig	190

Source: Milnor WR. 1989. *Hemodynamics*, 2nd ed., p. 235, Baltimore, Williams and Wilkins. With permission.

Note: All data are apparent pressure wave velocities (although the average of higher frequency harmonics approximates the true velocity in many cases), from relatively young subjects with normal cardiovascular systems, at approximately normal distending pressures. Ranges for each vessel and species taken from Table 9.1 of source.

17.3 Wave Propagation

The viscodasticity of blood vessels affects the hemodynamics of arterial flow. The primary function of arterial elasticity is to store blood during systole so that forward flow continues when the aortic valve is dosed. Elasticity also causes a finite wave propagation velocity, which is given approximately by the Moens–Korteweg relationship

$$c = \sqrt{\frac{Eh}{2\rho r}}$$

where E = wall elastic modulus, h = wall thickness, ρ = blood density, r = vessel radius.

Although Moens (1878) and Korteweg (1878) are credited with this formulation, Fung (1984, p. 107) has pointed out that the formula was first derived much earlier (Young, 1808). Wave speeds in arterial blood vessels from several species are given in Table 17.3. In general, wave speeds increase toward the periphery as vessel radius decreases and are considerably lower in the main pulmonary artery than in the aorta owing primarily to the lower pressure and consequently lower elastic modulus.

Wave reflections occur at branches where there is no perfect impedance matching of parent and daughter vessels. The input impedance of a network of vessels is the ratio of pressure to flow. For rigid vessels with laminar flow and negligible inertial effects, the input impedance is simply the resistance and is independent of pressure and flow rate. For elastic vessels, the impedance is dependent on the frequency of the fluctuations in pressure and flow. The impedance can be described by a complex function expressing the amplitude ratio of pressure to flow oscillations and the phase difference between the peaks.

$$\bar{Z}_i(\omega) = \frac{\bar{P}(\omega)}{\bar{Q}(\omega)}$$

$$|\bar{Z}_i(\omega)| = \left|\frac{\bar{P}(\omega)}{\bar{Q}(\omega)}\right|$$

$$\theta_i(\omega) = \theta[\bar{P}(\omega)] - \theta[\bar{Q}(\omega)]$$

where $\bar{Z}_i$ is the complex impedance, $|\bar{Z}_i|$ is the amplitude, and θ_i is the phase.

For an infinitely long straight tube with constant properties, input impedance will be independent of position in the tube and dependent only on vessel and fluid properties. The corresponding value of input impedance is called the *characteristic impedance Z*, given by

$$Z_0 = \frac{\rho c}{A}$$

where A = vessel cross-sectional area.

In general, the input impedance will vary from point to point in the network because of variations in vessel sizes and properties. If the network has the same impedance at each point (perfect impedance matching), there will be no wave reflections. Such a network will transmit energy most efficiently. The reflection coefficient R, defined as the ratio of reflected to incident wave amplitude is related to the relative characteristic impedance of the vessels at a junction. For a parent tube with characteristic impedance Z_0 branching into two daughter tubes with characteristic impedances Z_1 and Z_2, the reflection coefficient is given by

$$R = \frac{Z_0^{-1} - (Z_1^{-1} + Z_2^{-1})}{Z_0^{-1} + (Z_1^{-1} + Z_2^{-1})}$$

and perfect impedance matching requires

$$\frac{1}{Z_0} = \frac{1}{Z_1} + \frac{1}{Z_2}$$

The arterial circulation exhibits partial impedance matching; however, wave reflections do occur. At each branch point, local reflection coefficients typically are less than 0.2. Nonetheless, global reflection coefficients, which account for all reflections distal to a given site, can be considerably higher (Milnor, 1989, p. 217).

In the absence of wave reflections, the input impedance is equal to the characteristic impedance. Womersley's analysis predicts that impedance modulus will decrease monotonically with increasing frequency, whereas the phase angle is negative at low frequency and becomes progressively more positive with increasing frequency. Typical values calculated from Womersley's analysis are shown in Figure 17.1. In the actual circulation, wave reflections cause oscillations in the modulus and phase. Figure 17.2 shows input impedance measured in the ascending aorta of a human. Measurements of input resistance, characteristic impedance, and the frequency of the first minimum in the input impedance are summarized in Table 17.4.

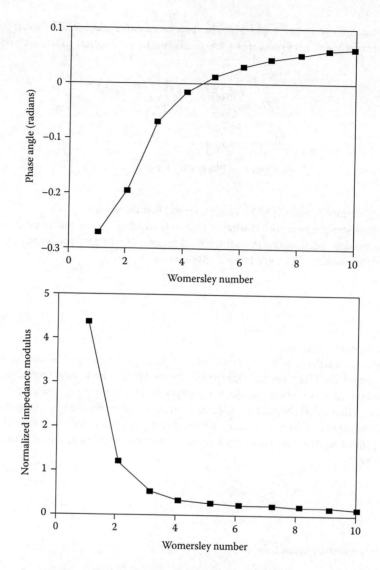

FIGURE 17.1 Characteristic impedance calculated from Womersley's analysis. The top panel contains the phase of the impedance and the bottom panel the modulus, both plotted as a function of the Womersley number N_w, which is promotional to frequency. The curves shown are for an unconstrained tube and include the effects of wall viscosity. The original figure has an inverted phase ordinate. (From Milnor, W.R. 1989. *Hemodynamics*, 2nd ed., p. 172, Baltimore, Williams and Wilkins. With permission.)

Typical pressure and velocity fluctuations throughout the cardiac cycle in man are shown in Figure 17.3. Although mean pressure decreases slightly toward the periphery due to viscous effects, peak pressure shows small increases in the distal aorta due to wave reflection and vessel taper. A rough estimate of mean pressure can be obtained as 1/3 of the sum of systolic pressure and twice the diastolic pressure. Velocity peaks during systole, with some backflow observed in the aorta early in diastole. Flow in the aorta is nearly zero through most of the diastole; however, more peripheral arteries such as the iliac and renal show forward flow throughout the cardiac cycle. This is a result of capacitive discharge of the central arteries as arterial pressure decreases.

Velocity varies across the vessel due to viscous and inertial effects as mentioned earlier. The velocities in Figure 17.3 were measured at one point in the artery. Velocity profiles are complex because the flow is

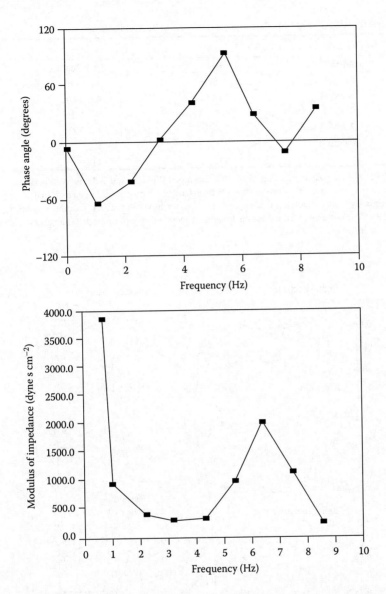

FIGURE 17.2 Input impedance derived from the pressure and velocity data in the ascending aorta of the pig. The top panel contains the phase and the bottom panel the modulus, both plotted as functions of frequency. The peripheral resistance (DC impedance) for this plot was 16,470 dyne s/cm². (From Mills CJ et al. 1970. Pressure–flow relationships and vascular impedance in man. *Cardiovasc Res* 4:405. With permission.)

pulsatile and vessels are elastic, curved, and tapered. Profiles measured in the thoracic aorta of a dog at normal arterial pressure and cardiac output are shown in Figure 17.4. Backflow occurs during diastole, and profiles are flattened even during peak systolic flow. The shape of the profiles varies considerably with mean aortic pressure and cardiac output (Ling et al., 1973).

In more peripheral arteries the profiles resemble parabolic ones as in fully developed laminar flow. The general features of these fully developed flow profiles can be modeled using Womersley's approach, although nonlinear effects may be important in some cases. The qualitative features of the profile depend on the Womersley number N_W. Unsteady effects become more important as N_W increases. Below a value

TABLE 17.4 Characteristic Arterial Impedances in Some Mammals: Average (±SE)

Species	Artery	R_m	Z_0	F_{min}
Dog	Aorta	2809–6830	125–288	6–8
Dog	Pulmonary	536–807	132–295	2–3.5
Dog	Femoral	110–162[a]	4.5–15.8[a]	8–13
Dog	Carotid	69[a]	7.0–9.4[a]	8–11
Rabbit	Aorta	20–50[a]	1.8–2.1[a]	4.5–9.8
Rabbit	Pulmonary		1.1[a]	3.0
Rat	Aorta	153[a]	11.2[a]	12

Source: Milnor WR. 1989. *Hemodynamics*, 2nd ed., p. 183, Baltimore, Williams and Wilkins. With permission.

Note: R_{in}, input resistance (mean arterial pressure/flow) in dyn s/cm⁵. Z_0 characteristic impedance, in dyn s/cm⁵, estimated by averaging high-frequency input impedances in aorta and pulmonary artery; value at 5 Hz for other arteries, f_{min}, frequency of first minimum of Z_i. Values estimated from published figures if averages were not reported. Ranges for each species and vessel taken from values in Table 7.2 of source.

[a] 10³ dyn s/cm⁵.

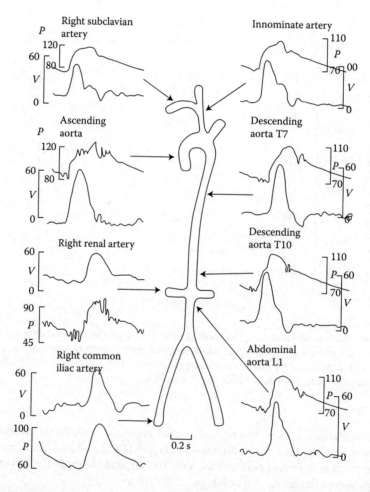

FIGURE 17.3 Simultaneous pressure and blood velocity patterns recorded at points in the systemic circulation of a human. Velocities were recorded with a catheter-tip electromagnetic flowmeter probe. The catheter included a lumen for simultaneous pressure measurement. V = velocity (cm/s), P = pressure (mm Hg). (From Mills CJ et al. 1970. *Cardiovac Res* 40:405. With permission.)

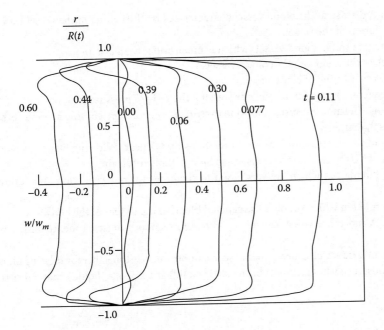

FIGURE 17.4 Velocity profiles obtained with a hot-film anemometer probe in the descending thoracic aorta of a dog at normal arterial pressure and cardiac output. The velocity at t = time/(cardiac period) is plotted as a function of radial position. Velocity w is normalized by the maximum velocity w_m and radial position at each time by the instantaneous vessel radius $R(t)$. The aortic valve opens at $t = 0$. Peak velocity occurs 11% of the cardiac period after aortic valve opening. (From Ling SC et al. 1973. *Circ Res* 33:198. With permission.)

of about 2 the instantaneous profiles are close to the steady parabolic shape. Profiles in the aortic arch are skewed due to curvature of the arch.

17.4 Pathology

Atherosclerosis is a disease of the arterial wall which appears to be strongly influenced by hemodynamics. The disease begins with a thickening of the intimal layer in locations which correlate with the shear stress distribution on the endothelial surface (Friedman et al., 1993). Over time the lesion continues to grow until a significant portion of the vessel lumen is occluded. The peripheral circulation will dilate to compensate for the increase in resistance of the large vessel, compromising the ability of the system to respond to increases in demand during exercise. Eventually the circulation is completely dilated, and resting flow begins to decrease. A blood clot may form at the site or lodge in a narrowed segment, causing an acute loss of blood flow. The disease is particularly dangerous in the coronary and carotid arteries due to the critical oxygen requirements of the heart and brain.

In addition to intimal thickening, the arterial wall properties also change with age. Most measurements suggest that arterial elastic modulus increases with age (hardening of the arteries); however, in some cases arteries do become more compliant (inverse of elasticity) (Learoyd and Taylor, 1966). Local weakening of the wall may also occur, particularly in the descending aorta, giving rise to an aneurysm, which, if ruptures, can cause sudden death.

Defining Terms

Aneurysm: A ballooning of a blood vessel wall either involving the whole circumference or only part of the circumference caused by weakening of the elastic material in the wall.

Atherosclerosis: A disease of the blood vessel characterized by thickening of the vessel wall and eventual occlusion of the vessel.

Collagen: A protein found in blood vessels which is much stiffer than elastin.

Elastin: A very elastic protein found in blood vessels.

Endothelial: The inner lining of blood vessels.

Impedance: A (generally) complex number expressing the ratio of pressure to flow.

Myogenic: A change in smooth-muscle tone due to stretch or relaxation, causing a blood vessel to resist changes in diameter.

Newtonian: A fluid whose stress-rate-of-strain relationship is linear, following Newton's law. The fluid will have a viscosity whose value is independent of rate of strain.

Pulmonary: The circulation which delivers blood to the lungs for reoxygenation and carbon dioxide removal.

Systemic: The circulation which supplies oxygenated blood to the tissues of the body.

Vasoconstrictor: A substance which causes an increase in smooth-muscle tone, thereby constricting blood vessels.

Vasodilator: A substance which causes a decrease in smooth-muscle tone, thereby dilating blood vessels.

Viscoelastic: A substance which exhibits both elastic (solid) and viscous (liquid) characteristics.

References

Chandran KB, Yoganathan AP, and Rittgers SE. 2007 *Biofluid Mechanics, the Human Circulation*. Taylor & Francis, Boca Raton, FL.

Friedman MH, Brinkman AM, Qin JJ, and Seed WA. 1993. Relation between coronary artery geometry and the distribution of early sudanophilic lesions. *Atherosclerosis* 98:193.

Fung YC. 1984. *Biodynamics: Circulation*. Springer-Verlag, New York.

Korteweg DJ. 1878. Uber die Fortpflanzungsgeschwindigkeit des Schalles in elastischen. *Rohren. Ann Phys Chem (NS)* 5:525.

Learoyd BM and Taylor MG. 1966. Alterations with age in the viscoelasdc properties of human arterial walls. *Circ Res* 18:278.

Liepsch D, Thurston G, and Lee M. 1991. Studies of fluids simulating blood-like rheological properties and applications in models of arterial branches. *Biorheology* 28:39.

Ling SC, Atabek WG, Letzing WG, and Patel DJ. 1973. Nonlinear analysis of aortic flow in living dogs. *Circ Res* 33:198.

Mills CJ, Gabe IT, Gault JN et al. 1970. Pressure–flow relationships and vascular impedance in man. *Cardiovasc Res* 4:405.

Milnor WR. 1989. *Hemodynamics*, 2nd ed. Baltimore, Williams and Wilkins.

Moens AI. 1878. *Die Pulskurve*, Leiden, E.J. Brill.

Nerem RM and Seed WA. 1972. An in-vivo study of aortic flow disturbances. *Cardiovasc Res* 6:1.

Womersley JR. 1957. The mathematical analysis of the arterial circulation in a state of oscillatory motion. Wright Air Development Center Technical Report WADC-TR-56-614.

Young T. 1808. Hydraulic investigations, subservient to an intended Croonian lecture on the motion of the blood. *Philos Trans Roy Soc London* 98:164.

Further Information

A good introduction to cardiovascular biomechanics, including arterial hemodynamics, is provided by K. B. Chandran et al. in *Biofluid Mechanics, the Human Circulation*. Y. C. Rung's *Biodynamics— Circulation* is also an excellent starting point, somewhat more mathematical than Chandran. Perhaps the most complete treatment of the subject is in *Hemodynamics* by W. R. Milnor, from which much of this chapter was taken. Milnor's book is quite mathematical and may be difficult for a novice to follow.

Current work in arterial hemodynamics is reported in a number of engineering and physiological journals, including the *Annals of Biomedical Engineering, Journal of Biomechanical Engineering, Circulation Research*, and *The American Journal of Physiology, Heart and Circulatory Physiology*. Symposia sponsored by the American Society of Mechanical Engineers, Biomedical Engineering Society, American Heart Association, and the American Physiological Society contain reports of current research.

18

Mechanics of Blood Vessels

18.1 Assumptions..18-1
Homogeneity of the Vessel Wall • Incompressibility of the Vessel
Wall • Inelasticity of the Vessel Wall • Residual Stress and Strain

18.2 Vascular Anatomy...18-2
18.3 Axisymmetric Deformation..18-3
18.4 Experimental Measurements..18-5
18.5 Equilibrium 18-5
18.6 Strain Energy Density Functions...18-7
Isotropic Blood Vessels • Anisotropic Blood Vessels

References..18-13

Thomas R. Canfield
*Argonne National
Laboratory*

Philip B. Dobrin
*Hines VA Hospital and
Loyola University Medical
Center*

18.1 Assumptions

This chapter is concerned with the mechanical behavior of blood vessels under static loading conditions and the methods required to analyze this behavior. The assumptions underlying this discussion are for *ideal* blood vessels that are at least regionally homogeneous, incompressible, elastic, and cylindrically orthotropic. Although physiologic systems are *nonideal*, much understanding of vascular mechanics has been gained through the use of methods based upon these ideal assumptions.

18.1.1 Homogeneity of the Vessel Wall

On visual inspection, blood vessels appear to be fairly homogeneous and distinct from the surrounding connective tissue. The inhomogeneity of the vascular wall is realized when one examines the tissue under a low-power microscope, where one can easily identify two distinct structures: the media and adventitia. For this reason, the assumption of vessel wall homogeneity is applied cautiously. Such an assumption may be valid only within distinct macroscopic structures. However, few investigators have incorporated macroscopic inhomogeneity into studies of vascular mechanics [1].

18.1.2 Incompressibility of the Vessel Wall

Experimental measurement of wall compressibility of 0.06% at 270 cm of H_2O indicates that the vessel can be considered incompressible when subjected to physiologic pressure and load [2]. In terms of the mechanical behavior of blood vessels, this is small relative to the large magnitude of the distortional strains that occur when blood vessels are deformed under the same conditions. Therefore, vascular compressibility may be important to understand other physiologic processes related to blood vessels, such as the transport of interstitial fluid.

18.1.3 Inelasticity of the Vessel Wall

That blood vessel walls exhibit inelastic behavior such as length–tension and pressure–diameter hysteresis, stress relaxation, and creep has been reported extensively [3,4]. However, blood vessels are able to maintain stability and contain the pressure and flow of blood under a variety of physiologic conditions. These conditions are dynamic but slowly varying with a large static component.

18.1.4 Residual Stress and Strain

Blood vessels are known to retract both longitudinally and circumferentially are excision. This retraction is caused by the relief of distending forces resulting from internal pressure and longitudinal tractions. The magnitude of retraction is influenced by several factors. Among these factors are growth, aging, and hypertension. Circumferential retraction of medium-caliber blood vessels, such as the carotid, iliac, and bracheal arteries, can exceed 70% following reduction of internal blood pressure to zero. In the case of the carotid artery, the amount of longitudinal retraction tends to increase during growth and to decrease in subsequent aging [5]. It would seem reasonable to assume that blood vessels are in a nearly stress-free state when they are fully retracted and free of external loads. This configuration also seems to be a reasonable choice for the reference configuration. However, this ignores residual stress and strain effects that have been the subject of current research [6–11].

Blood vessels are formed in a dynamic environment that gives rise to imbalances between the forces that tend to extend the diameter and length and the internal forces that tend to resist the extension. This imbalance is thought to stimulate the growth of elastin and collagen and to effectively reduce the stresses in the underlying tissue. Under these conditions, it is not surprising that a residual stress state exists when the vessel is fully retracted and free of external tractions. This process has been called *remodeling* [7]. Striking evidence of this remodeling is found when a cylindrical slice of the fully retracted blood vessel is cut longitudinally through the wall. The cylinder springs open, releasing bending stresses kept in balance by the cylindrical geometry [11].

18.2 Vascular Anatomy

A blood vessel can be anatomically divided into three distinct cylindrical sections when viewed under the optical microscope. Starting at the inside of the vessel, they are the intima, the media, and the adventitia. These structures have distinct functions in terms of the blood vessel physiology and mechanical properties.

The intima consists of a thin monolayer of endothelial cells that line the inner surface of the blood vessel. The endothelial cells have little influence on blood vessel mechanics but do play an important role in hemodynamics and transport phenomena. Because of their anatomical location, these cells are subjected to large variations in stress and strain as a result of pulsatile changes in blood pressure and flow.

The media represents the major portion of the vessel wall and provides most of the mechanical strength necessary to sustain structural integrity. The media is organized into alternating layers of interconnected smooth muscle cells and elastic lamellae. There is evidence of collagen throughout the media. These small collagen fibers are found within the bands of smooth muscle and may participate in the transfer of forces between the smooth muscle cells and the elastic lamellae. The elastic lamellae are principally composed of the fibrous protein elastin. The number of elastic lamellae depends upon the wall thickness and the anatomical location [12]. In the case of the canine carotid, the elastic lamellae account for a major component of the static structural response of the blood vessel [13]. This response is modulated by the smooth muscle cells, which have the ability to actively change the mechanical characteristics of the wall [14].

The adventitia consists of loose, more disorganized fibrous connective tissue, which may have less influence on mechanics.

18.3 Axisymmetric Deformation

In the following discussion, we will concern ourselves with the deformation of cylindrical tubes (see Figure 18.1). Blood vessels tend to be nearly cylindrical *in situ* and tend to remain cylindrical when a cylindrical section is excised and studied *in vitro*. Only when the vessel is dissected further does the geometry begin to deviate from cylindrical. For this deformation, there is a unique coordinate mapping

$$(R, \Theta, Z) \rightarrow (r, \theta, z) \tag{18.1}$$

where the undeformed coordinates are given by (R, Θ, Z) and the deformed coordinates are given by (r, θ, z). The deformation is given by a set of restricted functions

$$r = r(R) \tag{18.2}$$

$$\theta = \beta \Theta \tag{18.3}$$

$$z = \mu Z + C_1 \tag{18.4}$$

where the constants μ and β have been introduced to account for a uniform longitudinal strain and a symmetric residual strain that are both independent of the coordinate Θ.

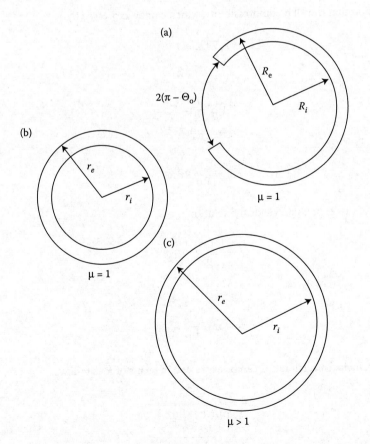

FIGURE 18.1 Cylindrical geometry of a blood vessel. (a) Stress-free reference configuration, (b) fully retracted vessel free of external traction, and (c) vessel *in situ* under longitudinal tether and internal pressurization.

If $\beta = 1$, there is no residual strain. If $\beta \neq 1$, residual stresses and strains are present. If $\beta > 1$, a longitudinal cut through the wall will cause the blood vessel to open up, and the new cross section will form a c-shaped section of an annulus with larger internal and external radii. If $\beta < 1$, the cylindrical shape is unstable, but a thin section will tend to overlap itself. In Choung and Fung's formulation, $\beta = \pi/\Theta_o$, where the angle Θ_o is half the angle spanned by the open annular section [6].

For cylindrical blood vessels, there are two assumed constraints. The first assumption is that the longitudinal strain is uniform through the wall and therefore

$$\lambda_z = \mu = \text{a constant} \tag{18.5}$$

for any cylindrical configuration. Given this, the principal stretch ratios are computed from the above function as

$$\lambda_r = \frac{dr}{dR} \tag{18.6}$$

$$\lambda_\theta = \beta \frac{r}{R} \tag{18.7}$$

$$\lambda_z = \mu \tag{18.8}$$

The second assumption is wall incompressibility, which can be expressed by

$$\lambda_r \lambda_\theta \lambda_z \equiv 1 \tag{18.9}$$

or

$$\beta\mu \frac{r}{R} \frac{dr}{dR} = 1 \tag{18.10}$$

and therefore

$$r\,dr = \frac{1}{\beta\mu} R\,dR \tag{18.11}$$

The integration of this expression yields the solution

$$r^2 = \frac{1}{\beta\mu} R^2 + c_2 \tag{18.12}$$

where

$$c_2 = r_e^2 - \frac{1}{\beta\mu} R_e^2 \tag{18.13}$$

As a result, the principal stretch ratios can be expressed in terms of R as follows:

$$\lambda_r = \frac{R}{\sqrt{\beta\mu(R^2 + \beta\mu c_2)}} \tag{18.14}$$

$$\lambda_\theta = \sqrt{\frac{1}{\beta\mu} + \frac{c_2}{R^2}} \tag{18.15}$$

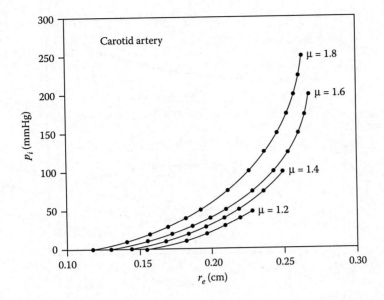

FIGURE 18.2 Pressure–radius curves for the canine carotid artery at various degrees of longitudinal extension.

18.4 Experimental Measurements

The basic experimental setup required to measure the mechanical properties of blood vessels *in vitro* is described in Reference 14. It consists of a temperature-regulated bath of physiologic saline solution to maintain immersed cylindrical blood vessel segments, devices to measure the diameter, an apparatus to hold the vessel at a constant longitudinal extension and to measure longitudinal distending force, and a system to deliver and control the internal pressure of the vessel with 100% oxygen. Typical data obtained from this type of experiment are shown in Figures 18.2 and 18.3.

18.5 Equilibrium

When blood vessels are excised, they retract both longitudinally and circumferentially. Restoration to natural dimensions requires the application of internal pressure, p_i, and a longitudinal tether force, F_T. The internal pressure and longitudinal tether are balanced by the development of forces within the vessel wall. The internal pressure is balanced in the circumferential direction by a wall tension, T. The longitudinal tether force and pressure are balanced by the retractive force of the wall, F_R

$$T = p_i r_i \tag{18.16}$$

$$F_R = F_T + p_i \pi r_i^2 \tag{18.17}$$

The first equation is the familiar law of Laplace for a cylindrical tube with internal radius r_i. It indicates that the force due to internal pressure, p_i, must be balanced by a tensile force (per unit length), T, within the wall. This tension is the integral of the circumferentially directed force intensity (or stress, σ_θ) across the wall

$$T = \int_{r_i}^{r_e} \sigma_\theta dr = \bar{\sigma}_\theta h \tag{18.18}$$

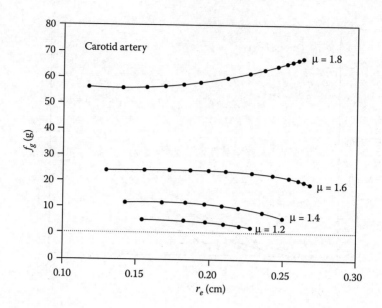

FIGURE 18.3 Longitudinal distending force as a function of radius at various degrees of longitudinal extension.

where $\bar{\sigma}_\theta$ is the mean value of the circumferential stress and h is the wall thickness. Similarly, the longitudinal tether force, F_T, and extending force due to internal pressure are balanced by a retractive internal force, F_R, due to axial stress, σ_z, in the blood vessel wall

$$F_R = 2\pi \int_{r_i}^{r_e} \sigma_z r\, dr = \bar{\sigma}_z\, \pi h(r_e + r_i) \tag{18.19}$$

where $\bar{\sigma}_z$ is the mean value of this longitudinal stress. The mean stresses are calculated from the above equation as

$$\bar{\sigma}_\theta = p_i \frac{r_i}{h} \tag{18.20}$$

$$\bar{\sigma}_z = \frac{F_T}{\pi h(r_e + r_i)} + \frac{p_i}{2} \frac{r_i}{h} \tag{18.21}$$

The mean stresses are a fairly good approximation for thin-walled tubes where the variations through the wall are small. However, the range of applicability of the thin-wall assumption depends upon the material properties and geometry. In a linear elastic material, the variation in σ_θ is less than 5% for $r/h > 20$. When the material is nonlinear or the deformation is large, the variations in stress can be more severe (see Figure 18.10).

The stress distribution is determined by solving the equilibrium equation

$$\frac{1}{r} \frac{d}{dr}(r\sigma_r) - \frac{\sigma_\theta}{r} = 0 \tag{18.22}$$

This equation governs how the two stresses are related and must change in the cylindrical geometry. For uniform extension and internal pressurization, the stresses must be functions of a single radial coordinate, r, subject to the two boundary conditions for the radial stress:

$$\sigma_r(r_i, \mu) = -p_i \qquad (18.23)$$

$$\sigma_r(r_e, \mu) = 0 \qquad (18.24)$$

18.6 Strain Energy Density Functions

Blood vessels are able to maintain their structural stability and contain steady oscillating internal pressures. This property suggests a strong elastic component, which has been called *pseudoelasticity* [4]. This elastic response can be characterized by a single potential function called the *strain energy density*. It is a scalar function of the strains that determines the amount of stored elastic energy per unit volume. In the case of a cylindrically orthotropic tube of incompressible material, the strain energy density can be written in the following functional form:

$$W = W^*(\lambda_r, \lambda_\theta, \lambda_z) + \lambda_r \lambda_\theta \lambda_z p \qquad (18.25)$$

where p is a scalar function of position, R. The stresses are computed from the strain energy by the following equation:

$$\sigma_i = \lambda_i \frac{\partial W^*}{\partial \lambda_i} + p \qquad (18.26)$$

We make the following transformation [15]:

$$\lambda = \frac{\beta r}{\sqrt{\beta \mu (r^2 - c_2)}} \qquad (18.27)$$

which upon differentiation gives

$$r \frac{d\lambda}{dr} = \beta^{-1}(\beta \lambda - \mu \lambda^3) \qquad (18.28)$$

After these expressions and the stresses in terms of the strain energy density function are introduced into the equilibrium equation, we obtain an ordinary differential equation for p

$$\frac{dp}{d\lambda} = \frac{\beta W^*_{\lambda_\theta} - W^*_{\lambda_r}}{\beta \lambda = \mu \lambda^3} - \frac{dW^*_{\lambda_r}}{d\lambda} \qquad (18.29)$$

subject to the boundary conditions

$$p(R_i) = p_i \qquad (18.30)$$

$$p(R_e) = 0 \qquad (18.31)$$

18.6.1 Isotropic Blood Vessels

A blood vessel generally exhibits anisotropic behavior when subjected to large variations in internal pressure and distending force. When the degree of anisotropy is small, the blood vessel may be treated as isotropic. For isotropic materials, it is convenient to introduce the strain invariants:

$$I_1 = \lambda_r^2 + \lambda_\theta^2 + \lambda_z^2 \qquad (18.32)$$

$$I_2 = \lambda_r^2\lambda_\theta^2 + \lambda_\theta^2\lambda_z^2 + \lambda_z^2\lambda_r^2 \tag{18.33}$$

$$I_3 = \lambda_r^2\lambda_\theta^2\lambda_z^2 \tag{18.34}$$

These are measures of strain that are independent of the choice of coordinates. If the material is incompressible

$$I_3 = j^2 \equiv 1 \tag{18.35}$$

and the strain energy density is a function of the first two invariants, then

$$W = W(I_1, I_2) \tag{18.36}$$

The least complex form for an incompressible material is the first-order polynomial, which was first proposed by Mooney to characterize rubber:

$$W^\star = \frac{G}{2}[(I_1 - 3) + k(I_2 - 3)] \tag{18.37}$$

It involves only two elastic constants. A special case, where $k = 0$, is the neo-Hookean material, which can be derived from thermodynamics principles for a simple solid. The exact solutions can be obtained for the cylindrical deformation of a thick-walled tube. In the case where there is no residual strain, we have the following equations:

$$P = -G(1 + k\mu^2)\left[\frac{\log \lambda}{\mu} + \frac{1}{2\mu^2\lambda^2}\right] + c_0 \tag{18.38}$$

$$\sigma_r = G\left[\frac{1}{\lambda^2\mu^2} + k\left(\frac{1}{\mu^2} + \frac{1}{\lambda^2}\right)\right] + p \tag{18.39}$$

$$\sigma_\theta = G\left[\lambda^2 + k\left(\frac{1}{\mu^2} + \lambda^2\mu^2\right)\right] + p \tag{18.40}$$

$$\sigma_z = G\left[\mu^2 + k\left(\lambda^2\mu^2 + \frac{1}{\lambda^2}\right)\right] + p \tag{18.41}$$

However, these equations predict stress softening for a vessel subjected to internal pressurization at fixed lengths, rather than the stress stiffening observed in experimental studies on arteries and veins (see Figures 18.4 and 18.5).

An alternative isotropic strain energy density function that can predict the appropriate type of stress stiffening for blood vessels is an exponential where the arguments are a polynomial of the strain invariants. The first-order form is given by

$$W^\star = \frac{G_0}{2k_1}\exp[k_1(I_1 - 3) + k_2(I_2 - 3)] \tag{18.42}$$

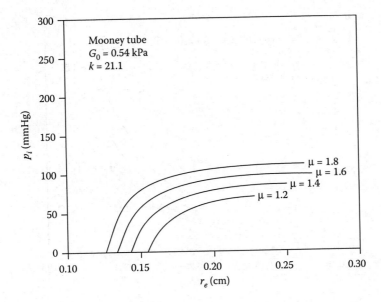

FIGURE 18.4   Pressure–radius curves for a Mooney–Rivlin tube with the approximate dimensions of the carotid.

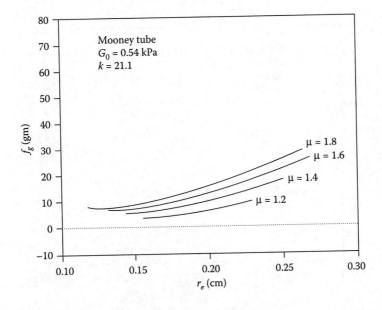

FIGURE 18.5   Longitudinal distending force as a function of radius for the Mooney–Rivlin tube.

This requires the determination of only two independent elastic constants. The third, G_0, is introduced to facilitate scaling of the argument of the exponent (see Figures 18.6 and 18.7). This exponential form is attractive for several reasons. It is a natural extension of the observation that biologic tissue stiffness is proportional to the load in simple elongation. This stress stiffening has been attributed to a statistical recruitment and alignment of tangled and disorganized long chains of proteins. The exponential forms resemble statistical distributions derived from these same arguments.

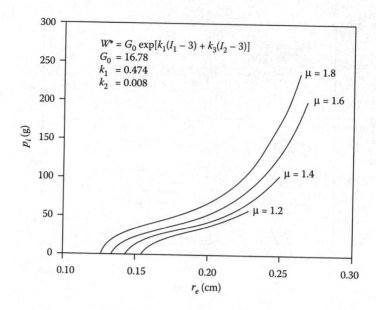

FIGURE 18.6 Pressure–radius curves for the tube with the approximate dimensions of the carotid calculated using an isotropic exponential strain energy density function.

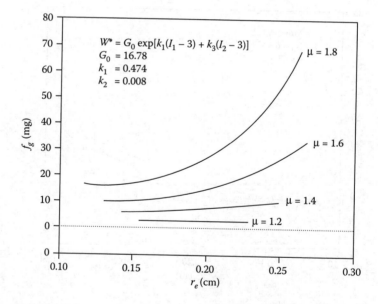

FIGURE 18.7 Longitudinal distending force as a function of radius for the isotropic tube.

18.6.2 Anisotropic Blood Vessels

Studies of the orthotropic behavior of blood vessels may employ polynomial or exponential strain energy density functions that include all strain terms or extension ratios. In particular, the strain energy density function can be of the form

$$W^\star = q_n(\lambda_r, \lambda_\theta, \lambda_z)$$

(18.43)

or

$$W^\star = e^{q_n(\lambda_r, \lambda_\theta, \lambda_z)} \tag{18.44}$$

where q_n is a polynomial of order n. Since the material is incompressible, the explicit dependence upon λ_r can be eliminated either by substituting $\lambda_r = \lambda_\theta^{-1}\lambda_z^{-1}$ or by assuming that the wall is thin and hence the contribution of these terms is small. Figures 18.8 and 18.9 illustrate how well the experimental data can be fitted to an exponential strain density function whose argument is a polynomial of order $n = 3$.

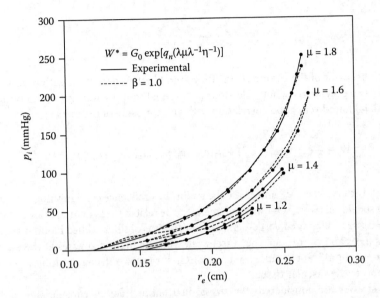

FIGURE 18.8 Pressure–radius curves for a fully orthotropic vessel calculated with an exponential strain energy density function.

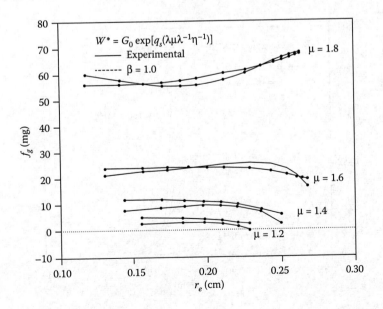

FIGURE 18.9 Longitudinal distending force as a function of radius for the orthotropic vessel.

Care must be taken to formulate expressions that will lead to stresses that behave properly. For this reason, it is convenient to formulate the strain energy density in terms of the Lagrangian strains

$$e_i = 1/2(\lambda_i^2 - 1) \tag{18.45}$$

and in this case, we can consider polynomials of the Lagrangian strains, $q_n(e_r, e_\theta, e_z)$.

Vaishnav et al. [16] proposed using a polynomial of the form

$$W^* = \sum_{i=2}^{n} \sum_{j=0}^{i} a_{ij-i} e_\theta^{i-j} e_z^j \tag{18.46}$$

to approximate the behavior of the canine aorta. They found better correlation with order-three polynomials over order-two polynomials, but order-four polynomials did not warrant the additional work.

Later, Fung et al. [4] found very good correlation with an expression of the form

$$W - \frac{C}{2} \exp[a_1(e_\theta^2 - e_z^{*2}) + a_2(e_z^2 - e_z^{*2}) + 2a_4(e_\theta e_z - e_\theta^* e_z^*)] \tag{18.47}$$

for the canine carotid artery, where e_θ^* and e_z^* are the strains in a reference configuration at *in situ* length and pressure. Why should this work? One answer appears to be related to residual stresses and strains.

When residual stresses are ignored, large-deformation analysis of thick-walled blood vessels predicts steep distributions in σ_θ and σ_z through the vessel wall, with the highest stresses at the interior. This prediction is considered significant because high tensions in the inner wall could inhibit vascularization and oxygen transport to the vascular tissue.

When residual stresses are considered, the stress distributions flatten considerably and become almost uniform at *in situ* length and pressure. Figure 18.10 shows the radial stress distributions computed for a vessel with $\beta = 1$ and $\beta = 1.11$. Takamizawa and Hayashi [9] have even considered the case where the strain distribution is uniform *in situ*. The physiologic implications are that the vascular tissue

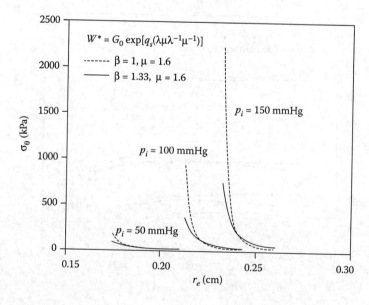

FIGURE 18.10 Stress distributions through the wall at various pressures for the orthotropic vessel.

is in a constant state of flux. The new tissue is synthesized in a state of stress that allows it to redistribute the internal loads more uniformly. There is probably no stress-free reference state [7,8,17]. Continuous dissection of the tissue into smaller and smaller pieces would continue to relieve residual stresses and strains [10].

References

1. Von Maltzahn, W.-W., Desdo, D., and Wiemier, W. 1981. Elastic properties of arteries: A nonlinear two-layer cylindrical model. *J. Biomech.* 4:389.
2. Carew, T.E., Vaishnav, R.N., and Patel, D.J. 1968. Compressibility of the arterial walls. *Circ. Res.* 23:61.
3. Bergel, D.H. 1961. The static elastic properties of the arterial wall. *J. Physiol.* 156:445.
4. Fung, Y.C., Fronek, K., and Patitucci, P. 1979. Pseudoelasticity of arteries and the choice of its mathematical expression. *Am. J. Physiol.* 237:H620.
5. Dobrin, P.B. 1978. Mechanical properties of arteries. *Physiol. Rev.* 58:397.
6. Choung, C.J. and Fung, Y.C. 1986. On residual stresses in arteries. *J. Biomed. Eng.* 108:189.
7. Fung, Y.C., Liu, S.Q., and Zhou, J.B. 1993. Remodeling of the constitutive equation while a blood vessel remodels itself under strain. *J. Biomech. Eng.* 115:453.
8. Rachev, A., Greenwald, S., Kane, T., Moore, J., and Meister, J.-J. 1994. Effects of age-related changes in the residual strains on the stress distribution in the arterial wall. In J. Vossoughi (ed.), *Proceedings of the 13th Society of Biomedical Engineering Recent Developments*, pp. 409–412, Washington DC, University of District of Columbia.
9. Takamizawa, K. and Hayashi, K. 1987. Strain energy density function and the uniform strain hypothesis for arterial mechanics. *J. Biomech.* 20:7.
10. Vassoughi, J. 1992. Longitudinal residual strain in arteries. *Proceedings of the 11th South Biomedical Engineering Conference*, Memphis, TN.
11. Vaishnav, R.N. and Vassoughi, J. 1983. Estimation of residual stresses in aortic segments. In C.W. Hall (ed.), *Biomedical Engineering II, Recent Developments*, pp. 330–333, New York, NY, Pergamon Press.
12. Wolinsky, H. and Glagov, S. 1969. Comparison of abdominal and thoracic aortic media structure in mammals. *Circ. Res.* 25:677.
13. Dobrin, P.B. and Canfield, T.R. 1984. Elastase, collagenase, and the biaxial elastic properties of dog carotid artery. *Am. J. Physiol.* 2547:H124.
14. Dobrin, P.B. and Rovick, A.A. 1969. Influence of vascular smooth muscle on contractile mechanics and elasticity of arteries. *Am. J. Physiol.* 217:1644.
15. Chu, B.M. and Oka, S. 1973. Influence of longitudinal tethering on the tension in thick-walled blood vessels in equilibrium. *Biorheology* 10:517.
16. Vaishnav, R.N., Young, J.T., Janicki, J.S., and Patel, D.J. 1972. Nonlinear anisotropic elastic properties of the canine aorta. *Biophys. J.* 12:1008.
17. Dobrin, P.D., Canfield, T., and Sinha, S. 1975. Development of longitudinal retraction of carotid arteries in neonatal dogs. *Experientia* 31:1295.
18. Doyle, J.M. and Dobrin, P.B. 1971. Finite deformation of the relaxed and contracted dog carotid artery. *Microvasc. Res.* 3:400.

19

The Venous System

19.1 Introduction **19**-1
19.2 Definitions **19**-2
  Capacitance • Compliance • Unstressed Volume • Stressed Volume • Capacity • Mean Filling Pressure • Venous Resistance • Venous Inertance
19.3 Methods to Measure Venous Characteristics........................... **19**-3
  Resistance • Capacitance • Compliance • Gravimetric Techniques • Outflow Occlusion • Integral of Inflow Minus Outflow
19.4 Typical Values.. **19**-5
Acknowledgments.. **19**-6
References... **19**-6

Artin A. Shoukas
Johns Hopkins University

Carl F. Rothe
Indiana University

19.1 Introduction

The venous system not only serves as a conduit for the return of blood from the capillaries to the heart but also provides a dynamic, variable blood storage compartment that influences cardiac output. The systemic (noncardiopulmonary) venous system contains more than 75% of the blood volume of the entire systemic circulation. Although the heart is the source of energy for propelling blood throughout the circulation, filling of the right heart before the subsequent beat is primarily passive. The subsequent amount of blood ejected is exquisitely sensitive to the transmural filling pressure (e.g., a change of right heart filling pressure of 1 cm water can cause the cardiac output to change by about 50%).

Because the blood vessels are elastic and have smooth muscle in their walls, contraction or relaxation of the smooth muscle can quickly redistribute blood between the periphery and the heart to influence cardiac filling and thus cardiac output. Even though the right ventricle is not essential for life, its functioning acts to reduce the central venous pressure to facilitate venous return [1]. It largely determines the magnitude of the cardiac output by influencing the degree of filling of the left heart. Dynamic changes in venous tone, by redistributing blood volume, can thus, at rest, change cardiac output over a range of more than ±20%. The dimensions of the vasculature influence both blood flow—by way of their resistive properties—and contained blood volume—by way of their capacitive properties. The arteries have about 10 times the resistance of the veins, and the veins are more than 10 times as compliant as the arteries.

The conduit characteristics of the venous system primarily depend on the anatomy of the system. Valves in the veins of the limbs are crucial for reducing the pressure in dependent parts of the body. Even small movements from skeletal muscle activity tend to compress the veins and move blood toward the heart. A competent valve then blocks back flow, thus relieving the pressure when the movement stops. Even a few steps can reduce the transmural venous pressure in the ankle from as much as 100 mmHg to about 20 mmHg. Without this mechanism, transcapillary movement of fluid into the extravascular spaces results in edema. Varicose (swollen) veins and peripheral pooling of blood can result from damage to the venous valves. During exercise, the rhythmic contraction of the skeletal muscles, in conjunction with venous valves, provides an important mechanism—the skeletal muscle pump—aiding the large increases in blood flow through the muscles without excessive increases in capillary pressure and blood pooling in the veins of the muscles. Without this mechanism, the increase in venous return leading to the dramatic increases in cardiac output would be greatly limited.

19.2 Definitions

19.2.1 Capacitance

Capacitance is a general term that relates the magnitude of contained volume to the transmural pressure across the vessel walls and is defined by the pressure–volume relationship. In living blood vessels, the pressure–volume relationship is complex and nonlinear. At transmural pressure near zero, there is a finite volume within the vessels (see definition of *unstressed volume*). If this volume is then removed from the vessels, there is only a small decrease in transmural pressure as the vessel collapses from a circular cross-section to an elliptical one. This is especially true for superficial or isolated venous vessels. However, for vessels which are tethered or embedded in tissue a negative pressure may result without appreciably changing the shape of the vessels. With increases in contained volume, the vessel becomes distended, and there is a concomitant increase in transmural pressure. The incremental change in volume to incremental change in transmural pressure is often relatively constant. At very high transmural pressures vessels become stiffer, and the incremental volume change to transmural pressure change is small. Because all blood vessels exhibit these nonlinearities, no single parameter can describe capacitance; instead the entire pressure–volume relationship must be considered.

19.2.2 Compliance

Vascular compliance (C) is defined as the slope of the pressure–volume relationship. It is the ratio of the change in incremental volume (ΔV) to a change in incremental transmural pressure (ΔP). Thus, $C = \Delta V/\Delta P$. Because the pressure–volume relationship is nonlinear, the slope of the relationship is not constant over its full range of pressures, and so the compliance should be specified at a given pressure. Units of compliance are those of volume divided by pressure, usually reported in mL/mmHg. Values are typically normalized to wet tissue weight or to total body weight. When the compliance is normalized by the total contained blood volume, it is termed the *vascular distensibility* and represents the fractional change in volume ($\Delta V/V$) per change in transmural pressure; $D = (\Delta V/V) \Delta P$, where V is the volume at control or at zero transmural pressure.

19.2.3 Unstressed Volume

Unstressed volume (V_0) is the volume in the vascular system when the transmural pressure is zero. It is a calculated volume obtained by extrapolating the relatively linear segment of the pressure–volume relationship over the normal operating range to zero transmural pressure. Many studies have shown that reflexes and drugs have quantitatively more influence on V_0 than on the compliance.

19.2.4 Stressed Volume

The *stressed volume* (V_s) is the volume of blood in the vascular system that must be removed to change the computed transmural pressure from its prevailing value to zero transmural pressure. It is computed as the product of the vascular compliance and transmural distending pressure: $V_s = V \times P$. The total contained blood volume at a specific pressure (P) is the sum of stressed and unstressed volume. The unstressed volume is then computed as the total blood volume minus the stressed volume. Because of the marked nonlinearity around zero transmural pressure and the required extrapolation, both V_0 and V_s are virtual volumes.

19.2.5 Capacity

Capacity refers to the amount of blood volume contained in the blood vessels at a specific distending pressure. It is the sum of the unstressed volume and the stressed volume, $V = V_0 + V_s$.

19.2.6 Mean Filling Pressure

If the inflow and outflow of an organ are suddenly stopped, and blood volume is redistributed so that all pressures within the vasculature are the same, this pressure is the *mean filling pressure* [2]. This pressure can be measured for the systemic or pulmonary circuits or the body as a whole. The arterial pressure often does not equal the venous pressure as flow is reduced to zero, because blood must move from the distended arterial vessels to the venous beds during the measurement maneuver, and the flow may stop before equilibrium occurs. This is because smooth-muscle activity in the arterial vessels, rheological properties of blood, or high interstitial pressures act to impede the flow. Thus, corrections must often be made [2,3]. The experimentally measured mean filling pressure provides a good estimate of P_v (the pressure in the minute venules), for estimating venous stressed volume.

19.2.7 Venous Resistance

Venous resistance (R) refers to the hindrance to blood flow through the venous vasculature caused by friction of the moving blood along the venous vascular wall. By definition it is the ratio of the pressure gradient between the entrance of the venous circulation, namely the capillaries, and the venous outflow divided by the venous flow rate. Thus,

$$R = \frac{(P_c = P_{ra})}{F} \tag{19.1}$$

where R is the venous resistance, P_c is the capillary pressure, P_{ra} is the right atrial pressure, and F is the venous flow. As flow is decreased to zero, arterial closure may occur, leading to a positive perfusion pressure at zero flow. With partial collapse of veins, a Starling resistor-like condition is present in which an increase in outlet pressure has no influence on flow until the outlet pressure is greater than the "waterfall" pressure.

19.2.8 Venous Inertance

Venous inertance (I_v) is the opposition to a change in flow rate related to the mass of the bolus of blood that is accelerated or decelerated. The inertance I_v for a cylindrical tube with constant cross-sectional area is $I_v = L\rho/A$, where L is the length of the vessel, ρ is the density of the blood, and A is the cross-sectional area [4].

19.3 Methods to Measure Venous Characteristics

Our knowledge of the nature and role of the capacitance characteristics of the venous system has been limited by the difficulty of measuring the various variables needed to compute parameter values. State-of-the-art equipment is often needed because of the low pressures and many disturbing factors present. Many of the techniques that have been used to measure venous capacitance require numerous assumptions that may not be correct or are currently impossible to evaluate [3].

19.3.1 Resistance

For the estimate of vascular resistance, the upstream to outflow pressure gradient across the tissues must be estimated along with a measure of flow. Pressures in large vessels are measured with a catheter connected to a pressure transducer, which typically involves measurement of minute changes in resistance elements attached to a stiff diaphragm which flexes proportionally to the pressure. For the veins in tissue, the upstream pressure, just downstream from the capillaries, is much more difficult to measure because of the minute size (~15 μm) of the vessels. For this a servo-null micropipette technique may be used. A glass micropipette with a tip diameter of about 2 μm is filled with a 1–2 mol saline solution. When the pipette is inserted into a vein, the pressure tends to drive the lower conductance blood plasma into the pipette. The conductance is measured using an AC-driven bridge. A servosystem, driven by the imbalance signal, is used to develop a counter pressure to maintain the interface between the low-conductance filling solution and the plasma near the tip of the pipette. This counter pressure, which equals the intravascular pressure, is measured with a pressure transducer. Careful calibration is essential.

Another approach for estimating the upstream pressure in the veins is to measure the mean filling pressure of the organ (see above) and assume that this pressure is the upstream venous pressure. Because this venous pressure must be less than the capillary pressure and because most of the blood in an organ is in the small veins and venules, this assumption, though tenuous, is not unreasonable. To measure flow many approaches are available, including electromagnetic, transit-time ultrasonic, or Doppler ultrasonic flowmeters. Usually the arterial inflow is measured with the assumption that the outflow is the same. Indicator dilution techniques are also used to estimate average flow. They are based on the principle that the reduction in concentration of infused indicator is inversely proportional to the rate of flow. Either a bolus injection or a continuous infusion may be used. Adequacy of mixing of indicator across the flow stream, lack of collateral flows, and adequately representative sampling must be considered [5].

19.3.2 Capacitance

For estimating the capacitance parameters of the veins, contained volume, rather than flow, and transmural pressure, rather than the longitudinal pressure gradient, must be measured. Pressures are measured as described above. For the desired pressure–volume relationship the total contained volume must be known.

The techniques used to measure total blood volume include *indicator dilution*. The ratio of the integral of indicator concentration time to that of concentration is used to compute the mean transit time (MTT) following the sudden injection of a bolus of indicator [3,5]. The active volume is the product of MTT and flow, with flow measured as outlined above. Scintigraphy provides an image of the distribution of radioactivity in tissues. A radioisotope, such as technetium-99 that is bound to red blood cells which in turn are contained within the vasculature, is injected and allowed to equilibrate. A camera, with many collimating channels sensitive to the emitted radiation, is placed over the tissue. The activity recorded is proportional to the volume of blood. Currently it is not possible to accurately calibrate the systems to provide measures of blood volume because of uncertain attenuation of radiation by the tissue and distance. Furthermore, delimiting a particular organ within the body and separating arterial and venous segments of the circulation are difficult.

19.3.3 Compliance

To estimate compliance, changes in volume are needed. This is generally easier than measuring the total blood volume. Using *plethysmography*, a rigid container is placed around the organ, and a servo system functions to change the fluid volume in the chamber to maintain the chamber pressure constant. The consequent volume change is measured and assumed to be primarily venous, because most of the vascular volume is venous. With a tight system and careful technique, at the end of the experiment both inflow and outflow blood vessels can be occluded and then the contained blood washed out and measured to provide a measure of the total blood volume [6].

19.3.4 Gravimetric Techniques

Gravimetric techniques can be used to measure changes in blood volume. If the organ can be isolated and weighed continuously with the blood vessels intact, changes in volume can be measured in response to drugs or reflexes. With an important modification, this approach can be applied to an organ or the systemic circulation; the tissues are perfused at a constant rate, and the outflow is emptied at a constant pressure into a reservoir. Because the reservoir is emptied at a constant rate for the perfusion, changes in reservoir volume reflect an opposite change in the perfused tissue blood volume [7]. To measure compliance, the outflow pressure is changed (2–5 mmHg) and the corresponding change in reservoir volume noted. With the inflow and outflow pressure held constant, the pressure gradients are assumed to be constant so that 100% of an outflow pressure change can be assumed to be transmitted to the primary capacitance vessels. Any reflex or drug-induced change in reservoir volume may be assumed to be inversely related to an active change in vascular volume [7–9]. If resistances are also changed by the reflex or drug, then corrections are needed and the interpretations are more complex.

19.3.5 Outflow Occlusion

If the outflow downstream from the venous catheter is suddenly occluded, the venous pressure increases, and its rate of increase is measured. The rate of inflow is also measured so that the compliance can be estimated as the ratio flow to rate of pressure rise: Compliance in mL/mmHg = (flow in mL/min)/(rate of venous pressure rise in mmHg/min). The method is predicated on the assumption that the inflow continues at a constant rate and that there is no pressure gradient between the pressure measuring point and the site of compliance for the first few seconds of occlusion when the rate of pressure rise is measured.

19.3.6 Integral of Inflow Minus Outflow

With this technique both inflow and outflow are measured and the difference integrated to provide the volume change during an experimental forcing. If there is a decrease in contained volume, the outflow will be transiently greater than the inflow. The volume change gives a measure of the response to drugs or reflexes. Following a change in venous pressure, the technique can be used to measure compliance. Accurate measures of flow are needed. Serious errors can result if the inflow is not measured but is only assumed to be constant during the experimental protocol. With all methods dependent on measured or controlled flow, small changes in zero offset, which is directly or indirectly integrated, leads to serious error after about 10 min, and so the methods are not useful for long-term or slow responses.

19.4 Typical Values

Cardiac output, the sine qua non of the cardiovascular system, averages about 100 mL/(min-kg). It is about 90 in humans, is over 110 mL/(min-kg) in dogs and cats, and is even higher on a body weight basis in small animals such as rats and mice. The mean arterial blood pressure in relaxed, resting, conscious mammals averages about 90 mmHg. The mean circulatory filling pressure averages about 7 mmHg, and the central venous pressure just outside the right heart about 2 mmHg. The blood volume of the body is about 75 mL/kg, but in humans it is about 10% less, and it is larger in small animals. It is difficult to measure accurately because the volume of distribution of the plasma is about 10% higher than that of the red blood cells.

Vascular compliance averages about 2 mL (mmHg-kg body weight). The majority is in the venules and veins. Arterial compliance is only about 0.05 mL/mmHg-kg. Skeletal muscle compliance is less than that of the body as a whole, whereas the vascular compliance of the liver is about 10 times that of other organs. The stressed volume is the product of compliance and mean filling pressure and so is about 15 mL/kg. By difference, the unstressed volume is about 60 mL/kg.

As flow is increased through a tissue, the contained volume increases even if the outflow pressure is held constant, because there is a finite pressure drop across the veins, which is increased as flow increases. This increase in upstream distending pressure acts to increase the contained blood volume. The volume sensitivity to flow averages about 0.1 mL per 1 mL/min change in flow [10]. For the body as a whole, the sensitivity is about 0.25 mL per 1 mL/min with reflexes blocked, and with reflexes intact it averages about 0.4 mL/min³. Using similar techniques, it appears that the passive compensatory volume redistribution from the peripheral toward the heart during serious left heart failure is similar in magnitude to a reflex-engendered redistribution from activation of venous smooth muscle [6].

The high-pressure carotid sinus baroreceptor reflex system is capable of changing the venous capacitance [9]. Over the full operating range of the reflex it is capable of mobilizing up to 7.5 mL/kg of blood by primarily changing the unstressed vascular volume with little or no changes in venous compliance [7,8]. Although this represents only a 10% change in blood volume, it can cause nearly a 100% change in cardiac output. It is difficult to say with confidence what particular organ and/or tissue is contributing to this blood volume mobilization. Current evidence suggests that the splanchnic vascular bed contributes significantly to the capacitance change, but this also may vary between species [11].

Acknowledgments

This work was supported by the National Heart Lung and Blood Institute grants HL 19039 and HL 07723.

References

1. Furey, S.A.I., Zieske, H., and Levy, M.N. 1984. The essential function of the right heart. *Am. Heart J.* 107: 404.
2. Rothe, C.F. 1993. Mean circulatory filling pressure: its meaning and measurement. *J. Appl. Physiol.* 74: 499.
3. Rothe, C.F. 1983. Venous system: Physiology of the capacitance vessels. In J.T. Shepherd, and F.M. Abboud (Eds.), *Handbook of Physiology: The Cardiovascular System*, sec. 2, Vol. 3, pt 1, pp. 397–452, Bethesda, MD, American Physiology Society.
4. Rose, W. and Shoukas, A.A. 1993. Two-port analysis of systemic venous and arterial impedances. *Am. J. Physiol.* 265 (*Heart Circ. Physiol.* 34): H1577.
5. Lassen, N.A. and Perl, W. 1979. *Tracer Kinetic Methods in Medical Physiology*. New York, Raven Press.
6. Zink, J., Delaive, J., Mazerall, E., and Greenway, C.V. 1976. An improved plethsmograph with servo control of hydrostatic pressure. *J. Appl. Physiol.* 41: 107.
7. Shoukas, A.A. and Sagawa, K. 1973. Control of total systemic vascular capacity by the carotid sinus baroreceptor reflex. *Circ. Res.* 33: 22.
8. Shoukas, A.A., MacAnespie, C.L., Brunner, M.J. et al. 1981. The importance of the spleen in blood volume shifts of the systemic vascular bed caused by the carotid sinus baroreceptor reflex in the dog. *Circ. Res.* 49: 759.
9. Shoukas, A.A. 1993. Overall systems analysis of the carotid sinus baroreceptor reflex control of the circulation. *Anesthesiology* 79: 1402.
10. Rothe, C.F. and Gaddis, M.L. 1990. Autoregulation of cardiac output by passive elastic characteristics of the vascular capacitance system. *Circulation* 81: 360.
11. Haase, E. and Shoukas, A.A. 1991. The role of the carotid sinus baroreceptor reflex on pressure and diameter relations of the microvasculature of the rat intestine. *Am. J. Physiol.* 260: H752.
12. Numao, Y. and Iriuchijima J. 1977. Effect of cardiac output on circulatory blood volume. *Jpn. J. Physiol.* 27: 145.

20

The Microcirculation Physiome

20.1 Introduction 20-1
20.2 Mechanics of Microvascular Blood Flow 20-2
    Mechanics of the Microvascular Wall • Capillary Blood
    Flow • Arteriolar and Venular Blood Flow • Microvascular
    Networks: Structure and Hemodynamics
20.3 Molecular Transport in the Microcirculation 20-7
    Transport of Oxygen, Carbon Dioxide, and Nitric
    Oxide • Transport of Solutes and Water
20.4 Regulation of Blood Flow 20-9
    Neurohumoral Regulation of Blood Flow • Local
    Regulation of Blood Flow • Coordination of Vasomotor
    Responses • Angiogenesis and Vascular Remodeling • Enabling
    Computational Tools and Methodologies for the Microcirculation
    Physiome Project
Defining Terms 20-12
Acknowledgments 20-12
References 20-13
Further Information 20-17

Aleksander S. Popel
Johns Hopkins University

Roland N. Pittman
*Virginia Commonwealth
University*

20.1 Introduction

The microcirculation comprises blood vessels (arterioles, capillaries, and venules) with diameters less than approximately 150 µm. The importance of the microcirculation is underscored by the fact that most of the hydrodynamic resistance of the circulatory system lies in the microvessels (especially in arterioles) and most of the exchange of nutrients and waste products occurs at the level of the smallest microvessels. The subjects of microcirculatory research are blood flow and molecular transport in microvessels, mechanical interactions and molecular exchange between these vessels and the surrounding tissue, and regulation of blood flow, pressure, and molecular transport [43]. This review focuses on quantitative aspects of microvascular research; thus, we frame it in terms of the microcirculation physiome, the quantitative and integrated description of physiological processes that involve the microcirculation in an animal or human, across multiple scales. To achieve a quantitative understanding of the complexity of these processes as well as understanding the relationships between the structure and functional behavior, it is necessary to build experiment-based mathematical and computational models. In addition to describing key experimental findings in the field, we will also review major accomplishments in mathematical and computational modeling and simulations. The experimental and theoretical information on the microcirculation can be organized in the form of databases encompassing anatomical, biophysical, and functional data; gene regulation; signaling and metabolic networks; regulation and control networks at different levels of biological organization; and computational models. This evolving effort is referred to as the Microcirculation Physiome Project, a subset of the Physiome Project [4,5,68].

Quantitative knowledge of microcirculatory blood flow, molecular transport, and their regulation has been accumulated primarily in the past 40 years owing to significant innovations in methods and techniques to measure microcirculatory parameters and analyze microcirculatory data. The development of these methods has required joint efforts of physiologists and biomedical engineers. Key innovations include significant improvements in intravital microscopy, the dual-slit method (Wayland–Johnson) for measuring velocity in microvessels, the servo-null method (Wiederhielm–Intaglietta) for measuring pressure in microvessels, the recessed oxygen microelectrode (Whalen) for polarographic measurements of partial pressure of oxygen, and the microspectrophotometric method (Pittman–Duling) for measuring oxyhemoglobin saturation in microvessels. The single-capillary cannulation method (Landis–Michel) has provided a powerful tool for studies of transport of water and solutes through the capillary endothelium. New experimental techniques have appeared, many adapted from cell biology and modified for *in vivo* studies, that are having a tremendous impact on the field. Examples include confocal and multiphoton microscopy for better three-dimensional resolution of microvascular structures, methods of optical imaging using fluorescent labels (e.g., labeling blood cells for velocity measurements), fluorescent dyes (e.g., calcium ion and nitric oxide sensitive dyes for measuring their dynamics in vascular smooth muscle, endothelium, and surrounding tissue cells *in vivo*), and quantum dots, development of sensors (glass filaments, optical and magnetic tweezers, atomic force microscopy (AFM)) for measuring forces in the nanonewton to piconewton range that are characteristic of cell–cell and molecular interactions, phosphorescence decay measurements as an indicator of oxygen tension and oxygen consumption, and methods of manipulating receptors on the surfaces of blood cells and endothelial cells. In addition to the dramatic developments in experimental techniques, quantitative knowledge and understanding of the microcirculation have been significantly enhanced by theoretical studies, perhaps having a larger impact than in other areas of physiology. Extensive theoretical work has been conducted on the mechanics of the red blood cell (RBC) and leukocyte, from the molecular to the cellular levels, mechanics of blood flow in single microvessels and microvascular networks, oxygen (O_2), carbon dioxide (CO_2), and nitric oxide (NO) exchange between microvessels and surrounding tissue, and water and solute transport through capillary endothelium and the surrounding tissue [81]. These theoretical studies not only aid in the interpretation of experimental data but in many cases also serve as a framework for quantitative testing of working hypotheses and as a guide in designing and conducting further experiments. The accumulated knowledge has led to significant progress in our understanding of mechanisms of regulation of blood flow and molecular exchange in the microcirculation in many organs and tissues under a variety of physiological and pathological conditions (e.g., hypoxia, hypertension, sickle cell anemia, diabetes, inflammation, hemorrhage, ischemia/reperfusion, sepsis, and cancer).

The goal of this chapter is to present an overview of the current status of research on systemic microcirculation. Issues of pulmonary microcirculation are not discussed. Because of space limitations, it is not possible to recognize numerous important contributions to the field of microcirculation. In most cases, we refer to recent reviews, when available, and journal articles where earlier references can be found. We discuss experimental and theoretical findings and point out gaps in our understanding of microcirculatory phenomena.

20.2 Mechanics of Microvascular Blood Flow

Vessel dimensions in the microcirculation are small enough so that the effects of the particulate nature of blood are significant [69]. Blood is a suspension of formed elements (RBCs, white blood cells (leukocytes), and platelets) in plasma. Plasma is an aqueous solution of mostly proteins (albumins, globulins, and fibrinogen) and electrolytes. Under static conditions, human RBCs are biconcave disks with a diameter ~7–9 μm. The main function of the RBC is delivery of O_2 to tissue. Most of the O_2 carried by the blood is chemically bound to hemoglobin inside the RBCs. The mammalian RBC comprises a viscoelastic membrane enveloping a viscous fluid, concentrated hemoglobin solution. The membrane consists of the plasma membrane and underlying cytoskeleton. The membrane can undergo deformations without changing its surface area, which is nearly conserved locally. RBCs are so easily deformable that they can flow through small pores with a diameter <3 μm. Leukocytes (grouped into several categories: granulocytes, monocytes, lymphocytes, macrophages, and phagocytes) are spherical cells with a diameter ~10–20 μm. They are stiffer than RBCs. The main function of these cells is immunologic, that is, protection of the body against microorganisms causing disease. In contrast to mammalian RBCs, leukocytes are nucleated and are endowed with an internal structural cytoskeleton. Leukocytes are capable of active ameboid motion, the property that allows their migration from the blood stream into the tissue. Platelets are disk-shaped blood elements with a diameter ~2–3 μm; they are devoid of a nucleus. Platelets play a key role in thrombogenic processes and blood coagulation. The normal volume fraction (hematocrit) of RBCs in humans is 40–45%. The total volume of RBCs in blood is much greater than the volume of leukocytes and platelets. Rheological properties of blood in arterioles and venules and larger vessels are determined primarily by RBCs; however, leukocytes play an important mechanical role in capillaries and small venules.

Blood plasma is a Newtonian fluid with viscosity of approximately 1.2 cP. The viscosity of whole blood in a rotational viscometer or a large-bore capillary viscometer exhibits shear-thinning behavior, that is, viscosity decreases when shear rate increases. At shear rates >100 s^{-1} and a hematocrit of 40%, typical viscosity values are 3–4 cP. The dominant mechanism of the non-Newtonian behavior is RBC aggregation and the secondary mechanism is RBC deformation under shear forces. The cross-sectional distribution of RBCs in vessels is nonuniform, with a core of concentrated RBC suspension and a cell-free or cell-depleted marginal layer, typically 2–5 μm thick, adjacent to the vessel wall. The nonuniform RBC distribution results in the *Fahraeus effect* (the microvessel hematocrit is smaller than the feed or discharge hematocrit) due to the fact that, on the average, RBCs move with a higher velocity than blood plasma, and the concomitant *Fahraeus–Lindqvist effect* (the apparent viscosity of blood is lower than the bulk viscosity measured with a rotational viscometer or a large-bore capillary viscometer at high shear rate). The *apparent viscosity* of a fluid flowing in a cylindrical vessel of radius R and length L under the influence of a pressure difference ΔP is defined as

$$\eta_a = \frac{\pi \Delta P R^4}{8QL}$$

where Q is the volumetric flow rate. For a Newtonian fluid, the apparent viscosity becomes the dynamic viscosity of the fluid and the above equation represents *Poiseuille's law*. The apparent viscosity is a function of hematocrit, vessel radius, blood flow rate, and other parameters. In the microcirculation, blood flows through a complex branching network of arterioles, capillaries, and venules. Arterioles are typically 10–150 μm in diameter, capillaries are 4–8 μm, and venules are 10–200 μm. Now, we will discuss vascular wall mechanics and blood flow in vessels of different size in more detail.

20.2.1 Mechanics of the Microvascular Wall

The wall of arterioles comprises the intima that contains a single layer of contiguous endothelial cells, the media that contains a single layer of smooth muscle cells in terminal and medium-size arterioles or several layers in the larger arterioles, and the adventitia that contains sympathetic nerve terminals and collagen fibers with occasional fibroblasts and mast cells. Fibers situated between the endothelium and the smooth muscle cells comprise the basement membrane. The single layer of smooth muscle cells terminates at the capillaries and reappears at the level of small venules; the capillary wall is devoid of smooth muscle cells, but instead contains pericytes loosely wrapped around endothelial cells. Venules typically have a larger diameter and smaller wall thickness-to-diameter ratio than arterioles of the corresponding branching order.

Most of our knowledge of the mechanics of the microvascular wall comes from *in vivo* or *in vitro* measurements of vessel diameter as a function of transmural pressure [25]. The development of isolated microvessel preparations has made it possible to precisely control the transmural pressure during experiments. In addition, these preparations allow one to separate the effects of metabolic factors and blood flow rate from the effect of pressure by controlling both the chemical environment and the flow rate through the vessel. Arterioles and venules exhibit vascular tone, that is, their diameter is maximal when smooth muscle is completely relaxed (inactivated). When the vascular smooth muscle is constricted, small arterioles may even completely close their lumen to blood flow, presumably by buckling endothelial cells. Arterioles exhibit a *myogenic response* not observed in other blood vessels, with the exception of cerebral arteries: within a certain physiological pressure range, the vessels constrict in response to elevation of transmural pressure and dilate in response to reduction of transmural pressure; in other words, in a certain range of pressures, the slope of the pressure–diameter relationship is negative [15]. Arterioles of different size exhibit different degrees of myogenic responsiveness. This effect has been documented in many tissues both *in vivo* and *in vitro* (in isolated arterioles) and has been shown to play an important role in the regulation of blood flow and capillary pressure (see Section 20.4 below).

The stress–strain relationship for a thin-walled microvessel can be derived from the experimentally obtained pressure–diameter relationship using the law of Laplace. Stress in the vessel wall can be decomposed into passive and active components. The passive component corresponds to the state of complete vasodilation. The active component determines the vascular tone and the myogenic response. Steady-state stress–strain relationships are, generally, nonlinear. For arterioles, diameter variations of 50% or even 100% under physiological conditions are not unusual, so that finite deformations have to be considered in formulating the constitutive relationship for the wall (relationship between stress, strain, and their temporal derivatives). Experiment-based mathematical models of microvessel mechanics have been formulated [15]. Pertinent to the question of microvascular mechanics is the mechanical interaction of a vessel with its environment, which consists of connective tissue, parenchymal and stromal cells, and extracellular fluid. There is ultrastructural evidence that blood vessels are tethered to the surrounding tissue, so that mechanical forces can be generated when the vessels constrict or dilate, or when the tissue is moving, for example, in contracting striated muscle, myocardium, or intestine. Little quantitative information is currently available about the magnitude of these forces, chiefly because of the difficulty of such measurements. Magnetic tweezers make it possible to probe the mechanics of the microvascular wall *in vivo* and its interaction with the surrounding tissue [38].

Under time-dependent conditions, microvessels exhibit viscoelastic behavior. In response to a stepwise change in the transmural pressure, arterioles typically respond with a fast "passive" change in diameter followed by a slow "active" response with a characteristic time of the order of tens of seconds. For example, when the pressure is suddenly increased, the vessel diameter will quickly increase, with subsequent vasoconstriction that may result in a lower value of steady-state diameter than that prior to the increase in pressure. Therefore, to accurately describe the time-dependent vessel behavior, the constitutive relationship between stress and strain or pressure and diameter must also contain temporal derivatives of these variables. Theoretical analysis of the resulting nonlinear equations shows that such constitutive equations lead to predictions of spontaneous oscillations of vessel diameter (*vasomotion*) under certain conditions [90] that can be characterized theoretically as "deterministic chaos." Theoretical analysis of Ca^{2+} oscillations in vascular smooth muscle cells also predicts spontaneous oscillations [62]. Vasomotion has been observed *in vivo* in various tissues and under various physiological conditions. Whether experimentally observed vasomotion and its effect on blood flow (flow motion) can be quantitatively described by the theoretical studies remains to be established. It should be noted that other mechanisms leading to spontaneous flow oscillations have been reported that are associated with blood rheology and not with vascular wall mechanics [16,48].

For most purposes, capillary compliance is not taken into account. However, in some situations, such as analysis of certain capillary water transport experiments or leukocyte motion in a capillary, this view is not adequate and capillary compliance has to be accounted for. Since the capillary wall is devoid of smooth muscle cells, much of this compliance is passive, and its magnitude is small. However, the presence of contractile proteins in the cytoskeleton of capillary endothelial cells and associated pericytes opens a possibility of active capillary constriction or dilation.

20.2.2 Capillary Blood Flow

Progress in this area is closely related to studies of mechanics of blood cells (described elsewhere in this book). In narrow capillaries, RBCs flow in a single file, separated by gaps of plasma. They deform and assume a parachute-like shape, generally nonaxisymmetric, leaving a submicron plasma sleeve between the RBC and endothelium. In the smallest capillaries, their shape is sausage-like. The hemoglobin solution inside an RBC is a Newtonian fluid. The constitutive relationship for the membrane is often expressed by the Evans–Skalak finite deformations model [69]; molecular-based models considering spectrin, actin, and other RBC cytoskeleton constituents have also been formulated [27,31,52]. The coupled mechanical problem of membrane and fluid motion has been extensively investigated using both analytical and numerical approaches [70]. An important result of the theoretical studies is the prediction of the apparent viscosity of blood. While these predictions are in good agreement with *in vitro* studies in glass tubes, they underestimate a few available *in vivo* capillary measurements of apparent viscosity. In addition, *in vivo* capillary hematocrit is typically lower than predicted from *in vitro* studies with tubes of the same size. To explain the low values of hematocrit, RBC interactions with the endothelial glycocalyx have been implicated [26]. Direct measurements of the glycocalyx thickness and microvascular resistance as well as theoretical analyses elucidate the role of the glycocalyx [93]. The endothelial glycocalyx and its associated macromolecules are often referred to, collectively, as the endothelial surface layer (ESL) [75]. The ESL appears to be exquisitely controlled, and it is affected by a variety of biochemical and mechanical factors [34,58,65].

The motion of leukocytes through blood capillaries has also been studied thoroughly. Because leukocytes are larger and stiffer than RBCs, under normal flow conditions, an increase in capillary resistance caused by a single leukocyte may be orders of magnitude greater than that caused by a single RBC [79]. Under certain conditions, flow stoppage may occur, caused by leukocyte plugging. After a period of ischemia, RBC and leukocyte plugging may prevent tissue reperfusion (ischemia–reperfusion injury) [37]. Chemical bonds between membrane-bound receptors and endothelial adhesion molecules play a crucial role in leukocyte–endothelium interactions. Methods of cell and molecular biology permit manipulation of the receptors and thus make it possible to study leukocyte microcirculatory mechanics at the molecular level; biophysical methods allow force measurements of single adhesion bonds. These methods open new and powerful ways to study cell micromechanics and cell–cell interactions.

20.2.3 Arteriolar and Venular Blood Flow

The cross-sectional distribution of RBCs in arterioles and venules is nonuniform. A concentrated suspension of RBCs forms a core surrounded by a cell-free or cell-depleted layer of plasma. This "lubrication" layer of lower viscosity fluid near the vessel wall results in lower values of the apparent viscosity of blood compared to its bulk viscosity, resulting in the Fahraeus–Lindqvist effect [69,71]. There is experimental evidence that velocity profiles of RBCs are generally symmetric in arterioles, except very close to vascular bifurcations, but may be asymmetric in venules; the profiles are close to parabolic in arterioles at normal flow rates, but are blunted in venules [9,30]. Moreover, flow in the venules may be stratified as the result of converging blood streams that do not mix rapidly. The key to understanding the pattern of arteriolar and venular blood flow is the mechanics of flow at vascular bifurcations, diverging for arteriolar flow and converging for venular flow [23]. An important question is under what physiological or pathological conditions do RBC aggregation affect arteriolar and venular velocity distribution and vascular resistance. Much is known about aggregation *in vitro*, but *in vivo* knowledge is incomplete

[3,12,53,69]. Under pathological conditions, such as sickle cell disease and diabetes, RBCs can interact with the endothelium via adhesion molecules [47].

Owing to recent advancements in computational fluid dynamics, including the application of lattice Boltzmann and dissipative particle dynamics methods, significant progress has been achieved in modeling multiple RBCs in narrow vessels and the formation of cell-free layer with or without the effects of RBC aggregation [32,59,95].

The problems of leukocyte distribution in the microcirculation and their interaction with the microvascular endothelium have attracted considerable attention in recent years [80]. Leukocyte rolling along the walls of venules, but not arterioles, has been demonstrated. This effect results from differences in the microvascular endothelium, mainly attributed to the differential expression of adhesion molecules on the endothelial surface [50]. Platelet distribution in the lumen is important because of platelets' role in blood coagulation. Detailed studies of platelet distribution in arterioles and venules show that the cross-sectional distribution of these disk-shaped blood elements is dependent on the blood flow rate and vessel hematocrit [94]; molecular details of platelet–endothelium interactions are available [86]. Considerable progress has been made in computational modeling of leukocytes in microvessels, and their interactions with the endothelium and with RBCs [13,42,59,61].

20.2.4 Microvascular Networks: Structure and Hemodynamics

Microvascular networks in different organs and tissues differ in their appearance and structural organization. Methods have been developed to quantitatively describe network angioarchitectonics and hemodynamics [69,71]. The microvasculature is an adaptable structure capable of changing its structural and functional characteristics in response to various stimuli [85]. *Angiogenesis*, rarefaction, and microvascular remodeling are important examples of this adaptive behavior that play important physiological and pathophysiological roles. Microvascular hydraulic pressure varies systematically between consecutive branching orders, decreasing from the systemic values down to 20–25 mm Hg in the capillaries and decreasing further by 10–15 mm Hg in the venules. Mean microvascular blood flow rate in arterioles decreases toward the capillaries, in inverse proportion to the number of "parallel" vessels, and increases from capillaries through the venules [53]. In addition to this longitudinal variation of blood flow and pressure among different branching orders, there are significant variations among vessels of the same branching order, referred to as flow heterogeneity. The heterogeneity of blood flow and RBC distribution in microvascular networks has been well documented in a variety of organs and tissues [74]. This phenomenon may have important implications for tissue exchange processes, so significant efforts have been devoted to the quantitative analysis of blood flow in microvascular networks. A mathematical model of blood flow in a network can be formulated as follows. First, network topology or vessel interconnections have to be specified. Second, the diameter and length of every vascular segment have to be known. Alternatively, vessel diameter can be specified as a function of transmural pressure and perhaps some other parameters; these relationships are discussed in the preceding section on wall mechanics. Third, the apparent viscosity of blood has to be specified as a function of vessel diameter, local hematocrit, and shear rate. Fourth, a relationship between RBC flow rates and bulk blood flow rates at diverging bifurcations has to be specified; this relationship is often referred to as the "bifurcation law." Finally, at the inlet vessel branches, boundary conditions have to be specified: bulk flow rate as well as RBC flow rate or hematocrit; alternatively, pressure can be specified at both inlet and outlet branches. This set of generally nonlinear equations can be solved to yield pressure at each bifurcation, blood flow rate through each segment, and discharge or microvessel hematocrit in each segment. These equations also predict vessel diameters if vessel compliance is taken into account. The calculated variables can then be compared with experimental data. Such a detailed comparison was reported for rat mesentery [71,74] and the scheme has been applied by many investigators to different tissues. The empirical relationships reflect the presence of the endothelial glycocalyx and its associated macromolecules, ESL [75]. Predictions of this flow model are also used in models of molecular transport.

20.3 Molecular Transport in the Microcirculation

20.3.1 Transport of Oxygen, Carbon Dioxide, and Nitric Oxide

One of the most important functions of the microcirculation is the delivery of O_2 to tissue and the removal of waste products, particularly of CO_2, from tissue. O_2 is required for aerobic intracellular respiration for the production of adenosine triphosphate (ATP). CO_2 is produced as a by-product of these biochemical reactions. Tissue metabolic rate can change drastically, for example, in aerobic muscle in the transition from rest to exercise, which necessitates commensurate changes in blood flow and O_2 delivery. One of the major issues studied is how O_2 delivery is matched to O_2 demand under different physiological and pathological conditions. This question arises for short-term or long-term regulation of O_2 delivery in an individual organism, organ, or tissue, as well as in the evolutionary sense, in phylogeny. The hypothesis of symmorphosis, a fundamental balance between structure and function, has been formulated for the respiratory and cardiovascular systems and tested in a number of animal species [92].

In the smallest exchange vessels (capillaries and small arterioles and venules), O_2 molecules are released from hemoglobin inside RBCs, diffuse through the plasma, cross the endothelium, the extravascular space, and parenchymal cells until they reach the mitochondria where they are utilized in the process of oxidative phosphorylation. The nonlinear relationship between hemoglobin saturation with O_2 and the local O_2 tension (PO_2) is described by the *oxyhemoglobin dissociation curve* (ODC). The theory of O_2 transport from capillaries to tissue was conceptually formulated by August Krogh in 1918 and it has dominated the thinking of physiologists for nine decades. The model he formulated considered a cylindrical tissue volume supplied by a single central capillary; this element was considered the building block for the entire tissue. A constant metabolic rate was assumed and PO_2 at the capillary–tissue interface was specified. The solution to the corresponding transport equation is the Krogh–Erlang equation describing the radial variation of O_2 tension in tissue. Over the years, the *Krogh tissue cylinder model* has been modified by many investigators to include transport processes in the capillary and PO_2-dependent consumption. However, in the past few years, new conceptual models of O_2 transport have emerged. First, it was discovered experimentally and subsequently corroborated by theoretical analysis that capillaries are not the only source of oxygen, but arterioles (*precapillary O_2 transport*) and to a smaller extent venules (postcapillary O_2 transport) also participate in tissue oxygenation; in fact, a complex pattern of O_2 exchange may exist among arterioles, venules, and adjacent capillary networks [64,87]. Second, theoretical analysis of intracapillary transport suggested that a significant part of the resistance to O_2 transport, on the order of 50%, is located within the capillary, primarily due to poor diffusive conductance of the plasma gaps between the erythrocytes; the consequence of this prediction, fluctuations of capillary PO_2, has been confirmed by recent experiments [36]. Third, the effect of *myoglobin-facilitated O_2 diffusion* in red muscle fibers and cardiac myocytes has been reevaluated; however, its significance must await additional experimental studies. Fourth, geometric and hemodynamic heterogeneities in O_2 delivery have been quantified experimentally and modeled theoretically. Theoretical analyses of oxygen transport have been applied to a variety of tissues and organs [24,35,67]. One important area of application of this knowledge is artificial oxygen carriers, hemoglobin-based and non-hemoglobin-based [60]; theoretical models of O_2 transport by blood substitutes have been developed [39,89] and used to guide experimental studies.

The transport of CO_2 is coupled to O_2 through the Bohr effect (effect of CO_2 tension on the blood O_2 content) and the Haldane effect (effect of PO_2 on the blood CO_2 content). The diffusion of CO_2 is faster than that of O_2 because CO_2 solubility in tissue is higher; theoretical studies predict that countercurrent exchange of CO_2 between arterioles and venules is of major importance so that equilibration of CO_2 tension with surrounding tissue should occur before capillaries are reached. Experiments are needed to test these theoretical predictions.

Nitric oxide (NO) is a diatomic gas that can be enzymatically synthesized from L-arginine by several isoforms of NO synthase (NOS). There are also nonenzymatic sources of NO. The isoforms of NO synthase are divided into inducible NOS (iNOS or NOS2) and constitutive NOS (cNOS), based on their nondependent and dependent, respectively, control of activity from intracellular calcium/calmodulin. Constitutive NOS are further classified as neuronal NOS (nNOS or NOS1) and endothelial NOS (eNOS or NOS3). Nitric oxide plays an important role in both autocrine and paracrine manners in a myriad of physiological processes, including regulation of blood pressure and blood flow, platelet aggregation, and leukocyte adhesion. In smooth muscle cells, NO activates the enzyme soluble guanylate cyclase (sGC) that catalyzes the conversion of guanosine triphosphate (GTP) to cyclic guanosine monophosphate (cGMP), thus causing vasodilation [8]. Traditionally, eNOS has been considered the principal source of bioavailable microvascular NO under most physiological conditions. Evidence exists that nNOS expressed in nerve fibers, which innervate arterioles, together with nNOS positive mast cells are also major sources of NO [46]. NO produced by endothelial cells diffuses to vascular smooth muscle and to the flowing blood, where it rapidly reacts with hemoglobin in RBCs and free hemoglobin present in pathological conditions, such as sickle cell disease, or during administration of free hemoglobin as a blood substitute. Other nonneuronal cell types, including cardiac and skeletal myocytes, also express nNOS. Direct measurements of NO concentration in the microcirculation with high spatial resolution have been performed with carbon fiber microsensors [10] and optical dyes [46], although recent criticism has been directed to current measurements of NO *in vivo* [40]. In addition to its vasodilatory effect, NO also inhibits mitochondrial respiration by its interaction with cytochrome *c* oxidase [19]. Mathematical models of NO transport have been developed that describe the transport of NO synthesized by eNOS and nNOS in and around microvessels [88]. Other mechanisms have been proposed and are under intense scrutiny, for example, NO reacting with thiols in blood to form long-lived *S*-nitrosothiols (SNOs) with vasodilatory activity [1], and nitrite being a source of NO [91]. There are significant discrepancies between experimental data and theoretical results that await resolution [17,40]; the sources of microvascular bioavailable NO also need to be revealed.

20.3.2 Transport of Solutes and Water

The movement of solute molecules across the capillary wall occurs primarily by two mechanisms: diffusion and solvent drag. Diffusion is the passive mechanism of transport that rapidly and efficiently transports small solutes over the small distances (tens of microns) between the blood supply (capillaries) and tissue cells. Solvent drag refers to the movement of solute that is entrained in the bulk flow of fluid across the capillary wall and is generally negligible, except in cases of large molecules with small diffusivities and high transcapillary fluid flow.

The capillary wall is composed of a single layer of endothelial cells about 1 μm thick. Lipid-soluble substances (e.g., O_2) can diffuse across the entire wall surface, whereas water-soluble substances are restricted to small aqueous pathways equivalent to cylindrical pores 8–9 nm in diameter (e.g., glucose in most capillaries); in capillaries with tight junctions and few fenestrations (brain, testes), glucose moves predominantly by carrier-mediated transport. Total pore area is about 0.1% of the surface area of a capillary. The permeability of the capillary wall to a particular substance depends upon the relative size of the substance and the pore ("restricted" diffusion). The efficiency of diffusive exchange can be increased by increasing the number of perfused capillaries (e.g., heart and muscle tissue from rest to exercise), since this increases the surface area available for exchange and decreases the distances across which molecules must diffuse.

The actual pathways through which small solutes traverse the capillary wall appear to be in the form of clefts between adjacent endothelial cells. Rather than being open slits, these porous channels contain a matrix of small cylindrical fibers (primarily glycosaminoglycans) that occupy about 5% of the volume of these pathways. The permeability properties of the capillary endothelium are modulated by a number of factors, among which are plasma protein concentration and composition, rearrangement of the endothelial cell glycocalyx, calcium influx into the endothelial cell and endothelial cell membrane potential. Many of the studies that have established our current understanding of the endothelial exchange barrier have been carried out on single perfused capillaries in the frog and in mammalian tissues [22,57]. There could be, in addition to the porous pathways, nonporous pathways that involve selective uptake of solutes and subsequent transcellular transport (of particular importance in endothelial barriers). To study such pathways, one must try to minimize the contributions to transcapillary transport from solvent drag.

The processes whereby water passes back and forth across the capillary wall are called filtration and absorption. The flow of water depends upon the relative magnitude of hydraulic and osmotic pressures across the capillary wall and is described quantitatively by the Kedem–Katchalsky equations (the particular form of the equations applied to capillary water transport is referred to as *Starling's law*). Recently, the physical mechanism of Starling's law has been reassessed [41]. Overall, in the steady state, there is an approximate balance between hydraulic and osmotic pressures, which leads to a small net flow of water. Generally, more fluid is filtered than is reabsorbed; the overflow is carried back to the vascular system by the lymphatic circulation. The lymphatic network is composed of a large number of small vessels, the terminal branches of which are closed. Flap valves (similar to those in veins) ensure unidirectional flow of lymph back to the central circulation. The smallest (terminal) vessels are very permeable, even to proteins that occasionally leak from systemic capillaries. Lymph flow is determined by interstitial fluid pressure and the lymphatic "pump" (one–way flap valves and skeletal muscle contraction). The control of interstitial fluid protein concentration is one of the most important functions of the lymphatic system. If more net fluid is filtered than can be removed by the lymphatics, the volume of interstitial fluid increases. This fluid accumulation is called edema. This circumstance is important clinically since solute exchange (e.g., O_2) decreases due to the increased diffusion distances produced when the accumulated fluid pushes the capillaries, tethered to the interstitial matrix, away from each other.

20.4 Regulation of Blood Flow

The cardiovascular system controls blood flow to individual organs (1) by maintaining arterial pressure within narrow limits and (2) by allowing each organ to adjust its vascular resistance to blood flow so that each receives an appropriate fraction of the cardiac output. There are three major mechanisms that control the function of the cardiovascular system: neural, humoral, and local [83]. The sympathetic nervous system and circulating hormones both provide overall vasoregulation, and thus coarse flow control, to all vascular beds. The local mechanisms provide finer regional control within a tissue, usually in response to local changes in tissue activity or local trauma. The three mechanisms can work independently of each other, but there are also interactions among them.

The classical view of blood flow control involved the action of vasomotor influences on a set of vessels called the "resistance vessels," generally arterioles and small arteries smaller than about 100–150 μm in diameter, which controlled flow to and within an organ [82]. The notion of "precapillary sphincters" that control flow in individual capillaries has been abandoned in favor of the current notion that the terminal arterioles control the flow in small capillary networks that branch off of these arterioles. In recent years, it has become clear that the resistance to blood flow is distributed over a wider range of vessel branching orders with diameters up to 500 μm. There are mechanisms to be discussed below that are available for coordinating the actions of local control processes over wider regions.

20.4.1 Neurohumoral Regulation of Blood Flow

The role of neural influences on the vasculature varies greatly from organ to organ. Although all organs receive sympathetic innervation, regulation of blood flow in the cerebral and coronary vascular beds occurs mostly through intrinsic local (metabolic) mechanisms. The circulations in skeletal muscle, skin, and some other organs, however, are significantly affected by the sympathetic nerves. In general, the level of intrinsic myogenic activity and sympathetic discharge sets the state of vascular smooth muscle contraction (basal vascular tone) and hence vascular resistance in organs. This basal tone is modulated by circulating and local vasoactive influences, for example, endothelium–derived relaxing factor (EDRF), identified as nitric oxide, endothelium-derived hyperpolarizing factor (EDHF) [11], prostacyclin (PGI2), endothelin, and vasoactive substances released from parenchymal cells.

20.4.2 Local Regulation of Blood Flow

In addition to neural and humoral mechanisms for regulating the function of the cardiovascular system, there are mechanisms intrinsic to the various tissues that can operate independently of neurohumoral influences. The site of local regulation is the microcirculation. Examples of local control processes are autoregulation of blood flow, reactive hyperemia, and active (or functional) hyperemia. The mechanisms of local regulation have been identified as (1) the myogenic mechanism based on the ability of vascular smooth muscle to actively contract in response to stretch; (2) the metabolic mechanism, based on a link between blood flow and tissue metabolism; and (3) the flow-dependent mechanism, primarily based on the release of NO by endothelial cells in response to shear forces. The effects are coordinated and integrated in the microvascular network via chemical and electrical signals propagating through gap junctions. Experimental evidence and theoretical models are discussed in References 14, 21, 44, 45, 66, 72, 82, and 83.

Cells have a continuous need for O_2 and also continuously produce metabolic wastes, some of which are vasoactive (usually vasodilators). Under normal conditions, there is a balance between O_2 supply and demand, but imbalances give rise to adjustments in blood flow that bring supply back into register with demand. Consider exercising skeletal muscle as an example. With the onset of exercise, metabolite production and O_2 requirements increase. The metabolites diffuse away from their sites of production and reach the vasculature. Vasodilation ensues, lowering resistance to blood flow. The resulting increase in blood flow increases the O_2 supply and finally a new steady state is achieved in which O_2 supply and demand are matched. This scenario operates for other tissues in which metabolic activity changes.

The following O_2–linked metabolites have been implicated as potential chemical mediators in the metabolic hypothesis: adenosine (from ATP hydrolysis: ATP → ADP → AMP → adenosine), H^+, and lactate (from lactic acid generated by glycolysis). Their levels are increased when there is a reduction in O_2 supply relative to demand (i.e., tissue hypoxia). The production of more CO_2 as a result of increased tissue activity (leading to increased oxidative metabolism) leads to vasodilation through increased H^+ concentration. Increased potassium ion and interstitial fluid osmolarity (i.e., more osmotically active particles) transiently cause vasodilation under physiological conditions associated with increased tissue activity.

It has also been established that the RBC itself could act as a mobile sensor for hypoxia [29]. The mechanism works as follows. Under conditions of low oxygen and pH, the RBC releases ATP, which binds to purinergic receptors on the endothelial cells. This leads to the production of the vasodilator NO in the endothelial cells. Since the most likely location for hypoxia would be in or near the venular network, the local vasodilatory response to NO is propagated to upstream vessels causing arteriolar vasodilation (see Section 20.4.3). The phenomenon has been described in a mathematical model [2].

20.4.3 Coordination of Vasomotor Responses

Communication via gap junctions between the two active cell types in the blood vessel wall, smooth muscle and endothelial cells, plays an important role in coordinating the responses among resistance elements in the vascular network [33,82,83]. There is chemical and electrical coupling between the cells of the vessel wall, and this signal, in response to locally released vasoactive substances (e.g., from vessel wall, RBCs, or parenchymal cells), can travel along a vessel in either direction with a length constant of about 2 mm. There are two immediate consequences of this communication. A localized vasodilatory stimulus of metabolic origin will be conducted to contiguous vessels, thereby lowering the resistance to blood flow in a larger region. In addition, this more generalized vasodilation should increase the homogeneity of blood flow in response to the localized metabolic event. The increase in blood flow produced as a result of this vasodilation will also cause flow to increase at upstream sites. The increased shear stress on the endothelium as a result of the flow increase will lead to vasodilation of these larger upstream vessels. Thus, the neurohumoral and local responses are linked together in a complex control system that matches regional perfusion to the local metabolic needs.

20.4.4 Angiogenesis and Vascular Remodeling

In addition to short-term regulation of blood flow operating on the time scale of tens of seconds to minutes, there are mechanisms that operate on the scales of hours, days, and weeks that result in angiogenesis (the capillary growth from preexisting microvessels) and microvascular remodeling or adaptation (structural and geometric changes in the vascular wall) [85]. Stimuli for angiogenesis and microvascular remodeling could be hypoxia, injury, inflammation, or neoplasia. The processes of angiogenesis and vascular remodeling are complex and knowledge at the molecular, cellular, and tissue level is being accumulated at a fast rate. Briefly, it is understood that low cellular oxygen is sensed through a transcription factor HIF1 (hypoxia-inducible factor) pathway, leading to activation of as many as 200 genes [84]. Among them is vascular endothelial growth factor (VEGF)—one of the most potent inducers of angiogenesis. Another VEGF-inducing factor is the transcription coactivator perixosome-proliferator-activated-receptor-gamma coactivator 1α (PGC1α) [49]. VEGF is secreted by parenchymal and stromal cells and diffuses through the extracellular space. Once it reaches endothelial cells, it activates them, causing hyperpermeability and expression of metalloproteinases (MMPs), which then participate in the proteolysis of the extracellular matrix. The activated endothelial cells migrate, proliferate, and differentiate, resulting in the formation of a capillary sprout. Subsequently, the endothelial cells secrete platelet-derived growth factor (PDGF) that participates in recruiting stromal fibroblasts and progenitor cells to the new capillaries. When these cells reach the vessels, they differentiate into pericytes and smooth muscle cells, thus stabilizing the vessels. Many of these processes are poorly understood. Therefore, quantitative computational approaches are particularly useful in gaining a better understanding of these processes; research in this area is rapidly evolving [56,63,77,78]. In parallel to modeling angiogenesis, theoretical models are being developed to describe long-term structural vascular remodeling and adaptation [73].

20.4.5 Enabling Computational Tools and Methodologies for the Microcirculation Physiome Project

Further progress in understanding the microcirculation physiome will benefit from the modeling and simulation infrastructure being developed around the world. These include methods for model development, storage, exchange, and integration. Below, we list some of the important elements of these methods; some of the aspects can be found in Reference 68.

Model types: A growing arsenal of modeling tools is available for building mathematical models: they include algebraic equations, deterministic ordinary and partial differential equations, probabilistic equations and stochastic Monte Carlo simulations, and rule-based agent-based models (ABM). All these tools have been used in describing microcirculatory phenomena.

Multiscale models: Many models span multiple spatial and temporal scales; such models are referred to as *multiscale* [6,31,77,78]. For example, a model of capillary flow (micrometer scale) may include a molecular-detailed model of the RBC membrane (nanometer scale) and endothelial glycocalyx (from nanometer to micrometer scale). A model of capillary sprouting during angiogenesis could include growth factor interactions with receptors (nanometer scale), endothelial cell proliferation, migration, and sprout formation (micrometer scale), and well as whole-body growth factor transport (meter scale);

in the same problem, ligand–receptor interactions occur at seconds to minutes scales, whereas vascular growth occurs at hours to days scale. Creating methodologies for multiscale modeling is an important goal of current research.

Modular design and module integration: Complex models might be composed of multiple modules at the same or different spatial and temporal scales; some of these modules may be commonly used by many investigators (e.g., MAPK—mitogen-activated protein kinases in signal transduction models, or the microcirculatory blood flow model in molecular transport models), whereas others maybe be custom designed for a particular application. These modules may represent different model types (e.g., differential equations versus ABM) and use different programming languages. There are several efforts to integrate multiple modules using a controller/integrator that controls the modules and data exchange between them [54,76]; this is also one of the goals of the Virtual Physiological Human project [20].

Markup languages: To facilitate model exchange among investigators, markup languages have been formulated that abide to the standards accepted by the modeling community. SBML (systems biology markup language) [28] and CellML [7] are the most common for processes described by ordinary differential equations, for example, signaling pathways. For spatial models, FieldML is being developed [18]. Together with modular design, markup languages will also facilitate the creation of public databases of computational models that can be used by different investigators.

Model databases: The BioModels database [51] based primarily on SBML (other formats are also available), and the CellML model repository [55] based on CellML contain hundreds of curated models.

Defining Terms

Angiogenesis: The growth of new capillaries from the preexisting microvessels.

Apparent viscosity: The viscosity of a Newtonian fluid that would require the same pressure difference to produce the same blood flow rate through a circular vessel as the blood.

Fahraeus effect: Microvessel hematocrit is smaller than hematocrit in the feed or discharge reservoir.

Fahraeus–Lindqvist effect: The apparent viscosity of blood in a microvessel is smaller than the bulk viscosity measured with a rotational viscometer or a large-bore capillary viscometer.

Krogh tissue cylinder model: A cylindrical volume of tissue supplied by a central cylindrical capillary.

Multiscale model: A model that considers processes at multiple spatial and/or temporal scales.

Myogenic response: Vasoconstriction in response to elevated transmural pressure and vasodilation in response to reduced transmural pressure.

Myoglobin-facilitated O_2 diffusion: An increase of O_2 diffusive flux as a result of myoglobin molecules acting as a carrier for O_2 molecules.

Oxyhemoglobin dissociation curve: The equilibrium relationship between hemoglobin oxygen saturation and O_2 tension.

Physiome: The quantitative and integrated description of the functional behavior of the physiological state of an animal or human.

Poiseuille's law: The relationship between volumetric flow rate and pressure difference for steady flow of a Newtonian fluid in a long circular tube.

Precapillary O_2 transport: O_2 diffusion from arterioles to the surrounding tissue.

Starling's law: The relationship between water flux through the endothelium and the difference between the hydraulic and osmotic transmural pressures.

Vasomotion: Spontaneous rhythmic variation of microvessel diameter.

Acknowledgments

This work was supported by National Institute of Health grants R01 HL18292, R01 HL101200, and R01 CA138264.

References

1. Allen BW, Stamler JS, and Piantadosi CA. Hemoglobin, nitric oxide and molecular mechanisms of hypoxic vasodilation. *Trends Mol Med* 15: 452–460, 2009.
2. Arciero JC, Carlson BE, and Secomb TW. Theoretical model of metabolic blood flow regulation: Roles of ATP release by red blood cells and conducted responses. *Am J Physiol Heart Circ Physiol* 295: H1562–1571, 2008.
3. Baskurt OK and Meiselman HJ. Blood rheology and hemodynamics. *Semin Thromb Hemost* 29: 435–450, 2003.
4. Bassingthwaighte JB. Microcirculation and the physiome projects. *Microcirculation* 15: 835–839, 2008.
5. Bassingthwaighte JB. Strategies for the physiome project. *Ann Biomed Eng* 28: 1043–1058, 2000.
6. Bassingthwaighte JB, Raymond GM, Butterworth E, Alessio A, and Caldwell JH. Multiscale modeling of metabolism, flows, and exchanges in heterogeneous organs. *Ann N Y Acad Sci* 1188: 111–120, 2009.
7. Beard DA, Britten R, Cooling MT, Garny A, Halstead MD, Hunter PJ, Lawson J et al. CellML metadata standards, associated tools and repositories. *Philos Transact A Math Phys Eng Sci* 367: 1845–1867, 2009.
8. Bian K, Doursout MF, and Murad F. Vascular system: Role of nitric oxide in cardiovascular diseases. *J Clin Hypertens (Greenwich)* 10: 304–310, 2008.
9. Bishop JJ, Nance PR, Popel AS, Intaglietta M, and Johnson PC. Effect of erythrocyte aggregation on velocity profiles in venules. *Am J Physiol Heart Circ Physiol* 280: H222–236, 2001.
10. Bohlen HG, Zhou X, Unthank JL, Miller SJ, and Bills R. Transfer of nitric oxide by blood from upstream to downstream resistance vessels causes microvascular dilation. *Am J Physiol Heart Circ Physiol* 297: H1337–1346, 2009.
11. Busse R, Edwards G, Feletou M, Fleming I, Vanhoutte PM, and Weston AH. EDHF: Bringing the concepts together. *Trends Pharmacol Sci* 23: 374–380, 2002.
12. Cabel M, Meiselman HJ, Popel AS, and Johnson PC. Contribution of red blood cell aggregation to venous vascular resistance in skeletal muscle. *Am J Physiol* 272: H1020–1032, 1997.
13. Caputo KE, Lee D, King MR, and Hammer DA. Adhesive dynamics simulations of the shear threshold effect for leukocytes. *Biophys J* 92: 787–797, 2007.
14. Carlson BE, Arciero JC, and Secomb TW. Theoretical model of blood flow autoregulation: Roles of myogenic, shear-dependent, and metabolic responses. *Am J Physiol Heart Circ Physiol* 295: H1572–1579, 2008.
15. Carlson BE and Secomb TW. A theoretical model for the myogenic response based on the length-tension characteristics of vascular smooth muscle. *Microcirculation* 12: 327–338, 2005.
16. Carr RT, Geddes JB, and Wu F. Oscillations in a simple microvascular network. *Ann Biomed Eng* 33: 764–771, 2005.
17. Chen K, Pittman RN, and Popel AS. Nitric oxide in the vasculature: Where does it come from and where does it go? A quantitative perspective. *Antioxid Redox Signal* 10: 1185–1198, 2008.
18. Christie GR, Nielsen PM, Blackett SA, Bradley CP, and Hunter PJ. FieldML: Concepts and implementation. *Philos Transact A Math Phys Eng Sci* 367: 1869–1884, 2009.
19. Cooper CE, Mason MG, and Nicholls P. A dynamic model of nitric oxide inhibition of mitochondrial cytochrome *c* oxidase. *Biochim Biophys Acta* 1777: 867–876, 2008.
20. Cooper J, Cervenansky F, De Fabritiis G, Fenner J, Friboulet D, Giorgino T, Manos S et al. The Virtual Physiological Human TOOLKIT. *Philos Transact A Math Phys Eng Sci* 368: 3925–3936, 2010.
21. Cornelissen AJ, Dankelman J, VanBavel E, and Spaan JA. Balance between myogenic, flow-dependent, and metabolic flow control in coronary arterial tree: A model study. *Am J Physiol Heart Circ Physiol* 282: H2224–2237, 2002.
22. Curry FR. Microvascular solute and water transport. *Microcirculation* 12: 17–31, 2005.
23. Das B, Enden G, and Popel AS. Stratified multiphase model for blood flow in a venular bifurcation. *Ann Biomed Eng* 25: 135–153, 1997.

24. Dash RK, Li Y, Kim J, Beard DA, Saidel GM, and Cabrera ME. Metabolic dynamics in skeletal muscle during acute reduction in blood flow and oxygen supply to mitochondria: In-silico studies using a multi-scale, top-down integrated model. *PLoS One* 3: e3168, 2008.

25. Davis MJ and Hill MA. Signaling mechanisms underlying the vascular myogenic response. *Physiol Rev* 79: 387–423, 1999.

26. Desjardins C and Duling BR. Heparinase treatment suggests a role for the endothelial cell glycocalyx in regulation of capillary hematocrit. *Am J Physiol* 258: H647–654, 1990.

27. Discher DE. New insights into erythrocyte membrane organization and microelasticity. *Curr Opin Hematol* 7: 117–122, 2000.

28. Drager A, Planatscher H, Motsou Wouamba D, Schroder A, Hucka M, Endler L, Golebiewski M, Muller W, and Zell A. SBML2 L(A)T(E)X: Conversion of SBML files into human-readable reports. *Bioinformatics* 25: 1455–1456, 2009.

29. Ellsworth ML, Ellis CG, Goldman D, Stephenson AH, Dietrich HH, and Sprague RS. Erythrocytes: Oxygen sensors and modulators of vascular tone. *Physiology (Bethesda)* 24: 107–116, 2009.

30. Ellsworth ML and Pittman RN. Evaluation of photometric methods for quantifying convective mass transport in microvessels. *Am J Physiol* 251: H869–879, 1986.

31. Fedosov DA, Caswell B, and Karniadakis GE. A multiscale red blood cell model with accurate mechanics, rheology, and dynamics. *Biophys J* 98: 2215–2225, 2010.

32. Fedosov DA, Caswell B, Popel AS, and Karniadakis GE. Blood flow and cell-free layer in microvessels. *Microcirculation* 17: 615–628, 2010.

33. Figueroa XF, Isakson BE, and Duling BR. Connexins: Gaps in our knowledge of vascular function. *Physiology (Bethesda)* 19: 277–284, 2004.

34. Gao L and Lipowsky HH. Composition of the endothelial glycocalyx and its relation to its thickness and diffusion of small solutes. *Microvasc Res* 80: 394–401, 2010.

35. Goldman D. Theoretical models of microvascular oxygen transport to tissue. *Microcirculation* 15: 795–811, 2008.

36. Golub AS and Pittman RN. Erythrocyte-associated transients in PO_2 revealed in capillaries of rat mesentery. *Am J Physiol Heart Circ Physiol* 288: H2735–2743, 2005.

37. Granger DN, Rodrigues SF, Yildirim A, and Senchenkova EY. Microvascular responses to cardiovascular risk factors. *Microcirculation* 17: 192–20 5, 2010.

38. Guilford WH and Gore RW. The mechanics of arteriole-tissue interaction. *Microvasc Res* 50: 260–287, 1995.

39. Gundersen SI, Chen G, and Palmer AF. Mathematical model of NO and O_2 transport in an arteriole facilitated by hemoglobin based O_2 carriers. *Biophys Chem* 143: 1–17, 2009.

40. Hall CN and Garthwaite J. What is the real physiological NO concentration *in vivo*? *Nitric Oxide* 21: 92–103, 2009.

41. Hu X and Weinbaum S. A new view of Starling's hypothesis at the microstructural level. *Microvasc Res* 58: 281–304, 1999.

42. Jadhav S, Eggleton CD, and Konstantopoulos K. A 3-D computational model predicts that cell deformation affects selectin-mediated leukocyte rolling. *Biophys J* 88: 96–104, 2005.

43. Johnson PC. Overview of the microcirculation. In: *Handbook of Physiology: Microcirculation*, edited by Tuma RF, Duran WN and Ley K: San Diego: Academic Press; 2008, p. xi–xxvi.

44. Kapela A, Bezerianos A, and Tsoukias NM. A mathematical model of vasoreactivity in rat mesenteric arterioles: I. Myoendothelial communication. *Microcirculation*: 16: 694–713, 2009.

45. Kapela A, Nagaraja S, and Tsoukias NM. A mathematical model of vasoreactivity in rat mesenteric arterioles. II. Conducted vasoreactivity. *Am J Physiol Heart Circ Physiol* 298: H52–65, 2010.

46. Kashiwagi S, Kajimura M, Yoshimura Y, and Suematsu M. Nonendothelial source of nitric oxide in arterioles but not in venules: Alternative source revealed *in vivo* by diaminofluorescein microfluorography. *Circ Res* 91: e55–64, 2002.

47. Kaul DK, Finnegan E, and Barabino GA. Sickle red cell-endothelium interactions. *Microcirculation* 16: 97–111, 2009.

48. Kiani MF, Pries AR, Hsu LL, Sarelius IH, and Cokelet GR. Fluctuations in microvascular blood flow parameters caused by hemodynamic mechanisms. *Am J Physiol* 266: H1822–1828, 1994.

49. Leick L, Hellsten Y, Fentz J, Lyngby SS, Wojtaszewski JF, Hidalgo J, and Pilegaard H. PGC-1alpha mediates exercise-induced skeletal muscle VEGF expression in mice. *Am J Physiol Endocrinol Metab* 297: E92–103, 2009.

50. Ley K. The role of selectins in inflammation and disease. *Trends Mol Med* 9: 263–268, 2003.

51. Li C, Donizelli M, Rodriguez N, Dharuri H, Endler L, Chelliah V, Li L et al. BioModels Database: An enhanced, curated and annotated resource for published quantitative kinetic models. *BMC Syst Biol* 4: 92, 2010.

52. Li J, Lykotrafitis G, Dao M, and Suresh S. Cytoskeletal dynamics of human erythrocyte. *Proc Natl Acad Sci USA* 104: 4937–4942, 2007.

53. Lipowsky HH. Microvascular rheology and hemodynamics. *Microcirculation* 12: 5–15, 2005.

54. Liu G, Qutub AA, Vempati P, Mac Gabhann F, and Popel AS. Module-based multiscale simulation of angiogenesis in skeletal muscle. *Theor Biol Med Model.* 8: 6, 2011.

55. Lloyd CM, Lawson JR, Hunter PJ, and Nielsen PF. The CellML model repository. *Bioinformatics* 24: 2122–2123, 2008.

56. Mac Gabhann F and Popel AS. Systems biology of vascular endothelial growth factors. *Microcirculation* 15: 715–738, 2008.

57. Michel CC and Curry FE. Microvascular permeability. *Physiol Rev* 79: 703–761, 1999.

58. Mulivor AW and Lipowsky HH. Inflammation- and ischemia-induced shedding of venular glycocalyx. *Am J Physiol Heart Circ Physiol* 286: H1672–1680, 2004.

59. Munn LL and Dupin MM. Blood cell interactions and segregation in flow. *Ann Biomed Eng* 36: 534–544, 2008.

60. Napolitano LM. Hemoglobin-based oxygen carriers: First, second or third generation? Human or bovine? Where are we now? *Crit Care Clin* 25: 279–301, 2009.

61. Pappu V and Bagchi P. 3D computational modeling and simulation of leukocyte rolling adhesion and deformation. *Comput Biol Med* 38: 738–753, 2008.

62. Parthimos D, Edwards DH, and Griffith TM. Minimal model of arterial chaos generated by coupled intracellular and membrane Ca^{2+} oscillators. *Am J Physiol* 277: H1119–1144, 1999.

63. Peirce SM. Computational and mathematical modeling of angiogenesis. *Microcirculation* 15: 739–751, 2008.

64. Pittman RN. Oxygen transport and exchange in the microcirculation. *Microcirculation* 12: 59–70, 2005.

65. Platts SH and Duling BR. Adenosine A3 receptor activation modulates the capillary endothelial glycocalyx. *Circ Res* 94: 77–82, 2004.

66. Pohl U and de Wit C. A unique role of NO in the control of blood flow. *News Physiol Sci* 14: 74–80, 1999.

67. Popel AS. Theory of oxygen transport to tissue. *Crit Rev Biomed Eng* 17: 257–321, 1989.

68. Popel AS and Hunter PJ. Systems biology and physiome projects. *Wiley Interdisciplinary Reviews: Systems Biology and Medicine* 1: 153–158, 2009.

69. Popel AS and Johnson PC. Microcirculation and hemorheology. *Ann Rev Fluid Mechanics* 37: 43–69, 2005.

70. Pozrikidis C. *Computational Hydrodynamics of Capsules and Biological Cells.* Taylor & Francis, 2010, p. 1–327.

71. Pries AR and Secomb TW. Blood flow in microvascular networks. In: *Handbook of Physiology. Microcirculation.* (2nd Edition ed.), edited by Tuma RF, Duran WN and Ley K: San Diego: Academic Press; 2008, pp. 3–36.

72. Pries AR and Secomb TW. Control of blood vessel structure: Insights from theoretical models. *Am J Physiol Heart Circ Physiol* 288: H1010–1015, 2005.

73. Pries AR and Secomb TW. Modeling structural adaptation of microcirculation. *Microcirculation* 15: 753–764, 2008.

74. Pries AR and Secomb TW. Origins of heterogeneity in tissue perfusion and metabolism. *Cardiovasc Res* 81: 328–335, 2009.

75. Pries AR, Secomb TW, and Gaehtgens P. The endothelial surface layer. *Pflugers Arch* 440: 653–666, 2000.

76. Qutub AA, Liu G, Vempati P, and Popel AS. Integration of angiogenesis modules at multiple scales: From molecular to tissue. *Pac Symp Biocomput* 316–327, 2009.

77. Qutub AA, Mac Gabhann F, Karagiannis ED, and Popel AS. In silico modeling of angiogenesis at multiple scales: From nanoscale to organ system. In: *Multiscale Modeling of Particle Interactions: Applications in Biology and Nanotechnology.* edited by King MR and Gee DJ: Wiley, Hoboken, NJ, 2010, p. 287–320.

78. Qutub AA, Mac Gabhann F, Karagiannis ED, Vempati P, and Popel AS. Multiscale models of angiogenesis. *IEEE Eng Med Biol Mag* 28: 14–31, 2009.

79. Schmid-Schonbein GW. Biomechanics of microcirculatory blood perfusion. *Annu Rev Biomed Eng* 1: 73–102, 1999.

80. Schmid-Schonbein GW and Granger DN. *Molecular Basis for Microcirculatory Disorders.* Springer-Verlag, Paris, France 2003.

81. Secomb TW, Beard DA, Frisbee JC, Smith NP, and Pries AR. The role of theoretical modeling in microcirculation research. *Microcirculation* 15: 693–698, 2008.

82. Segal SS. Integration of blood flow control to skeletal muscle: Key role of feed arteries. *Acta Physiol Scand* 168: 511–518, 2000.

83. Segal SS. Regulation of blood flow in the microcirculation. *Microcirculation* 12: 33–45, 2005.

84. Semenza GL. Hydroxylation of HIF-1: Oxygen sensing at the molecular level. *Physiology (Bethesda)* 19: 176–182, 2004.

85. Skalak TC. Angiogenesis and microvascular remodeling: A brief history and future roadmap. *Microcirculation* 12: 47–58, 2005.

86. Tailor A, Cooper D, and Granger D. Platelet-vessel wall interactions in the microcirculation. *Microcirculation* 12: 275–285, 2005.

87. Tsai AG, Johnson PC, and Intaglietta M. Oxygen gradients in the microcirculation. *Physiol Rev* 83: 933–963, 2003.

88. Tsoukias NM. Nitric oxide bioavailability in the microcirculation: Insights from mathematical models. *Microcirculation* 15: 813–834, 2008.

89. Tsoukias NM, Goldman D, Vadapalli A, Pittman RN, and Popel AS. A computational model of oxygen delivery by hemoglobin-based oxygen carriers in three-dimensional microvascular networks. *J Theor Biol* 248: 657–674, 2007.

90. Ursino M, Colantuoni A, and Bertuglia S. Vasomotion and blood flow regulation in hamster skeletal muscle microcirculation: A theoretical and experimental study. *Microvasc Res* 56: 233–252, 1998.

91. van Faassen EE, Bahrami S, Feelisch M, Hogg N, Kelm M, Kim-Shapiro DB, Kozlov AV et al. Nitrite as regulator of hypoxic signaling in mammalian physiology. *Med Res Rev* 29: 683–741, 2009.

92. Weibel ER and Hoppeler H. Exercise-induced maximal metabolic rate scales with muscle aerobic capacity. *J Exp Biol* 208: 1635–1644, 2005.

93. Weinbaum S, Tarbell JM, and Damiano ER. The structure and function of the endothelial glycocalyx layer. *Annu Rev Biomed Eng* 9: 121–167, 2007.

94. Woldhuis B, Tangelder GJ, Slaaf DW, and Reneman RS. Concentration profile of blood platelets differs in arterioles and venules. *Am J Physiol* 262: H1217–1223, 1992.

95. Zhang J, Johnson PC, and Popel AS. Effects of erythrocyte deformability and aggregation on the cell free layer and apparent viscosity of microscopic blood flows. *Microvasc Res* 77: 265–272, 2009.

Further Information

Handbook of Physiology. Microcirculation (2nd ed.), edited by Tuma RF, Duran WN and Ley K: Elsevier, American Physiological Society, 2008, 949 pp.

Original research articles on microcirculation can be found in academic journals: *Microcirculation, Microvascular Research, American Journal of Physiology (Heart and Circulatory Physiology), Journal of Vascular Research,* and *Biorheology.*

21

Mechanics and Deformability of Hematocytes

21.1 Introduction 21-1
21.2 Fundamentals.. 21-2
Stresses and Strains in Two Dimensions • Basic Equations for
Newtonian Fluid Flow
21.3 Red Cells.. 21-3
Size and Shape • Red Cell Cytosol • Membrane Area
Dilation • Membrane Shear Deformation • Stress Relaxation and
Strain Hardening • New Constitutive Relations for the Red Cell
Membrane • Bending Elasticity
21.4 Leukocytes 21-7
Size and Shape • Mechanical Behavior • Cortical
Tension • Apparent Viscosity
21.5 Summary.. 21-10
Definition of Terms 21-11
References..21-11
Further Information... 21-13

Richard E. Waugh
University of Rochester

Robert M.
Hochmuth
Duke University

21.1 Introduction

The term "hematocytes" refers to the circulating cells of the blood. These are divided into two main classes: erythrocytes, or red cells, and leukocytes, or white cells. In addition to these, there are specialized cell-like structures called platelets. The mechanical properties of these cells are of special interest because of their physiological role as circulating corpuscles in the flowing blood. The importance of the mechanical properties of these cells and their influence on blood flow is evident in a number of hematological pathologies. The properties of the two main types of hematocytes are distinctly different. The essential character of a red cell is that of an elastic bag enclosing a Newtonian fluid of comparatively low viscosity. The essential behavior of leukocytes is that of a highly viscous fluid drop with a more or less constant cortical (surface) tension. Under the action of a given force, red cells deform much more readily than white cells. In this chapter, we focus on descriptions of the behavior of the two cell types separately, concentrating on the viscoelastic characteristics of the red cell membrane and the fluid characteristics of the white cell cytosol.

21.2 Fundamentals

21.2.1 Stresses and Strains in Two Dimensions

The description of the mechanical deformation of the membrane is cast in terms of principal *force resultants* and *principal extension ratios* of the surface. The force resultants, like conventional three-dimensional strain, are generally expressed in terms of a tensorial quantity, the components of which depend on coordinate rotation. For the purposes of describing the constitutive behavior of the surface, it is convenient to express the surface resultants in terms of rotationally invariant quantities. These can be either the principal force resultants N_1 and N_2, or the isotropic resultant $\overline{N}$ and the maximum shear resultant N_s. The surface strain is also a tensorial quantity but may be expressed in terms of the principal extension ratios of the surface λ_1 and λ_2. The *rate* of surface shear deformation is given by (Evans and Skalak 1979)

$$V_s = \left(\frac{\lambda_1}{\lambda_2}\right)^{1/2} \frac{d}{dt}\left(\frac{\lambda_1}{\lambda_2}\right)^{1/2} \tag{21.1}$$

The membrane deformation is calculated from observed macroscopic changes in cell geometry, usually with the use of simple geometric shapes to approximate the cell shape. The membrane force resultants are calculated from force balance relationships. For example, in the determination of the *area expansivity modulus* of the red cell membrane or the *cortical tension* in neutrophils, the force resultants in the plane of the membrane of the red cell or the cortex of a white cell are isotropic. In this case, as long as the membrane surface of the cell does not stick to the pipette, the membrane force resultant can be calculated from the law of Laplace:

$$\Delta P = 2\overline{N}\left(\frac{1}{R_p} - \frac{1}{R_c}\right) \tag{21.2}$$

where R_p is the radius of the pipette, R_c is the radius of the spherical portion of the cell outside the pipette, $\overline{N}$ is the isotropic force resultant (tension) in the membrane, and ΔP is the aspiration pressure in the pipette.

21.2.2 Basic Equations for Newtonian Fluid Flow

The constitutive relations for fluid flow in a sphere undergoing axisymmetric deformation can be written as

$$\sigma_{rr} = -p + 2\eta\frac{\partial V_r}{\partial r} \tag{21.3}$$

$$\sigma_{r\theta} = \eta\left[\frac{1}{r}\frac{\partial V_r}{\partial \theta} + r\frac{\partial}{\partial r}\left(\frac{V_\theta}{r}\right)\right] \tag{21.4}$$

where σ_{rr} and $\sigma_{r\theta}$ are components of the stress tensor, p is the hydrostatic pressure, r is the radial coordinate, θ is the angular coordinate in the direction of the axis of symmetry in spherical coordinates, and V_r and V_θ are components of the fluid velocity vector. These equations effectively define the material viscosity, η. The second term in Equation 21.3 contains the radial strain rate $\dot{\varepsilon}_{rr}$ and the bracketed term in Equation 21.4 corresponds to $\dot{\varepsilon}_{r\theta}$. In general, η may be a function of the strain rate. For the purposes of evaluating this dependence, it is convenient to define the mean shear rate $\dot{\gamma}_m$ averaged over the cell volume and duration of the deformation process t_e:

$$\dot{\gamma}_m = \left(\frac{3}{4} \frac{1}{t_e} \int_0^{t_e} \int_0^{R(t)} \int_0^{\pi} \frac{r^2}{R^3} (\dot{\varepsilon}_{ij} \dot{\varepsilon}_{ij}) \sin\theta \; d\theta dr dt \right)^{1/2} \tag{21.5}$$

where repeated indices indicate summation.

21.3 Red Cells

21.3.1 Size and Shape

The normal red cell is a biconcave disk at rest. The average human cell is approximately 7.7 μm in diameter and varies in thickness from ~2.8 μm at the rim to ~1.4 μm at the center (Fung et al. 1981). However, red cells vary considerably in size even within a single individual. The mean surface area is ~130 μm² and the mean volume is 98 μm³ (Table 21.1), but the range of sizes within a population is Gaussian distributed with standard deviations (S.D.) of ~15.8 μm² for the area and ~16.1 μm³ for the volume (Fung et al. 1981). Cells from different species vary enormously in size, and tables for different species have been tabulated elsewhere (Hawkey et al. 1991).

Red cell deformation takes place under two important constraints: fixed surface area and fixed volume. The constraint of fixed volume arises from the impermeability of the membrane to cations. Even though the membrane is highly permeable to water, the inability of salts to cross the membrane prevents significant water loss because of the requirement for colloidal osmotic equilibrium (Lew and Bookchin 1986). The constraint of fixed surface area arises from the large resistance of bilayer membranes to changes in area per molecule (Needham and Nunn 1990). These two constraints place strict limits on the kinds of deformations that the cell can undergo and the size of the aperture that the cell can negotiate. Thus, a major determinant of red cell deformability is its ratio of surface area to volume. One measure of this parameter is the *sphericity*, defined as the dimensionless ratio of the two-thirds power of the cell volume to the cell area times a constant that makes its maximum value 1.0:

$$S = \frac{4\pi}{(4\pi/3)^{2/3}} \cdot \frac{V^{2/3}}{A} \tag{21.6}$$

The mean value of sphericity of a normal population of cells was measured by interference microscopy to be 0.79 with an S.D. of 0.05 at room temperature (Fung et al. 1981). Similar values were obtained using micropipettes: mean = 0.81, S.D. = 0.02 (Waugh and Agre 1988). The membrane area increases with temperature, and the membrane volume decreases with temperature, so the sphericity at physiological temperature is expected to be somewhat smaller. Based on measurements of the thermal area expansivity of 0.12%/°C (Waugh and Evans 1979), and a change in volume of −0.14%/°C (Waugh and Evans 1979), the mean sphericity at 37°C is estimated to be 0.76–0.78 (see Table 21.1).

TABLE 21.1 Parameter Values for a Typical Red Blood Cell (37°C)

Area	132 μm²
Volume	96 μm³
Sphericity	0.77
Membrane area modulus	400 mN/m
Membrane shear modulus	0.006 mN/m
Membrane viscosity	0.00036 mN · s/m
Membrane bending stiffness	0.2×10^{-18} J
Thermal area expansivity	0.12%/°C
$\dfrac{1}{V}\dfrac{dV}{dT}$	−0.14%/°C

TABLE 21.2   Viscosity of Red Cell Cytosol (37°C)

Hemoglobin Concentration (g/L)	Measured Viscosity[a] (mPa · s)	Best Fit Viscosity[b] (mPa · s)
290	4.1–5.0	4.2
310	5.2–6.6	5.3
330	6.6–9.2	6.7
350	8.5–13.0	8.9
370	10.8–17.1	12.1
390	15.0–23.9	17.2

[a] Data taken from Cokelet and Meiselman (1968) and Chien et al. (1970).
[b] Fitted curve from Ross and Minton (1977).

21.3.2 Red Cell Cytosol

The interior of a red cell is a concentrated solution of hemoglobin, the oxygen-carrying protein, and it behaves as a Newtonian fluid (Cokelet and Meiselman 1968). In a normal population of cells, there is a distribution of hemoglobin concentrations in the range of 29–39 g/dl. The viscosity of the cytosol depends on the hemoglobin concentration as well as the temperature (see Table 21.2). Based on theoretical models (Ross and Minton 1977), the temperature dependence of the cytosolic viscosity is expected to be the same as that of water, that is, the ratio of cytosolic viscosity at 37°C to the viscosity at 20°C is the same as the ratio of water viscosity at those same temperatures. In most cases, even in the most dense cells, the resistance to flow of the cytosol is small compared with the viscoelastic resistance of the membrane when membrane deformations are appreciable.

21.3.3 Membrane Area Dilation

The large resistance of the membrane to area dilation has been characterized in micromechanical experiments. The changes in surface area that can be produced in the membrane are small, and so they can be characterized in terms of a simple Hookean elastic relationship between the isotropic force resultant $\overline{N}$ and the fractional change in surface area $\alpha = A/Ao - 1$:

$$\overline{N} = K\alpha \tag{21.7}$$

The proportionality constant K is called the *area compressibility modulus* or the *area expansivity modulus*. Early estimates placed its value at room temperature at ~450 mN/m (Evans and Waugh 1977) and showed a dependence of the modulus on temperature, its value changing from ~300 mN/m at 45°C to a value of ~600 mN/m at 5°C (Waugh and Evans 1979). Subsequently, it was shown that the measurement of this parameter using micropipettes is affected by extraneous electric fields, and the value at room temperature was corrected upward to ~500 mN/m (Katnik and Waugh 1990). The values in Table 21.3 are based on this measurement, and the fractional change in the modulus with temperature is based on the original micropipette measurements (Waugh and Evans 1979).

21.3.4 Membrane Shear Deformation

The shear deformations of the red cell surface can be large, and so a simple linear relationship between force and extension is not adequate for describing the membrane behavior. The large resistance of the membrane composite to area dilation led early investigators to postulate that the membrane maintained constant surface density during shear deformation, that is, the surface was two-dimensionally incompressible. Most of what exists in the literature about the shear deformation of the red cell membrane is based on this assumption. Indeed, even a recent three-dimensional neo-Hookean relationship proposed

TABLE 21.3 Temperature Dependence of Viscoelastic Coefficients of the Red Cell Membrane

Temperature (°C)	K (mN/m)[a]	μ_m (mN/m)[b]	η (mN·s/m)[c]
5	660	0.0078	0.0021
15	580	0.0072	0.0014
25	500	0.0065	0.00074
37	400	0.0058	0.00036
45	340	0.0053	—

[a] Based on a value of the modulus at 25°C of 500 mN/m and the fractional change in modulus with temperature measured by Waugh and Evans (1979).
[b] Based on linear regression to the data of Waugh and Evans (1979).
[c] Data from Hochmuth et al. (1980).

by Dao et al. (2003) applies the constant area constraint in modeling extensional deformation of red cells by optical tweezers. In the mid-1990s, experimental evidence emerged that this assumption is an over-simplification of the true cellular behavior, and that deformation produces changes in the local surface density of the membrane elastic network (Discher et al. 1994). Nevertheless, the older simpler relationships provide a reliable description of the cell behavior that can be useful for many applications, and so the properties of the cell defined under that assumption are summarized here.

For a simple, two-dimensional, incompressible, hyperelastic material, the relationship between the membrane shear force resultant N_s and the material deformation is (Evans and Skalak 1979)

$$N_s = \frac{\mu_m}{2}\left(\frac{\lambda_1}{\lambda_2} - \frac{\lambda_2}{\lambda_1}\right) + 2\eta_m V_s \tag{21.8}$$

where λ_1 and λ_2 are the principal extension ratios for the deformation and V_s is the rate of surface shear deformation (Equation 21.1). The *membrane shear modulus* μ_m and the *membrane viscosity* η_m are defined by this relationship. Values for these coefficients at different temperatures are given in Table 21.3.

21.3.5 Stress Relaxation and Strain Hardening

Subsequent to these original formulations, a number of refinements to these relationships have been proposed. Observations of persistent deformations after micropipette aspiration for extended periods of time formed the basis for the development of a model for long-term stress relaxation (Markle et al. 1983). The characteristic times for these relaxations were on the order of 1–2 h, and they are thought to correlate with permanent rearrangements of the membrane elastic network.

Another type of stress relaxation is thought to occur over very short times (~0.1 s) after rapid deformation of the membrane either by micropipette (Chien et al. 1978) or in cell extension experiments (Waugh and Bisgrove, unpublished observations). This phenomenon is thought to be due to transient entanglements within the deforming network. Whether or not the phenomenon actually occurs remains controversial. The stresses relax rapidly, and it is difficult to account for inertial effects of the measuring system and to reliably assess the intrinsic cellular response. In a more recent report, magnetic twisting cytometry was used to measure storage and loss moduli over a wide range of frequencies. The strains in these studies were small, and the elastic deformation dominated by bending, so it is unclear if the lack of frequency dependence of the storage modulus observed in that study has implications here, but the membrane behavior at low frequencies was consistent with the moduli determined from cell extension.

Finally, there has been some evidence that the coefficient for shear elasticity may be a function of the surface extension, increasing with increasing deformation. This was first proposed by Fischer in an effort to resolve discrepancies between theoretical predictions and observed behavior of red cells undergoing dynamic deformations in fluid shear (Fischer et al. 1981). Increasing elastic resistance with extension has also been proposed as an explanation for discrepancies between theoretical predictions based on a constant modulus and measurements of the length of a cell projection into a micropipette (Waugh and Marchesi 1990). However, owing to the approximate nature of the mechanical analysis of cell deformation in shear flow, and the limits of optical resolution in micropipette experiments, the evidence for a dependence of the modulus on extension is not clear-cut, and this issue remains unresolved.

21.3.6 New Constitutive Relations for the Red Cell Membrane

More recent descriptions of membrane deformation recognize that the membrane is a composite of two layers with distinct mechanical behavior. The membrane bilayer, composed of phospholipids and integral membrane proteins, exhibits a large elastic resistance to area dilation but is fluid in surface shear. The membrane skeleton, composed of a network of structural proteins at the cytoplasmic surface of the bilayer, is locally compressible and exhibits an elastic resistance to surface shear. The assumption that the membrane skeleton is locally incompressible is no longer applied. This assumption had been challenged over the years on the basis of theoretical considerations, but only very recently has experimental evidence emerged that shows definitively that the membrane skeleton is compressible. This led to a model for membrane behavior (Mohandas and Evans 1994) where the principal stress resultants in the membrane skeleton are related to the membrane deformation by

$$N_1 = \mu_N\left(\frac{\lambda_1}{\lambda_2} - 1\right) + K_N\left(\lambda_1\lambda_2 - \frac{1}{(\lambda_1\lambda_2)^2}\right) \tag{21.9}$$

and

$$N_2 = \mu_N\left(\frac{\lambda_2}{\lambda_1} - 1\right) + K_N\left(\lambda_1\lambda_2 - \frac{1}{(\lambda_1\lambda_2)^2}\right) \tag{21.10}$$

where μ_N and K_N are the shear and isotropic moduli of the membrane skeleton, respectively. Values for the coefficients determined from fluorescence measurements of skeletal density distributions during micropipette aspiration studies are $\mu_N \approx 0.01$ mN/m and $K_N \approx 0.02$ mN/m (Discher et al. 1994). These new concepts for membrane constitutive behavior have yet to be explored thoroughly. The temperature dependence of these moduli is unknown, and the implications such a model will have on interpretation of dynamic deformations of the membrane remain to be resolved.

An important new area of development involves attempts to derive constitutive behavior from molecular-level models of the membrane skeleton. These approaches have led to reliable predictions of cell elastic behavior in micropipette aspiration (Discher et al. 1998) and cell extension using optical tweezers (Li et al. 2005). The most recent models also capture many of the dynamic behaviors of the red cell (Fedosov et al. 2010), although this most recent analysis did not allow for local changes in the density of the elastic network that have been well documented experimentally (Discher et al. 1994). Thus, while there are a number of mathematical descriptions that do an excellent job of capturing the essential characteristics of the cell, one that completely and accurately captures all aspects of the cell behavior remains an unmet goal.

21.3.7 Bending Elasticity

Even though the membrane is very thin, it has a high resistance to surface dilation. This property, coupled with the finite thickness of the membrane gives the membrane a small but finite resistance to bending. This resistance is characterized in terms of the *membrane bending modulus*. The bending resistance of biological membranes is inherently complex because of their lamellar structure. There is a local resistance to bending due to the inherent stiffness of the individual leaflets of the membrane bilayer. (Because the membrane skeleton is compressible, it is thought to contribute little if anything to the membrane bending stiffness.) In addition to this local stiffness, there is a *nonlocal bending resistance* due to the net compression and expansion of the adjacent leaflets resulting from the curvature change. The nonlocal contribution is complicated by the fact that the leaflets may be redistributed laterally within the membrane capsule to equalize the area per molecule within each leaflet. The situation is further complicated by the likely possibility that molecules may exchange between leaflets to alleviate curvature-induced dilation/compression. Thus, the bending stiffness measured by different approaches probably reflects contributions from both local and nonlocal mechanisms, and the measured values may differ because of different contributions from the two mechanisms. Estimates based on buckling instabilities during micropipette aspiration give a value of $\sim 0.18 \times 10^{-18}$ J (Evans 1983), measurements based on the mechanical formation of lipid tubes from the cell surface give a value of $0.2 \pm 0.02 \times 10^{-18}$ J (Butler et al. 2008, Hwang and Waugh 1997), and estimates based on thermal fluctuations of the membrane yield similar values.

21.4 Leukocytes

While red cells account for approximately 40% of the blood volume, leukocytes occupy less than 1% of the blood volume. Yet, because leukocytes are less deformable, they can have a significant influence on blood flow, especially in the microvasculature. Unlike red cells, which are very similar to each other, as are platelets, there are several different kinds of leukocytes. Originally, leukocytes were classified into groups according to their appearance when viewed with the light microscope. Thus, there are *granulocytes*, *monocytes*, and *lymphocytes* (Alberts et al. 2002). The granulocytes with their many internal granules are separated into *neutrophils*, *basophils*, and *eosinophils* according to the way each cell stains. The neutrophil, also called a *polymorphonuclear leukocyte* because of its segmented or "multilobed" nucleus, is the most common white cell in the blood (see Table 21.4). The lymphocytes, which constitute 20–40% of the white cells and which are further subdivided into *B lymphocytes* and *killer* and *helper T lymphocytes*, are the smallest of the white cells. The other types of leukocytes are found with much less frequency. Most of the geometric and mechanical studies of white cells reported below have focused on the neutrophil because it is the most common cell in the circulation, although the lymphocyte has also received attention.

21.4.1 Size and Shape

White cells at rest are spherical. The surfaces of white cells contain many folds, projections, and "microvilli" to provide the cells with sufficient membrane area to deform as they enter capillaries with

TABLE 21.4 Size and Appearance of White Cells in the Circulation

	Occurrence[a] (% of WBCs)	Cell Volume[b] (μm³)	Cell Diameter[b] (μm)	Nucleus[c] % Cell Volume	Cortical Tension (mN/m)
Granulocytes					
Neutrophils	50–70	300–310	8.2–8.4	21	0.024–0.035[d]
Basophils	0–1	—			—
Eosinophils	1–3	—		18	—
Monocytes	1–5	400	9.1	26	0.06[e]
Lymphocytes	20–40	220	7.5	44	0.035[e]

[a] Diggs et al. (1985).
[b] Ting-Beall et al. (1993, 1995).
[c] Schmid-Schönbein et al. (1980).
[d] Evans and Yeung (1989), Needham and Hochmuth (1992), Tsai et al. (1993, 1994).
[e] Hochmuth, Zhelev, and Ting-Beall, unpublished data.

diameters much smaller than the resting diameter of the cell. (Without the reservoir of membrane area in these folds, the constraints of constant volume and membrane area would make a spherical cell essentially undeformable.) The excess surface area of the neutrophil, when measured in a wet preparation, is slightly more than twice the apparent surface area of a smooth sphere with the same diameter (Evans and Yeung 1989, Ting-Beall et al. 1993). It is interesting to note that each type of white cell has its own unique surface topography, which allows one to readily determine if a cell is, for example, a neutrophil or monocyte or lymphocyte (Hochmuth et al. 1994).

The cell volumes listed in Table 21.4 were obtained with the light microscope, either by measuring the diameter of the spherical cell or by aspirating the cell into a small glass pipette with a known diameter and then measuring the resulting length of the cylindrically shaped cell. Other values for cell volume obtained using transmission electron microscopy are somewhat smaller, probably because of cell shrinkage due to fixation and drying prior to measurement (Schmid-Schonbein et al. 1980, Ting-Beall et al. 1995). Although the absolute magnitude of the cell volume measured with the electron microscope may be erroneous, if it is assumed that all parts of the cell dehydrate equally when they are dried in preparation for viewing, then this approach can be used to determine the volume occupied by the nucleus (Table 21.4) and other organelles of various white cells. The volume occupied by the granules in the neutrophil and eosinophil (recall that both are granulocytes) is 15% and 23%, respectively, whereas the granular volume in monocytes and lymphocytes is less than a few percent.

21.4.2 Mechanical Behavior

The early observations of Bagge et al. (1977) led them to suggest that the neutrophil behaves as a simple viscoelastic solid with a Maxwell element (an elastic and viscous element in series) in parallel with an elastic element. This elastic element in the model was thought to pull the unstressed cell into its spherical shape. Subsequently, Evans and colleagues (Evans and Kukan 1984, Evans and Yeung 1989) showed that the cells flow continuously into a pipette, with no apparent approach to a static limit, when a constant suction pressure was applied. Thus, the cytoplasm of the neutrophil should be treated as a liquid rather than a solid, and its surface has a persistent *cortical tension* that causes the cell to assume a spherical shape.

21.4.3 Cortical Tension

Using a micropipette and a small suction pressure to aspirate a hemispherical projection from a cell body into the pipette, Evans and Yeung (1989) measured a value for the cortical tension of 0.035 mN/m. Needham and Hochmuth (1992) measured the cortical tension of individual cells that were driven down a tapered pipette in a series of equilibrium positions. In many cases, the cortical tension increased as the cell moved further into the pipette, which means that the cell has an apparent area expansion modulus (Equation 21.7). They obtained an average value of 0.04 mN/m for the expansion modulus and an extrapolated value for the cortical tension (at zero area dilation) in the resting state of 0.024 mN/m. Herant (Herant et al. 2005) examined cortical tension as a cell engulfed a bead, and found a lower resting value but a much higher dependence on surface dilation. For dilations of the surface up to 25%, they found $T = T_o + k(A - A_o)/A_o$, where $T_o = 0.010$ mN/m and $k = 0.16$ mN/m. The importance of the actin cytoskeleton in maintaining cortical tension was demonstrated by Tsai et al. (1994). The treatment of the cells with a drug that disrupts actin filament structure (CTB = cytochalasin B) resulted in a decrease in cortical tension from 0.027 to 0.022 mN/m at a CTB concentration of 3 μM and to 0.014 mN/m at 30 μM.

Unpublished measurements in one of our laboratories (RMH) indicate that the value for the cortical tension of a monocyte is about double that for a granulocyte, that is, 0.06 mN/m, and the value for a lymphocyte is about 0.035 mN/m.

21.4.4 Apparent Viscosity

Using their model of the neutrophil as a Newtonian liquid drop with a constant cortical tension and (as they showed) a negligible surface viscosity, Yeung and Evans (1989) analyzed the flow of neutrophils into a micropipette and obtained a value for the *cytoplasmic viscosity* of about 200 Pa · s. In their experiments, the aspiration pressures were on the order of 10–1000 Pa. Similar experiments by Needham and Hochmuth (1990) using the same Newtonian model (with a negligible surface viscosity) but using higher aspiration pressures (ranging from 500 to 2000 Pa) gave an average value for the cytoplasmic viscosity of 135 Pa · s for 151 cells from five individuals. The apparent discrepancy between these two sets of experiments was resolved to a large extent by Tsai and colleagues (Tsai et al. 1993), who demonstrated that the neutrophil viscosity decreases with an increasing rate of deformation. They proposed a model of the cytosol as a *power law fluid*:

$$\eta = \eta_c \left(\frac{\dot{\gamma}_m}{\dot{\gamma}_c} \right)^{-b} \tag{21.11}$$

where $b = 0.52$, $\dot{\gamma}_m$ is defined by Equation 21.5, and η_c is a characteristic viscosity of 130 Pa · s when the characteristic mean shear rate, $\dot{\gamma}_c$, is 1 s^{-1}. These values are based on an approximate method for calculating the viscosity from measurements of the total time it takes for a cell to enter a micropipette. Because of different approximations used in the calculations, the values of viscosity reported by Tsai (Tsai et al. 1993) tend to be somewhat smaller than those reported by Evans and coworkers or Hochmuth and coworkers. Nevertheless, the shear rate dependence of the viscosity is the same, regardless of the method of calculation. Values for the viscosity are given in Table 21.5.

In addition to the dependence of the viscosity on shear rate, there is evidence that values estimated using these approximate models also depend on the extent of deformation. In micropipette experiments, the initial rate at which the cell enters the pipette is significantly faster than predicted, even when the shear rate dependence of the viscosity is taken into account. In a separate approach, the cytosolic viscosity was estimated from the observation of the time course of the cell's return to a spherical geometry after expulsion from a micropipette. When the cellular deformations were large, a viscosity of 150 Pa · s was estimated (Tran-Son-Tay et al. 1991), but when the deformations were small, the estimated viscosity was only 60 Pa · s (Dong et al. 1988, Hochmuth et al. 1993). Thus, it appears that the viscosity is smaller when the magnitude of the deformation is small, and increases as deformations become large.

Although it is clear that the essential behavior of the cell is fluid, the simple fluid drop model with a constant and uniform viscosity does not match the observed time course of cell deformation in detail. In addition to variations in viscosity with magnitude and rate of deformation, there is a rapid initial entry phase that is not predicted by the fluid drop model. One approach that was considered to address this was the application of a *Maxwell fluid* model with a constant cortical tension (Dong et al. 1988). While

TABLE 21.5 Viscous Parameters of White Blood Cells

Cell Type	Range of Viscosities (Pa · s)[a]		Characteristic Viscosity (Pa · s)	Shear Rate Dependence (b)
	Minimum	Maximum		
Neutrophil	50	500	130[b]	0.52[b]
in 30 μM CTB	41	52	54[b]	0.26[b]
Monocyte	70	1000	—	—
HL60 (G1)	—	—	220[c]	0.53[c]
HL60 (S)	—	—	330[c]	0.56[c]

[a] Evans and Yeung (1989), Needham and Hochmuth (1992), Tsai et al. (1993, 1994).
[b] Tsai et al. (1993, 1994).
[c] Tsai and Waugh (1996a,b).

the model worked well for the shape recovery of neutrophils following small deformations, attempts to apply this model for continuous, finite-deformation flow of a neutrophil into a pipette required continuous adjustment of the material coefficients over time (Dong and Skalak 1992). A more successful approach was taken by Drury and Dembo, who developed a finite element analysis of a cell using a model having substantial cortical dissipation with shear thinning and a shear thinning cytoplasm (Drury and Dembo 2001). Their model matches cellular behavior during micropipette aspiration over a wide range of pipette diameters and entry rates, except for the initial rapid entry phase. To account for this phenomenon, a model was introduced in which the cell interior comprised two distinct phases: the cytoskeleton and the cytosol (Herant et al. 2003). Inclusion of all of these characteristics accurately captures most of the fine details of cell behavior, and has been used in subsequent extensions of this approach to examine phagocytosis (Herant et al. 2006). Unfortunately, these advanced models are complex and not easily summarized, and the reader is referred to the original reports for further details.

Although the mechanical properties of the neutrophil have been studied extensively as discussed above, the other white cells have not been studied in depth. Unpublished results from one of our laboratories (RMH) indicate that monocytes are somewhat more viscous (from roughly 30% to a factor of two) than neutrophils under similar conditions in both recovery experiments and experiments in which the monocyte flows into a pipette. A lymphocyte, when aspirated into a small pipette so that its relatively large nucleus is deformed, behaves as an elastic body in that the projection length into the pipette increases linearly with the suction pressure. This elastic behavior appears to be due to the deformation of the nucleus, which has an apparent area elastic modulus of 2 mN/m. A lymphocyte recovers its shape somewhat more quickly than the neutrophil does, although this recovery process is driven by both the cortical tension and the elastic nucleus. These preliminary results are discussed by Tran-Son-Tay et al. (1994). Finally, the properties of a human myeloid leukemic cell line (HL60) thought to resemble immature neutrophils of the bone marrow have also been characterized, as shown in Table 21.5. The apparent cytoplasmic viscosity varies both as a function of the cell cycle and during maturation toward a more neutrophil-like cell. The characteristic viscosity $\dot{\gamma}_c = 1\,s^{-1}$ is 200 Pa·s for HL60 cells in the G1 stage of the cell cycle. This value increases to 275 Pa·s for cells in the S phase, but decreases with maturation, so that 7 days after induction, the properties approach those of neutrophils (150 Pa·s) (Tsai et al. 1996a,b).

It is important to note in closing that the characteristics described above apply to passive leukocytes. It is the nature of these cells to respond to environmental stimulation and engage in active movements and shape transformations. *White cell activation* produces significant heterogeneous changes in cell properties. The cell projections that form as a result of stimulation (called pseudopodia) are extremely rigid, whereas other regions of the cell may retain the characteristics of a passive cell. In addition, the cell may produce large protrusive or contractile forces. The changes in cellular mechanical properties that result from cellular activation are complex, but are being addressed in computational models of the cell that include cortical dynamics and a multiphase cell interior. Such models have been used to obtain insights into the mechanisms of phagocytosis, and good agreement between model predictions and cell behavior has been demonstrated (Herant et al. 2005, 2006).

21.5 Summary

Constitutive equations that capture the essential features of the responses of red blood cells and passive leukocytes have been formulated, and material parameters characterizing the cellular behavior have been measured. The red cell response is dominated by the cell membrane, which can be described as a hyperviscoelastic, two-dimensional continuum. The passive white cell behaves like a highly viscous fluid drop, and its response to external forces is dominated by the large viscosity of the cytosol. Refinements of these constitutive models and extension of mechanical analysis to activated white cells is anticipated as the ultrastructural events that occur during cellular deformation are delineated in increasing detail.

Definition of Terms

Area expansivity modulus: A measure of the resistance of a membrane to area dilation. It is the proportionality between the isotropic force resultant in the membrane and the corresponding fractional change in membrane area (units: 1 mN/m = 1 dyn/cm = 1000 pN/μm).

Cortical tension: Analogous to surface tension of a liquid drop, it is a persistent contractile force per unit length at the surface of a white blood cell (units: 1 mN/m = 1 dyn/cm).

Cytoplasmic viscosity: A measure of the resistance of the cytosol to flow (units: 1 Pa·s = 10 poise).

Force resultant: The stress in a membrane integrated over the membrane thickness. It is the two-dimensional analog of stress with units of force/length (units: 1 mN/m = 1 dyn/cm = 1000 pN/μm).

Maxwell fluid: A constitutive model in which the response of the material to applied stress includes both an elastic and viscous response in series. In response to a constant applied force, the material will respond elastically at first, then flow. At fixed deformation, the stresses in the material will relax to zero.

Membrane bending modulus: The intrinsic resistance of the membrane to changes in curvature. It is usually construed to exclude nonlocal contributions. It relates the moment resultants (force times length per unit length) in the membrane to the corresponding change in curvature (inverse length) (units: 1 N m = 1 joule = 10^7 erg = 10^{18} pN μm).

Membrane shear modulus: A measure of the elastic resistance of the membrane to surface shear deformation, that is, changes in the shape of the surface at constant surface area (Equation 21.8) (units: 1 mN/m = 1 dyn/cm = 1000 pN/μm).

Membrane viscosity: A measure of the resistance of the membrane to surface shear flow, that is, to the rate of surface shear deformation (Equation 21.8) (units: 1 mN·s/m = 1 mPa·s m = 1 dyn·s/cm = 1 surface poise).

Nonlocal bending resistance: A resistance to bending resulting from the differential expansion and compression of the two adjacent leaflets of a lipid bilayer. It is termed nonlocal because the leaflets can move laterally relative to one another to relieve local strains such that the net resistance to bending depends on the integral of the change in curvature of the entire membrane capsule.

Power law fluid: A model to describe the dependence of the cytoplasmic viscosity on rate of deformation (Equation 21.11).

Principal extension ratios: The ratios of the deformed length and width of a rectangular material element (in principal coordinates) to the undeformed length and width.

Sphericity: A dimensionless ratio of the cell volume (to the 2/3 power) to the cell area. Its value ranges from near zero to one, the maximum value corresponding to a perfect sphere (Equation 21.6).

White cell activation: The response of a leukocyte to external stimuli that involves reorganization and polymerization of the cellular structures and is typically accompanied by changes in cell shape and cell movement.

References

Alberts, B., Johnson, A., Lewis, J., Raff, M., Roberts, K., and Walter, P., 2002. *Molecular Biology of the Cell* Garland Science, New York.

Bagge, U., Skalak, R., and Attefors, R., 1977. Granulocyte rheology, *Adv. Microcirc.* 7, 29–48.

Butler, J., Mohandas, N., and Waugh, R. E., 2008. Integral protein linkage and the bilayer-skeletal separation energy in red blood cells, *Biophys. J.* 95, 1826–1836.

Chien, S., Sung, K. L. P., Skalak, R., and Usami, S., 1978. Theoretical and experimental studies on viscoelastic properties of erythrocyte membrane, *Biophys. J.* 24, 463–487.

Cokelet, G. R. and Meiselman, H. J., 1968. Rheological comparison of hemoglobin solutions and erythrocyte suspensions, *Science* 162, 275–277.

Dao, M., Lim, C. T., and Suresh, S., 2003. Mechanics of the human red blood cell deformed by optical tweezers, *J. Mech. Phys. Solid* 51, 2259–2280.

Diggs, L. W., Sturm, D., and Bell, A., 1985. *The Morphology of Human Blood Cells*. Abbott Laboratories, Abbott Park, IL.

Discher, D. E., Boal, D. H., and Boey, S. K., 1998. Simulations of the erythrocyte cytoskeleton at large deformation. II. Micropipette aspiration, *Biophys. J.* 75, 1584–1597.

Discher, D. E., Mohandas, N., and Evans, E. A., 1994. Molecular maps of red cell deformation: hidden elasticity and *in situ* connectivity, *Science* 266, 1032–1035.

Dong, C. and Skalak, R., 1992. Leukocyte deformability: Finite element modeling of large viscoelastic deformation, *J. Theor. Biol.* 158, 173–193.

Dong, C., Skalak, R., Sung, K. L. P., Schmid-Schonbein, G. W., and Chien, S., 1988. Passive deformation analysis of human leukocytes, *J. Biomech. Eng.* 110, 27–36.

Drury, J. L. and Dembo, M., 2001. Aspiration of human neutrophils: Effects of shear thinning and cortical dissipation, *Biophys. J.* 81, 3166–3177.

Evans, E. and Kukan, B., 1984. Passive material behavior of granulocytes based on large deformation and recovery after deformation tests, *Blood* 64, 1028–1035.

Evans, E. and Yeung, A., 1989. Apparent viscosity and cortical tension of blood granulocytes determined by micropipet aspiration, *Biophys. J.* 56, 151–160.

Evans, E. A., 1983. Bending elastic modulus of red blood cell membrane derived from buckling instability in micropipet aspiration tests, *Biophys. J.* 43, 27–30.

Evans, E. A. and Skalak, R., 1979. Mechanics and thermodynamics of biomembranes, *CRC Crit. Rev. Bioeng.* 3, 181–418.

Evans, E. A. and Waugh, R., 1977. Osmotic correction to elastic area compressibility measurements on red cell membrane, *Biophys. J.* 20, 307–313.

Fedesov, D. A., Caswell, B., and Karniadakis, G. E., 2010. A multiscale red blood cell model with accurate mechanics, rheology and dynamics, *Biophys. J.* 98, 2215–2225.

Fischer, T. M., Haest, C. W. M., Stohr-Liesen, M., Schmid-Schonbein, H., and Skalak, R., 1981. The stress-free shape of the red blood cell membrane, *Biophys. J.* 34, 409–422.

Fung, Y. C., Tsang, W. C. O., and Patitucci, P., 1981. High-resolution data on the geometry of red blood cells, *Biorheol.* 18, 369–385.

Hawkey, C. M., Bennett, P. M., Gascoyne, S. C., Hart, M. G., and Kirkwood, J. K., 1991. Erythrocyte size, number and haemoglobin content in vertebrates, *Br. J. Haematol.* 77, 392–397.

Herant, M., Heinrich, V., and Dembo, M., 2005. Mechanics of neutrophil phagocytosis: Behavior of the cortical tension, *J. Cell Sci.* 118, 1789–1797.

Herant, M., Heinrich, V., and Dembo, M., 2006. Mechanics of neutrophil phagocytosis: Experiments and quantitative models, *J. Cell Sci.* 119, 1903–1913.

Herant, M., Marganski, W. A., and Dembo, M., 2003. The mechanics of neutrophils: Synthetic modeling of three experiments, *Biophys. J.* 84, 3389–3413.

Hochmuth, R. M., Buxbaum, K. L., and Evans, E. A., 1980. Temperature dependence of the viscoelastic properties of red cell membrane, *Biophys. J.* 29, 177–182.

Hochmuth, R. M., Ting-Beall, H. P., Beaty, B. B., Needham, D., and Tran-Son-Tay, R., 1993. Viscosity of passive human neutrophils undergoing small deformations, *Biophys. J.* 64, 1596–1601.

Hochmuth, R. M., Ting-Beal, H. P., and Zhelev, D. V., 1994. The mechanical properties of individual passive neutrophils *in vitro*, in *Physiology and Pathophysiology of Leukocyte Adhesion*, Granger, D. N. and Schmid-Schoenbein, G. W. Oxford University Press, London.

Hwang, W. C. and Waugh, R. E., 1997. Energy of dissociation of lipid bilayer from the membrane skeleton of red blood cells, *Biophys. J.* 72, 2669–2678.

Katnik, C. and Waugh, R., 1990. Alterations of the apparent area expansivity modulus of red blood cell membrane by electric fields, *Biophys. J.* 57, 877–882.

Lew, V. L. and Bookchin, R. M., 1986. Volume, pH and ion content regulationin human red cells: Analysis of transient behavior with an integrated model, *J. Membr. Biol.* 10, 311–330.

Li, J., Dao, M., Lim, C. T., and Suresh, S., 2005. Spectrin-level modeling of the cytoskeleton and optical tweezers stretching of the erythrocyte, *Biophys. J.* 88, 3707–3719.

Markle, D. R., Evans, E. A., and Hochmuth, R. M., 1983. Force relaxation and permanent deformation of erythrocyte membrane, *Biophys. J.* 42, 91–98.

Mohandas, N. and Evans, E. A., 1994. Mechanical properties of the red cell membrane in relation to molecular structure and genetic defects, *Annu. Rev. Biophys. Biomol. Struct.* 23, 787–818.

Needham, D. and Hochmuth, R. M., 1990. Rapid flow of passive neutrophils into a 4 micron pipet and measurement of cytoplasmic viscosity, *J. Biomech. Eng.* 112, 269–276.

Needham, D. and Hochmuth, R. M., 1992. A sensitive measure of surface stress in the resting neutrophil, *Biophys. J.* 61, 1664–1670.

Needham, D. and Nunn, R. S., 1990. Elastic deformation and failure of lipid bilayer membranes containing cholesterol, *Biophys. J.* 58, 997–1009.

Ross, P. D. and Minton, A. P., 1977. Hard quasispherical model for the viscosity of hemoglobin solutions, *Biochem. Biophys. Res. Commun.* 76, 971–976.

Schmid-Schonbein, G. W., Usami, S., Skalak, R., and Chien, S., 1980. The interaction of leukocytes and erythrocytes in capillary and postcapillary vessels, *Microvasc. Res.* 19, 45–70.

Ting-Beall, H. P., Needham, D., and Hochmuth, R. M., 1993. Volume and osmotic properties of human neutrophils., *Blood* 81, 2774–2780.

Ting-Beall, H. P., Zhelev, D. V., and Hochmuth, R. M., 1995. Comparison of different drying procedures for scanning electron microscopy using human leukocytes, *Microsc. Res. Tech.* 32, 357–361.

Tran-Son-Tay, R., Kirk, T. F., 3rd, Zhelev, D. V., and Hochmuth, R. M., 1994. Numerical simulation of the flow of highly viscous drops down a tapered tube, *J. Biomech. Eng.* 116, 172–177.

Tran-Son-Tay, R., Needham, D., Yeung, A., and Hochmuth, R. M., 1991. Time-dependent recovery of passive neutrophils after large deformation, *Biophys. J.* 60, 856–866.

Tsai, M. A., Frank, R. S., and Waugh, R. E., 1993. Passive mechanical behavior of human neutrophils: Power-law fluid, *Biophys. J.* 65, 2078–2088.

Tsai, M. A., Frank, R. S., and Waugh, R. E., 1994. Passive mechanical behavior of human neutrophils: Effect of cytochalasin B, *Biophys. J.* 66, 2166–2172.

Tsai, M. A., Waugh, R. E., and Keng, P. C., 1996a. Cell cycle-dependence of HL-60 cell deformability, *Biophys. J.* 70, 2023–2029.

Tsai, M. A., Waugh, R. E., and Keng, P. C., 1996b. Changes in HL-60 cell deformability during differentiation induced by DMSO, *Biorheol.* 33, 1–15.

Waugh, R. and Evans, E. A., 1979. Thermoelasticity of red blood cell membrane, *Biophys. J.* 26, 115–132.

Waugh, R. E. and Agre, P., 1988. Reductions of erythrocyte membrane viscoelastic coefficients reflect spectrin deficiencies in hereditary spherocytosis, *J. Clin. Invest.* 81, 133–141.

Waugh, R. E. and Marchesi, S. L., 1990. Consequences of structural abnormalities on the mechanical properties of red blood cell membrane, in *Cellular and Molecular Biology of Normal and Abnormal Erythrocyte Membranes*, Cohen, C. M. and Palek, J. UCLA Symposia, Alan R. Liss, New York, NY, pp. 185–199.

Yeung, A. and Evans, E., 1989. Cortical shell-liquid core model for passive flow of liquid-like spherical cells into micropipets, *Biophys. J.* 56, 139–49.

Further Information

The basic information on the mechanical analysis of biomembrane deformation can be found in Evans and Skalak (1979), which also appeared as a book under the same title (CRC Press, Boca Raton, 1980).

A more recent work that focuses more closely on the structural basis of the membrane properties is Evans and Mohandas, 1994. Mechanical properties of the red cell membrane in relation to molecular structure and genetic defects. *Annual Review of Biophysics & Biomolecular Structure* 23: 787–818. We are unaware of more recent reviews of red cell mechanics, and readers are referred to the primary literature.

The basic information about white blood cell biology can be found in the book by Alberts et al. (1989). A more thorough review of white blood cell structure and response to stimulus can be found in two reviews by T. P. Stossel, one titled "The mechanical response of white blood cells," in the book *Inflammation: Basic Principles and Clinical Correlates*, edited by J. I. Galin et al. Raven Press, New York, 1988, pp. 325–342, and the second titled "The molecular basis of white blood cell motility," in the book *The Molecular Basis of Blood Diseases*, edited by G. Stamatoyannopoulos et al., W. B. Saunders, Philadelphia, 1994, pp. 541–562. Additional information about white cell rheology can be found in the book, *Cell Mechanics and Cellular Engineering*, edited by Van C. Mow et al., Springer Verlag, New York, 1994.

22

Mechanics of Tissue/
Lymphatic Transport

22.1 Introduction 22-1
22.2 Basic Concepts of Tissue/Lymphatic Transport 22-2
   Transcapillary Filtration • Starling Pressures and Edema
   Prevention • Interstitial Fluid Transport • Lymphatic
   Architecture • Lymphatic Morphology • Lymphatic Network
   Display • Mechanics of Lymphatic Valves • Lymph Formation and
   Pump Mechanisms • Tissue Mechanical Motion and Lymphatic
   Pumping
22.3 Conclusion 22-12
Defining Terms 22-13
Acknowledgments 22-13
References 22-13
Further Reading 22-17

Geert W.
Schmid-Schönbein
University of California,
San Diego

Alan R. Hargens
University of California,
San Diego

22.1 Introduction

The transport of fluid and metabolites from the blood to the tissue is critically important for maintaining the viability and function of cells within tissues. Similarly, the transport of fluid, biological signaling molecules, microorganisms, and cell disposal products from the tissue to the lymphatic system of vessels and nodes is also crucial to maintain immune surveillance and tissue and organ health. Therefore, it is important to understand the mechanisms for transporting fluid containing micro- and macromolecules or colloidal materials from the blood to the tissue and the drainage of this fluid into the lymphatic system. Because of the abbreviated nature of this chapter, readers are encouraged to consult more complete reviews of blood/tissue/lymphatic transport by Kawai and Ohhashi (2009), Aukland and Reed (1993), Hargens and Akeson (1986), Jain (1987), Lai-Fook (1986), Schmid-Schönbein (1990), Schmid-Schönbein and Zweifach (1994), Staub (1988), Staub et al. (1987), Wei et al. (2003), and Zweifach and Silverberg (1985) and on lymphangiogenesis and its biological and biophysical control factors (Adams and Alitalo, 2007; Swartz and Fleury, 2007; Tammela and Alitalo, 2010). Muthuchamy and Zawieja (2008) have summarized the contractile protein machinery of the lymphatic smooth muscle.

Many previous studies of blood/tissue/lymphatic transport have used isolated organs or whole animals under general anesthesia. Under these conditions, the transport of fluid and metabolites is artificially low in comparison to animals that are actively moving. In some cases, investigators employed passive motion by connecting an animal's limb to a motor to facilitate studies of blood to lymph transport and lymphatic flow. However, new methods and technology allow studies of physiologically active animals so that a better understanding of the importance of transport phenomena in moving tissues is now apparent, especially in the skeletal muscle, skin, and subcutaneous tissue. Therefore, the major focus of this chapter is on the recent developments in the understanding of the mechanics of tissue/lymphatic transport.

The majority of the fluid that is filtered from the microcirculation into the interstitial space is carried out of the tissue via the lymphatic network. This unidirectional transport system originates with a set of blind channels in distal regions of the microcirculation. It carries a variety of interstitial molecules, proteins, metabolites, colloids, and even cells along channels deeply embedded in the tissue parenchyma toward a set of sequential lymph nodes and eventually back into the venous system via the right and left thoracic ducts. The lymphatics are the pathways for immune surveillance and thus, they are one of the important pathways of the immune system (Wei et al., 2003). For example, antigen-presenting dendritic cells, present in small quantities in tissues that are in contact with the external environment (mainly the skin), often acquire foreign antigens. The optimal encounter with naive T cells for presenting these antigens requires that the dendritic cells migrate to draining lymph nodes through lymphatic vessels (Randolph et al., 2005). Their delivery to the lymph nodes depends on the flow into the initial lymphatics (Miteva et al., 2010).

In the following section, we describe basic transport and tissue morphology as related to lymph flow. We also present recent evidence for a two-valve system in lymphatics that offers an updated view of lymph transport.

22.2 Basic Concepts of Tissue/Lymphatic Transport

22.2.1 Transcapillary Filtration

Since lymph is formed from the fluid filtered from the blood, an understanding of transcapillary exchange must be gained first. Usually, pressure parameters favor filtration of the fluid across the capillary wall to the interstitium (J_c) according to the Starling–Landis Equation 22.1:

$$J_c = L_p A[(P_c - P_t) - \sigma_p(\pi_c - \pi_t)] \tag{22.1}$$

where J_c is the net transcapillary fluid transport, L_p is the hydraulic conductivity of the capillary wall, A is the capillary surface area, P_c is the capillary blood pressure, P_t is the interstitial fluid pressure, σ_p is the reflection coefficient for protein, π_c is the capillary blood colloid osmotic pressure, and π_t is the interstitial fluid colloid osmotic pressure.

In the tissue, the fluid transported out of the capillaries is passively carried in the interstitial space via a percolation process around interstitial matrix proteins. According to Darcy's law, the average interstitial fluid velocity

$$q = -(k/\mu) \, \text{grad}(p) \tag{22.2a}$$

where $\text{grad}(p)$ is the pressure gradient, μ is the fluid coefficient of viscosity, and k is an empirical coefficient (it is a tensor in a three-dimensional tissue) whose value depends on the porosity ϕ of the fluid interstitial space. The fluid velocity, v, in the fluid phase around cells and in between solid fibers of the extracellular matrix is related to q by the relation

$$v = q/\phi \tag{22.2b}$$

In the normal tissue (e.g., not swollen), the majority of the fluid that enters the interstitial space is either reabsorbed by the capillary and/or venous vasculature or drained by the initial lymphatic vessels. If all filtered fluid is drained by the lymphatics

$$J_c = J_l \tag{22.3}$$

where J_l is the lymph flow. The fluid flow into the initial lymphatics depends on periodic compression and expansion of the initial lymphatics (microvessels that have a single layer of endothelium with highly specialized cell junctions that form the primary valve system in the lymphatics; see below). The primary valves permit the entry of fluid across the lymphatic endothelium into the initial lymphatics but prevent retrograde flow of fluid back into the interstitial space. Therefore, lymph fluid formation requires that the pressure within the initial lymphatic vessels P_L is lower than the adjacent interstitial fluid pressure P_t for establishing lymph flow:

$$P_t > P_L \tag{22.4}$$

The initial lymphatics have a set of specialized primary valves at the junction between their endothelial cells, so that the fluid can enter if $P_t > P_L$ (which occurs when the initial lymphatic channel expands) but there is no fluid flow when $P_t < P_L$ (when an initial lymphatic vessel is being compressed). The uptake of fluid from the interstitial fluid into the lymphatic channels therefore depends on the periodic mechanical expansion and the expansion of the initial lymphatics and process that is facilitated by a variety of organ-specific intrinsic and extrinsic tissue motions.

Fluid flow inside the lymphatics with Newtonian viscous fluid (which is incompressible at the stresses encountered in the lymphatics) due to low cell concentrations and at low Reynolds number is governed by the Stokes approximation of the equation of motion for incompressible fluid. The fluid is propelled forward by the compression of the initial lymphatics (in the contractile lymphatics by the contraction of the lymphatic smooth muscle), and retrograde flow is prevented by valves.

Each lymphatic compartment (in the initial and the downstream contractile lymphatics) requires a pair of valves to achieve forward flow: one upstream to allow the entry of fluid into the compartment and one downstream to prevent the return of fluid that has been discharged downstream. In the initial lymphatics, the primary valves formed by the endothelial junctions serve as upstream valves, the traditional intraluminal valves serve as secondary downstream valves. In contractile lymphatics, a pair of traditional intraluminal valves, one upstream and one downstream of each lymph compartment ("lymphangion"), serve to provide unidirectional flow toward the lymph nodes.

22.2.2 Starling Pressures and Edema Prevention

Hydrostatic and colloid osmotic pressures within the blood and interstitial fluid primarily govern transcapillary fluid shifts (Figure 22.1). Although input arterial pressure averages about 100 mm Hg at the heart level, capillary blood pressure P_c is significantly reduced due to resistance R, according to the Poiseuille Equation 22.4

$$R = \frac{8\,\eta l}{\pi r^4} \tag{22.5}$$

where η is the blood viscosity, l is the vessel length between feed artery and capillary, and r is the radius.

Therefore, normally at the heart level, P_c is approximately 30 mm Hg. However, during upright posture, P_c at the foot level is about 90 mm Hg and only about 25 mm Hg at the head level (Parazynski et al., 1991). The differences in P_c between capillaries of the head and feet are due to gravitational variation of the blood pressure such that the pressure $p = \rho g h$. Although myogenic vasoconstriction decreases local capillary pressure below the heart level, volumes of transcapillary filtration and lymph flows are generally higher in tissues of the lower body as compared to those of the upper body. Moreover, one might expect much more sparse distribution of lymphatic vessels in the upper body tissues. The brain has no lymphatics, but most other vascular tissues have lymphatics. In fact, tissues of the lower body of humans and other tall animals have efficient skeletal muscle pumps, prominent lymphatic systems, and noncompliant skin and fascial boundaries to prevent dependent edema (Hargens et al., 1987).

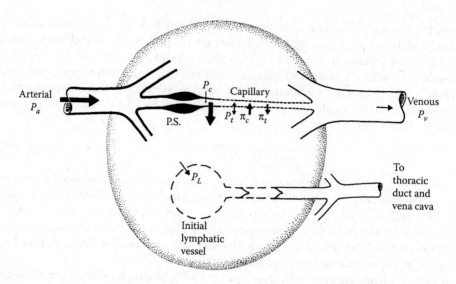

FIGURE 22.1 Starling pressures that regulate transcapillary fluid balance. The pressure parameters that determine the direction and the magnitude of transcapillary exchange include capillary blood pressure P_c, interstitial fluid pressure P_t (directed into the capillary when positive or directed into the tissue when negative), plasma colloidal osmotic pressure π_c, and interstitial fluid colloidal osmotic pressure π_t. Precapillary sphincters (PS) regulate P_c, capillary flow, and capillary surface area A. It is generally agreed that a hydrostatic pressure gradient (P_t > lymph pressure P_l) drains off excess interstitial fluid under conditions of net filtration. The relative magnitudes of pressures are depicted by the size of arrows. (From Hargens AR. 1986. *Handbook of Bioengineering*, vol. 19, pp. 1–35, New York, McGraw-Hill. With permission.)

Other pressure parameters in the Starling–Landis Equation 22.1 such as P_t, π_c, and π_t are not as sensitive to changes in body posture as is P_c. The typical values for P_t range from −2 to 10 mm Hg depending on the tissue or organ under investigation (Wiig, 1990). However, during movement, P_t in the skeletal muscle increases to 150 mm Hg or higher (Murthy et al., 1994), providing a mechanism to promote lymphatic flow and venous return via the skeletal pump (Figure 22.2). Blood colloid osmotic pressure π_c usually ranges between 25 and 35 mm Hg and is the other major force for retaining plasma within the vascular system and preventing edema. Interstitial π_t depends on the reflection coefficient of the capillary wall (σ_p ranges from 0.5 to 0.9 for different tissues) as well as washout of interstitial proteins during high filtration rates (Aukland and Reed, 1993). Typically, π_t ranges between 8 and 15 mm Hg with higher values in the upper body tissues compared to those in the lower body (Aukland and Reed, 1993; Parazynski et al., 1991). Precapillary sphincter activity (see Figure 22.1) also decreases blood flow, decreases capillary filtration area A, and reduces P_c in dependent tissues of the body to help prevent edema during upright posture (Aratow et al., 1991).

The conventional view of Starling's principle should be reconsidered in light of the role of glycocalyx as the semipermeable layer of endothelium. The low rate of transcapillary filtration and lymph formation in many tissues is explained by standing plasma protein gradients within the intercellular cleft of continuous capillaries (glycocalyx model) and around fenestrations (Levick and Michel, 2010). Narrow breaks in the junctional strands of the cleft create high local outward fluid velocities, which may cause a disequilibrium between the subglycocalyx space π and π_t. The recent review of interstitial–lymph transport by Levick and Michel (2010) suggests that the effect of π_t on the filtration of fluid from the capillary to the interstitium (J_c) is less than that predicted by the conventional Starling equation. Hu and Weinbaum (1999) introduced a new analysis of the fluid flow through endothelial gaps by proposing that the glycocalyx serves as the primary molecular sieve required to maintain colloid osmotic pressures. They predict lower filtration rates than predicted by the traditional Starling model.

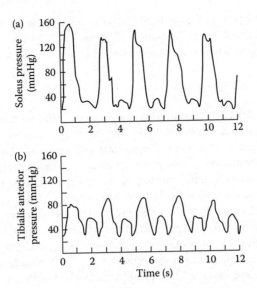

FIGURE 22.2 Simultaneous intramuscular pressure oscillations in the soleus (a) and the tibialis anterior (b) muscles during plantar- and dorsiflexion exercise. Soleus muscle is an integral part of the calf muscle pump. (From Murthy G et al. 1994. *J Appl Physiol* 76:2742. Modified with permission.)

22.2.3 Interstitial Fluid Transport

Interstitial flow of proteins and other macromolecules occurs by two mechanisms: diffusion and convection. During simple diffusion according to Fick's Equation 22.5

$$J_p = -D \frac{\partial c_p}{\partial x} \tag{21.6}$$

where J_p is the one-dimensional protein flux, D is the diffusion coefficient, and $\partial cp/\partial x$ is the concentration gradient of protein through the interstitial space.

For most macromolecules such as proteins, the diffusional transport is limited. It serves to disperse molecules, but it does not effectively serve to transport large molecules, especially if their diffusion is restricted by interstitial matrix proteins, membrane barriers, or other structures that limit their free thermal motion. Instead, both experimental and theoretical evidence highlights the dependence of volume and solute flows on hydrostatic and osmotic pressure gradients (Hammel, 1994; Hargens and Akeson, 1986) and suggests that convective flow plays the dominating role in interstitial flow and transport of nutrients to tissue cells. For example, in the presence of osmotic or hydrostatic pressure gradients, protein transport J_p is coupled to fluid transport according to

$$J_p = \overline{c}_p J_v \tag{22.7}$$

where $\overline{c}_p$ is the average protein concentration and J_v is the volume flow of fluid.

The transport of interstitial fluid toward the lymphatics requires convective flow since it depends on relatively few channels in the interstitium. Diffusion cannot serve such a purpose because diffusion merely disperses fluid and proteins. Lymph formation and flow greatly depend upon tissue movement or activity related to muscle contraction and tissue deformations. It is also generally agreed that the formation of the initial lymph depends solely on the composition of nearby interstitial fluid and pressure gradients across the interstitial/lymphatic boundary (Hargens, 1986; Zweifach and Lipowsky, 1984). For this reason, lymph formation and flow can be quantified by measuring the disappearance of isotope-labeled albumin from subcutaneous tissue or skeletal muscle (Reed et al., 1985).

22.2.4 Lymphatic Architecture

To understand lymph transport in engineering terms, it is paramount that we develop a detailed picture of the lymphatic network topology and vessel morphology. This task is facilitated by a number of morphological and ultrastructural studies from past decades that give a general picture of the morphology and location of lymphatic vessels in different tissues. Lymphatics are studied by injections of macroscopic and microscopic contrast media and by light and electron microscopic sections. The display of the lymphatics is organ specific and there are many variations in lymphatic architecture (Schmid-Schönbein, 1990). In this chapter, we will focus our discussion predominantly on skeletal muscle, intestine, and skin. However, the mechanisms outlined below may in part be also relevant to other tissues and organs.

In the skeletal muscle, lymphatics are positioned in the *immediate* proximity of the arterioles. The majority of feeder arteries in the skeletal muscle and most, but not all, of the arcade arterioles are closely accompanied by a lymphatic vessel (Figure 22.3). Lymphatics can be traced along the entire length of the arcade arterioles, but they can be traced only over relatively short distances (less than about 50 μm) into the side branches of the arcades, the transverse (terminal) arterioles that supply the blood into the capillary network. Systematic reconstructions of the lymphatics in skeletal muscle have yielded little evidence for lymphatic channels that enter into the capillary network per se (Skalak et al., 1984). Thus, the network density of lymphatics is quite low compared to the high density of the capillary network in muscle, a characteristic feature of lymphatics in most organs (Skalak et al., 1986). The close association between lymphatics and vasculature is also present in the skin (Ikomi and Schmid-Schönbein, 1995) and in other organs, and may extend into the central vasculature. Saharinen et al. (2004) reviewed lymphatic vasculature development and molecular regulation in tumor metastasis and inflammation. It is

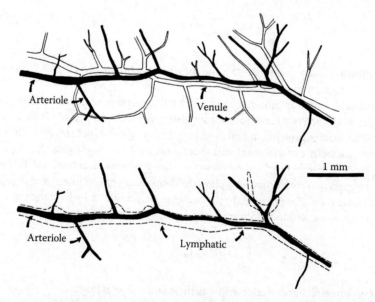

FIGURE 22.3 Tracing of a typical lymphatic channel (bottom panel) in rat spinotrapezius muscle after injection with a micropipette of a carbon contrast suspension. All lymphatics are of the initial type and are closely associated with the arcade arterioles. Few lymphatics follow the path of the arcade venules, or their side branches, the collecting venules, or the transverse arterioles. (With kind permission from Springer Science+Business Media: *Tissue Nutrition and Viability*, Lymph transport in skeletal muscle, 1986, pp. 243–262, Skalak TC, Schmid-Schönbein GW, and Zweifach BW.)

apparent that the current understandings of lymphatic growth factors and strategies to limit lymphatic vessel growth may allow the manipulation of lymphatic growth in disease.

Interstitial fluid flow is itself a major determinant of the growth of lymphatic vessels and their directionality (Boardman and Swartz, 2003; Ng et al., 2004). This consideration is important in the design of tissue engineering approaches for lymphatic vessels (Helm et al., 2007).

22.2.5 Lymphatic Morphology

Histological sections of the lymphatics permit its classification into two distinct subsets: *initial* lymphatics and *collecting* lymphatics. The initial lymphatics (sometimes also denoted as terminal or capillary lymphatics) form a set of blind endings in the tissue that feed into the collecting lymphatics, and that in turn, are the conduits into the lymph nodes. While both initial and collecting lymphatics are lined by a highly attenuated endothelium, only the collecting lymphatics have smooth muscle in their media. In accordance, contractile lymphatics exhibit spontaneous narrowing of their lumen, while there is no evidence for contractility (in the sense of a smooth muscle contraction) in the initial lymphatics. Contractile lymphatics are capable of peristaltic smooth muscle contractions that in conjunction with periodic opening and closing of the intraluminal valves permit unidirectional fluid transport. The lymphatic smooth muscle has adrenergic innervation (Ohhashi et al., 1982), it exhibits myogenic contraction (Hargens and Zweifach, 1977; Mizuno et al., 1997), and it reacts with a variety of vasoactive stimuli (Ohhashi et al., 1978; Benoit, 1997), including signals that involve nitric oxide (Bohlen and Lash, 1992; Ohhashi and Takahashi, 1991; Yokoyama and Ohhashi, 1993). Recently, Kawai and Ohhashi (2009) and Zawieja (2009) reviewed the important intrinsic pump function of the collecting lymphatics with a specialized set of contractile proteins in the smooth muscle.

The lymphatic endothelium has a number of similarities with vascular endothelium. It forms a continuous lining and has typical cytoskeletal fibers such as microtubules, intermediate fibers, and actin in both fiber bundle form and matrix form. There are numerous caveolae, Weibel-Palade bodies, but lymphatic endothelium has fewer interendothelial adhesion complexes and a discontinuous basement membrane. The residues of the basement membrane are attached to interstitial collagen via anchoring filaments (Leak and Burke, 1968) that provide relatively firm attachment of the endothelium to interstitial structures.

22.2.6 Lymphatic Network Display

One of the interesting aspects regarding lymphatic transport in skeletal muscle is the fact that all lymphatics *inside* the muscle parenchyma are of the noncontractile, *initial* type (Skalak et al., 1984). The *collecting* lymphatics can only be observed outside the muscle fibers as conduits to adjacent lymph nodes. The fact that all lymphatics inside the tissue parenchyma are of the initial type is not unique to skeletal muscle, but has been demonstrated in other organs (Unthank and Bohlen, 1988; Yamanaka et al., 1995). The initial lymphatics are positioned in the adventitia of the arcade arterioles surrounded by collagen fibers (Figure 22.4). In this position, they are in immediate proximity to the arteriolar smooth muscle, and adjacent to myelinated nerve fibers and a set of mast cells that accompany the arterioles. The initial lymphatics are frequently sandwiched between arteriolar smooth muscle and their paired venules, and they in turn are embedded between the skeletal muscle fibers (Skalak et al., 1984). The initial lymphatics are firmly attached to the adjacent basement membrane and collagen fibers via anchoring filaments (Leak and Burke, 1968). The basement membrane of the lymphatic endothelium is discontinuous, especially at the interendothelial junctions, so that macromolecules and even cells and particles enter the initial lymphatics (Bach and Lewis, 1973; Bollinger et al., 1981; Casley-Smith, 1962; Ikomi et al., 1996; Strand and Persson, 1979).

The lumen cross section of the initial lymphatics is highly irregular in contrast to the overall circular cross section of the collecting lymphatics (Figure 22.4). The lumen cross section of the initial lymphatics

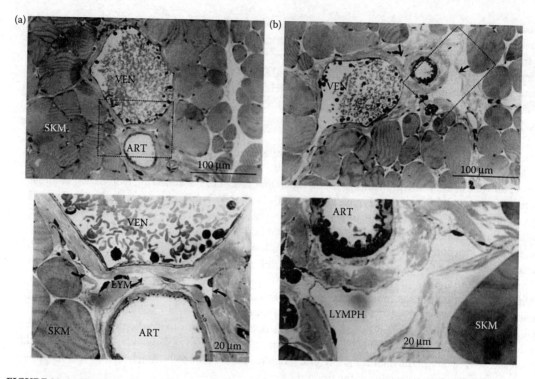

FIGURE 22.4 Histological cross sections of lymphatics (LYM) in rat skeletal muscle before (a) and after (b) contraction of the paired arcade arterioles (ART). The lymphatic channel is of the initial type with a single attenuated endothelial layer (curved arrows). Note that in the dilated arteriole, the lymphatic is essentially compressed (a) whereas the lymphatic is expanded after arteriolar contraction (b) that is noticeable by the folded endothelial cells in the arteriolar lumen. In both cases, the lumen cross-sectional shape of the initial lymphatic channels is highly irregular. All lymphatics in the skeletal muscle have these characteristic features. (Adapted from Skalak TC, Schmid-Schönbein GW, and Zweifach BW. 1984. *Microvasc Res* 28: 95.)

is partially or completely collapsed and may frequently span around the arcade arteriole. In fact, we have documented cases in which the arcade arteriole is completely surrounded by an initial lymphatic channel, highlighting the fact that the activity of the lymphatics is closely linked to that of the arterioles (Ikomi and Schmid-Schönbein, 1995).

Direct labeling of lymphatic and vascular endothelium shows that there exist numerous direct vascular connections between lymphatic and microvascular endothelial vessels with membrane contacts but no detectable fluid exchange between the two systems (Robichaux et al., 2010).

22.2.6.1 Intraluminal (Secondary) Lymphatic Valves

The initial lymphatics in the skeletal muscle have intraluminal valves that consist of bileaflets and a funnel structure (Mazzoni et al., 1987). The leaflets are flexible structures and are opened and closed by a viscous pressure drop along the valve funnel. In the closed position, these leaflets can support considerable pressures (Eisenhoffer et al., 1995; Ikomi et al., 1997). This arrangement preserves normal valve function even in the initial lymphatics with irregularly shaped lumen cross sections.

22.2.6.2 Primary Lymphatic Valves

The lymphatic endothelial cells are attenuated and have many of the morphological characteristics of vascular endothelium, including expression of P-selectin, von Willebrand factor (Di Nucci et al., 1996), and factor VIII (Schmid-Schönbein, 1990). The identity of the lymphatic endothelium involves the transcription factor PROX1 (Johnson et al., 2008). An important difference between vascular and lymphatic endothelium lies in the arrangement of the endothelial junctions. In the initial lymphatics, the endothelial cells lack tight junctions (Schneeberger and Lynch, 1984) and are frequently encountered in an overlapping but open position, so that proteins, large macromolecules, and even chylomicron particles can readily pass through the junctions (Casley-Smith, 1962, 1964; Leak, 1970). Examination of the junctions with scanning electron microscopy shows that there exists a periodic *interdigitating* arrangement of endothelial extensions. Individual extensions are attached via anchoring filaments to the underlying basement membrane and connective tissue, but the two extensions of adjacent endothelial cells resting on top of each other are not attached by interendothelial adhesion complexes. Mild mechanical stretching of the initial lymphatics shows that the endothelial extensions can be separated in part from each other, indicating that the membranes of two neighboring lymphatic endothelial cells are not attached to each other, but are firmly attached to the underlying basement membrane (Castenholz, 1984). Lymphatic endothelium does not exhibit continuous junctional complexes, and instead has a "streak and dot"-like immunostaining pattern of VE-cadherin and associated intracellular proteins desmoplakin and plakoglobulin (Schmelz et al., 1994). VE-cadherin and platelet endothelial cell adhesion molecule (PECAM-1) form an interlaced labeling pattern with minimal overlap, in contrast to vascular endothelium (Baluk et al., 2007; Murfee et al., 2007). But the staining pattern is nonuniform along the initial lymphatics; in larger lymphatics, a more continuous pattern is present. This highly specialized arrangement has been referred to as the *lymphatic endothelial microvalves* (Schmid-Schönbein, 1990) or primary lymphatic valves. They are *"primary"* because fluid from the interstitium must first pass across these valves before entering the lymphatic lumen and then pass across the intraluminal, that is, secondary valves. The particles deposited into the interstitial space adjacent to the initial lymphatics pass across the endothelium of the initial lymphatics. However, once the particles are inside the initial lymphatic lumen, they cannot return back into the interstitial space unless the endothelium is injured. Indeed, the endothelial junctions of the initial lymphatics serve as a functional valve system (Trzewik et al. 2001). Similar to vascular endothelium, the lymphatic endothelial junctions also serve as a signaling mechanism as reviewed by Dejana et al. (2009).

22.2.7 Mechanics of Lymphatic Valves

In contrast to the central large valves in the heart that are closed by inertial fluid forces, the lymphatic valves are small and the fluid Reynolds number is almost zero. Thus, because no inertial forces are available to open and close these valves, a different valve morphology has evolved in these small valves. The valves form long funnel-shaped channels that are inserted into the lymph conduits and attached at their base. The funnel is prevented from inversion by attachment via a buttress to the lymphatic wall. The valve wall structure consists of a collagen layer sandwiched between two endothelial layers and the entire structure is quite deformable under mild physiological fluid pressures. The funnel structure allows a *viscous pressure gradient* that is sufficient to generate a pressure drop during forward fluid motion to open, and upon flow reversal to close the valves (Mazzoni et al., 1987). The primary lymphatic valves also open as passive structures at the peripheral endothelial cell extensions. They require sites where they are free to bend into the lumen of the initial lymphatics and where they are *not* attached by anchoring filaments to the adjacent extracellular matrix (Mendoza and Schmid-Schönbein, 2003).

22.2.8 Lymph Formation and Pump Mechanisms

One of the important questions fundamental to lymphology is: How do fluid and large particles in the interstitium find their way into the initial lymphatics? In light of the relative sparse existence of the initial lymphatics, a directed convective transport is required that can be provided by either a hydrostatic or a colloid osmotic pressure drop (Zweifach and Silberberg, 1979). However, the exact mechanism of this unidirectional flow has remained an elusive target. Several proposals have been advanced and these are discussed in detail in Schmid-Schönbein (1990). Briefly, a number of authors have postulated that there exists a constant pressure drop from the interstitium into the initial lymph, which may support a steady fluid flow into the lymphatics. But repeated measurements with different techniques have uniformly failed to provide supporting evidence for a *steady* pressure drop to transport fluid into the initial lymphatics (Clough and Smaje, 1978; Zweifach and Prather, 1975). Under steady-state conditions, no steady pressure drop exists in the vicinity of the initial lymphatics in skeletal muscle within the resolution of the measurement technique (about 0.2 cm H_2O) (Skalak et al., 1984). An order of magnitude estimate of the pressure drop expected at the relatively slow flow rates of the lymphatics shows, however, that the pressure drop from the interstitium may be significantly lower (Schmid-Schönbein, 1990). Furthermore, the assumption of a *steady* pressure drop is not in agreement with the substantial evidence that lymph flow rate is enhanced under unsteady conditions (see below). Some investigators have postulated an osmotic pressure in the lymphatics to aspirate fluid into the initial lymphatics (Casley-Smith, 1972) due to ultrafiltration across the lymphatic endothelium, a mechanism referred to as "bootstrap effect" (Perl, 1975). Critical tests of this hypothesis, such as the microinjection of hyperosmotic protein solutions, have not led to a uniformly accepted hypothesis for lymph formation involving an osmotic mechanism. Others have suggested a retrograde aspiration mechanism, such that the recoil in the collecting lymphatics serves to lower the pressure in the initial lymphatics upstream of the collecting lymphatics (Reddy, 1986; Reddy and Patel, 1995), or an electric charge difference across the lymphatic endothelium (O'Morchoe et al., 1984).

22.2.9 Tissue Mechanical Motion and Lymphatic Pumping

An intriguing feature is that lymphatic flow rates depend on tissue motion. In a resting tissue, the lymph flow rate is relatively small. But different forms of tissue motion serve to enhance lymph flow. This was originally demonstrated for pulsatile pressures in the rabbit ear. Perfusion of the ear with steady pressure (even at the same mean pressure) stops lymph transport, whereas pulsatile pressures promote lymph transport (Parsons and McMaster, 1938). In light of the paired arrangement of the arterioles and lymphatics, periodic expansion of the arterioles compresses adjacent lymphatics, and vice versa, a reduction of arteriolar diameter during the pressure reduction phase expands adjacent lymphatics (Skalak et al., 1984) (Figure 22.4). Vasomotion, associated with a slower contraction of the arterioles, but with a larger amplitude than pulsatile pressure, increases lymph formation (Colantuoni et al., 1984; Intaglietta and Gross, 1982). In addition, muscle contractions, simple walking (Olszewski and Engeset, 1980), respiration, intestinal peristalsis, skin compression (Ohhashi et al., 1991), and other tissue motions are associated with increased lymph flow rates. Periodic tissue motions are significantly more effective to enhance the lymph flow than elevation of the venous pressure (Ikomi et al., 1996), which is also associated with enhanced fluid filtration (Renkin et al., 1977).

A requirement for lymph fluid flow is the periodic expansion and compression of the initial lymphatics. Since the initial lymphatics do not have their own smooth muscle, the expansion and compression of the initial lymphatics depends on the motion of the tissue in which they are embedded. In skeletal muscle, the strategic location of the initial lymphatics in the adventitia of the arterioles provides the milieu for expansion and compression via several mechanisms: arteriolar pressure pulsations or vasomotion, active or passive skeletal muscle contractions, or external muscle compression. Direct measurements of the cross-sectional area of the initial lymphatics during arteriolar contractions or during skeletal muscle shortening support this hypothesis (Mazzoni et al., 1990; Skalak et al., 1984) (Figure 22.5). The different lymph pump mechanisms are additive. The resting skeletal muscle has much lower lymph flow rates (provided largely by the arteriolar pressure pulsation and vasomotion) than the skeletal muscle during exercise (produced by a combination of intramuscular pressure pulsations and skeletal muscle shortening) (Ballard et al., 1998).

Measurements of lymph flow rates in an afferent lymph vessel (diameter of about 300–500 μm, proximal to the popliteal node) in the hind leg (Ikomi and Schmid-Schönbein, 1996) demonstrate that lymph fluid formation is influenced by passive or active motion of the surrounding tissue. Lymphatics in this tissue region drain the muscle and skin of the hind leg, and the majority is of the *initial* type,

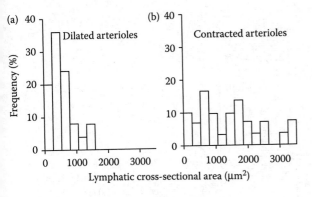
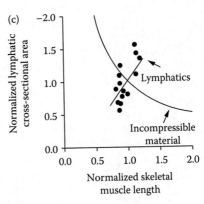

FIGURE 22.5 Histograms of initial lymphatic cross-sectional area in rat spinotrapezius muscle before (a) and after (b) contraction of the paired arteriole with norepinephrine. Lymphatic cross-sectional area as a function of muscle length during active contraction or passive stretch (c). Cross-sectional area and muscle length are normalized with respect to the values *in vivo* in resting muscle. Note the expansion of the initial lymphatics with contraction of the arterioles or muscle stretch. (Adapted from Skalak TC, Schmid-Schönbein GW, and Zweifach BW. 1984. *Microvasc Res* 28: 95; Mazzoni MC, Skalak TC, and Schmid-Schönbein GW. 1990. *Am J Physiol* 259: H1860.)

whereas the collecting lymphatics are detected outside the tissue parenchyma in the fascia proximal to the node. Without whole leg rotation, lymph flow remains at low but nonzero values. If the pulse pressure is stopped, lymph flow falls to values below detectable limits (less than about 10% of the values during pulse pressure). The introduction of whole leg passive movement causes strong, frequency-dependent lymph flow rates that increase linearly with the logarithm of frequency between 0.03 and 1.0 Hz (Figure 22.6). The elevation of venous pressure, which enhances fluid filtration from the vasculature and elevates flow rates, does not significantly alter the dependency of lymph flow on periodic tissue motion (Ikomi et al., 1996).

Similarly, the application of passive tissue compression on the skin elevates the lymph flow rate in a frequency-dependent manner. Lymph flow rates are determined to a significant degree by the *local* action of the lymph pump because the arrest of the heartbeat and the reduction of the central blood pressure to zero do not stop lymph flow. Instead, cardiac arrest reduces lymph flow rate only about 50% during continued leg motion or application of periodic shear stress to the skin for several hours (Ikomi and Schmid-Schönbein, 1996). Periodic compression of the initial lymphatics also enhances proteins and lymphocyte counts in the lymphatics (Ikomi et al., 1996) (Figure 22.7). Thus, either arteriolar smooth muscle or parenchymal skeletal muscle activity expands and compresses the initial lymphatics in skeletal muscle. These mechanisms serve to adjust lymph flow rates according to organ activity such that a resting skeletal muscle has a very low lymph flow rate. During normal daily activity or mild or strenuous exercise, lymph flow rates as well as protein and cell transport into the lymphatics increases (Olszewski et al., 1977).

22.2.9.1 Lymph Pump Mechanism with Primary and Secondary Valves

Regular expansion and compression of the initial lymphatic channels requires a set of valves to achieve unidirectional flow. Such valves open and close with each expansion and compression of the lymphatics to permit entry at the upstream end of the lymphatics and discharge downstream toward the lymph nodes. There is a cycle of valve opening and closing with every expansion and compression of the lymphatic channels. During expansion, the upstream primary lymphatics are open and permit entry of interstitial fluid. The secondary valves are closed to prevent retrograde flow along the lymphatic channels. During compression, the primary valves are closed, whereas the secondary valves are open to permit discharge along the lymphatic channels into the contractile lymphatics and toward the lymph nodes.

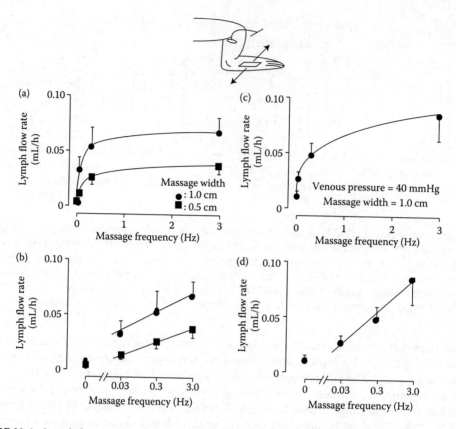

FIGURE 22.6 Lymph flow rates in a prenodal afferent lymphatic draining the hind leg as a function of the frequency of a periodic surface shear motion (massage) without (panels a, b) and with (panels c, d) elevation of the venous pressure by placement of a cuff. Zero frequency refers to a resting leg with a lymph flow rate that depends on pulse pressure. The amplitudes of the tangential skin shear motion were 1 and 0.5 cm (panels a, b) and 1 cm in the presence of the elevated venous pressure (panels c, d). Note that the ordinates in panels c and d are larger than those in panels a and b. (Adapted from Ikomi and Schmid-Schönbein, 1996. *Am J Physiol* 271: H173.)

Thus, we view lymphatic transport as having a robust mechanism that requires the presence of two-valve systems. In fact, all compartments that rely on a repeated cycle of expansion and compression require two-valve systems, the lymphangions along the contractile lymphatics, and even larger structures such as the ventricles of the heart, the blower in the fireplace, or even the shipping locks in the Panama Canal. None of these structures can provide unidirectional transport if one of the valves is removed, irrespective of whether it is located upstream or downstream (Schmid-Schönbein, 2003). In inflammation, the primary lymphatic valves may fail due to apoptosis of the lymphatic endothelium (Lynch et al., 2007). This leads to the failure of the fluid transport into the initial lymphatics and into contractile lymphatics (Zawieja, 1996), eventually forming tissue edema and possibly amplifying the inflammatory process. The strategies to control tissue edema formation need to take into consideration the delicate primary lymphatic endothelium and its specialized junctions by preventing their failure or restoring their function after failure.

22.3 Conclusion

The lymphatic vessels are a unique transport system that is present even in primitive physiological systems. These vessels carry out a multitude of functions, many of which have yet to be discovered.

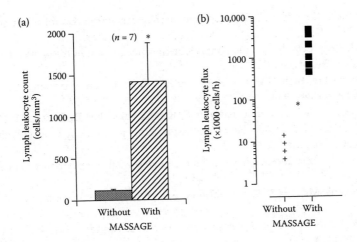

FIGURE 22.7 Lymph leukocyte count (a) and leukocyte flux (b) before and after application of periodic hind leg skin shear motion (massage) at a frequency of about 1 Hz and amplitude of 1 cm. The flux rates were computed from the product of lymph flow rates and the lymphocyte counts. *Statistically significant different from the case without massage. (Adapted from Ikomi and Schmid-Schönbein, 1996. *Am J Physiol* 271: H173.)

Lymphatics have a two-valve system: a primary valve system at the level of the lymphatic endothelium and a secondary valve system in the lumen of the lymphatics, facilitating unidirectional transport toward the lymphatic nodes and thoracic duct. The details of lymphatic growth kinetics are subject to initial molecular analysis designed to identify key growth factors and their molecular control (Lohela et al., 2003). A more detailed bioengineering analysis, especially at the molecular level (Jeltsch et al., 1997), is a fruitful area for future exploration.

Defining Terms

Capillary: The smallest blood vessel of the body that provides oxygen and other nutrients to nearby cells and tissues.

Colloid osmotic pressure: A negative pressure that depends on protein concentration (mainly of albumin and globulins) and prevents excess filtration across the capillary wall.

Edema: Excess fluid or swelling within a given tissue.

Interstitium: The space between cells of various tissues of the body. Normally fluid and proteins within this space are transported from the capillary to the initial lymphatic vessel.

Lymphatic system: The clear network of vessels that return excess fluid and proteins to the blood via the thoracic duct.

Acknowledgments

This work was supported by NASA grants NNX10AM18G and NNX09AP11G as well as NIH grants HL 10881.

References

Adams RH and Alitalo K. 2007. Molecular regulation of angiogenesis and lymphangiogenesis. *Nat Rev Mol Cell Biol* 8: 464–478.

Aratow M, Hargens AR, Meyer J-U et al. 1991. Postural responses of head and foot cutaneous microvascular flow and their sensitivity to bed rest. *Aviat Space Environ Med* 62: 246.

Aukland K and Reed RK. 1993. Interstitial–lymphatic mechanisms in the control of extracellular fluid volume. *Physiol Rev* 73: 1.

Bach C and Lewis GP. 1973. Lymph flow and lymph protein concentration in the skin and muscle of the rabbit hind limb. *J Physiol (Lond)* 235: 477.

Ballard RE, Watenpaugh DE, Breit GA et al. 1998. Leg intramuscular pressures during locomotion in humans. *J Appl Physiol* 84: 1976.

Baluk P, Fuxe J, Hashizume H, Romano T, Lashnits E, Butz S, Vestweber D, Corada M, Molendini C, Dejana E, and McDonald DM. 2007. Functionally specialized junctions between endothelial cells of lymphatic vessels. *J Exp Med* 204: 2349–2362.

Benoit JN. 1997. Effects of alpha-adrenergic stimuli on mesenteric collecting lymphatics in the rat. *Am J Physiol* 273: R331.

Boardman KC and Swartz MA. 2003. Interstitial flow as a guide for lymphangiogenesis. *Circ Res* 92: 801–808.

Bohlen HG and Lash JM. 1992. Intestinal lymphatic vessels release endothelial-dependent vasodilators. *Am J Physiol* 262: H813.

Bollinger A, Jäger K, Sgier F et al. 1981. Fluorescence microlymphography. *Circulation* 64: 1195.

Casley-Smith JR. 1962. The identification of chylomicra and lipoproteins in tissue sections and their passage into jejunal lacteals. *J Cell Biol* 15: 259.

Casley-Smith JR. 1964. Endothelial permeability—The passage of particles into and out of diaphragmatic lymphatics. *Quart J Exp Physiol* 49: 365.

Casley-Smith JR. 1972. The role of the endothelial intercellular junctions in the functioning of the initial lymphatics. *Angiologica* 9: 106.

Castenholz A. 1984. Morphological characteristics of initial lymphatics in the tongue as shown by scanning electron microscopy. *Scanning Electr Microsc* 1984: 1343.

Clough G and Smaje LH. 1978. Simultaneous measurement of pressure in the interstitium and the terminal lymphatics of the cat mesentery. *J Physiol (Lond)* 283: 457.

Colantuoni A, Bertuglia S, and Intaglietta M. 1984. A quantification of rhythmic diameter changes in arterial microcirculation. *Am J Physiol* 246: H508.

Dejana E, Orsenigo F, Molendini C, Baluk P, and McDonald DM. 2009. Organization and signaling of endothelial cell-to-cell junctions in various regions of the blood and lymphatic vascular trees. *Cell Tissue Res* 335: 17–25.

Di Nucci A, Marchetti C, Serafini S et al. 1996. P-selectin and von Willebrand factor in bovine mesenteric lymphatics: An immunofluorescent study. *Lymphology* 29: 25.

Eisenhoffer J, Kagal A, Klein T et al. 1995. Importance of valves and lymphangion contractions in determining pressure gradients in isolated lymphatics exposed to elevations in outflow pressure. *Microvasc Res* 49: 97.

Hammel HT. 1994. How solutes alter water in aqueous solutions. *J Phys Chem* 98: 4196.

Hargens AR. 1986. Interstitial fluid pressure and lymph flow. In: R Skalak, S Chien (eds.), *Handbook of Bioengineering*, 19: pp. 1–35, New York, McGraw-Hill.

Hargens AR and Akeson WH. 1986. Stress effects on tissue nutrition and viability. In: AR Hargens (ed.), *Tissue Nutrition and Viability*, pp. 1–24, New York, Springer-Verlag.

Hargens AR, Millard RW, Pettersson K et al. 1987. Gravitational haemodynamics and oedema prevention in the giraffe. *Nature* 329: 59.

Hargens AR and Zweifach BW. 1977. Contractile stimuli in collecting lymph vessels. *Am J Physiol* 233: H57.

Helm CL, Zisch A, and Swartz MA. 2007. Engineered blood and lymphatic capillaries in 3-D VEGF-fibrin-collagen matrices with interstitial flow. *Biotechnol Bioeng* 96: 167–176.

Hu X and Weinbaum S. 1999. A new view of Starling's hypothesis at the microstructural level. *Microvasc Res* 58: 281–304.

Ikomi F, Hunt J, Hanna G et al. 1996. Interstitial fluid, protein, colloid and leukocyte uptake into interstitial lymphatics. *J Appl Physiol* 81: 2060.

Ikomi F and Schmid-Schönbein GW. 1995. Lymph transport in the skin. *Clin Dermatol* 13(5): 419.

Ikomi F and Schmid-Schönbein GW. 1996. Lymph pump mechanics in the rabbit hind leg. *Am J Physiol* 271: H173.

Ikomi F, Zweifach BW, and Schmid-Schönbein GW. 1997. Fluid pressures in the rabbit popliteal afferent lymphatics during passive tissue motion. *Lymphology* 30: 13.

Intaglietta M and Gross JF. 1982. Vasomotion, tissue fluid flow and the formation of lymph. *Int J Microcirc Clin Exp* 1: 55.

Jain RK. 1987. Transport of molecules in the tumor interstitium: A review. *Cancer Res* 47: 3039.

Jeltsch M, Kaipainen A, Joukov V et al. 1997. Hyperplasia of lymphatic vessels in VEGF-C transgenic mice. *Science* 276: 1423.

Johnson NC, Dillard ME, Baluk P, McDonald DM, Harvey NL, Frase SL, and Oliver G. 2008. Lymphatic endothelial cell identity is reversible and its maintenance requires Prox1 activity. *Genes Dev* 22: 3282–3291.

Kawai Y and Ohhashi T. 2009. Topics of physiological and pathophysiological functions of lymphatics. *Curr Mol Med* 9(8): 942.

Lai-Fook SJ. 1986. Mechanics of lung fluid balance. *Crit Rev Biomed Eng* 13: 171.

Leak LV. 1970. Electron microscopic observations on lymphatic capillaries and the structural components of the connective tissue–lymph interface. *Microvasc Res* 2: 361.

Leak LV and Burke JF. 1968. Ultrastructural studies on the lymphatic anchoring filaments. *J Cell Biol* 36: 129.

Levick JR and Michel CC. 2010. Microvascular fluid exchange and the revised Starling principle. *Cardiovasc Res* 87(2): 198–210.

Lohela M, Saaristo A, Veikkola T, and Alitalo K. 2003. Lymphangiogenic growth factors, receptors and therapies. *Thromb Haemost* 90: 167–184.

Lynch PM, DeLano FA, and Schmid-Schönbein GW. 2007. The primary valves in the initial lymphatics during inflammation. *Lymphat Res Biol* 5: 3–10.

Mazzoni MC, Skalak TC, and Schmid-Schönbein GW. 1987. The structure of lymphatic valves in the spinotrapezius muscle of the rat. *Blood Vessels* 24: 304.

Mazzoni MC, Skalak TC, and Schmid-Schönbein GW. 1990. The effect of skeletal muscle fiber deformation on lymphatic volume. *Am J Physiol* 259: H1860.

Mendoza E and Schmid-Schönbein GW. 2003. A model for mechanics of primary lymphatic valves. *J Biomech Eng* 125: 407–413.

Miteva DO, Rutkowski JM, Dixon JB, Kilarski W, Shields JD, and Swartz MA. 2010. Transmural flow modulates cell and fluid transport functions of lymphatic endothelium. *Circ Res* 106: 920–931.

Mizuno R, Dornyei G, Koller A et al. 1997. Myogenic responses of isolated lymphatics: Modulation by endothelium. *Microcirculation* 4: 413.

Murfee WL, Rappleye JW, Ceballos M, and Schmid-Schönbein GW. 2007. Discontinuous expression of endothelial cell adhesion molecules along initial lymphatic vessels in mesentery: The primary valve structure. *Lymphat Res Biol* 5: 81–90.

Murthy G, Watenpaugh DE, Ballard RE et al. 1994. Supine exercise during lower body negative pressure effectively simulates upright exercise in normal gravity. *J Appl Physiol* 76: 2742.

Muthuchamy M and Zawieja D. 2008. Molecular regulation of lymphatic contractility. *Ann N Y Acad Sci* 1131: 89–99.

Ng CP, Helm CL, and Swartz MA. 2004. Interstitial flow differentially stimulates blood and lymphatic endothelial cell morphogenesis *in vitro*. *Microvasc Res* 68: 258–264.

Ohhashi T, Kawai Y, and Azuma T. 1978. The response of lymphatic smooth muscles to vasoactive substances. *Plügers Arch* 375: 183.

Ohhashi T, Kobayashi S, Tsukahara S et al. 1982. Innervation of bovine mesenteric lymphatics: From the histochemical point of view. *Microvasc Res* 24: 377.

Ohhashi T and Takahashi N. 1991. Acetylcholine-induced release of endothelium-derived relaxing factor from lymphatic endothelial cells. *Am J Physiol* 260: H1172.

Ohhashi T, Yokoyama S, and Ikomi F. 1991. Effects of vibratory stimulation and mechanical massage on micro- and lymph-circulation in the acupuncture points between the paw pads of anesthetized dogs. In: H Niimi, FY Zhuang (eds.), *Recent Advances in Cardiovascular Diseases*, pp. 125–133, National Cardiovascular Center, Osaka.

Olszewski WL and Engeset A. 1980. Intrinsic contractility of prenodal lymph vessels and lymph flow in human leg. *Am J Physiol* 239: H775.

Olszewski WL, Engeset A, Jaeger PM et al. 1977. Flow and composition of leg lymph in normal men during venous stasis, muscular activity and local hyperthermia. *Acta Physiol Scand* 99: 149.

O'Morchoe CCC, Jones WRI, Jarosz HM et al. 1984. Temperature dependence of protein transport across lymphatic endothelium *in vitro*. *J Cell Biol* 98: 629.

Parazynski SE, Hargens AR, Tucker B et al. 1991. Transcapillary fluid shifts in tissues of the head and neck during and after simulated microgravity. *J Appl Physiol* 71: 2469.

Parsons RJ and McMaster PD. 1938. The effect of the pulse upon the formation and flow of lymph. *J Exp Med* 68: 353.

Perl W. 1975. Convection and permeation of albumin between plasma and interstitium. *Microvasc Res* 10: 83.

Randolph GJ, Angeli V, and Swartz MA. 2005. Dendritic-cell trafficking to lymph nodes through lymphatic vessels. *Nat Rev Immunol* 5(8): 617.

Reddy NP. 1986. Lymph circulation: Physiology, pharmacology, and biomechanics. *Crit Rev Biomed Sci* 14: 45.

Reddy NP and Patel K. 1995. A mathematical model of flow through the terminal lymphatics. *Med Eng Phy* 17: 134.

Reed RK, Johansen S, and Noddeland H. 1985. Turnover rate of interstitial albumin in rat skin and skeletal muscle. Effects of limb movements and motor activity. *Acta Physiol Scand* 125: 711.

Renkin EM, Joyner WL, Sloop CH et al. 1977. Influence of venous pressure on plasma–lymph transport in the dog's paw: Convective and dissipative mechanisms. *Microvasc Res* 14: 191.

Robichaux JL, Tannol E, Rappleye JW, CeballosM, Schmid-Schönbein GW, and Murfee WL. 2010. Lymphatic/blood endothelial cell connections at the capillary level in the adult rat mesentery. *Anat Rec* 293: 1629–1638.

Saharinen P, Tammela T, Karkkainen MJ, and Alitalo K. 2004. Lymphatic vasculature: Development, molecular regulation and role in tumor metastasis and inflammation. *Trends Immunol* 25: 387.

Schmelz M, Moll R, Kuhn C et al. 1994. Complex adherentes, a new group of desmoplakin-containing junctions in endothelial cells: II. Different types of lymphatic vessels. *Differentiation* 57: 97.

Schmid-Schönbein GW. 1990. Microlymphatics and lymph flow. *Physiol Rev* 70: 987.

Schmid-Schönbein GW. 2003. The second valve system in lymphatics. *Lymphat Res Biol* 1: 25–31.

Schmid-Schönbein GW and Zweifach BW. 1994. Fluid pump mechanisms in initial lymphatics. *News Physiol Sci* 9: 67.

Schneeberger EE and Lynch RD. 1984. Tight junctions: Their structure, composition and function. *Circ Res* 5: 723.

Skalak TC, Schmid-Schönbein GW, and Zweifach BW. 1984. New morphological evidence for a mechanism of lymph formation in skeletal muscle. *Microvasc Res* 28: 95.

Skalak TC, Schmid-Schönbein GW, and Zweifach BW. 1986. Lymph transport in skeletal muscle. In: AR Hargens (ed.), *Tissue Nutrition and Viability*, pp. 243–262, Springer-Verlag, New York.

Staub NC. 1988. New concepts about the pathophysiology of pulmonary edema. *J Thorac Imaging* 3: 8.

Staub NC, Hogg JC, and Hargens AR. 1987. *Interstitial-Lymphatic Liquid and Solute Movement*, pp. 1–290, Basel, Karger.

Strand S-E and Persson BRR. 1979. Quantitative lymphoscintigraphy I: Basic concepts for optimal uptake of radiocolloids in the parasternal lymph nodes of rabbits. *J Nucl Med* 20: 1038.

Swartz MA and Fleury ME. 2007. Interstitial flow and its effects in soft tissues. *Annu Rev Biomed Eng* 9: 229–256.

Tammela T and Alitalo K. 2010. Lymphangiogenesis: Molecular mechanisms and future promise. *Cell* 140: 460–476.

Trzewik J, Mallipattu, SR, Artmann, GM et al. 2001. Evidence for a second valve system in lymphatics: Endothelial microvalves. *FASEB J* 15: 1711.

Unthank JL and Bohlen HG. 1988. Lymphatic pathways and role of valves in lymph propulsion from small intestine. *Am J Physiol* 254: G389.

Wei SH, Parker I, Miller MJ, and Cahalan MD. 2003. A stochastic view of lymphocyte motility and trafficking within the lymph node. *Immunol Rev* 195: 136.

Wiig H. 1990. Evaluation of methodologies for measurement of interstitial fluid pressure (P_i): Physiological implications of recent P_i data. *Crit Rev Biomed Eng* 18: 27.

Yamanaka Y, Araki K, and Ogata T. 1995. Three-dimensional organization of lymphatics in the dog small intestine: A scanning electron microscopic study on corrosion casts. *Arch Hist Cyt* 58: 465.

Yokoyama S and Ohhashi T. 1993. Effects of acetylcholine on spontaneous contractions in isolated bovine mesenteric lymphatics. *Am J Physiol* 264: H1460.

Zawieja DC. 1996. Lymphatic microcirculation. *Microcirculation* 3: 241–243.

Zawieja DC. 2009. Contractile physiology of lymphatics. *Lymphat Res Biol* 7(2): 87–96.

Zweifach BW and Lipowsky HH. 1984. Pressure-flow relations in blood and lymph microcirculation. In: E Renkin and C Michel (eds), *Handbook of Physiology: The Cardiovascular System: Microcirculation*, sec 2, vol. 4, pt 1, pp. 251–307, Bethesda, MD, American Physiological Society.

Zweifach BW and Prather JW. 1975. Micromanipulation of pressure in terminal lymphatics of the mesentary. *J Appl Physiol* 228: 1326.

Zweifach BW and Silberberg A. 1979. The interstitial–lymphatic flow system. In: AC Guyton, DB Young (eds.), *International Review of Physiology—Cardiovascular Physiology III*, pp. 215–260, University Park Press, Baltimore.

Zweifach BW and Silverberg A. 1985. The interstitial–lymphatic flow system. In: MG Johnston, CC Michel (eds.), *Experimental Biology of the Lymphatic Circulation*, pp. 45–79, Elsevier, Amsterdam.

Further Reading

Drinker, C.K. and J.M. Yoffey. 1941. *Lymphatics, Lymph and Lymphoid Tissue: Their Physiological and Clinical Significance.* Harvard University Press, Cambridge, Massachusetts. This is a classic treatment of the lymphatic circulation by two pioneers in the field of lymphatic physiology.

Yoffey, J.M. and F.C. Courtice. 1970. *Lymphatics, Lymph and the Lymphomyeloid Complex.* Academic Press, London, New York. This is a classic book in the field of lymphatic physiology. The book contains a comprehensive review of pertinent literature and experimental physiology on the lymphatic system.

23

Modeling in Cellular Biomechanics

23.1 Introduction 23-1
23.2 Mechanical Properties of the Cell..23-2
    Constitutive Relations • Interpretation of Experiments • Properties
    of Cellular Components
23.3 Cell Motility...23-6
    Cell Spreading and Interaction with the Extracellular Matrix • Cell
    Rolling and Adhesion • Cell Crawling • Cell Swimming and
    Gliding
23.4 Mechano-, Mechanoelectrical, and Electromechanical
    Transduction 23-13
    Mechanotransduction • Mechanoelectrical Transduction,
    Mechanosensitive Channels, and Electromechanical Transduction
23.5 Modeling Cells in Disease 23-15
    Cancer • Malaria • Nuclear Envelope Deficiency
Acknowledgments...23-17
References...23-17
Further Information..23-22

Alexander A.
Spector
Johns Hopkins University

Roger Tran-Son-Tay
University of Florida

23.1 Introduction

Mechanical forces, stresses, strains, and velocities play a critical role in many important aspects of cell physiology, such as adhesion, motility, and signal transduction. Cellular mechanics is now considered an important indicator of pathological conditions, including the state of the disease (e.g., Diez-Silva et al., 2010).

The modeling of cellular mechanics is a challenging task because of the interconnection of mechanical, electrical, and biochemical processes; involvement of different structural cellular components; and multiple timescales. It can involve nonlinear mechanics and thermodynamics, and because of its complexity, it will most likely require the use of computational techniques. Typical requirements in the development of cell models include the constitutive relations describing the state or evolution of the cell and its components, mathematical solution or transformation of the corresponding equations and boundary conditions, and computational implementation of the model.

Modeling is a powerful tool in the simulation of the processes in cells dealing with different temporal and spatial scales. It is effective in the interpretation and design of experiments, as well as in the prediction of new effects and phenomena. It is clear that modeling will play an increased role in improving our understanding of complex cell biology and physiology, under both normal and pathological conditions, and, ultimately, in helping in the treatment of various diseases (Bao and Suresh, 2003; Heidemann and Wirtz, 2004; Kamm and Mofrad, 2006; Discher et al., 2009).

In this chapter, we focus on several important features of cell behavior and cell modeling where cell mechanics plays a crucial role. They include constitutive relationships for the cell and its components (cytoskeleton, nucleus, cellular membrane) and their applications to major experiments to probe cellular mechanical properties. We also consider cell spreading, adhesion, and interaction with the extracellular matrix (ECM). We discuss various forms of cell motility, such as rolling, crawling, swimming, and gliding. Then, we review several forms of mechanotransduction in cells. Finally, we discuss the latest results on the modeling of cells in disease and consider important examples of cancer, malaria, and nuclear envelope deficiency. Some areas where mechanics also plays an important role, such as cell growth and division, are left for further reading.

23.2 Mechanical Properties of the Cell

23.2.1 Constitutive Relations

The basis of the modeling of cell mechanics is the relationships between the applied (internal) forces (stresses) and the corresponding strains or velocities. Under appropriate timescales, cells can be treated as elastic. In this case, the stresses can be expressed in terms of strains (displacement gradients). If a cell undergoes large deformation under physiological or experimental conditions, such as red blood cells (RBCs) in narrow capillaries or cells in the micropipette aspiration experiment (Evans and Skalak, 1980), the corresponding equations become nonlinear. If a cell and the applied forces are such that cellular properties are direction-independent, then the cell can be considered as isotropic. If the properties of the cell or its components are different depending on the direction (e.g., the cylindrical cochlear outer hair cell is softer in the longitudinal direction), then the cell is considered as anisotropic. Cells can acquire anisotropy as a result of structural rearrangements in response to application of certain stimuli (e.g., cytoskeletal reorganization in endothelial cells in response to exposure to blood-related shear stresses or cyclic stretches of the blood vessel). To simulate various time-dependent processes in cells, viscoelastic (viscous) models are used. Although most of the earlier work on cell rheology were focused on RBCs, knowledge of the rheological properties of white blood cells (WBCs) or leukocytes is also important in the comprehension of microcirculation flow dynamics. There are strong evidences (Tran-Son-Tay et al., 1991) that WBCs exhibit behavior similar to liquid drops. However, it is known that they cannot be modeled as simple Newtonian drops because the apparent viscosity of the cells changes with the rate and the extent of deformation. Kan et al. (1999b), using a three-layer model, were able to explain the inconsistencies reported in the literature. In their model, the outer layer is the cortical region surrounding the second layer (cytoplasm), and the third layer is the nucleus. They found that to understand the rheological behavior of WBCs, it is essential to have information on the deformation of the nucleus. Assigning apparent viscosity to cells can be misleading without accounting for the shape of the cell/nucleus under deformation, and can lead to incorrect estimates of the WBC material properties. For example, Kan et al. (1998) found that a compound drop (cell) behaves like a homogeneous simple liquid drop only if the core (nucleus) is sufficiently deformed and the timescale of the core, related to the combination of its viscosity and capillarity, is comparable to that of the shell layer (membrane). In other words, the apparent viscosity depends not only on the rheological properties of the cell but also on the flow dynamics surrounding it. Unless the presence and possible deformation of the nucleus are explicitly accounted for, neither Newtonian nor non-Newtonian models can adequately predict the hydrodynamics of WBCs.

Yamada et al. (2000) developed a method of laser tracking particles embedded in the cytoskeletal components inside living cells. The authors applied this method to measuring the complex modulus of the cellular content within a broad frequency range, and they showed that the frequency dependence of the modulus is close to a power law.

Previously, a number of experiments on adherent cells were interpreted from the standpoint of Maxwell, Voight, and standard linear solid models. More recently, a viscoelastic model with a weak-power dependence of the complex modulus on the frequency (strain rate) was proposed (e.g., Fabry et al., 2001; Lenormand et al., 2007). Like in the engineering structural damping model, the loss tangent in this model is independent of frequency but the weak-power behavior transforms into frequency-linear (fluid-type) behavior for higher frequencies (shorter timescales). The parameters of the power law model have been shown to be applicable to a variety of cells within several orders of the frequency magnitude. It was, however, lately noticed that for slow cellular processes, such as cell differentiation or apoptosis (very low frequencies), the power law changes: thus, there are timescales that are characterized by different power law parameters (Stamenovic et al., 2007).

Purely elastic or viscoelastic models treat the cellular material as a single phase. While the cell has several components, its content can be treated as a biphasic medium where one (solid) phase is associated with the cytoskeleton, and the other (fluid) is related to the cytoplasm. This approach can be further developed to include more phases important to the cell behavior, such as triphasic (solid–fluid–ion) models of cell mechanics (Guilak et al., 2006).

Long molecules that compose the cellular cytoskeleton can be treated from the standpoint of polymer mechanics where the response of the material to the application of a force is associated with changes in entropy (transition from disorder to more order). The cytoskeleton fiber are considered either as chains of segments that are completely free to move in three directions (freely joined chain model) or as flexible slender rods (worm-like chain model).

Similar constitutive relations have been developed for cellular components, such as the cytoskeleton and nucleus. Modeling the cell membrane has the main distinct feature because it has to be treated as an intrinsically two-dimensional (2-D) continuum.

23.2.2 Interpretation of Experiments

There are several major techniques that are used to extract the mechanical properties of cells. The models and experiments are interconnected: the experiments provide free parameters for the models, and, in turn, the models are the basis for the interpretation of the experiments. One of the most common techniques is micropipette aspiration, where a pipette is sealed on the surface of a cell, negative pressure is applied inside the pipette, and a portion of the cell is aspirated inside the pipette (Hochmuth, 2000 for review). The height of the aspirated portion of the cell can be considered as an inverse measure of cell stiffness. The same technique is used to observe the time response of the cell, and in this case, the corresponding relaxation time(s) is a measure of the cell's viscoelastic properties. The experiment with micropipette aspiration of an RBC was interpreted by considering the cell membrane (including the cytoskeleton) as a nonlinear (neo-Hookean) elastic half-space characterized by two parameters, an area expansion modulus and shear modulus. Earlier continuum models of the RBC membrane were summarized in the monograph by Evans and Skalak (1980). Later, Discher et al. (1998) developed an analysis of the micropipette aspiration by considering the RBC cytoskeleton as a polymer network. Each RBC cytoskeletal spectrin was treated as a worm-like chain, and the state of the whole network inside the micropipette was determined by a Monte Carlo simulation (Figure 23.1).

Theret et al. (1988) analyzed the micropipette experiment with endothelial cells. The cell was interpreted as a linear elastic incompressible isotropic half-space, and the pipette was considered as an axisymmetric rigid punch. This approach was later extended (Sato et al., 1990) to consider the cell as a linear viscoelastic incompressible material obeying the standard linear solid model. Haider and Guilak (2002) have applied an axisymmetric boundary integral model to estimate elastic parameters of chondrocytes, assuming the cell to have the shape of a finite sphere. Baaijens et al. (2005) have applied the finite element method to analyze the micropipette aspiration experiment with chondrocytes by assuming them to be nonlinear viscoelastic and biphasic. Zhou et al. (2005) have developed a finite element analysis of the micropipette experiment in the case of large viscoelastic deformations where the cell was treated as a standard neo-Hookean viscoelastic solid. Spector et al. (1998) analyzed the application of the micropipette to a cylindrical cochlear outer hair cell. The cell composite membrane

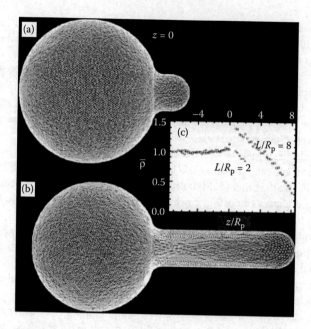

FIGURE 23.1 Simulation of the micropipette aspiration of the red blood cell cytoskeletal network for different ratios, (a) and (b), of the aspiration length, L, to the radius of the pipette, R_p. (c) The profiles of the network element density along the z-axis of the pipette. (From Discher, D.E., Boal, D.H., and Boey, S.K. *Biophys. J.*, 75, 1584, 1998. With permission.)

(wall) was treated as an orthotropic elastic shell, and the corresponding problem was solved by using the Fourier series.

Another technique widely used in the estimation of the properties of cells is atomic force microscopy, where the sample is probed by a rigid tip located at the end of a cantilever of a prescribed stiffness, and the displacement of the tip is tracked with a laser. The cell/tip contact force versus cell deflection characterizes the cell (cellular components) mechanical properties. A traditional interpretation of this experiment is based on the Hertz theory of frictionless contact of a rigid tip with an elastic isotropic half-space (e.g., Radmacher et al., 1996). Mahaffy et al. (2004) have refined this interpretation by interpreting the cell (fibroblast) as a layer of a finite thickness with two types of boundary conditions between the bottom of the cell and the substrate, full slip or full adhesion. The authors applied this approach to capture different properties of different parts of the fibroblast, including the cell's thickest central part as well as thinner areas of the lamellipodia. Unnikrishnan et al. (2007) have used a numerical finite element method to interpret the atomic force microscopy (AFM)-obtained measurements of cellular micromechanical properties.

Magnetocytometry is also a popular method for the characterization of cellular mechanical properties. In this method, a magnetic bead specifically coated to adhere to a targeted area is perturbed by a magnetic field. The properties of the cell are extracted by using the resulting force or torque versus the displacement or rotation angle of the bead. Wang and Ingber (1994) used this technique to analyze how the viscoelastic properties of the cytoskeleton of endothelial cells are controlled by cell shape and the cell's interaction with the ECM. Mijailovich et al. (2002) have developed a finite element interpretation of the experiment. Karcher et al. (2003) considered a bead under the action of a magnetic force on the surface of a cellular monolayer. On the basis of a linear viscoelastic model and finite element solution, the authors found the force/displacement relationship for the bead.

Many methods measure the mechanical properties of cells using probes in contact with the plasma membrane as opposed to probes placed within the cytoplasm. Therefore, these methods assess apparent mechanical properties that are dominated by the cortical cytoskeleton, which is enriched in acto-myosin stress fibers. In contrast, particle tracking microrheology probes the viscoelastic properties of the intracellular milieu by probing the spontaneous displacements of nanoparticles lodged in the cytoplasm of living cells (Wirtz, 2009). This approach allows probing the local, frequency-dependent viscoelastic moduli of cells by analyzing the mean-squared displacements of the cytoplasm-embedded nanoparticles (Tseng et al., 2002).

Other techniques used to probe cellular mechanical properties include laser/optical tweezers, deformation by two plates, and application of shear flow in the microchamber (Van Vilet et al., 2003; Janmey and Schmidt, 2006; Suresh, 2007 for review).

23.2.3 Properties of Cellular Components

There are a number of different approaches to the modeling of the cellular cytoskeleton. The continuum constitutive relations include viscoelastic monophasic, multiphasic, and polymer models (Mofrad et al., 2006). There are also structural models of the cytoskeleton, including an important one that is based on the concept of tensegrity, where the structure is supported by a system of prestressed components balanced by another system whose components are under compression. Ingber (1993, 2003a,b) have proposed to apply this concept to the mechanics of adherent cells, where the prestress is associated with the contractile machinery of actin fibers, and it is balanced by compression in microtubules and traction forces at cellular adhesions. This concept was incorporated into a computational model and applied to the prediction of the rheological behavior of living cells (Sultan et al., 2004). Another example of structural models of the cytoskeleton is the foam-like model proposed by Satcher and Dewey (1996) that was applied to the estimation of the elastic properties of endothelial cell's cytoskeleton. Some cells have naturally anisotropic cytoskeleton; Spector et al. (2001) have considered the 2-D cylindrical cytoskeleton of the cochlear outer hair cell and estimated its anisotropic properties. Fletcher and Mullins (2010) recently reviewed cell mechanics focusing on how the cell cytoskeleton generate, transmit, and respond to mechanical signals for short and long timescales.

The mechanical properties of the nucleus, the stiffest component of the cell, are important for those of the cell as a whole. Also, the mechanotransduction pathway connecting the adhesion sites, the cytoskeleton, and the nucleus results in the alteration of gene expression and protein synthesis. Recently, Lee et al. (2007) and Hale et al. (2008) showed that the molecular interconnections between the nuclear envelope and the cytoskeleton mediated by linkers of nucleus and cytoskeleton (linker nucleoskeleton and cytoskeleton (LINC) complexes) play a critical role in cytoplasmic rheology.

Guilak et al. (2000) have probed the nuclear properties by using the micropipette aspiration experiment and its interpretation on the basis of the standard linear viscoelastic model. Dahl et al. (2005) applied atomic force microscopy and found weak-power law viscoelastic relationships for the nuclear mechanics. Caille et al. (2002) have used two-plate compression of endothelial cells and interpreted the nucleus and cytoplasm as two different hyperelastic materials. Tseng et al. (2004) have applied the particle nanotracking method to estimate the viscoelastic properties of cellular nuclei. A direct force transduction can contribute to the adhesion–cytoskeleton–nucleus mechanotransduction pathway (Maniotis et al., 1997; Thomas et al., 2002). It has also been discovered that there is a mechanism of the cytoskeletal modulation of nuclear shape. In this regard, Jean et al. (2005) have developed a model of force transmission through the cytoskeleton to the nucleus that resulted from endothelial cell rounding. Cell rounding was caused by the alteration of cell adhesion via the application of trypsin. A review of the nuclear mechanics and methods was recently published by Lammerding et al. (2007).

The starting point of modeling cellular membranes is constitutive relations in 2-D space. Some cellular membranes (e.g., the RBC membrane), where the plasma membrane is attached to the underlying 2-D cytoskeleton, can be treated as elastic or viscoelastic solids (Evans and Skalak, 1980). The constitutive relations for the RBC can include bending because this mode of deformation is important to this cell's shape under physiological and experimental conditions (Evans, 1974, 1980). Pure plasma membrane has to be considered as a special liquid whose primary properties are tension and bending.

Helfrich (1973) has proposed energy functional as a function of membrane curvature and its original (spontaneous) curvature. In axisymmetric cases, the Euler–Lagrange equation for the bending energy functional can be explicitly derived in the form of nonlinear fourth-order ordinary differential equation (ODE) and solved by the finite difference method (e.g., Derenyi et al., 2002; Powers et al., 2002; Lim and Huber, 2009). Alternatively, Feng and Klug (2006) have developed a finite element method to directly minimize the bending energy functional. Atilgan and Sun (2007) have developed a coarse-grain triangular element model to analyze membranes and membranes with embedded proteins and found equilibrium states by using the Monte Carlo method. From the standpoint of general continuum mechanics, Steigmann (1999) has shown that the liquid membrane strain energy functional (function) is determined by curvatures and local area compressibility. In many cases, liquid membranes are considered as fully incompressible, and the area preservation condition is introduced via a Lagrange multiplier. Membrane tethers (narrow tubes) are a general phenomenon in liquid membranes. Such tethers can form naturally for cell–cell communication or for the slowing down of moving cells (such as leukocytes). Pulling membrane tethers is also an effective method to probe the local membrane properties. An approach based on thermodynamic balance of the tether system was previously applied to estimate the membrane bending modulus, membrane–cytoskeleton adhesion energy, and tension (e.g., Waugh and Hochmuth, 1987; Bozic et al., 1992; Dai and Sheetz, 1999). The details of the shape of a narrow tether are often unavailable in light microscopy. Alternatively, membrane shape in the whole tether region can be computed from the analysis of the equilibrium (steady-state deformation) of the tether. Calladine and Greenwood (2002) have proposed a version of the shell theory to determine the shape of the membrane in the tether region. Schumacher et al. (2009) have extended this approach and modeled tether shape in different cells, taking into account particular arrangement of bonds between the membrane and the cytoskeleton near the tether.

23.3 Cell Motility

Cell motility refers to the ability of a cell to move spontaneously and actively. All cell movements are a manifestation of mechanical work; they require a fuel (ATP) and proteins that convert the energy stored in ATP into motion. The cytoskeleton plays a critical role in cell motility. It can undergo constant rearrangement, which can produce movements. There are several types of cell motility and some of them are reviewed below.

23.3.1 Cell Spreading and Interaction with the Extracellular Matrix

When a cell is in contact with a proper substrate, it deforms and spreads onto the surface, and this action is called cell spreading. The cell spreading involves many events such as intracellular signaling, reorganization of cytoskeleton, and bond formation among adhesion molecules. In the later stages of cell spreading, actin polymerization pushes the cell membrane outward, making the cell more flattened. Actin polymerization and depolymerization are also responsible for the protrusion and the contraction of lamellipodium in cell crawling.

As an investigation of the early stages of cell spreading, which are considered as a rather passive process, Cuvelier et al. (2007) measured the contact radius with time using reflection interference microscopy for various combinations of cell and substrate types. They observed a universal power law behavior regardless of the experimental conditions, and to explain the behavior, they proposed a model in which a cell is modeled as a viscous adhesive cortical shell enclosing a less viscous interior. They concluded that the cell spreading is limited by its mesoscopic structure and material properties.

Cell spreading (shape), adhesion, and traction force generation as a result of cell interaction with the ECM are critically important for intracellular signaling, cell cycle, and cell fate under normal conditions and in disease. The same factors can determine the lineage commitment of stem cells (Engler et al., 2006; Guilak et al., 2009). Out of the factors determining stem cell lineage commitment, the stiffness of the substrate (ECM) plays an important role. While the physics of this phenomenon has not been fully understood, Walcott and Sun (2010) and Zemel et al. (2010) recently proposed models of this mechanism and related the substrate stiffness to the contractile (traction) forces generated by the cell cytoskeleton. It has also been noticed that the cell interaction with 2-D surfaces (including stem cells) can be quite different from that with three-dimensional (3-D) extracellular matrices (Cukierman et al., 2001; Fraley et al., 2010). Li et al. (2010) proposed a cell spreading model that includes molecular mechanisms of actin polymerization and integrin binding between cell and ECM, and predicted the change of contact radius with time. Their results agree well with experimental data, and confirmed the general power law behavior observed by Cuvelier et al. (2007). Their model also enables the examination of the effects of ECM stiffness and bond density on the cell spreading. Sun et al. (2009) proposed a continuum model of cell spreading in which specific interaction, long-range recruiting interaction, and diffusion of binders are included. The specific interactions between receptors on cell membrane and ligands on substrate surface are described by a chemical reaction equation, and long-range recruiting interactions are simplified by a traction-separation law. Their model identified different stages of cell spreading mediated by different mechanisms. Using a model of evolution of stress fibers and its finite element implementation, McGarry et al. (2009) have simulated the traction forces generated by cells, including fibroblast and mesenchymal stem cells, spread over a system of elastic microposts. Pathak et al. (2008) applied a similar approach to the simulation of cell spreading over a surface micropatterned with ligand-coated patches. Sengers et al. (2007) have presented a review of computational modeling of cell spreading and tissue regeneration in porous scaffolds. Dallon et al. (1999) have developed a model of cells interacting with the ECM where the cells were modeled as discrete objects and the matrix was modeled as a continuum. Using computational simulation, the authors considered the effects of changing cellular properties on fiber alignment.

23.3.2 Cell Rolling and Adhesion

Cell rolling can be described as a decrease in the velocity of cells (occurring only with leukocytes) in preparation to adhere to an endothelial wall. It is an essential part of a larger process of the immune system, which allows leukocytes to travel and bind to trauma-induced tissues. A factor that influences the effectiveness of rolling is cell velocity. As leukocyte velocity decreases (slow rolling), the chance of adhesion rises. Another contributing factor to this phenomenon is time. Leukocytes are viscoelastic bodies, which means that they are susceptible to deformation when a given force is applied over a specific time. As this interval grows, the shape of the leukocyte changes even more, causing an increase in the contact area of the cell. As the contact area increases, so does its chance of adhesion.

As noted earlier, there is much evidence to support the statement that rolling is an absolute prerequisite to leukocyte adhesion. Although this is certainly true for muscle and skin tissue, this is not conclusive for all tissues. The liver, lung, and heart are examples where rolling may not be necessary for leukocyte recruitment. In the lung's alveolar capillaries and the liver's sinusoids, rolling is not observed because the volume of each is extremely small, which allows for adhesion to occur straight from tethering.

The recent cell adhesion paradigm has been developed to emphasize the role of kinetics. Conceptualized by Bell (1978) and refined by several authors (Hammer and Lauffenburger, 1987; Dembo et al., 1988), the reaction kinetics approach integrates the adhesive interaction of the cells with the surface into the adhesion mechanism. Several physicochemical properties can affect the adhesion of a cell, such as rates of reaction, affinity, mechanical elasticity, kinetic response to stress, and length of adhesion molecules.

Several models have been proposed for describing the interaction of the leukocyte with the endothelium cells. Mathematical models of cell rolling/adhesion can be classified into two classes based on equilibrium (Evans, 1985; Alon et al., 1995) and kinetics concepts (Dembo et al., 1988; Alon et al., 1998; Kan et al., 1999a). The kinetic approach is more capable of handling the dynamics of cell adhesion and rolling. In this approach, the formation and dissociation of bonds occur according to the reverse and forward rate constants.

Using this concept, Hammer and Lauffenburger (1987) studied the effect of external flow on cell adhesion. The cell is modeled as a solid sphere, and the receptors at the surface of the sphere are assumed to diffuse and to convect into the contact area. The main finding is that the adhesion parameters, such as the reverse and forward reaction rates and the receptor number, have a strong influence on the peeling of the cell from the substrate.

Dembo et al. (1988) developed a model based on the ideas of Evans (1985) and Bell (1978). In this model, a piece of membrane is attached to the wall, and a pulling force is exerted on one end while the other end is held fixed. The cell membrane is modeled as a thin inextensible membrane. The model of Dembo et al. (1988) was subsequently extended via a probabilistic approach for the formation of bonds by Cozens-Roberts et al. (1990). Other authors used the probabilistic approach and Monte Carlo simulation to study the adhesion process as reviewed by Zhu (2000). Dembo's model has also been extended to account for the distribution of microvilli on the surface of the cell and to stimulate the rolling and the adhesion of a cell on a surface under shear flow. Hammer and Apte (1992) modeled the cell as a microvilli-coated hard sphere covered with adhesive springs. The binding and breakage of bonds and the distribution of the receptors on the tips of the microvilli are computed using a probabilistic approach.

To take into account the cell deformability, which has shown to be necessary for calculating the magnitude of the adhesion force, Dong and Lei (2000) have modeled the cell as a liquid drop encapsulated into an elastic ring. They show how the deformability and the adhesion parameters affect the leukocyte and adhesion process in shear flow. However, only a small portion of the adhesion length is allowed to peel away from the vessel wall. This constraint is not physically sound, and a more sophisticated model was developed by N'Dri et al. (2003).

Chang et al. (2000) used computer simulation of cell adhesion to study the initial tethering and rolling process based on Bell's model, and constructed a state diagram for cell adhesion under viscous flows under an imposed shear rate of 100 s^{-1}. This shear rate corresponds to the experimental value where rolling of the cell occurs. To create the state diagrams, the ratio of rolling velocity V to the hydrodynamic velocity V_H (velocity of nonadherent cells translating near the wall), V/V_H, is computed as a function of the reverse reaction rate, k_{ro}, for a given value of r_o using the Bell equation

$$k_r = k_{ro} \exp\left(\frac{r_o f}{k_B T}\right) \tag{23.1}$$

Here, k_{ro} is the unstressed dissociation rate constant, $k_B T$ the thermal energy, r_o the reactive compliance, and f represents the bond force. From the graph of V/V_H versus k_{ro}, the values of k_{ro} for a given value of r_o are estimated. The estimated values are used to plot k_{ro} as a function of r_o for a given ratio of V/V_H. From these curves, different dynamic states of adhesion can be identified. The first state, where cells move at a velocity greater than 95% of the hydrodynamic velocity V_H, is defined as no adhesion state. The second state, where $0 < V/V_H < 0.5$, is considered as the rolling domain and consists of fast and transient adhesion regimes. The first adhesion state, where $V/V_H = 0.0$ for a given period of time, defines the final state. Figure 23.2 shows the computed values of k_{ro} as a function of r_o.

Adhesion occurs for high values of k_{ro} and low values of r_o, as indicated by the wide area between the no- and firm-adhesion zones in Figure 23.3. As r_o increases, k_{ro} has to decrease for adhesion to take place. In the simulation (Figure 23.3), both association rate k_f and wall shear rate are kept constant. Varying k_f does not change the shape of the state diagram but shifts the location of the rolling envelope in the k_{ro}–r_o plane. The shear rate used in Chang et al. (2000) is in the range of the physiological flow for postcapillary venules and lies between 30 and 400 s^{-1}. They found that as the shear rate increases, there is an abrupt change from firm adhesion to no adhesion without rolling motion. As r_o increases, k_{ro} has to decrease in order for adhesion to take place. In the simulation, both association rate k_f and wall shear rate are kept constant. For values of r_o less than 0.1 Å and high reverse rate constant values k_{ro}, the rolling velocity is independent of the spring constant.

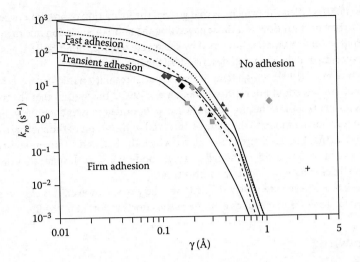

FIGURE 23.2 State diagram for adhesion. Four different states are shown. The dotted curve represents a velocity of 0.3 V_H and the dashed curve represents a velocity of 0.1 V_H. (From Chang, K.C., Tees, D.F.J., and Hammer, D.A., *Proc. Natl. Acad. Sci. USA*, 97, 11262, 2000. With permission.)

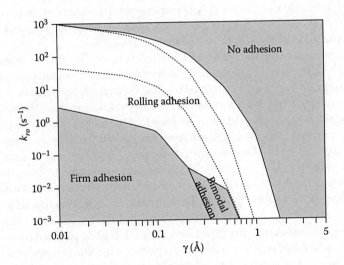

FIGURE 23.3 State diagram for shear rate ranging from 30 to 400 s^{-1}. The dotted curves indicate the boundaries of the rolling state at shear rate $G = 100$ s^{-1}. The rolling adhesion area represents the region where rolling motion occurs over shear rate ranging from 30 to 400 s^{-1}. In the bimodal adhesion regime, cells display either firm adhesion or no adhesion, without rolling motion, as the applied shear rate is altered from 100 to 400 s^{-1}. (From Chang, K.C., Tees, D.F.J., and Hammer, D.A., *Proc. Natl. Acad. Sci. USA*, 97, 11262, 2000. With permission.)

Tees et al. (2002) used the approach described in Chang et al. (2000) to study the effect of particle size on adhesion. They observed that an increase of the particle size raises the rolling velocity. This is consistent with the experimental findings of Shinde Patil et al. (2001). In both studies, the Bell model is used to construct the state diagram but the same results can be achieved using the spring model.

Using leukocytes, Alon et al. (1995) showed that the Bell equation and the spring model both fit the experimental data better than the linear relationship, suggesting an exponential dependence of k_r on f_b.

Chen and Springer (1999) studied the principles that govern the formation of bonds between a cell moving freely over a substrate in shear flow and those governing the bond dissociation due to hydrodynamic forces, and found that bond formation is governed by shear rate whereas bond breakage is governed by shear stress. This experimental data are well described by the Bell equation.

In the study of Smith et al. (1999), a high temporal and spatial resolution microscopy is used to reveal features that previous studies could not capture (Alon et al., 1995). They found that the measured dissociation constants for neutrophil tethering events at 250 pN/bond are lower than the values predicted by the Bell and Hookean spring models. The plateau observed in the graph of the shear stress versus the reaction rate K_r suggests that there is a force value above which the Bell and spring models are not valid. Since the model proposed so far considers the cell as a rigid body, whether the plateau is due to molecular, mechanical, or cell deformation is not clear at this time.

Cell rolling/adhesion has been extensively studied over the years. However, it is clear that much further studies are needed. Table 23.1 summarizes some of the efforts reported in the literature.

23.3.3 Cell Crawling

The process of cell crawling consists of three major stages: (1) pushing the leading edge, (2) establishing new adhesions in the front area and weakening of the exiting adhesions in the trailing area, and (3) pulling the back of the cell. Polymerization of the actin fibers in the protruded area of the crawling cell is considered the main mechanism of pushing the cell ahead. Thus, the modeling of the production of the pushing force is based on the polymerization/depolymerization analysis of actin fibers. There are two main approaches to the modeling of the polymerization-based active forces. In the first approach, the kinetics of a single fiber or array of fibers is considered. In the second, which is the continuum-type model, the fibers are treated as one phase of a two-phase reacting cytosol.

Peskin et al. (1993) have proposed the Brownian Ratchet theory for the active force production. The main component of that theory was the interaction between a rigid protein and a diffusing object in front of it. If the object undergoes a Brownian motion, and the fiber undergoes polymerization, there are rates at which the polymer can push the object and overcome the external resistance. The problem was formulated in terms of a system of reaction–diffusion equations for the probabilities of the polymer to have a certain number of monomers. Two limiting cases, fast diffusion and fast polymerization, were treated analytically that resulted in an explicit force/velocity relationship. This theory was subsequently extended to elastic objects and to the transient attachment of the filament to the object. The correspondence of these models to recent experimental data is discussed in the article by Mogilner and Oster (2003).

Mogilner and Edelstein-Keshet (2002) modeled the protrusion of the leading edge of a cell by considering an array of actin fibers inclined with respect to the cell membrane. The authors have considered the main sequence of events associated with the actin dynamics, including polymerization of the barbed edge of actin polymer and depolymerization at the protein pointed edge. The barbed edges assemble actin monomers with molecules of ATP attached. The new barbed edges are activated by Arp2/3 complexes and they branch to start new actin filaments. The rate of polymerization is controlled by capping of the barbed edges. The problem reduced to a system of reaction–diffusion equations and was solved in the steady-state case. As a result of this solution, the force/velocity relationships corresponding to different regimes were obtained. More recently, Bindschadler et al. (2004) have constructed a comprehensive model of actin cycle that can be used in various problems of cell motility. The authors took into account the major actin-binding protein, regulating actin assembly and disassembly and solved the problem as a steady-state case.

An alternative to the explicit analysis of actin fibers is a continuum approach where the cytoskeletal fibers are treated as one of the two phases of the cytosol. Dembo and Harlow (1986) have proposed a general model of contractile biological polymer networks based on the analysis of reactive interpenetrating flow. In that model, the cytoplasm was viewed as a mixture of a contractile network of randomly oriented cytoskeletal filaments and an aqueous solution. Both phases were treated as homogeneous Newtonian fluids. Alt and Dembo (1999) have applied a similar approach to the modeling of the motion

TABLE 23.1 Overview of Some Fundamental Adhesion Kinetic Models

Kinetic Model	Main Assumptions/Features	Major Findings
Point attachment (Hammer and Lauffenberger, 1987)	Bonds are equally stressed in the contact area (flat)	Adhesion occurrence depends on values of dimensionless quantities that characterize the interaction between the cell and the surface
	Binding and dissociation occur according to characteristic rate constants	
	Receptors diffuse and convect into the binding area of contact	
Peeling (Dembo et al., 1988)	Clamped elastic membrane	Critical tension to overcome the tendency of the membrane to spread over the surface can be calculated
	Bond stress and chemical rate constants are related to bond strain	
	Bonds are linear springs fixed in the plane of the membrane	Predictions of model depend on whether the bonds are catch bonds or slip bonds
	Chemical reaction of bond formation and breakage is reversible	
	Diffusion of adhesion molecules is negligible	If adhesion is mediated by catch bonds, then no matter how much tension is applied, it is impossible to separate the membrane and the surface
Microvilli-coated hard sphere covered with adhesive springs (Hammer and Apte, 1992)	Combined point attachment model with peeling model	Model can describe rolling, transit attachment, and firm adhesion
	Binding determined by a random statistical sampling of a probablility distribution that describes the binding (or unbinding)	A critical adhesion modulator is the spring slippage (it relates the strain of a bond to its rate of breakage; the higher the slippage, the faster the breakage for the same strain)
Two-dimensional elastic ring (Dong et al., 1999)	Bond density related to the kinetics of bond formation	Shear forces acting on the entire cortical shell of the cell are transmitted on a relatively small "peeling zone" at the cell's trailing edge
	Bonds are elastic springs	
	Interaction between moving fluid and adherent cell	
Two-dimensional cell modeled as a liquid and a compound drop (N'Dri et al., 2003)	Cell deforms with nucleus inside	Results compare well with numerical and experimental results found in the literature for simple liquid drop
	Bonds are elastic springs	Cell viscosity and surface tension affect leukocyte rolling velocity
	Macro/micro model for cell deformation	
	Kinetics model based on Dembo (1988). Nanoscale model for ligand–receptor	Nucleus increases the bond lifetime and decreases leukocyte rolling velocity
	Uniform flow at the inlet as in parallel-flow chamber assay	Cell with larger diameter rolls faster. Uniform flow at the inlet as in parallel flow chamber assay

of ameboid cell. The authors paid special attention to the boundary conditions. They introduced three boundary surfaces: the area of contact between the cell and the substrate, the surface separating the cell body and the lamellipodium, and they specified particular boundary conditions along each of these surfaces. The numerical solution of the problem resulted in cellular responses in the form of waves along the direction of the cellular movement. Recently, a two-phase continuum model has been applied to two problems of motility of the active neutrophil. In the first problem, the neutrophil was stimulated with the chemoattractant fMLP and the generation of the pseudopod was modeled, and in the second, the cell moved inside the micropipette toward the same chemoattractant. Two models, a cytoskeletal swelling force and a polymerization force, were used for the active force production. A finite difference method in terms of the time variable and a Galerkin finite element treatment in terms of the special variables were used to obtain numerical solutions.

Bottino et al. (2002) used a version of the continuum two-phase method and studied the crawling of the nematode sperm. This process is also driven by polymerization of another (not actin) protein, called the major sperm protein (MSP). The proposed model considers the major stages of crawling, including filament polymerization and generation of the force for the lamellipodial extension, storage of elastic energy, and finally the production of the contraction that pulls the rear of the cell. The total stresses consisted of two parts, the passive elastic stresses and active tensile stresses. In the acidic environment near the leading edge of the cell, the cytosol solates, and the elastic energy is released to push the cell forward. The solation was modeled by the removal of the active stresses. The solation rate was modeled by a pH gradient with lower pH at the rear part of the cell (Figure 23.4). The finite element method was used in the implementation of a 2-D version of the model.

23.3.4 Cell Swimming and Gliding

Most bacteria move by swimming by which they use helical flagella. In the bacteria with a left-handed helix (e.g., *Escherichia coli* and *Salmonella*), counterclockwise rotation generates a force pushing the cell forward. In contrast, clockwise rotation results in instability of the cell motion: the flagella fly apart, and the cell is not pushed in any particular direction. In the former case, the cell movement looks like smooth swimming, and in the latter case, the cell tumbles. In general, bacteria alternate between these two regimes of movement. The rotation of flagella is controlled by the molecular motor embedded in the bacterial membrane and driven by the transmembrane proton gradient. The movement of the bacterium can be changed by the addition of chemoattractants, which results in the suppression of tumbling and swimming toward a food source.

In contrast to bacterial swimming, many microorganisms, including myxobacteria, cyanobacteria, and flexobacteria, move via gliding. Nozzle-like structures were found in some of these bacteria. Slime is extruded through the nozzle pores, and this fact leads to a hypothesis that bacterial sliding is driven by a slime-related propulsion mechanism. In earlier models of torque and switching in the bacterial flagellar motor, the motor consisted of two, rotating and stationary, parts. The rotating part had tilted positively and negatively charged strips along its surface. The stationary part of the motor included several channels conducting protons. Each channel had two binding sides, and, therefore, could be in four states. The electrostatic energy of the interaction between the charges along the rotation part and protons bound to the channels was converted into the corresponding torque acting on the moving part. Further development and review of the models of this type can be found in Elston and Oster (1996).

CheY is one of the proteins controlling the motor in the flagella in chemotaxis. Phosphorylation of this protein results in tumbling of the bacterium. Mogilner et al. (2002) have modeled the process of switching of the bacterial molecular motor in response to binding CheY. The motor was assumed being in one of the two states that correspond to the two directions of rotation of the flagella. The kinetic equations for the probabilities of the motor being in each state included a rate constant proportional to the concentration of CheY. In addition, the free energy profile with two minima that depends on the CheY concentration was introduced. As a result, the fraction of time that the motor rotates clockwise

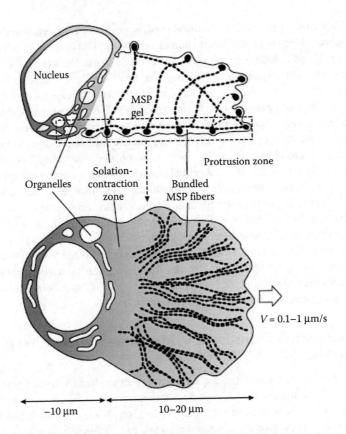

FIGURE 23.4 The model of locomotion of the nematode cell. At the leading edge of the cell, the growing MSP filaments bundle into thick fibers that push the cell front out, and at the same time, store elastic energy. In the acidic environment at the rear part of the cell, the interfilament interaction weakens, the filaments unbundle and contract, providing the contractile force up the cell body. (From Mogilner, A. and Oster, G. *Curr. Biol.*, 13, R721, 2003. With permission.)

was found as a function of the CheY concentration. The function described by a sigmoidal curve was checked against experimental data and good agreement was found. Wolgemuth et al. (2002) have proposed a model of myxobacteria gliding. The authors assumed that the area inside the cell near the nozzle is filled with a polyelectrolyte gel that consists of cross-linked fibers. When the bacterium interacts with its liquid environment, the gel swells and releases from the nozzle. This results in the generation of a propulsive force pushing the bacterium forward. The authors showed that the extrusion of the gel through 50 nozzles produces a force sufficient to drive the bacterium through the viscous environment at velocities observed in the experiment.

23.4 Mechano-, Mechanoelectrical, and Electromechanical Transduction

23.4.1 Mechanotransduction

Cells of all types are constantly exposed to external forces within their physiological environment. In mechanotransduction, cells convert the external mechanical signals into biochemical, morphological, biophysical, and other similar responses. As an example, endothelial cells respond to shear stresses acting on the cell's surface. Under physiological conditions, these stresses are associated with blood flow. In another example, the external stress (compression) causes mechanotransduction in chondrocytes, which is important both for the functioning of natural cartilage and for the design of artificial cartilage. Adhesion (traction) forces along the area of interaction of a cell with ECM determine cell shape, growth, and division (Chen et al., 1997, 2004 for review). General models that include biochemical aspect of signaling are complex, and their philosophy is discussed in the article by Asthagiri and Lauffenburger (2000). Here, we concentrate on some mechanical and mechanoelectrical aspects of the problem. One common phenomenon that accompanies mechanotransduction is a rearrangement of the cellular cyto-skeleton in response to external forces. Suciu et al. (1997) have modeled the process of reorientation of the actin filaments in response to shear stresses acting on the membrane of endothelial cells. The authors assumed that the filament angular drift velocity is proportional to the applied shear stress and reduced the problem to a system of integro-differential equations in terms of the partial concentration of actin filaments being in different states (free, attached to the membrane, etc.). The same mathematical approach was later used to model the actin filaments in endothelial cells subjected to a cyclic stretch (simulation of the effect of the circumferential cyclic stretch of blood vessels). Thoumine et al. (1999) have analyzed such changes that occur during fibroblast spreading and they found a significant stiffening of the cell. Sato et al. (2000) have reported significant changes in the viscoelastic properties of endothelial cells as a result of the action of shear stresses. Kaunas et al. (2010) have proposed a kinematic model of fiber dynamics resulting from ECM stretching. Ingber (2006) and Poirier et al. (2007) have presented recent reviews of mechanotransduction and its models.

23.4.2 Mechanoelectrical Transduction, Mechanosensitive Channels, and Electromechanical Transduction

During mechanoelectrical transduction, the mechanical stimuli applied to the cell membrane result in (in-) activation of ionic currents through mechanosensitive channels. In eukaryotic cells, such channels are typically connected to the cell cytoskeleton. In several examples, stretch-activated channels modulate cell volume in cardiac ventricular myocytes, have a functional role in electrical and mechanical activity of smooth muscles, are involved in bone response to mechanical loading, produce a Ca^{2+} influx that leads to waves of calcium-induced calcium release, and so on. One of the features of mechanosensitive channels is the sensing not only of the stimulus itself but also its time history (Sachs and Morris, 1998). The main technique of studying the physiology of mechanosensitive channels is the patch pipette, and it was found that a full opening of the channel requires several cmHg of pressure, or several thousandth of Newton per meter of the equivalent membrane force (resultant). In the modeling of mechanosensitive channels, the channel has several states, and the probability of the channel being open is determined by free energy barriers that depend on the mechanical stimulus. Usually, this stimulus is represented by isotropic tension in the cell membrane, which, in the expression of free energy, is multiplied by a typical change in the area of the channel. Bett and Sachs (2000) have analyzed the mechanosensitive channels in the chick heart, and, to reflect the observed inactivation of ionic current, used a three—closed, open, and inactivated—state model of the channel. The authors have also proposed that inactivation consists of two stages: reorganization of the cytoskeleton and blocking action of an agent released by the cell. A quantitative description of this two-step process was based on a viscoelastic-type model that reflected the mechanical properties of the cortical layer underlying the channel. Auditory hair cells and vestibular cells receive mechanical stimuli and sense them via transducer channels located in the sterocilia bundle on the top of the cell. The channels in hair cells that receive acoustic signals are very fast (Corey and Hudspeth, 1979). A theoretical interpretation of the behavior of these channels is based on gating-spring concept that relates the local tension to the transition probability of the channel to be in open and close states. The latest results on the arrangement of the bundle components involved in mechanotransduction were obtained by Beurg et al. (2009) (also, Gillespie and Muller, 2009 for review). Note that the protein responsible for stereocilia bundle mechanotransduction has not been identified. In was also recently found that, in addition to "passive" mechanotransduction, the stereocilia bundle has active (motor) properties by amplifying input mechanical signals. A mathematical model of such phenomena in the form of dynamical systems was discussed by Nadrowski et al. (2004). One more mode of electromechanical transduction can be found in biological membranes whose curvature is coupled in a bidirectional way to the applied electric field (Petrov, 1999). Physical models of this membrane phenomenon, called flexoelectricity, that related membrane curvature–electric field coupling to a redistribution of electrical charges associated with the bilayer were proposed by Hristova et al. (1991) and, recently, by Harland et al. (2010). Zhang et al. (2001) have explained voltage-induced membrane movement in terms of a redistribution of bilayer charges resulting in changes in membrane tension.

Electromechanical transduction, a special form of signal transduction, was found in outer hair cells in the mammalian cochlea. The hearing process in vertebrates is associated only with the mechano-electric form of transduction via transducer channels in the stereocilia of a single type of sensory cells (see above). However, mammals have a special arrangement with two types of sensory cells, inner and outer hair cells. The outer hair cell provides a positive feedback in the processing of sound where its unique form of motility, called electromotility, plays a critical role. The main features of this phenomenon are cell length (and radius) changes, active force generation, and transfer of an electric charge, all in response to changes in the transmembrane potential. Deformation of the cell causes electric (displacement) current in the cell membrane. These features constitute the direct and converse piezoelectric-like effect. Tolomeo and Steele (1995) have proposed a linear piezoelectric model to describe the outer hair cell mechanics and electromotility. Spector (2001) (also, Spector and Jean, 2004) has proposed a thermodynamically based nonlinear model of electromechanical coupling in the outer hair cell. The membrane protein that plays a key role in the outer hair cell electromotility, named prestin, has been identified. Other cells, such as HEK cells, transfected with prestin acquire major features of the outer hair cell electromotility. Thus, modeling piezoelectric cellular membranes is now a more general area where one of the major goals is to combine cellular-level continuous constitutive relations with emerging molecular details of the structure of prestin.

23.5 Modeling Cells in Disease

23.5.1 Cancer

When a normal healthy cell's genetic material is altered, the cell responds differently to the host's growth regulators, leading to an uncontrolled growth of abnormal tumor cells. Like the normal cells, the tumor cells obtain glucose and oxygen and other nourishments, allowing a regular proliferation rate of tumor cells. A solid tumor arises as the growing spheroid of cells expands, making the core region inaccessible to nutrients. Cancer cells have different cytoskeletal structures from those of normal cells after oncogene transformed the normal cell to cancer cell. As a result, cancer cells can have different deformability and motility. Cancer cells have been reported to be more deformable than normal cells (Lee and Lim, 2007).

Individual cancer cell models have been often considered in tumor modeling using cellular automata or agent-based modeling approaches (Hwang et al., 2009). Jiang et al. (2005) used a lattice Monte Carlo model to describe tumor cell dynamics such as proliferation, adhesion, and viability. At the subcellular level, a network model regulates the expression of proteins that control the cell cycle. Their model predicts the microenvironmental conditions required for tumor cell survival and spheroid growth curve under different nutrient supply conditions. Gerlee and Anderson (2007) proposed a cellular automaton model of tumor growth in which each cell is equipped with a microenvironment network that takes environment variables as an input and determines cellular behavior as an output. They found that the tissue oxygen concentration affects the tumor at both the morphological level and the phenotype level. Gerlee and Anderson (2009) also investigated the emergence of a motile invasive phenotype of cancer cell in a tumor using an individual-based modeling approach, and found that a motile subclone can emerge in a wide range of microenvironmental growth conditions.

Tumor often spreads to other parts of the body by metastasis. Cancer cells often leave the tumor, enter into and circulate through the vascular system, leave the circulation, and form another tumor at a location distant from the original site. There have been efforts to model the cancer cell's motility and interactions with tissues during the process of metastasis. Ramis-Conde et al. (2009) presented a mathematical model of cancer cell intravasation. They used an individual force-based multiscale approach for cellular protein pathways and physical properties of the cell. They studied the influence of different protein pathways on transendothelial migration and obtained the simulation results comparable with experimental data. Gerisch and Chaplain (2008) developed a continuum model of cancer cell invasion of tissue in the form of a system of partial differential equations. Their model converges to a system of reaction–diffusion–taxis equations when the sensing radius that cells use to detect their environment goes to zero.

23.5.2 Malaria

Malaria is caused by the infection of RBCs by parasites of which *Plasmodium falciparum* is known to be the deadliest. When RBC is infected by *P. falciparum*, the RBC's biomechanical properties change such that it becomes less deformable and more adhesive. More rigid RBCs tend to block microcirculation, preventing oxygen supply to organs in the body. There have been efforts to model the biomechanical behavior of malaria-infected RBCs. Suresh et al. (2005) incorporated a 3-D hyperelastic constitutive model into a finite element code, and compared with experimental data. They found that the stiffness increases with the maturation of the parasite. By matching the computational model with experimental data, they estimated the shear modulus of RBC infected with different stages of the *P. falciparum* parasite. Jiao et al. (2009) developed a multicomponent model to account for the parasite within the infected RBC. They found that the membrane shear elastic modulus obtained from their multicomponent model is different from the ones obtained from hemispherical cap model and homogeneous half-space model due to the nonnegligible volume occupied by the parasite inside the infected cell. Kondo et al. (2009) developed a numerical model of blood flow with malaria-infected RBCs based on conservation laws of fluid dynamics. They modeled the deformability of infected RBC using springs governed by Hook's law. They simulated the rolling motion resulting from the interactions with endothelial cells and healthy RBCs, which increased the flow resistance. Ferrer et al. (2007) presented an individual-based model of *P. falciparum*-infected erythrocyte *in vitro* cultures. Cells are arranged in a 3-D grid and the rules of behavior are applied to each individual cell and culture medium. They reproduced several published experimental cultures from simulations of the model.

23.5.3 Nuclear Envelope Deficiency

The nucleus in the eukaryotic cell is enclosed by a nuclear envelope that consists of inner and outer nuclear membranes. Beneath the inner nuclear membrane lies the nuclear lamina, which is a network of filaments consisting of lamin proteins. The nuclear lamina is believed to be responsible for the structural integrity of the nucleus. When the genes encoding nuclear envelop proteins are mutated, structural changes occur in the nuclear envelope, which leads to various diseases, such as Emeri–Dreifus muscular dystrophy and Hutchinson–Gilford progeria (early aging) syndrome. Rowat et al. (2005, 2006) used a micropipette aspiration technique and showed that the nuclear envelope undergoes deformations, maintaining structural stability when exposed to mechanical stress. They developed a theory for a 2-D elastic material to characterize the elastic behavior of nuclear membranes. They also found that the nuclear envelopes in mouse embryo fibroblasts lacking the inner nuclear membrane protein, emerin, are more fragile than those in wild-type cells. They presented a model of nucleus stabilization in the pipette, combining their experimental results and theoretical considerations. Yokokawa et al. (2008) characterized the mechanical properties of the nuclear envelope of living HeLa cells in a culture medium by combining AFM imaging and force measurement. Their elasticity measurement showed that the nuclear envelope is soft enough to absorb a large deformation by the AFM probe. Dahl et al. (2004) established swelling conditions that separate the nuclear envelope from the nucleoplasm, and performed micro-pipette aspiration of swollen and unswollen nuclear envelopes of *Xenopus* oocyte. They measured the network elastic modulus of the nuclear envelope to be 25 mN/m. They found that the nuclear envelope is much stiffer and more resilient than the plasma membranes of cells.

Acknowledgments

The authors are thankful to Drs. Denis Wirtz, Alex Mogilner, and Sean Sun who reviewed the chapter and provided valuable comments. We also acknowledge funding supporting our research, R01 DC 002775 to A.S. and R01 HL 095508 and R01 HL 091005 to R.T.S.T.

References

Alon, R., Chen, S., Fuhlbrigge, R., Puri, K.D., and Springer, T.A. The kinetics and shear threshold of transient and rolling interactions of L-selectin with its ligand on leukocytes, *Proc. Natl. Acad. Sci. USA*, 95, 11631, 1998.

Alon, R., Hammer, D.A., and Springer, T.A. Lifetime of the P-selectin-carbohydrate bond and its response to tensile force in hydrodynamic flow, *Nature (London)*, 374, 539, 1995.

Alt, W. and Dembo, M. Cytoplasm dynamics and cell motion: Two-phase flow model, *Math. Biosci.*, 156, 207, 1999.

Asthagiri, A.R. and Lauffenburger, D.A. Bioengineering models of cell signaling, *Ann. Biomed. Eng.*, 2, 31, 2000.

Atilgan, E. and Sun, S.X. Shape transitions in lipid membranes and protein mediated vesicle fusion and fission, *J. Chem. Phys.*, 126, Art. 095102, 2007.

Baaijens, F.P.T., Triskey, W.R., and Laursen, T.A. Large deformation finite element analysis of micropipette aspiration to determine the mechanical properties of the chondrocyte, *Ann. Biomed. Eng.*, 33, 494, 2005.

Bao, G. and Suresh, S. Cell and molecular mechanics of biological materials, *Nat. Mater.*, 2, 715, 2003.

Bell, G.I. Models for the specific adhesion of cells to cells, *Science*, 200, 618, 1978.

Bett, G.C. and Sachs, F. Activation and inactivation of mechanosensitive currents in the chick heart, *J. Memb. Biol.*, 173, 237, 2000.

Beurg, M., Fettiplace, R., Nam J.H., and Ricci, A.J. Location of inner hair cell mechanotransducer using high-speed calcium imaging, *Nat. Neurosci.*, 12, 553, 2009.

Bindschadler, M., Osborn, E.A., Dewey, C.F. et al. A mechanistic model of the actin cycle, *Biophys. J.*, 86, 2720, 2004.

Bottino, D., Mogilner, A., Roberts, T. et al. How nematode sperm crawl, *Cell Sci.*, 115, 367, 2002.

Bozic, B., Svetina, S., Zeks, B. et al. Role of lamellar membrane structure in tether formation from bilayer vesicles, *Biophys. J.*, 61, 963, 1992.

Caille, N., Thuomine, O., Tardy, Y. et al. Contribution of the nucleus to the mechanical properties of endothelial cells, *J. Biomech.*, 33, 177, 2002.

Calladine, C.R. and Greenwood, J.A. Mechanics of tether formation in liposomes, *J. Biomech. Eng.*, 124, 576, 2002.

Chang, K.C., Tees, D.F.J., and Hammer, D.A. The state diagram for cell adhesion under flow: Leukocyte rolling and firm adhesion, *Proc. Natl. Acad. Sci. USA*, 97, 11262, 2000.

Chen, C.S., Mrksich, M., Huang, S. et al. Geometric control of cell life and death, *Science*, 276, 1425, 1997.

Chen, C.S., Tan, J., and Tien, J. Mechanotransduction of cell-matrix and cell-cell contacts, *Annu. Rev. Biomed. Eng.*, 6, 275, 2004.

Chen, S. and Springer, T.A. An automatic breaking system that stabilizes leukocyte rolling by an increase in selectin bond number with shear, *J. Cell Biol.*, 144, 185, 1999.

Corey, D.P. and Hudspeth, A.J. Response latency of vertebrate hair cells, *Biophys. J.*, 26, 499, 1979.

Cozens-Roberts, C., Lauffenburger, D.A., and Quinn, J.A. A receptor-mediated cell attachment and detachment kinetics; I. Probabilistic model and analysis, *Biophys. J.*, 58, 841, 1990.

Cukierman, E., Pankov, R., Stevens, D.R. et al. Taking cell-matrix adhesions to the third dimension, *Science*, 294, 1708, 2001.

Cuvelier, D., Théry, M., Chu, Y.-S. et al. The universal dynamics of cell spreading, *Curr. Biol.*, 17,694, 2007.

Dahl, K.N., Engler, A.J., Pajerowski, J.D. et al. Power-law rheology of isolated nuclei with deformation mapping of nuclear substructures, *Biophys. J.*, 89, 2855, 2005.

Dahl, K.N., Kahn, S.M., Wilson, K.L. et al. The nuclear envelope lamina network has elasticity and a compressibility limit suggestive of a molecular shock absorber, *J. Cell. Sci.*, 117, 4779, 2004.

Dai J. and Sheetz, M.P. Membrane tether formation from blebbing cells, *Biophys. J.*, 77, 1999.

Dallon, J.C., Sherratt, J.A., and Maini, P.K. Mathematical modelling of extracellular matrix dynamics using discrete cells: Fiber orientation and tissue regeneration, *J. Theor. Biol.*, 199, 449, 1999.

Dembo, M. and Harlow, F. Cell motility, contractile networks, and the physics of interpenetrating reactive flow, *Biophys. J.*, 50, 109, 1986.

Dembo, M., Torney, D.C., Saxaman, K., and Hammer D. The reaction-limited kinetics of membrane-to-surface adhesion and detachment, *Proc. R. Soc. Lond. B*, 234, 55, 1988.

Derenyi, I., Julecher, F., and Prost, J. Formation and interaction of membrane tubes, *Phys. Rev. E*, 88, Art 238101, 2002.

Diez-Silva, M., Dao, M., Han, J.Y. et al. Shape and biomechanical characteristics of human red blood cells in health and disease, *MRS Bull.*, 35, 382, 2010.

Discher, D., Dong, C., Fredberg, J.J. et al. Biomechanics: Cell research and applications for the next decade, *Ann. Biomed. Eng.*, 37, 847, 2009.

Discher, D.E., Boal, D.H., and Boey, S.K. Simulation of the erythrocyte cytoskeleton at large deformation. II. Micropipette aspiration, *Biophys. J.*, 75, 1584, 1998.

Dong, C. and Lei, X.X. Biomechanics of cell rolling: Shear flow, cell-surface adhesion, and cell deformability, *J. Biomech.*, 33, 35, 2000.

Elston, T.C. and Oster, G. Protein turbines! The bacterial flagellar motor, *Biophys. J.*, 73, 703, 1996.

Engler, A.J., Sen, S., Sweeney, H.L. et al. Matrix elasticity directs stem cell lineage specification, *Cell*, 126, 677, 2006.

Evans, E.A. Bending resistance and chemically induced moments in membrane bilayers, *Biophys. J.*, 14, 923, 1974.

Evans, E.A. Detailed mechanics of membrane-membrane adhesion and separation. I. Continuum of molecular cross-bridges, *Biophys. J.*, 48, 175, 1985.

Evans, E.A. Minimum energy analysis of membrane deformation applied to pipet aspiration and surface adhesion of red blood cells, *Biophys. J.*, 30, 265, 1980.

Evans, E.A. and Skalak, R. *Mechanics and Thermodynamics of Biomembranes*, CRC Press, Boca Raton, FL, 1980.

Fabry, B., Maksym, G.N., Butler, J.P. et al. Scaling the microrheology of living cells, *Physiol. Rev. Lett.*, 87, 148102, 2001.

Feng, F. and Klug, W.S. Finite element modeling of lipid bilayer membranes, *J. Comput. Phys.*, 220, 394, 2006.

Ferrer, J., Vidal, J., Prats, C. et al. Individual-based model and simulation of *Plasmodium falciparum* infected erythrocyte *in vitro* cultures, *J. Theor. Biol.*, 248, 448, 2007.

Fletcher, D.A. and Mullins, R.D. Cell mechanics and the cytoskeleton, *Proc. Natl. Acad. Sci. USA*, 463, 485, 2010.

Fraley, S.I., Feng, Y.F., Krishnamurthy, R. et al. A distinctive role for focal adhesion proteins in three-dimensional cell motility, *Nat. Cell Biol.*, 12, 598, 2010.

Gerisch, A. and Chaplain, M.A.J. Mathematical modeling of cancer cell invasion of tissue: Local and non-local models and the effect of adhesion, *J. Theor. Biol.*, 250, 684, 2008.

Gerlee, P. and Anderson, A.R.A. An evolutionary hybrid cellular automaton model of solid tumour growth, *J. Theor. Biol.*, 246, 583, 2007.

Gerlee, P. and Anderson, A.R.A. Evolution of cell motility in an individual-based model of tumour growth, *J. Theor. Biol.*, 259, 67, 2009.

Gillespie, P.G. and Muller, U. Mechanotransduction by hair cells: Models, molecules, and mechanisms, *Cell*, 139, 33, 2009.

Guilak, F., Cohen, D.M., Estes, B.T. et al. Control of stem cell fate by physical interactions with the extracellular matrix, *Cell Stem Cell*, 5, 17, 2009.

Guilak, F., Haider, M.A., Karcher, E. et al. Mutiphasic models of cell mechanics, In *Cytoskeletal Mechanics. Models and Measurements*, Eds, R. Kamm and Mofrad M.R.K., pp. 84–102, 2006.

Guilak, F., Tedrow, J.R., and Burgkart, R. Viscoelastic properties of the cell nucleus, *Biochem. Biophys. Res. Comm.*, 269, 781, 2000.

Haider M.A. and Guilak, F. An axisymmetric boundary integral model for assessing elastic cell properties in the micropipette aspiration contact problem, *J. Biomech. Eng.*, 124, 586, 2002.

Hale, C.M., Shrestha, A.L., Khatau, S.B. et al. Dysfunctional connections between the nucleus and the actin and microtubule networks in laminopathic models, *Biophys. J.*, 11, 5462, 2008.

Hammer, D.A. and Apte, S.M. Simulation of cell rolling and adhesion on surfaces in shear-flow—General results and analysis of selectin-mediated neutrophil adhesion, *Biophys. J.*, 63, 35, 1992.

Hammer, D.A. and Lauffenburger, D.A. A dynamical model for receptor-mediated cell adhesion to surfaces, *Biophys. J.*, 52, 475, 1987.

Harland, B., Brownell, W.E., Spector, A.A. et al. Voltage-induced bending and electromechanical coupling in lipid bilayers, *Phys. Rev. E*, 81, Art. 031907, 2010.

Heidemann, S.R. and Wirtz, D. Cell and molecular mechanics of biological materials, *Trends Cell Biol.*, 14, 160, 2004.

Helfrich, W. Elastic properties of lipid bilayers: Theory and possible experiments, *Z. Naturforsch.*, C28, 693, 1973.

Hochmuth, R.M. Micropipette aspiration of living cells, *J. Biomech.*, 33, 15, 2000.

Hristova., K. Bivas, I., Petrov, A.G., and Derzanski, A. Influence of the electric double layers of the membrane on the value of its flexoelectric coefficient, *Mol. Cryst. Liq. Cryst.*, 200, 71, 1991.

Hwang, M., Garbey, M., Berceli, S.A. et al. Rule-based simulation of multi-cellular biological systems-A review of modeling techniques, *Cell. Mol. Bioeng.*, 2, 285, 2009.

Ingber, D.E., Cellular mechanotransduction: Putting all the pieces together again, *FASEB J.*, 20, 811, 2006.

Ingber, D.E. Cellular tensegrity-defining new rules of biological design that govern the cytoskeleton, *J. Cell Sci.*, 104, 613, 1993.

Ingber, D.E. Tensegrity I. Cell structure and hierarchical systems biology. *J. Cell Sci.*, 116, 1157, 2003a.

Ingber, D.E. Tensegrity II. How structural networks influence cellular information processing networks, *J. Cell Sci.*, 116, 1397, 2003b.

Janmey, P. and Schmidt, C. Experimental measurements of intracellular mechanics, In *Cytoskeletal Mechanics. Models and Measurements*, Eds, R. Kamm and Mofrad M.R.K., pp. 1–17, Cambridge University Press, Cambridge, 2006.

Jean, R.P., Chen, C.S., and Spector, A.A. Finite-element analysis of the adhesion-cytoskeleton-nucleus mechanotransduction pathway during endothelial cell rounding: Axisymmetric model, *J. Biomech. Eng.*, 127, 594, 2005.

Jiang, Y., Pjesivac-Grbovic, J., Cantrell, C. et al. A multiscale model for avascular tumor growth, *Biophys. J.*, 89, 3884, 2005.

Jiao, G.Y., Tan, K.S.W., Sow, C.H. et al. Computational modeling of the micropipette aspiration of malaria infected erythrocytes, *ICBME 2008, Proceedings*, 23, 1788, 2009.

Kamm, R. and Mofrad, M.R.K. Introduction, with the biological basis for cell mechanics, In *Cytoskeletal Mechanics. Models and Measurements*, Eds, R. Kamm and Mofrad M.R.K., pp. 1–17, Cambridge University Press, Cambridge, 2006.

Kan, H.-C., Udaykumar, H.S., Shyy, W., and Tran-Son-Tay, R. Hydrodynamics of a compound drop with application to leukocyte modeling, *Phys. Fluids*, 10, 760, 1998.

Kan, H.-C., Udaykumar, H.S., Shyy, W., and Tran-Son-Tay, R. Numerical analysis of the deformation of an adherent drop under shear flow, *J. Biomech. Eng.*, 121, 160, 1999a.

Kan, H.-C., Udaykumar H.S., Shyy W. et al. Effects of nucleus on leukocyte recovery, *Ann. Biomed. Eng.*, 27, 648, 1999b.

Karcher, H., Lammerding, J., Huang, H. et al. A three-dimensional viscoelastic model for cell deformation with experimental verification, *Biophys. J.*, 85, 3336, 2003.

Kaunas, R., Huang, Z.Y., and Hahn, J. A kinematic model coupling stress fiber dynamics with JNK activation in response to matrix stretching, *J. Theor. Biol.* 264, 593, 2010.

Kondo, H., Imai, Y., Ishikawa, T. et al. Hemodynamic analysis of microcirculation in malaria infection, *Ann. Biomed. Eng.*, 37, 702, 2009.

Lammerding, J., Dahl, K.N., Discher, D.E. et al. Nuclear mechanics and methods, *Cell Mechanics*, 83, 269, 2007.

Lee, G.Y.H. and Lim, C.T. Biomechanics approaches to studying human diseases, *Trends Biotechnol.*, 25, 111, 2007.

Lee, J.S.H., Hale, C.M., Panorchan, P. et al. Nuclear lamin A/C deficiency induces defects in cell mechanics, polarization, and migration, *Biophys. J*, 93, 2542, 2007.

Lenormand, G., Bursac, P., and Butler, J.P. Out-of-equilibrium dynamics in the cytoskeleton of the living cell, *Phys. Rev. E.*, 76, Art 041901, 2007.

Li, Y., Xu, G.-K., Li, B. et al. A molecular mechanisms-based biophysical model for two-phase cell spreading, *Appl. Phys. Lett.*, 96, 043703, 2010.

Lim, G.H.W. and Huber, G. The tether infinitesimal tori and spheres algorithm: A versatile calculator for axisymmetric problems in equilibrium membrane mechanics, *Biophys. J.*, 96, 2064, 2009.

Mahaffy, R.E., Park, S., Gerde, E. et al. Quantitative analysis of the viscoelastic properties of thin regions of fibroblasts using atomic force microscopy, *Biophys. J.*, 86, 1777, 2004.

Maniotis, A.J., Chen, C.S., and Ingber, D.E. Demonstration of mechanical connections between integrinscy to skeletal filaments, and nucleoplasm that stabilize nuclear structure, *Proc. Natl. Acad. Sci. USA*, 94, 849, 1997.

McGarry, J.P., Fu, J., Yang, M.T. et al. Simulation of the contractile response of cells on an array of microposts, *Phil. Trans. Royal Soc. Phys. Eng Sci.*, 367, 3477, 2009.

Mijailovich, S.M., Kojic, M., Zivkovic, M. et al. A finite element model of cell deformation during magnetic bead twisting, *J. Appl. Physiol*, 93, 1429, 2002.

Mofrad, M.R.K., Karcher, H., and Kamm, R.D. Continuum elastic and viscoelastic models of the cell. In *Cytoskeletal Mechanics. Models and Measurements*, Eds, R. Kamm and Mofrad M.R.K., Cambridge University Press, Cambridge, pp. 71–83, 2006.

Mogilner, A. and Edelstein-Keshet, L. Regulation of actin dynamics in rapidly moving cells: A quantitative analysis, *Biophys. J.*, 83, 1237, 2002.

Mogilner, A., Elston, T.C., Wang, H. et al. Switching in the bacterial flagellar motor, In *Computational Cell Biology*, Fall, C.P., Marland, E.S., Wagner, J.M. et al. Eds. Springer, New York, 2002, chap. 13.

Mogilner, A. and Oster, G. Polymer motors: Pushing out the front and pulling up the back, *Curr. Biol.*, 13, R721, 2003.

Nadrowski, B., Martin, P., and Julicher, F. Active hair-bundle motility harnesses noise to operate near an optimum of mechano sensitivity, *Proc. Natl. Acad. Sci. USA*, 33, 12195, 2004.

N'Dri, N.A., Shyy, W., and Tran-Son-Tay, R., Computational modeling of cell adhesion and movement using a continuum-kinetics approach, *Biophys. J.*, 85, 2273, 2003.

Pathak, A., Deshpande, V.S., McMeeking, R.M., and Evans, A.G.J. The simulation of stress fibre and focal adhesion development in cells on patterned substrates, *Royal Soc. Interface*, 5, 507, 2008.

Peskin, C.S., Odell, G.M., and Oster, G. Cellular motors and thermal fluctuation: The Brownian ratchet, *Biophys. J.*, 65, 316, 1993.

Petrov, A.G. *The Lyotropic State of Matter. Molecular Physics and Living Matter Physics.* Gordon and Breach Publ., Australia, 1999.

Poirier, C.C. and Iglesias, P.A. An integrative approach to understanding mechanosensation. *Brief. Bioinform.*, 8, 258, 2007.

Powers, T.R., Huber, G., Goldstein, R.E. Fluid-membrane tethers: Minimal surfaces and elastic boundary layers, *Phys. Rev. E.*, 65, Art 041901, 2002.

Radmacher, M., Fritz, M., Kacher, C.M. et al. Measuring the viscoelastic properties of human platelets with the atomic force microscope, *Biophys. J.*, 70, 556, 1996.

Ramis-Conde, I., Chaplain M.A.J., Anderson, A.R.A. et al. Multi-scale modeling of cancer cell intravasation: The role of cadherins in metastasis, *Phys. Biol.*, 6, 016008, 2009.

Rowat, A.C., Foster, L.J., Nielsen, M.M. et al. Characterization of the elastic properties of the nuclear envelope, *J. R. Soc. Interface*, 2, 63, 2005.

Rowat, A.C., Lammerding, J., and Ipsen, J.H. Mechanical properties of the cell nucleus and the effect of emerin deficiency, *Biophys. J.*, 91, 4649, 2006.

Sachs, F. and Morris, C.E. Mechanosensitive ion channels in non-specialized cells, In *Reviews of Physiology, Biochemistry, and Pharmacology*, Blausten, M.P. et al., Eds. pp. 1–78, Springer, Berlin, 1998.

Satcher, R.L. and Dewey, C.F. Theoretical estimates of mechanical properties of the endothelial cell cytoskeleton, *Biophys. J.*, 71, 109, 1996.

Sato, M., Nagayama, K., Kataoka, N. et al. Local mechanical properties measured by atomic force microscopy for cultured bovine endothelial cells exposed to shear stress, *J. Biomech.*, 33, 127, 2000.

Sato M., Theret, D.P, Wheeler, L.T. et al. Application of the micropipette technique to the measurement of cultured porcine aortic endothelial cell viscoelastic properties, *J. Biomech. Eng.*, 112, 263, 1990.

Schumacher, K.R., Popel, A.S., Anvari, B. et al. Computational analysis of the tether-pulling experiment to probe plasma membrane-cytoskeleton interaction in cells, *Phys. Rev. E*, 80, Article 041905, 2009.

Sengers, B.G., Taylor, M., Please, C.P. et al. Computational modelling of cell spreading and tissue regeneration in porous scaffolds, *Biomaterials*, 28, 1926, 2007.

Shinde Patil, V.R., Campbell, C.J., Yun, Y.H., Slack, S.M., and Goetz, D.J. Particle diameter influences adhesion under flow, *Biophys. J.*, 80, 1733, 2001.

Smith Mcrae, J., Berg, E.L., and Lawrence, M.B. A direct comparison of selectin-mediated transient, adhesive events using high temporal resolution, *Biophys. J.*, 77, 3371, 1999.

Spector, A.A. A nonlinear electroelastic model of the auditory outer hair cell, *Int. J. Solids Struct.*, 38, 2115, 2001.

Spector, A.A., Ameen, M., and Popel, A.S. Simulation of motor-driven cochlear outer hair cell electromotility, *Biophys. J.*, 81, 11, 2001.

Spector, A.A., Brownell, W.E., and Popel, A.S. Analysis of the micropipette experiment with the anisotropic outer hair cell wall, *J. Acoust. Soc. Am.*, 103, 1001, 1998.

Spector, A.A. and Jean, R.P. Models and balance of energy in the piezoelectric cochlear outer hair cell wall, *J. Biomech. Eng.*, 126, 17, 2004.

Stamenovic, D., Rosenblatt, N., and Montoya-Zavala, M. Rheological behavior of living cells is time scale-dependent, *Biophys. J.*, 93, L39, 2007.

Steigmann, D.J. Fluid films with curvature elasticity, *Arch. Rat. Mech. Anal.*, 150, 127, 1999.

Suciu, A., Civelekoglu, G., Tardy, Y. et al. Model of the alignment of actin filaments in endothelial cells subjected to fluid shear stress, *Bull. Math. Biol.*, 59, 1029, 1997.

Sultan, C., Stamenovic, D., and Ingber, D.E. A computational tensegrity model predicts dynamic rheological behaviors in living cells, *Ann. Biomed. Eng.*, 32, 520, 2004.

Sun, L., Cheng, Q.H., Gao, H.J. et al. Computational modeling for cell spreading on a substrate mediated by specific interactions, long-range recruiting interactions, and diffusion of binders, *Phys. Rev. E*, 79, 061907, 2009.

Suresh, S. Biomechanics and biophysics of cancer cells, *Acta Biomater.*, 3, 413, 2007.

Suresh, S., Spatz, J., Mills, J.P. et al. Connections between single-cell biomechanics and human disease states: Gastrointestinal cancer and malaria, *Acta Biomater.*, 1, 15, 2005.

Tees, D.F.J., Chang, K.C., Rodgers, S.D., and Hammer, D.A. Simulation of cell adhesion to bioreactive surfaces in shear: The effect of cell size, *Ind. Eng. Chem. Res.*, 41, 486, 2002.

Theret, D.P., Levesque, M.J., Sato, M. et al. The application of a homogeneous half-space model in the analysis of endothelial cell micropipette measurements, *J. Biomech. Eng.*, 110, 190, 1988.

Thomas, C.H., Colllier, J.H., Sfeir, C. et al. Engineering gene expression and protein synthesis by modulation of nuclear shape, *Proc. Natl. Acad. Sci. USA*, 99, 1972, 2002.

Thoumine, O., Cardoso, O, and Meister, J.J. Changes in the mechanics of fibroblast during spreading: A micromanipulation study, *Eur. Biophys. J.*, 27, 222, 1999.

Tolomeo, J.A. and Steele, C.R. Orthotropic piezoelectric properties of the cochlear outer hair cell wall. *J. Acoust. Soc. Am.*, 97, 3006, 1995.

Tran-Son-Tay, R., Needham, D., Yeung, A., and Hochmuth, R.M. Time dependent recovery of passive neutrophils after large deformation, *Biophys. J.*, 60, 856, 1991.

Tseng, Y., Kole, T.P., and Wirtz, D. Micro mechanical mapping of live cells by multiple-particle-tracking microrheology, *Biophys. J.*, 83, 3162, 2002.

Tseng, Y., Lee, J.S.H., Kole, T.P. et al. Micro-organization and visco-elasticity of the interphase nucleus revealed by particle nanotracking, *J. Cell Sci.*, 117, 2159, 2004.

Unnikrishnan, G.U., Unnikirishnan, V.U., and Reddy, J.N. Constitutive material modeling of cell: A micromechanics approach, *J. Biomech. Eng.*, 129, 315, 2007.

Van Vilet, K.L., Bao, G., and Suresh, S. The biomechanics toolbox: Experimental approaches for living cells and biomolecules, *Acta Mater.*, 51, 5881, 2003.

Walcott, S. and Sun, S.X. A mechanical model of actin stress fiber formation and substrate elasticity sensing in adherent cells, *Proc. Natl. Acad. Sci. USA*, 107, 7757, 2010.

Wang, N and Ingber, D.E. Control of cytoskeletal mechanics by extracellular matrix, cell shape, and mechanical tension, *Biophys. J.*, 66, 2181, 1994.

Waugh, R.E. and Hochmuth, R.M. Mechanical equilibrium of thick, hollow, liquid membrane cylinders, *Biophys. J.*, 52, 391, 1987.

Wirtz, D. Particle-tracking microrheology of living cells: Principles and applications, *Annu. Rev. Biophys.*, 38, 301, 2009.

Wolgemuth, C., Holczyk, E., Kaiser, D. et al. How Myxobacteria glide, *Curr. Biol.*, 12, 369, 2002.

Yamada, S., Wirtz, D., and Kuo, S.C. Mechanics of living cells measured by laser tracking microrheology, *Biophys. J.*, 78, 1736, 2000.

Yokokawa, M., Takeyasu, K., and Yoshimura S.H. Mechanical properties of plasma membrane and nuclear envelope measured by scanning probe microscope, *J. Microsc.*, 232, 82, 2008.

Zemel, A., Rehfeldt, F., Brown, A.E.X. et al. Optimal matrix rigidity for stress-fibre polarization in stem cells, *Nat. Phys.*, 6, 468, 2010.

Zhang, P.C., Keleshian, A.M., and Sachs, F. Voltage-induced membrane movement, *Nature*, 413, 428, 2001.

Zhou, E.H., Lim, C.T., and Quek, S.T. Finite element simulation of the micropipette aspiration of a living cell under going large viscoelastic deformation, *Mech. Advanced Mater. Struct.*, 12, 501, 2005.

Zhu, C. Kinetics and mechanics of cell adhesion, *J. Biomech.*, 33, 23, 2000.

Further Information

Fall, C.P., Marland, E.S., Wagner, J.M., and Tyson, J.I. Eds. *Computational Cell Biology*, Springer, New York, 2002 (this book consists of several sections written by leading experts in the mathematical and computational analysis of cell physiology; the material includes exercises, necessary mathematics, and software, and it can be used for teaching advanced graduate courses).

Mogilner, A., Wollman, R., Civelekoglu-Scholey, G., and Scholey, J. Modeling mitosis, *Trends Cell Biol.*, 16, 88, 2006.

Zaman, M.H. Ed. *Statistical Mechanics of Cellular Systems and Processes*, Cambridge University Press, Cambridge, 2009 (a collection of chapters on statistical models of molecules, cells, and cellular systems).

24

Cochlear Mechanics

24.1 Anatomy...24-2
  Components • Material Properties
24.2 Passive Models...24-5
  Resonators • Traveling Waves • One-Dimensional Model •
  Two-Dimensional Model • Three-Dimensional Model
24.3 Active Process...24-10
  Outer Hair Cell Electromotility • Hair Bundle Transduction
  Process
24.4 Active Models...24-12
  Push-Forward/Pull-Backward Active Model • Summary of Some
  Issues • Traveling Wave • Motility versus Beating • OHC Roll-
  Off • Tectorial Membrane Properties: Resonance? • Multiple
  Traveling Wave Modes • Stiffness Change along the Cochlea
24.5 Concluding Comments...24-19
References...24-19
Further Information...24-22

Charles R. Steele
Stanford University

Sunil Puria
Stanford University

The inner ear is a transducer of mechanical force to an appropriate neural excitation. The key element is the receptor cell, or hair cell, which has stereocilia on the apical surface and afferent (and sometimes efferent) neural synapses on the lateral walls and base. Generally, for hair cells, mechanical displacement of the stereocilia in the forward direction toward the tallest stereocilia causes the generation of electrical impulses in the nerves, while backward displacement causes the inhibition of spontaneous neural activity. Displacement in the lateral direction has no effect. For moderate frequencies of sinusoidal stereociliary displacement (20–200 Hz), the neural impulses are in synchrony with the mechanical displacement, one impulse for each cycle of excitation. Such impulses are transmitted to the higher centers of the brain and can be perceived as sound. For lower frequencies, however, neural impulses in synchrony with the excitation are apparently confused with the spontaneous, random firing of the nerves. Consequently, there are three mechanical devices in the inner ear of vertebrates that provide perception in the different frequency ranges. At zero frequency, that is, linear acceleration, the otolithic membrane provides a constant force acting on the stereocilia of hair cells. For low frequencies associated with the rotation of the head, the semicircular canals provide the proper force on the stereocilia. For frequencies in the hearing range, the cochlea provides the proper force on the stereocilia. In nonmammalian vertebrates, the equivalent of the cochlea is a bent tube, and the upper frequency of hearing is at most 12 kHz. For mammals, the upper frequency is considerably higher, 20 kHz for man but extending to almost 200 kHz for toothed whales and some bats. Other creatures, such as certain insects, as well as some frogs and birds living in noisy environments, can perceive high frequencies, but may not have the frequency discrimination of mammals.

Auditory research is a broad field (Keidel and Neff 1976). This chapter provides a brief guide of a restricted view, focusing on the fluid-elastic aspects of the transfer of the input sound pressure into the correct stimulation of hair cell stereocilia in the cochlea. In a general sense, the mechanical functions of the semicircular canals and the otoliths are clear, as are the functions of the outer ear and middle ear; however, the cochlea continues to elude a complete explanation. It is evident that the normal function of the cochlea requires a full integration of mechanical, electrical, and chemical effects on the milli-, micro-, and nanometer scales. Texts that include details of the anatomy are by Pickles (1988), Gulick et al. (1989), and Geisler (1998). Surveys specifically on the cochlea are by Steele (1987), Hudspeth (1989), de Boer (1991), Dallos (1992), Ruggero (1993), and Nobili et al. (1998). Today, many laboratories have excellent websites that contain both introductory information and other details. Nevertheless, because of the immensity of his contributions, Békésy (1960) remains the required reading for anyone embarking on a serious work on the cochlea.

24.1 Anatomy

The cochlea is a coiled tube in the shape of a snail shell (cochlea = schnecke = snail), with a length of about 35 mm and a radius of about 1 mm in human. Figure 24.1 shows a finite element (FE) model that is based entirely on three-dimensional (3D) reconstruction from micro-computed tomography (micro-CT) imaging. This shows the eardrum, middle ear, vestibular canals, as well as the cochlea. Böhnke and Arnold (1999) apparently presented the first construction of an FE model from a CT image. Presently, a number of laboratories possess this capability.

There is not a large size difference across species: the length of the cochlea is 60 mm in elephant and 7 mm in mouse. There are two and a half turns of the coil in man and dolphin, and five turns in guinea pig. There is a correlation of the coiling with the hearing capability of land animals (West 1985). Manoussaki et al. (2008) also consider sea mammals, and find that the ratio of curvature at the base to the curvature at the apex is a feature that correlates strongly with low-frequency hearing limits. However, any benefit of the coiling, which is so striking in mammals, is yet to be found for higher frequency. The default explanation is that the coiling is just for packaging.

Consequently, the cochlea is often modeled as a straight box shown in Figure 24.2, which includes the minimum essential mechanical features. The box is filled with fluid, with mechanical properties close to water. The box is divided into two fluid chambers by a partition, a portion of which, the *basilar membrane* (BM), is thin and tapered. At the left end, representing the basal end of the cochlea, is a piston, the *stapes*, through which sound pressure is applied to the upper fluid chamber. Since the walls

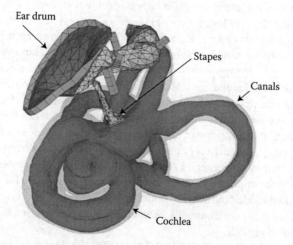

FIGURE 24.1 Finite element model of middle ear, vestibular apparatus, and cochlea. The mesh is generated from a micro-CT image of a human temporal bone.

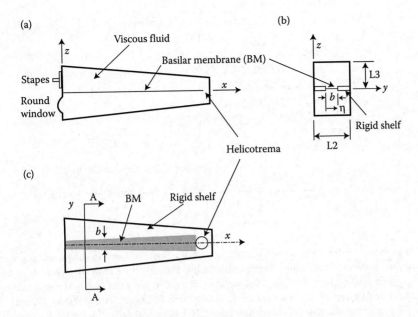

FIGURE 24.2 The standard straight box model of the cochlear with the organ of Corti removed. The Cartesian coordinates $\{x, y, z\}$ represent the distance from the stapes, the distance across the scala width, and the height above the partition, respectively. (a) Side, (b) cross section (A–A), and (c) top views.

are stiff bone and the fluid is nearly incompressible, there is a relief window, the *round window* (RW), at the basal end of the lower fluid region. At the right end, representing the apex of the cochlea, there is a hole in the partition, the helicotrema, so fluid can flow between the two chambers without obstruction. With realistic physical values for the BM dimensions and elasticity, this box model yields rather good agreement with the cochlear response.

24.1.1 Components

Figure 24.3 shows some details of the BM and the organ of Corti. The partition shown in Figure 24.3 consists of three segments: on the one side, the *bony shelf* (or *primary spiral osseous lamina*), in the middle, the BM, and on the other side, a thick support (*spiral ligament*). A second partition (not shown) is the *Reissner's membrane*, attached at one side above the edge of the bony shelf and attached at the other side to the wall of the cochlea. *Scala media* is the region between the Reissner's membrane and the BM, and is filled with *endolymphatic fluid*. This fluid has an ionic content similar to intracellular fluid, high in potassium and low in sodium, but with a resting positive electrical potential of around +80 mV. The electrical potential is supplied by the *stria vascularis* on the wall in scala media. The region above the Reissner's membrane is *scala vestibuli*, and the region below the main partition is *scala tympani*. Scala vestibuli and scala tympani are connected at the apical end of the cochlea by the *helicotrema*, and are filled with *perilymphatic fluid*. This fluid is similar to extracellular fluid, low in potassium and high in sodium with zero electrical potential. Distributed along the scala media side of the BM is the sensory epithelium, the *organ of Corti*. This contains one row of *inner hair cells* and three rows of *outer hair cells*. In humans, each row contains about 4000 cells. Each of the inner hair cells has about 20 afferent synapses; these are considered to be the primary receptors. In comparison, the outer hair cells are sparsely innervated but have both afferent (5%) and efferent (95%) synapses.

The BM is divided into two sections. Connected to the edge of the bony shelf, on the left in Figure 24.3, is the *arcuate zone*, consisting of a single layer of transverse fibers. Connected to the edge of the

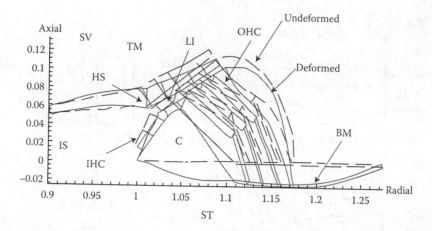

FIGURE 24.3 Shell model for the cross section of cochlea with the organ of Corti in the guinea pig apex (*y–z* plane). The dashed lines show the undeformed configuration, while the solid lines show the deformed configuration due to static pressure loading toward ST, greatly amplified. The radial and axial distances are in millimeters. SV, scala vestibule; ST, scala tympani; IS, inner sulcus; C, cortilymph; TM, tectorial membrane; IP, inner pillar; OP, outer pillar; BM, basilar membrane; IHC, inner hair cells; OHC, outer hair cells; HS, Hensen's stripe; L1, sub-tectorial membrane fluid region. The OHC stereocilia are sheared by the motion of the pillars of Corti and reticular lamina relative to the TM. The basilar membrane is supported on the left by the bony shelf and on the right by the spiral ligament. The IHC are the primary receptors, each with about 20 afferent synapses. The IC is a fluid region in contact with the IHC stereocilia.

spiral ligament, on the right in Figure 24.3, is the *pectinate zone,* consisting of a double layer of transverse fibers in an amorphous ground substance. The *arches of Corti* form a truss over the arcuate zone, which consist of two rows of *pillar cells.* The foot of the inner pillar is attached at the point of connection of the bony shelf to the arcuate zone, while the foot of the outer pillar cell is attached at the common border of the arcuate zone and pectinate zone. The heads of the inner and outer pillars are connected and form the support point for the *reticular lamina.*The other edge of the reticular lamina is attached to the top of *Henson cells,* which have bases connected to the BM. The inner hair cells are attached on the bony shelf side of the inner pillars, while the three rows of outer hair cells are attached to the reticular lamina. The region bounded by the inner pillar cells, the reticular lamina, the Henson cells, and the BM forms another fluid region. This fluid is considered to be perilymph since it appears that ions can flow freely through the arcuate zone of the BM. The stereocilia of the hair cells protrude into the endolymph. Thus, the outer hair cells are immersed in perilymph at 0 mV, have an intracellular potential of −70 mV, and have stereocilia at the upper surface immersed in endolymph at a potential of +80 mV. In some regions of the ears of some vertebrates (Freeman and Weiss 1990), the stereocilia are freestanding. However, mammals always have a *tectorial membrane,* originating near the edge of the bony shelf and overlying the rows of hair cells parallel to the reticular lamina. The tallest rows of stereocilia of the outer hair cells are attached to the tectorial membrane. Under the tectorial membrane and inside the inner hair cells is a fluid space, the *inner sulcus,* filled with endolymph. The stereocilia of the inner hair cells are not attached to the overlying tectorial membrane, so the motion of the fluid in the inner sulcus must provide the mechanical input to these primary receptor cells. Since the inner sulcus is found only in mammals, the fluid motion in this region generated by acoustic input may be crucial to high-frequency discrimination capability.

With a few exceptions of specialization, the dimensions of all the components in the cross section of the mammalian cochlea change smoothly and slowly along the length, in a manner consistent with high stiffness at the base, or input end, and low stiffness at the apical end. For example, in the cat, the BM width increases from 0.1 to 0.4 mm while the thickness of the fiber layers decreases from 13 to 5 μm.

TABLE 24.1 Typical Values and Estimates for Young's Modulus E

Compact bone	20	GPa
Keratin	3	GPa
Basilar membrane fibers	1.9	GPa
Microtubules	1.2	GPa
Actin	1	GPa
Collagen	1	GPa
Reissner's membrane	60	MPa
Red blood cell, extended (assuming thickness = 10 nm)	45	MPa
Rubber, elastin	4	MPa
Basilar membrane ground substance	200	kPa
Tectorial membrane	30	kPa
Jell-O	3	kPa
Henson's cells	1	kPa

The density of transverse collagen fibers decreases more than the thickness, from about 6000 fibers per μm at the base to 500 fibers per μm at the apex (Cabezudo 1978).

24.1.2 Material Properties

Both the perilymph and the endolymph have the viscosity and density of water. The bone of the wall and the bony shelf appear to be similar to a compact bone, with a density approximately twice that of water. The remaining components of the cochlea are a soft tissue with a density near to that of water. The stiffnesses of the components vary over a wide range, as indicated by the values of the Young's modulus listed in Table 24.1. These values are taken directly or estimated from many sources, including the stiffness measurements in the cochlea by Békésy (1960), Gummer et al. (1981), Strelioff and Flock (1984), Miller (1985), Zwislocki and Cefaratti (1989), and Olson and Mountain (1994).

24.2 Passive Models

The anatomy of the cochlea is complex. By modeling, one attempts to isolate and understand the essential features. The following is an indication of proposition and controversy associated with a few such models.

24.2.1 Resonators

The ancient Greeks suggested that the ear consisted of a set of tuned resonant cavities. As each component in the cochlea was discovered subsequently, it was proposed to be the tuned resonator. The most well-known resonance theory is by Helmholtz. According to this theory, the transverse fibers of the BM are under tension and respond like the strings of a piano. The short strings at the base respond to high frequencies and the long strings toward the apex respond to low frequencies. The important feature of the Helmholtz theory is the *place principle*, according to which the receptor cells at a certain *place* along the cochlea are stimulated by a certain frequency. Thus, the cochlea provides a real-time frequency separation (Fourier analysis) of any complex sound input. This aspect of the Helmholtz theory has since been validated, since each of the some 30,000 fibers exiting the cochlea in the auditory nerve is sharply tuned to a particular frequency. A basic difficulty with such a resonance theory is that sharp tuning requires small damping, which is associated with a long ringing after the excitation ceases. Yet the cochlea is remarkable for combining sharp tuning with short time delay for the onset of reception and the same short time delay for the cessation of reception. A particular problem with the

Helmholtz theory arises from the equation for the resonant frequency for a plate consisting of a set of unidirectional fibers (strings) under tension:

$$f = \frac{1}{2b}\sqrt{\frac{T}{\rho_p h}} \tag{24.1}$$

where T is the tensile force per unit width, ρ_p is the density of the plate, b is the length, and h is the thickness of the plate. In man, the frequency range over which the cochlea operates is $f = 200\text{–}20{,}000$ Hz, a factor of 100, while the change in length b is only a factor of 5 and the thickness of the BM h varies the wrong way by a factor of 2 or so. Thus, to produce the necessary range of frequency, the tension T would have to vary by a factor of about 800. In fact, the spiral ligament, which would supply such tension, varies in area by a factor of only 10.

Instead of the plate under tension, it is better to consider the *bending stiffness* of the BM with the mass from inviscid fluid on both sides. The resonant frequency is

$$f = \frac{1}{2\pi}\sqrt{\frac{4k}{\pi\rho}} \tag{24.2}$$

where ρ is the density of the fluid and k is the volume stiffness (pressure divided by area displacement) of the plate. For a plate with simply supported edges, we have

$$k = \frac{120 c_f EI}{b^5} \approx \frac{10 c_f Et^3}{b^5} \tag{24.3}$$

where c_f is the volume fraction of fibers, E is the Young's modulus, t is the thickness, and b is the width. For a frequency of 1000 Hz, Equation 24.2 indicates the stiffness of $k = 3 \times 10^{10}$ N/m^5, which is within an order of magnitude of values given by Békésy (1960, Figure 12-37) for chicken, mouse, rat, guinea pig, and cow (but not for elephant, which has the specialization of a porous bony shelf). The measurement was on *ex vivo* preparations and it was difficult (no one has attempted to repeat it), and his measured stiffness along the cochlea varies over three orders of magnitude. Consequently, the agreement with Equation 24.2 is considered as reasonable, so Equations 24.2 and 24.3 can be used for an approximation for the location of the maximum amplitude for a given frequency, the best frequency for a point (BF). Table 24.2 shows values at the base and apex of the guinea pig cochlea. The frequency from the tension model (Equation 24.1) and from the bending model (Equations 24.2 and 24.3) show the effectiveness of the bending. For modest ratios of geometry, the variation in frequency is a factor of 400. Of course, in the cochlea, the BF from Equations 24.2 and 24.3 marks not a resonance but rather a transition region.

TABLE 24.2 Frequency Range Capability of BM Pectinate Zone (for Guinea Pig) for Bending Stiffness and Tension Stiffness

	Base	Apex	Ratio
Elastic modulus E	1 GPa	1 GPa	1
BM fiber volume fraction c_f	0.08	0.01	7
BM width b	80 μm	180 μm	0.44
BM fiber layer thickness t	7 μm	1 μm	7
Spiral ligament width c	200 μm	40 μm	5
Frequency tension	247 Hz	130 Hz	1.9
Frequency bending	52,000 Hz	130 Hz	400

24.2.2 Traveling Waves

No theory predicted the actual behavior found in the cochlea in 1928 by Békésy (1960). He observed *traveling waves* moving along the cochlea from the base toward the apex, which have a maximum amplitude at a certain place for a given frequency. The place depends on the frequency, as in the Helmholtz theory, but the amplitude envelope in not very localized. In Békésy's experimental models, and in subsequent mathematical and experimental models, the anatomy of the cochlea is greatly simplified. The coiling, Reissner's membrane, and the organ of Corti are all ignored, so the cochlea is treated as a straight tube with a single partition (Figure 24.2). (An exception is in Fuhrmann et al. 1987.) The gradient in the BM stiffness gives beautiful traveling waves in both experimental and mathematical models.

24.2.3 One-Dimensional Model

A majority of work has been based on the assumption that the fluid motion is one-dimensional (1D). With this simplification, the governing equations are similar to those for an electrical transmission line and for the long wavelength response of an elastic tube containing fluid. The equation for the pressure p in a tube with constant cross-sectional area A and with constant frequency of excitation is

$$\frac{d^2p}{d^2x} + \frac{2\rho\omega^2}{AK}p = 0 \tag{24.4}$$

where x is the distance along the tube, and K is the generalized partition stiffness, equal to the net pressure divided by the displaced area of the cross section. The factor of 2 accounts for fluid on both sides of the elastic partition. Often, K is represented in the form of a single-degree-of-freedom oscillator

$$K = k + i\omega d - m\omega^2 \tag{24.5}$$

where k is the static stiffness, d is the damping, and m is the mass density

$$m = \rho_P \frac{h}{b} \tag{24.6}$$

A good approximation is to treat the pectinate zone of the BM as transverse beams with simply supported edges, for which Equation 24.2 gives the stiffness. The solution of Equation 24.4 can be obtained by numerical or asymptotic (called Wentzel-Kramers-Brillouin (WKB) or combined local-global (CLG)) methods. The result is traveling waves for which the amplitude of the BM displacement builds to a maximum and then rapidly diminishes. The parameters of K are adjusted to obtain an agreement with the measurements of the dynamic response in the cochlea. Often, all the material of the organ of Corti is assumed to be rigidly attached to the BM so that h is relatively large and the effect of mass m is large. Then, the maximum response is near the *in vacua* resonance of the partition given by

$$\omega^2 = \frac{bp}{h\rho} \tag{24.7}$$

The following are the objections to the 1D model (e.g., Siebert 1974): (1) The solutions of Equation 24.4 show wavelengths of response in the region of maximum amplitude that are small in comparison with the size of the cross section, violating the basic assumption of 1D fluid flow. (2) In the drained cochlea, Békésy (1960) observed no resonance of the partition, so there is no significant partition mass. The significant mass is entirely from the fluid and therefore Equation 24.7 is not correct. This is consistent with the observations of experimental models. (3) In model studies by Békésy (1960) and others, the localization of response is independent of the area A of the cross section. Thus, Equation 24.4 cannot govern the most interesting part of the response, the region near the maximum amplitude for a given frequency BF. (4) Mechanical and neural measurements in the cochlea show dispersion, which is incompatible with the 1D model (Lighthill 1991). (5) The 1D model fails badly in comparison with experimental measurements in models for which the parameters of geometry, stiffness, viscosity, and density are known. Nevertheless, the simplicity of Equation 24.4 and the analogy with the transmission line have made the 1D model popular. We note that there is interest in utilizing the principles in an analog model built on a silicon chip because of the high performance of the actual cochlea. Watts (1993) reports on the first model with an electrical analog of 2D fluid in the scali. An observation is that the transmission line hardware models are sensitive to failure of one component, while the two-dimensional (2D) model is not. In experimental models, Békésy found that a hole at one point in the membrane had little effect on the response at other points.

24.2.4 Two-Dimensional Model

The pioneering work with 2D fluid motion was begun in 1931 by Ranke, as reported in Ranke (1950) and discussed by Siebert (1974). Analysis of 2D and 3D fluid motion without the *a priori* assumption of long or short wavelengths and for physical values of all parameters is discussed by Steele (1987). The first of the two major benefits derived from the 2D model is the allowance of short-wavelength behavior, that is, the variation in fluid displacement and pressure in the duct height direction. Localized fluid motion near the elastic partition generally occurs near the point of maximum amplitude and the exact value of A becomes immaterial. The second major benefit of a 2D model is the admission of a stiffness-dominated elastic partition (i.e., massless) that better approximates the physiological properties of the BM. The two benefits together address all the objections the 1D model discussed previously. 2D models start with the Navier–Stokes and continuity equations governing the fluid motion, and an anisotropic plate equation governing the elastic partition motion. The displacement potential φ for the incompressible and inviscid fluid must satisfy Laplace's equation:

$$\varphi_{,xx} + \varphi_{,zz} = 0 \tag{24.8}$$

where x is the distance along the partition, z is the distance perpendicular to the partition, and the subscripts with commas denote partial derivatives. The displacement components and pressure are

$$u = \varphi_{,x} \quad w = \varphi_{,z} \quad p = \rho\omega^2\varphi \tag{24.9}$$

The traveling wave solution is assumed in the WKB form:

$$\varphi(x,z,t) \approx \Psi(x)\frac{\cosh n(z-H)}{-n\sinh nH}e^{i\theta} \quad \theta = \omega t - \int_0^x n(x)\,dx \tag{24.10}$$

where θ is the phase, n is the local wave number, Ψ is the "amplitude" function, and H is the height of the fluid chamber. We use the method of Whitham (Jimenez and Whitham 1976) to obtain the wave number and amplitude function, which has been used on the cochlea (e.g., Taber and Steele 1979, Yoon et al. 2009). Lagrangean density is the difference in the kinetic and potential energy densities:

$$\Lambda = T - V = \rho b\int_0^H (\varphi_{,x}^2 + \varphi_{,z}^2)\,dz - \frac{1}{2}k(bw)^2 \tag{24.11}$$

The kinetic energy is doubled for fluid on both sides of the BM. With the assumed form of Equation 24.10, the time-averaged value becomes

$$\Lambda = \Psi^2(x)F(n,x) \quad F(n,x) = \frac{b}{2}\left(\frac{2\rho\omega^2}{n\tanh nH} - kb\right) \tag{24.12}$$

Then the variational problem yields the Euler equations:

$$\frac{\partial\Lambda}{\partial\Psi} = 0 \tag{24.13}$$

The solution of Equation 24.13 is just

$$F(n,x) = \frac{b}{2}\left(\frac{2\rho\omega^2}{n\tanh nH} - kb\right) = 0 \tag{24.14}$$

which is the eikonal equation, or local dispersion relation. The second Euler equation is

$$\left(\frac{\partial\Lambda}{\partial\theta_{,x}}\right)_{,x} = 0 \tag{24.15}$$

which gives the relation for the amplitude function Ψ:

$$\Psi^2(x)F_{,n}(n,x) = \text{constant} \tag{24.16}$$

For a given frequency, Equation 24.14 must be solved numerically for the wave number n at each point x. The stiffness k, height of the fluid chamber H, and width of the BM b all vary slowly with the distance x. For physiological values of the parameters, the stiffness is large at the stapes $x = 0$, and becomes small toward the apex. Consequently, the wave number is small at the stapes (long wavelength) and becomes large (i.e., short wavelength) as x increases. For small values of the wave number $nH = 1$, the results, Equations 24.14 and 24.16, reduce to the 1D problem, Equation 24.4.

24.2.4.1 Fluid Viscosity

The fluid viscosity is important. There is a viscous boundary layer that is generally smaller than the width of the BM. Taking this into account yields the modified eikonal equation:

$$F(n,x) = \frac{b}{2}\left(\frac{2\rho\omega^2}{n\left[\tanh nH - (1 + (i\omega\rho/\mu n^2))^{-1/2}\right]} - kb\right) = 0 \tag{24.17}$$

where μ is the fluid viscosity. The viscous term produces a small imaginary part of the wave number. This has little effect in the long wavelength region and the location of the peak amplitude, but causes a rapid decrease of the wave amplitude past the peak.

24.2.5 Three-Dimensional Model

A further improvement in the agreement with experimental models can be obtained by adding the component of fluid motion in the direction across the membrane for a full 3D model. The importance

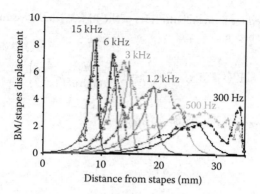

FIGURE 24.4 Comparison of 3D model calculations (solid curves) with experimental results of Zhou et al. (1994) (dashed curves) for the amplitude envelopes for different frequencies. This is the first life-sized model, but with an isotropic BM and fluid viscosity 28 times that of water. The agreement is reasonable for the higher frequencies but rough for the lower frequencies.

of the third dimension is discussed by Kolston (2000). The solution by direct numerical means is computationally intensive, and was first carried out by Raftenberg (1990), who reports a portion of his results for the fluid motion around the organ of Corti. Böhnke et al. (1996) used FE for the most accurate description to date of the structure of the organ of Corti. However, the fluid is not included and only a restricted segment of the cochlea is considered. Both the inviscid fluid and the details of the structure are considered with a simplified element description and simplified geometry by Kolston and Ashmore (1996). Today, a number of laboratories have the capability for treating the actual geometry obtained from micro-CT scans such as shown in Figure 24.1. However, the viscosity of the fluid is not considered, which reduces the computing time with standard FE programs to a reasonable value. Givelberg and Bunn (2003) provide the first numerical solution for a coiled box model with viscous fluid, using forward integration in time. Cheng et al. (2008) use a modified FE approach for the straight box model also with viscous fluid. Computer times are given in hours for the linear response for a single frequency.

An efficient approach for computing the 3D viscous fluid motion is offered by the asymptotic WKB solution, which yields results for computer times of 1 s per frequency. The procedure is the same as for the 2D analysis, except that 10–40 harmonics of motion in the y-direction in Figure 24.2 are added. The best verification of the mathematical model and calculation procedure comes from comparison with measurements in experimental models for which the parameters are known (Taber and Steele 1979). Zhou et al. (1994) provide the first life-sized experimental model, designed to be similar to the human cochlea, but with a fluid viscosity 28 times that of water to facilitate optical imaging. Results are shown in Figures 24.4 and 24.5. An improved life-sized model is by White and Grosh (2005), which has fluid on one side of the BM. Fluid is on both sides of the life-sized model by Wittbrodt et al. (2006), and a good agreement was found between the WKB calculation and the experimental measurements. In that model, polyimide is used for the BM, with a layer of 9000 transverse aluminum ribs to achieve a semblance of the orthotropic construction of the actual BM.

As shown by Taber and Steele (1979), the 3D fluid motion has a significant effect on the pressure distribution. This is confirmed by the measurements by Olson (1998) for the pressure at different depths in the cochlea, which show a substantial increase near the partition.

24.3 Active Process

Before around 1980, it was thought that the processing may have two levels. Initially, the BM and the fluid provide the correct place for a given frequency (a purely mechanical "first filter"). Subsequently, the

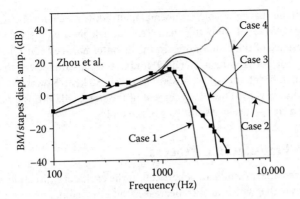

FIGURE 24.5 Comparison of 3D model calculations with experimental results of Zhou et al. (1994) for amplitude at the place $x = 19$ mm as a function of frequency. The scales are logarithmic (20 dB is a factor of 10 in amplitude). Case 1 shows a direct comparison with the physical parameters of the experiment, with isotropic BM and viscosity 28 times that of water. Case 2 is computed for the viscosity reduced to that of water. Case 3 is computed for the BM made of transverse fibers. Case 4 shows the effect of active OHC feed-forward, with the pressure gain $\alpha = 0.21$ and feed-forward distance $\Delta x = 25$ μm. Thus, lower viscosity, BM orthotropy, and active feed-forward all contribute to higher amplitude and increased localization of the response.

micromechanics and electrochemistry in the organ of Corti, with possible neural interactions, perform a further sharpening (a physiologically vulnerable "second filter").

A hint that the two-filter concept had difficulties was in the measurements of Rhode (1971), who found significant nonlinear behavior of the BM in the region of the maximum amplitude at moderate amplitudes of tone intensity. Passive models cannot explain this, since the usual mechanical nonlinearities are significant only at very high intensities, that is, at the threshold of pain. Russell and Sellick (1977) made the first *in vivo* mammalian intracellular hair cell recordings and found that the cells are as sharply tuned as the nerve fibers. Subsequently, improved measurement techniques in several laboratories found that the BM is actually as sharply tuned as the hair cells and the nerve fibers. Thus, the sharp tuning occurs at the BM. No passive cochlear model, even with physically unreasonable parameters, has yielded amplitude and phase response similar to such measurements. Measurements in a damaged or dead cochlea show a response similar to that of a passive model. Further evidence for an active process comes from Kemp (1978), who discovered that sound pulses into the ear caused echoes coming from the cochlea at delay times corresponding to the travel time to the place for the frequency and back. Spontaneous emission of sound energy from the cochlea has now been measured in the external ear canal in all vertebrates (Probst 1990). Some of the emissions can be related to the hearing disability of tinnitus (ringing in the ear). The conclusion drawn from these discoveries is that normal hearing involves an active process in which the energy of the input sound is greatly enhanced. A widely accepted concept is that spontaneous emission of sound energy occurs when the local amplifiers are not functioning properly and enter some sort of limit cycle (Zweig and Shera 1995). However, there remains a doubt about the nature of this process (Allen and Neely 1992, Hudspeth 1989, Nobili et al. 1998).

24.3.1 Outer Hair Cell Electromotility

The hair cell is covered extensively elsewhere in this book. Here, we mention a few important points. Since the outer hair cells have sparse afferent innervation, they have long been suspected of serving a basic motor function, perhaps beating and driving the subtectorial membrane fluid. Nevertheless, it was surprising when Brownell et al. (1985) found that the outer hair cells have *electromotility*: The cell expands and contracts in an oscillating electric field, either extra- or intracellular. The electromotility exists at frequencies far higher than possible for normal contractile mechanisms (Ashmore 1987). The sensitivity is about 20 nm/mV (about 10^5 better than PZT-2, a widely used piezoelectric ceramic). The motility is due to the presence of the protein prestin in the outer hair cell (OHC) plasma membrane, and found nowhere else in the body. Frank et al. (1999) find in the constrained cell that the ratio of axial force generation to transmembrane voltage is constant to nearly 80 kHz. However, it is established that the intracellular voltage change due to the displacement of the stereocilia drops off at a low frequency. Ashmore (2008) provides a comprehensive summary of the topic.

24.3.2 Hair Bundle Transduction Process

A displacement of the stereociliary bundle on a hair cell in the excitatory direction causes an opening of ion channels in the stereocilia, which in turn decreases the intracellular potential. This depolarization causes neural excitation, and in the piezoelectric OHC, a decrease of the cell length. However, in nonmammalian vertebrates, there is no prestin and no electromotility of hair cells. Furthermore, it is well established that the hair bundle can go into spontaneous oscillation. Thus, the resonance of the hair bundle itself can supply energy into the motion. This enhances the reception for sounds of low amplitude. Spontaneous and evoked emissions are similar in character to those from mammalian ears.

Schwander et al. (2010) survey the recent advances in understanding the hair bundle particularly related to the genes linked to deafness. They suggest that both hair bundle motility and somatic electromotility may be needed for mammalian hearing. From a different perspective, Peng and Ricci (2010) also come to this conclusion. It is clear from Dallos et al. (2008) that prestin, which causes the OHC motility, is necessary for normal mammalian hearing. How this operates for high frequencies has been the subject of numerous investigations, including the consideration of the extracellular electrical field by Dallos and Evans (1995), and theoretical treatment of detail of the stereocilia by consideration of Breneman et al. (2009).

24.4 Active Models

De Boer (1991), Geisler (1993), and Hubbard (1993) discuss models in which the electromotility of the outer hair cells feeds energy into the BM. The partition stiffness K is expanded from Equation 24.3 into a transfer function, containing a number of parameters and delay times. These are classed as phenomenological models, for which the physiological basis of the parameters is not of primary concern. The displacement gain may be defined as the ratio of stereociliary shearing displacement to cell expansion. For these models, the gain used is larger by orders of magnitude than the maximum found in laboratory measurements of isolated hair cells.

24.4.1 Push-Forward/Pull-Backward Active Model

Another approach (Steele et al. 1993, Geisler and Sang 1995) appears promising. Because of the inclinations, the OHC, the phalangeal process (PhP), and the reticular lamina form a stiff triangular structure, connected to the BM by Deiters rod (D), as seen in Figure 24.6a. As indicated in Figure 24.6b, a downward force on the BM at the distance x from the stapes causes a shear on the stereocilia at that point. Through the transduction process, the OHC expands, but because of the inclination of the OHC, the push down on the BM occurs at the distance $x + \Delta x_1$. This is the "push-forward" or the "positive feed-forward."

The force of OHC expansion is equal and opposite at the cell ends. The cantilever arrangement of the reticular lamina and the tectorial membrane provides little resistance to this upward force. All that remains to carry this force is the upper end of the PhP. In Figure 24.6b, the shear of the OHC at $x + \Delta x_2$ causes a tension in the PhP connected at that point and an upward force on D located at $x + \Delta x_1$. This is the "pull-backward" or the "negative feed backward." So, the expansion of an OHC causes the push down at the distance Δx_1 in the forward (apical) direction and a pull up at the distance $\Delta x_2 - \Delta x_1$ in the

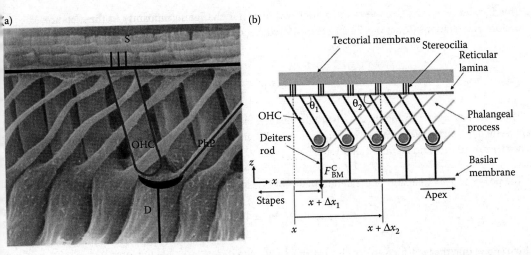

FIGURE 24.6 Scanning electron micrograph (SEM) of the longitudinal view of organ of Corti of the mole rat cochlea (Raphael et al. 1991). Outer hair cell, Deiters cell, phalangeal process, and stereocilia are labeled as OHC, D, PhP, and S, respectively (a). Schematic of the longitudinal view of the organ of Corti (b), showing the tilt of the outer hair cells (OHC) based on SEM image. For one hair cell whose apex lies at a distance x, the base is located at distance $x + \Delta x_1$, while the phalangeal process connected to the base of the hair cell is attached to the upper surface of the reticular lamina at $x + \Delta x_2$. θ_1: the OHC angle with respect to reticular lamina, θ_2: the phalangeal process angle with respect to the reticular laminar. The force on the BM through the Deiters rod is F_{BM}^C, which consists of the downward push due to an expansion of the hair cell at x and an upward pull through the phalangeal process due to an expansion of the hair cell at $x + \Delta x_2$.

backward (basal) direction. There is also a ripple effect, extending in both directions, but we consider only the primary push and pull. Of course, for the response for a given frequency, all the quantities vary sinusoidally, so we refer to this as feed-forward/backward.

The total force acting on the BM (F_{BM}) is twice the fluid force (F_{BM}^f), for fluid on both sides of the BM, plus the OHC force acting through the Deiters rods F_{BM}^C.

$$F_{BM} = 2F_{BM}^f + F_{BM}^C \tag{24.18}$$

The fluid force is the same as for the 3D passive box model. For small amplitudes, the transduction and OHC motility are linear, so the cell force is proportional to the total force on the BM. Thus, the cell force acting on the BM at the point $x + \Delta x_1$ in Figure 24.6b depends on the total force on the BM at x and the total force acting on the BM at $x + \Delta x_2$, as expressed by the difference equation:

$$F_{BM}^C(x + \Delta x_1, t) = \alpha\left[F_{BM}(x,t)\right] - \alpha_2\left[F_{BM}(x + \Delta x_2, t)\right] \tag{24.19}$$

The constants of proportionality or "gains" from the OHC push and the PhP pull are α_1 and α_2, respectively. The details of OC compliance, OHC transduction, and motility are all lumped into the gains. Because of the small resistance to the vertical force of the reticular lamina and tectorial membrane, the net push and pull must be equal, so $\alpha_1 = \alpha_2 = \alpha$.

With the WKB approximation, all quantities are in the form of an exponential multiplied by a slowly varying function (Equation 24.10). Therefore, the spatial difference can be approximated as

$$F_{BM}^C(x + \Delta x_1, t) = F_{BM}^C(x,t)e^{-in\Delta x_1} \tag{24.20}$$

This is valid when the (complex) wavenumber n does not change significantly in the distance Δx_1. Therefore, the relations Equations 24.18 and 24.19 reduce to

$$F_{BM} = 2F_{BM}^f + F_{BM}^C = \frac{2F_{BM}^f}{1 - \alpha_1 e^{in\Delta x_1} + \alpha_2 e^{-in(\Delta x_2 - \Delta x_1)}} \qquad (24.21)$$

Thus, the box model in Figure 24.2 is used, with the elaborate OC shown in Figures 24.3 and 24.6 represented by the simple terms in the denominator of Equation 24.21. This denominator multiplies the denominator of the fluid term in Equation 24.17 for the 2D model and the equivalent for the 1D or 3D models.

The power series expansion of the denominator of Equation 24.21 is

$$1 - \alpha e^{in\Delta x_1} + \alpha e^{-in(\Delta x_2 - \Delta x_1)} = 1 - \alpha in\Delta x_2 + \cdots \qquad (24.22)$$

which shows that the feed-forward/backward effect is negligible for long wavelengths, when $n\Delta x_2$ is very small. Since the fluid loading in Equation 24.17 is primarily mass-like, the first effect for shorter wavelength in Equation 24.22 is negative damping. For a reversed traveling wave, with n negative, the effect is an increase in the damping.

The full behavior is not transparent from Equation 24.21 but can be seen from the numerical results. For modest values of the gain, $\alpha < 0.2$, the real part of n, which gives the phase, is little affected by the push–pull terms. The imaginary part of n can be substantially modified. Generally, it is determined by the viscosity of the fluid and causes the rapid decrease in amplitude in the region past the maximum response. However, the push–pull terms of Equation 24.21 can overcome the viscosity effect and a region near "best frequency" (BF), where the sign of the imaginary part of n is reversed, that is, a region of "negative damping." Apically, the fluid viscosity resumes dominance and the amplitude decreases exponentially. So, for a given frequency, the push–pull is negligible for a long wavelength (small n) and a very short wavelength (large n) but very significant for a band of wavelengths near BF.

The feed-forward/backward model for the OC involves just the three parameters. Reasonable values for the distances Δx_1 and Δx_2 are used, while the gain α is adjusted for a best fit with the experiments.

The comparison of the 3D calculations and measurements for the (passive) life-sized model in the configuration of Figure 24.2 are shown in Figure 24.4. Various modifications are shown in Figure 24.5 for the frequency response at a particular point. Case 1 is for the experimental situation of an isotropic BM and high fluid viscosity. In Case 2, the viscosity is reduced to that of water, which causes a shift of the peak response to a higher frequency and an increase in peak amplitude. Case 3 shows the effect of reducing the longitudinal stiffness of the BM to zero, corresponding to the transverse fibers in the actual cochlea. The peak amplitude and location do not change, but the high-frequency roll-off is substantially sharper. Finally, Case 4 shows the effect of adding just the feed-forward term of Equation 24.20. The peak amplitude increases by an order of magnitude and the location shifts by an octave, but the high-frequency roll-off remains the same.

A comparison with measurements in the chinchilla cochlea is shown in Figure 24.7, modified from Narayan et al. (1998). In the box model representation of Figure 24.2, the BM properties of width, thickness, elastic modulus, and fiber volume fraction are taken as close as possible to the actual values for the BM pectinate zone. In Figure 24.7a, the amplitude of the BM velocity is normalized to the stapes velocity. So, for a linear system, the response would be independent of input amplitude. Instead, the measured response for a low sound pressure of 20 dB is greater than that for a high sound pressure of 80 dB by two orders of magnitude. This amplification occurs in a narrow frequency band near BF and is due to the active process. When the animal dies, the passive response is close to that for 80 dB. Thus, the active process greatly enhances the response for low sound intensity and is negligible for high intensity. The 3D model results are also shown in Figure 24.7, calculated with values shown in Table 24.3. The simple

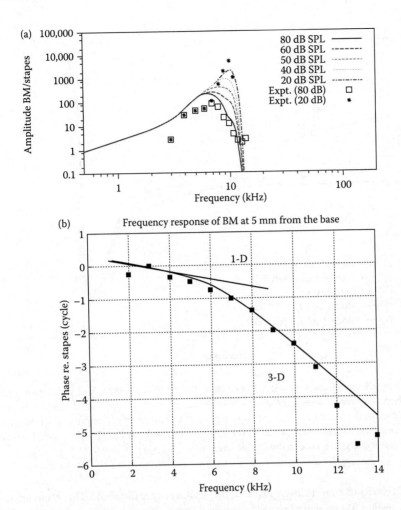

FIGURE 24.7 Experiments in chinchilla (Ruggero et al. 1997) and computed with 3D model (Lim and Steele 2002, modified by Yoon). (a) Amplitude of BM displacement and (b) phase response. The amplitude is normalized to the stapes displacement. Experimental points are shown for 20 and 80 dB SPL. The active process increases the relative amplitude for low-input sound levels.

TABLE 24.3 Properties for Chinchilla Cochlea

Length of the cochlea (mm)	18	Fiber volume fraction (%)	3~0.7
Stapes footplate area (mm²)	0.7	OHC angle (θ_1)	75°
SV area (mm²) (base to apex)	0.6–0.2	Phalangeal process angle (θ_2)	22°
Length of outer hair cell (μm)	25–65	Gain factor (α) for 20 dB SPL	0.11
BM width (mm)	0.15–0.48	Distance from the stapes (x^*) in mm	4
BM thickness (μm)	3–1	Passive best frequency (BF)	7 kHz

push–pull approximation in Equation 24.21 does well in simulating the measurements. The gain varies from 0 for the high intensity to 0.11 for 20 dB. Both the push and the pull are included, which gives a shift of about half an octave of the passive peak to the active, similar to the measurements.

The question remains about how the motion of the BM is transferred to the excitation of the IHC. A remarkable result is by Narayan et al. (1998), who measured the auditory nerve fiber threshold and the BM response in one animal. From the BM measurements, they then determined the fixed amplitude of BM

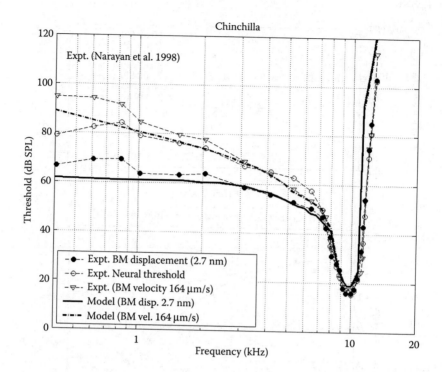

FIGURE 24.8 Comparisons of auditory nerve fiber neural threshold with BM velocity and displacement for chinchilla. The threshold curve for one fiber (open circles connected by a thin solid line) is compared to constant-amplitude BM displacement and velocity reponses as measured in one animal by Narayan et al. (1998). The calculations for the displacement and velocity response of the feed-forward/backward model (thick solid lines and thick dash-dotted lines, respectively) are close to the measurements.

displacement and velocity that most closely matched the auditory nerve threshold. The results are shown in Figure 24.8. The constant BM velocity is close to the neural threshold. Added to Figure 24.8 are the results from the 3D model calculation for constant BM displacement and velocity, which are in good agreement with the measurements. Since the stereocilia of the IHC in Figure 24.3 are not attached to the overlying tectorial membrane, the cells must be excited by the fluid motion. The drag force is due to the fluid velocity. Thus, it is not surprising that there is a better relation of BM velocity, rather than displacement, to neural excitation. In fact, the situation is more complicated. Legan et al. (2005) found that in a mouse mutant, the OHC arrangement is perfectly normal, giving sharp tuning of the BM and normal emissions. The neural threshold is, however, elevated by 60 dB. In this mutant, only the tectorial membrane appears to be altered. In particular, the Hensen stripe that is located near the stereocilia of the IHC is missing. In addition, the outer margin of the tectorial membrane is also missing. Therefore, the proper arrangement of the tectorial membrane is necessary to deliver the proper excitation to the IHC. Steele and Puria (2005) find that the phase of IHC excitation depends on the details of stiffness and geometry of the tectorial membrane.

The significant nonlinear effect is the saturation of the active process at high amplitudes. In Figures 24.7 and 24.8, this is taken into account by letting the gain be a function of the input sound level. It is more realistic to have the gain be a function of the amplitude of the force during the cycle of motion, which introduces substantial nonlinearity (Lim and Steele 2002, 2003). This produces two-tone interaction, the generation of combination tones, and the ringing from a click excitation, all from the simple feed-forward/backward approximation of Equation 24.19. A variety of alternate considerations for the active nonlinear behavior have been proposed. In particular, Dierkes et al. (2008) show that an array of hair cell bundles can provide a substantial sharpening of the response.

24.4.2 Summary of Some Issues

Rapid development in the measurement and computational technique related to auditory biomechanics is ongoing. The following are a few of the open issues.

24.4.2.1 Bone Conduction

Hearing by bone conduction is of high clinical significance. There are many measurements showing that the volume displacements of oval and RW are exactly out of phase for air-conducted acoustic excitation. Because the fluid is nearly incompressible and the walls are stiff bone, the input inward displacement of the stapes in Figure 24.2 will cause a nearly equal volume outward displacement of the RW. All existing theories assume that this is also the case for bone-conducted sound. As shown by Békésy (1960) in models, any sort of excitation, whether through the stapes or through shaking the entire cochlea, will cause the same traveling wave. However, measurements by Stenfeld et al. (2004) indicate that this is not the case for bone conduction. Indeed, for some frequencies, the two windows are in phase. Thus, there must be compliance in the cochlea not yet explained (often referred to as a "third window") that for some reason is more significant for bone conduction.

24.4.3 Traveling Wave

The traveling wave observed in the cochlea by Békésy (1960) was not anticipated by any theoretical consideration. There remain contrary opinions, for example, Sohmer and Freeman (2004) consider their measurements as evidence against the significance of any traveling wave. The traveling wave does not occur in lizards and turtles, but most likely occurs in bird. For mammals, the evidence for the existence and importance of the traveling wave seems overwhelming. We mention the direct *in vivo* observation of waves by Ren (2002), the close relation of BM displacement and neural excitation found in the same animal by Narayan et al. (1998), and the agreement in calculations for the traveling wave and experiment for the BM motion (Figure 24.8). This issue should be at an end.

24.4.4 Motility versus Beating

In nonmammalian hearing organs, there are no pillars, Deiters cells, or inner sulcus as shown in Figure 24.3. Furthermore, the cells similar to OHCs cannot have somatic motility. Nevertheless, in the responsive frequency range, the neural tuning is as sharp as in mammals, and evoked and spontaneous emissions occur very similar to those in mammals (Manley 2006). Crawford and Fettiplace (1985) discovered that the cilia on turtle hair cells have spontaneous activity, that is, they beat without external excitation. This mechanotransducer (MET) channel phenomenon is described as a Hopf bifurcation. In all vertebrates, the cilia and transduction channels are similar. Is the energy of the active process generated by MET instability or somatic motility of the cell, or is it a combination? This is a subject of current investigation. The consensus seems to be building that both are needed for mammalian hearing (Peng and Ricci 2010, Schwander et al. 2010).

24.4.5 OHC Roll-Off

The feed-forward/backward discussed here depends on the force of motility of the OHC to be independent of frequency. However, the electrical properties of the OHC appear to be such that for a fixed amplitude of shear force on the cilia, there is a significant decrease in the intracellular potential at a frequency much less than BF. Several laboratories propose more detailed analysis of intracellular or extracellular behavior that would maintain the effect of the motility for high frequency. Dallos and Evans (1995) find that the extracellular electric field can enhance the motility for high frequency. Another consideration is the stiffness of the OHC, which Zheng et al. (2007) show plays a role. In any case, it is clear that the motility operates at high frequency. Frank et al. (1999) show that the constrained isolated OHC generates force proportional to the transmembrane voltage well past 80 kHz. Grosh et al. (2004) find in the intact guinea pig cochlea, which has an upper limit of hearing of 50 kHz, that mechanical response can be elicited by electrical signals up to 100 kHz. Dallos (2008) provides an overall perspective.

24.4.6 Tectorial Membrane Properties: Resonance?

Many authors have used OC models with a strong resonance of the tectorial membrane (TM), for example, Gummer et al. (1996). It has the effect of overcoming the OHC low-frequency roll-off problem. Several laboratories have measured the properties of the TM, including Gueta et al. (2006), Masaki et al. (2006), and Gavara and Chadwick (2009). Details are different, but the general conclusion is that the TM is a rather soft tissue, with an elastic Young's modulus in the range of 0.5–30 kPa. Different animals have a great difference in TM size. Such a difference for animals that have roughly the same frequency range makes a resonant TM seem to be an unlikely key feature. Nowotny and Gummer (2006) measure the TM response due to electrical stimulation and find no resonance for frequencies well past BF. So, there are indications that the TM does not have a strong resonance.

24.4.7 Multiple Traveling Wave Modes

The box model Figure 24.2 has the traveling wave. In addition, there is a symmetric wave with equal pressure in the fluid regions. Consequently, there is no loading of the BM, so this wave travels with the speed of sound in water. Peterson and Bogert (1950) first formulated the split of the response into the symmetric "fast" wave and asymmetric "slow" wave. The measurements of Olson (1998) confirm the presence of the slow traveling wave and the fast pressure wave in the cochlea. In the cochlea, each of the fluid spaces in the organ of Corti (Figure 24.3) can support an independent wave. Karavitaki (2002) offers measurements of motion of the fluid in the OC that support the notion of multiple waves. As discussed by de Boer (2006), recent models, for example, Mountain and Hubbard (2006), have such capability. The goal remains for a model of the OC with physically realistic geometric and stiffness properties and with 3D viscous fluid, which can simulate the environment of the cilia for all frequencies. The expectation is that additional waves in the inner sulcus (IS) and the fluid spaces of the organ of Corti do play a significant role.

24.4.8 Stiffness Change along the Cochlea

Almost every component of the cochlear cross section has been proposed at one time or another as the fundamental resonance element. Most probably agree with Békésy (1960) that the BM has the strongest stiffness gradient and is the most likely candidate. Modest variation in values of width, thickness, and fiber volume fraction of the pectinate zone work together to explain the frequency range of the Guinea Pig (GP) cochlea. The change in the volume stiffness is five orders of magnitude. The direct measurement of the GP cochlea by Békésy (1960) shows a change of three orders of magnitude, with a reasonable extrapolation to four orders of magnitude. However, Naidu and Mountain (1998) find that the point load stiffness variation is totally inadequate to explain the frequency range in gerbil. With a different preparation, Emadi et al. (2004) find much more compliance in the apical region, which seems to correspond to a reasonable frequency range. This discrepancy in the measurements from the two laboratories has not yet been explained. The gerbil has a very specialized BM. Generally, in mammals, the pectinate zone of the BM in Figure 24.3 consists of two parallel layers of collagen fibers. For gerbil, however, the lower layer is in the form of an arch. It appears that the stiffness measured by both laboratories is in the postbuckling range of this arch. The conclusion is that the soft cells covering the BM make point load or volume compliance measurements difficult to make and interpret. As is often the case, a combination of theoretical mechanics and experimental approaches is needed.

24.5 Concluding Comments

The cochlea (Figure 24.1) is a complex organ with a remarkable capability for the transduction of the input mechanical sound pressure into electrical activity of the auditory nerve fibers. The simple box model (Figure 24.2) represents the passive behavior of the cochlea. Experimental models and 3D calculations based on the physiological values for tissue properties and geometry do well in showing the development of the main traveling wave. The peak of this wave for a particular frequency corresponds to the place of most significant neural excitation. Discrete resonators have the disadvantage that low damping is required for sharp tuning, but high damping is required for quick onset and offset. In contrast, the fluid-elastic behavior of the box in Figure 24.2 provides high frequency selectivity with excellent transient response. A click as well as the onset and offset of a pure tone cause a wave that propagates along the BM with little refection from the far end. So, the basic features of localization and timing are described well by the fluid-elastic response of the box model. A variety of approximations and solution methods have been used. The focus here is on the WKB approach, which is the most efficient method for dealing with the 3D fluid-elastic interaction and has been verified by comparison with experimental models.

Adding to the passive behavior is the active process, which greatly improves the reception of low-intensity sounds for all creatures, including insects. For the mammalian cochlea, this increases the amplitude of response by two orders of magnitude and increases the sharpness of response, without having a big effect on the localization and the phase. In general consideration of dynamic systems, this may seem impossible. A key is the electromotility of the outer hair cells, which can be interpreted as a piezoelectric property of the cell plasma membrane. The active process has been the subject of intense research activity for the last 30 years. A variety of approaches have been developed to explain this phenomenon. The focus here is on the simplest model, based on the geometry of the sensory organ of Corti. This provides a spatial finite difference relation and is referred to as feed-forward/backward. This is not the same as a time delay, and provides a significant input of energy into the traveling wave without disrupting the stability. The rather complex features of the sensory organ make sense with the feed-forward/backward. However, the calculation assumes that the motility persists to frequencies at least for that of the place. How this might occur has not been resolved. Consequently, many consider that the motility may work in combination with the resonance features of the hair bundle. We anticipate that these issues may not be resolved soon.

References

Allen JB and Neely ST. 1992. Micromechanical models of the cochlea. *Phys Today* 45:40–47.

Ashmore J. 2008. Cochlear outer hair cell motility. *Physiol Rev* 88:173–210.

Ashmore JF. 1987. A fast motile response in guinea-pig outer hair cells: The cellular basis of the cochlear amplifier. *J Physiol* 388:323–347.

Békésy G von. 1960. *Experiments in Hearing*. McGraw-Hill, New York.

Böhnke F and Arnold W. 1999. 3D-finite element model of the human Cochlea including fluid-structure couplings. *ORL* 61(5):305–310.

Böhnke F, von Mikusch-Buchberg J, and Arnold W. 1996. 3D finite elemente modell des cochleären Verstärkers. *Biomedizinische Technik* 42:311–312.

Breneman KD, Brownell WE, and Rabbitt RD. 2009. Hair cell bundles: Flexoelectric motors of the inner ear. *PLoS ONE* 4(4):e5201.

Brownell WE, Bader CR, Bertrand D, and de Ribaupierre Y. 1985. Evoked mechanical responses of isolated cochlear outer hair cells. *Science* 227:194–196.

Cabezudo LM. 1978. The ultrastructure of the basilar membrane in the cat. *Acta Otolaryngol* 86:160–175.

Cheng L, White RD, and Grosh K. 2008. Three-dimensional viscous finite element formulation for acoustic fluid–structure interaction. *Comput Methods Appl Mech Eng* 197(49–50):4160–4172.

Crawford AC and Fettiplace R. 1985. The mechanical properties of ciliary bundles of turtle cochlear hair cells. *J Physiol* 364:359–79.

Dallos P. 1992. The active cochlea. *J Neurosci* 12(12):4575–4585.

Dallos P. 2008. Cochlear amplification, outer hair cells and prestin. *Curr Opin Neurobiol* 18(4):370–376.

Dallos P and Evans B. 1995. High-frequency motility of outer hair cells and the cochlear amplifier. *Science* 267:2006–2009.

Dallos P, Wu X, Cheatham MA, Gao J, Zheng J, Anderson CT, Jia S et al. 2008. Prestin-based outer hair cell motility is necessary for Mammalian cochlear amplification. *Neuron* 58(3):333–339.

de Boer E. 1991. Auditory physics. Physical principles in hearing theory. III. *Phys Rep* 203(3):126–231.

de Boer E. 2006. Cochlear activity in perspective. *Auditory Mechanisms, Processes and Models*, Eds. AL Nuttall, T Ren, P Gillespie, K Grosh, and E de Boer, World Scientific, New Jersey, pp. 393–409.

Dierkes K, Lindner B, and Jülicher F. 2008. Enhancement of sensitivity gain and frequency tuning by coupling of active hair bundles. *Proc Natl Acad Sci USA* 105(48):18669–18674.

Emadi G, Richter CP, and Dallos P. 2004. Stiffness of the gerbil basilar membrane: Radial and longitudinal variations. *J Neurophysiol* 91(1):474–488.

Evans BN and Dallos P. 1993. Stereocilia displacement induced somatic motility of cochlear outer hair cells. *Proc Natl Acad Sci* 90:8347–8391.

Frank G, Hemmert W, and Gummer AW. 1999. Limiting dynamics of high-frequency electromechanical transduction of outer hair cells. *Proc Natl Acad Sci USA* 96(8):4420–4425.

Freeman DM and Weiss TF. 1990. Hydrodynamic analysis of a two-dimensional model for micromechanical resonance of free-standing hair bundles. *Hear Res* 48:37–68.

Fuhrmann E, Schneider W, and Schultz M. 1987. Wave propagation in the cochlea (inner ear): Effects of Reissner's membrane and non-rectangular cross section. *Acta Mech* 70:15–30.

Gavara N and Chadwick RS 2009. Collagen-based mechanical anisotropy of the tectorial membrane: Implications for inter-row coupling of outer hair cell bundles. *PLoS ONE* 4(3):e4877.

Geisler CD. 1993. A realizable cochlear model using feedback from motile outer hair cells. *Hear Res* 68:253–262.

Geisler CD. 1998. *From Sound to Synapse: Physiology of the Mammalian Ear*. Oxford University Press, New York.

Geisler CD and C. Sang 1995. A cochlear model using feed-forword outer-hair-cell forces. *Hear Res* 85:132–146.

Givelberg E and Bunn J. 2003. A comprehensive three-dimensional model of the cochlea. *J Comput Phys* 191(2):377–391.

Grosh K, Zheng J, and Zou Y. 2004. High-frequency electromotile responses in the cochlea. *J Acoust Soc Am* 115(5):2178–2184.

Gueta R, Barlam D, Shneck RZ, and Rousso I. 2006. Measurement of the mechanical properties of isolated tectorial membrane using atomic force microscopy. *Proc Natl Acad Sci USA* 103(40):14790–14795.

Gulick WL, Gescheider GA, and Fresina RD 1989. *Hearing: Physiological Acoustics, Neural Coding, and Psychoacoustics*. Oxford University Press, London.

Gummer AW, Hemmert W, and Zenner HP. 1996. Resonant tectorial membrane motion in the inner ear: Its crucial role in frequency tuning. *Proc Natl Acad Sci USA* 93:8727–8732.

Gummer AW, Johnston BM, and Armstrong NJ. 1981. Direct measurements of basilar membrane stiffness in the guinea pig. *J Acoust Soc Am* 70:1298–1309.

Hubbard AE. 1993. A traveling wave-amplifier model of the cochlea. *Science* 259:68–71.

Hudspeth AJ. 1989. How the ear's works work. *Nature* 34:397–404.

Jimenez J and Whitham GB. 1976. An averaged Lagrangian method for dissipative *wavetrains, Proc R Soc Lond A* 349(1658):277–287.

Keidel WD and Neff WD (eds). 1976. *Handbook of Sensory Physiology, Volume V: Auditory System*. Springer-Verlag, Berlin.

Kemp DT. 1978. Stimulated acoustic emissions from within the human auditory system. *J Acoust Soc Am* 64:1386–1391.

Kolston PJ. 2000. The importance of phase data and model dimensionality to cochlear mechanics. *Hear Res* 145(1–2):25–36.

Kolston PJ and Ashmore JF 1996. Finite element micromechanical modeling of the cochlea in three dimensions. *J Acoust Soc Am* 99:455–467.

Karavitaki KD. 2002. Measurements and models of electrically-evoked motion in the gerbil organ of Corti. Boston University. PhD. Thesis.

Legan PK, Lukashkina VA, Goodyear RJ, Lukashkin AN, Verhoeven K, Van Camp G, Russell IJ, and Richardson GP. 2005. A deafness mutation isolates a second role for the tectorial membrane in hearing. *Nat Neurosci* 8(8):1035–1042.

Lighthill J. 1991. Biomechanics of hearing sensitivity. *J Vib Acoust* 113:1–13.

Lim KM and Steele CR. 2002. A three-dimensional nonlinear active cochlear model analyzed by the WKB-numeric method. *Hear Res* 170(1–2):190–205.

Lim KM and Steele CR. 2003. Response suppression and transient behavior in a nonlinear active cochlear model with feed-forward. *Int J Solids Struct* 40(19):5097–5107.

Manley GA. 2006. Spontaneous otoacoustic emissions from free-standing stereovillar bundles of ten species of lizard with small papillae. *Hear Res* 212(1–2):33–47.

Manoussaki D, Chadwick RS, Ketten DR, Arruda J, Dimitriadis EK, and O'Malley JT. 2008. The influence of cochlear shape on low-frequency hearing. *Proc Natl Acad Sci USA* 105(16):6162–6166.

Masaki K, Weiss TF, and Freeman DM. 2006. Poroelastic bulk properties of the tectorial membrane measured with osmotic stress. *Biophys J* 91(6):2356–2370.

Miller CE. 1985. Structural implications of basilar membrane compliance measurements. *J Acoust Soc Am* 77:1465–1474.

Mountain DC and Hubbard AE. 2006. What stimulates the inner hair cell? *Auditory Mechanisms, Processes and Models*, Eds. AL Nuttall, T Ren, P Gillespie, K Grosh, and E de Boer, World Scientific, New Jersey, pp. 466–473.

Naidu RC and Mountain DC. 1998. Measurements of the stiffness map challenge a basic tenet of cochlear theories. *Hear Res* 124:124–131.

Narayan SS, Temchin AN, Recio A, and Ruggero MA. 1998. Frequency tuning of basilar membrane and auditory nerve fibers in the same cochleae. *Science* 282(5395):1882–1884.

Nobili R, Mommano F, and Ashmore J. 1998. How well do we understand the cochlea? *TINS* 21(4):159–166.

Nowotny M and Gummer AW. 2006. Nanomechanics of the subtectorial space caused by electromechanics of cochlear outer hair cells. *Proc Natl Acad Sci USA* 103(7):2120–2125.

Olson ES. 1998. Observing middle and inner ear mechanics with novel intracochlear pressure sensors. *J Acoust Soc Am* 103(6):3445–3463.

Olson ES and Mountain DC. 1994. Mapping the cochlear partition's stiffness to its cellular architecture. *J Acoust Soc Am* 95(1):395–400.

Peng AW and Ricci AJ. 2010. Somatic motility and hair bundle mechanics, are both necessary for cochlear amplification? *Hear Res* 273(1–2):109–122.

Peterson LC and Bogert BP 1950. A dynamical theory of the Cochlea. *J Acoust Soc Am* 22(3):369–381.

Pickles JO. 1988. *An Introduction to the Physiology of Hearing*, 2nd ed. Academic Press, London.

Probst R. 1990. Otoacoustic emissions: An overview. *Adv Oto-Rhino-Laryngol* 44:1–91.

Raftenberg MN. 1990. Flow of endolymph in the inner spiral sulcus and the subtectorial space. *J Acoust Soc Am* 87(6):2606–2620.

Ranke OF. 1950. Theory of operation of the cochlea: A contribution to the hydrodynamics of the cochlea. *J Acoust Soc Am* 22:772–777.

Raphael Y, Lenoir M, Wroblewski R, and Pujol R. 1991. The sensory epithelium and its innervation in the mole rat cochlea. *J Comp Neurol* 314:367–382.

Ren T. 2002. Longitudinal pattern of basilar membrane vibration in the sensitive cochlea. *Proc Natl Acad Sci USA* 99(26):17101–17106.

Rhode WS. 1971. Observations of the vibration of the basilar membrane in squirrel monkeys using the Mössbauer technique. *J Acoust Soc Am* 49:1218–1231.

Ruggero MA. 1993. Distortion in those good vibrations. *Curr Biol* 3(11):755–758.

Ruggero MA, Narayan SS, Temchin AN and Recio A. 2000. Mechanical bases of frequency tuning and neural excitation at the base of the cochlea: Comparison of basilar-membrane vibrations and auditory-nerve-fiber responses in chinchilla. *Proc Natl Acad Sci USA* 97(22):11744–11750.

Ruggero MA, Rich NC, Recio A, Narayan SS, and Robles L. 1997. Basilar-membrane responses to tones at the base of the chinchilla cochlea. *J. Acoust. Soc. Am.* 101(4):2151–2163.

Russell IJ and Sellick PM. 1977. Tuning properties of cochlear hair cells. *Nature* 267:858–860.

Schwander M, Kachar B, and Müller U. 2010. The cell biology of hearing. *J Cell Biol* 190(1):9–20.

Siebert WM. 1974. Ranke revisited—A simple short-wave cochlear model. *J Acoust Soc Am* 56(2):594–600.

Sohmer H and Freeman S. 2004. Further evidence for a fluid pathway during bone conduction auditory stimulation. *Hear Res* 193(1–2):105–110.

Steele CR. 1987. Cochlear Mechanics. *Handbook of Bioengineering*, Eds. R Skalak and S Chien, pp. 30.11–30.22, McGraw-Hill, New York.

Steele CR, Baker G, Tolomeo JA, and Zetes DE. 1993. Electro-mechanical models of the outer hair cell, *Biophysics of Hair Cell Sensory Systems*. Eds. H Duifhuis, JW Horst, P van Dijk, and SM van Netten, World Scientific Press, Singapore, pp. 207–214.

Steele CR and Puria S. 2005. Force on inner hair cell cilia. *Int J Solids Struct* 42(21–22):5887–5904.

Stenfelt S, Hato N, and Goode RL. 2004. Fluid volume displacement at the oval and round windows with air and bone conduction stimulation. *J Acoust Soc Am* 115(2):797–812.

Strelioff D and Flock Å. 1984. Stiffness of sensory-cell hair bundles in the isolated guinea pig cochlea. *Hear Res* 15:19–28.

Taber LA and Steele CR. 1979. Comparison of 'WKB' and experimental results for three-dimensional cochlear models. *J Acoust Soc Am* 65:1007–1018.

Watts L. 1993. *Cochlear Mechanics: Analysis and Analog VLSI*. PhD Thesis, California Institute of Technology.

West CD. 1985. The relationship of the spiral turns of the cochlea and the length of the basilar membrane to the range of audible frequencies in ground dwelling mammals. *J Acoust Soc Am* 77(3):1091–1101.

White RD and Grosh K. 2005. Microengineered hydromechanical cochlear model. *Proc Natl Acad Sci USA* 102(5):1296–1301.

Wittbrodt MJ, Puria S, and Steele CR. 2006. Developing a physical model of the human cochlea using micro-fabrication methods. *Audiol Neurotol* 11:104–112.

Yoon YJ, Puris S, and Steele CR. 2009. A cochlear model using the time-averaged Lagrangean and the push-pull mechanism in the organ of Corti. *J Mechanics Mater Struct* 4(5):977–986.

Zheng J, Deo N, Zou Y, Grosh K, and Nuttall AL. 2007. Alters Cochlear mechanics and amplification: *In vivo* evidence for a role of stiffness modulation in the organ of Corti. *J Neurophysiol* 97:994–1004.

Zhou G, Bintz L, Anderson DZ, and Bright KE. 1994. A life-sized physical model of the human cochlea with optical holographic readout. *J Acoust Soc Am* 93(3):1516–1523.

Zweig G and Shera CA. 1995. The origin of periodicity in the spectrum of evoked otoacoustic emissions. *J Acoust Soc Am* 98(4):2018–2047.

Zwislocki JJ and Cefaratti LK. 1989. Tectorial membrane II: Stiffness measurements *in vivo*. *Hear Res* 42:211–227.

Further Information

The following are workshop proceedings that document many of the developments:

Allen JB, Hall JL, Hubbard A, Neely ST, and Tubis A. (eds). 1985. *Peripheral Auditory Mechanisms*. Springer, Berlin.

Cooper NP and Kemp DT (eds). 2008. *Concepts and Challenges in the Biophysics of Hearing.* World Scientific, Singapore.

Dallos P, Geisler CD, Matthews JW, Ruggero MA, and Steele CR (eds). 1990. *The Mechanics and Biophysics of Hearing.* Springer, Berlin.

De Boer E and Viergever MA (eds). 1983. *Mechanics of Hearing.* Nijhoff, The Hague.

Duifhuis H, Horst JW, van Kijk P, and van Netten SM (eds). 1993. *Biophysics of Hair Cell Sensory Systems.* World Scientific, Singapore.

Gummer AW (ed). 2002. *Biophysics of the Cochlea.* World Scientific, Singapore.

Lewis ER, Long GR, Lyon RF, Narins PM, Steele CR, and Hecht-Poinar E (eds). 1997. *Diversity in Auditory Mechanics.* World Scientific, Singapore.

Nuttal AL, Ren T, Gillespie P, Grosh K, and deBoer E. 2006. *Auditory Mechanismx, Processes and Models.* World Scientific, Singapore.

Wada T, Koike T, Takasada T, Ikeda K, and Ohyama K (eds). 2000. *Recent Developments in Auditory Mechanics.* World Scientific, Singapore.

Wilson JP and Kemp DT (eds). 1988. *Cochlear Mechanisms: Structure, Function, and Models.* Plenum, New York.

25

Inner Ear Hair Cell Bundle Mechanics

25.1 Introduction 25-1
25.2 Hair Cell Bundle Structure 25-1
25.3 Hair Bundle Mechanical Stiffness.................................25-3
25.4 Analytical Models..25-4
25.5 Computational Model...25-5
    Finite Element Models • Fluid Flow Stimulation • Transduction Channel Kinetics
25.6 Mechanical Properties of Hair Bundle Structures.....25-7
25.7 Hair Bundle Response to Different Types of Stimuli....25-9
25.8 Effect of Different Bundle Shapes...............................25-10
25.9 Concluding Remarks...25-11
References...25-11

Jong-Hoon Nam
University of Rochester

Wally Grant
Virginia Polytechnic Institute and State University

25.1 Introduction

Hair cells are the sensory receptors in the inner ear. Auditory hair cells in the cochlea detect pressure waves to mediate hearing. Vestibular hair cells in *semicircular canals*, *utricule*, and *saccule* detect head movement and orientation. The hair cells are named so because of their characteristic structure at the apical surface of the cell called the hair bundle (see Figure 25.1). Mechanical stimuli such as sound pressure, acceleration, or gravity arrive through the extracellular structure at the hair bundle where it is turned into neural spike-train signals. How different mechanical stimuli are captured, amplified, and encoded by hair cells is an important question in the inner ear science. The hair bundles have sophisticated structure and characteristic shapes depending on different inner ear organs (Figure 25.1). Even within the same sensory organ, the hair bundle shapes vary considerably and systematically. Considering such diverse and systematically arranged bundle shapes, it is logical to assume that the hair bundle mechanics play a crucial role on the hair cell's function.

25.2 Hair Cell Bundle Structure

Histological studies have enhanced the knowledge on the hair bundle structure. Among the findings are the various linkages that connect the *cilia*, and the more prominent of these are *tip links*. These connect the tip of a *stereocilium* to the shaft of the neighboring stereocilium. Tip links have inspired many biophysical theories (Pickles et al. 1984). Figure 25.2 illustrates structural components of a hair bundle such as stereocilia, *kinocilium*, tip link, and other fine filamentous links.

A hair cell bundle has dozens of stereocilia, and the numbers range from as few as 10 up to 150. Each stereocilium looks like a sharpened pencil. Its rootlet is inserted into the *cuticular plate*, a dense matrix

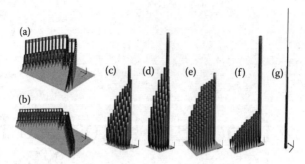

FIGURE 25.1 Various hair bundles from (a) rat cochlea apical turn, (b) rat cochlea basal turn, (c) mouse utricle striolar region, (d) mouse utricle extrastriolar region, (e) turtle utricle striolar region, (f) turtle utricle medial extrastriolar region, and (g) turtle semicircular canal. Scale bars are 1 mm in (a–f) and 5 mm in (g). A hair bundle is composed of hexagonally packed hairs (stereocilia) with unidirectional height gradient. Other than that, the bundles have a great variance in morphology depending on the organ and the location. The consequence of the variance is not yet fully understood.

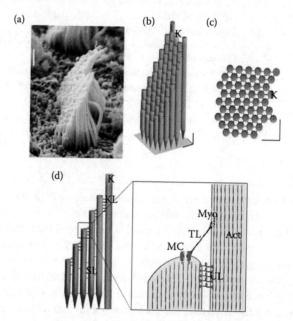

FIGURE 25.2 Structure of a hair bundle. (a) Scanning electron microscopic image of a hair bundle in turtle utricle. Note that wavy-looking stereocilia are preparation artifacts of the SEM; stereocilia *in vivo* are straight. (SEM from E. H. Peterson.) (b) Computer-rendered image of a similar hair bundle in (a). (c) Cross-sectional view of a hair bundle. Kinocilium (K) is at the taller end of bundle. The tip links (TL) are unidirectional along the height gradient of stereocilia. (d) Vertical view of a column of stereocilia, including the kinocilium. A stereocilium is packed with actin fibers (Act), while the kinocilium has a 9 + 2 microtubule structure. The stereocilia are tightly bound by various filaments such as kinocilial link (KL), upper lateral link (UL), tip link (TL), and shaft link (SL). The upper end of the tip link is pulled by myosin motors (Myo) and the bottom end is tethered to mechanotransduction ion channels (MC).

of *actin* fibers in the hair *cell apex*. In the transverse plane, the stereocilia in the bundle are arranged hexagonally (Figure 25.2c). In the sagittal section, stereocilia are arranged in ascending height similar to a staircase (Figure 25.2d). There is one kinocilium at the tallest end of the bundle. The kinocilium in the auditory hair cells disappears as they fully develop while that of vestibular hair cells persists.

Each stereocilium is packed with crystallized *f-actin* fibers. There are 300–400 actin fibers in the shaft region while the number of fibers reduces as the stereocilium tapers into the root (Tilney et al. 1980). The actin fibers are bound together by cross-linking proteins such as *espin* and *fimbrin* (Loomis et al. 2003). The diameter of stereocilia shaft ranges from 200 to 600 nm, and the rootlet of stereocilia is about 50 nm in diameter. The height of stereocilia has a range from 1 to 100 μm. Stereocilia in semicircular canals are approximately 100 μm tall while those in the basal turn of the cochlea are as short as 1 μm.

Various fine filaments tightly bind the stereocilia into a bundle. They are parallel to the cuticular plate and aligned with all three axes of the hexagonal array. In vestibular hair bundles, there are *kinocilial links, upper lateral links, shaft links,* and *ankle links* (Figure 25.2d). The kinocilial links bind the kinocilium to the rest of the bundle, and like tip links, they are composed of *protocadherin15* and *cadherin23* proteins. The upper lateral links bind the tips of stereocilia, and their molecular identity is unknown. The shaft links and ankle links are found only at the earlier developing stage in the auditory hair cell bundles. Because of their location, which is inefficient as a bundle binder, their mechanical or physiological role is unclear.

Tip links obliquely connect the tips of shorter stereocilia to the shaft of the next taller stereocilia (Figure 25.2d). Unlike other interciliary filaments, the tip links run along the gradient of stereociliary height, which defines the *excitatory–inhibitory* (E–I) direction of the cell. They are 8–11 nm thick and 150–200 nm long (Kachar et al. 2000). The tip link is composed of two proteins, protocadherin15 and cadherin23 (Kazmierczak et al. 2007). The bottom end of a tip link is mechanically coupled to a mechanotransduction ion channel (Beurg et al. 2009). The upper end of a tip link is connected to myosin motors (Holt et al. 2002). The myosin motors run up and down the actin of the stereocilia. Mechanical stimulation is delivered to the transduction channel through tip links and the channel's chance of opening is regulated by the tension maintained by myosin motors at the tip link's upper end. These myosin motors also adjust the tip link tension during the activation process and are responsible for adaptation in the bundle.

25.3 Hair Bundle Mechanical Stiffness

Hair bundles in the inner ear are subject to various mechanical stimuli such as gravity, head acceleration, or sound pressure that produce deflection of the hair bundles. Deflection of a hair bundle results in: stretching of the tip links, opening of the ion channels, that allows a depolarizing inward ion current flow into the hair cell, which in turn initiates neural signals. The study of the transfer function between mechanical stimulus and bundle deformation has centered on hair bundle *mechanical stiffness* (force/unit deflection). Furthermore, the *tonotopic arrangement* (systematic variation of characteristic frequencies along cochlear epithelium) of the hair bundle stiffness together with the mass carried by the bundle can explain its frequency map in lower vertebrates such as a lizard (Manley and Köppl 2008). In mammalian cochlea, the consequence of the variation of bundle stiffness is not yet understood.

The earliest stiffness measurements of hair bundles were made using the guinea pig cochlea (Strelioff and Flock 1984), turtle cochlea (Crawford and Fettiplace 1985), and bullfrog sacculus (Howard and Ashmore 1986). Measured hair bundle stiffness ranges from 0.2 mN/m in bullfrog saccule to 5 mN/m in rat cochlea. Because physiologically meaningful bundle deformation does not exceed 2° in angular rotation of stereocilia, the bundle mechanics was initially assumed to be linear. However, the hair bundle stiffness is nonlinear and it depends on displacement (Howard and Hudspeth 1988), measurement timing (Géléoc et al. 1997), stimulus direction (Szymko et al. 1992), and extracellular calcium concentration (Marquis and Hudspeth 1997, Lumpkin et al. 1997). Among these variations in stiffness, the dependence of the stiffness on the transduction channel activity has provided much insight into inner ear mechanoelectric transduction. It was consistently observed across various types of hair cells that the passive hair bundle without transduction channel activity becomes linear in force–displacement relations (bullfrog saccule: Howard and Hudspeth 1988; turtle cochlea: Ricci et al. 2000; mouse cochlea: Russell et al. 1992). Based on this finding, it is now believed that the hair bundle not only receives external stimulus but also provides a mechanical feedback by generating an active force (Kennedy et al. 2005, Chan and Hudspeth 2005). Because this active feedback disappears with the disruption of tip links, or the inactivation of channels, hair bundle force must originate from the transduction channels. This force from the transduction channel has been named the single channel gating force by Howard and Hudspeth (Howard and Hudspeth 1988). The single channel gating force ranges from 0.6 to 3.0 pN. A hair bundle can generate forces up to several hundred pN on a sub-millisecond timescale (Kennedy et al. 2005).

25.4 Analytical Models

A hair cell is most sensitive when the hair bundle deflects along the bilateral symmetric line, called the E–I axis (Shotwell et al. 1981). In other words, it has a primary direction of response. Although under some experimental conditions it has been observed otherwise (Stauffer and Holt 2007, Nam and Fettiplace 2008), stereocilia in a bundle are bound so tightly that they deform in unison (Karavitaki and Corey 2006, Kozlov et al. 2007). This observation has been used as grounds for simplifying the hair bundle mechanics to a *single-degree-of-freedom system*.

A single-degree-of-freedom model (Howard and Hudspeth 1987) for the hair bundle mechanics was represented by two elastic springs and a damper as a Maxwell–Kelvin–Voigt model. The single variable was the displacement of bundle tip along the E–I axis. In the simplest form of bundle mechanics, the force applied to the bundle F_{HB} is expressed as

$$F_{HB} = K_S X - N p_o z + F_0 \qquad (25.1)$$

where K_S is the stiffness of the bundle without the tip link additional stiffness included, N is the number of transduction channels in the bundle, p_o is the ratio of open channels to the total number of channels, and z is the single channel gating force. The last term F_0 is a constant to secure $F_{HB} = 0$ at $X = 0$. Without the last two terms, the equation is simply a Hooke's law. The second term in the right-hand side implies the interaction between the transduction channel and the bundle. The channel open probability p_o, is described using first-order Boltzmann relations

$$p_o = \frac{1}{(1 + \exp[(-z(X - X_0)/k_B T)])} \qquad (25.2)$$

where k_B is the Boltzmann's constant, T is the absolute temperature, and X_0 is the bundle displacement at 50% open probability. This equation implies that as X increases, the open probability approaches one, and as X decreases, it becomes zero. The single channel gating force z is defined as $z = \gamma k_{GS} b$, where k_{GS} is the spring constant of putative transduction channel complex and b is the gating swing (conformational change of transduction channel between open and closed state). Geometric gain γ is defined as the gating spring elongation divided by the bundle tip displacement and is approximated by the ratio of the interciliary distance and the bundle height. Because of its virtue of simplicity, this single-degree-of-freedom model of hair cell mechanotransduction has been widely adopted and modified for various purposes. For example, Cheung and Corey (2006) compared different adaptation theories of hair cells. Nadrowski and his colleagues (Nadrowski et al. 2004) suggested the positive role of ambient noise to hair cell sensitivity. Martin et al. (2000) explained the spontaneous oscillations of bullfrog saccule hair bundles.

While the single-degree-of-freedom model contributed to the improvement and the understanding of hair cell mechanotransduction, there were approaches more focused on hair bundle mechanics itself. An early study of hair bundles represented the stereocilia by two rigid bars, elastically hinged at their rootlets (Geisler 1993). This model presented ideas on how the stereociliar rotational displacement delivers tension to the tip link by the relative shear between stereocilia. Some studies represent hair bundles as a hinged plate, hemisphere, or array of cylinders, to investigate the fluid mechanics activation of hair bundles (Zetes and Steele 1997, Freeman and Weiss 1988, Shatz 2000). *Finite element* (FE) analysis of hair bundle was first introduced to analyze the mechanical behavior of a single stereocilium (Duncan and Grant 1997). The FE method was further applied to analyze a column of stereocilia (Cotton and Grant 2004) and whole three-dimensional bundles (Silber et al. 2004). This continuum mechanics-based approach was further developed to study hair bundle's dynamic interaction with channel kinetics of utricular hair cell (Nam et al. 2007) and cochlear hair cell (Beurg et al. 2008). The remainder of this chapter introduces the examples of recent progresses in understanding the bundle mechanics and mechanotransduction using the FE method.

25.5 Computational Model

25.5.1 Finite Element Models

The hair bundle is a sophisticated structure, and the geometry of many different hair bundles has been well documented (Duncan et al. 2001, Xue et al. 2005). This information was obtainable with current electron and confocal microscopic techniques. A mechanical consequence of various hair bundle shapes can be better understood with a model that reflects their real structure. The FE method serves such a purpose. It is an efficient and well-established method to analyze the mechanics of complicated structures. Grant and his colleagues introduced the FE methods to analyze hair bundle mechanics (Duncan and Grant 1997, Cotton and Grant 2000, 2004, Nam et al. 2005, 2006, 2007a,b).

The hair bundle FE model is composed of two different element types. Stereocilia and kinocilium are represented by shear deformable Timoshenko beams. For interciliary filaments, link elements were used. Ankle links were neglected in the model as they contribute little structurally. The range of element mesh size for stereocilia was from 0.05 to 1.0 μm, after considering the real geometry of hair bundle, the matrix condition number, and the computational efficiency.

The equation of motion at time t is

$$\mathbf{M}\left[{}^{t+\Delta t}\ddot{\mathbf{U}}^{(k)}\right] + {}^{t}\mathbf{C}\left[{}^{t+\Delta t}\dot{\mathbf{U}}^{(k)}\right] + {}^{t}\mathbf{K}\left[\Delta\mathbf{U}^{(k)}\right] = {}^{t+\Delta t}\mathbf{R} - {}^{t+\Delta t}\mathbf{F}^{(k-1)} \tag{25.3}$$

where $\mathbf{M}$, $\mathbf{C}$, and $\mathbf{K}$ are the mass, damping, and stiffness matrix and $\mathbf{U}$, $\mathbf{R}$, and $\mathbf{F}$ are the displacement, applied force, and internal force vectors. Over-dot variables denote the differentiation with respect to time. Superscripts to the left of the variable t denote time, while those to the right k indicate the iterative step within each time step. For the damping, a proportional damping was used such as

$$^{t}\mathbf{C} = \alpha_c\mathbf{M} + \beta_c{}^{t}\mathbf{K} \tag{25.4}$$

where α_c and β_c are scalar constants. This relation represents the bundle's internal damping—between stereocilia or within stereocilia. There is another fluid friction caused by the fluid flow on the surface of the hair bundle. This external damping was considered as an external force and included in the external force term $\mathbf{R}$. The damping coefficients α_c and β_c were chosen so that the overall effective damping of the hair bundle matches the experimentally measured values (100–200 nN · s/m).

At each time step, an incremental displacement vector $\Delta\mathbf{U}^{(k)}$ is computed and the displacement updated by

$$^{t+\Delta t}\mathbf{U}^{(k)} = {}^{t+\Delta t}\mathbf{U}^{(k-1)} + \Delta\mathbf{U}^{(k)} \tag{25.5}$$

Iterations of k for that time step continue until the internal force distribution converges.

For the solution of the dynamic structural analysis, the direct Newmark integration method was used. This method was chosen because it is a single-step, implicit method that is unconditionally stable.

The velocity and displacement vectors at time step $t + \Delta t$ are calculated by solving the equations below using two coefficients β and γ:

$$^{t+\Delta t}\dot{\mathbf{U}} = {}^{t}\dot{\mathbf{U}} + \Delta t\left\{(1-\gamma)\,{}^{t}\ddot{\mathbf{U}} + \gamma\,{}^{t+\Delta t}\ddot{\mathbf{U}}\right\} \tag{25.6}$$

$$^{t+\Delta t}\mathbf{U} = {}^{t}\mathbf{U} + {}^{t}\dot{\mathbf{U}}\Delta t + \Delta t^{2}\left\{\left(\frac{1}{2}-\beta\right){}^{t}\ddot{\mathbf{U}} + \beta\,{}^{t+\Delta t}\ddot{\mathbf{U}}\right\} \tag{25.7}$$

A typical time step size is 1–10 μs. With a proper choice of Newmark coefficients ($\gamma \geq 0.5$ and $\beta \leq 0.5$), the analysis is stable.

25.5.2 Fluid Flow Stimulation

Fluid mechanics around the hair bundle was considered as follows. For a vestibular hair cell bundle that is subject to relative fluid velocity of less than 1 μm/ms, and a viscosity near 1 mPa-s, results in a Reynolds number range of 10^{-5}–10^{-3}. With such low Reynolds number, the convective terms in the Navier–Stokes equations are eliminated. Nondimensional analysis of the Navier–Stokes equations, for an incompressible fluid, and without body forces, shows that transient effects are small and can be considered negligible (Nam et al. 2005). This same analysis shows that pressure and viscous force effects are important. These are incorporated in Oseen's improvement to Stokes drag at low Reynolds number flow. This drag formulation was used to simulate the drag force acting on individual stereocilia in this work. The Oseen formulation allows for interrupted flow around the cylindrical stereocilia body and is a much better approximation to the actual flow situation encountered by hair cell bundles than Stoke's formulation. The drag formulation used here should be considered as a first-order primary effect, and may underestimate the actual drag force. This underestimation may occur due to the fluid flow encountered after the endolymph flows past the stereocilia.

The drag force D on a cylindrical shape caused by the flow of a viscous fluid is given as

$$D = C_{D}\frac{1}{2}\rho A|V|V \tag{25.8}$$

where C_{D} is the drag coefficient, the velocity magnitude V is the relative velocity between the stereocilium and the fluid, A is the projected bundle area normal to the fluid flow, and ρ is the fluid density. Since the stereocilia have long cylindrical shapes and the Reynolds number (Rn) is much less than 1.0, the drag coefficient, C_{D}, will be approximated by Oseen's drag formulation

$$C_{D} = \frac{8\pi}{Rn\log(7.4/Rn)} \tag{25.9}$$

The fluid drag on the extracellular links was ignored. Because the hair bundle deflects infinitesimally (angular displacement is less than 2°), no disturbance by the bundle on the fluid flow is considered, that is, the fluid applies force to the bundle, but the bundle does not disturb the fluid. Further details of dynamic analysis and parameter values can be found in Nam et al. (2005).

25.5.3 Transduction Channel Kinetics

The mechanotransduction channel interacts with the hair bundle. In this simulation, the interaction can be achieved by adjusting the original (unstained) length of the tip link. As the channel state changes from closed to open, the length of the tip link was increased by the gating swing and vice versa.

Literature values for the gating swing are estimated between 1 and 10 nm (Cheung and Corey 2006). The upper attachment point of the tip link moves according to the work or myosin, which is termed slow adaptation. Because it is computationally costly to remesh according to the slow adaptation, in the computer model, the slow adaptation was reflected in the length change of the tip link. Therefore, the change of length in the tip link is due to an active process and is described by

$$\Delta x = nb + x_A \tag{25.10}$$

where b is the gating swing length, n is the channel state (0 when closed, 1 when open), and x_A is the movement of upper attachment due to the slow adaptation.

The transduction channel kinetics is assumed to have four states. This is the minimum number of channel states to consider the calcium effect on channel kinetics. There are open and closed configuration and each configuration has calcium bound and unbound states. Rate coefficients between the states are defined by four rate constants. Two coefficients describe the calcium binding and unbinding rate:

$$k_{01} = k_b C_{FA} \tag{25.11}$$

$$k_{10} = k_b K_D \tag{25.12}$$

where k_b is the calcium binding coefficient, C_{FA} is the calcium concentration at the binding site, and K_D is the dissociation constant of calcium. The channel state of opened (k_{CO}) or closed (k_{OC}) is described by the following two expressions, where two additional rate coefficients are utilized

$$k_{CO} = k_F \exp(\eta \Delta E / k_B T) \tag{25.13}$$

$$k_{OC} = k_R \exp(-(1 - \eta)) \Delta E / k_B T \tag{25.14}$$

where ΔE is the energy difference between open and closed state of the channel. ΔE is defined by the tension in the tip link f, gating swing b, and calcium-binding modification f_{Ca} such as

$$\Delta E = b(f - f_{ca} - f_0) \tag{25.15}$$

When positive, f_{Ca} facilitates the channel closure and stabilizes the closed state (Crawford et al. 1989, Cheung and Corey 2006). The myosin motor provided the resting tension of the tip link. Further details of channel kinetics, including the myosin-regulated adaptation, can be found in Beurg et al. (2008).

25.6 Mechanical Properties of Hair Bundle Structures

There are experiments that can be used to arrive at hair bundle mechanical properties. Bashtanov et al. (2004) selectively removed the tip link or shaft links and measured the bundle stiffness by treating hair bundle solutions that contained BAPTA (to remove tip links) or subtilisin (to remove shaft links). They used chicken utricular hair cells for this study. The bundle stiffness was measured by analyzing the frequency of the freely standing bundle's Brownian motion.

Spoon et al. (2007) implemented a similar experiment protocol—removal of tip links or shaft links. Different from Bashtanov et al., they used the glass fiber technique for the stiffness measurement of turtle utricular hair bundles. Computer simulations of similar bundles to those tested complemented the experiment. Simulated bundle is shown in Figure 25.2. The geometric information is from the *striolar region* in the turtle utricle. The striolar region is a narrow crescent-shaped region in the utricular epithelium where the hair bundles' polarity reverses. Like the experiment, four cases were simulated to determine the structural contribution of different link types and to estimate the mechanical properties of the bundle structural components (Figure 25.2d). Link structures of a hair bundle include the tip link assemblies (TLA), the upper lateral links (UL), the kinocilial links (KL), and the shaft links (SL). In addition to these links, the flexibility of stereocilia roots affects the bundle compliance. Here, the TLA includes any proteins in series with the tip link from actin core to actin core, including the tip link itself.

To obtain the stiffness of the hair bundle in a resting state, a small point load of 1.0 pN in the excitatory direction (toward taller edge) is applied at the tip of the kinocilium. The deflection at the tip of the kinocilium is computed and the bundle stiffness is defined as the applied load divided by the tip deflection. The hair bundle without tip links represents the BAPTA-treated hair bundle. The hair bundle missing SL represents the subtilisin-treated hair bundle. A hair bundle washed with BAPTA and subtilisin has no tip or SL.

Four mechanical parameter values were sought in the study: (1) stereocilia Young's modulus E_S, (2) stiffness of the TL k_{TL}, (3) UL stiffness k_{UL}, and (4) SL stiffness k_{SL}. A set of optimal mechanical parameters (E_S^*, k_{TL}^*, k_{UL}^*, and k_{SL}^*) were found that minimize the difference between the modeled results and the three experimental outcomes (Spoon et al. 2007, namely, 66 ± 9% and 63 ± 10% stiffness reduction after tip and shaft link removal, and the intact bundle stiffness of 42 ± 25 pN/μm ($n = 28$). Initial values of E_S, k_{TL}, k_{UL}, and k_{SL} were taken from the previous study (Nam et al. 2006). Then, three of the parameters were held constant and the value of the fourth was found that minimized the difference. This process was repeated for the other three parameters in turn, and then the entire process was repeated until the values converged. After the optimal mechanical properties were identified (E_S^*, k_{TL}^*, k_{UL}^*, and k_{SL}^*), a series of parametric studies was performed to observe the effects of each individual mechanical parameter on the whole bundle stiffness. In each of the four parametric studies, three of the optimal mechanical properties were fixed and the remaining parameter varied.

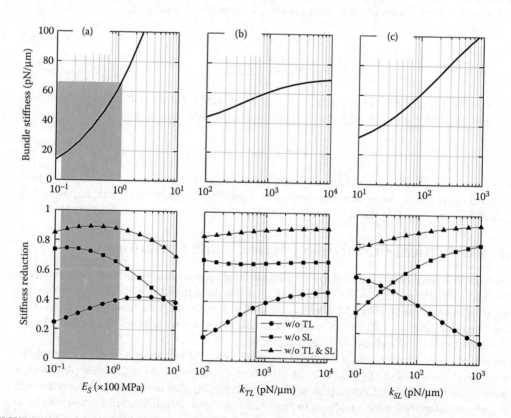

FIGURE 25.3 Identifying the mechanical property of hair bundle structures. The shaded area indicates the measured stiffness range of 42 ± 25 pN/μm ($n = 28$). Top row: stiffness change due to change of (a) Young's modulus of stereocilia E_S, (b) stiffness of tip link k_{TL}, and (c) stiffness of shaft link k_{SL}. Bottom row: fraction of stiffness reduction when TL (circle), SL (square), or both TL and SL (triangle) were removed.

Figure 25.3 shows the simulation results. The shaded area is the range of experimental results. When the Young's modulus of stereocilia E_S = 100 MPa, the stiffness of the TLA k_{TL} = 1000 pN/μm, and the stiffness of SL k_{SL} = 100 pN/μm, the simulated results became close to experimental results. Simulated bundle stiffness was 60 pN/μm. Stiffness reductions due to the removal of TL and SL were 65% and 40%, respectively.

25.7 Hair Bundle Response to Different Types of Stimuli

In experiments, to observe single cell response, the overlying acellular matrix such as *tectorial membrane* in cochlea or otoconial layer in vestibular organs is removed. Then, the mechanical stimulus is delivered by a glass probe or fluid jet. It is unclear how different stimulus types affect a hair cell response. Such different stimulus conditions were simulated using a computer model (Figure 25.4).

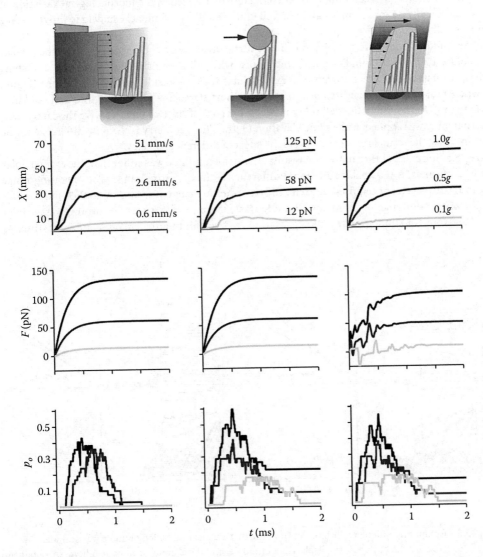

FIGURE 25.4 Hair bundle response to different stimulation types. The top row depicts the stimulus conditions of each column. Below three rows are the time response of hair bundle displacement (X), reaction force at the bundle tip (F), and fraction of open channels (p_o). The columns are the three different stimulus methods: fluid jet, flexible glass fiber, and *in vivo*.

To simulate the flexible glass fiber condition, step forces were applied to the three tallest cilia of the bundle. To simulate the fluid jet condition, the ambient fluid was given velocities ramped from zero to a steady-state value. The time constants and magnitudes of the *in vitro* stimuli were adjusted to achieve $X(t)$ curves similar to the following *in vivo* conditions. To simulate the *in vivo* condition, the bundle was subjected to both a ramped displacement and a shear flow from the ambient fluid. The time course of displacements was selected to match the whole utricle analysis results (Davis et al. 2007). Three stimulus levels were simulated: 0.1*g*, 0.5*g*, and 1.0*g*, where *g* is the acceleration due to gravity.

25.8 Effect of Different Bundle Shapes

As shown in Figure 25.1, there are strikingly diverse hair bundles. While auditory hair bundles change their height monotonically according to their characteristic frequency, the morphological variation in the vestibular organs is more complex and not well understood. An FE model can help to provide some idea on this matter.

Two hair bundles from different locations in the turtle utricle were chosen. One is from the striolar region (Figure 25.2), where bundles are round shaped with tall stereocilia (up to ~10 µm) and short kinocilium (~10 µm). The other is from the extrastriolar region (outside the striolar region) (Figure 25.1f), where bundles are in elongated oval shape with short stereocilia (up to ~4.5 µm) and tall kinocilium (>10 µm). In the simulation, all other model properties of the two bundles were the same. Even the external force was applied at the same elevation (9 µm). The geometry is the only difference in the simulation. Thus, the results reflect exclusively the effect of different geometry.

Figure 25.5 summarizes the simulation results. The striolar bundle was stiffer than the extrastriolar bundle by five times. A noticeable functional difference is the operating range. The operating range is the bundle displacement required to excite the transduction current from 10% to 90% of its maximum. The operating range of the striolar bundle was 188 nm, while it was 697 nm in extrastriolar bundle. Therefore, the simulation results suggest that the two hair bundles encode a different stimulus range.

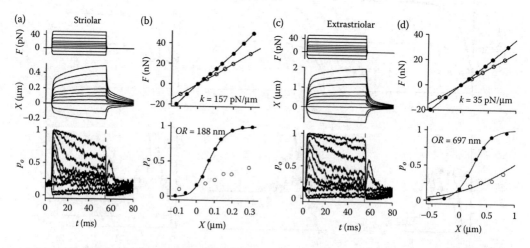

FIGURE 25.5 Comparing different hair bundles from the turtle utricle. (a) Striolar bundle was stimulated with a family of step forces (top). The bundle tip displacement (middle) and the channel open probability were obtained (bottom). (b) F–X relations (top) and p_o–X relations (bottom) of the striolar hair bundle. (c) Extrastriolar bundle was simulated. (d) F–X relations (top) and p_o–X relations (bottom) of the extrastriolar hair bundle. The displacement and the open probability in (b) and (d) were measured at the onset of stimulation (the vertical broken lines in the left of p_o–t plots).

25.9 Concluding Remarks

The understanding of hair cell mechanics, electrophysiology, and the basics of its neural science and mechanical behaviors has made great strides over the past two decades. The interdisciplinary nature of these studies will continue and true hybrid investigators (those with neural, electrophysiology, mechanics backgrounds) will be needed in the future. Biomedical engineers can contribute to this field in two ways. First, their study helps to understand hearing and balancing disorders. Second, their study can provide new insights for the design of biologically inspired mechanotransduction sensors and prosthetics.

References

Bashtanov, M. E., R. J. Goodyear, G. P. Richardson, and I. J. Russell. 2004. The mechanical properties of chick (*Gallus domesticus*) sensory hair bundles: Relative contributions of structures sensitive to calcium chelation and subtilisin treatment. *J Physiol* **559**(Pt 1): 287–99.

Beurg, M., R. Fettiplace, J. H. Nam, and A. J. Ricci. 2009. Localization of inner hair cell mechanotransducer channels using high-speed calcium imaging. *Nat Neurosci* **12**(5): 553–8.

Beurg, M., J. H. Nam, A. Crawford, and R. Fettiplace. 2008. The actions of calcium on hair bundle mechanics in mammalian cochlear hair cells. *Biophys J* **94**(7): 2639–53.

Chan, D. K. and A. J. Hudspeth. 2005. Ca^{2+} current-driven nonlinear amplification by the mammalian cochlea *in vitro*. *Nat Neurosci* **8**(2): 149–55.

Cheung, E. L. and D. P. Corey. 2006. Ca^{2+} changes the force sensitivity of the hair-cell transduction channel. *Biophys J* **90**(1): 124–39.

Cotton, J. and W. Grant. 2004. Computational models of hair cell bundle mechanics: II. Simplified bundle models. *Hear Res* **197**(1–2): 105–11.

Cotton, J. R. and J. W. Grant. 2000. A finite element method for mechanical response of hair cell ciliary bundles. *J Biomech Eng* **122**(1): 44–50.

Crawford, A. C., M. G. Evans, and R. Fettiplace. 1989. Activation and adaptation of transducer currents in turtle hair cells. *J Physiol* **419**: 405–34.

Crawford, A. C. and R. Fettiplace. 1985. The mechanical properties of ciliary bundles of turtle cochlear hair cells. *J Physiol* **364**: 359–79.

Davis, J. L., J. Xue, E. H. Peterson, and J. W. Grant. 2007. Layer thickness and curvature effects on otoconial membrane deformation in the utricle of the red-ear slider turtle: Static and modal analysis. *J Vestib Res* **17**(4): 145–62.

Duncan, R. K. and J. W. Grant. 1997. A finite-element model of inner ear hair bundle micromechanics. *Hear Res* **104**(1–2): 15–26.

Duncan, R. K., K. E. Ile, M. G. Dubin, and J. C. Saunders. 2001. Hair bundle profiles along the chick basilar papilla. *J Anat* **198**(Pt 1): 103–16.

Freeman, D. M. and T. F. Weiss. 1988. The role of fluid inertia in mechanical stimulation of hair cells. *Hear Res* **35**(2–3): 201–7.

Geisler, C. D. 1993. A model of stereociliary tip-link stretches. *Hear Res* **65**(1–2): 79–82.

Geleoc, G. S., G. W. Lennan, G. P. Richardson, and C. J. Kros. 1997. A quantitative comparison of mechanoelectrical transduction in vestibular and auditory hair cells of neonatal mice. *Proc Biol Sci* **264**(1381): 611–21.

Holt, J. R., S. K. Gillespie, and D. W. Provance. 2002. A chemical-genetic strategy implicates myosin-1c in adaptation by hair cells. *Cell* **108**(3): 371–81.

Howard, J. and J. F. Ashmore. 1986. Stiffness of sensory hair bundles in the sacculus of the frog. *Hear Res* **23**(1): 93–104.

Howard, J. and A. J. Hudspeth. 1987. Mechanical relaxation of the hair bundle mediates adaptation in mechanoelectrical transduction by the bullfrog's saccular hair cell. *Proc Natl Acad Sci USA* **84**(9): 3064–8.

Howard, J. and A. J. Hudspeth. 1988. Compliance of the hair bundle associated with gating of mechano-electrical transduction channels in the bullfrog's saccular hair cell. *Neuron* **1**(3): 189–99.

Kachar, B., M. Parakkal, M. Kurc, Y. Zhao, and P. G. Gillespie. 2000. High-resolution structure of hair-cell tip links. *Proc Natl Acad Sci USA* **97**(24): 13336–41.

Karavitaki, K. D. and D. P. Corey. 2006. Hair bundle mechanics at high frequencies: A test of series or parallel transduction. Singapore, World Scientific.

Kazmierczak, P., H. Sakaguchi, and J. Tokita. 2007. Cadherin 23 and protocadherin 15 interact to form tip-link filaments in sensory hair cells. *Nature* **449**(7158): 87–91.

Kennedy, H. J., A. C. Crawford, and R. Fettiplace. 2005. Force generation by mammalian hair bundles supports a role in cochlear amplification. *Nature* **433**(7028): 880–3.

Kozlov, A. S., T. Risler, and A. J. Hudspeth. 2007. Coherent motion of stereocilia assures the concerted gating of hair-cell transduction channels. *Nat Neurosci* **10**(1): 87–92.

Loomis, P. A., L. Zheng, and G. Sekerkova. 2003. Espin cross-links cause the elongation of microvillus-type parallel actin bundles in vivo. *J Cell Biol* **163**(5): 1045–55.

Lumpkin, E. A., R. E. Marquis, and A. J. Hudspeth. 1997. The selectivity of the hair cell's mechanoelectrical-transduction channel promotes Ca^{2+} flux at low Ca^{2+} concentrations. *Proc Natl Acad Sci USA* **94**(20): 10997–1002.

Manley, G. A. and C. Köppl. 2008. What have lizard ears taught us about auditory physiology? *Hear Res* **238**(1–2): 3–11.

Marquis, R.E. and A. J. Hudspeth. 1997. Effects of extracellular Ca^{2+} concentration on hair-bundle stiffness and gating-spring integrity in hair cells. *Proc Natl Acad Sci USA.* **94**(22): 11923–8.

Martin, P., A. D. Mehta, and A. J. Hudspeth. 2000. Negative hair-bundle stiffness betrays a mechanism for mechanical amplification by the hair cell. *Proc Natl Acad Sci USA* **97**(22): 12026–31.

Nadrowski, B., P. Martin, and F. Jülicher. 2004. Active hair-bundle motility harnesses noise to operate near an optimum of mechanosensitivity. *Proc Natl Acad Sci USA* **101**(33): 12195–200.

Nam, J.-H., J. R. Cotton, and J. W. Grant. 2005. Effect of fluid forcing on vestibular hair bundles. *J Vestib Res* **15**(5–6): 263–78.

Nam, J. H., J. R. Cotton, and W. Grant. 2007a. A virtual hair cell, I: addition of gating spring theory into a 3-D bundle mechanical model. *Biophys J* **92**(6): 1918–28.

Nam, J. H., J. R. Cotton, and W. Grant. 2007b. A virtual hair cell, II: evaluation of mechanoelectric transduction parameters. *Biophys J* **92**(6): 1929–37.

Nam, J. H., J. R. Cotton, E. H. Peterson, and W. Grant. 2006. Mechanical properties and consequences of stereocilia and extracellular links in vestibular hair bundles. *Biophys J* **90**(8): 2786–95.

Nam, J. H. and R. Fettiplace. 2008. Theoretical conditions for high-frequency hair bundle oscillations in auditory hair cells. *Biophys J* **95**(10): 4948–62.

Pickles, J. O., S. D. Comis, and M. P. Osborne. 1984. Cross-links between stereocilia in the guinea pig organ of Corti, and their possible relation to sensory transduction. *Hear Res* **15**(2): 103–12.

Ricci, A. J., A. C. Crawford, and R. Fettiplace. 2000. Active hair bundle motion linked to fast transducer adaptation in auditory hair cells. *J Neurosci* **20**(19): 7131–42.

Russell, I. J., M. Kossl, and G. P. Richardson. 1992. Nonlinear mechanical responses of mouse cochlear hair bundles. *Proc Biol Sci* **250**(1329): 217–27.

Shatz, L. F. 2000. The effect of hair bundle shape on hair bundle hydrodynamics of inner ear hair cells at low and high frequencies. *Hear Res* **141**(1–2): 39–50.

Shotwell, S. L., R. Jacobs, and A. J. Hudspeth. 1981. Directional sensitivity of individual vertebrate hair cells to controlled deflection of their hair bundles. *Ann N Y Acad Sci* **374**: 1–10.

Silber, J., J. Cotton, J. H. Nam, E. H. Peterson, and W. Grant. 2004. Computational models of hair cell bundle mechanics: III. 3-D utricular bundles. *Hear Res* **197**(1–2): 112–30.

Spoon C., J. H. Nam, and W. Grant. 2007. Experimental and computational analysis of hair bundle mechanics at different macular locations in the turtle utricle. Abstract No. 736, Association for Research in Otolaryngology 30th Midwinter Meeting, Denver, CO.

Stauffer, E. A. and J. R. Holt. 2007. Sensory transduction and adaptation in inner and outer hair cells of the mouse auditory system. *J Neurophysiol* **98**(6): 3360–9.

Strelioff, D. and A. Flock. 1984. Stiffness of sensory-cell hair bundles in the isolated guinea pig cochlea. *Hear Res* **15**(1): 19–28.

Szymko, Y. M., P. S. Dimitri, and J. C. Saunders. 1992. Stiffness of hair bundles in the chick cochlea. *Hear Res* **59**(2): 241–9.

Tilney, L. G., D. J. Derosier, and M. J. Mulroy. 1980. The organization of actin filaments in the stereocilia of cochlear hair cells. *J Cell Biol* **86**(1): 244–59.

Xue, J. and E. H. Peterson. 2006. Hair bundle heights in the utricle: Differences between macular locations and hair cell types. *J Neurophysiol* **95**: 171–186.

Zetes, D. E. and C. R. Steele. 1997. Fluid-structure interaction of the stereocilia bundle in relation to mechanotransduction. *J Acoust Soc Am* **101**(6): 3593–601.

26

Exercise Physiology

26.1 Introduction 26-1
26.2 Muscle Energetics 26-1
26.3 Cardiovascular Adjustments 26-3
26.4 Maximum Oxygen Uptake 26-4
26.5 Respiratory Responses 26-6
26.6 Optimization 26-8
26.7 Thermoregulatory Response 26-8
26.8 Applications 26-8
Defining Terms 26-10
References...26-10
Further Information...26-10

Cathryn R. Dooly
Lander University

Arthur T. Johnson
University of Maryland

26.1 Introduction

The study of exercise physiology should be important to medical and biological engineers because many of the principles and laws of nature are relevant to the homeostasis of the human body. Cognizance of the acute and chronic responses to exercise gives an insight and an understanding of the physiological stresses to which the human body is subjected. To appreciate exercise responses requires a true systems approach to physiology, because during exercise, all physiological responses contribute to a highly integrated and totally supportive mechanism toward the performance of the physical stress of exercise. Unlike the study of pathology and disease, the study of exercise physiology clarifies the way the human body is supposed to function while performing at its healthy best.

For exercise involving resistance, physiological and psychological adjustments begin even before the start of exercise. The central nervous system (CNS) anticipates the task before it, assessing how much muscular force to apply and computing trial limb trajectories to accomplish the required movement. Heart rate, blood pressure, and respiration begin rising in anticipation of increased oxygen demands.

26.2 Muscle Energetics

Human muscle fibers convert chemical energy from the food that we eat into mechanical energy. Energy transfer occurs from the release of energy trapped within chemical bonds. Adenosine triphosphate (ATP), the fundamental energy source for muscle cells, is stored at maximal levels, as well as significant amounts of creatine phosphate (CP) and glycogen, the stored form of glucose.

When the muscle proteins actin and myosin engage in response to high-intensity, short-duration muscular activity, the ATP-CP system (or phosphagan system) is activated in the sarcoplasm of the muscle cell. CP is catabolized by creatine kinase to creatine and inorganic phosphate (Pi), yielding free energy. This energy can be used in turn to generate ATP from adenosine diphosphate (ADP) and Pi. During high-intensity, short-duration muscular activity, as in a one repetition maximum, ATP generation declines rapidly as CP stores are depleted. If physical exertion continues after PC depletion, ATP generation must be accomplished by other pathways, though slower. Maximally contracting skeletal muscle uses approximately 1.7×10^{-5} mole of ATP per gram per second (White et al. 1959). ATP stores in skeletal muscle tissue amount to 5×10^{-6} mole per gram of tissue, or enough to meet muscular energy demands for no longer than 0.5 s. Resting muscle contains 4–6 times as much CP as it does ATP, but the total supply of high-energy phosphate cannot sustain muscular activity for more than a few seconds.

Glycogen is a polysaccharide present in muscle tissue in large amounts. Glycogen is catabolized to glucose and pyruvic acid in the sarcoplasm, which in turn becomes lactic acid in a deoxygenated environment. These reactions, collectively known as *anaerobic* glycolysis, generate ATP in the absence of oxygen.

When sufficient oxygen is available (*aerobic* conditions) in the mitochondria of the muscle cell or other tissues, these processes are reversed. ATP is reformed from ADP and AMP (adenosine monophosphate), CP is reformed from creatine and phosphate, and glycogen is reformed from glucose or lactic acid. Energy to fuel these processes is derived from the complete oxidation of carbohydrates, fatty acids, or amino acids to form carbon dioxide and water. These reactions are summarized by the following equations:

$$ATP \leftrightarrow ADP + P + \text{free energy}$$

$$CP + ADP \leftrightarrow \text{creatine} + ATP$$

$$\text{Glycogen or glucose} + P + ADP \leftrightarrow \text{lactate} + ATP$$

Aerobic:

$$\text{Glycogen or fatty acids} + P + ADP + O_2 \rightarrow CO_2 + H_2O + ATP$$

All conditions:

$$2\,ADP \leftrightarrow ATP + AMP$$

The most intense levels of exercise occur anaerobically (Mole 1983) and can be maintained for only a minute or two (see Figure 26.1).

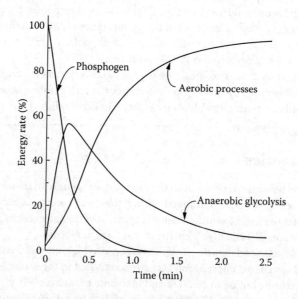

FIGURE 26.1 Energy transfer mechanics. (From Mole, P.A. 1983. Exercise metabolism. In A.A. Bove and D.T. Lowenthal (Eds.), *Exercise Medicine*, pp. 43–48. New York, Academic Press.)

26.3 Cardiovascular Adjustments

Skeletal muscle ergoreceptors and metaboreceptors in muscles, tendons, and joints relay information regarding vibrations and stretch, and the chemical status (O_2, CO_2, electrolytes, glucose, pH) of the muscle, respectively, and relay information to the CNS that the muscles have begun movement (exercise pressor reflex). The CNS processes this information to increase heart rate, stroke volume, and blood pressure via the sympathetic nervous system (SNS). Cardiac output, the amount of blood pumped by the heart per minute, is the product of heart rate and stroke volume (the amount of blood pumped per heart beat). Heart rate increases nearly exponentially at the beginning of exercise with a time constant of about 30 s. Stroke volume does not change immediately but lags a bit until cardiac output completes the loop back to the heart. The increase in stroke volume with exercise is accomplished by Starling's law of the heart, which states that the greater the volume of blood entering the heart during diastole (filling phase), the greater the force of contraction and volume of blood ejected during systole (emptying phase).

At rest, a large volume of blood is stored in the veins, especially in the extremities. When exercise begins, this blood is transferred from the venous side of the heart to the arterial side of the heart. The driving force of blood at the initiation of exercise against the resistance of the arteries causes a rise in both systolic (heart ventricular contraction) and diastolic (the pause between heart contractions when heart chambers fill with blood) blood pressures. These increased blood pressures are detected by cardiac, aortic arch, and carotid arterial baroreceptors (arterial and cardiopulmonary baroreflexes) (see Figure 26.2).

As a consequence, small sphincter muscles encircling the entrance to the arterioles (small arteries) are stimulated to relax via the CNS and locally produced nitric oxide. Using Poiseuille's law, the resistance to blood flow can be calculated as

$$\text{Resistance} = \frac{8\,L\mu}{\pi\,r^4}$$

where R is the resistance of the vessel ($\text{N} \cdot \text{s/m}^5$), L is the length of the vessel (m), μ is the viscosity of the blood ($\text{kg/(m} \cdot \text{s)}$ or N s/m^2), and r is the radius of the vessel (m) raised to fourth power.

Blood flow is proportional to the pressure difference across the system, and inversely proportional to resistance. This can be illustrated with the following:

$$\text{Blood flow} = \Delta\text{pressure/resistance}$$

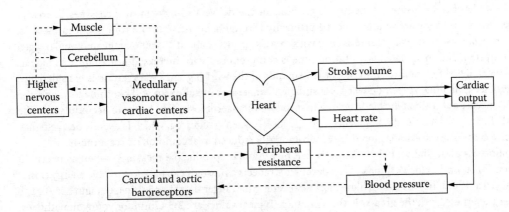

FIGURE 26.2 General scheme for blood pressure regulation. (From Johnson, A.T. 2007. *Biomechanics and Exercise Physiology: Quantitative Modeling*, Taylor & Francis, Boca Raton, FL.)

Note that blood flow can be increased by a change in the pressure difference (Δpressure), a decrease in resistance, or a combination of the two. The most favorable way to increase blood flow is through a change in resistance, since small adjustments in blood vessel radius result in significant changes in resistance (attributed to the relationship between vascular resistance and vessel radius). Change in resistance is largely accomplished by changes in blood vessel radius or diameter, as blood viscosity and vessel length do not change appreciably under normal conditions. Thus, blood flow to the various organs in the body can be regulated by small changes in blood vessel radius via vasoconstriction and vasodilatation. The advantage to this is that blood can be easily diverted to areas where it is needed the most during exercise performance, that is, the exercising muscles.

To meet the oxygen demands of the exercising muscles, blood is diverted away from tissues and organs not directly involved with exercise performance. Blood flow is thus reduced to the gastrointestinal tract and kidneys, and increased not only to exercising skeletal muscle but also to cardiac muscle and the skin. Most resistance to blood flow occurs in the arterioles. These vessels account for as much as 70–80% of the drop in mean arterial pressure across the entire cardiovascular system due to their vasoconstrictive and vasodilatative properties. Increasing the arteriole radius by 19% will decrease the resistance to one-half. Thus, systolic blood pressure returns to baseline, and diastolic blood pressure may actually fall, following recovery from exercise.

The heart operates as two pumping systems in a series. The left heart pumps blood throughout the systemic blood vessels (aorta, arteries, arterioles, capillaries, venules, and veins), whereas the right heart pumps blood throughout the pulmonary blood vessels (pulmonary arteries, veins, capillaries, and venules). Blood pressures in the systemic vessels are higher than blood pressures in the pulmonary system.

Two chambers comprise each pump of the heart. The atria are like an assist device that produces some suction and collects blood from the veins. Their main purpose is to deliver blood to the ventricle of each pump, which is the more powerful chamber that develops blood pressure. The myocardium (middle muscular layer of the heart wall) of the left ventricle is considerably thicker and stronger than the myocardium of the right ventricle. With two pumps and four chambers in a series, matching flow rates among them could be challenging. If the flow rate is not properly matched, blood is at risk of accumulating downstream from the most powerful chamber and upstream from the weakest chamber.

Myocardial tissue exerts a more forceful contraction if it is stretched prior to heart contraction (systole). This property, previously referred to as Starling's law, serves to equalize the flow rates between the two pumps, resulting in a more powerful ejection of blood from the heart during systole, and greater blood volume accumulation during filling (diastole).

26.4 Maximum Oxygen Uptake

The heart has been considered the limiting factor for the delivery of oxygen to the tissues. Increases in heart rate during exercise are achieved primarily through a decrease in the time spent in diastole. Thus, the increase in stroke volume as seen with exercise peaks at about 40–60% of the maximal oxygen consumption, and then plateaus, as filling time is compromised with increased heart rates. As long as the oxygen delivery is sufficient to meet the demands of the working muscles, exercise is considered to be aerobic. When the oxygen delivery is insufficient, anaerobic metabolism will continue to supply the energy needs, but ultimately, lactic acid, a by-product of anaerobiosis, will begin to accumulate in the blood. To remove lactic acid and resynthesize glucose, oxygen is required, which is usually delayed until exercise ceases, or the exercise intensity is substantially reduced to accommodate resynthesis.

The fitness of an individual is characterized by a highly reproducible measure known as maximal oxygen consumption (or VO_2 max). This parameter reflects a person's capacity for aerobic energy transfer as well as the ability to sustain high-intensity exercise for longer than 4 or 5 min (see Figure 26.3). The higher the fitness level, the greater is the VO_2 max. Typical values are 2.5 L/min for young nonathletes, 5.0 L/min for well-trained male athletes, with females having VO_2 max values of 70–80% that of males. Maximal oxygen consumption declines steadily with age at a rate of about 1% per year.

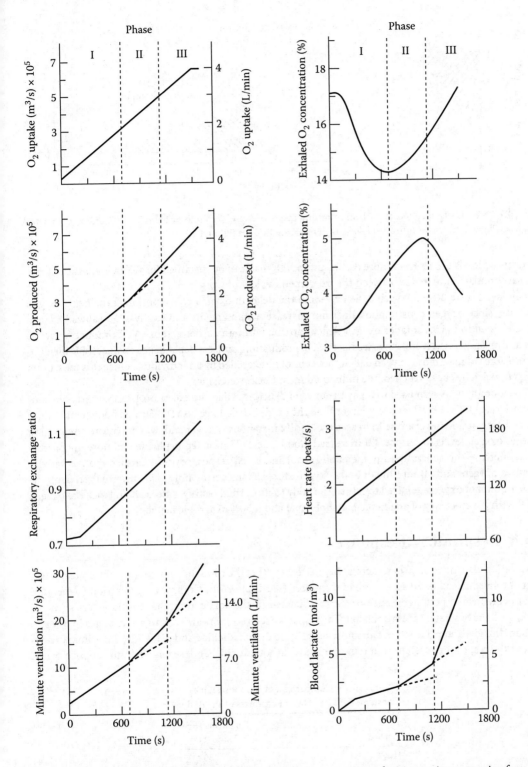

FIGURE 26.3 Concurrent typical changes in blood and respiratory parameters during exercise progressing from rest to maximum. Two transitions shown are the aerobic threshold and the anaerobic threshold. (From Skinner, J.S. and McLellan, T.H. 1980. *Res. Q. Exerc. Sport.* 51: 234.)

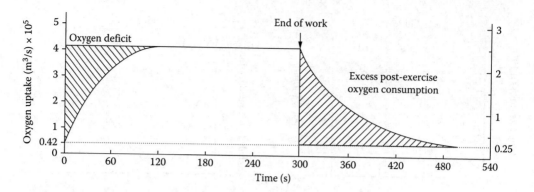

FIGURE 26.4 Oxygen uptake at the beginning and end of exercise. (From Johnson, A.T. 2007. *Biomechanics and Exercise Physiology: Quantitative Modeling*, Taylor & Francis, Boca Raton, FL.)

Exercise levels higher than those that result in VO_2 max can be sustained for various lengths of time. The accumulated difference between the oxygen equivalent of work and VO_2 max is called the oxygen deficit (see Figure 26.4). Oxygen deficit refers to the delay in oxygen consumption at the beginning of exercise, since oxygen consumption does not increase instantaneously to steady-state values. Trained athletes tend to have a smaller oxygen deficit, attributed to an earlier aerobic ATP production at the beginning of exercise, resulting in less lactic acid production, and less dependence on anaerobic metabolism. There is a maximum oxygen deficit that cannot be exceeded by an individual. Once this maximum oxygen deficit has been reached, the individual must cease exercising.

The amount of oxygen used to repay the oxygen deficit is called the excess post-exercise oxygen consumption (EPOC). EPOC is always larger than the oxygen deficit because (1) elevated body temperature immediately following exercise increases the bodily metabolism in general, which requires more than resting oxygen levels to service, (2) increased blood catecholamine (epinephrine and norepinephrine) levels increase the general bodily metabolism, (3) increased respiratory and cardiac muscle activity requires oxygen, and (4) refilling of body oxygen stores. Considering only lactic acid oxygen debt, the total amount of oxygen required to return the body to its normal resting state is about twice the oxygen debt, with the efficiency of anaerobic metabolism at about 50% of aerobic metabolism.

26.5 Respiratory Responses

Respiration also increases when exercise begins, except that the time constant for respiratory responses is about 45 s instead of 30 s for cardiac responses (see Table 26.1). Control of respiration (see Figure 26.5) begins when peripheral chemoreceptors located in the aortic arch, the carotid arteries (in the neck), and the brainstem are stimulated. These specialized receptors are sensitive to changes in oxygen, carbon dioxide, and pH levels but are most sensitive to carbon dioxide and pH. Thus, the primary function of the respiratory system is to remove excess carbon dioxide, and, secondarily, to supply oxygen.

TABLE 26.1 Comparison of Response Time Constants for Four Major Responses of the Body

System	Dominant Time Constant (s)
Heart	30
Respiratory system	45
Oxygen uptake	49
Thermal system	3600

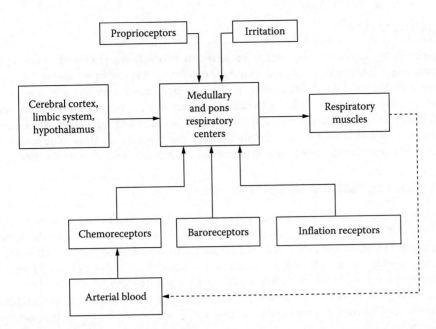

FIGURE 26.5 General scheme of respiratory control. (From Johnson, A.T. 2007. *Biomechanics and Exercise Physiology: Quantitative Modeling,* Taylor & Francis, Boca Raton, FL.)

Perhaps this is because excess carbon dioxide has narcotic effects, but insufficient oxygen does not produce severe reactions until oxygen levels in the inhaled air fall to one-half of normal. However, trained runners have demonstrated exercise-induced hypoxemia (low oxygen levels in the blood) at very high cardiac outputs, resulting in a mismatch in the ventilation–perfusion ratio in the lung, as well as diffusion limitations due to the reduced time red blood cells spend in the pulmonary capillaries.

Oxygen is conveyed by convection (warm air molecules that are replaced by cooler molecules) in the upper airways and by diffusion in the lower airways to the alveoli (air sacs in the lower reaches of the lung where gas is exchanged at the blood–gas barrier). Oxygen must diffuse from the alveoli, through the extremely thin alveolocapillary membrane, composed of a thin layer of endothelial cells, into solution in the blood. Oxygen diffuses further into red blood cells where it is bound chemically to hemoglobin molecules. The order of each of these processes is reversed in the working muscles where the concentration gradient for oxygen is in the opposite direction. The complete transfer of oxygen between alveolar air and pulmonary blood requires about 0.75 s. Carbon dioxide requires somewhat less time, about 0.15 s. Thus, alveolar air more closely reflects the levels of blood carbon dioxide than oxygen.

Both respiration rate and tidal volume (known as ventilation, or the amount of air moved per breath) increase with exercise, but above the lactate threshold, the tidal volume no longer increases (it remains at about 2–2.5 L). From that point, increases in ventilation are accomplished by increases in respiration rate. A similar limitation occurs for stroke volume in the heart (limited to about 120 mL).

The work of respiration, representing only about 1–2% of the body's oxygen consumption at rest increases to 8–10% or more of the body's oxygen consumption during exercise. Contributing greatly to this is the work to overcome resistance to the movement of air in the airways, lung tissue, and chest wall tissue. Turbulent air flow in the upper airways (those nearest and including the mouth and nose) contributes a great deal of pressure drop. The lower airways are not as rigid as the upper airways and are influenced by the stretching and contraction of the lung tissue that surrounds them. High exhalation pressures external to the airways coupled with low static pressures inside (due to high flow rates inside) tend to close these airways somewhat and limit exhalation airflow rates. The resistance of these airways becomes very high, and the respiratory system appears like a flow source, but only during extreme exhalation.

26.6 Optimization

Energy demands during exercise are so great that optimal courses of action are followed for many physiological responses (see Table 26.2). Walking occurs most naturally at a pace that represents the smallest energy expenditure. The transition from walking to running occurs when running expends less energy than walking; ejection of blood from the left ventricle appears to be optimized to minimize energy expenditure; heart rate variation centers around the most efficient rate; and respiratory rate, breathing waveforms, the ratio of inhalation time to exhalation time, airways resistance, tidal volume, and other respiratory parameters all appear to be regulated to minimize energy expenditure (Johnson 1993, 2009).

26.7 Thermoregulatory Response

When exercise is prolonged, heat begins to accumulate in the body. For heat to become stored, exercise must be performed at a relatively low rate. Increased body temperature stimulates neurons in the respiratory center to exert some control over ventilation, but only during prolonged exercise. Acute exercise is too vigorous and ends too abruptly for significant heat accumulation. The energy to fuel muscular activities amounts to, at most, a 20–25% efficiency, and, in general, the smaller the muscle mass, the less efficient it is. Muscle fibers convert chemical energy (from the food we eat) into the mechanical energy required to produce the movement of skeletal muscles. The remaining 75–80% of the total energy expenditure is lost as heat.

The thermal challenges to exercise are met in several ways. Blood sent to the limbs and blood returning from the limbs is normally conveyed by arteries and veins in close proximity deep inside the limb. This tends to conserve heat by countercurrent heat exchange between the arteries and the veins. Thermal stress causes blood to return via surface veins rather than from deep veins. The skin surface temperature increases and the heat loss by convection and radiation (transfer of heat between two objects not in direct contact) also increases. Additionally, vasodilatation of cutaneous blood vessels augments surface heat loss but places an additional burden on the heart to deliver added blood to the skin as well as to the exercising muscles. Plasma volume is thus reduced from excessive sweating to cool the body, and consequently, stroke volume decreases with a concomitant increase in heart rate. Ultimately, cardiac output is reduced since cardiac output equals the product of heart rate and stroke volume. This phenomenon is referred to as the cardiovascular drift.

As the body temperature rises, the hypothalamus stimulates the vasodilatation of skin blood vessels and sweat gland activity to increase evaporative (conversion of a liquid to a gas) heat loss. Different areas of the body begin sweating earlier than others, but eventually the entire body is involved. If the evaporation of sweat occurs on the skin surface, then the full cooling power of evaporating sweat (670 W · h/kg) is felt. If the sweat is absorbed by clothing, then the full benefit of sweat evaporation is not realized at the skin. If the sweat falls from the skin, as is commonly experienced in very humid conditions, no cooling benefit transpires.

Prolonged sweating leads to plasma volume losses, as already stated, with some hemoconcentration (decreased blood volume in relation to number of red blood cells of 2% or more). This increased red cell concentration leads to increased blood viscosity, and cardiac work becomes even greater.

26.8 Applications

The knowledge of exercise physiology imparts to the medical or biological engineer the ability to design devices to be used with or by humans or animals, or to borrow from human physiology to apply to other situations. There is a continual need for engineers to design equipment used by athletes, sports, and health enthusiasts, for diagnostic evaluation, to modify prostheses or devices for the handicapped to allow for performance of greater than light levels of work and exercise, to alleviate physiological stresses caused by personal protective equipment and other occupational ergonometric gear, to design human-powered

TABLE 26.2 Summary of Exercise Responses for a Normal Young Male

	Rest	Light Exercise	Moderate Exercise	Heavy Exercise	Maximal Exercise
Oxygen uptake (L/min)	0.30	0.60	2.2	3.0	3.2
Maximal oxygen uptake (%)	10	20	70	95	100
Physical work rate (W)	0	10	140	240	430
Aerobic fraction (%)	100	100	98	85	50
Performance time (min)	α	480	5	9.3	3.0
Carbon dioxide production (L/min)	0.18	1.5	2.3	2.8	3.7
Respiratory exchange ratio	0.72	0.84	0.94	1.0	1.1
Blood lactic acid (mmol/L)	1.0	1.8	4.0	7.2	9.6
Heart rate (beats/min)	70	130	160	175	200
Stroke volume (L)	0.075	0.100	0.105	0.110	0.110
Cardiac output (L/min)	5.2	13	17	19	22
Minute volume (L/min)	6	22	50	80	120
Tidal volume (L)	0.4	1.6	2.3	2.4	2.4
Respiration rate (breaths/min)	15	26	28	57	60
Peak flow (L/min)	216	340	450	480	480
Muscular efficiency (%)	0	5	18	20	20
Aortic hemoglobin saturation (%)	98	97	94	93	92
Inhalation time (s)	1.5	1.25	1.0	0.7	0.5
Exhalation time (s)	3.0	2.0	1.1	0.75	0.5
Respiratory work rate (W)	0.305	0.705	5.45	12.32	20.03
Cardiac work rate (W)	1.89	4.67	9.61	11.81	14.30
Systolic pressure (mmHg)	120	134	140	162	172
Diastolic pressure (mmHg)	80	85	90	95	100
End-inspiratory lung volume (L)	2.8	3.2	4.6	4.6	4.6
End-expiratory lung volume (L)	2.4	2.2	2.1	2.1	2.1
Gas partial pressures (mmHg)					
Arterial pCO_2	40	41	45	48	50
pO_2	100	98	94	93	92
Venous pCO_2	44	57	64	70	72
pO_2	36	23	17	10	9
Alveolar pCO_2	32	40	28	20	10
pO_2	98	94	110	115	120
Skin conductance [W/($m^2 \cdot$ °C)]	5.3	7.9	12	13	13
Sweat rate (kg/s)	0.001	0.002	0.008	0.007	0.002
Walking/running speed (m/s)	0	1.0	2.2	6.7	7.1
Ventilation/perfusion of the lung	0.52	0.50	0.54	0.82	1.1
Respiratory evaporative water loss (L/min)	1.02×10^{-5}	4.41×10^{-5}	9.01×10^{-4}	1.35×10^{-3}	2.14×10^{-3}
Total body convective heat loss (W)	24	131	142	149	151
Mean skin temperature (°C)	34	32	30.5	29	28
Heat production (W)	105	190	640	960	1720
Equilibrium rectal temperature (°C)	36.7	38.5	39.3	39.7	500
Final rectal temperature (°C)	37.1	38.26	39.3	37.4	37

machines that are compatible with the capabilities of its operators, and to invent systems to establish and maintain locally benign surroundings in otherwise harsh environments. Recipients of these efforts include athletes, the handicapped, laborers, public safety and military personnel, space and deep sea explorers, farmers, power plant workers, construction workers, and many others where the rate of work is externally imposed or environmentally challenged. The study of exercise physiology, especially in the medical and biological engineer lexicon, can potentially enhance engineering paradigms.

Defining Terms

Anaerobic threshold: The transition between exercise levels that can be sustained through nearly complete aerobic metabolism and those that rely on at least partially anaerobic metabolism. Above the anaerobic threshold, blood lactate increases and the relationship between ventilation and oxygen uptake becomes nonlinear.

Baroreceptors: Stretch receptors located within the cardiovascular system that detect changes in blood pressure.

Cardiovascular drift: Plasma volume losses due to excessive sweating causes an increase in the heart rate during prolonged exercise to compensate for the decrease in stroke volume. This compensation helps to maintain cardiac output.

Chemoreceptors (and metaboreceptors): These sensory organs send information regarding the chemical/metabolic state of muscles (oxygen, carbon dioxide, glucose, electrolytes).

Excess post-exercise oxygen consumption (EPOC): It is the difference between resting oxygen consumption and the accumulated rate of oxygen consumption following exercise termination. EPOC relates to the replacement cost of creatine phosphate, lactic acid resynthesis to glucose, elevated body temperature, catecholamine action, and the cost of elevated heart and breathing rates.

Maximal oxygen consumption: It is the maximum rate of oxygen utilized by the human body during severe dynamic exercise. The amount of oxygen consumed is determined, in part, by age, gender, maximal cardiac output, maximal arterial–mixed venous oxygen difference, and physical condition.

Mechanoreceptors: An end organ that responds to changes in mechanical stress such as stretch, vibration, pressure, compression, or distension.

Oxygen deficit: The accumulated difference between actual oxygen consumption at the beginning of exercise and the rate of oxygen consumption that would exist if oxygen consumption rose immediately to its steady-state level corresponding to exercise level.

References

Johnson, A.T. 1993. How much work is expended for respiration? *Front. Med. Biol. Eng.* 5: 265.

Johnson, A.T. 2007. *Biomechanics and Exercise Physiology: Quantitative Modeling,* Taylor & Francis, Boca Raton, FL.

Mole, P.A. 1983. Exercise metabolism. In A.A. Bove and D.T. Lowenthal (Eds.), *Exercise Medicine,* pp. 43–48. New York, Academic Press.

Skinner, J.S. and McLellan, T. H. 1980. The transition from aerobic to anaerobic metabolism. *Res. Q. Exerc. Sport.* 51: 234.

White, A. Handler, P., Smith, E.L., and Stetten, D. 1959. *Principles of Biochemistry,* New York, McGraw-Hill.

Further Information

Biological Foundations of Biomedical Engineering, edited by J. Kline (Little Brown and Company, 1976) is a very good textbook of physiology written for engineers.

Exercise Physiology: Theory and Application to Fitness and Performance, by S. Powers and E. Howley (McGraw-Hill, 2009) is intended for those persons interested in exercise physiology, clinical exercise physiology, kinesiology, exercise science, and physical therapy. The book contains numerous clinical applications sporting performance and health-related physical fitness.

Physiology of Sport and Exercise, by J. Wilmore, D. Costill and W.L. Kenny (Human Kinetics, 2008) is an excellent additional reference on the physiology of sport and exercise.

Textbook of Work Physiology: Physiological Bases of Exercise by P. O. Astrand, K. Rodahl, H. Dahl and S. Stromme (Human Kinetics, 2003) contains a great deal of updated information on exercise physiology and is generally considered the standard textbook on the subject.

27

Factors Affecting Mechanical Work in Humans

Ben F. Hurley
University of Maryland

Arthur T. Johnson
University of Maryland

27.1 Exercise Biomechanics...27-1
      Equilibrium • Muscular Movement • Muscular
      Efficiency • Locomotion
References...27-9

High technology has entered our diversions and leisure activities. Sports, exercise, and training are no longer just physical activities but include machines and techniques attuned to individual capabilities and needs. This chapter considers several factors related to exercise and training that help in understanding human performance.

Physiological work performance is determined by energy transformation that begins with the process of photosynthesis and ends with the production of biological work (Figure 27.1). Energy in the form of nuclear transformations is converted into radiant energy, which then transforms the energy from carbon dioxide and water into oxygen and glucose through photosynthesis. In plants, the glucose can also be converted into fats and proteins. Upon ingesting plants or other animals that eat plants, humans convert this energy through cellular respiration (the reverse of photosynthesis) into chemical energy in the form of adenosine triphosphate (ATP). The endergonic reactions (energy absorbed from the surroundings) that produce ATP are followed by exergonic reactions (energy released to the surroundings) that release energy through the breakdown of ATP to produce chemical and mechanical work in the human body. The steps involved in the synthesis and breakdown of carbohydrates, fats, and proteins produce chemical work and provide energy for the mechanical work produced from muscular contractions. The purpose of this chapter is to provide a brief summary of some factors that can affect mechanical work in humans.

27.1 Exercise Biomechanics

27.1.1 Equilibrium

Any body, including the human body, remains in stable equilibrium if the vectorial sum of all forces and torques acting on the body is zero. An unbalanced force results in linear acceleration and an unbalanced torque results in rotational acceleration. Static equilibrium requires that

$$\sum F = 0 \tag{27.1}$$

$$\sum T = 0 \tag{27.2}$$

where F is vectorial forces (N) and T is vectorial torques (N m).

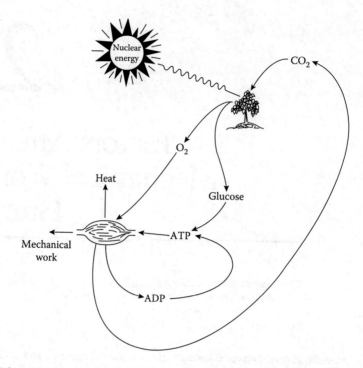

FIGURE 27.1 Schematic of energy transformations leading to muscular mechanical work.

TABLE 27.1 Fraction of Body Weights for Various Parts of the Body

Body Part	Fraction
Head and neck	0.07
Trunk	0.43
Upper arms	0.07
Forearms and hands	0.06
Thighs	0.23
Lower legs and feet	0.14
	1.00

Some sports activities, such as wrestling, weight lifting, and fencing, require stability, whereas other activities, such as running, jumping, and diving, cannot be performed unless there is managed instability. Shifting the body position allows for proper control. The mass of the body is distributed as in Table 27.1, and the center of mass is located at approximately 56% of a person's height and midway from side to side and front to back. The center of mass can be made to shift by extending the limbs or by bending the torso.

27.1.2 Muscular Movement

Mechanical movement results from the contraction of muscles that are attached at each end to bones that can move relative to each other. The arrangement of this combination is commonly known as a class 3 lever (Figure 27.2), where one joint acts as the fulcrum (Figure 27.3), the other bone acts as the load, and the muscle provides the force interposed between the fulcrum and the load. This arrangement requires that the muscle force be greater than the load, sometimes by a very large amount, but the distance through which the muscle moves is made very small. These characteristics match muscle

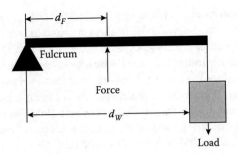

FIGURE 27.2 Class 3 lever is arranged with the applied force interposed between the fulcrum and the load. Most skeletal muscles are arranged in this fashion.

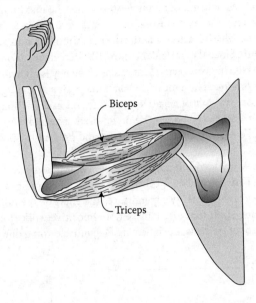

FIGURE 27.3 Biceps muscle of the arm is arranged as a class 3 lever. The load is located at the hand and the fulcrum is located at the elbow.

capabilities well (muscles can produce 7×10^5 N/m², but cannot move far). Since the distance is made smaller, the speed of shortening of the contracting muscle is also slower than it would be if the arrangement between the force and the load was different:

$$\frac{S_L}{S_M} = \frac{d_L}{d_M} \tag{27.3}$$

where S is the speed (m/s), d is the distance from the fulcrum (m), and L and M denote the load and the muscle, respectively.

27.1.3 Muscular Efficiency

Efficiency relates the external, or physical, work produced to the total chemical energy consumed:

$$\eta = \frac{\text{External work produced}}{\text{Chemical energy consumed}} \tag{27.4}$$

Muscular efficiencies range from close to zero to about 20–25%. The larger numbers would be obtained for leg exercises that involve lifting the body weight. In carpentry and foundry work, where both arms and legs are used, the average mechanical efficiency is approximately 10% (Johnson, 1991). For finer movements that require exquisite control, small muscles are often arranged in an antagonistic fashion, that is, the final movement is produced as a result of the difference between two or more muscles working against each other. In this case, efficiencies approach zero. Isometric muscular contraction, where a force is produced but no movement results, has an efficiency of zero (Johnson et al., 2002).

Generally, muscles are able to exert the greatest force when the velocity of muscle contraction is zero. The power produced by this muscle would be zero. When the velocity of muscle contraction is about 8 m/s, the force produced by the muscle becomes zero, and the power produced by this muscle again becomes zero. Somewhere in between the above conditions stated, the power produced and the efficiency become the maximum (Figure 27.4).

The isometric length–tension relationship of a muscle shows that the maximum force developed by a muscle is exerted at its resting length (the length of a slightly stretched muscle attached by its tendons to the skeleton) and decreases to zero at twice its resting length. The maximum force also decreases to zero at the shortest possible muscular length. Since the muscular contractile force depends on the length of the muscle and since the length changes during contraction, muscular efficiency is always changing (Figure 27.5).

Negative (eccentric) work is produced by a muscle when it maintains a force against an external force tending to stretch the muscle. An example of negative work is found in the action of the leg muscle during a descent of a flight of stairs. Since the body is being lowered, external work is less than zero. The muscles are using physiological energy to control the descent and prevent the body from accumulating kinetic energy as it descends.

Muscular efficiencies for walking downhill approach 120% (McMahon, 1984). Since heat produced by the muscle is the difference between 100% and the percent efficiency, the heat produced by muscles walking downhill is about 220% of their energy expenditure. The energy expenditure of muscles undergoing negative work is about one-sixth that of a muscle doing positive work (Johnson, 1991); so, a leg muscle going uphill produces about twice as much heat as a leg muscle going downhill.

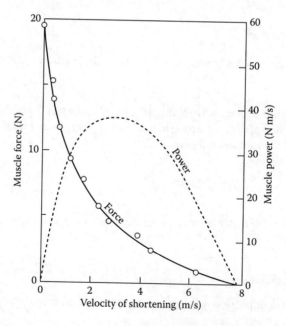

FIGURE 27.4 Force and power output of a muscle as a function of velocity. (Adapted and used with permission from Milsum, J. H. *Biological Control Systems Analysis*, McGraw-Hill, New York, 1966.)

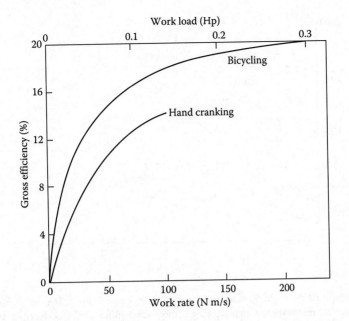

FIGURE 27.5 Gross efficiency for hand cranking or bicycling is a function of the rate of work. (From Goldman, R.F., 1978. *Safety in Manual Materials Handling*, National Institute for Occupational Safety and Health (NIOSH), Cincinnati, OH, pp. 110–116.)

27.1.4 Locomotion

The act of locomotion involves both positive and negative work. There are four successive stages of a walking stride. In the first stage, both feet are on the ground, with one foot ahead of the other. The trailing foot pushes forward and the front foot is pushing backward. In the second stage, the trailing foot leaves the ground and the front foot applies a braking force. The center of mass of the body begins to lift over the front foot. In the third stage, the trailing foot is brought forward and the supporting foot applies a vertical force. The center of mass of the body is at its highest point above the supporting foot. In the last stage, the body's center of mass is lowered and the trailing foot provides an acceleration force.

This alteration of the raising and lowering of the body's center of mass, along with the pushing and braking provided by the feet, makes walking a low-efficiency maneuver. Walking has been likened to alternatively applying the brakes and accelerator while driving a car. Just as the fuel efficiency of the car would suffer from this mode of propulsion, so does the energy efficiency of walking suffer from the way walking is performed.

There is an optimum speed of walking. If the walking speed is more than this optimum speed, additional muscular energy is required to propel the body forward. Moving slower than the optimal speed requires additional muscular energy to retard the leg movement. Thus, the optimal speed is related to the rate at which the leg can swing forward. A simple analysis of the leg as a physical pendulum shows that the optimal walking speed is related to the length of the leg:

$$S \propto \sqrt{L} \tag{27.5}$$

Unlike walking, there is a stage of running during which both feet leave the ground. The center of mass of the body does not rise and fall as much during running as during walking; so, the efficiency for running can be greater than for walking.

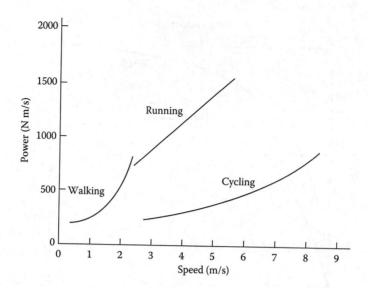

FIGURE 27.6 Power required for walking, running, and cycling by an adult male. The curves for walking and running interact at about 2.3 m/s and show that walking is more efficient below the intersection and running is more efficient above the intersection. (Redrawn with permission from Alexander, R.M. *Am. Sci.*, 72: 348, 1984.)

At a speed of about 2.5 m/s, running appears to be more energy efficient than walking, and the transition is usually made between these forms of locomotion (Figure 27.6). Unlike walking, there does not appear to be a functional relationship between speed and the length of the leg; so, running power expenditure is linearly related to speed alone.

Why would anyone want to propel the extra weight of a bicycle in addition to body weight? On the surface, it would appear that cycling would cost more energy than running or walking. However, the center of mass of the body does not move vertically as long as the cyclist sits on the seat. Without the positive and negative work associated with walking or running, cycling is a much more efficient form of locomotion than the other two (Figure 27.6), and the cost of moving the additional weight of the bicycle can be easily supplied.

Many sports or leisure activities have a biomechanical basis. An understanding of the underlying biomechanical processes can lead to improved performance. Yet, there are limits to performance that cause frustrations for competitive athletes. Hence, additional factors are sometimes employed to expand these limits. A brief discussion of some of these factors is given here.

27.1.4.1 Age

It is well established that structural and functional deterioration occurs to most physiological systems in the body with aging, independent of disease or inactivity (Juckett, 2010). There are both primary aging (i.e., age-dependent or normal aging) effects and secondary aging (i.e., temporally associated with age, but not necessarily due to the aging process) effects (Brody and Schneider, 1986). Both adversely influence the mechanical and physiological work performance. Aging effects on the cardiovascular, neuromuscular, and musculoskeletal systems have a particularly high impact on mechanical work capacity. Age-associated deterioration of these systems results in a decline in maximal oxygen consumption (aerobic capacity), and a loss of muscle mass, strength, power, fatigue resistance, and bone mineral density, as well as a gain in body fat, particularly in the abdominal region (Kyle et al., 2001; Kuk et al., 2009). These changes also lead to greater disease prevalence and a volitional decline in physical activity. For this reason, with advanced age, it is difficult to determine how much of the loss in work capacity can be attributed to primary aging versus inactivity.

Young athletes who continue to train to an older age maintain a large portion of their aerobic capacity with age, but still experience some losses due to both primary and secondary aging. Although the declines in aerobic capacity (Pollack et al., 1997) and skeletal muscle function (Kyle et al., 2001) with age can be considerable, regular exercise (training) results in substantial slowing of the age-associated declines in most systems. Many of the aging effects on both the cardiovascular (Bortz, 2010) and musculoskeletal (Lynch et al., 1999) systems can be at least partly reversed within the first couple of months of exercise training (Hurley and Kostek, 2001; Walts et al., 2008).

The loss of aerobic capacity with aging and inactivity is primarily due to losses in cardiac output, which in turn results from decreases in maximal heart rate, whereas the maximal capacity to extract oxygen from the peripheral blood does not change much with aging. Thus, aging results in a reduced blood flow to the active muscles during exercise as a result of a loss of cardiac output. Although inactivity can also result in loss of cardiac output, it appears to be largely the result of a loss in plasma volume, with reductions in heart volume and heart contractility playing a smaller role.

Maximal force production (muscular strength) is maintained for a much longer time period throughout aging than aerobic capacity. For example, significant declines in aerobic capacity (Fleg et al., 2005) is already observed in the thirties, whereas strength is maintained until the sixties (Lynch et al., 1999). Losses in aerobic capacity, though not linear, can be greater than 10% per decade (Buskirk and Hodgson, 1987), whereas age-associated strength losses occur at a rate of ~12–14% per decade (Lynch et al., 1999). Likewise, the loss of muscle mass occurs at a rate of ~6% per decade, again beginning in the sixties for men, but two decades earlier in women (Lynch et al., 1999). Muscle power has a faster rate of decline than strength (Kostka 2005) and appears to be more closely related to the functional abilities in the elderly than strength (Puthoff et al., 2008), presumably due to the relative importance of movement velocity in many activities of daily living.

27.1.4.2 Regular Exercise

For the purpose of this chapter, regular exercise will be divided into two training modalities: aerobic exercise training and resistance (strength) training. Aerobic training consists of regular muscular activities that use large amounts of oxygen for energy production. These include exercises such as walking, jogging, swimming, and cycling. Strength training (ST) refers to exercising regularly against an external load, such as during isotonic (same tension), isokinetic (same movement velocity), or isometric (same muscle length) ST. Isotonic and isokinetic ST can be divided into the shortening and lengthening phases (often incorrectly named concentric and eccentric phases) (Faulkner, 2003), and can be performed with free weights such as barbells and dumbbells, machines, or by just using one's body mass for resistance, such as is done with certain kinds of calisthenics.

27.1.4.2.1 Aerobic Exercise Training

When aerobic exercise is performed regularly, it stimulates many biochemical reactions that raise the critical threshold level of exercise intensity at which metabolic homeostasis (equilibrium) can be maintained. Many compensatory reactions allow the body to adapt to minor stresses, such as mild aerobic exercise, so that homeostasis (equilibrium) can be maintained. For example, the increased energy demands of aerobic exercise stimulate an increase in heart rate, respiration, blood flow, and many other cardiovascular and metabolic reactions that allow the body to maintain homeostasis. As the intensity of exercise increases, it becomes more difficult for compensatory mechanisms to maintain homeostasis. After exceeding about 80% of an untrained person's maximal exercise capacity, homeostasis can no longer be maintained for more than a few minutes before exhaustion results.

Regular aerobic exercise (training) elevates the threshold level that a single exercise session can be performed before disturbing and eventually losing homeostasis. It does this by elevating the maximal physiological capacity for homeostasis so that the same intensity of aerobic exercise may no longer disrupt homeostasis due to a lower percentage of maximal capacity. In addition, training produces specific adaptations during submaximal exercise that permit greater and longer amounts of work before losing homeostasis (Hurley and Hagberg, 1998). A good example of this is when blood lactate rises with increased intensity of exercise. Prior to training, blood lactate concentration rises substantially when the intensity of exercise exceeds ~75% of maximal oxygen consumption (VO_2max). Following training, the same intensity of exercise results in a lower concentration of blood lactate, resulting in a higher fraction of the untrained VO_2max before blood lactate reaches the same level as before training during exercise. This adaptation is so profound that blood lactate levels are often only slightly above the resting values after training, when performing submaximal exercise (e.g., <65% of VO_2max). Thus, exercise training allows an individual to perform a much greater amount of work during exercise before homeostasis is disturbed to the point at which fatigue ensues.

27.1.4.2.2 Strength Training

Muscular strength declines with age (Lindle et al., 1997; Lynch et al., 1999), disease, and as a consequence of the administration of some medications used for the treatment of the disease (Fiatarone-Singh, 2002; Hurley and Hanson, 2009). However, strength can be increased substantially in a relatively short time period with ST (Walts et al., 2008). Muscle power can also be increased with ST, but the magnitude of increase depends on the movement velocity of training used during the muscle shortening phase of exercise.

The typical training modalities of ~2 s during the shortening phase and ~4 s during the muscle lengthening phase of movement result in ~30% increase in strength (Lemmer et al., 2000) and ~25% increase in power (Jozsi et al., 1999; Delmonico et al., 2005). However, increases of almost 100% have been reported when high-velocity training has been incorporated (Fielding et al., 2002). Our group has reported increases in muscle mass of ~12% with ST, within the first couple of months of training, based on magnetic resonance imaging (MRI) measurements of the entire volume of the muscle being trained (Ivey et al., 2000) and about half that amount when the male sex hormone, testosterone, has been obliterated (Hanson and Hurley, unpublished data, 2010). The amount of force per unit of muscle volume, known as muscle quality, also increases substantially with ST (Tracey et al., 1999). We have shown that ~3 decades of age-related strength loss and two decades of age-related muscle mass loss can be recovered/reversed within the first couple of months of ST (Ivey et al., 2000; Lemmer et al., 2000).

27.1.4.3 Sex Differences

Cardiovascular fitness and muscular strength are substantially higher in men compared to women. The aerobic capacity in men is about 40–50% higher than women. In addition, the upper body strength is ~100% higher and the lower body strength is ~50% higher in men (Lynch et al., 1999). However, these differences are diminished substantially when body composition is taken into consideration. For example, when VO_2max is expressed with reference to body mass (mL/kg of body weight/min), this difference narrows to ~20% and to ~10% when differences in muscle mass are taken into consideration.

The differences in muscular strength between men and women are also narrowed when normalized for fat-free mass (Lynch et al., 1999). There does not appear to be any significant difference in responses to training between men and women when expressed on a relative basis (% change), but men appear to have greater muscle mass gains than women in response to ST when expressed in absolute terms (Ivey et al., 2000).

Women can be less fatigable than men for some muscle groups during isometric contractions, but sex differences vary substantially depending on the task, muscle groups involved, and age of the participant (Hunter, 2009). This conditional explanation is based on the fact that task differences are limited by different physiological systems.

27.1.4.4 Genetics

There appears to be evidence that genetic factors contribute significantly to whether one chooses to be sedentary or physically active, to aerobic capacity, and to muscular power, but the specific genes responsible for these influences are still not known (Rankinen et al., 2010). We have observed great interindividual variability in the loss of both muscle strength and mass with age (Lindle et al., 1997; Lynch et al., 1999), as well as the gain in muscle strength and muscle mass with exercise training (Ivey et al., 2000; Walts et al., 2008).

Seeman et al. (1996) reported that genetic factors accounted for 60–80% of the interindividual differences in lean body mass, whereas Huygens et al. (2004) reported the heritability of skeletal muscle mass of up to 90%. These data provide strong support that genetic factors may influence sarcopenia (i.e., alterations in strength and muscle mass with age), as well as strength and muscle mass response to ST. However, none of these studies assessed the effects of specific candidate genes or candidate gene variations (polymorphisms) on strength or muscle mass response to training.

The heritability of muscle mass and strength indicates that specific genes contribute to differences in muscle phenotype. More importantly, specific polymorphisms could at least partly explain the interindividual variability in sarcopenia and muscle response to ST. Moreover, our research group and others have explored the relationship of gene polymorphisms to muscle phenotypes in genes thought to have a plausible physiological connection to changes in strength and muscle mass. Unfortunately, however, this work has been largely unsuccessful in identifying either single genes or gene interactions that explain more than about 5% of training responses in these muscle phenotypes. Thus, despite the knowledge of important relationships between genetics and muscle function, little is known about the specific gene variations that may explain this genetic contribution (Rankinen et al., 2010).

References

Alexander, R.M. Walking and running. *Am. Sci.*, 72: 348, 1984.

Bortz, W. Disuse and aging. *J. Gerontol. A Biol. Sci. Med. Sci.*, 65(4): 382–385, 2010.

Brody, J. A., and Schneider, E. L. Diseases and disorders of aging: An hypothesis. *J. Chronic. Dis.*, 39: 871–876, 1986.

Buskirk, E. R., and Hodgson, J. L. Age and aerobic power: The rate of change in men and women. *Fed. Proc.*, 46: 1824–1829, 1987.

Delmonico, M. J., Kostek, M. C., Doldo, N. A., Hand, B. D., Bailey, J. A., Rabon-Stith, K. M., Conway, J. M., and Hurley, B. F. The effect of moderate velocity strength training on peak muscle power, velocity, and muscle power quality in older men and women. *J. Appl. Physiol.*, 99: 1712–1718, 2005.

Faulkner, J. A. Terminology for contractions of muscles during shortening, while isometric, and during lengthening. *J. Appl. Physiol.*, 95: 455–459, 2003.

Fiatarone-Singh, M. A. Exercise comes of age: Rationale and recommendations for a geriatric exercise prescription. *J. Geronto: Med. Sci.*, 57A: M262–M282, 2002.

Fielding R. A., LeBrasseur, N. K., Cuoco, A., Bean, J., Mizer, K., and Fiatarone-Singh, M. A. High-velocity resistance training increases skeletal muscle peak power in older women. *J. Am. Geriatr. Soc.*, 50: 655–662, 2002.

Fleg, J. L., Morrell, C. H., Bos, A. G., Brant, L. J., Talbot, L. A., Wright, J. G., and Lakatta, E. G. Accelerated longitudinal decline of aerobic capacity in healthy older adults. *Circulation*, 112(5): 674–682, 2005.

Hunter, S. K. Sex differences and mechanisms of task specific muscle fatigue. *Exerc. Sport Sci. Rev.*, 37: 113–122, 2009.

Hurley, B. F. and Hagberg, J.M. Optimizing health in older persons: Aerobic or strength training? In *Exerc. Sport Sci. Rev.*, 26: 61–89, Williams & Wilkins, Baltimore, MD, 1998.

Hurley, B. F. and Hanson, E. D. Can strength training reverse the side effects of cancer treatment? *J. Act. Aging*, Nov/Dec: 44–52, 2009.

Hurley, B. F. and Kostek, M. C. Exercise interventions for seniors. What training modality is best for health? *Orthop. Phys. Ther. Clin. North Am.*, 10: 213–225, 2001.

Huygens, W., Thomis, M. A., Peeters, M. W., Vlietinck, R. F., and Beunen, G. P. Determinants and upper-limit heritabilities of skeletal muscle mass and strength. *Can. J. Appl. Physiol.*, 29: 186–200, 2004.

Ivey, F. M., Tracy, B. L., Lemmer, J. T., Hurlbut, D. E., Martel, G. F., Roth, S. M., Fozard, J. L., Metter, E. J., and Hurley, B. F. The effects of age, gender and myostatin genotype on the hypertrophic response to heavy resistance strength training. *J Gerontol: Med. Sci.*, 55A: M641–M648, 2000.

Johnson, A. T. *Biomechanics and Exercise Physiology*, John Wiley, New York, 1991.

Johnson, A. T., Benjamin, M. B., and Silverman, N. Oxygen consumption, heat production, and muscular efficiency during uphill and downhill walking. *Appl. Ergon.*, 33: 485–491, 2002.

Jozsi, A. C., Campbell, W. W., Joseph, L., Davey, S. L., and Evans, W. J. Changes in power with resistance training in older and younger men and women. *J. Gerontol.*, 54A: M591–M596, 1999.

Juckett, D. A. What determines age-related disease: Do we know all the right questions? *Age (Dordr.)*, 32(2): 155–160, 2010.

Kostka, T. Quadriceps maximal power and optimal shortening velocity in 335 men aged 23–88 years. *Eur. J. Appl. Physiol.*, 95: 140–145, 2005.

Kuk, J. L., Saunders, T. J., Davidson, L. E., and Ross, R. Age-related changes in total and regional fat distribution. *Ageing Res. Rev.*, 8: 339–348, 2009.

Kyle, U. G., Genton, L., Hans, D., Karsegard, L., Slosman, D. O., and Pichard, C. Age-related differences in fat-free mass, skeletal muscle, body cell mass and fat mass between 18 and 94 years. *Eur. J. Clin. Nutr.*, 55: 663–672, 2001.

Lemmer, J. T., Hurbut, D. E., Martel, G. F., Tracy, B. L., Ivey, F. M., Metter, E. J., Fozard, J. L., Fleg, J. L., and Hurley, B. F. Age and gender responses to strength training and detraining. *Med. Sci. Sports Exerc.*, 32: 1505–1512, 2000.

Lindle, R., Metter, E., Lynch, N., Fleg, J., Fozard, J., Tobin, J., Roy, T., and Hurley, B. Age and gender comparisons of muscle strength in 654 women and men aged 20–93. *J. Appl. Physiol.*, 83: 1581–1587, 1997.

Lynch, N. A., Metter, E. J., Lindle, R. S., Fozard, J. L., Tobin, J. D., Roy, T. A., Fleg, J. L., and Hurley, B. F. Muscle quality I: Age-associated differences in arm vs. leg muscle groups. *J. Appl. Physiol.*, 86: 188–194, 1999.

McMahon, T. A. *Muscles, Reflexes, and Locomotion*, Princeton University Press, Princeton, NJ, 1984.

Milsum, J. H. *Biological Control Systems Analysis*, McGraw-Hill, New York, 1966.

Pollack, M. L., Mengelkoch, L. F., Graves, J. S., Lowenthal, D. T., Limacher, M. C., Foster, C., and Wilmore, J. H. Twenty year follow-up of aerobic power and body composition of older track athletes. *J. Appl. Physiol.*, 82: 1508–1516, 1997.

Puthoff, M. L., Janz, K. F., and Nielson, D. The relationship between lower extremity strength and power to everyday walking behaviors in older adults with functional limitations. *J. Geriatr. Phys. Ther.*, 31: 24–31, 2008.

Rankinen, T., Roth, S. M., Bray, M. S., Loos, R., Perusse, L., Wolfarth, B., Hagberg, J. M., and Bouchard, C. Advances in exercise, fitness, and performance genomics. *Med. Sci. Sports Exerc.*, 42: 835–846, 2010.

Seeman, E., Hopper, J., Young, N., Formica, C., Goss, P., and Tsalamandris, C. Do genetic factors explain associations between muscle strength, lean mass, and bone density? A twin study. *Am. J. Physiol.*, 270: E320–E327, 1996.

Tracy, B.L., Ivey, F.M., Hurlbut, D., Martel, G. F., Lemmer, J.T., Siegel, E. L., Metter, E. J., Fozard, J. L., Fleg, J. L., and Hurley, B. F. 1999. Muscle quality II: Effects of strength training in 65–75 year old men and women, *J. Appl. Physiol.* 86: 195–201.

Walts, C. T., Hanson, E. D., Delmonico, M. J., Yao, L., Wang, M. Q., and Hurley, B. F. Do sex or race differences influence strength training effects on muscle or fat? *Med. Sci. Sports Exerc.*, 40(4): 669–676, 2008.

III

Biomaterials

Joyce Y. Wong
Boston University

28 Metallic Biomaterials *Joon B. Park and Young Kon Kim*.............................. **28**-1
Introduction • Stainless Steels • CoCr Alloys • Ti Alloys • Dental Metals • Other
Metals • Corrosion of Metallic Implants • Manufacturing of Implants • Defining
Terms • References • Further Reading

29 Ceramic Biomaterials *W. G. Billotte*.. **29**-1
Introduction • Nonabsorbable or Relatively Bioinert Bioceramics • Biodegradable
or Resorbable Ceramics • Bioactive or Surface-Reactive Ceramics • Deterioration of
Ceramics • Bioceramic Manufacturing Techniques • Defining Terms • In Memory
Of • Acknowledgments • References • Further Information

30 Polymeric Biomaterials *Hai Bang Lee, Gilson Khang, and Jin Ho Lee*..................... **30**-1
Introduction • Polymerization and Basic Structure • Polymers Used as
Biomaterials • Sterilization • Surface Modifications for Improving
Biocompatibility • Chemogradient Surfaces for Cell and Protein
Interaction • Defining Terms • Acknowledgments • References

31 Composite Biomaterials *Roderic S. Lakes*...**31**-1
Structure • Bounds on Properties • Anisotropy of
Composites • Particulate Composites • Fibrous Composites • Porous
Materials • Biocompatibility • Summary • References

32 Biodegradable Polymeric Biomaterials: An Updated Overview *C. C. Chu*.............. **32**-1
Introduction • Glycolide/Lactide-Based Biodegradable Linear
Aliphatic Polyesters • Nonglycolide/Lactide-Based Linear Aliphatic
Polyesters • Nonaliphatic Polyester-Type Biodegradable Polymers • Biodegradation
Properties of Synthetic Biodegradable Polymers • Role of Linear Aliphatic Biodegradable
Polyesters in Tissue Engineering and Regeneration • Supercritical Carbon Dioxide
Sterilization • Defining Terms • References • Further Information

33 Biologic Biomaterials: Tissue-Derived Biomaterials (Collagen) *Shu-Tung Li*.......... **33**-1
Structure and Properties of Collagen and Collagen-Rich Tissues • Biotechnology of
Collagen • Design of a Resorbable Collagen-Based Medical Implant • Tissue Engineering
for Tissue and Organ Regeneration • Defining Terms • References

34 Biologic Biomaterials: Silk *Biman Mandal and David L. Kaplan* 34-1
Structure and Properties • Sources of Silk Proteins • Processing
Silk Proteins • Engineered Silk Matrices for Cell-Based Engineering
and Drug Delivery • Applications of Silkworm Silk for Bone and
Cartilage Tissue Engineering • Silk Degradation • Silk Immunological
Responses • Conclusions • Acknowledgments • References

35 Biofunctional Hydrogels *Melissa K. McHale and Jennifer L. West* 35-1
Introduction • Synthetic Hydrogels • Hydrogel Biofunctionality • Importance
of Physical Properties of Hydrogels • Design of Complex Biofunctional
Hydrogels • Summary • References

36 Soft Tissue Replacements *K. B. Chandran, K. J. L. Burg, and S. W. Shalaby* 36-1
Blood-Interfacing Implants • Defining Terms • References • Nonblood-Interfacing
Implants for Soft Tissues • References • Further Information

37 Hard Tissue Replacements *Sang-Hyun Park, Adolfo Llinás, and Vijay K. Goel* 37-1
Long Bone Repair • Joint Replacements • Total Joint Replacements • Defining
Terms • References

28

Metallic Biomaterials

28.1 Introduction 28-1
28.2 Stainless Steels 28-2
28.3 CoCr Alloys 28-4
28.4 Ti Alloys 28-6
  Pure Ti and Ti6Al4V • TiNi Alloys
28.5 Dental Metals 28-12
28.6 Other Metals 28-13
28.7 Corrosion of Metallic Implants 28-14
  Electrochemical Aspects • Pourbaix Diagrams in Corrosion • Rate
  of Corrosion and Polarization Curves • Corrosion of Available
  Metals • Stress Corrosion Cracking
28.8 Manufacturing of Implants 28-18
  Stainless Steels • Co–Cr Alloys • Ti and Its Alloys
Defining Terms 28-19
References 28-20
Further Reading 28-22

Joon B. Park
University of Iowa

Young Kon Kim
Inje University

28.1 Introduction

Metals are used as biomaterials because of their excellent electrical and thermal conductivity and mechanical properties. Since some electrons are independent in metals, they can quickly transfer an electric charge and thermal energy. The mobile free electrons act as the binding force to hold the positive metal ions together. This attraction is strong, as evidenced by the closely packed atomic arrangement resulting in high specific gravity and high melting points of most metals. Since the metallic bond is essentially nondirectional, the position of the metal ions can be altered without destroying the crystal structure resulting in a plastically deformable solid.

Some metals are used as passive substitutes for hard tissue replacement such as total hip and knee joints, for fracture healing aids as bone plates and screws, spinal fixation devices, and dental implants because of their excellent mechanical properties and *corrosion* resistance. Some metallic alloys are used for more active roles in devices such as vascular stents, catheter guide wires, orthodontic archwires, and cochlea implants.

The first metal alloy developed specifically for human use was the "vanadium steel," which was used to manufacture bone fracture plates (Sherman plates) and screws. Most metals such as iron (Fe), chromium (Cr), cobalt (Co), nickel (Ni), titanium (Ti), tantalum (Ta), niobium (Nb), molybdenum (Mo), and tungsten (W) that were used to make alloys for manufacturing implants can only be tolerated by the body in minute amounts. Sometimes these metallic elements, in naturally occurring forms, are essential for the function of red blood cells (Fe) or synthesis of vitamin B_{12} (Co), but cannot be tolerated in large amounts in the body (Black, 1992). The biocompatibility of the metallic implant is of considerable concern because these implants can corrode in an *in vivo* environment (Williams, 1982). The consequences of corrosion are the disintegration of the implant material *per se*, which will weaken the implant, and the harmful effect of corrosion products on the surrounding tissues and organs.

28.2 Stainless Steels

The first stainless steel utilized for implant fabrication was the 18-8 (type 302 in modern classification), which is stronger and more resistant to corrosion than the vanadium steel. Vanadium steel is no longer used in implants because its corrosion resistance is inadequate *in vivo*. Later, 18-8sMo stainless steel was introduced, which contains a small percentage of molybdenum to improve the corrosion resistance in chloride solution (salt water). This alloy became known as *type 316 stainless steel*. In the 1950s, the carbon content of 316 stainless steel was reduced from 0.08 to a maximum amount of 0.03% (all are weight percent unless specified) for better corrosion resistance to chloride solution and to minimize the sensitization and hence became known as type *316L stainless steel*. The minimum effective concentration of chromium is 11% to impart corrosion resistance in stainless steels. Despite being a reactive element, chromium and its alloys can be *passivated* by 30% nitric acid to give excellent corrosion resistance.

The *austenitic stainless steels*, especially types 316 and 316L, are most widely used for implant fabrication. These cannot be hardened by heat treatment but can be hardened by cold working. This group of stainless steels is nonmagnetic and possesses better corrosion resistance than any other group. The inclusion of molybdenum enhances resistance to *pitting corrosion* in salt water. The American Society of Testing and Materials (ASTM) recommends type 316L rather than type 316 for implant fabrication. The specifications for 316L stainless steel are given in Table 28.1. The only difference in composition between the 316L and 316 stainless steels is the maximum content of carbon, that is, 0.03% and 0.08%, respectively, as noted earlier.

Nickel stabilizes the austenitic phase [γ, face-centered cubic crystal (fcc) structure] at room temperature and enhances corrosion resistance. The austenitic phase formation can be influenced by both the Ni and Cr contents as shown in Figure 28.1 for 0.10% carbon stainless steels. The minimum amount of Ni for maintaining austenitic phase is approximately 10%.

Table 28.2 gives the mechanical properties of 316L stainless steel. A wide range of properties exist depending on the heat treatment (annealing to obtain softer materials) or cold working (for greater strength and hardness). Figure 28.2 shows the effect of cold working on the yield and ultimate tensile strength of 18-8 stainless steels. The engineer must consequently be careful when selecting materials of this type. Even the 316L stainless steels may corrode inside the body under certain circumstances in a highly stressed and oxygen-depleted region, such as the contacts under the screws of the bone fracture plate. Thus, these stainless steels are suitable for use only in temporary implant devices such as fracture plates, screws, and hip nails. Surface modification methods such as anodization, passivation, and

TABLE 28.1 Compositions of 316L Stainless Steel

Element	Composition (%)
Carbon	0.03 max.
Manganese	2.00 max.
Phosphorus	0.03 max.
Sulfur	0.03 max.
Silicon	0.75 max.
Chromium	17.00–20.00
Nickel	12.00–14.00
Molybdenum	2.00–4.00

Source: Adapted from ASTM. 1992. *Annual Book of ASTM Standards*, Vol. 13, *Medical Devices and Services*, F139–F86, p. 61. Philadelphia, PA: ASTM.

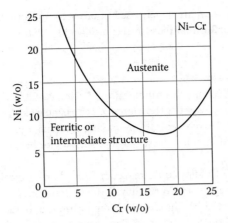

FIGURE 28.1 The effect of Ni and Cr contents on the austenitic phase of stainless steels containing 0.1% C. (Adapted from Keating, F.H. 1956. *Chromium–Nickel Austenitic Steels*. London: Butterworths.)

TABLE 28.2 Mechanical Properties of 316L Stainless Steel for Implants

Condition	Ultimate Tensile Strength, min. (MPa)	Yield Strength (0.2% offset), min. (MPa)	Elongation 2 in. (50.8 mm) min.%	Rockwell Hardness
Annealed	485	172	40	95 HRB
Cold-worked	860	690	12	—

Source: Adapted from ASTM. 1992. *Annual Book of ASTM Standards*, Vol. 13, *Medical Devices and Services*, F139–F86, p. 61. Philadelphia, PA: ASTM.

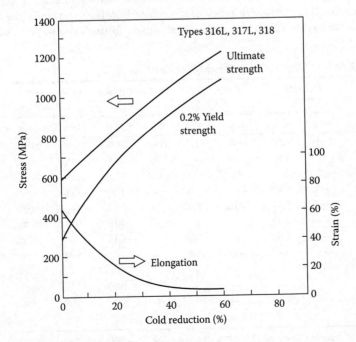

FIGURE 28.2 Effect of cold work on the yield and ultimate tensile strength of 18-8 stainless steel. (Adapted from ASTM. 1980. *Annual Book of ASTM Standards*. Philadelphia, PA: ASTM.)

glow-discharge nitrogen implantation are widely used in order to improve corrosion resistance, wear resistance, and fatigue strength of 316L stainless steel (Bordiji et al., 1996).

28.3 CoCr Alloys

There are basically two types of cobalt–chromium alloys: (1) the castable CoCrMo alloy and (2) the CoNiCrMo alloy, which is usually *wrought* by (hot) *forging*. The castable CoCrMo alloy has been used for many decades in dentistry and, relatively recently, in making artificial joints. The wrought CoNiCrMo alloy is relatively new, now used for making the stems of prostheses for heavily loaded joints such as the knee and hip.

The ASTM lists four types of CoCr alloys that are recommended for surgical implant applications: (1) cast CoCrMo alloy (F75), (2) wrought CoCrWNi alloy (F90), (3) wrought CoNiCrMo alloy (F562), and (4) wrought CoNiCrMoWFe alloy (F563). The chemical compositions of these alloys are summarized in Table 28.3. Currently only two of the four alloys are used extensively in implant fabrications: the castable CoCrMo and the wrought CoNiCrMo alloy. As can be noticed from Table 28.3, the compositions of these alloys are quite different from one another.

The two basic elements of the CoCr alloys form a solid solution of up to 65% Co. Molybdenum is added to produce finer grains which results in higher strengths after casting or forging. Chromium enhances corrosion resistance as well as solid solution strengthening of the alloy.

The CoNiCrMo alloy originally called MP35N (Standard Pressed Steel Co.) contains approximately 35% Co and Ni each. This alloy is highly corrosion resistant to seawater (containing chloride ions) under stress. Cold working can increase the strength of this alloy considerably as shown in Figure 28.3. However, there is a considerable difficulty of cold working on this alloy, especially when making large devices such as hip joint stems. Only hot forging can be used to fabricate a large implant with this alloy.

The abrasive wear properties of the wrought CoNiCrMo alloy are similar to those of cast CoCrMo alloy (about 0.14 mm/year in joint simulation tests with ultra-high-molecular-weight polyethylene acetabular cup); however, the former is not recommended for the bearing surfaces of joint prosthesis because of its poor frictional properties with itself or other materials. The superior fatigue and ultimate tensile strength of the wrought CoNiCrMo alloy make it suitable for such applications, which require

TABLE 28.3 Chemical Compositions of Co–Cr Alloys

Element	CoCrMo (F75) Min.	Max.	CoCrWNi (F90) Min.	Max.	CoNiCrMo (F562) Min.	Max.	CoNiCrMoWFe (F563) Min.	Max.
Cr	27.0	30.0	19.0	21.0	19.0	21.0	18.00	22.00
Mo	5.0	7.0	—	—	9.0	10.5	3.00	4.00
Ni	—	2.5	9.0	11.0	33.0	37.0	15.00	25.00
Fe	—	0.75	—	3.0	—	1.0	4.00	6.00
C	—	0.35	0.05	0.15	—	0.025	—	0.05
Si	—	1.00	—	1.00	—	0.15	—	0.50
Mn	—	1.00	—	2.00	—	0.15	—	1.00
W	—	—	14.0	16.0	—	—	3.00	4.00
P	—	—	—	—	—	0.015	—	—
S	—	—	—	—	—	0.010	—	—
Ti	—	—	—	—	—	1.0	0.50	3.50
Co		Balance						

Source: Adapted from ASTM. 1992. *Annual Book of ASTM Standards*, Vol. 13, *Medical Devices and Services*, F75–F87, p. 42; F90–F87, p. 47; F562–F84, p. 150. Philadelphia, PA: ASTM.

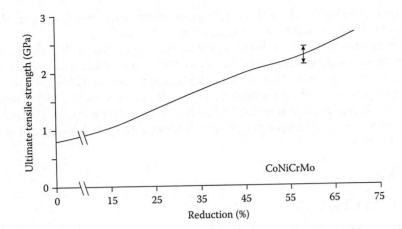

FIGURE 28.3 Relationship between ultimate tensile and the amount of cold work for CoNiCrMo alloy. (Adapted from Devine, T.M. and Wulff, J. 1975. *J. Biomed. Mater. Res.* 9, 151–167.)

long service life without fracture or stress fatigue. Such is the case for the stems of the hip joint prostheses. This advantage is better appreciated when the implant has to be replaced, since it is quite difficult to remove the failed piece of implant embedded deep in the femoral medullary canal. Furthermore, the revision arthroplasty is usually inferior to the primary surgery in terms of its function due to poorer fixation of the implant.

The mechanical properties required for CoCr alloys are given in Table 28.4. As with the other alloys, the increased strength is accompanied by decreased ductility. Both the cast and wrought alloys have excellent corrosion resistance.

Experimental determination of the rate of release of nickel from the CoNiCrMo alloy and 316L stainless steel in 37°C Ringer's solution showed an interesting result. Although the cobalt alloy has more initial release of nickel ions into the solution, the rate of release was about the same (3×10^{-10} g/cm²/day) for both alloys (Richards Manufacturing Company, 1980). This is rather surprising since the nickel content of the CoNiCrMo alloy is about three times that of 316L stainless steel.

The metallic products released from the prosthesis because of wear, corrosion, and fretting may impair organs and local tissues. *In vitro* studies have indicated that particulate Co is toxic to human osteoblast-like cell lines and inhibits synthesis of type-I collagen, osteocalcin, and alkaline phosphatase in the culture medium. However, particulate Cr and CoCr alloys are well tolerated by cell lines without significant toxicity. The toxicity of metal extracts *in vitro* have indicated that Co and Ni extracts at 50%

TABLE 28.4 Mechanical Property Requirements of Co–Cr Alloys

Property	Cast CoCrMo (F75)	Wrought CoCrWNi (F90)	Wrought CoNiCrMo (F562) Solution Annealed	Wrought CoNiCrMo (F562) Cold-Worked and Aged
Tensile strength (MPa)	655	860	793–1000	1793 min.
Yield strength (0.2% offset) (MPa)	450	310	240–655	1585
Elongation (%)	8	10	50.0	8.0
Reduction of area (%)	8	—	65.0	35.0
Fatigue strength (MPa)[a]	310	—	—	—

Source: Adapted from ASTM. 1992. *Annual Book of ASTM Standards*, Vol. 13, *Medical Devices and Services*, F75–F87, p. 42; F90–F87, p. 47; F562–F84, p. 150. Philadelphia, PA: ASTM.

[a] From Semlitch, M. 1980. *Eng. Med.* 9, 201–207.

concentration appear to be highly toxic since all viability parameters were altered after 24 h. However, Cr extract seems to be less toxic than Ni and Co (Granchi et al., 1996).

The modulus of elasticity for the CoCr alloys does not change with the changes in their ultimate tensile strength. The values range from 220 to 234 GPa, which are higher than other materials such as stainless steels. This may have some implications of different load transfer modes to the bone in artificial joint replacements, although the effect of the increased modulus on the fixation and longevity of implants is not clear. Low wear (average linear wear on the MeKee–Farrar component was 4.2 µm/year) has been recognized as an advantage of metal-on-metal hip articulations because of its hardness and toughness (Schmalzried et al., 1996).

28.4 Ti Alloys

28.4.1 Pure Ti and Ti6Al4V

Attempts to use titanium for implant fabrication dates back to the late 1930s. It was found that titanium was tolerated in cat femurs, as was stainless steel and Vitallium® (CoCrMo alloy). Its lightness (4.5 g/cm³, see Table 28.5) and good mechanochemical properties are salient features for implant application.

There are four grades of unalloyed, commercially pure (cp) titanium for surgical implant applications as shown in Table 28.6. The impurity contents separate them; oxygen, iron, and nitrogen should be controlled carefully. Oxygen, in particular, has a great influence on the ductility and strength.

One titanium alloy (Ti6Al4V) is widely used to manufacture implants, and its chemical requirements are given in Table 28.7. The main alloying elements of the alloy are aluminum (5.5%–6.5%) and vanadium (3.5%–4.5%). The Ti6Al4V alloy has approximately the same fatigue strength (550 MPa) of CoCr alloy after rotary bending fatigue tests (Imam et al., 1983). Titanium is an allotropic material, which exists as a hexagonal close-packed structure (hcp, α-Ti) up to 882°C and body-centered cubic structure (bcc, β-Ti) above this temperature. Titanium alloys can be strengthened and mechanical properties varied by

TABLE 28.5 Specific Gravities of Some Metallic Implant Alloys

Alloys	Density (g/cm³)
Ti and its alloys	4.5
316 Stainless steel	7.9
CoCrMo	8.3
CoNiCrMo	9.2
NiTi	6.7

TABLE 28.6 Chemical Compositions of Titanium and Its Alloy

Element	Grade 1	Grade 2	Grade 3	Grade 4	Ti6Al4V[a]
Nitrogen	0.03	0.03	0.05	0.05	0.05
Carbon	0.10	0.10	0.10	0.10	0.08
Hydrogen	0.015	0.015	0.015	0.015	0.0125
Iron	0.20	0.30	0.30	0.50	0.25
Oxygen	0.18	0.25	0.35	0.40	0.13
Titanium			Balance		

Source: Adapted from ASTM. 1992. *Annual Book of ASTM Standards*, Vol. 13, *Medical Devices and Services*, F67–F89, p. 39; F136–F84, p. 55. Philadelphia, PA: ASTM.

[a] Aluminum 6.00% (5.50–6.50), vanadium 4.00% (3.50–4.50), and other elements 0.1% maximum or 0.4% total. All are maximum allowable weight percent.

TABLE 28.7   Mechanical Properties of Ti and Its Alloys

Properties	Grade 1	Grade 2	Grade 3	Grade 4	Ti6Al4V	Ti13Nb13Zr
Tensile strength (MPa)	240	345	450	550	860	1030
Yield strength (0.2% offset) (MPa)	170	275	380	485	795	900
Elongation (%)	24	20	18	15	10	15
Reduction of area (%)	30	30	30	25	25	45

Source: Adapted from ASTM. 1992. *Annual Book of ASTM Standards*, Vol. 13, *Medical Devices and Services*, F67–F89, p. 39; F136–F84, p. 55. Philadelphia, PA: ASTM; Davidson, J.A. et al. 1994. *Biomed. Mater. Eng.* 4, 231–243.

controlled composition and thermomechanical processing techniques. Addition of alloying elements to titanium enables it to have a wide range of properties: (1) Aluminum tends to stabilize the α-phase, that is, increase the transformation temperature from α- to β-phase (Figure 28.4). (2) Vanadium stabilizes the β-phase by lowering the temperature of the transformation from α to β.

The α-alloy has a single-phase microstructure (Figure 28.5a) that promotes good weldability. The stabilizing effect of the high aluminum content of these groups of alloys makes excellent strength characteristics and oxidation resistance at high temperature (300–600°C). These alloys cannot be heat-treated for precipitation hardening since they are single-phased.

Addition of controlled amounts of β-stabilizers causes the higher-strength β-phase to persist below the transformation temperature, which results in the two-phase system. The precipitates of β-phase will appear by heat treatment in the solid solution temperature and subsequent quenching, followed by aging at a somewhat lower temperature. The aging cycle causes the coherent precipitation of some fine α particles from the metastable β, imparting α structure may produce local strain field capable of absorbing deformation energy. Cracks are stopped or deterred at the α particles, so that the hardness is higher than for the solid solution (Figure 28.5b).

The higher percentage of β-stabilizing elements (13% V in Ti13V11Cr3Al alloy) results in a microstructure that is substantially β, which can be strengthened by heat treatment (Figure 28.5c). Another Ti alloy (Ti13Nb13Zr) with 13% Nb and 13% Zr showed *martensite* structure after water-quenched and

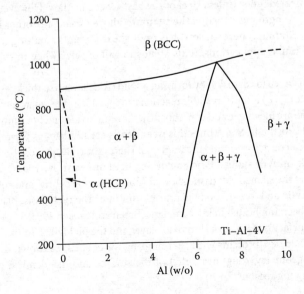

FIGURE 28.4   Part of phase diagram of Ti–Al–V at 4 w/o V. (Adapted from Smith, C.J.E. and Hughes, A.N. 1966. *Eng. Med.* 7, 158–171.)

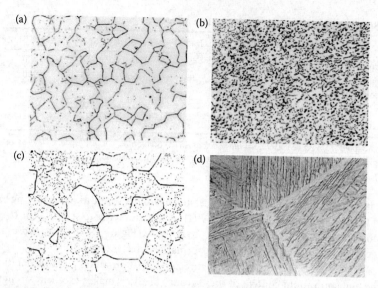

FIGURE 28.5 Microstructure of Ti alloys (all are ×500). (a) Annealed α-alloy. (b) Ti6Al4V, α–β alloy, annealed. (c) β-alloy, annealed. (d) Ti6Al4V, heat-treated at 1650°C and quenched. (Adapted from Hille, G.H. 1966. *J. Mater.* 1, 373–383; Imam, M.A. et al. 1983. *Titanium Alloys in Surgical Implants.* Philadelphia, PA: ASTM Special Technical Publication 796, pp. 105–119.)

aged, which showed high corrosion resistance with low modulus ($E = 79$ MPa) (Davidson et al., 1994). The formation of plates of martensite induces considerable elastic distortion in the parent crystal structure and increases strength (Figure 28.5d).

The mechanical properties of the cp titanium and its alloys are given in Table 28.7. The modulus of elasticity of these materials is about 110 GPa except 13Nb13Zr alloy. From Table 28.7, one can see that the higher impurity content of the cp-Ti leads to higher strength and reduced ductility. The strength of the material varies from a value much lower than that of 316 stainless steel or the CoCr alloys to a value about equal to that of annealed 316 stainless steel of the cast CoCrMo alloy. However, when compared for the specific strength (strength per density), the titanium alloys exceed any other implant materials as shown in Figure 28.6. Titanium, nevertheless, has poor shear strength, making it less desirable for bone screws, plates, and similar applications. It also tends to gall or seize when in sliding contact with itself or other metals.

Titanium derives its resistance to corrosion by forming a solid oxide layer to a thickness of 10 nm. Under *in vivo* conditions, the oxide (TiO_2) is the only stable reaction product. However, micromotion at the cement-prosthesis and cement-bone are inevitable and consequently, titanium oxide and titanium alloy particles are released in cemented joint prosthesis. Sometimes this wear debris accumulates as periprosthetic fluid collections and triggers giant cell response around the implants. This cystic collection continued to enlarge and aspiration revealed a "dark" heavily stained fluid containing titanium wear particles and histiocytic cells. Histological examination of the stained soft tissue showed "fibrin necrotic debris" and collagenous, fibrous tissue containing a histiocytic and foreign body giant cell infiltrate. The metallosis, black staining of the periprosthetic tissues, has been implicated in knee implant (Breen and Stoker, 1993).

The titanium implant surface consists of a thin oxide layer and the biological fluid of water molecules, dissolved ions, and biomolecules (proteins with surrounding water shell) as shown in Figure 28.7. The microarchitecture (microgeometry, roughness, etc.) of the surface and its chemical compositions are important due to the following reasons:

1. Physical nature of the surface either at the atomic, molecular, or higher level relative to the dimensions of the biological units may cause different contact areas with biomolecules, cells, and so on.

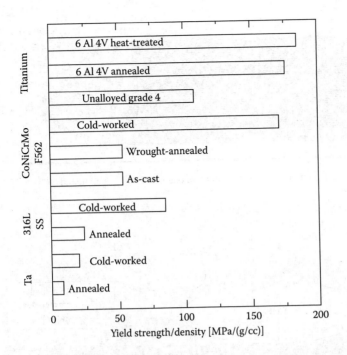

FIGURE 28.6 Yield strength-to-density ratio of some implant materials. (Adapted from Hille, G.H. 1966. *J. Mater.* 1, 373–383.)

The different contact areas, in turn, may produce different perturbations and types of bonding of the biological units, which may influence their conformation and function.

2. Chemical composition of the surface may produce different types of bonding to the biomolecules, which may then also affect their properties and function. Metals undergo chemical reactions at the surface depending on the environment which cause the difficulties of understanding the exact nature of the interactions.

The surface–tissue interaction is dynamic rather than static, that is, it will develop into new stages as time passes, especially during the initial period after implantation. During the initial few seconds after implantation, there will be only water, dissolved ions, and free biomolecules in the closest proximity of the surface but no cells. The composition of biofluid will then change continuously as inflammatory and healing processes proceed, which in turn also probably causes changes in the composition of the adsorbed layer of biomolecules on the implant surface until quasiequilibrium sets in. Eventually, cells and tissues will approach the surface and, depending on the nature of the adsorbed layer, they will respond in specific ways that may further modify the adsorbed biomolecules. The type of cells closest to the surface and their activities will change with time. For example, depending on the type of initial interaction, the final results may be fibrous capsule formation or tissue integration (Kasemo and Lausma, 1988; Hazan et al., 1993; Takatsuka et al., 1995; Takeshita et al., 1997; Yan et al., 1997).

Osseointegration is defined as direct contact without intervening soft tissue between viable remodeled bone and an implant. Surface roughness of titanium alloys has a significant effect on the bone apposition to the implant and on the bone implant interfacial pullout strength. The average roughness increased from 0.5 to 5.9 μm and the interfacial shear strength increased from 0.48 to 3.5 MPa (Feighan et al., 1995). Highest levels of osteoblast cell attachment are obtained with rough sand blast surfaces where cells differentiated more than those on the smooth surfaces (Keller et al., 1994). Chemical changes of the titanium surface following heat treatment is thought to form a TiO_2 hydrogel layer on top of the TiO_2 layer as shown in Figure 28.8. The TiO_2 hydrogel layer may induce the apatite crystal formation (Kim et al., 1996).

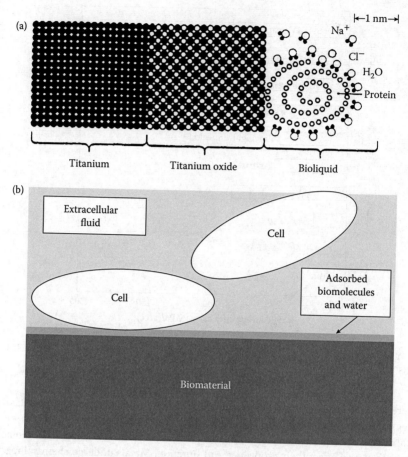

FIGURE 28.7 (a) Interface between a titanium implant and bioliquid and (b) the cell surface interaction. (Adapted from Kasemo, B. and Lausma, J. 1988. *Int. J. Oral Maxillofac Implant.* 3, 247–259.)

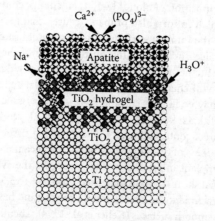

FIGURE 28.8 Chemical change of titanium implant surface of alkali following heat treatment. (Adapted from Kim, H. et al. 1996. *J. Biomed. Mater. Res.* 32, 409–417.)

In general, on the rougher surfaces there are lower cell numbers, decreased rate of cellular proliferation, and increased matrix production compared to smooth surface. Bone formation appears to be strongly related to the presence of transforming growth factor β_1 in the bone matrix (Kieswetter et al., 1996).

28.4.2 TiNi Alloys

The *titanium–nickel* alloys show unusual properties, that is, after deformation the material can snap back to its previous shape following heating of the material. This phenomenon is called *shape memory effect* (SME). The SME of TiNi alloy was first observed by Buehler and Wiley at the U.S. Naval Ordnance Laboratory (Buehler et al., 1963). The equiatomic TiNi or NiTi alloy (Nitinol) exhibits an exceptional SME near room temperature: if it is plastically deformed below the transformation temperature, it reverts back to its original shape as the temperature is raised. The SME can be generally related to a diffusionless martensitic phase transformation which is also thermoelastic in nature, the thermoelasticity being attributed to the ordering in the parent and martensitic phases (Wayman and Shimizu, 1972). Another unusual property is the *superelasticity*, which is shown schematically in Figure 28.9. As can be seen, the stress does not increase with increased strain after the initial elastic stress region and upon release of the stress or strain the metal springs back to its original shape in contrast to other metals such as stainless steel. The superelastic property is utilized in orthodontic archwires since the conventional stainless-steel wires are too stiff and harsh for the tooth. In addition, the SME can also be utilized.

Some possible applications of shape memory alloys are orthodontic dental archwire, intracranial aneurysm clip, *vena cava* filter, contractile artificial muscles for an artificial heart, vascular stent, catheter guide wire, and orthopedic staple (Duerig et al., 1990).

In order to develop such devices, it is necessary to understand fully the mechanical and thermal behavior associated with the martensitic phase transformation. A widely known NiTi alloy is 55-Nitinol (55 wt% or 50 at% Ni), which has a single phase and the mechanical memory plus other properties, for example, high acoustic damping, direct conversion of heat energy into mechanical energy, good fatigue properties, and low-temperature ductility. Deviation from the 55-Nitinol (near stoichiometric NiTi) in the Ni-rich direction yields a second group of alloys which are also completely nonmagnetic but differ from 55-Nitinol in their ability to be thermally hardened to higher hardness levels. Shape recovery

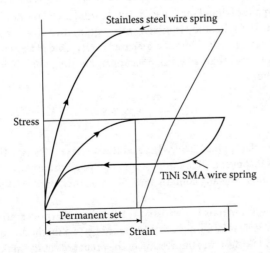

FIGURE 28.9 Schematic illustration of the stainless steel wire and TiNi SMA wire springs for orthodontic archwire behavior. (Modified from Wayman, C.M. and Duerig, T.W. 1990. *Engineering Aspects of Shape Memory Alloys.* London: Butterworth-Heinemann, pp. 3–20.)

TABLE 28.8 Chemical Composition of Ni–Ti Alloy Wire

Element	Composition (%)
Ni	54.01
Co	0.64
Cr	0.76
Mn	0.64
Fe	0.66
Ti	Balance

capability decreases and heat treatability increases rapidly as the Ni content approaches 60%. Both 55- and 60-Nitinols have relatively low modulus of elasticity and can be tougher and more resilient than stainless steel, NiCr, or CoCr alloys.

Efficiency of 55-Nitinol shape recovery can be controlled by changing the final annealing temperatures during preparation of the alloy device (Lee et al., 1988). For the most efficient recovery, the shape is fixed by constraining the specimen in a desired configuration and heating to 482°C–510°C. If the annealed wire is deformed at a temperature below the shape recovery temperature, shape recovery will occur upon heating, provided the deformation has not exceeded crystallographic strain limits (~8% strain in tension). The NiTi alloys also exhibit good biocompatibility and corrosion resistance *in vivo*.

There is no significant difference between titanium and NiTi in the inhibition of mitosis in human fibroblasts. NiTi showed lower percentage bone and bone contact area than titanium and the Ti6Al4V alloy (Takeshita et al., 1997).

The mechanical properties of NiTi alloys are especially sensitive to the stoichiometry of composition (typical composition is given in Table 28.8) and the individual thermal and mechanical history. Although much is known about the processing, mechanical behavior, and properties relating to the SME, considerably less is known about the thermomechanical and physical metallurgy of the alloy.

28.5 Dental Metals

Dental *amalgam* is an alloy made of liquid mercury, and other solid metal particulate alloys are made of silver, tin, copper, and so on. The solid alloy is mixed with (liquid) mercury in a mechanical vibrating mixer and the resulting material is packed into the prepared cavity. One of the solid alloys is composed of at least 65% silver, and not more than 29% tin, 6% copper, 2% zinc, and 3% mercury. The reaction during setting is thought to be

$$\gamma + Hg \rightarrow \gamma + \gamma_1 + \gamma_2 \tag{28.1}$$

in which the γ phase is Ag_3Sn, the γ_1 phase is Ag_2Hg_3, and the γ_2 phase is Sn_7Hg. The phase diagram for the Ag–Sn–Hg system shows that over a wide compositional range all three phases are present. The final composition of dental amalgams typically contain 45%–55% mercury, 35%–45% silver, and about 15% tin after fully set in about 1 day.

Gold and gold alloys are useful metals in dentistry as a result of their durability, stability, and corrosion resistance (Nielsen, 1986). Gold fillings are introduced by two methods: casting and malleting. *Cast* restorations are made by taking a wax impression of the prepared cavity, making a mold from this impression in a material such as gypsum silica, which tolerates high temperature, and casting molten gold in the mold. The patient is given a temporary filling for the intervening time. Gold *alloys* are used for cast restorations, since they have mechanical properties which are superior to those of pure gold.

Corrosion resistance is retained in these alloys provided they contain 75% or more of gold and other noble metals. Copper, alloyed with gold, significantly increases its strength. Platinum also improves the strength, but no more than about 4% can be added, or the melting point of the alloy is elevated excessively. Silver compensates for the color of copper. A small amount of zinc may be added to lower the melting point and to scavenge oxides formed during melting. Gold alloys of different composition are available. Softer alloys containing more than 83% gold are used for inlays which are not subjected to much stress. Harder alloys containing less gold are chosen for crowns and cusps which are more heavily stressed.

Malleted restorations are built up in the cavity from layers of *pure* gold foil. The foils are welded together by pressure at ambient temperature. In this type of welding, the metal layers are joined by thermal diffusion of atoms from one layer to the other. Since intimate contact is required in this procedure, it is particularly important to avoid contamination. The pure gold is relatively soft, so this type of restoration is limited to areas not subjected to much stress.

28.6 Other Metals

Several other metals have been used for a variety of specialized implant applications. *Tantalum* has been subjected to animal implant studies and has been shown very biocompatible. Due to its poor mechanical properties (Table 28.9) and high density (16.6 g/cm^3), it is restricted to few applications such as wire sutures for plastic surgeons and neurosurgeons and a radioisotope for bladder tumors.

Platinum group metals such as Pt, Pd, Rh, Ir, Ru, and Os are extremely corrosion resistant but have poor mechanical properties (Wynblatt, 1986). They are mainly used as alloys for electrodes such as pacemaker tips because of their high resistance to corrosion and low threshold potentials for electrical conductivity.

Thermoseeds made of 70% Ni and 30% Cu have been produced which possess Curie points in the therapeutic *hyperthermia* range, approximately 40°C–50°C (Ferguson et al., 1992). Upon the application of an alternating magnetic field, eddy currents are induced, which will provide a continuous heat source through resistive heating of the material. As the temperature of a ferromagnetic substance nears its Curie point, however, there is a loss of ferromagnetic properties and a resulting loss of heat output. Thus, self-regulation of temperature is achieved and can be used to deliver a constant hyperthermic temperature extracorporeally at any time and duration.

Surface modifications of metal alloys such as coatings by plasma spray, physical or chemical vapor deposition, ion implantation, and fluidized-bed deposition have been used in industry (Smith, 1993). Coating implants with tissue-compatible materials such as hydroxyapatite, oxide ceramics, Bioglass®, and pyrolytic carbon are typical applications in implants. Such efforts have been ineffective if the implants are permanent in general, and if the implants are subjected to a large loading, in particular. The main problem is the delamination of the coating or eventual wear of the coating. The added cost of coating or ion implanting hinders the use of such techniques unless the technique shows unequivocal superiority compared to the nontreated implants.

TABLE 28.9   Mechanical Properties of Tantalum

Properties	Annealed	Cold-Worked
Tensile strength (MPa)	207	517
Yield strength (0.2% offset) (MPa)	138	345
Elongation (%)	20–30	2
Young's modulus (GPa)	—	190

Source: Adapted from ASTM. 1992. *Annual Book of ASTM Standards*, Vol. 13, *Medical Devices and Services*, F560–F86, p. 143. Philadelphia, PA: ASTM.

28.7 Corrosion of Metallic Implants

Corrosion is the unwanted chemical reaction of a metal with its environment, resulting in its continued degradation to oxides, hydroxides, or other compounds. Tissue fluid in the human body contains water, dissolved oxygen, proteins, and various ions such as chloride and hydroxide. As a result, the human body presents a very aggressive environment for metals used for implantation. Corrosion resistance of a metallic implant material is consequently an important aspect of its biocompatibility.

28.7.1 Electrochemical Aspects

The lowest free energy state of many metals in an oxygenated and hydrated environment is that of the oxide. Corrosion occurs when metal atoms become ionized and go into solution, or combine with oxygen or other species in solution to form a compound which flakes off or dissolves. The body environment is very aggressive in terms of corrosion since it is not only aqueous, but also contains chloride ions and proteins. A variety of chemical reactions occur when a metal is exposed to an aqueous environment, as shown in Figure 28.10. The electrolyte, which contains ions in solution, serves to complete the electric circuit. In the human body, the required ions are plentiful in the body fluids. Anions are negative ions which migrate toward the *anode*, and cations are positive ions which migrate toward the *cathode*. At the anode, or the positive electrode, the metal oxidizes by losing valence electrons as in the following:

$$M \rightarrow M^{n+} + ne^- \tag{28.2}$$

At the cathode, or the negative electrode, the following reduction reactions are important:

$$M^{n+} + ne^- \rightarrow M \tag{28.3}$$

$$M^{2+} + OH^- + 2e^- \rightarrow MOH \tag{28.4}$$

$$2H_3O^+ + 2e^- \rightarrow H_2 \uparrow + 2H_2O \tag{28.5}$$

$$\frac{1}{2}O_2 + H_2O + 2e^- \rightarrow 2OH^- \tag{28.6}$$

The tendency of metals to corrode is expressed most simply in the standard electrochemical series of *Nernst potentials*, as shown in Table 28.10. These potentials are obtained in electrochemical measurements in which one electrode is a standard hydrogen electrode formed by bubbling hydrogen through a layer of finely divided platinum black. The potential of this reference electrode is defined to be zero.

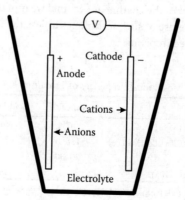

FIGURE 28.10 Electrochemical cell.

TABLE 28.10 Standard Electrochemical Series

Reaction	ΔE_o (V)
Li $\leftrightarrow$ Li$^+$	−3.05
Na $\leftrightarrow$ Na$^+$	−2.71
Al $\leftrightarrow$ Al^{3+}	−1.66
Ti $\leftrightarrow$ Ti^{3+}	−1.63
Cr $\leftrightarrow$ Cr^{2+}	−0.56
Fe $\leftrightarrow$ Fe^{2+}	−0.44
Cu $\leftrightarrow$ Cu^{2+}	−0.34
Co $\leftrightarrow$ Co^{2+}	−0.28
Ni $\leftrightarrow$ Ni^{2+}	−0.23
H$_2$ $\leftrightarrow$ 2H$^+$	−0.00
Ag $\leftrightarrow$ Ag$^+$	+0.80
Au $\leftrightarrow$ Au$^+$	+1.68

Noble metals are those which have a potential higher than that of a standard hydrogen electrode; base metals have lower potentials.

If two dissimilar metals are present in the same environment, the one which is most negative in the *galvanic series* will become the anode, and bimetallic (or galvanic) corrosion will occur. *Galvanic corrosion* can be much more rapid than the corrosion of a single metal. Consequently, implantation of dissimilar metals (mixed metals) is to be avoided. Galvanic action can also result in corrosion within a single metal, if there is inhomogeneity in the metal or in its environment, as shown in Figure 28.11.

The potential difference, E, actually observed depends on the concentration of the metal ions in solution according to the Nernst equation

$$E = E_o + \left(\frac{RT}{nF} \right) \ln[M^{n+}] \tag{28.7}$$

in which R is the gas constant, E_o is the standard electrochemical potential, T is the absolute temperature, F is Faraday's constant (96,487 C/mol), and n is the number of moles of ions.

The order of nobility observed in actual practice may differ from that predicted thermodynamically. The reasons are that some metals become covered with a *passivating* film of reaction products which protects the metal from further attack. The dissolution reaction may be strongly irreversible so that a potential barrier must be overcome. In this case, corrosion may be inhibited even though it

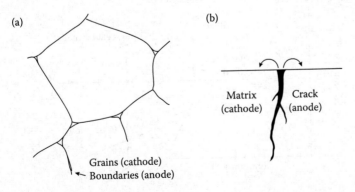

(a)

(b)

Grains (cathode)
Boundaries (anode)

Matrix (cathode)   Crack (anode)

FIGURE 28.11 Micro-corrosion cells. (a) Grain boundaries are anodic with respect to the grain interior. (b) Crevice corrosion due to oxygen-deficient zone in metal's environment.

remains energetically favorable. The kinetics of corrosion reactions are not determined by the thermodynamics alone.

28.7.2 Pourbaix Diagrams in Corrosion

The *Pourbaix diagram* is a plot of regions of *corrosion*, *passivity*, and *immunity* as they depend on electrode potential and pH (Pourbaix, 1974). The Pourbaix diagrams are derived from the Nernst equation and from the solubility of the degradation products and the equilibrium constants of the reaction. For the sake of definition, the *corrosion region* is set arbitrarily at a concentration greater than 10^{-6} g atom/L (molar) or more of metal in the solution at equilibrium. This corresponds to about 0.06 mg/L for metals such as iron and copper, and 0.03 mg/L for aluminum. *Immunity* is defined as equilibrium between metal and its ions at less than 10^{-6} M. In the region of immunity, the corrosion is energetically impossible. Immunity is also referred to as cathodic protection. In the passivation domain, the stable solid constituent is an oxide, hydroxide, hydride, or a salt of the metal. *Passivity* is defined as equilibrium between a metal and its reaction products (oxides, hydroxides, etc.) at a concentration of 10^{-6} M or less. This situation is useful if reaction products are adherent. In the biomaterials setting, passivity may or may not be adequate; disruption of a passive layer may cause an increase in corrosion. The equilibrium state may not occur if reaction products are removed by the tissue fluid. Materials differ in their propensity to reestablish a passive layer which has been damaged. This layer of material may protect the underlying metal if it is firmly adherent and nonporous; in this case, further corrosion is prevented. Passivation can also result from a concentration polarization due to a buildup of ions near the electrodes. This is not likely to occur in the body since the ions are continually replenished. Cathodic depolarization reactions can aid in the passivation of a metal by virtue of an energy barrier which hinders the kinetics. Equations 28.5 and 28.6 are examples.

There are two diagonal lines in the diagrams shown in Figure 28.12. The top oxygen line represents the upper limit of the stability of water and is associated with oxygen-rich solutions or electrolytes near oxidizing materials. In the region above this line, oxygen is evolved according to $2H_2O \rightarrow O_2 \uparrow +4H^+ + 4e^-$. In the human body, saliva, intracellular fluid, and interstitial fluid occupy regions near the oxygen line, since they are saturated with oxygen. The lower hydrogen diagonal line represents the lower limit of the stability of water. Hydrogen gas is evolved according to Equation 28.5. Aqueous corrosion occurs in the region between these diagonal lines on the Pourbaix diagram. In the human body, urine, bile, the lower gastrointestinal tract, and secretions of ductless glands occupy a region somewhat above the hydrogen line.

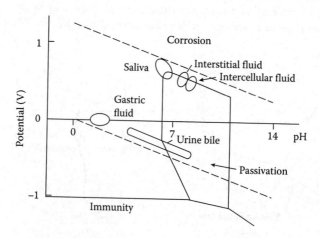

FIGURE 28.12 Pourbaix diagram for chromium, showing regions associated with various body fluids. (Modified from Black, J. 1992. *Biological Performance of Materials*, 2nd ed. New York: Marcel Dekker.)

The significance of the Pourbaix diagram is as follows. Different parts of the body have different pH values and oxygen concentrations. Consequently, a metal which performs well (is immune or passive) in one part of the body may suffer an unacceptable amount of corrosion in another part. Moreover, pH can change dramatically in tissue that has been injured or infected. In particular, normal tissue fluid has a pH of about 7.4, but in a wound it can be as low as 3.5, and in an infected wound the pH can increase to 9.0.

Pourbaix diagrams are useful, but do not tell the whole story; there are some limitations. Diagrams are made considering equilibrium among metal, water, and reaction products. The presence of other ions, for example, chloride, may result in very much different behavior, and large molecules in the body may also change the situation. Prediction of passivity may in some cases be optimistic, since reaction rates are not considered.

28.7.3 Rate of Corrosion and Polarization Curves

The regions in the Pourbaix diagram specify whether corrosion will take place, but they do not determine the rate. The rate, expressed as an electric current density (current per unit area), depends on electrode potential as shown in the polarization curves in Figure 28.13. From such curves, it is possible to calculate the number of ions per unit time liberated into the tissue, as well as the depth of metal removed by corrosion in a given time. An alternative experiment is one in which the weight loss of a specimen of metal due to corrosion is measured as a function of time.

The rate of corrosion also depends on the presence of synergistic factors, such as those of mechanical origin (uneven distribution of mechanical stress). The stressed alloy failures occur due to the propagation of cracks in corrosive environments. For example, in corrosion fatigue (stress corrosion cracking), repetitive deformation of a metal in a corrosive environment results in acceleration of both the corrosion and the fatigue microdamage. Since the body environment involves both repeated mechanical loading and a chemically aggressive environment, fatigue testing of implant materials should always be performed under physiological environmental conditions, under Ringer's solution at body temperature. In *fretting corrosion*, rubbing of one part on another disrupts the passivation layer, resulting in accelerated corrosion. In *pitting*, the corrosion rate is accelerated in a local region. Stainless steel is vulnerable to pitting. Localized corrosion can occur if there is inhomogeneity in the metal or in the environment. *Grain boundaries* in the metal may be susceptible to the initiation of corrosion, as a result of their higher

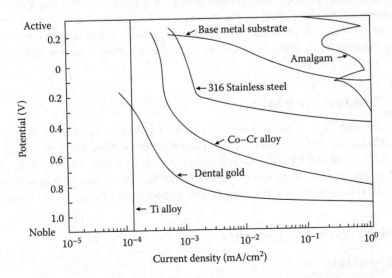

FIGURE 28.13 Potential–current density curves for some biomaterials. (Adapted from Greener, E.H., Harcourt, J.K., and Lautenschlager, E.P. 1972. *Materials Science in Dentistry*. Baltimore, MD: Williams & Wilkins.)

energy level. *Crevices* are also vulnerable to corrosion, since the chemical environment in the crevice may differ from that in the surrounding medium. The area of contact between a screw and a bone plate, for example, can suffer *crevice corrosion*.

28.7.4 Corrosion of Available Metals

Choosing a metal for implantation should take into account the corrosion properties discussed above. Metals which are in current use as biomaterials include gold, cobalt–chromium alloys, type 316 stainless steel, cp-titanium, titanium alloys, nickel–titanium alloys, and silver–tin–mercury amalgam.

The noble metals are immune to corrosion and would be ideal materials if corrosion resistance were the only concern. Gold is widely used in dental restorations and in that setting it offers superior performance and longevity. Gold is not, however, used in orthopedic applications because of its high density, insufficient strength, and high cost.

Titanium is a base metal in the context of the electrochemical series; however, it forms a robust passivating layer and remains passive under physiological conditions. Corrosion currents in normal saline are very low: 10^{-8} A/cm^2. Titanium implants remain virtually unchanged in appearance. Ti offers superior corrosion resistance but is not as stiff or strong as steel or Co–Cr alloys.

Cobalt–chromium alloys, like titanium, are passive in the human body. They are widely in use in orthopedic applications. They do not exhibit pitting corrosion.

Stainless steels contain enough chromium to confer corrosion resistance by passivity. The passive layer is not as robust as in the case of titanium or the cobalt chrome alloys. Only the most corrosion resistant of the stainless steels are suitable for implants. These are the austenitic types: 316, 316L, and 317, which contain molybdenum. Even these types of stainless steel are vulnerable to pitting and to crevice corrosion around screws.

The phases of dental amalgam are passive at neutral pH, the transpassive potential for the γ_2 phase is easily exceeded, due to interphase galvanic couples or potentials due to differential aeration under dental plaque. Amalgam, therefore, often corrodes and is the most active (corrosion prone) material used in dentistry.

Corrosion of an implant in the clinical setting can result in symptoms such as local pain and swelling in the region of the implant, with no evidence of infection, cracking or flaking of the implant as seen on x-ray films, and excretion of excess metal ions. At surgery, gray or black discoloration of the surrounding tissue may be seen and flakes of metal may be found in the tissue. Corrosion also plays a role in the mechanical failures of orthopedic implants. Most of these failures are due to fatigue, and the presence of a saline environment certainly exacerbates fatigue. The extent to which corrosion influences fatigue in the body is not precisely known.

28.7.5 Stress Corrosion Cracking

When an implant is subjected to stress, the corrosion process could be accelerated due to the mechanical energy. If the mechanical stress is repeated, then fatigue stress corrosion takes place such as in the femoral stem of the hip joint and hip nails made of stainless steels (Dobbs and Scales, 1979; Sloter and Piehler, 1979). However, other mechanisms of corrosion such as fretting may also be involved at the point of contact such as in the counter-sink of the hip nail or bone fracture plate for the screws.

28.8 Manufacturing of Implants

28.8.1 Stainless Steels

The austenitic stainless steels work-harden very rapidly as shown in Figure 28.2 and, therefore, cannot be cold-worked without intermediate heat treatments. The heat treatments should not induce, however, the formation of chromium carbide (CCr_4) in the grain boundaries; this may cause corrosion. For the same reason, the austenitic stainless-steel implants are not usually welded.

The distortion of components by the heat treatments can occur but this problem can be solved by controlling the uniformity of heating. Another undesirable effect of the heat treatment is the formation of surface oxide scales which have to be removed either chemically (acid) or mechanically (sand-blasting). After the scales are removed, the surface of the component is polished to a mirror or mat finish. The surface is then cleaned, degreased, and passivated in nitric acid (ASTM Standard F86). The component is washed and cleaned again before packaging and sterilizing.

28.8.2 Co–Cr Alloys

The CoCrMo alloy is particularly susceptible to work-hardening so that the normal fabrication procedure used with other metals cannot be employed. Instead, the alloy is cast by a lost wax (or investment casting) method which involves making a wax pattern of the desired component. The pattern is coated with a refractory material, first by a thin coating with a slurry (suspension of silica in ethyl silicate solution) followed by complete investing after drying (1) the wax is then melted out in a furnace (100°C–150°C), (2) the mold is heated to a high temperature burning out any traces of wax- or gas-forming materials, (3) molten alloy is poured with gravitational or centrifugal force, and (4) the mold is broken after cooled. The mold temperature is about 800°C–1000°C and the alloy is at 1350°C–1400°C.

Controlling the mold temperature will have an effect on the grain size of the final cast; coarse ones are formed at higher temperatures which will decrease the strength. However, high processing temperature will result in larger carbide precipitates with greater distances between them resulting in a less brittle material. Again there is a complementary (trade off) relationship between strength and toughness.

28.8.3 Ti and Its Alloys

Titanium is very reactive at high temperature and burns readily in the presence of oxygen. Therefore, it requires an inert atmosphere for high-temperature processing or is processed by vacuum melting. Oxygen diffuses readily in titanium and the dissolved oxygen embrittles the metal. As a result, any hot working or forging operation should be carried out below 925°C. Machining at room temperature is not the solution to all the problems since the material also tends to gall or seize the cutting tools. Very sharp tools with slow speeds and large feeds are used to minimize this effect. Electrochemical machining is an attractive means.

Defining Terms

Amalgam: An alloy obtained by mixing silver tin alloy with mercury.
Anode: A positive electrode in an electrochemical cell.
Cathode: A negative electrode in an electrochemical cell.
Corrosion: Unwanted reaction of metal with environment. In a Pourbaix diagram, it is the region in which the metal ions are present at a concentration of more than 10^{-6} M.
Crevice corrosion: A form of localized corrosion in which concentration gradients around preexisting crevices in the material drive corrosion processes.
Curie temperature: Transition temperature of a material from ferromagnetic to paramagnetic.
Galvanic corrosion: Dissolution of metal driven by macroscopic differences in electrochemical potential, usually as a result of dissimilar metals in proximity.
Galvanic series: Table of electrochemical potentials (voltage) associated with the ionization of metal atoms. These are called Nernst potentials.
Hyperthermia: Application of high enough thermal energy (heat) to suppress the cancerous cell activities. Above 41.5°C (but below 60°C) is needed to have any effect.

Immunity: Resistance to corrosion by an energetic barrier. In a Pourbaix diagram, it is the region in which the metal is in equilibrium with its ions at a concentration of less than 10^{-6} M. Noble metals resist corrosion by immunity.

Martensite: A metastable structure formed by quenching of austenite (g) structure in alloys such as steel and Ti alloys. They are brittle and hard and, therefore, are further heated to make tougher.

Nernst potential: Standard electrochemical potential measured with respect to a standard hydrogen electrode.

Noble: Type of metal with a positive standard electrochemical potential.

Passivation: Production of corrosion resistance by a surface layer of reaction products. (Normally oxide layer which is impervious to gas and water.)

Passivity: Resistance to corrosion by a surface layer of reaction products. In a Pourbaix diagram, it is the region in which the metal is in equilibrium with its reaction products at a concentration of less than 10^{-6} M.

Pitting: A form of localized corrosion in which pits form on the metal surface.

Pourbaix diagram: Plot of electrical potential versus pH for a material in which the regions of corrosion, passivity, and immunity are identified.

Shape memory effect (SME): Thermoelastic behavior of some alloys which can revert back to their original shape when the temperature is greater than the phase transformation temperature of the alloy.

Superelasticity: Minimal stress increase beyond the initial strain region resulting in very low modulus in the region for some shape memory alloys.

References

ASTM. 1980. *Annual Book of ASTM Standards*. Philadelphia, PA: ASTM.

ASTM. 1992. *Annual Book of ASTM Standards*, Vol. 13, *Medical Devices and Services*. Philadelphia, PA: ASTM.

Black, J. 1992. *Biological Performance of Materials*, 2nd ed. New York: Marcel Dekker.

Bordiji, K., Jouzeau, J., Mainard, D., Payan, E., Delagoutte, J., and Netter, P. 1996. Evaluation of the effect of three surface treatments on the biocompatibility of 316L stainless steel using human differentiated cells. *Biomaterials* 17, 491–500.

Breen, D.J. and Stoker, D.J. 1993. Titanium lines: A manifestation of metallosis and tissue response to titanium alloy megaprostheses at the knee. *Clin. Radiol.* 43, 274–277.

Buehler, W.J., Gilfrich, J.V., and Wiley, R.C. 1963. Effect of low-temperature phase changes on the mechanical properties of alloys near composition Ti–Ni. *J. Appl. Phys.* 34, 1475–1477.

Davidson, J.A., Mishra, A.K., Kovacs, P., and Poggie, R.A. 1994. New surface hardened, low-modulus, corrosion-resistant Ti–13Nb–13Zr alloy for total hip arthroplasty. *Biomed. Mater. Eng.* 4, 231–243.

Devine, T.M. and Wulff, J. 1975. Cast vs. wrought cobalt–chromium surgical implant alloys. *J. Biomed. Mater. Res.* 9, 151–167.

Dobbs, H.S. and Scales, J.T. 1979. Fracture and corrosion in stainless steel hip replacement stems. In *Corrosion and Degradation of Implant Materials*, Syrett, B.C. and Acharya, A. eds. Philadelphia, PA: ASTM, pp. 245–258.

Duerig, T.W., Melton, K.N., Stockel, D., and Wayman, C.M. 1990. *Engineering Aspects of Shape Memory Alloys*. London: Butterworth-Heinemann.

Feighan, J.E., Goldberg, V.M., Davy, D., Parr, J.A., and Stevenson, S. 1995. The influence of surface-blasting on the incorporation of titanium-alloy implants in a rabbit intramedullary model. *J. Bone. Joint. Surg. Am.* 77A, 1380–1395.

Ferguson, S.D., Paulus, J.A., Tucker, R.D., Loening, S.A., and Park, J.B. 1992. Effect of thermal treatment on heating characteristics of Ni–Cu alloy for hyperthermia: Preliminary studies. *J. Appl. Biomater.* 4, 55–60.

Granchi, D., Ciapetti, G., Savarino, L., Cavedagna, D., Donati, M.E., and Pizzoferrato, A. 1996. Assessment of metal extract toxicity on human lymphocytes cultured *in vitro*. *J. Biomed. Mater. Res.* 31, 183–191.

Greener, E.H., Harcourt, J.K., and Lautenschlager, E.P. 1972. *Materials Science in Dentistry*. Baltimore, MD: Williams & Wilkins.

Hazan, R., Brener, R., and Oron, U. 1993. Bone growth to metal implants is regulated by their surface chemical properties. *Biomaterials* 14, 570–574.

Hille, G.H. 1966. Titanium for surgical implants. *J. Mater.* 1, 373–383.

Imam, M.A., Fraker, A.C., Harris, J.S., and Gilmore, C.M. 1983. Influence of heat treatment on the fatigue lives of Ti–6Al–4V and Ti–4.5Al–5Mo–1.5CR. In *Titanium Alloys in Surgical Implants*, Luckey, H.A. and Kubli, F.E. eds. Philadelphia, PA: ASTM Special Technical Publication 796, pp. 105–119.

Kasemo, B. and Lausma, J. 1988. Biomaterial and implant surface: A surface science approach. *Int. J. Oral Maxillofac Implant.* 3, 247–259.

Keating, F.H. 1956. *Chromium–Nickel Austenitic Steels*. London: Butterworths.

Keller, J.C., Stanford, C.M., Wightman, J.P., Draughn, R.A., and Zaharias, R. 1994. Characterizations of titanium implant surfaces. III. *J. Biomed. Mater. Res.* 28, 939–946.

Kieswetter, K., Schwartz, Z., Hummert, T.W., Cochran, D.L., Simpson, J., and Boyan, B.D. 1996. Surface roughness modulates the local production of growth factors and cytokines by osteoblast-like MG-63 cells. *J. Biomed. Mater. Res.* 32, 55–63.

Kim, H., Miyaji, F., Kokubo, T., and Nakamura, T. 1996. Preparation of bioactive Ti and its alloys via simple chemical surface treatment. *J. Biomed. Mater. Res.* 32, 409–417.

Lee, J.H., Park, J.B., Andreasen, G.F., and Lakes, R.S. 1988. Thermomechanical study of Ni–Ti alloys. *J. Biomed. Mater. Res.* 22, 573–588.

Nielsen, J.P. 1986. Dental noble-metal casting alloys: Composition and properties. In *Encyclopedia of Materials Science and Engineering*, Bever, M.B. ed. Oxford, Cambridge: Pergamon Press, pp. 1093–1095.

Pourbaix, M. 1974. *Atlas of Electrochemical Equilibria in Aqueous Solutions*, 2nd ed. Houston/CEBELCOR, Brussels: NACE.

Richards Manufacturing Company. 1980. Biophase implant material. Technical Information Publication 3846, Memphis, TN.

Schmalzried, T.P., Peters, P.C., Maurer, B.T., Bragdon, C.R., and Harris, W.H. 1996. Long-duration metal-on-metal total hip arthroplasties with low wear of the articulating surfaces. *J. Arthroplasty* 11, 322–331.

Semlitch, M. 1980. Properties of wrought CoNiCrMo alloy Protasul-10, a highly corrosion and fatigue resistant implant material for joint endoprostheses. *Eng. Med.* 9, 201–207.

Sloter, L.E. and Piehler, H.R. 1979. Corrosion-fatigue performance of stainless steel hip nails—Jewett type. In *Corrosion and Degradation of Implant Materials*, Syrett, B.C. and Acharya, A. eds. Philadelphia, PA: ASTM, pp. 173–195.

Smith, W.F. 1993. *Structure and Properties of Engineering Alloys*, 2nd ed. New York: McGraw-Hill.

Smith, C.J.E. and Hughes, A.N. 1966. The corrosion-fatigue behavior of a titanium-6w/o aluminum-4w/o vanadium alloy. *Eng. Med.* 7, 158–171.

Takatsuka, K., Yamamuro, T., Nakamura, T., and Kokubo, T. 1995. Bone-bonding behavior of titanium alloy evaluated mechanically with detaching failure load. *J. Biomed. Mater. Res.* 29, 157–163.

Takeshita, F., Ayukawa, Y., Iyama, S., Murai, K., and Suetsugu, T. 1997. Long-term evaluation of bone-titanium interface in rat tibiae using light microscopy, transmission electron microscopy, and image processing. *J. Biomed. Mater. Res.* 37, 235–242.

Wayman, C.M. and Duerig, T.W. 1990. An introduction of martensite and shape memory. In *Engineering Aspects of Shape Memory Alloys*, Duerig, T.W., Melton, K.N., Stockel, D., and Wayman, C.M. eds. London: Butterworth-Heinemann, pp. 3–20.

Wayman, C.M. and Shimizu, K. 1972. The shape memory ('Marmem') effect in alloys. *Metal Sci. J.* 6, 175–183.

Williams, D.F. 1982. *Biocompatibility in Clinical Practice*. Boca Raton, FL: CRC Press.

Wynblatt, P. 1986. Platinum group metals and alloys. In *Encyclopedia of Materials Science and Engineering*, Bever, M.B. ed. Oxford, Cambridge: Pergamon Press, pp. 3576–3579.

Yan, W., Nakamura, T., Kobayashi, M., Kim, H., Miyaji, F., and Kokubo, T. 1997. Bonding of chemically treated titanium implants to bone. *J. Biomed. Mater. Res.* 37, 267–275.

Further Reading

Bardos, D.I. 1977. Stainless steels in medical devices, In *Handbook of Stainless Steels.* Peckner, D. and Bernstein, I.M., eds., pp. 1–10, McGraw-Hill, New York.

Bechtol, C.O., Ferguson, A.B., Jr., and Laing, P.G. 1959. *Metals and Engineering in Bone and Joint Surgery,* Williams & Wilkins, Baltimore, MD.

Comte, T.W. 1984. Metallurgical observations of biomaterials, In *Contemporary Biomaterials,* Boretos, J.W. and Eden, M., eds., pp. 66–91, Noyes, Park Ridge, NJ.

Dumbleton, J.H. and Black, J. 1975. *An Introduction to Orthopaedic Materials,* C. Thomas, Springfield, IL.

Fontana, M.G. and Greene, N.O. 1967. *Corrosion Engineering,* pp. 163–168, McGraw-Hill, New York.

Hildebrand, H.F. and Champy, M., Eds. 1988. *Biocompatibility of Co–Cr–Ni Alloys,* Plenum Press, New York.

Levine, S.N., Ed. 1968. *Materials in Biomedical Engineering,* Vol. 146, Annals of New York Academy of Science, New York.

Luckey H.A., Ed. 1983. *Titanium Alloys in Surgical Implants,* ASTM Special Technical Publication 796, Philadelphia, PA.

Mears, D.C. 1979. *Materials and Orthopaedic Surgery,* Williams & Wilkins, Baltimore, MD.

Park, J.B. 1984. *Biomaterials Science and Engineering,* Plenum Press, New York.

Perkins, J., Ed. 1975. *Shape Memory Effects in Alloys,* Plenum Press, New York.

Puckering, F.B., Ed. 1979. *The Metallurgical Evolution of Stainless Steels,* pp. 1–42, American Society for Metals and the Metals Society, Metals Park, OH.

Weinstein, A., Horowitz, E., and Ruff, A.W., Eds. 1977. *Retrieval and Analysis of Orthopaedic Implants,* NBS, U.S. Department of Commerce, Washington, DC.

Williams, D.F. and Roaf, R. 1973. *Implants in Surgery,* W.B. Sauders Co., Ltd, London.

29

Ceramic Biomaterials

29.1 Introduction 29-1
29.2 Nonabsorbable or Relatively Bioinert Bioceramics...................29-2
    Relatively Bioinert Ceramics • Alumina (Al_2O_3) • Zirconia
    (ZrO_2) • Carbons
29.3 Biodegradable or Resorbable Ceramics......................................29-8
    Calcium Phosphate • Aluminum–Calcium–Phosphate (ALCAP)
    Ceramics • Coralline • Tricalcium Phosphate Ceramics • Zinc-
    Calcium–Phosphorous Oxide Ceramics • Zinc–Sulfate–Calcium–
    Phosphate Ceramics • Ferric–Calcium–Phosphorous Oxide
    Ceramics
29.4 Bioactive or Surface-Reactive Ceramics 29-16
    Glass Ceramics • Ceravital
29.5 Deterioration of Ceramics..29-20
29.6 Bioceramic Manufacturing Techniques....................................29-23
    Hard Tissue Replacement • Tissue Integration • Hydroxyapatite
    Synthesis Method
Defining Terms 29-26
In Memory Of...29-26
Acknowledgments..29-26
References...29-26
Further Information..29-32

W. G. Billotte
University of Dayton

29.1 Introduction

Ceramics are defined as the art and science of making and using solid articles with inorganic nonmetallic materials as their essential component (Kingery et al., 1976). Ceramics are refractory, polycrystalline compounds, usually inorganic, including silicates, metallic oxides, carbides and various refractory hydrides, sulfides, and selenides. Oxides such as Al_2O_3, MgO, SiO_2, and ZrO_2 contain metallic and nonmetallic elements and ionic salts such as $NaCl$, $CsCl$, and ZnS (Park and Lakes, 1992). Exceptions to the former include covalently bonded ceramics such as diamond and carbonaceous structures such as graphite and pyrolized carbons (Park and Lakes, 1992).

Ceramics in the form of pottery have been used by humans for thousands of years. Until recently, their use was somewhat limited because of their inherent brittleness, susceptibility to notches or micro-cracks, low tensile strength, and low impact strength. However, in the past 100 years, innovative techniques for fabricating ceramics have led to their use as "high-tech" materials. In recent years, humans have realized that ceramics and their composites can also be used to augment or replace various parts of the body, particularly bone. Thus, the ceramics used for the latter purposes are classified as *bioceramics*. Their relative inertness to the body fluids, high compressive strength, and esthetically pleasing appearance led to the use of ceramics in dentistry as dental crowns. Some carbons have found use as implants

29-1

TABLE 29.1   Desired Properties of Implantable Bioceramics

1. Nontoxic
2. Noncarcinogenic
3. Nonallergic
4. Noninflammatory
5. Biocompatible
6. Biofunctional for its lifetime in the host

especially for blood interfacing applications such as heart valves. Due to their high specific strength as fibers and their biocompatibility, ceramics are also being used as reinforcing components of composite implant materials and for tensile loading applications such as artificial tendon and ligaments (Park and Lakes, 1992).

Unlike metals and polymers, ceramics are difficult to shear plastically due to the (ionic) nature of the bonding and minimum number of slip systems. These characteristics make the ceramics nonductile and are responsible for almost zero creep at room temperature (Park and Lakes, 1992). Consequently, ceramics are very susceptible to notches or microcracks because instead of undergoing plastic deformation (or yield) they will fracture elastically on initiation of a crack. At the crack tip, the stress could be many times higher than the stress in the material away from the tip, resulting in a *stress concentration* which weakens the material considerably. The latter makes it difficult to predict the tensile strength of the material (ceramic). This is also the reason why ceramics have low tensile strength compared to compressive strength. If a ceramic is flawless, it is very strong even when subjected to tension. Flawless glass fibers have twice the tensile strengths of high strength steel (~7 GPa) (Park and Lakes, 1992).

Ceramics are generally hard; in fact, the measurement of hardness is calibrated against ceramic materials. Diamond is the hardest, with a hardness index of 10 on Moh's scale, and talc ($Mg_3Si_3O_{10}COH$) is the softest ceramic (Moh's hardness 1), while ceramics such as *alumina* (Al_2O_3; hardness 9), quartz (SiO_2; hardness 8), and apatite ($Ca_5P_3O_{12}F$; hardness 5) are in the middle range. Other characteristics of ceramic materials are: (1) high melting temperatures and (2) low conductivity of electricity and heat. These characteristics are due to the chemical bonding within ceramics.

In order to be classified as a bioceramic, the ceramic material must meet or exceed the properties listed in Table 29.1. The number of specific ceramics currently in use or under investigation cannot be accounted for in the space available for bioceramics in this book. Thus, this chapter will focus on a general overview of the relatively bioinert, bioactive or surface-reactive ceramics, and biodegradable or resorbable bioceramics.

Ceramics used in fabricating implants can be classified as nonabsorbable (relatively inert), bioactive or surface reactive (semi-inert) (Hench, 1991, 1993), and biodegradable or resorbable (non-inert) (Hentrich et al., 1971; Graves et al., 1972). Alumina, zirconia, silicone nitrides, and carbons are inert bioceramics. Certain *glass ceramics* and dense *hydroxyapatites* are semi-inert (bioreactive) and *calcium phosphates* and calcium aluminates are resorbable ceramics (Park and Lakes, 1992).

29.2 Nonabsorbable or Relatively Bioinert Bioceramics

29.2.1 Relatively Bioinert Ceramics

Relatively bioinert ceramics maintain their physical and mechanical properties while in the host. They resist corrosion and wear and have all the properties listed for bioceramics in Table 29.1. Examples of relatively bioinert ceramics are dense and porous aluminum oxides, zirconia ceramics, and single-phase calcium aluminates (Table 29.2). Relatively bioinert ceramics are typically used as structural-support implants. Some of these are bone plates, bone screws, and femoral heads (Table 29.3). Examples of

TABLE 29.2 Examples of Relatively Bioinert Bioceramics

Bioinert Ceramics	References
1. Pyrolitic carbon-coated devices	Adams and Williams (1978)
	Bokros et al. (1972)
	Bokros (1972)
	Chandy and Sharma (1991)
	Dellsperger and Chandran (1991)
	Kaae (1971)
	More and Silver (1990)
	Shimm and Haubold (1980)
	Shobert (1964)
2. Dense and nonporous aluminum oxides	Hench (1991)
	Hentrich et al. (1971)
	Krainess and Knapp (1978)
	Park (1991)
	Ritter et al. (1979)
	Shackelford (1988)
3. Porous aluminum oxides	Hench (1991)
	Hentrich et al. (1971)
	Park (1991)
	Ritter et al. (1979)
	Shackelford (1988)
4. Zirconia ceramics	Barinov and Bashenko (1992)
	Drennan and Steele (1991)
	Hench (1991)
	Kumar et al. (1989)
5. Dense hydroxyapatites	Bajpai (1990)
	Cotell et al. (1992)
	Fulmer et al. (1992)
	Huaxia et al. (1992)
	Kijima and Tsutsumi (1979)
	Knowles et al. (1993)
	Meenen et al. (1992)
	Niwa et al. (1980)
	Posner et al. (1958)
	Schwartz et al. (1993)
	Valiathan et al. (1993)
	Whitehead et al. (1993)
6. Calcium aluminates	Hammer et al. (1972)
	Hentrich et al. (1971)
	Hulbert and Klawitter (1971)

nonstructural support uses are ventilation tubes, sterilization devices (Feenstra and de Groot, 1983), and drug-delivery devices (see Table 29.3).

29.2.2 Alumina (Al_2O_3)

The main source of high-purity alumina (aluminum oxide, Al_2O_3) is bauxite and native corundum. The commonly available alumina (alpha, α) can be prepared by calcining alumina trihydrate. The chemical composition and density of commercially available "pure" calcined alumina are given in Table 29.4. The American Society for Testing and Materials (ASTM) specifies that alumina for implant use should contain 99.5% pure alumina and less than 0.1% combined SiO_2 and alkali oxides (mostly Na_2O) (F603-78).

Alpha alumina has a rhombohedral crystal structure ($a = 4.758$ Å and $c = 12.991$ Å). Natural alumina is known as sapphire or ruby, depending on the types of impurities which give rise to color. The

TABLE 29.3 Uses of Bioinert Bioceramics

Bioinert Ceramics	References
1. In reconstruction of acetabular cavities	Boutin (1981)
	Dorlot et al. (1988)
2. As bone plates and screws	Zimmerman et al. (1991)
3. In the form of ceramic–ceramic composites	Boutin (1981)
	Chignier et al. (1987)
	Sedel et al. (1991)
	Terry et al. (1989)
4. In the form of ceramic–polymer composites	Hulbert (1992)
5. As drug delivery devices	Buykx et al. (1992)
6. As femoral heads	Boutin (1981)
	Dörre (1991)
	Ohashi et al. (1988)
	Oonishi (1992)
7. As middle ear ossicles	Grote (1987)
8. In the reconstruction of orbital rims	Heimke (1992)
9. As components of total and partial hips	Feenstra and de Groot (1983)
10. In the form of sterilization tubes	Feenstra and de Groot (1983)
11. As ventilation tubes	Feenstra and de Groot (1983)
12. In the repair of the cardiovascular area	Chignier et al. (1987)
	Ely and Haubald (1993)

single-crystal form of alumina has been used successfully to make implants (Kawahara, 1989; Park, 1991). Single-crystal alumina can be made by feeding fine alumina powders onto the surface of a seed crystal which is slowly withdrawn from an electric arc or oxy-hydrogen flame as the fused powder builds up. Single crystals of alumina up to 10 cm in diameter have been grown by this method (Park and Lakes, 1992).

The strength of polycrystalline alumina depends on its grain size and porosity. Generally, the smaller the grains, the lower the porosity and the higher the strength (Park and Lakes, 1992). The ASTM standards (F603-78) requires a flexural strength greater than 400 MPa and elastic modulus of 380 GPa (Table 29.5).

Aluminum oxide has been used in the area of orthopedics for more than 25 years (Hench, 1991). Single-crystal alumina has been used in orthopedics and dental surgery for almost 20 years. Alumina is usually a quite hard material with hardness varies from 20 to 30 GPa. This high hardness permits its use as an abrasive (emery) and as bearings for watch movements (Park and Lakes, 1992). Both polycrystalline and single-crystal alumina have been used clinically. The high hardness is accompanied by low friction and wear and inertness to the *in vivo* environment. These properties make alumina an ideal

TABLE 29.4 Chemical Composition of Calcined Alumina

Chemicals	Composition (wt%)
Al_2O_3	99.6
SiO_2	0.12
Fe_2O_3	0.03
Na_2O	0.04

Source: Adapted from Park J.B. and Lakes R.S. 1992. *Biomaterials—An Introduction.* 2nd ed., p. 121, Plenum Press, New York.

TABLE 29.5 Physical Property Requirements of Alumina and Partially Stabilized Zirconia

Properties	Alumina	Zirconia
Elastic modulus (GPa)	380	190
Flexural strength (GPa)	>0.4	1.0
Hardness, Mohs	9	6.5
Density (g/cm³)	3.8–3.9	5.95
Grain size (μm)	4.0	0.6

Source: Adapted from Park J.B. 1993. Personal communication.

Note: Both the ceramics contain 3 mol% Y_2O_3.

candidate for use in joint replacements (Park and Lakes, 1992). Aluminum oxide implants in bones of rhesus monkeys have shown no signs of rejection or toxicity for 350 days (Hentrich et al., 1971; Graves et al., 1972). One of the most popular uses for aluminum oxide is in total hip protheses. Aluminum oxide hip protheses with an ultra-high-molecular-weight polyethylene (UHMWPE) socket have been claimed to be a better device than a metal prostheses with a UHMWPE socket (Oonishi, 1992). However, the key for success of any implant, besides the correct surgical implantation, is the highest possible quality control during fabrication of the material and the production of the implant (Hench, 1991).

29.2.3 Zirconia (ZrO_2)

Pure zirconia can be obtained from chemical conversion of zircon ($ZrSiO_4$), which is an abundant mineral deposit (Park and Lakes, 1992). Zirconia has a high melting temperature ($T_m = 2953$ K) and chemical stability with $a = 5.145$ Å, $b = 0.521$ Å, $c = 5.311$ Å, and $\beta = 99°14$ (Park and Lakes, 1992). It undergoes a large volume change during phase changes at high temperature in pure form; therefore, a dopant oxide such as Y_2O_3 is used to stabilize the high-temperature (cubic) phase. We have used 6 mol% Y_2O_3 as dopant to make zirconia for implantation in bone (Hentrich et al., 1971). Zirconia produced in this manner is referred to as *partially stabilized* zirconia (Drennan and Steele, 1991). However, the physical properties of zirconia are somewhat inferior to that of alumina (Table 29.5).

High-density zirconia oxide showed excellent compatibility with autogenous rhesus monkey bone and was completely nonreactive to the body environment for the duration of the 350-day study (Hentrich et al., 1971). Zirconia has shown excellent biocompatibility and good wear and friction when combined with UHMWPE (Kumar et al., 1989; Murakami and Ohtsuki, 1989).

29.2.4 Carbons

Carbons can be made in many allotropic forms: crystalline diamond, graphite, noncrystalline glassy carbon, and quasicrystalline pyrolitic carbon. Among these, only pyrolitic carbon is widely utilized for implant fabrication; it is normally used as a surface coating. It is also possible to coat surfaces with diamond. Although the techniques of coating with diamond have the potential to revolutionize medical device manufacturing, it is not yet commercially available (Park and Lakes, 1992).

The crystalline structure of carbon, as used in implants, is similar to the graphite structure shown in Figure 29.1. The planar hexagonal arrays are formed by strong covalent bonds in which one of the valence electrons or atoms is free to move, resulting in high but anisotropic electric conductivity. Since the bonding between the layers is stronger than the van der Waals force, it has been suggested that the layers are *cross-linked*. However, the remarkable lubricating property of graphite cannot be attained unless the cross-links are eliminated (Park and Lakes, 1992).

The poorly crystalline carbons are thought to contain unassociated or unoriented carbon atoms. The hexagonal layers are not perfectly arranged, as shown in Figure 29.2. Properties of individual crystallites

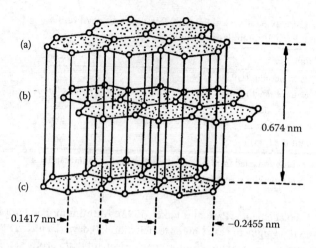

FIGURE 29.1 Crystal structure of graphite. (From Shobert E.I. II. 1964. *Carbon and Graphite*. Academic Press, New York. With permission.)

seem to be highly anisotropic. However, if the crystallites are randomly dispersed, the aggregate becomes isotropic (Park and Lakes, 1992).

The mechanical properties of carbon, especially pyrolitic carbon, are largely dependent on its density, as shown in Figures 29.3 and 29.4. The increased mechanical properties are directly related to increased density, which indicates that the properties of pyrolitic carbon depend mainly on the aggregate structure of the material (Park and Lakes, 1992).

Graphite and glassy carbon have a much lower mechanical strength than pyrolitic carbon (Table 29.6). However, the average modulus of elasticity is almost the same for all carbons. The strength of pyrolitic carbon is quite high compared to graphite and glassy carbon. Again, this is due to the fewer number of flaws and unassociated carbons in the aggregate.

A composite carbon which is reinforced with carbon fiber has been considered for making implants. However, the carbon–carbon composite is highly anisotropic, and its density is in the range 1.4–1.45 g/cm^3 with a porosity of 35%–38% (Table 29.7).

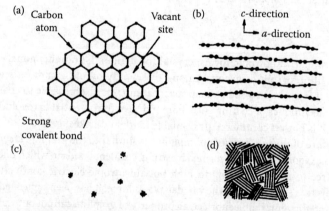

FIGURE 29.2 Schematic presentation of poorly crystalline carbon. (a) Single-layer plane, (b) parallel layers in a crystallite, (c) unassociated carbon, and (d) an aggregate of crystallites, single layers and unassociated carbon. (From Bokros J.C. 1972. *Chem. Phys. Carbon*. 5:70–81. With permission.)

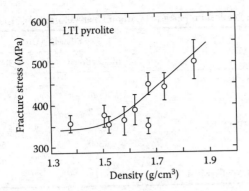

FIGURE 29.3 Fracture stress versus density for unalloyed LTI pyrolite carbons. (From Kaae J.L. 1971. *J. Nucl. Mater.* 38:42–50. With permission.)

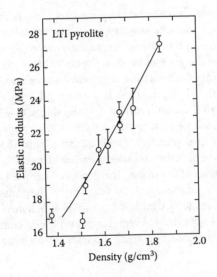

FIGURE 29.4 Elastic modulus versus density for unalloyed LTI pyrolite carbons. (From Kaae J.L. 1971. *J. Nucl. Mater.* 38:42–50. With permission.)

TABLE 29.6 Properties of Various Types of Carbon

| | Types of Carbon | | |
Properties	Graphite	Glassy	Pyrolitica[a]
Density (g/cm³)	1.5–1.9	1.5	1.5–2.0
Elastic modulus (GPa)	24	24	28
Compressive strength (MPa)	138	172	517 (575[a])
Toughness (mN/cm³)[b]	6.3	0.6	4.8

Source: Adapted from Park J.B. and Lakes R.S. 1992. *Biomaterials—An Introduction.* 2nd ed., p. 133. Plenum Press, New York.

[a] 1.0 w/o Si-alloyed pyrolitic carbon, Pyrolite™ (Carbomedics, Austin, TX).

[b] 1 mN/cm³ = 1.45 × 10⁻³ in.lb/in.³.

TABLE 29.7 Mechanical Properties of Carbon Fiber-Reinforced Carbon

Property	Fiber Lay-Up	
	Unidirectional	0–90° Crossply
Flexural modulus (GPa)		
Longitudinal	140	60
Transverse	7	60
Flexural strength (MPa)		
Longitudinal	1200	500
Transverse	15	500
Interlaminar shear strength (MPa)	18	18

Source: Adapted from Adams D. and Williams D.F. 1978. *J. Biomed. Mater. Res.* 12:38.

Carbons exhibit excellent compatibility with tissue. Compatibility of pyrolitic carbon-coated devices with blood has resulted in extensive use of these devices for repairing diseased heart valves and blood vessels (Park and Lakes, 1992).

Pyrolitic carbons can be deposited onto finished implants from hydrocarbon gas in a *fluidized bed* at a controlled temperature and pressure. The anisotropy, density, crystallite size, and structure of the deposited carbon can be controlled by temperature, composition of the fluidized gas, the bed geometry, and the residence time (velocity) of the gas molecules in the bed. The microstructure of deposited carbon should be highly controlled, since the formation of growth features associated with uneven crystallization can result in a weaker material (Figure 29.5). It is also possible to introduce various elements into the fluidized gas and co-deposit them with carbon. Usually silicon (10–20 w/o) is co-deposited (or alloyed) to increase hardness for applications requiring resistance to abrasion, such as heart valve disks.

Recently, success was achieved in depositing pyrolitic carbon onto the surfaces of blood vessel implants made of polymers. This type of carbon is called ultra-low-temperature isotropic (ULTI) carbon instead of low-temperature isotropic (LTI) carbon. The deposited carbon has excellent compatibility with blood and is thin enough not to interfere with the flexibility of the grafts (Park and Lakes, 1992).

The vitreous or glassy carbon is made by controlled pyrolysis of polymers such as phenolformaldehyde, Rayon (cellulose), and polyacrylonitrite at high temperature in a controlled environment. This process is particularly useful for making carbon fibers and textiles which can be used alone or as components of composites.

29.3 Biodegradable or Resorbable Ceramics

Although Plaster of Paris was used in 1892 as a bone substitute (Peltier, 1961), the concept of using synthetic resorbable ceramics as bone substitutes was introduced in 1969 (Hentrich et al., 1969; Graves et al., 1972). *Resorbable ceramics*, as the name implies, degrade upon implantation in the host. The resorbed material is replaced by endogenous tissues. The rate of degradation varies from material to material. Almost all bioresorbable ceramics except Biocoral and Plaster of Paris (calcium sulfate dihydrate) are variations of calcium phosphate (Table 29.8). Examples of resorbable ceramics are aluminum calcium phosphate, coralline, Plaster of Paris, hydroxyapatite, and tricalcium phosphate (Table 29.8).

29.3.1 Calcium Phosphate

Calcium phosphate has been used in the form of artificial bone. This material has been synthesized and used for manufacturing various forms of implants, as well as for solid or porous coatings on other implants (Table 29.9).

Calcium phosphate can be crystallized into salts such as hydroxyapatite and β-whitlockite depending on the Ca:P ratio, presence of water, impurities, and temperature. In a wet environment and at

(a)

(b)

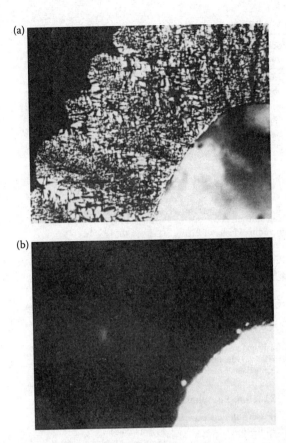

FIGURE 29.5 Microstructure of carbons deposited in a fluidized bed. (a) A granular carbon with distinct growth features. (b) An isotropic carbon without growth features. Both under polarized light. ×240. (From Bokros J.C., LaGrange L.D., and Schoen G.J. 1972. *Chem. Phys. Carbon.* 9:103–171. With permission.)

lower temperatures (<900°C), it is more likely that hydroxyl- or hydroxyapatite will form, while in a dry atmosphere and at a higher temperature, β-whitlockite will be formed (Park and Lakes, 1992). Both forms are very tissue-compatible and are used as bone substitutes in a granular form or a solid block. The apatite form of calcium phosphate is considered to be closely related to the mineral phase of bone and teeth.

The mineral part of bone and teeth is made of a crystalline form of calcium phosphate similar to hydroxyapatite $[Ca_{10}(PO_4)_6(OH)_2]$. The apatite family of mineral $[A_{10}(BO_4)_6X_2]$ crystallizes into hexagonal rhombic prisms and has unit cell dimensions $a = 9.432$ Å and $c = 6.881$ Å. The atomic structure of hydroxyapatite projected down the c-axis onto the basal plane is shown in Figure 29.6. Note that the hydroxyl ions lie on the corners of the projected basal plane and they occur at equidistant intervals (3.44 Å) along the columns perpendicular to the basal plane and parallel to the c-axis. Six of the 10 calcium ions in the unit cell are associated with the hydroxyls in these columns, resulting in strong interactions among them (Park and Lakes, 1992).

The ideal Ca:P ratio of hydroxyapatite is 10:6 and the calculated density is 3.219 g/cm³. Substitution of OH with fluoride gives apatite greater chemical stability due to the closer coordination of fluoride (symmetric shape) when compared to the hydroxyl (asymmetric, two atoms) by the nearest calcium. This is why fluoridation of drinking water helps in resisting caries of the teeth (Park and Lakes, 1992).

The mechanical properties of synthetic calcium phosphates vary considerably (Table 29.10). The wide variations in properties of polycrystalline calcium phosphates are due to the variations in the structure

TABLE 29.8 Examples of Biodegradable Bioceramics

Biodegradable or Resorbable Bioceramics	References
1. Aluminum–calcium–phosphorous oxides	Bajpai et al. (1985)
	Mattie and Bajpai (1988)
	Wyatt et al. (1976)
2. Glass fibers and their composites	Alexander et al. (1987)
	Zimmerman et al. (1991)
3. Corals	Bajpai (1983)
	Guillemin et al. (1989)
	Khavari and Bajpai (1993)
	Sartoris et al. (1986)
	Wolford et al. (1987)
4. Calcium sulfates, including Plaster of Paris	Bajpai (1983)
	Peltier (1961)
	Scheidler and Bajpai (1992)
5. Ferric–calcium–phosphorous oxides	Fuski et al. (1993)
	Larrabee et al. (1993)
	Stricker et al. (1992)
6. Hydroxyapatites	Bajpai and Fuchs (1985)
	Bajpai (1983)
	Jenei et al. (1986)
	Ricci et al. (1986)
7. Tricalcium phosphate	Bajpai (1983)
	Bajpai et al. (1988)
	Lemons et al. (1988)
	Morris and Bajpai (1989)
8. Zinc–calcium–phosphorous oxides	Arar et al. (1989)
	Bajpai (1988)
	Binzer and Bajpai (1987)
	Gromofsky et al. (1988)
9. Zinc–sulfate–calcium–phosphorous oxides	Scheidler and Bajpai (1992)

and manufacturing processes. Depending on the final firing conditions, calcium phosphate can be calcium hydroxyapatite or β-whitlockite. In many instances, both types of structures exist in the same final product (Park and Lakes, 1992).

Polycrystalline hydroxyapatite has a high elastic modulus (40–117 GPa). Hard tissues such as bone, dentin, and dental enamel are natural composites which contain hydroxyapatite (or a similar mineral), as well as protein, other organic materials, and water. Enamel is the stiffest hard tissue, with an elastic modulus of 74 GPa, and contains the most mineral. Dentin ($E = 21$ GPa) and compact bone ($E = 12$–18 GPa) contain comparatively less mineral. The Poisson ratio for the mineral or synthetic hydroxyapatite is about 0.27 which is close to that of bone (≈ 0.3) (Park and Lakes, 1992).

Hontsu et al. (1997) were able to deposit an amorphous HA film on Ti, α-Al_2O_3, SiO//Si(100), and $SrTiO_3$ using a pulsed ArF excimer laser. Upon heat treatment, the amorphous film was converted into the crystalline form of HA. The HA film's electrical properties were measured for the first time (Table 29.11).

The most important property of hydroxyapatite as a biomaterial is its excellent biocompatibility. Hydroxyapatite appears to form a direct chemical bond with hard tissues (Piattelli and Trisi, 1994). On implantation of hydroxyapatite particles or porous blocks in bone, new lamellar cancellous bone forms within 4–8 weeks (Bajpai and Fuchs, 1985). Scanning electron micrograph ($\times 500$) of a set and hardened hydroxyapatite–cysteine composite is shown in Figure 29.7. The composite sets and hardens on addition of water.

TABLE 29.9 Uses of Biodegradable Bioceramics

Biodegradable or Resorbable Ceramics	References
1. As drug delivery devices	Abrams and Bajpai (1994)
	Bajpai (1992)
	Bajpai (1994)
	Benghuzzi et al. (1991)
	Moldovan and Bajpai (1994)
	Nagy and Bajpai (1994)
2. For repairing damaged bone due to disease or trauma	Bajpai (1990)
	Gromofsky et al. (1988)
	Khavari and Bajpai (1993)
	Morris and Bajpai (1987)
	Scheidler and Bajpai (1992)
3. For filling space vacated by bone screws, donor bone, excised tumors, and diseased bone loss	Bajpai and Fuchs (1985)
	Ricci et al. (1986)
4. For repairing and fusion of spinal and lumbo-sacral vertebrae	Bajpai et al. (1984)
	Yamamuro et al. (1988)
5. For repairing herniated disks	Bajpai et al. (1984)
6. For repairing maxillofacial and dental defects	Freeman et al. (1981)
7. Hydroxyapatite ocular implants	De Potter et al. (1994)
	Shields et al. (1993)

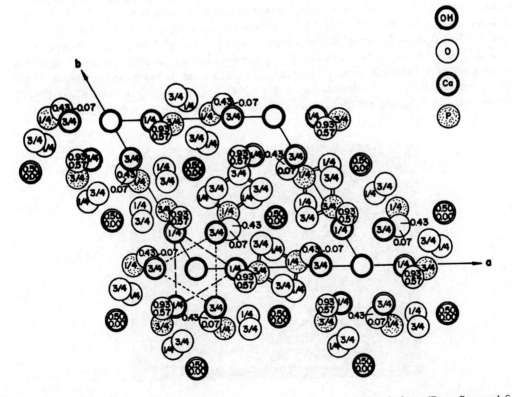

FIGURE 29.6 Hydroxyapatite structure projected down the *c*-axis onto the basal plane. (From Posner A.S., Perloff A., and Diorio A.D. 1958. *Acta Cryst.* 11:308–309.)

TABLE 29.10 Physical Properties of Calcium Phosphate

Properties	Values
Elastic modulus (GPa)	4.0–117
Compressive strength (MPa)	294
Bending strength (MPa)	147
Hardness (Vickers, GPa)	3.43
Poisson's ratio	0.27
Density (theoretical, g/cm³)	3.16

Source: Adapted from Park J.B. and Lakes R.S. 1992. *Biomaterials—An Introduction.* 2nd ed., p. 125. Plenum Press, New York.

TABLE 29.11 Electrical Properties of an HA Film

Dielectric constant (ε_r)	5.7 (25°C 1 MHz)
Loss tangent (tan δ)	<2%
Breakdown electric field	10^4 V cm^{-1}

Source: Adapted from Hontsu S. et al. 1997. *Thin Solid Films* 295:214–217.

Many different methods have been developed to make precipitates of hydroxyapatite from an aqueous solution of $Ca(NO_3)_2$ and NaH_2PO_4. There has been successful use of modifications to wet precipitation procedure of Jarcho and colleagues for synthesizing hydroxyapatites for use as bone implants (Jarcho et al., 1979; Bajpai and Fuchs, 1985), and drug delivery devices (Bajpai, 1992, 1994; Parker and Bajpai, 1993; Abrams and Bajpai, 1994). The dried, filtered precipitate is placed in a high-temperature furnace and calcined at 1150°C for 1 h. The calcined powder is then ground in a ball mill, and the particles are separated by an automatic sieve shaker and sieves. The sized particles are then pressed in a die and sintered at 1200°C for 36 h for making drug delivery devices (Bajpai, 1989, 1992; Abrams and Bajpai, 1994). Above 1250°C, hydroxyapatite shows a second precipitation phase along the grain boundaries (Park and Lakes, 1992).

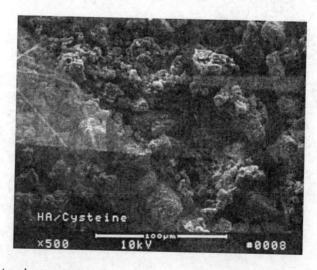

FIGURE 29.7 Scanning electron micrograph (×500) of a set and hardened hydroxyaptite (HA)-cysteine composite. The small white cysteine particles can be seen on the larger HA particles.

29.3.2 Aluminum–Calcium–Phosphate (ALCAP) Ceramics

Initially we fabricated a calcium aluminate ceramic containing phosphorous pentoxide (Hentrich et al., 1969, 1971; Graves et al., 1972). Aluminum–calcium–phosphorous oxide (ALCAP) ceramic was developed later (Bajpai and Graves, 1980). ALCAP has insulating dielectric properties but no magnetic or piezoelectric properties (Allaire et al., 1989). ALCAP ceramics are unique because they provide a multipurpose crystallographic system where one phase of the ceramic on implantation can be more rapidly resorbed than the others (Wyatt et al., 1976; Bajpai, 1983; Mattie and Bajpai, 1988). ALCAP is prepared from stock powders of aluminum oxide, calcium oxide, and phosphorous pentoxide. A ratio of 50:34:16 by weight of AlO_2:CaO:P_2O_5 is used to obtain the starting mixture for calcination at 1350°C in a high-temperature furnace for 12 h. The calcined material is ground in a ball mill and sieved by an automatic siever to obtain particles of the desired size. The particulate powder is then pressed into solid blocks or hollow cylinders (green shape) and sintered at 1400°C for 36 h to increase the mechanical strength. ALCAP ceramic implants have given excellent results in terms of biocompatibility and gradual replacement of the ceramic material with endogenous bone (Mattie and Bajpai, 1988; Bajpai, 1992). A scanning electron micrograph (×1000) of sintered porous ALCAP is shown in Figure 29.8.

29.3.3 Coralline

Coral is a natural substance made by marine invertebrates. According to Holmes et al. (1984), the marine invertebrates live in the limestone exostructure, or coral. The porous structure of the coral is unique for each species of marine invertebrate (Holmes et al., 1984). Corals for use as bone implants are selected on the basis of structural similarity to bone (Holmes et al., 1984). Coral provides an excellent structure for the ingrowth of bone, and the main component, calcium carbonate, is gradually resorbed by the body (Khavari and Bajpai, 1993). Corals can also be converted into hydroxyapatite by a hydrothermal exchange process. Interpore 200, a coral hydroxyapatite, resembles cancellous bone (Sartoris et al., 1986). Both pure coral (Biocoral) and coral transformed to hydroxyapatite are currently used to repair traumatized bone, to replace diseased bone, and to correct various bone defects.

Biocoral is composed of crystalline calcium carbonate or aragonite, the metastable form of calcium carbonate. The compressive strength of Biocoral varies from 26 (50% porous) to 395 MPa (dense)

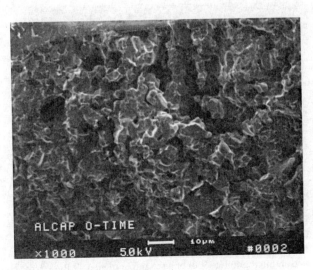

FIGURE 29.8 Scanning electron micrograph (×1000) of porous sintered ALCAP.

and depends on the porosity of the ceramic. Likewise, the modulus of elasticity (Young's modulus) of Biocoral varies from 8 (50% porous) to 100 GPa (dense) (Biocoral, 1989).

29.3.4 Tricalcium Phosphate Ceramics

A multicrystalline porous form of β-tricalcium phosphate [β-$Ca_3(PO_4)_2$] has been used successfully to correct periodontal defects and augment bony contours (Metsger et al., 1982). X-ray diffraction of β-tricalcium phosphate shows an average interconnected porosity of over 100 μm (Lemons et al., 1988). Often tribasic calcium phosphate is mistaken for β-tricalcium phosphate. According to Metsger et al. (1982), tribasic calcium phosphate is a nonstoichiometric compound often bearing the formula of hydroxyapatite [$Ca_{10}(PO_4)_6(OH)_2$].

β-Tricalcium phosphate is prepared by a wet precipitation procedure from an aqueous solution of $Ca(NO_3)_2$ and NaH_2PO_4 (Bajpai et al., 1988). The precipitate is calcined at 1150°C for 1 h, ground, and sieved to obtain the desired size particles for use as bone substitutes (Bajpai et al., 1988; Bajpai, 1990) and for making ceramic matrix drug delivery systems (Morris and Bajpai, 1989; Nagy and Bajpai, 1994; Moldovan and Bajpai, 1994). These particles are used as such or pressed into cylindrical shapes and sintered at 1150°C–1200°C for 36 h to achieve the appropriate mechanical strength for use as drug delivery devices (Bajpai, 1989, 1992, 1994; Benghuzzi et al., 1991). A scanning electron micrograph (500×) of a set and hardened TCP–cysteine composite is shown in Figure 29.9. The composite sets and hardens on the addition of water. TCP is usually more soluble than synthetic hydroxyapatite and, on implantation, allows for good bone ingrowth and eventually is replaced by endogenous bone.

29.3.5 Zinc–Calcium–Phosphorous Oxide Ceramics

Zinc is essential for human metabolism and is a component of at least 30 metalloenzymes (Pories and Strain, 1970). In addition, zinc may also be involved in the process of wound healing (Pories and Strain 1970). Thus zinc–calcium–phosphorous oxide polyphasic (ZCAP) ceramics were synthesized to repair bone defects and deliver drugs (Binzer and Bajpai, 1987; Bajpai, 1988, 1993; Arar and Bajpai, 1992). ZCAP is prepared by thermal mixing of zinc oxide, calcium oxide, and phosphorous pentoxide powders (Bajpai, 1988). ZCAP, like ALCAP, has insulating dielectric properties but no magnetic or piezoelectric properties (Allaire et al., 1989). Various ratios of these powders have been used to produce the desired material

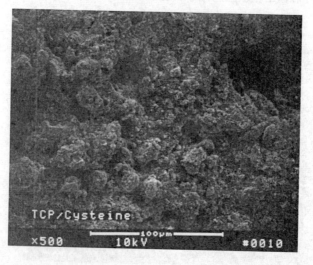

FIGURE 29.9 Scanning electron micrograph (×500) of a set and hardened TCP–cysteine composite. The small white cysteine particles can be seen on the larger TCP particles.

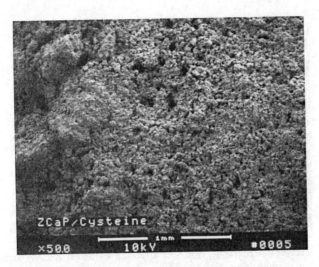

FIGURE 29.10 Scanning electron micrograph (×500) of a set and hardened ZCAP–cysteine composite. The small white cysteine particles have blended with the ZCAP particles.

(Bajpai, 1988). The oxide powders are mixed in a ball mill and subsequently calcined at 800°C for 24 h. The calcined ceramic is then ground and sieved to obtain the desired size particles. Scanning electron micrograph (×500) of a set and hardened ZCAP–cysteine composite is shown in Figure 29.10. The composite sets and hardens upon addition of water. To date, ZCAP ceramics have been used to repair experimentally induced defects in bone and for delivering drugs (Binzer and Bajpai, 1987; Bajpai, 1993).

29.3.6 Zinc–Sulfate–Calcium–Phosphate Ceramics

Zinc–sulfate–calcium–phosphate polyphasic (ZSCAP) ceramics are prepared from stock powders of zinc sulfate, zinc oxide, calcium oxide, and phosphorous pentoxide (Bajpai, 1988). A ratio of 15:30:30:25 by weight of $ZnSO_4$:ZnO:CaO:P_2O_5 is mixed in a crucible and allowed to cool for 30 min after the exothermal reaction has subsided. The cooled mixture is calcined in a crucible at 650°C for 24 h. The calcined ceramic is ground in a ball mill and the particles of the desired size are separated by sieving in an automatic siever. Scanning electron micrograph (×2000) of set and hardened ZSCAP particles (45–63 μm) is shown in Figure 29.11. ZSCAP sets and hardens upon addition of water. ZSCAP particles, on implantation in bone, set and harden on contact with blood and have been used to repair experimentally induced defects in bone (Scheidler and Bajpai, 1992).

29.3.7 Ferric–Calcium–Phosphorous Oxide Ceramics

Ferric–calcium–phosphorous oxide polyphasic (FECAP) ceramic is prepared from powders of ferric (III) oxide, calcium oxide, and phosphorous pentoxide (Stricker et al., 1992; Fuski et al., 1993; Larrabee et al., 1993). The powders are combined in various ratios by weight and mixed in a blender. Blocks of the mixture are then pressed in a die by means of a hydraulic press and calcined at 1100°C for 12 h. The calcined ceramic blocks are crushed and ground in a ball mill. The calcined ceramic is ground in a ball mill and the particles of the desired size are separated by sieving in an automatic siever. A scanning electron micrograph (×1000) of a set and hardened FECAP-α ketoglutaric acid composite is shown in Figure 29.12. The composite sets and hardens on the addition of water. Studies conducted to date suggest complete resorption of FECAP particles implanted in bone within 60 days (Larrabee et al., 1993). This particular ceramic could be used in patients suffering from anemia and similar diseases (Fuski et al., 1993).

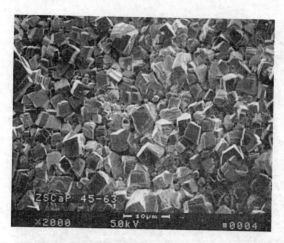

FIGURE 29.11 Scanning electron micrograph (×2000) of a set and hardened ZSCAP particles (45–63 μm). Sulfate is hardly visible between the cube-shaped ZCAP particles.

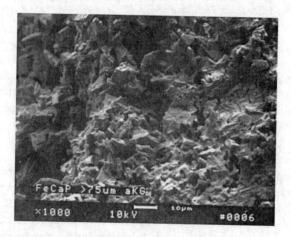

FIGURE 29.12 Scanning electron micrograph (×1000) of a set and hardened FECAP–α-ketoglutaric acid composite. Plate-shaped FECAP particles have been aggregated by the acid.

29.4 Bioactive or Surface-Reactive Ceramics

Upon implantation in the host, surface-reactive ceramics form strong bonds with adjacent tissues. Examples of surface-reactive ceramics are dense nonporous glasses, Bioglass and Ceravital, and hydroxyapatites (Table 29.12). One of their many uses is the coating of metal prostheses. This coating provides a stronger bonding to the adjacent tissues, which is very important for prostheses. A list of the uses of surface-reactive ceramics is shown in Table 29.13.

29.4.1 Glass Ceramics

Several variations of Bioglass and Ceravital glass ceramics have been used by various workers within the last decade. Glass ceramics used for implantation are silicon oxide-based systems with or without phosphorous pentoxide.

Glass ceramics are polycrystalline ceramics made by controlled crystallization of glasses developed by S.D. Stookey of Corning Glass Works in the early 1960s (Park and Lakes, 1992). Glass ceramics were

TABLE 29.12　Examples of Surface-Reactive Bioceramics

Surface-Reactive Bioceramics	References
1. Bioglasses and Ceravital™	Ducheyne (1985)
	Gheyson et al. (1983)
	Hench (1991)
	Hench (1993)
	Ogino et al. (1980)
	Ritter et al. (1979)
2. Dense and nonporous glasses	Andersson et al. (1992)
	Blencke et al. (1978)
	Li et al. (1991)
	Ohtsuki et al. (1992)
	Ohura et al. (1992)
	Schepers et al. (1993)
	Takatsuko et al. (1993)
3. Hydroxyapatite	Bagambisa et al. (1993)
	Bajpai (1990)
	Fredette et al. (1989)
	Huaxia et al. (1992)
	Knowles and Bonfield (1993)
	Niwa et al. (1980)
	Park and Lakes (1992)
	Posner et al. (1958)
	Schwartz et al. (1993)
	Whitehead et al. (1993)

TABLE 29.13　Uses of Surface-Reactive Bioceramics

Surface-Reactive Bioceramics	References
1. For coating of metal prostheses	Cotell et al. (1992)
	Huaxia et al.(1992)
	Ritter et al. (1979)
	Takatsuko et al. (1993)
	Whitehead et al. (1993)
2. In reconstruction of dental defects	Hulbert et al. (1987)
	Gheysen et al. (1983)
	Schepers et al. (1988)
	Schepers et al. (1989)
3. For filling space vacated by bone screws, donor bone, excised tumors, and diseased bone loss	Hulbert et al. (1987)
	Schepers et al. (1993)
	Terry et al. (1989)
4. As bone plates and screws	Doyle (1990)
	Ducheyne and McGuckin (1990)
	Yamamuro et al. (1988)
5. As replacements of middle ear ossicles	Feenstra and de Groot (1983)
	Grote (1987)
	Hench (1991)
	Hench (1993)
	Reck et al. (1988)
6. For lengthening of rami	Feenstra and de Groot (1983)
7. For correcting periodontal defects	Feenstra and de Groot (1983)
8. In replacing subperiosteal teeth	Hulbert (1992)

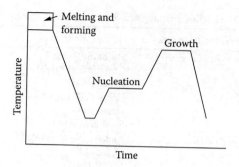

FIGURE 29.13 Temperature–time cycle for a glass ceramic. (From Kingery W.D., Bowen H.K., and Uhlmann D.R. *Introduction to Ceramics*. 2nd ed., p. 368. 1976. New York. Copyright Wiley-VCH Verlag GmbH & Co. KGaA. Reproduced with permission.)

first utilized in photosensitive glasses, in which small amounts of copper, silver, and gold are precipitated by ultraviolet light irradiation. These metallic precipitates help to nucleate and crystallize the glass into a fine-grained ceramic which possesses excellent mechanical and thermal properties. Both Bioglass and Ceravital glass ceramics have been used as implants (Yamamuro et al., 1990).

The formation of glass ceramics is influenced by the nucleation and growth of small (<1 μm diameter) crystals as well as the size distribution of these crystals. It is estimated that about 10^{12}–10^{15} nuclei/cm^3 are required to achieve such small crystals. In addition to the metallic agents already mentioned, Pt groups, TiO_2, ZrO_2, and P_2O_5 are widely used for nucleation and crystallization. The nucleation of glass is carried out at temperatures much lower than the melting temperature. During processing the melt viscosity is kept in the range of 10^{11} and 10^{12} Poise for 1–2 h. In order to obtain a larger fraction of the microcrystalline phase, the material is further heated to an appropriate temperature for maximum crystal growth. Deformation of the product, phase transformation within the crystalline phases, or redissolution of some of the phases should be avoided. The crystallization is usually more than 90% complete with grain sizes 0.1–1 μm. These grains are much smaller than those of conventional ceramics. Figure 29.13 shows a schematic representation of temperature–time cycle for a glass ceramic (Park and Lakes, 1992).

The glass ceramics developed for implantation are SiO_2–CaO–Na_2O–P_2O_5 and Li_2O–ZnO–SiO_2 systems. Two major groups are experimenting with the SiO_2–CaO–Na_2O–P_2O_5 glass ceramic. One group varied the compositions (except for P_2O_5) in order to obtain the best glass ceramic composition for

TABLE 29.14 Compositions of Bioglass and Ceravital Glass Ceramics

Type	Code	SiO_2	CaO	Na_2O	P_2O_5	MgO	K_2O
Bioglass	42S5.6	42.1	29.0	26.3	2.6	—	—
	(45S5)46S5.2	46.1	26.9	24.4	2.6	—	—
	49S4.9	49.1	25.3	23.8	2.6	—	—
	52S4.6	52.1	23.8	21.5	2.6	—	—
	55S4.3	55.1	22.2	20.1	2.6	—	—
	60S3.8	60.1	19.6	17.7	2.6	—	—
Ceravital	Bioactive[a]	40–50	30–35	5–10	10–15	2.5–5	0.5–3
	Nonbioactive[b]	30–35	25–30	3.5–7.5	7.5–12	1–2.5	0.5–2

Source: From Park J.B. and Lakes R.S. 1992. *Biomaterials—An Introduction*. 2nd ed., p. 127. Plenum Press, New York. With permission.

[a] The Ceravital® composition is in wt%, while the Bioglass® compositions are in mol%.

[b] In addition, Al_2O_3 (5.0–15.0), TiO_2 (1.0–5.0), and Ta_2O_5 (5–15) are added.

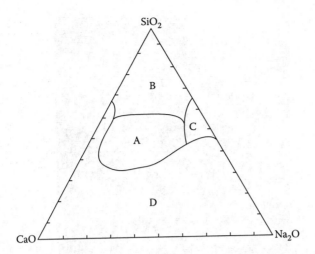

FIGURE 29.14 Approximate regions of the tissue–glass–ceramic bonding for the SiO_2–CaO–Na_2O system. A: Bonding within 30 days. B: Nonbonding; reactivity is too low. D: Bonding does not form glass. (From Hench L.L. and Ethridge E.C. 1982. *Biomaterials: An Interfacial Approach*, p. 147. Academic Press, New York. With permission.)

inducing direct bonding with bone (Table 29.14). The bonding to bone is related to the simultaneous formation of a calcium phosphate and SiO_2-rich film layer on the surface, as exhibited by the 46S5.2-type Bioglass. If a SiO_2-rich layer forms first and a calcium phosphate film develops later (46–55 mol% SiO_2 samples) or no phosphate film is formed (60 mol% SiO_2), then direct bonding with bone does not occur (Park and Lakes, 1992). The approximate region of the SiO_2–CaO–Na_2O system for the tissue–glass–ceramic reaction is shown in Figure 29.14. As can be seen, the best region (region A) for good tissue bonding is the composition given for 46S5.2-type Bioglass (see Table 29.14) (Park and Lakes, 1992).

29.4.2 Ceravital

The composition of Ceravital is similar to that of Bioglass in SiO_2 content but differs somewhat in other components (see Table 29.14). In order to control the dissolution rate, Al_2O_3, TiO_2, and Ta_2O_5 are added in Ceravital glass ceramic. The mixtures, after melting in a platinum crucible at 1500°C for 3 h, are annealed and cooled. The nucleation and crystallization temperatures are 680°C and 750°C, respectively, each for 24 h. When the size of crystallites reaches approximately 4 Å and the characteristic needle structure is not formed, the process is stopped to obtain a fine-grain structured glass ceramic (Park and Lakes, 1992).

Glass ceramics have several desirable properties compared to glasses and ceramics. The thermal coefficient of expansion is very low, typically 10^{-7}–10^{-5}°C^{-1}, and in some cases it can even be made negative. Due to the controlled grain size and improved resistance to surface damage, the tensile strength of these materials can be increased by at least a factor of 2, from about 100 to 200 MPa. The resistance to scratching and abrasion of glass ceramics is similar to that of sapphire (Park and Lakes, 1992).

A transmission electron micrograph of Bioglass glass ceramic implanted in the femur of rats for 6 weeks showed intimate contacts between the mineralized bone and the Bioglass (Figure 29.15). The mechanical strength of the interfacial bond between bone and Bioglass ceramic is on the same order of magnitude as the strength of the bulk glass ceramic (850 kg/cm^2 or 83.3 MPa), which is about three-fourths that of the host bone strength (Park and Lakes, 1992).

A negative characteristic of the glass ceramic is its brittleness. In addition, limitations on the compositions used for producing a biocompatible (or osteoconductive) glass ceramic hinders the production of a glass ceramic which has substantially higher mechanical strength. Thus, glass ceramics cannot be

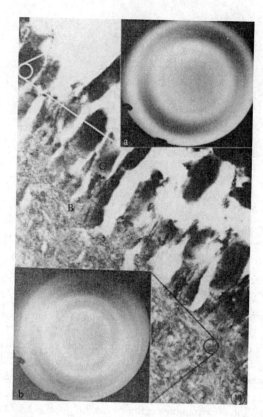

FIGURE 29.15 Transmission electron micrograph of well-mineralized bone (B) juxtaposed to the glass-ceramic (C) which fractured during sectioning (×51,500). Inset (a) is the diffraction pattern from ceramic area and (b) is from bone area. (From Beckham C.A., Greenlee T.K. Jr, and Crebo A.R. 1971. *Calc. Tiss. Res.* 8:165–171. With permission.)

used for making major load-bearing implants such as joint implants. However, they can be used as fillers for bone cement, dental restorative composites, and coating material (see Table 29.13). A glass ceramic containing 36 wt% of magnetite in a β-wollastonite- and $CaOSiO_2$-based glassy matrix has been synthesized for treating bone tumors by hyperthermia (Kokubo et al., 1992).

29.5 Deterioration of Ceramics

It is of great interest to know whether the inert ceramics such as alumina undergo significant static or dynamic fatigue. Even for the biodegradable ceramics, the rate of degradation *in vivo* is of paramount importance. Controlled degradation of an implant with time on implantation is desirable. Above a critical stress level, the fatigue strength of alumina is reduced by the presence of water. This is due to the delayed crack growth, which is accelerated by the water molecules (Park and Lakes, 1992). Reduction in strength occurs if water penetrates the ceramic. Decrease in strength was not observed in samples which did not show water marks on the fractured surface (Figure 29.16). The presence of a small amount of silica in one sample lot may have contributed to the permeation of water molecules that is detrimental to the strength (Park and Lakes, 1992). It is not clear whether the static fatigue mechanism operates in single-crystal alumina. It is reasonable to assume that static fatigue will occur if the ceramic contains flaws or impurities, because these will act as the source of crack initiation and growth under stress (Park and Lakes, 1992).

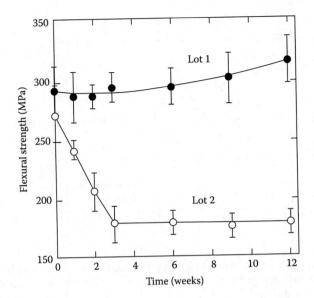

FIGURE 29.16 Flexural strength of dense alumina rods after aging under stress in Ringer's solution. Lots 1 and 2 are from different batches of production. (From Krainess F.E. and Knapp W.J. 1978. *J. Biomed. Mater. Res.* 12:245. With permission.)

Studies of the fatigue behavior of vapor-deposited pyrolitic carbon fibers (with a thickness of 4000–5000 Å) onto a stainless-steel substrate showed that the film does not break unless the substrate undergoes plastic deformation at 1.3×10^{-2} strain and up to 1 million cycles of loading. Therefore, the fatigue is closely related to the substrate, as shown in Figure 29.17. Similar substrate–carbon adherence is the basis for the pyrolitic carbon-deposited polymer arterial grafts (Park and Lakes, 1992).

The fatigue life of ceramics can be predicted by assuming that the fatigue fracture is due to the slow growth of preexisting flaws. Generally, the strength distribution, σ_i, of ceramics in an inert environment can be correlated with the probability of failure F by the following equation:

$$\mathrm{Ln}\,\mathrm{Ln}\!\left(\frac{1}{1-F}\right) = m\,\mathrm{Ln}\!\left(\frac{s_i}{s_o}\right) \tag{29.1}$$

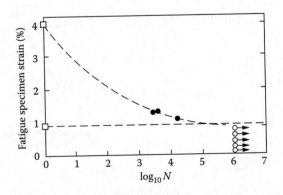

FIGURE 29.17 Strain versus number of cycles to failure (○ = absence of fatigue cracks in carbon film; ● = fracture of carbon film due to fatigue failure of substrates; □ = data from substrate determined in a single-cycle tensile test). (From Shimm H.S. and Haubold A.D. 1980. *Biomater. Med. Dev. Art. Org.* 8:333–344. With permission.)

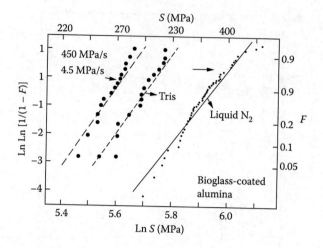

FIGURE 29.18 Plot of Ln Ln[1/(1 − *F*)] versus Ln *S* for Bioglass-coated alumina in a Tris–hydroxyaminomethane buffer and liquid nitrogen. *F* is the probability of failure and *S* is strength. (From Ritter J.E. Jr et al. 1979. *J. Biomed. Mater. Res.* 13:260. With permission.)

Both *m* and s_o are constants in the equation. Figure 29.18 shows a good fit for Bioglass-coated alumina (Park and Lakes, 1992).

A minimum service life (t_{min}) of a specimen can be predicted by means of a proof test wherein it is subjected to stresses that are greater than those expected in service. Proof tests also eliminate the weaker pieces. This minimum life can be predicted from the following equation:

$$t_{min} = B\sigma_p^{N-2}\sigma_a^{-N}$$

(29.2)

Here σ_p is the proof test stress, σ_a is the applied stress, and *B* and *N* are constants.

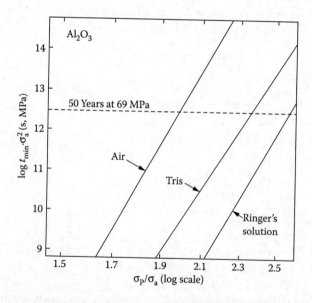

FIGURE 29.19 Plot of Equation 29.3 for alumina after proof testing. *N* = 43.85, *m* = 13.21, and σ_o = 55728 psi. (From Ritter J.E. Jr. et al. 1979. *J. Biomed. Mater. Res.* 13:261. With permission.)

Equation 29.2, after rearrangement, reads as follows:

$$t_{min}\sigma_a^2 = B\left(\frac{\sigma_p}{\sigma_a}\right)^{N-2}$$

(29.3)

Figure 29.19 shows the plot of Equation 29.3 for alumina on a logarithmic scale (Park and Lakes, 1992).

29.6 Bioceramic Manufacturing Techniques

To fabricate bioceramics in more and more complex shapes, scientists are investigating the use of old and new manufacturing techniques. These techniques range from the adaptation of an age-old pottery technique to the latest manufacturing methods for high-temperature ceramic parts for airplane engines. No matter where the technique is perfected, the ultimate goal is the fabrication of bioceramic particles or devices in a desired shape in a consistent manner with the desired properties. The technique used to fabricate the bioceramic device will depend greatly on the ultimate application of the device, whether it is for hard tissue replacement or for the integration of the device within the surrounding tissue.

29.6.1 Hard Tissue Replacement

Hard tissue replacement implies that the bioceramic device will be used for load-bearing applications. Although it is desirable to have a device with a sufficient porosity for the surrounding tissue to infiltrate and attach to the device, the most important and immediate property is the strength of the device. In order to accomplish this, one must manufacture a bioceramic implant with a density and strength sufficient to mimic that of bone. However, if the bioceramic part is significantly stronger than the surrounding bone, one runs into the common problem seen with metals called *stress shielding*. The density of the bioceramic greatly determines its overall strength. As the density increases, so does the overall strength of the bioceramic. Some of the techniques used to manufacture dense bioceramics are injection molding, gel casting, bicontinuous microemulsion, inverse microemulsion, emulsion, and additives.

Injection molding is a common technique used to form plastic parts for many commercial applications such as automobile parts. Briefly, the process involves forcing a heated material into a die and then ejecting the formed piece from the die. Injection molding allows for making complex shapes. Cihlar and Trunec (1996) found that by calcining (1273 K, 3 h) and milling the HA prior to mixing with a binder, an ethylene vinyl acetate copolymer (EVA)/HA mixture of 63% HA, they achieved 98% relative density with only 16% shrinkage using injection molding. The maximum flexural strength was 60 MPa for HA products sintered at 1473 K. However, this is still not strong enough for load-bearing applications. They also observed that HA decomposed to α-TCP at temperatures greater than 1573 K (Cihlar and Trunec, 1996).

In gel casting, HA is formed using the standard chemical precipitation. The calcium phosphate precipitant (30%, w/v) is then mixed with glycerol and filtered. The "gel cake" is sintered at 1200°C for 2 h. This yielded a density of >99% and a highly uniform microstructure (Varma and Sivakumar, 1996).

Bicontinuous microemulsion, inverse microemulsion, and emulsion are all wet chemistry-based methods to produce nanometer-sized HA powders. All three methods yield >97% relative density upon sintering at 1200°C for 2 h. The biocontinuous and inverse microemulsion resulted in the two smallest HA particle sizes, 22 and 24 nm, respectively (Lim et al., 1997).

Another strategy to increase the density of ceramics is to use additives or impurities in small weight percents during sintering. The major disadvantages of this technique are: (1) the possible decomposition of the original pure bioceramic and (2) results may end in all or portions of the bioceramic being nonbiocompatible.

Suchanek et al. (1997) studied the addition of several different additives to HA in 5 wt% amounts. The additives studied were K_2CO_3, Na_2CO_3, H_3BO_3, KF, $CaCl_2$, KCl, KH_2PO_4, $(KPO_3)_n$, $Na_2Si_2O_5$, $Na_2P_2O_7$, Na_3PO_4, $(NaPO_3)_n$, $Na_5P_3O_{10}$, and β-NaCaPO$_4$. HA has a fracture toughness of 1 MPa m$^{1/2}$, whereas human bone has a fracture toughness of 2–12 MPa m$^{1/2}$. One of the ways to improve the mechanical properties is to improve the densification of HA. Suchanek et al. (1997) found that the following additives (5 wt%) did not improve the densification of HA: H_3BO_3, $CaCl_2$, KCl, KH_2PO_4, $(KPO_3)_n$, and $Na_2Si_2O_5$. The densification of HA was improved through the addition (5 wt%) of K_2CO_3, Na_2CO_3, KF, $Na_2P_2O_7$, Na_3PO_4, $(NaPO_3)_n$, $Na_5P_3O_{10}$, and β-NaCaPO$_4$. However, H_3BO_3, $CaCl_2$, KH_2PO_4, $(KPO_3)_n$, $Na_2Si_2O_5$, K_2CO_3, Na_2CO_3, and KF produced the formation of β-TCP or CaO. Sodium phosphates used in this study were added to HA without the formation of β-TCP or CaO. The only compound that improved densification, did not cause formation of β-TCP or CaO, and provided a weak interface for HA was β-NaCaPO$_4$.

Another additive that has been investigated to improve the performance of HA is lithium (Li). Addition of lithium can increase the microhardness and produces a fine microstructure in HA. Fanovich et al. (1998) found that addition of 0.2 wt% of Li to HA produced the maximum microhardness (5.9 GPa). However, addition of high amounts of Li to HA results in abnormal grain growth and large pores. Furthermore, Li addition to HA results in the formation of β-TCP upon sintering.

Zirconia has been used as an additive to HA in order to improve its mechanical strength. Kawashima et al. (1997) found that addition of partially stabilized zirconia (PSZ) to HA can be used to increase the fracture toughness to 2.8 MPa m$^{1/2}$. Bone has a fracture toughness of 2–12 MPa m$^{1/2}$ (Suchanek et al., 1997). PSZ was added to HA in different percentages (17, 33, 50 wt%) and it was found that 50 wt% PSZ had the highest fracture toughness. The surface energy of the PSZ-HA was not significantly different from HA alone. This suggests that the PSZ-HA composite could be biocompatible because of the similarity of the surface with HA (Kawashima et al., 1997).

29.6.2 Tissue Integration

The porosity is a critical factor for growth and integration of a tissue into the bioceramic implant. In particular, the open porosity that is connected to the outside surface is critical to the integration of tissue into the ceramic especially if the bioceramic is inert. Several methods have been developed to form porous ceramics: two of these are starch consolidation and drip casting.

In starch consolidation (Table 29.15), starch powders of a specific size are mixed with a bioceramic slurry at a predetermined weight percent. Upon heating, the starch will uptake water from the slurry mixture and swell. Upon sintering of the starch—bioceramic mixture, the starch is burned out and the pores are left in their place. Starch consolidation has been used to form complex shapes in alumina with ultimate porosities between 23 and 70 vol%. By controlling the starch content, one can control the ultimate porosity and resulting pore sizes. Large pores formed using starch consolidation in alumina were in the size range 10–80 μm, whereas small pores varied between 0.5 and 9.5 μm (Lyckfeldt and Ferreira, 1998).

Liu (1996) used a drip casting technique (Table 29.15) to form porous HA granules with pore sizes from 95 to 400 μm. The granules had a total porosity from 24 to 76 vol%. The HA was made into a slurry using water and poly(vinyl butyral) powders. The slurry was then dripped onto a spherical mold surface. This technique is similar to that of drip casting by dripping an HA slurry into a liquid nitrogen bath. In both instances, calcining and sintering procedures are used to produce the final product (Liu, 1996).

29.6.3 Hydroxyapatite Synthesis Method

The following solutions have been prepared:

Solution 1: Dissolve 157.6 g of calcium nitrate tetrahydrate [Ca(NO$_3$)$_2$4H$_2$O] in 500 mL of DI water. Bring the solution to a pH of 11 by adding ≈70 mL of ammonium hydroxide (NH$_4$OH). Bring the solution to 800 mL with DI water.

TABLE 29.15 Bioceramic Manufacturing Techniques for Hard Tissue Replacement or Tissue Integration

Manufacturing Technique	References
Hard Tissue Replacement	
Injection molding	Cihlar and Trunec (1996)
Bicontinuous microemulsion	Lim et al. (1997)
Inverse microemulsion	
Emulsion	
Additives	Fanovich et al. (1998); Kawashima et al. (1997); Suchanek et al. (1997)
Tissue Integration	
Drip casting	Liu (1996); Lyckfeldt and Ferreira (1998)
Starch consolidation	Lyckfeldt and Ferreira (1998)
Polymeric sponge method	
Foaming method	
Organic additives	
Gel casting	
Slip casting	
Direct coagulation consolidation	
Hydrolysis-assisted solidification	
Freezing	

Solution 2: Dissolve 52.8 g of ammonium phosphate dibasic [$(NH_4)_2HPO_4$] in 500 mL of DI water. Bring the solution to a pH of 11 by adding ≈150 mL of ammonium hydroxide (NH_4OH). Add DI water until the precipitate is completely dissolved, 250–350 mL.

29.6.3.1 Special Note

If you use calcium nitrate [$Ca(NO_3)_2 \cdot nH_2O$] instead of calcium nitrate tetrahydrate you need to recalculate the amount of calcium nitrate to add to make Solution 1 on the basis of the absence of the extra four waters. If you do not, you will have to add a large amount of ammonium hydroxide to pH the solution:

1. Add one-half of Solution 1 to a 2-L separatory funnel
2. Add one-half of Solution 2 to a 2-L separatory funnel
3. Titrate both solutions into a 4-L beaker under heat and constant stirring
4. Boil gently for 30 min
5. Repeat steps 1–4 for the rest of Solutions 1 and 2
6. Let cool completely allowing precipitate to settle to bottom of the beaker
7. Pour contents of beaker into 250 mL of polypropylene bottles
8. Centrifuge bottles for 10 min at (10,000 rpm) 16,000g
9. Collect precipitate from the six bottles into two and resuspend with DI water
10. Fill the four empty bottles with the reaction mixture and centrifuge all six as before
11. Collect precipitant from the two bottles that were resuspended with DI water
12. Combine remaining four bottles into two bottles and resuspend with DI water
13. Repeat steps 10–12 as necessary
14. Dry precipitate for 24–48 h at 70°C
15. Calcine the precipitate for 1 h at 1140°C
16. Grind and sieve product as desired

Defining Terms

Alumina: Aluminum oxide (Al_2O_3) which is very hard (Mohs hardness is 9) and strong. Single crystals are called sapphire or ruby depending on the color. Alumina is used to fabricate hip-joint-socket components or dental root implants.

Calcium phosphate: A family of calcium phosphate ceramics including aluminum calcium phosphate, ferric calcium phosphate, hydroxyapatite and tricalcium phosphate (TCP), and zinc calcium phosphate which are used to substitute or augment bony structures and deliver drugs.

Glass ceramics: A glass crystallized by heat treatment. Some of these have the ability to form chemical bonds with hard and soft tissues. Bioglass and Ceravital are well-known examples.

Hydroxyapatite: A calcium phosphate ceramic with a calcium-to-phosphorus ratio of 5/3 and a nominal composition $Ca_1O(PO_4)_6(OH)_2$. It has good mechanical properties and excellent biocompatibility. Hydroxyapatite is the mineral constituent of bone.

LTI carbon: A silicon-alloyed pyrolitic carbon deposited onto a substrate at low temperature with isotropic crystal morphology. It is highly compatible with blood and used for cardiovascular implant fabrication such as artificial heart valve.

Maximum radius ratio: The ratio of atomic radii computed by assuming the largest atom or ion which can be placed in a crystal's unit cell structure without deforming the structure.

Mohs scale: A hardness scale in which 10 (diamond) is the hardest and 1 (talc) is the softest.

In Memory Of

In memory of Dr. P.K. Bajpai who left us early in 1998, I would like to share our laboratory's recipe for hydroxyapatite. Dr. Bajpai's lab and research at the University of Dayton have ended after 30 plus years, but I felt it would be fitting to share this recipe as a way to encourage other scientists to continue exploring the possibilities of bioceramics.

Acknowledgments

The author is grateful to Dr. Joon B. Park for inviting him to write this chapter and providing the basic shell from his book to expand upon. The author thanks his wife, Zoe, for her patience and understanding. The author also thanks Dr. M.C. Hofmann for her support and help.

References

Abrams L. and Bajpai P.K. 1994. Hydroxyapatite ceramics for continuous delivery of heparin. *Biomed. Sci. Instrum.* 30:169–174.

Adams D. and Williams D.F. 1978. Carbon fiber-reinforced carbon as a potential implant material. *J. Biomed. Mater. Res.* 12:35–42.

Alexander H., Parsons J.R., Ricci J.L., Bajpai P.K., and Weiss A.B. 1987. Calcium-based ceramics and composites in bone reconstruction. *Crit. Rev.* 4:43–47.

Allaire M., Reynolds D., and Bajpai P.K. 1989. Electrical properties of biocompatible ALCAP and ZCAP ceramics. *Biomed. Sci. Instrum.* 25:163–168.

Andersson O.H., Guizhi L., Kangasniemi K., and Juhanoja J. 1992. Evaluation of the acceptance of glass in bone. *J. Mater. Sci.: Mater. Med.* 3:145–150.

ASTM. 1980. *Annual Book of ASTM Standards, part 46, F603-78.* American Society for Testing and Materials, Philadelphia, PA.

Arar H.A. and Bajpai P.K. 1992. Insulin delivery by zinc calcium phosphate (ZCAP) ceramics. *Biomed. Sci. Instrum.* 28:172–178.

Bagambisa F.B., Joos U., and Schilli W. 1993. Mechanisms and structure of the bond between bone and hydroxyapatite ceramics. *J. Biomed. Mater. Res.* 27:1047–1055.

Bajpai P.K. 1983. Biodegradable scaffolds in orthopedic, oral, and maxillofacial surgery. In: *Biomaterials in Reconstructive Surgery*. L.R. Rubin (Ed.), pp. 312–328. C.V. Mosby Co., St. Louis, MO.

Bajpai P.K. 1988. ZCAP Ceramics. US. Patent No. 4778471.

Bajpai P.K. 1989. Ceramic implantable drug delivery system. *T.I.B. & A.O.* 3:203–211.

Bajpai P.K. 1990. Ceramic amino acid composites for repairing traumatized hard tissues. In: *Handbook of Bioactive Ceramics*, Vol. II. *Calcium Phosphate and Hydroxyapatite Ceramics*. T. Yamamuro, L.L. Hench, and J. Wilson-Hench (Eds.), pp. 255–270. CRC Press, Baton Raton, FL.

Bajpai P.K. 1992. Ceramics: A novel device for sustained long term delivery of drugs. In: *Bioceramics*, Vol. 3, J.A. Hulbert and S.F. Hulbert (Eds.), pp. 87–99. Rose-Hulman Institute of Technology, Terra Haute, IN.

Bajpai P.K. 1993. Zinc based ceramic cysteine composite for repairing vertebral defects. *J. Instrum. Sci.* 6:346.

Bajpai P.K. 1994. Ceramic drug delivery systems. In: *Biomedical Materials Research in the Far East (I)*. Xingdong Zhang and Yoshito Ikada (Eds.), pp. 41–42. Kobunshi Kankokai Inc., Kyoto, Japan.

Bajpai P.K. and Fuchs C.M. 1985. Development of a hydroxyapatite bone grout. In: *Proceedings of the First Annual Scientific Session of the Academy of Surgical Research*, San Antonio, TX. C.W. Hall (Ed.), pp. 50–54. Pergamon Press, New York, NY.

Bajpai P.K., Fuchs C.M., and McCullum D.E. 1988. *Development of tricalcium phosphate ceramic cements*. In: *Quantitative Characterization and Performance of Porous Implants for Hard Tissue Applications*, ASTM STP 953, J.E. Lemons (Ed.), pp. 377–388. American Society for Testing and Materials, Philadelphia, PA.

Bajpai P.K., Fuchs C.M., and Strnat M.A.P. 1985. Development of alumino-calcium phosphorous oxide (ALCAP) ceramic cements. In: *Biomedical Engineering IV Recent Developments. Proceedings of the Fourth Southern Biomedical Engineering Conference*, Jackson, M.S. and B. Sauer (Eds.), pp. 22–25. Pergamon Press, New York, NY.

Bajpai P.K. and Graves G.A. Jr. 1980. Porous Ceramic Carriers for Controlled Release of Proteins, Polypeptide Hormones and other Substances within Human and/or Mammalian Species. US. Patent No. 4218255.

Bajpai P.K., Graves G.A. Jr, Wilcox L.G., and Freeman M.J. 1984. Use of resorbable alumino-calcium-phosphorous-oxide ceramics (ALCAP) in health care. *Trans. Soc. Biomater.* 7:353.

Barinov S.M. and Bashenko Yu.V. 1992. Application of ceramic composites as implants: Result and problem. In: *Bioceramics and the Human Body*. A. Ravaglioli and A. Krajewski (Eds.), pp. 206–210. Elsevier Applied Science, London.

Beckham C.A., Greenlee T.K. Jr, and Crebo A.R. 1971. Bone formation at a ceramic implant interface. *Calc. Tiss. Res.* 8:165–171.

Benghuzzi H.A., Giffin B.F., Bajpai P.K., and England B.G. 1991. Successful antidote of multiple lethal infections with sustained delivery of difluoromethylornithine by means of tricalcium phosphate drug delivery devices. *Trans. Soc. Biomater.* 24:53.

Binzer T.J. and Bajpai P.K. 1987. The use of zinc–calcium–phosphorous oxide (ZCAP) ceramics in reconstructive bone surgery. *Digest of Papers, Sixth Southern Biomedical Engineering Conference*, Dallas, TX. R.C. Eberhart (Ed.), pp. 182–185. McGregor and Werner, Washington, DC.

Biocoral. 1989. *From Coral to Biocoral*, p. 46. Innoteb, Paris, France.

Blencke B.A., Bromer H., and Deutscher K.K. 1978. Compatibility and long-term stability of glass–ceramic implants. *J. Biomed. Mater. Res.* 12:307–318.

Bokros J.C. 1972. Deposition structure and properties of pyrolitic carbon. *Chem. Phys. Carbon.* 5:70–81.

Bokros J.C., LaGrange L.D., and Schoen G.J. 1972. Control of structure of carbon for use in bioengineering. *Chem. Phys. Carbon.* 9:103–171.

Boutin P. 1981. T.H.R. using alumina–alumina sliding and a metallic stem: 1330 cases and an 11-year follow-up. In: *Orthopaedic Ceramic Implants*, Vol. 1. H. Oonishi and H.Y. Ooi (Eds.), Japanese Society of Orthopaedic Ceramic Implants, Tokyo.

Buykx W.J., Drabarek E., Reeve K.D., Anderson N., Mathivanar R., and Skalsky M. 1992. Development of porous ceramics for drug release and other applications. In: *Bioceramics*, Vol. 3. J.E. Hulbert and S.F. Hulbert (Eds.), pp. 349–354. Rose Hulman Institute of Technology, Terre Haute, IN.

Chandy T. and Sharma C.P. 1991. Biocompatibility and toxicological screening of materials. In: *Blood Compatible Materials and Devices*. C.P. Sharma and M. Szycher (Eds.), pp. 153–166. Technomic Publishing Co., Lancaster, PA.

Chignier E., Monties J.R., Butazzoni B., Dureau G., and Eloy R. 1987. Haemocompatibility and biological course of carbonaceous composites for cardiovascular devices. *Biomaterials* 8:18–23.

Cihlar J. and Trunec M. 1996. Injection moulded hydroxyapatite ceramics. *Biomaterials* 17:1905–1911.

Cotell C.M., Chrisey D.B., Grabowski K.S., Sprague J.A., and Gossett C.R. 1992. Pulsed laser deposition of hydroxyapatite thin films on Ti–6Al–4V. *J. Appl. Biomater.* 3:87–93.

de Groot K. 1983. *Bioceramics of Calcium Phosphate*. CRC Press, Boca Raton, FL.

De Potter P., Shields C.L., Shields J.L., and Singh A.D. 1994. Use of the hydroxyapatite ocular implant in the pediatric population. *Arch. Opthalmol.* 112:208–212.

Dellsperger K.C. and Chandran K.B. 1991. Prosthetic heart valves. In: *Blood Compatible Materials and Devices*. C.P. Sharma and M. Szycher (Eds.), Technomic Publishing Co., Lancaster, PA.

Dorlot J.M., Christel P., and Meunier A. 1988. Alumina hip prostheses: Long term behaviors. In: *Bioceramics. Proceedings of First International Symposium on Ceramics in Medicine*. H. Oonishi, H. Aoki, and K. Sawai (Eds.), pp. 236–301. Ishiyaku EuroAmerica, Inc., Tokyo.

Dörre E. 1991. Problems concerning the industrial production of alumina ceramic components for hip prosthesis. In: *Bioceramics and the Human Body*. A. Ravaglioli and A. Krajewski (Eds.), pp. 454–460. Elsevier Applied Science, London.

Doyle C. 1990. Composite bioactive ceramic–metal materials. In: *Handbook of Bioactive Ceramics*. T. Yamamuro, L.L. Hench, and J. Wilson (Eds.), pp. 195–208. CRC Press, Boca Raton, FL.

Drennan J. and Steele B.C.H. 1991. Zirconia and hafnia, In: *Concise Encyclopedia of Advanced Ceramic Materials*. R.J. Brook (Ed.), pp. 525–528. Pergamon Press, Oxford, NY.

Ducheyne P. 1985. Bioglass coatings and bioglass composites as implant materials. *J. Biomed. Mater. Res.* 19:273–291.

Ducheyne P. and McGuckin, J.F. Jr. 1990. Composite bioactive ceramic–metal materials. In: *Handbook of Bioactive Ceramics*. T. Yamamuro, L.L. Hench, and J. Wilson (Eds.), pp. 75–86. CRC Press, Boca Raton, FL.

Ely J.L. and Haubald A.O. 1993. Static fatigue and stress corrosion in pyrolitic carbon. In: *Bioceramics*, Vol. 6. P. Ducheyne and D. Christiansen (Eds.), pp. 199–204. Butterworth-Heinemann, Boston, MA.

Fanovich M.A., Castro M.S., and Porto Lopez J.M. 1998. Improvement of the microstructure and micro-hardness of hydroxyapatite ceramics by addition of lithium. *Mater. Lett.* 33:269–272.

Feenstra L and de Groot K. 1983. Medical use of calcium phosphate ceramics. In: *Bioceramics of Calcium Phosphate*. K. de Groot (Ed.), pp. 131–141. CRC Press, Boca Raton, FL.

Fredette S.A., Hanker J.S., Terry B.C., and Beverly L. 1989. Comparison of dense versus porous hydroxy-apatite (HA) particles for rat mandibular defect repair. *Mater. Res. Soc. Symp. Proc.* 110:233–238.

Freeman M.J., McCullum D.E., and Bajpai P.K. 1981. Use of ALCAP ceramics for rebuilding maxillo-facial defects. *Trans. Soc. Biomater.* 4:109.

Fulmer M.T., Martin R.I., and Brown P.W. 1992. Formation of calcium deficient hydroxyapatite at near-physiological temperature. *J. Mater. Sci.: Mater. Med.* 3:299–305.

Fuski M.P., Larrabee R.A., and Bajpai P.K. 1993. Effect of ferric calcium phosphorous oxide ceramic implant in bone on some parameters of blood. *T.I.B. & A.O.* 7:16–19.

Gheysen G., Ducheyne P., Hench L.L., and de Meester P. 1983. Bioglass composites: A potential material for dental application. *Biomaterials* 4:81–84.

Graves G.A. Jr, Hentrich R.L. Jr, Stein H.G., and Bajpai P.K. 1972. Resorbable ceramic implants in bioc-eramics. In: *Engineering and Medicine (Part I)*. C.W. Hall, S.F. Hulbert, S.N. Levine, and F.A. Young (Eds.), pp. 91–115. Interscience Publishers, New York, NY.

Gromofsky J.R., Arar H., and Bajpai P.K. 1988. Development of zinc calcium phosphorous oxide ceramic–organic acid composites for repairing traumatized hard tissue. In: *Digest of Papers, Seventh Southern Biomedical Engineering Conference*. Greenville, S.C. and D.D. Moyle (Eds.), pp. 20–23. Mcgregor and Werner, Washington, DC.

Grote J.J. 1987. Reconstruction of the ossicular chain with hydroxyapatite prostheses. *Am. J. Otol.* 8:396–401.

Guillemin G., Meunier A., Dallant P., Christel P., Pouliquen J.C., and Sedel L. 1989. Comparison of coral resorption and bone apposition with two natural corals of different porosities. *J. Biomed. Mater. Res.* 23:765–779.

Hammer J. III, Reed O., and Greulich R. 1972. Ceramic root implantation in baboons. *J. Biomed. Mater. Res.* 6:1–13.

Heimke G. 1992. Use of alumina ceramics in medicine. In: *Bioceramics*, Vol. 3. J.E. Hulbert and S.F. Hulbert (Eds.), pp. 19–30. Rose Hulman Institute of Technology, Terre Haute, IN.

Hench L.L. 1991. Bioceramics: From concept to clinic. *J. Am. Ceram. Soc.* 74:1487–1510.

Hench L.L. 1993. Bioceramics: From concept to clinic. *Am. Ceram. Soc. Bull.* 72:93–98.

Hench L.L. and Ethridge E.C. 1982. *Biomaterials: An Interfacial Approach*, p. 147. Academic Press, New York.

Hentrich R.L. Jr, Graves G.A. Jr, Stein H.G., and Bajpai P.K. 1969. An evaluation of inert and resorbable ceramics for future clinical applications. *Fall Meeting, Ceramics-Metals Systems*, Division of the American Ceramic Society, Cleveland, OH.

Hentrich R.L. Jr, Graves G.A. Jr, Stein H.G., and Bajpai P.K. 1971. An evaluation of inert and resorbable ceramics for future clinical applications. *J. Biomed. Mater. Res.* 5:25–51.

Holmes R., Mooney V., Bucholz R., and Tencer A. 1984. A coralline hydroxyapatite bone graft substitute. *Clin. Orthopaed. Relat. Res.* 188:252–262.

Hontsu S., Matsumoto T., Ishii J., Nakamori M., Tabata H., and Kawai T. 1997. Electrical properties of hydroxyapatite thin films grown by pulsed laser deposition. *Thin Solid Films* 295:214–217.

Huaxia J.I., Ponton C.B., and Marquis P.M. 1992. Microstructural characterization of hydroxyapatite coating on titanium. *J. Mater. Sci.: Mater. Med.* 3:283–287.

Hulbert S.F. 1992. Use of ceramics in medicine. In: *Bioceramics*, Vol. 3. J.E. Hulbert and S.F. Hulbert (Eds.), pp. 1–18. Rose Hulman Institute of Technology, Terre Haute, IN.

Hulbert S.F., Bokros J.C., Hench L.L., Wilson J., and Heimke G. 1987. Ceramics in clinical applications: Past, present, and future. In: *High Tech Ceramics*. P. Vincezini (Ed.), pp. 189–213. Elsevier, Amsterdam, the Netherlands.

Hulbert S.F. and Klawitter J.J. 1971. Application of porous ceramics for the development of load-bearing internal orthopedic applications. *Biomed. Mater. Symp.* pp. 161–229.

Jarcho M., Salsbury R.L., Thomas M.B., and Doremus R.H. 1979. Synthesis and fabrication of β-tricalcium phosphate (whitlockite) ceramics for potential prosthetic applications. *J. Mater. Sci.* 14:142–150.

Jenei S.R., Bajpai P.K., and Salsbury R.L. 1986. Resorbability of commercial hydroxyapatite in lactate buffer. *Proceedings of the Second Annual Scientific Session of the Academy of Surgical Research*. S.C. Clemson and D.N. Powers (Ed.), pp. 13–16. Clemson University Press, Clemson, SC.

Kaae J.L. 1971. Structure and mechanical properties of isotropic pyrolitic carbon deposited below 1600°C. *J. Nucl. Mater.* 38:42–50.

Kawahara H. Ed. 1989. *Oral Implantology and Biomaterials*. Elsevier, Amsterdam, the Netherlands.

Kawashima N., Soetanto K., Watanabe K., Ono K., and Matsuno T. 1997. The surface characteristics of the sintered body of hydroxyapatite–zirconia composite particles. *Coll. Surf. B: Biointerf.* 10:23–27.

Khavari F. and Bajpai P.K. 1993. Coralline–sulfate bone substitutes. *Biomed. Sci. Instrum.* 29:65–69.

Kijima T. and Tsutsumi M. 1979. Preparation and thermal properties of dense polycrystalline oxyhydroxyapatite. *J. Am. Cer. Soc.* 62:954–960.

Kingery W.D., Bowen H.K., and Uhlmann D.R. 1976. *Introduction to Ceramics*. 2nd ed., p. 368. Wiley, New York.

Knowles J.C. and Bonfield W. 1993. Development of a glass reinforced hydroxyapatite with enhanced mechanical properties. The effect of glass composition on mechanical properties and its relationship to phase changes. *J. Biomed. Mater. Res.* 27:1591–1598.

Kokubo T., Kushitani H., Ohtsuki C., Sakka S., and Yamamuro T. 1992. Chemical reaction of bioactive glass and glass-ceramics with a simulated body fluid. *J. Mat. Sci.: Mater. Med.* 3:79–83.

Krainess F.E. and Knapp W.J. 1978. Strength of a dense alumina ceramic after aging *in vitro*. *J. Biomed. Mater. Res.* 12:241–246.

Kumar P., Shimizu K., Oka M., Kotoura Y., Nakayama Y., Yamamuro T., Yanagida T., and Makinouchi K. 1989. Biological reaction of zirconia ceramics. In: *Bioceramics. Proceedings of 1st International Symposium on Ceramics in Medicine*. H. Oonishi, H. Aoki, and K. Sawai (Eds.), pp. 341–346, Ishiyaku Euroamerica, Inc., Tokyo.

Larrabee R.A., Fuski M.P., and Bajpai P.K. 1993. A ferric–calcium–phosphorous–oxide ceramic for rebuilding bone. *Biomed. Sci. Instrum.* 29:59–64.

Lemons J.E., Bajpai P.K., Patka P., Bonel G., Starling L.B., Rosenstiel T., Muschler G, Kampnier S., and Timmermans T. 1988. Significance of the porosity and physical chemistry of calcium phosphate ceramics orthopaedic uses. In: *Bioceramics: Material Characteristics Versus In Vivo Behavior*. P. Ducheyne (Ed.), Vol. 523, pp. 190–197, The New York Academy of Sciences, New York.

Lemons J.E. and Niemann K.M.W. 1979. *Porous Tricalcium Phosphate Ceramic for Bone Replacement. 25th Annual O.R.S.*, Meetings, San Francisco, CA, February 20–22, p. 162.

Li R., Clark A.E., and Hench L.L. 1991. An investigation of bioactive glass powders by sol–gel processing, *J. Appl. Biomater.* 2:231–239.

Lim G.K., Wang J., Ng S.C., Chew C.H., and Gan L.M. 1997. Processing of hydroxyapatite via microemulsion and emulsion routes. *Biomaterials* 18:1433–1439.

Liu D. 1996. Fabrication and characterization of porous hydroxyapatite granules. *Biomaterials* 17:1955–1957.

Lyckfeldt O. and Ferreira J.M.F. 1998. Processing of porous ceramics by starch consolidation. *J. Eur. Cer. Soc.* 18:131–140.

Mattie D.R. and Bajpai P.K. 1988. Analysis of the biocompatibility of ALCAP ceramics in rat femurs. *J. Biomed. Mater. Res.*, 22:1101–1126.

Meenen N.M., Osborn J.F., Dallek M., and Donath K. 1992. Hydroxyapatite-ceramic for juxta-articular implantation. *J. Mat. Sci.: Mater. Med.* 3:345–351.

Metsger S., Driskell T.D., and Paulsrud J.R. 1982. Tricalcium phosphate ceramic— A resorbable bone implant: Review and current status. *JADA* 105:1035–1038.

Moldovan K. and Bajpai P.K. 1994. A ceramic system for continuous release of aspirin. *Biomed. Sci. Instrum.* 30:175–180.

More R.B. and Silver M.D. 1990. Pyrolitic carbon prosthetic heart valve occluder wear: *In vitro* results for the Bjork–Shiley prosthesis. *J. Appl. Biomater.* 1:267–278.

Morris L.M. and Bajpai P.K. 1989. Development of a resorbable tricalcium phosphate (TCP) amine antibiotic composite. *Mat. Res. Soc. Symp.* 110:293–300.

Murakami T. and Ohtsuki N. 1989. Friction and wear characteristics of sliding pairs of bioceramics and polyethylene. In: *Bioceramics. Proceedings of 1st International Symposium on Ceramics in Medicine*. H. Oonishi, H. Aoki, and K. Sawai (Eds.), pp. 225–230. Ishiyaku Euroamerica, Inc., Tokyo.

Nagy E.A. and Bajpai P.K. 1994. Development of a ceramic matrix system for continuous delivery of azidothymidine. *Biomed. Sci. Instrum.* 30:181–186.

Niwa S., Sawai K., Takahashie S., Tagai H., Ono M., and Fukuda Y. 1980. *Experimental Studies on the Implantation of Hydroxyapatite in the Medullary Canal of Rabbits, Trans. First World Biomaterials Congress*, Baden, Austria. p. 4.10.4.

Ogino M., Ohuchi F., and Hench L.L. 1980. Compositional dependence of the formation of calcium phosphate film on bioglass, *J. Biomed. Mater. Res.* 12:55–64.

Ohashi T., Inoue S., Kajikawa K., Ibaragi K., Tada T., Oguchi M., Arai T., and Kondo K. 1988. The clinical wear rate of acetabular component accompanied with alumina ceramic head. In: *Bioceramics*.

Proceedings of 1st International Symposium on Ceramics in Medicine. H. Oonishi, H. Aoki, and K. Sawai (Eds.), pp. 278–283. Ishiyaku EuroAmerica, Inc. Tokyo.

Ohtsuki C., Kokubo T., and Yamamuro T. 1992. Compositional dependence of bioactivity of glasses in the system $CaO-SiO_2-Al_2O_3$: Its *in vitro* evaluation. *J. Mat. Sci.: Mater. Med.* 3:119–125.

Ohura K., Nakamura T., Yamamuro T., Ebisawa Y., Kokubo T., Kotoura Y., and Oka M. 1992. Bioactivity of $Cao-SiO_2$ glasses added with various ions. *J. Mat. Sci.: Mater. Med.* 3:95–100.

Oonishi H. 1992. Bioceramic in orthopaedic surgery—Our clinical experiences. In: *Bioceramics*, Vol. 3. J.E. Hulbert and S.F. Hulbert (Eds.), pp. 31–42. Rose Hulman Institute of Technology, Terre Haute, IN.

Park J.B. 1991. Aluminum oxides: Biomedical applications. In: *Concise Encyclopedia of Advanced Ceramic Materials*, R.J. Brook (Ed.), pp. 13–16. Pergamon Press, Oxford.

Park J.B. 1993. Personal communication.

Park J.B. and Lakes R.S. 1992. Ceramic Implant Materials. In: *Biomaterials—An Introduction*. 2nd ed., Plenum Press, New York.

Parker D.R. and Bajpai P.K. 1993. Effect of locally delivered testosterone on bone healing. *Trans. Soc. Biomater.* 26:293.

Peltier L.F. 1961. The use of plaster of Paris to fill defects in bone. *Clin. Orthop.* 21:1–29.

Piattelli A. and Trisi P. 1994. A light and laser scanning microscopy study of bone/hydroxyapatite-coated titanium implants interface: Histochemical evidence of unmineralized material in humans. *J. Biomed. Mater. Res.* 28:529–536.

Pories W.J. and Strain W.H. 1970. Zinc and wound healing. In: *Zinc Metabolism*, A.S. Prasad (Ed.), pp. 378–394. Thomas, Springfield, IL.

Posner A.S., Perloff A., and Diorio A.D. 1958. Refinement of hydroxyapatite structure. *Acta Cryst.* 11:308–309.

Reck R., Störkel S, and Meyer A. 1988. Bioactive glass-ceramics in middle ear surgery: An eight year review. In: *Bioceramics: Material Characteristics Versus In Vivo Behavior. Ann. NY Acad. Sci.* 253:100–106.

Ricci J.L., Bajpai P.K., Berkman A., Alexander H., and Parsons J.R. 1986. Development of a fast-setting ceramic based grout material for filling bone defects. In: *Biomedical Engineering V Recent Developments. Proceedings of the Fifth Southern Biomedical Engineering Conference.* Shreveport L.A. and S. Saha (Eds.), pp. 475–481. Pergamon Press, New York.

Ritter J.E. Jr, Greenspan D.C., Palmer R.A., and Hench L.L. 1979. Use of fracture of an alumina and bioglass coated alumina, *J. Biomed. Mater. Res.* 13:251–263.

Sartoris D.J., Gershuni D.H., Akeson W.H., Holmes R.E., and Resnick D. 1986. Coralline hydroxyapatite bone graft substitutes: Preliminary report of radiographic evaluation. *Radiology* 159:133–137.

Scheidler P.A. and Bajpai P.K. 1992. Zinc sulfate calcium phosphate (ZSCAP) composite for repairing traumatized bone. *Biomed. Sci. Instrum.* 28:183–188.

Schepers E., De Clercq M., and Ducheyne P. 1988. Interfacial behavior of bulk bioactive glass and fiber-reinforced bioactive glass dental root implants. *Ann. NY Acad. Sci.* 523:178–189.

Schepers E.J.G, Ducheyne P., Barbier L., and Schepers S. 1993. Bioactive glass particles of narrow size range: A new material for the repair of bone defects. *Impl. Dent.* 2:151–156.

Schepers E., Ducheyne P., and De Clercq M. 1989. Interfacial analysis of fiber-reinforced bioactive dental root implants. *J. Biomed. Mater. Res.* 23:735–752.

Schwartz Z., Braun G., Kohave D., Brooks B., Amir D., Sela J., and Boyan B. 1993. Effects of hydroxyapatite implants on primary mineralization during rat tibial healing: Biochemical and morphometric analysis. *J. Biomed. Mater. Res.* 27:1029–1038.

Sedel L., Meunier A., Nizard R.S., and Witvoet J. 1991. Ten year survivorship of cemented ceramic–ceramic total hip replacement. In: *Bioceramics* Vol. 4. *Proceedings of the 4th International Symposium on Ceramics in Medicine.* W. Bonfield, G.W. Hastings, and K.E. Tanner (Eds.), pp. 27–37. Butterworth-Heinemann Ltd., London, UK.

Shackelford J.F. 1988. *Introduction to Materials Science for Engineers*, 2nd ed., Macmillan Publishing Co., New York.

Shields J.A., Shields C.L., and De Potter P. 1993. Hydroxyapatite orbital implant after enucleation-experience with 200 cases. *Mayo Clinic Proc.* 68:1191–1195.

Shimm H.S. and Haubold A.D. 1980. The fatigue behavior of vapor deposited carbon films. *Biomater. Med. Dev. Art. Org.* 8:333–344.

Shobert E.I. II. 1964. *Carbon and Graphite.* Academic Press, New York.

Stricker N.J., Larrabee R.A., and Bajpai P.K. 1992. Biocompatibility of ferric calcium phosphorous oxide ceramics. *Biomed. Sci. Instrum.* 28:123–128.

Suchanek W., Yashima M., Kakihana M., and Yoshimura M. 1997. Hydroxyapatite ceramics with selected sintering additives. *Biomaterials* 18:923–933.

Takatsuko K., Yamamuro T., Kitsugi T., Nakamura T., Shibuya T., and Goto T. 1993. A new bioactive glass-ceramic as a coating material on titanium alloy. *J. Appl. Biomater.* 4:317–329.

Terry B.C., Baker R.D., Tucker M.R., and Hanker J.S. 1989. Alveolar ridge augmentation with composite implants of hydroxyapatite and plaster for correction of bony defects, deficiencies and related contour abnormalities. *Mat. Res. Soc. Symp.* 110:187–198.

Valiathan A., Randhawa G.S., and Randhawa A. 1993. Biomaterial aspects of calcium hydroxyapatite. *T.I.B. & A.O.* 7:1–7.

Varma H.K. and Sivakumar R. 1996. Dense hydroxyapatite ceramics through gel casting technique. *Mater. Lett.* 29:57–61.

Whitehead R.Y., Lacefield W.R., and Lucas L.C. 1993. Structure and integrity of a plasma sprayed hydroxyapatite coating on titanium. *J. Biomed. Mater. Res.* 27:1501–1507.

Wolford L.M., Wardrop R.W., and Hartog J.M. 1987. Coralline porous hydroxyapatite as a bone graft substitute in orthognathic surgery. *J. Oral. Maxillofacial. Surg.* 45:1034–1042.

Wyatt D.F., Bajpai P.K., Graves G.A. Jr, and Stull P.A. 1976. Remodelling of calcium aluminate phosphorous pentoxide ceramic implants in bone. *IRCS. Med. Sci.* 4:421.

Yamamuro T., Hench L.L., and Wilson J. 1990. *Handbook of Bioactive Ceramics I and II.* CRC Press, Boca Raton, FL.

Yamamuro T., Shikata J., Kakutani Y., Yoshii S., Kitsugi T., and Ono K. 1988. Novel methods for clinical applications of bioactive ceramics. In: *Bioceramics: Material Characteristics Versus in vivo Behavior.* *Ann. NY Acad. Sci.* 523:107–114.

Zimmerman M.C., Alexander H., Parsons J.R., and Bajpai P.K. 1991. The design and analysis of laminated degradable composite bone plates for fracture fixation. In: *High-Tech Textiles*, T.L. Vigo and A.F. Turbak (Eds.), pp. 132–148. ACS Symposium Series 457, American Chemical Society, Washington, DC.

Further Information

Bajpai P.K. 1987. *Surgical Cements.* US Patent No. 4668295.

Bajpai P.K. 1988. *ZCAP Ceramics.* US Patent No. 4778471.

Bonfield W., Hastings G.W., and Tanner K.E. 1991. *Bioceramics, Vol. 4. Proceedings of the 4th International Symposium on Ceramics in Medicine.* Butterworth-Heinemann, London, UK.

Brook J. 1991. *Concise Encyclopedia of Advanced Ceramic Materials.* Pergamon Press, Oxford.

de Groot K. 1983. *Bioceramics of Calcium Phosphate.* CRC Press, Boca Raton, FL.

Ducheyne P. and Christiansen D. 1993. *Bioceramics*, Vol. 6. Butterworth-Heinemann, Boston, MA.

Ducheyne P. and Lemons J.E. 1988. Bioceramics: material characteristics versus *in vivo* behavior. *Ann. NY Acad. Sci.*, New York, NY.

Filgueiras M.R.T., LaTorre G., and Hench L.L. 1993. Solution effects on the surface reactions of three bioactive glass compositions. *J. Biomed. Mater. Res.* 27:1485–1493.

Frank R.M., Wiedemann P., Hemmerle J., and Freymann M. 1991. Pulp capping with synthetic hydroxyapatite in human premolars. *J. Appl. Biomater.* 2:243–250.

Fulmer M.T. and Brown P.W. 1993. Effects of Na_2HPO_4 and NaH_2PO_4 on hydroxyapatite formation. *J. Biomed. Mater. Res.* 27:1095–1102.

Garcia R. and Doremus R.H. 1992. Electron microscopy of the bone–hydroxyapatite interface from a human dental implant. *J. Mater. Sci.: Mater. Med.* 3:154–156.

Hall C.W., Hulbert S.F., Levine S.N., and Young F.A. 1972. *Engineering and Medicine.* Interscience, New York.

Hench L.L. 1991. Bioceramics: From concept to clinic. *J. Am. Ceram. Soc.* 74:1487–1510.

Hench L.L. and Ethridge E.C. 1982. *Biomaterials: An Interfacial Approach.* Academic Press, New York.

Hulbert J.A. and Hulbert S.F. 1992. *Bioceramics*, Vol. 3. *Proceedings of the Third International Symposium on Ceramics in Medicine*, Rose-Hulman Institute of Technology, Terra Haute, IN.

Kawahara H. Ed. 1989. *Oral Implantology and Biomaterials.* Elsevier, Amsterdam, the Netherlands.

Kingery W.D., Bowen H.K., and Uhlmann D.R. 1976. *Introduction to Ceramics*, 2nd ed., p. 368. Wiley, New York.

Lemons J.E. 1988. *Quantitative Characterization and Performance of Porous Implants for Hard Tissue Applications*, ASTM STP 953. American Society for Testing and Materials, Philadelphia, PA.

Mattie D.R. and Bajpai P.K. 1986. Biocompatibility testing of ALCAP ceramics. *IRCS Med. Sci.* 14:641–643.

Neo M., Nakamura T., Ohtsuki C., Kokubo T., and Yamamuro T. 1993. Apatite formation on three kinds of bioactive material at an early stage *in vivo*: A comparative study by transmission electron microscopy. *J. Biomed. Mater. Res.* 27:999–1006.

Oonishi H. and Ooi Y. 1981. *Orthopaedic ceramic implants*, Vol. I. *Proceedings of Japanese Society of Orthopaedic Ceramic Implants.*

Oonishi H., Aoki H., and Sawai K. 1988. *Bioceramics*, Vol. 1. *Proceedings of First International Symposium on Ceramics in Medicine.* Ishiyaku EuroAmerica, Inc., Tokyo.

Ravaglioli A. and Krajewski A. 1992. *Bioceramics and the Human Body.* Elsevier Applied Science, London and New York.

Rubin L.R. 1983. *Biomaterials in Reconstructive Surgery.* C.V. Mosby Co., St. Louis, MO.

Sharma C.P. and Szycher M. 1991. *Blood Compatible Materials and Devices: Perspectives Toward 21st Century.* Technomic Publishing Co., Lancaster, PA.

Signs S.A., Pantano C.G., Driskell T.D., and Bajpai P.K. 1979. *In vitro* dissolution of synthos ceramics in an acellular physiological environment. *Biomater. Med. Dev. Art. Org.* 7:183–190.

Stea S., Tarabusi C., Ciapetti G., Pizzoferrato A., Toni A., and Sudanese A. 1992. Microhardness evaluations of the bone growing into porous implants. *J. Mater. Sci.: Mater. Med.* 3:252–254.

van Blitterswijk C.A. and Grote J.J. 1989. Biological performance of ceramics during inflammation and infection. *Crit. Rev. Biocompatib.* 5:13–43.

Wilson J. and Low S.B. 1992. Bioactive ceramics for periodontal treatment: Comparative studies in the patus monkey. *J. Appl. Biomater.* 3:123–129.

Yamamuro T., Hench L.L., and Wilson J. 1990. *Handbook of Bioactive Ceramics.* CRC Press, Boca Raton, FL.

Zhang X. and Ikada Y. 1994. *Biomedical Materials Research in the Far East (I).* Kobunshi Kankokai Inc., Kyoto, Japan.

30

Polymeric Biomaterials

30.1 Introduction 30-1
30.2 Polymerization and Basic Structure 30-1
    Polymerization • Basic Structure • Effect of Structural
    Modification on Properties
30.3 Polymers Used as Biomaterials...30-8
    Polyvinylchloride • Polyethylene • Polypropylene •
    Polymethylmethacrylate • PS and Its Copolymers • Polyesters •
    Polyamides (Nylons) • Fluorocarbon Polymers • Rubbers •
    Polyurethanes • Polyacetal, Polysulfone, and Polycarbonate •
    Biodegradable Polymers
30.4 Sterilization..30-13
30.5 Surface Modifications for Improving Biocompatibility.........30-14
30.6 Chemogradient Surfaces for Cell and Protein Interaction 30-16
Defining Terms 30-20
Acknowledgments...30-22
References..30-22

Hai Bang Lee
*Korea Research
Institute of Chemical
Technology*

Gilson Khang
*Chonbuk National
University*

Jin Ho Lee
Hannam University

30.1 Introduction

Synthetic polymeric materials have been widely used in medical disposable supply, prosthetic materials, dental materials, implants, dressings, extracorporeal devices, encapsulants, polymeric drug delivery systems, and orthodoses as that of metal and ceramic substituents (Lee, 1989). The main advantages of the polymeric *biomaterials* compared to metal or ceramic materials are ease of manufacturability to produce various shapes (latex, film, sheet, fibers, etc.), ease of secondary processability, reasonable cost, and availability with desired mechanical and physical properties. The required properties of polymeric biomaterials are similar to other biomaterials, that is, *biocompatibility*, sterilizability, adequate mechanical and physical properties, and manufacturability as given in Table 30.1.

The objectives of this chapter are: (1) the review of basic chemical and physical properties of the synthetic polymers, (2) the sterilization of the polymeric biomaterials, (3) the importance of the surface treatment for improving biocompatibility, and (4) the application of the *chemogradient surface* for the study on cell-to-polymer interactions.

30.2 Polymerization and Basic Structure

30.2.1 Polymerization

To link the small molecules, one has to force them to lose their electrons through the chemical processes of condensation and addition. By controlling the reaction temperature, pressure, and time in the presence of catalyst(s), the degree to which *repeating units* are put together into chains can be manipulated.

TABLE 30.1 Requirements for Biomedical Polymers

Properties	Description
Biocompatibility	Noncarcinogenesis, nonpyrogenicity, nontoxicity, and nonallergic response
Sterilizability	Autoclave, dry heating, ethyleneoxide gas, and radiation
Physical property	Strength, elasticity, and durability
Manufacturability	Machining, molding, extruding, and fiber forming

Source: Modified from Lewin, M. and Preston, J. Eds. 1989. *Handbook of Fiber Science and Technology Volume III: High Technology Fibers, Part B*, 332 pp, Marcel Dekker, Inc., New York. With permission.

30.2.1.1 Condensation or Step Reaction Polymerization

During *condensation polymerization*, a small molecule such as water will be condensed out by the chemical reaction. For example,

$$\underset{\text{(amine)}}{\text{R-NH}_2} + \underset{\text{(carboxylic acid)}}{\text{R}'\text{COOH}} \rightarrow \underset{\text{(amide)}}{\text{R}'\text{CONHR}} + \underset{\text{(condensed molecule)}}{\text{H}_2\text{O}} \tag{30.1}$$

This particular process is used to make polyamides (Nylons). Nylon was the first commercial polymer, made in the 1930s.

Some typical condensation polymers and their interunit linkages are given in Table 30.2. One major drawback of condensation polymerization is the tendency for the reaction to cease before the chains grow to a sufficient length. This is due to the decreased mobility of the chains and reactant chemical species as polymerization progresses. This results in short chains. However, in the case of Nylon, the chains are polymerized to a sufficiently large extent before this occurs and the physical properties of the polymer are preserved.

Natural polymers such as polysaccharides and proteins are also made by condensation polymerization. The condensing molecule is always water (H_2O).

TABLE 30.2 Typical Condensation Polymers

Type	Interunit Linkage
Polyester	$\overset{\displaystyle O}{\overset{\displaystyle \|}{-\text{C}-\text{O}-}}$
Polyamide	$\overset{\displaystyle O \quad H}{\overset{\displaystyle \| \quad \|}{-\text{C}-\text{N}-}}$
Polyurea	$\overset{\displaystyle H \quad O \quad H}{\overset{\displaystyle \| \quad \| \quad \|}{-\text{N}-\text{C}-\text{N}-}}$
Polyurethane	$\overset{\displaystyle O \quad H}{\overset{\displaystyle \| \quad \|}{-\text{O}-\text{C}-\text{N}-}}$
Polysiloxane	$\overset{\displaystyle R}{\underset{\displaystyle R}{-\text{Si}-\text{O}-}}$
Protein	$\overset{\displaystyle O \quad H}{\overset{\displaystyle \| \quad \|}{-\text{C}-\text{N}-}}$

30.2.1.2 Addition or Free Radical Polymerization

Addition polymerization can be achieved by rearranging the bonds within each monomer. Since each "mer" has to share at least two covalent electrons with other mers, the monomer should have at least one double bond, for example, the case of ethylene:

$$
n \{C = C\} \rightarrow - C -(C - C -) C - \tag{30.2}
$$

The breaking of a double bond can be made with an *initiator*. This is usually a free radical such as benzoyl peroxide ($H_5C_6COO–OOCC_6H_5$). The initiation can be activated by heat, ultraviolet light, and other chemicals. The free radicals (initiators) can react with monomers and this free radical can react with another monomer and the process can continue on. This process is called propagation. The propagation process can be terminated by combining two free radicals, by transfer, or by disproportionate processes. Some of the free radical polymers are given in Table 30.3. There are three more types

TABLE 30.3　Monomers for Addition Polymerization and Suitable Process

		Polymerization Mechanism			
Monomer Names	Chemical Structure	Radical	Cationic	Anionic	Coordination
Acrylonitrile	$CH_2=CH$ $\mid$ $C\equiv N$	+	−	+	+
Ethylene	$CH_2–CH_2$	+	+	−	−
Methacrylate	$CH_2=CH$ $\mid$ $COOCH_3$	+	−	+	+
Methylmethacrylate	$CH_2=CCH_3$ $\mid$ $COOCH_3$	+	−	+	+
Propylene	$CH_2=CH$ $\mid$ CH_3	−	−	−	−
Styrene	$CH_2=CH$ $\mid$ C_6H_5	+	+	+	+
Vinylchloride	$CH_2=CH$ $\mid$ Cl Cl	+	−	−	+
Vinylidenechloride	Cl $\mid$ $CH_2=C$ $\mid$ Cl				

Source:　Modified form Billmeyer, F.W. Jr. *Text Book of Polymer Science*, 3rd ed. 1984. New York. Copyright Wiley-VCH Verlag GmbH & Co. KGaA. Reproduced with permission.

Note:　+, high polymer former; −, no reaction or oligomers only.

of initiating species for addition polymerization beside free radicals: cations, anions, and coordination (stereospecific) catalysts. Some monomers can use two or more of the initiation processes but others can use only one process as given in Table 30.3.

30.2.2 Basic Structure

Polymers have very long-chain molecules which are formed by *covalent bonding* along the backbone chain. The long chains are held together either by secondary bonding forces such as van der Waals and hydrogen bonds or primary covalent bonding forces through crosslinks between chains. The long chains are very flexible and can be tangled easily. In addition, each chain can have *side groups*, branches, and copolymeric chains or blocks which can also interfere with the long-range ordering of chains. For example, paraffin wax has the same chemical formula as polyethylene (PE) $[(CH_2CH_2)_n]$, but will crystallize almost completely because of its much shorter chain lengths. However, when the chains become extremely long (from 40 to 50 repeating units $[-CH_2CH_2-]$ to several thousands as in linear PE), they cannot be crystallized completely (up to 80–90% crystallization is possible). Also, branched PE in which side chains are attached to the main backbone chain at positions normally occupied by a hydrogen atom will not crystallize easily due to the *steric hindrance* of side chains resulting in a more noncrystalline structure. The partially crystallized structure is called semicrystalline which is the most commonly occurring structure for linear polymers. The semicrystalline structure is represented by disordered noncrystalline (amorphous) regions and ordered crystalline regions which may contain folded chains as shown in Figure 30.1.

The degree of polymerization (DP) is defined as an average number of mers, or repeating units, per molecule, that is, chain. Each chain may have a different number of mers depending on the condition of polymerization. Also, the length of each chain may be different. Therefore, it is assumed that there is an average DP or average molecular weight (MW). The relationship between MW and DP can be expressed as

$$\text{MW of a polymer} = \text{DP} \times \text{MW of mer (or repeating unit)} \tag{30.3}$$

The two average MWs most commonly used are defined in terms of the numbers of molecules, Ni, having molecular weight, Mi; or wi, the weight of species with molecular weights Mi as follows:

1. The number-average molecular weight, Mn, is defined by

$$\text{Mn} = \frac{\Sigma NiMi}{\Sigma NiMi} = \Sigma niMi = \frac{\Sigma Wi}{\Sigma(Wi/Mi)} = \frac{1}{\Sigma(wiMi)} \tag{30.4}$$

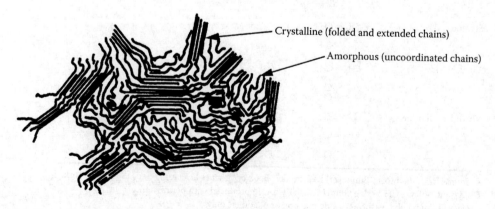

FIGURE 30.1 Fringed-micelle model of a linear polymer with semicrystalline structure.

2. The weight average molecular weight, Mw, is defined by

$$Mw = \frac{\Sigma WiMi}{\Sigma Wi} = \Sigma wiMi = \frac{\Sigma NiMi^2}{\Sigma NiMi} \qquad (30.5)$$

An absolute method of measuring the molecular weight is one that depends on theoretical considerations, counting molecules and their weight directly. The relative methods require calibration based on an absolute method and include intrinsic viscosity and gel permeation chromatography. Absolute methods of determining the number-average molecular weight (Mn) include osmometry and other colligative methods, and end group analysis. Light-scattering yields an absolute weight-average molecular weight (Mw).

As the molecular chains become longer by the progress of polymerization, their relative mobility decreases. The chain mobility is also related to the physical properties of the final polymer. Generally, the higher the molecular weight, the less the mobility of chains which results in higher strength and greater thermal stability. The polymer chains can be arranged in three ways: linear, branched, and a cross-linked (or 3-D) network as shown in Figure 30.2. Linear polymers such as polyvinyls, polyamides, and polyesters are much easier to crystallize than the cross-linked or branched polymers. However, they cannot be crystallized 100% as with metals. Instead, they become semicrystalline polymers. The arrangement of chains in crystalline regions is believed to be a combination of folded and extended chains. The chain folds, which are seemingly more difficult to form, are necessary to explain observed single-crystal structures in which the crystal thickness is too small to accommodate the length of the

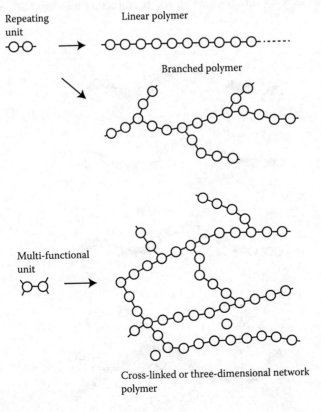

FIGURE 30.2 Arrangement of polymer chains into linear, branched, and network structure depending on the functionality of the repeating units.

chain as determined by electron and x-ray diffraction studies. The classical "fringed-micelle" model in which the amorphous and crystalline regions coexist has been modified to include chain folds in the crystalline regions. The cross-linked or 3-D network polymers such as polyphenolformaldehyde cannot be crystallized at all and they become noncrystalline, amorphous polymers.

Vinyl polymers have a repeating unit $-CH_2-CHX-$, where X is some monovalent side group. There are three possible arrangements of side groups (X): (1) atactic, (2) isotactic, and (3) syndiotactic. In atactic arrangements, the side groups are randomly distributed, while in syndiotactic and isotactic arrangements they are either in alternating positions or on one side of the main chain. If side groups are small like PE (X = H) and the chains are linear, the polymer crystallizes easily. However, if the side groups are large as in polyvinyl chloride (X = Cl) and polystyrene (PS) (X = C_6H_5, benzene ring) and are randomly distributed along the chains (atactic), then a noncrystalline structure will be formed. The isotactic and syndiotactic polymers usually crystallize even when the side groups are large.

Copolymerization, in which two or more homopolymers (one type of repeating unit throughout its structure) are chemically combined, always disrupts the regularity of polymer chains, thus promoting the formation of a noncrystalline structure. Possible arrangement of the different copolymerization is shown in Figure 30.3. The addition of *plasticizers* to prevent crystallization by keeping the chains separated from one another will result in more flexible polymers, a noncrystalline version of a polymer which normally crystallizes. An example is celluloid which is normally made of crystalline nitrocellulose plasticized with camphor. Plasticizers are also used to make rigid noncrystalline polymers like polyvinylchloride (PVC) into a more flexible solid (a good example is Tygon® tubing).

Elastomers, or rubbers, are polymers which exhibit large stretchability at room temperature and can snap back to their original dimensions when the load is released. The elastomers are noncrystalline polymers which have an intermediate structure consisting of long-chain molecules in 3-D

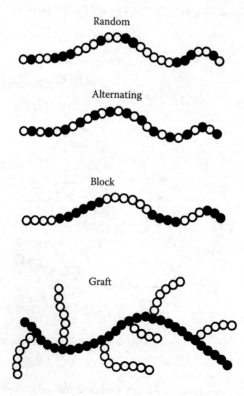

FIGURE 30.3 Possible arrangements of copolymers.

networks (see Section 30.2.3 for more details). The chains also have "kinks" or "bends" in them which straighten when a load is applied. For example, the chains of *cis*-polyisoprene (natural rubber) are bent at the double bond due to the methyl group interfering with the neighboring hydrogen in the repeating unit $[-CH_2-C(CH_3)=CH-CH_2-]$. If the methyl group is on the opposite side of the hydrogen, then it becomes *trans*-polyisoprene which will crystallize due to the absence of the steric hindrance present in the *cis* form. The resulting polymer is a very rigid solid called gutta percha which is not an elastomer. Below the *glass transition temperature* (T_g; second-order transition temperature between viscous liquid and solid), natural rubber loses its compliance and becomes a glass-like material. Therefore, to be flexible, all elastomers should have T_g well below room temperature. What makes the elastomers not behave like liquids above T_g is in fact due to the cross-links between chains which act as pinning points. Without cross-links, the polymer would deform permanently. An example is latex which behaves as a viscous liquid. Latex can be cross-linked with sulfur (*vulcanization*) by breaking double bonds (C=C) and forming C−S−S−C bonds between the chains. The more the cross-links are introduced, the more rigid the structure becomes. If all the chains are cross-linked together, the material will become a 3-D rigid polymer.

30.2.3 Effect of Structural Modification on Properties

The physical properties of polymers can be affected in many ways. In particular, the chemical composition and arrangement of chains will have a great effect on the final properties. By such means, the polymers can be tailored to meet the end use.

30.2.3.1 Effect of Molecular Weight and Composition

The molecular weight and its distribution have a great effect on the properties of a polymer since its rigidity is primarily due to the immobilization or entanglement of the chains. This is because the chains are arranged like cooked spaghetti strands in a bowl. By increasing the molecular weight, the polymer chains become longer and less mobile and a more rigid material results as shown in Figure 30.4. Equally important is that all chains should be equal in length since if there are short chains they will act as plasticizers. Another obvious way of changing properties is to change the chemical composition of the backbone or side chains. Substituting the backbone carbon of a PE with divalent oxygen or sulfur will decrease the melting and glass transition temperatures since the chain becomes more flexible due to the increased rotational freedom. On the other hand, if the backbone chains can be made more rigid, then a stiffer polymer will result.

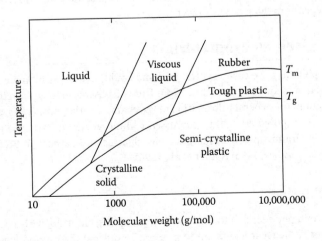

FIGURE 30.4 Approximate relations among molecular weight, T_g, T_m, and polymer properties.

TABLE 30.4   Effect of Side-Chain Substitution
on Melting Temperature in PE

Side Chain	T_m (°C)
–H	140
–CH$_3$	165
–CH$_2$CH$_3$	124
–CH$_2$CH$_2$CH$_3$	75
–CH$_2$CH$_2$CH$_2$CH$_3$	−55
–CH$_2$CHCH$_2$CH$_3$	196
$\quad\quad\quad$|$\quad\quad$CH$_3$	
$\quad\quad\quad\quad$CH$_3$	350
$\quad\quad\quad\quad$|	
–CH$_2$CCH$_2$CH$_3$	
$\quad\quad\quad\quad$|	
$\quad\quad\quad\quad$–CH$_3$	

30.2.3.2 Effect of Side-Chain Substitution, Cross-Linking, and Branching

Increasing the size of side groups in linear polymers such as PE will decrease the melting temperature due to the lesser perfection of molecular packing, that is, decreased crystallinity. This effect is seen until the side group itself becomes large enough to hinder the movement of the main chain as shown in Table 30.4. Very long side groups can be thought of as being branches.

Cross-linking of the main chains is, in effect, similar to the side-chain substitution with a small molecule, that is, it lowers the melting temperature. This is due to the interference of the cross-linking which causes decreased mobility of the chains resulting in further retardation of the crystallization rate. In fact, a large degree of cross-linking can prevent crystallization completely. However, when the cross-linking density increases for a rubber, the material becomes harder and the glass transition temperature also increases.

30.2.3.3 Effect of Temperature on Properties

Amorphous polymers undergo a substantial change in their properties as a function of temperature. The glass transition temperature, T_g, is a boundary between the glassy region of behavior in which the polymer is relatively stiff and the rubbery region in which it is very compliant. T_g can also be defined as the temperature at which the slope of volume change versus temperature has a discontinuity in slope as shown in Figure 30.5. Since polymers are noncrystalline or at most semicrystalline, the value obtained in this measurement depends on how fast it is taken.

30.3 Polymers Used as Biomaterials

Although hundreds of polymers are easily synthesized and could be used as biomaterials, only 10–20 polymers are mainly used in medical device fabrications from disposable to long-term implants as given in Table 30.5. In this section, the general information of the characteristics, properties, and applications of the most commonly used polymers will be discussed (Billmeyer, 1984; Park, 1984; Leininger and Bigg, 1986; Shalaby, 1988; Brandrup and Immergut, 1989; Sharma and Szycher, 1991; Park and Lakes, 1992; Dumitriu, 1993; Lee and Lee, 1995; Ratner et al., 1996).

30.3.1 Polyvinylchloride

PVC is an amorphous, rigid polymer due to the large side group (Cl, chloride) with a T_g of 75–105°C. It has a high melting viscosity, hence it is difficult to process. To prevent the thermal degradation of the polymer (HCl could be released), thermal stabilizers such as metallic soaps or salts are incorporated.

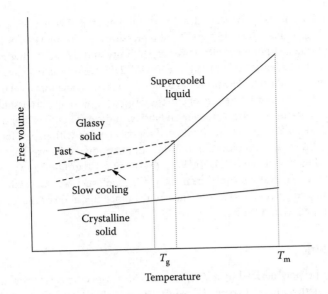

FIGURE 30.5 Change of volume versus temperature of a solid. The glass transition temperature (T_g) depends on the rate of cooling and below T_g, the material behaves as a solid like a window glass.

Lubricants are formulated on PVC compounds to prevent adhesion to metal surfaces and facilitate the melt flow during processing. Plasticizers are used in the range 10–100 parts per 100 parts of PVC resin to make it flexible. Di-2-ethylhexylphthalate is used in medical PVC formulation. However, the plasticizers of trioctyltrimellitate, polyester, azelate, and phosphate ester are also used to prevent extraction by blood, aqueous solution, and hot water during autoclaving sterilization.

PVC sheets and films are used in blood and solution storage bags and surgical packaging. PVC tubing is commonly used in intravenous (IV) administration, dialysis devices, catheters, and cannulae.

30.3.2 Polyethylene

PE is available commercially in five major grades: (1) high density (HDPE), (2) low density (LDPE), (3) linear low density (LLDPE), (4) very low density (VLDPE), and (5) ultra-high-molecular weight (UHMWPE). HDPE is polymerized at a low temperature (60–80°C) and at a low pressure (~10 kg/cm²) using metal

TABLE 30.5 Biomedical Application of Polymeric Biomaterials

Synthetic Polymers	Applications
Polyvinylchloride (PVC)	Blood and solution bag, surgical packaging, IV sets, dialysis devices, catheter bottles, connectors, and cannulae
Polyethylene (PE)	Pharmaceutical bottle, nonwoven fabric, catheter, pouch, flexible container, and orthopedic implants
Polypropylene (PP)	Disposable syringes, blood oxygenator membrane, suture, nonwoven fabric, and artificial vascular grafts
Polymethylmethacrylate (PMMA)	Blood pump and reservoirs, membrane for blood dialyzer, implantable ocular lens, and bone cement
Polystyrene (PS)	Tissue culture flasks, roller bottles, and filterwares
Polyethyleneterephthalate (PET)	Implantable suture, mesh, artificial vascular grafts, and heart valve
Polytetrafluoroethylene (PTFE)	Catheter and artificial vascular grafts
Polyurethane (PU)	Film, tubing, and components
Polyamide (Nylon)	Packaging film, catheters, sutures, and mold parts

catalysts. A highly crystalline, linear polymer with a density ranging from 0.94 to 0.965 g/cm³ is obtained. LDPE is derived from a high temperature (150–300°C) and pressures (1000–3000 kg/cm²) using free radical initiators. A highly branched polymer with lower crystallinity and densities ranging from 0.915 to 0.935 g/cm³ is obtained. LLDPE (density: 0.91–0.94 g/cm³) and VLDPE (density: 0.88–0.89 g/cm³), which are linear polymers, are polymerized under low pressures and temperatures using metal catalysts with comonomers such as 1-butene, 1-hexene, or 1-octene to obtain the desired physical properties and density ranges.

HDPE is used in pharmaceutical bottles, nonwoven fabrics, and caps. LDPE is found in flexible container applications, nonwoven-disposable and laminated (or coextruded with paper) foil, and polymers for packaging. LLDPE is frequently employed in pouches and bags due to its excellent puncture resistance and VLDPE is used in extruded tubes. UHMWPE (MW > 2 × 10⁶ g/mol) has been used for orthopedic implant fabrications, especially for load-bearing applications such as an acetabular cup of total hip and the tibial plateau and patellar surfaces of knee joints. Biocompatibility tests for PE are given by ASTM standards in F981, F639, and F755.

30.3.3 Polypropylene

Polypropylene (PP) can be polymerized by a Ziegler–Natta stereospecific catalyst which controls the isotactic position of the methyl group. Thermal (T_g: −12°C, T_m: 125–167°C and density: 0.85–0.98 g/cm³) and physical properties of PP are similar to PE. The average molecular weight of commercial PP ranges from 2.2 to 7.0 × 10⁵ g/mol and has a wide molecular weight distribution (polydispersity) which is from 2.6 to 12. Additives for PP such as antioxidants, light stabilizer, nucleating agents, lubricants, mold release agents, antiblock, and slip agents are formulated to improve the physical properties and processability. PP has an exceptionally high flex life and excellent environment stress-cracking resistance, hence it had been tried for finger joint prostheses with an integrally molded hinge design (Park, 1984). The gas and water vapor permeability of PP are in-between those of LDPE and HDPE. PP is used to make disposable hypothermic syringes, blood *oxygenator* membrane, packaging for devices, solutions, and drugs, *suture*, artificial vascular *grafts*, nonwoven fabrics, and so on.

30.3.4 Polymethylmethacrylate

Commercial polymethylmethacrylate (PMMA) is an amorphous (T_g: 105°C and density: 1.15–1.195 g/cm³) material with good resistance to dilute alkalis and other inorganic solutions. PMMA is best known for its exceptional light transparency (92% transmission), high *refractive index* (1.49), good weathering properties, and as one of the most biocompatible polymers. PMMA can be easily machined with conventional tools, molded, surface coated, and plasma etched with glow or corona discharge. PMMA is used broadly in medical applications such as a blood pump and reservoir, an IV system, membranes for blood dialyzer, and in *in vitro* diagnostics. It is also found in contact lenses and implantable ocular lenses due to excellent optical properties, dentures, and maxillofacial prostheses due to good physical and coloring properties, and *bone cement* for joint prostheses fixation (ASTM standard F451).

Another acrylic polymer such as polymethylacrylate, polyhydroxyethyl-methacrylate (PHEMA), and polyacrylamide (PAAm) are also used in medical applications. PHEMA and PAAm are *hydrogels*, lightly cross-linked by ethyleneglycoldimethylacrylate to increase their mechanical strength. The extended wear soft contact lenses are synthesized from PMMA and *N*-vinylpyrrolidone or PHEMA which have high water content (above 70%) and a high oxygen permeability.

30.3.5 PS and Its Copolymers

The PS is polymerized by free radical polymerization and is usually atactic. Three grades are available: unmodified general purpose PS (general purpose polystyrene (GPPS), T_g: 100°C), high impact PS (HIPS), and PS foam. GPPS has good transparency, lack of color, ease of fabrication, thermal stability, ow specific gravity (1.04–1.12 g/cm³), and relatively high modulus. HIPS contains a rubbery modifier which forms chemical bonding with the growing PS chains. Hence, the ductility and impact strength are increased and the resistance to environmental stress cracking is also improved. PS is mainly processed by injection molding at 180–250°C. To improve processability, additives such as stabilizers, lubricants, and mold releasing agents are formulated. GPPS is commonly used in tissue culture flasks, roller bottles, vacuum canisters, and filterware.

Acrylonitrile–butadiene–styrene (ABS) *copolymers* are produced by three monomers: acrylonitrile, butadiene, and styrene. The desired physical and chemical properties of ABS polymers with a wide range of functional characteristics can be controlled by changing the ratio of these monomers. They are resistant to the common inorganic solutions, have good surface properties, and dimensional stability. ABS is used for IV sets, clamps, blood dialyzers, diagnostic test kits, and so on.

30.3.6 Polyesters

Polyesters such as polyethyleneterephthalate (PET) are frequently found in medical applications due to their unique chemical and physical properties. PET is so far the most important of this group of polymers in terms of biomedical applications such as artificial vascular graft, sutures, and meshes. It is highly crystalline with a high melting temperature (T_m: 265°C), hydrophobic, and resistant to hydrolysis in dilute acids. In addition, PET can be converted by conventional techniques into molded articles such as luer filters, check valves, and catheter housings. Polycaprolactone is crystalline and has a low melting temperature (T_m: 64°C). Its use as a soft matrix or coating for conventional polyester fibers was proposed by recent investigation (Leininger and Bigg, 1986).

30.3.7 Polyamides (Nylons)

Polyamides are known as Nylons and are designated by the number of carbon atoms in the repeating units. Nylons can be polymerized by step reaction (or condensation) and ring-scission polymerization. They have excellent fiber-forming ability due to interchain *hydrogen bonding* and a high degree of crystallinity, which increases strength in the fiber direction.

The presence of –CONH– groups in polyamides attracts the chains strongly toward one another by hydrogen bonding. Since the hydrogen bond plays a major role in determining properties, the number and distribution of –CONH– groups are important factors. For example, T_g can be decreased by decreasing the number of –CONH– groups. On the other hand, an increase in the number of –CONH– groups improves physical properties such as strength as one can see that Nylon 66 is stronger than Nylon 610, and Nylon 6 is stronger than Nylon 11.

In addition to the higher Nylons (610 and 11), there are aromatic polyamides named aramids. One of them is poly(p-phenyleneterephthalate) commonly known as Kevlar®, made by DuPont. This material can be made into fibers. The specific strength of such fibers is five times that of steel and, therefore, it is most suitable for making composites.

Nylons are hygroscopic and lose their strength *in vivo* when implanted. The water molecules serve as plasticizers which attack the amorphous region. Proteolytic enzymes also aid in hydrolyzing by attacking the amide group. This is probably due to the fact that the proteins also contain the amide group along their molecular chains which the proteolytic enzymes could attack.

30.3.8 Fluorocarbon Polymers

The best known fluorocarbon polymer is polytetrafluoroethylene (PTFE), commonly known as Teflon® (DuPont). Other polymers containing fluorine are polytrifluorochloroethylene, polyvinylfluoride, and fluorinated ethylene propylene. Only PTFE will be discussed here since the others have rather inferior chemical and physical properties and are rarely used for implant fabrication.

PTFE is made from tetrafluoroethylene under pressure with a peroxide catalyst in the presence of excess water for removal of heat. The polymer is highly crystalline (over 94% crystallinity) with an average molecular weight of $0.5–5 \times 10^6$ g/mol. This polymer has a very high density ($2.15–2.2$ g/cm³), low modulus of elasticity (0.5 GPa), and tensile strength (14 MPa). It also has a very low surface tension (18.5 erg/cm²) and friction coefficient (0.1).

Standard specifications for the implantable PTFE are given by ASTM F754. PTFE also has an unusual property of being able to expand on a microscopic scale into a microporous material which is an excellent thermal insulator. PTFE cannot be injection molded or melt extruded because of its very high melting viscosity and it cannot be plasticized. Usually the powders are sintered to above 327°C under pressure to produce implants.

30.3.9 Rubbers

Silicone, natural, and synthetic rubbers have been used for the fabrication of implants. Natural rubber is made mostly from the latex of the *Hevea brasiliensis* tree and the chemical formula is the same as that of *cis*-1,4 polyisoprene. Natural rubber was found to be compatible with blood in its pure form. Also, cross-linking by x-ray and organic peroxides produces rubber with superior blood compatibility compared with rubbers made by the conventional sulfur vulcanization.

Synthetic rubbers were developed to substitute for natural rubber. The Ziegler–Natta types of stereo-specific polymerization techniques have made this variety possible. The synthetic rubbers have rarely been used to make implants. The physical properties vary widely due to the wide variations in preparation recipes of these rubbers.

Silicone rubber, developed by Dow Corning Company, is one of the few polymers developed for medical use. The repeating unit is dimethyl siloxane which is polymerized by a condensation polymerization. Low-molecular-weight polymers have low viscosity and can be cross-linked to make a higher molecular weight, rubber-like material. Medical-grade silicone rubbers contain stannous octate as a catalyst and can be mixed with a base polymer at the time of implant fabrication.

30.3.10 Polyurethanes

Polyurethanes are usually thermosetting polymers: they are widely used to coat implants. Polyurethane rubbers are produced by reacting a prepared prepolymer chain with an aromatic di-isocyanate to make very long chains possessing active isocyanate groups for cross-linking. The polyurethane rubber is quite strong and has good resistance to oil and chemicals.

30.3.11 Polyacetal, Polysulfone, and Polycarbonate

These polymers have excellent mechanical, thermal, and chemical properties due to their stiffened main backbone chains. Polyacetals and polysulfones are being tested as implant materials, while polycarbonates have found their applications in the heart/lung assist devices, food packaging, and so on.

Polyacetals are produced by reacting formaldehyde. These are also sometimes called polyoxymethylene and known widely as Delrin® (DuPont). These polymers have a reasonably high molecular weight ($>2 \times 10^4$ g/mol) and have excellent mechanical properties. More importantly, they display an excellent resistance to most chemicals and to water over wide temperature ranges.

Polysulfones were developed by Union Carbide in the 1960s. These polymers have a high thermal stability due to the bulky side groups (therefore, they are amorphous) and rigid main backbone chains. They are also highly stable to most chemicals but are not so stable in the presence of polar organic solvents such as ketones and chlorinated hydrocarbons.

Polycarbonates are tough, amorphous, and transparent polymers made by reacting bisphenol A and diphenyl carbonate. It is noted for its excellent mechanical and thermal properties (high T_g: 150°C), hydrophobicity, and antioxidative properties.

30.3.12 Biodegradable Polymers

Recently, several biodegradable polymers such as polylactide (PLA), polyglycolide (PGA), poly(glycolide-*co*-lactide) (PLGA), poly(dioxanone), poly(trimethylene carbonate), poly(carbonate), and so on are extensively used or tested on a wide range of medical applications due to their good biocompatibility, controllable biodegradability, and relatively good processability (Khang et al., 1997a). PLA, PGA, and PLGA are bioresorbable polyesters belonging to the group of poly-α-hydroxy acids. These polymers degrade by nonspecific hydrolytic scission of their ester bonds. The hydrolysis of PLA yields lactic acid which is a normal byproduct of anaerobic metabolism in the human body and is incorporated in the tricarboxylic acid (TCA) cycle to be finally excreted by the body as carbon dioxide and water. PGA biodegrades by a combination of hydrolytic scission and enzymatic (esterase) action producing glycolic acid which can either enter the TCA cycle or is excreted in urine and can be eliminated as carbon dioxide and water. The degradation time of PLGA can be controlled from weeks to over a year by varying the ratio of monomers and the processing conditions. It might be a suitable biomaterial for use in tissue-engineered repair systems in which cells are implanted within PLGA films or scaffolds and in drug delivery systems in which drugs are loaded within PLGA microspheres. PGA (T_m: 225–230°C, T_g: 35–40°C) can be melt spun into fibers which can be converted into bioresorbable sutures, meshes, and surgical products. PLA (T_m: 173–178°C, T_g: 60–65°C) exhibit high tensile strength and low elongation resulting in a high modulus suitable for load-bearing applications such as in bone fracture fixation. Poly-*p*-dioxanone (T_m: 107–112°C, T_g: ~10°C) is a bioabsorbable polymer which can be fabricated into flexible monofilament surgical sutures.

30.4 Sterilization

Sterilizability is an important aspect of the biomedical polymers because they have lower thermal and chemical stability than other materials such as ceramics and metals; consequently, they are also more difficult to sterilize using conventional techniques. Commonly used sterilization techniques are dry heat, autoclaving, radiation, and ethylene oxide gas (Block, 1977).

In dry heat sterilization, the temperature varies between 160°C and 190°C. This is above the melting and softening temperatures of many linear polymers such as PE and PMMA. In the case of polyamide (Nylon), oxidation will occur at the dry sterilization temperature although this is below its melting temperature. The only polymers which can safely be dry-sterilized are PTFE and silicone rubber.

Steam sterilization (autoclaving) is performed under high steam pressure at relatively low temperatures (125–130°C). However, if the polymer is subjected to attack by water vapor, this method cannot be employed. PVC, polyacetals, PE (low-density variety), and polyamides belong to this category.

Chemical agents such as ethylene and propylene oxide gases (Glaser, 1979) and phenolic and hypochloride solutions are widely used for sterilizing polymers since these can be used at low temperatures. Chemical agents sometimes cause polymer deterioration even when sterilization takes place at room temperature. However, the time of exposure is relatively short (overnight), and most polymeric implants can be sterilized with this method.

Radiation sterilization (Sato, 1983) using the isotopic ^{60}Co can also deteriorate polymers since at high dosage the polymer chains can be dissociated or cross-linked according to the characteristics of the chemical structures, as shown in Table 30.6. In the case of PE, at high dosage (above 10^6 Gy), it becomes a brittle and hard material. This is due to a combination of random chain scission cross-linking. PP articles will often discolor during irradiation giving the product an undesirable tint color but the more

TABLE 30.6 Effect of Gamma Irradiation on Polymers Which Could Be Cross-Linked or Degraded

Cross-Linking Polymers	Degradable Polymers
Polyethylene	Polyisobutylene
Polypropylene	Poly-α-methylstyrene
Polystyrene	Polymethylmethacrylate
Polyarylates	Polymethacrylamide
Polyacrylamide	Polyvinylidenechloride
Polyvinylchloride	Cellulose and derivatives
Polyamides	Polytetrafluoroethylene
Polyesters	Polytrifluorochloroethylene
Polyvinylpyrrolidone	
Polymethacrylamide	
Rubbers	
Polysiloxanes	
Polyvinylalcohol	
Polyacroleine	

severe problem is the embrittlement resulting in flange breakage, luer cracking, and tip breakage. The physical properties continue to deteriorate with time, following irradiation. These problems of coloration and changing physical properties are best resolved by avoiding the use of any additives which discolor at the sterilizing dose of radiation (Khang et al., 1996c).

30.5 Surface Modifications for Improving Biocompatibility

Prevention of *thrombus* formation is important in clinical applications, where blood is in contact, such as hemodialysis membranes and tubes, artificial heart and heart–lung machines, prosthetic valves, and artificial vascular grafts. In spite of the use of anticoagulants, considerable platelet deposition and thrombus formation take place on the artificial surfaces (Branger et al., 1990).

Heparin, one of the complex carbohydrates known as mucopolysaccharides or glycosaminoglycan, is currently used to prevent formation of clots. In general, heparin is well tolerated and devoid of serious consequences. However, it allows platelet adhesion to foreign surfaces and may cause hemorrhagic complications such as subdural hematoma, retroperitoneal hematoma, gastrointestinal bleeding, hemorrhage into joints, ocular, and retinal bleeding, and bleeding at surgical sites (Lazarus, 1980). These difficulties give rise to an interest in developing new methods of hemocompatible materials.

Many different groups have studied immobilization of heparin (Kim and Feijen, 1985; Park et al., 1988) on the polymeric surfaces, heparin analogs, and heparin–prostaglandin or heparin–fibrinolytic enzyme conjugates (Jozefowicz and Jozefowicz, 1985). The major drawback of these surfaces is that they are not stable in the blood environment. It has not been firmly established that a slow leakage of heparin is needed for it to be effective as an immobilized antithrombogenic agent, if not its effectiveness could be hindered by being "coated over" with an adsorbed layer of more common proteins such as albumin and *fibrinogen*. Fibrinolytic enzymes, urokinase, and various prostaglandins have also been immobilized by themselves in order to take advantage of their unique fibrin dissolution or antiplatelet aggregation actions (Oshiro, 1983).

Albumin-coated surfaces have been studied because surfaces that resisted platelet adhesion *in vitro* were noted to adsorb albumin preferentially (Keogh et al., 1992). Fibronectin coatings have been used in *in vitro* endothelial cell (EC) seeding to prepare a surface similar to the natural blood vessel lumen (Lee et al., 1989). Also, algin-coated surfaces have been studied due to their good biocompatibility and biodegradability (Lee et al., 1990b, 1997b). Recently, plasma gas discharge (Khang et al., 1997a) and corona treatment (Khang et al., 1996d) with reactive groups introduced on the polymeric surfaces have emerged as other ways to modify biomaterial surfaces (Lee et al., 1991, 1992).

Hydrophobic coatings composed of silicon- and fluorine-containing polymeric materials as well as polyurethanes have been studied because of the relatively good clinical performances of Silastic®, Teflon, and polyurethane polymers in cardiovascular implants and devices. Polymeric fluorocarbon coatings deposited from a tetrafluoroethylene gas discharge have been found to greatly enhance resistance to both acute thrombotic occlusion and embolization in small-diameter Dacron® grafts.

Hydrophilic coatings have also been popular because of their low interfacial tension in biological environments (Hoffman, 1981). Hydrogels as well as various combinations of hydrophilic and hydrophobic monomers have been studied on the premise that there will be an optimum polar-dispersion force ratio which could be matched on the surfaces of the most passivating proteins. The passive surface may induce less clot formation. PE oxide-coated surfaces have been found to resist protein adsorption and cell adhesion and have therefore been proposed as potential "blood-compatible" coatings (Lee et al., 1990a). General physical and chemical methods to modify the surfaces of polymeric biomaterials are listed in Table 30.7 (Ratner et al., 1996).

Another way of making antithrombogenic surfaces is the saline perfusion method, which is designed to prevent direct contacts between blood and the surface of biomaterials by means of perfusing saline solution through the porous wall which is in contact with blood (Park and Kim, 1993; Khang et al., 1996a, b). It has been demonstrated that the adhesion of the blood cells could be prevented by the saline perfusion through PE, alumina, sulfonated/nonsulfonated PS/ styrene butadiene rubber (SBR), expanded PTFE, and polysulfone porous tubes.

TABLE 30.7 Physical and Chemical Surface Modification Methods for Polymeric Biomaterials

To modify blood compatibility	Octadecyl group attachment to surface
	Silicon containing block copolymer additive
	Plasma fluoropolymer deposition
	Plasma siloxane polymer deposition
	Radiation-grafted hydrogels
	Chemically modified PS for heparin-like activity
To influence cell adhesion and growth	Oxidized PS surface
	Ammonia plasma-treated surface
	Plasma-deposited acetone or methanol film
	Plasma fluoropolymer deposition
To control protein adsorption	Surface with immobilized polyethyelene glycol
	Treated enzyme-linked immunosorbent assay dish surface
	Affinity chromatography particulates
	Surface cross-linked contact lens
To improve lubricity	Plasma treatment
	Radiation-grafted hydrogels
	Interpenetrating polymeric networks
To improve wear resistance and corrosion resistance	Ion implantation
	Diamond deposition
	Anodization
To alter transport properties	Plasma deposition (methane, fluoropolymer, siloxane)
To modify electrical characteristics	Plasma deposition
	Solvent coatings
	Parylene coatings

Source: Adapted from Ratner, B.D. et al. 1996. *Biomaterials Science: An Introduction to Materials in Medicine*, Academic Press, New York, p. 106.

30.6 Chemogradient Surfaces for Cell and Protein Interaction

The behavior of the adsorption and desorption of blood proteins or adhesion and proliferation of different types of mammalian cells on polymeric materials depends on the surface characteristics such as wettability, hydrophilicity/hydrophobicity ratio, bulk chemistry, surface charge and charge distribution, surface roughness, and rigidity.

Many research groups have studied the effect of the surface wettability on the interactions of biological species with polymeric materials. Some have studied the interactions of different types of cultured cells or blood proteins with various polymers with different wettabilities to correlate the surface wettability and blood or tissue compatibility (Baier et al., 1984). One problem encountered from the study using different kinds of polymers is that the surfaces are heterogeneous, both chemically and physically (different surface chemistry, roughness, rigidity, crystallinity, etc.), which caused widely varying results. Some others have studied the interactions of different types of cells or proteins with a range of methacrylate copolymers with different wettabilities and have the same kind of chemistry but are still physically heterogeneous (van Wachem et al., 1985). Another methodological problem is that such studies are often tedious, laborious, and time-consuming because a large number of samples must be prepared to characterize the complete range of the desired surface properties.

Many studies have been focused on the preparation of surfaces whose properties are changed gradually along the material length. Such chemogradient surfaces are of particular interest in basic studies of the interactions between biological species and synthetic material surfaces since the effect of a selected property can be examined in a single experiment on one surface preparation. A chemogradient of methyl groups was formed by diffusion of dimethyldichlorosilane through xylene on flat hydrophilic silicon dioxide surfaces (Elwing et al., 1989). The wettability chemogradient surfaces were made to investigate hydrophilicity-induced changes of adsorbed proteins.

Recently, a method for preparing wettability chemogradients on various polymer surfaces was developed (Lee et al., 1989, 1990a; Khang et al., 1997b). The wettability chemogradients were produced via radio frequency and plasma discharge treatment by exposing the polymer sheets continuously to the plasma (Lee et al., 1991). The polymer surfaces oxidized gradually along the sample length with increasing plasma exposure time and thus the wettability chemogradient was created. Another method for preparing a wettability chemogradient on polymer surfaces using corona discharge treatment has been developed as shown in Figure 30.6 (Lee et al., 1992). The wettability chemogradient was produced by treating the polymer sheets with corona from a knife-type electrode whose power was gradually changed along the sample length. The polymer surface gradually oxidized with the increasing power and the wettability chemogradient was created. Chemogradient surfaces with different functional groups such

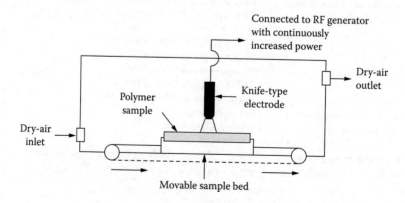

FIGURE 30.6 Schematic diagram showing corona discharge apparatus for the preparation of wettability chemogradient surfaces.

s –COOH, –CH$_2$ OH, –CONH$_2$, and –CH$_2$ NH$_2$ were produced on PE surfaces by the above corona reatment followed by vinyl monomer grafting and substitution reactions (Kim et al., 1993; Lee et al., 1994a,b). We have also prepared chargeable functional groups (Lee et al., 1997c,d, 1998), comb-like polyethyleneoxide (PEO) (Jeong et al., 1996; Lee et al., 1997a), and phospholipid polymer chemogradient surfaces (Iwasaki et al., 1997) by the corona discharge treatment, followed by graft copolymerization with subsequent substitution reaction of functional vinyl monomers such as acrylic acid, sodium p-sulfonic styrene, and N,N-dimethyl aminopropyl acrylamide, poly(ethyleneglycol) mono-methacrylate, and ω-methacryloyloxyalkyl phosphorylcholine, respectively.

The water contact angles of the corona-treated PE surfaces gradually decrease along the sample length with increasing corona power (from about 95° to about 45°) as shown in Figure 30.7. The decrease in contact angles, that is, the increase in wettability along the sample length was due to the oxygen-based polar functionalities incorporated on the surface by the corona treatment. It was also confirmed by Fourier transform infrared spectroscopy in the attenuated total reflectance mode and electron spectroscopy for chemical analysis (ESCA).

In order to investigate the interaction of different types of cells in terms of the surface hydrophilicity/ hydrophobicity of polymeric materials, Chinese hamster ovaries (CHO), fibroblasts, and bovine aortic EC were cultured for 1 and 2 days on the PE wettability chemogradient surfaces. The maximum adhesion and growth of the cells appeared around a water contact angle of 50–55° as shown in Figure 30.8. The observation of scanning electron microscopy (SEM) also verified that the cells are more adhered, spread, and grown onto the sections with moderate hydrophilicity as shown in Figure 30.9.

To determine the cell proliferation rates, the migration of fibroblasts on PE wettability chemogradient surfaces was observed (Khang et al., 1999b). After the change of culture media at 24 h, cell growth morphology was recorded for 1 or 2 h intervals at the position of 0.5, 1.5, 2.5, and 4.5 cm for the counting of grown cells and the observation of cell morphology with a video tape recorder. The proliferation rates of fibroblast cells were calculated from the slopes of Figure 30.10 as given in Table 30.8. The proliferation rates on the PE surfaces with wettability chemogradient showed that as the surface wettability increased, it increased and then decreased. The maximum proliferation rate of the cells as 1111 cells/h cm^2 appeared at around the position 2.5 cm.

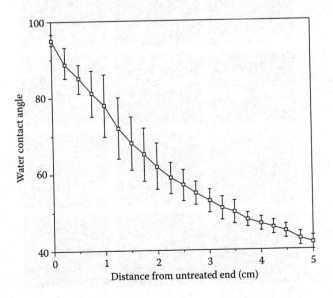

FIGURE 30.7 Changes in water contact angle of corona-treated PE surface along the sample length. Sample numbers, $n = 3$.

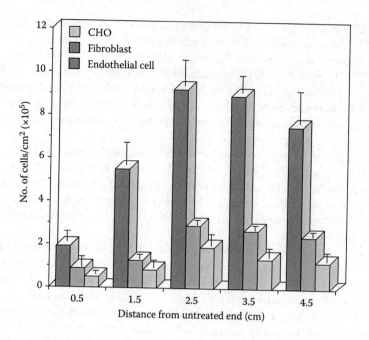

FIGURE 30.8 CHO, fibroblast, and EC growth on wettability chemogradient PE surfaces after 2-day culture (number of seeded cells, $4 \times 10^4/cm^2$). $n = 3$.

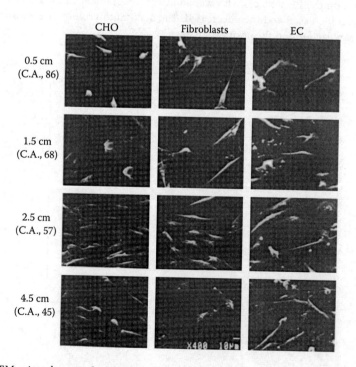

FIGURE 30.9 SEM microphotographs of CHO, fibroblast, and ECs grown on PE wettability chemogradient surface along the sample length after 2-day culture (original magnification; ×400).

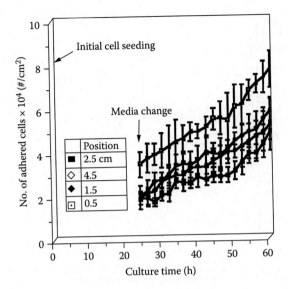

FIGURE 30.10 Fibroblast cell proliferation rates on wettability chemogradient PE surfaces (24–60 h culture).

To observe the effect of serum proteins on the cell adhesion and growth behaviors, fetal bovine serum, which contains more than 200 kinds of different proteins, was adsorbed onto the wettability gradient PE surfaces for 1 h at 37°C. Figure 30.11 shows the relative adsorbed amount of serum proteins on the wettability gradient surfaces determined by ESCA. The maximum adsorption of the proteins appeared at around the 2.5 cm position, which is the same trend as the cell adhesion, growth, and migration behaviors. It can be explained that preferential adsorption of some serum proteins, like fibronectin and vitronectin from culture medium, onto the moderately wettable surfaces may be a reason for better cell adhesion, spreading, and growth. Proteins like fibronectin and vitronectin are well known as cell-adhesive proteins. Cells attached on surfaces are spread only when they are compatible on the surfaces. It seems that surface wettability plays an important role for cell adhesion, spreading, and migration.

Also investigated were (1) platelet adhesion on wettability chemogradient (Lee and Lee, 1998), (2) cell interaction on microgrooved PE surfaces (groove depth, 0.5 μm; groove width, 0.45 μm; and pitch, 0.9 μm) with wettability chemogradient (Khang et al., 1997c), (3) detachment of human endothelial under flow from wettability gradient surface with different functional groups (Raurdy et al., 1997), (4) cell interaction on microporous polycarbonate membrane with wettability chemogradient (Lee et al., 1999b), and (5) cell interaction on poly(lactide-*co*-glycolide) surface with wettability chemogradient (Khang et al., 1999a).

During the last several years, "chemogradient surfaces" have evolved into easier and more popular tools for the study of protein adsorption and platelet or cell interactions continuously which relate to

TABLE 30.8 Proliferation Rates of Fibroblast Cells on Wettability Gradient PE Surfaces

Positions (cm)	Contact Angle (°)	Cell Proliferation Rate (#cell/h cm²)
2.5	55	1111
4.5	45	924
1.5	67	838
0.5	85	734

Note: 24–60 h culture.

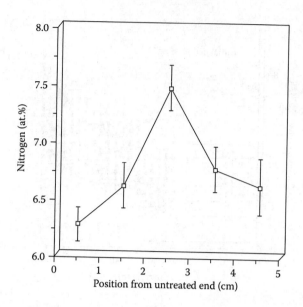

FIGURE 30.11 Serum protein adsorption on PE wettability chemogradient surface (1 h adsorption). $n = 3$.

the surface properties such as wettability, chemistry and charge, or dynamics of polymeric materials. In many studies, different kinds of polymeric materials with widely varying surface chemistries are used and the explanation of the results is often controversial due to the surface heterogeneity. In addition, these studies are tedious, laborious, and time-consuming, and biological variations are more likely to occur. The application of chemogradient surfaces for these studies can reduce these discomforts and problems, and eventually save time and money. Also, chemogradient surfaces are valuable in investigating the basic mechanisms by which complicated systems such as proteins or cells interact with surfaces, since a continuum of selected and controlled physical–chemical properties can be studied in one experiment on the polymeric surface.

The possible applications of chemogradient surfaces in the near future are: (1) separation devices of cells and/or biological species by different surface properties, (2) column packing materials for separation, (3) biosensing, and so on.

Defining Terms

Acetabulum: The socket portion of the hip joint.

Addition (or free radical) polymerization: Polymerization in which monomers are added to the growing chains, initiated by free radical agents.

Biocompatibility: Acceptance of an artificial implant by the surrounding tissues and as a whole. The implant should be compatible with tissues in terms of mechanical, chemical, surface, and pharmacological properties.

Biomaterials: Synthetic materials used to replace part of a living system or to function in intimate contact with living tissue.

Bone cement: Mixture of polymethylmethacrylate powder and methylmethacrylate monomer liquid to be used as a grouting material for the fixation of orthopedic joint implants.

Branching: Chains grown from the sides of the main backbone chains.

Chemogradient surface: The surface whose properties such as wettability, surface charge, and hydrophilicity/hydrophobicity ratio are changed gradually along the length of the material.

Condensation (step reaction) polymerization: Polymerization in which two or more chemicals are reacted to form a polymer by condensing out small molecules such as water and alcohol.

Copolymers: Polymers made from two or more monomers which can be obtained by grafting, block, alternating, or random attachment of the other polymer segment.

Covalent bonding: Bonding of atoms or molecules by sharing valence electrons.

Dacron®: Polyethyleneterephthalate polyester that is made into fiber. If the same polymer is made into a film, it is called Mylar.

Delrin®: Polyacetal made by Union Carbide.

Elastomers: Rubbery materials. The restoring force comes from uncoiling or unkinking of coiled or kinked molecular chains. They can be highly stretched.

Embolus: Any foreign matter, as a blood clot or air bubble, carried in the blood stream.

Fibrinogen: A plasma protein of high molecular weight that is converted into fibrin through the action of thrombin. This material is used to make (absorbable) tissue adhesives.

Filler: Materials added as a powder to a rubber to improve its mechanical properties.

Free volume: The difference in volume occupied by the crystalline state (minimum) and noncrystalline state of a material for a given temperature and a pressure.

Glass transition temperature: Temperature at which solidification without crystallization takes place from viscous liquid.

Grafts: A transplant.

Heparin: A substance found in various body tissues, especially in the liver, that prevents the clotting of blood.

Hydrogel: Polymer which can absorb 30% or more of its weight in water.

Hydrogen bonding: A secondary bonding through dipole interactions in which the hydrogen ion is one of the dipoles.

Hydroquinone: Chemical inhibitor added to the bone cement liquid monomer to prevent accidental polymerization during storage.

Initiator: Chemical used to initiate the addition polymerization by becoming a free radical which in turn reacts with a monomer.

Ionic bonding: Bonding of atoms or molecules through electrostatic interaction of positive and negative ions.

Kevlar®: Aromatic polyamides made by DuPont.

Lexan®: Polycarbonate made by General Electric.

Oxygenator: An apparatus by which oxygen is introduced into blood during circulation outside the body, as during open-heart surgery.

Plasticizer: Substance made of small molecules, mixed with (amorphous) polymers to make the chains slide more easily past each other, making the polymer less rigid.

Refractive index: Ratio of speed of light in vacuum to speed of light in a material. It is a measure of the ability of a material to refract (bend) a beam of light.

Repeating unit: Basic molecular unit which can represent a polymer backbone chain. The average number of repeating units is called the degree of polymerization.

Repeating unit: The smallest unit representing a polymer molecular chain.

Semicrystalline solid: Solid which contains both crystalline and noncrystalline regions and usually occurs in polymers due to their long-chain molecules.

Side group: Chemical group attached to the main backbone chain. It is usually shorter than the branches and exists before polymerization.

Steric hindrance: Geometrical interference which restrains movements of molecular groups such as side chains and main chains of a polymer.

Suture: Material used in closing a wound with stitches.

Tacticity: Arrangement of asymmetrical side groups along the backbone chain of polymers. Groups could be distributed at random (atactic), one side (isotactic), or alternating (syndiotactic).

Teflon®: Polytetrafluoroethylene made by DuPont.

Thrombus: The fibrinous clot attached at the site of thrombosis.

Udel®: Polysulfone made by General Electric.

Valence electrons: The outermost (shell) electrons of an atom.

van der Waals bonding: A secondary bonding arising through the fluctuating dipole–dipole interactions.

Vinyl polymers: Thermoplastic linear polymers synthesized by free radical polymerization of vinyl monomers having a common structure of $CH_2=CHR$.

Vulcanization: Cross-linking of a (natural) rubber by adding sulfur.

Ziegler–Natta catalyst: Organometallic compounds which have the remarkable capacity of polymerizing a wide variety of monomers to linear and stereoregular polymers.

Acknowledgments

This work was supported by grants from the Korean Ministry of Health and Welfare (grant Nos. HMP-95-G-2-33 and HMP-97-E-0016) and the Korean Ministry of Science and Technology (grant No. 97-N1-02-05-A-02).

References

Baier, R.E., Meyer, A.E., Natiella, J.R., Natiella, R.R., and Carter, J.M. 1984. Surface properties determine bioadhesive outcomes: methods and results, *J. Biomed. Mater. Res.*, 18: 337–355.

Billmeyer, F.W. Jr. 1984. *Textbook of Polymer Science*, 3rd ed. Wiley, New York.

Block, S.S. (Ed.) 1977. *Disinfection, Sterilization, and Preservation*, 2nd ed. Rea and Febiger, Philadelphia, PA.

Brandrup, J. and Immergut, E.H. (Eds.) 1989. *Polymer Handbook*, 3rd ed. Wiley-Interscience, New York.

Branger, B., Garreau, M., Baudin, G., and Gris, J.C. 1990. Biocompatibility of blood tubings, *Int. J. Artif. Organs*, 13: 697–703.

Dumitriu, S. (Ed.) 1993. *Polymeric Biomaterials*, Marcel Dekker, New York.

Elwing, E., Askendal, A., and Lundstorm, I. 1989. Desorption of fibrinogen and γ-globulin from solid surfaces induced by a nonionic detergent, *J. Colloid Interface Sci.*, 128: 296–300.

Glaser, Z.R. 1979. Ethylene oxide: Toxicology review and field study results of hospital use, *J. Environ. Pathol. Toxicol.*, 2: 173–208.

Hoffman, A.S. 1981. Radiation processing in biomaterials: A review, *Radiat. Phys. Chem.*, 18: 323–340.

Iwasaki, Y., Ishihara, K., Nakabayashi, N., Khang, G., Jeon, J.H., Lee, J.W., and Lee, H.B. 1997. Preparation of gradient surfaces grafted with phospholipid polymers and evaluation of their blood compatibility. In: *Advances in Biomaterials Science*, Vol. 1, T. Akaike, T. Okano, M. Akashi, M. Terano, and N. Yui, Eds. pp. 91–100, CMC Co., Ltd., Tokyo.

Jeong, B.J., Lee, J.H., and Lee, H.B. 1996. Preparation and characterization of comb-like PEO gradient surfaces. *J. Colloid Interface Sci.*, 178: 757–763.

Jozefowicz, M. and Jozefowicz, J. 1985. New approaches to anticoagulation: Heparin-like biomaterials. *J. Am. Soc. Art. Intern. Org.* 8: 218–222.

Keogh, J.R., Valender, F.F., and Eaton, J.W. 1992. Albumin-binding surfaces for implantable devices, *J. Biomed. Mater. Res.*, 26: 357–372.

Khang, G., Park J.B., and Lee, H.B. 1996a. Prevention of platelet adhesion on the polysulfone porous catheter by saline perfusion, I. *In vitro* investigation, *Bio-Med. Mater. Eng.*, 6: 47–66.

Khang, G., Park, J.B., and Lee, H.B. 1996b. Prevention of platelet adhesion on the polysulfone porous catheter by saline perfusion, II. *Ex vivo* and *in vivo* investigation, *Bio-Med. Mater. Eng.*, 6: 123–134.

Khang, G., Lee, H.B., and Park, J.B. 1996c. Radiation effects on polypropylene for sterilization, *Bio-Med. Mater. Eng.*, 6: 323–334.

Khang, G., Kang, Y.H., Park, J.B., and Lee, H.B. 1996d. Improved bonding strength of polyethylene/polymethylmethacrylate bone cement—A preliminary study, *Bio-Med. Mater. Eng.*, 6: 335–344.

Khang, G., Jeon, J.H., Lee, J.W., Cho, S.C., and Lee, H.B. 1997a. Cell and platelet adhesion on plasma glow discharge-treated poly(lactide-co-glycolide), *Bio-Med. Mater. Eng.*, 7: 357–368.

Khang, G., Lee, J.H., and Lee, H.B. 1997b. Cell and platelet adhesion on gradient surfaces, In: *Advances in Biomaterials Science*, Vol. 1, T. Akaike, T. Okano, M. Akashi, Terano, and N. Yui, Eds. pp. 63–70, CMC Co., Ltd., Tokyo.

Khang, G., Lee, J.W., Jeon, J.H., Lee, J.H., and Lee, H.B. 1997c. Interaction of fibroblasts on microgrooved polyethylene surfaces with wettability gradient, *Biomat. Res.*, 1: 1–6.

Khang, G., Lee, S.J., Lee, J.H., Kim, Y.S., and Lee, H.B. 1999a. Interaction of fibroblast cells on poly(lactide-co-glycolide) surface with wettability gradient, *Biomed. Mater. Eng.*, 9: 179–187.

Khang, G., Lee, S.J., Lee, J.H., and Lee, H.B. 1999b. Interaction of fibroblast cells onto fibers with different diameter, *Korea Polym. J.*, 7: 102–107.

Kim, S.W. and Feijen, J. 1985. Surface modification of polymers for improved blood biocompatibility, *CRC Crit. Rev. Biocompat.*, 1: 229–260.

Kim, H.G., Lee, J.H., Lee, H.B., and Jhon, M.S. 1993. Dissociation behavior of surface-grafted poly(acrylic acid): Effects of surface density and counterion size, *J. Colloid Interface Sci.*, 157: 82–87.

Lazarus, J.M. 1980. Complications in hemodialysis: An overview, *Kidney Int.*, 18: 783–796.

Lee, H.B. 1989. Application of synthetic polymers in implants. In: *Frontiers of Macromolecular Science*, T. Seagusa, T., Higashimura, and A. Abe, Eds. pp. 579–584, Blackwell Scientific Publications, Oxford.

Lee, H.B. and Lee, J.H. 1995. Biocompatibility of solid substrates based on surface wettability. In: *Encyclopedic Handbook of Biomaterials and Bioengineering: Materials*, Vol. 1., D.L. Wise, D.J. Trantolo, D.E. Altobelli, M.J. Yasemski, J.D. Gresser, and E.R. Schwartz, pp. 371–398, Marcel Dekker, New York.

Lee, J.H. and Lee, H.B. 1998. Platelet adhesion onto wettability gradient surfaces in the absence and presence of plasma protein, *J. Biomed. Mater. Res.*, 41: 304–311.

Lee, J.H., Khang, G., Park, K.H., Lee, H.B., and Andrade, J.D. 1989. Polymer surfaces for cell adhesion: I. Surface modification of polymers and ESCA analysis. *J. Korea Soc. Med. Biol. Eng.*, 10: 43–51.

Lee, J.H., Khang, G., Park, J.W., and Lee, H.B. 1990a. Plasma protein adsorption on polyethyleneoxide gradient surfaces, *33rd IUPAC International Symposium on Macromolecules*, July 8–13, Montreal, Canada.

Lee, J.H., Shin, B.C., Khang, G., and Lee, H.B. 1990b. Algin impregnated vascular graft: I. *In vitro* investigation. *J. Korea Soc. Med. Biol. Eng.*, 11: 97–104.

Lee, J.H., Park, J.W., and Lee, H.B. 1991. Cell adhesion and growth on polymer surfaces with hydroxyl groups prepared by water vapor plasma treatment, *Biomaterials*, 12: 443–448.

Lee, J.H., Kim, H.G., Khang, G., Lee, H.B., and Jhon, M.S. 1992. Characterization of wettability gradient surfaces prepared by corona discharge treatment, *J. Colloid Interface Sci.*, 151: 563–570.

Lee, J.H., Kim, H.W., Pak, P.K., and Lee, H.B. 1994a. Preparation and characterization of functional group gradient surfaces, *J. Polym. Sci., Part A, Polym. Chem.*, 32: 1569–1579.

Lee, J.H., Jung, H.W., Kang, I.K., and Lee, H.B. 1994b. Cell behavior on polymer surfaces with different functional groups, *Biomaterials*, 15: 705–711.

Lee, J.H., Jeong, B.J., and Lee, H.B. 1997a. Plasma protein adsorption and platelet adhesion onto comb-like PEO gradient surface, *J. Biomed. Mater. Res.*, 34: 105–114.

Lee, J.H., Kim, W.G., Kim, S.S., Lee, J.H., and Lee, H.B. 1997b. Development and characterization of an alginate-impregnated polyester vascular graft, *J. Biomed. Mater. Res.*, 36: 200–208.

Lee, J.H., Khang, G., Lee, J.H., and Lee, H.B. 1997c. Interactions of protein and cells on functional group gradient surfaces, *Macromol. Symp.*, 118: 571–576.

Lee, J.H., Khang, G., Lee, J.H., and Lee, H.B. 1997d. Interactions of cells on chargeable functional group gradient surfaces, *Biomaterials*, 18: 351–358.

Lee, J.H., Khang, G., Lee, J.H., and Lee, H.B. 1998. Platelet adhesion onto chargeable functional group gradient surfaces, *J. Biomed. Mater. Res.*, 40: 180–186.

Lee, J.H., Lee, S.J., Khang, G., and Lee, H.B. 1999. Interaction of fibroblasts on polycarbonate membrane surfaces with different micropore sizes and hydrophilicity, *J. Biomater. Sci. Polym. Ed.*, 10: 283–294.

Leininger, R.I. and Bigg, D.M. 1986. Polymers. In: *Handbook of Biomaterials Evaluation*, pp. 24–37, Macmillan Publishing Co., New York.

Lewin, M. and Preston, J. Eds. 1989. *Handbook of Fiber Science and Technology Volume III: High Technology Fibers, Part B*, 332 pp, Marcel Dekker, Inc., New York.

Oshiro, T. 1983. Thrombosis, antithrombogenic characteristics of immobilized urokinase on synthetic polymers, In: *Biocompatible Polymers, Metals, and Composites*, M. Szycher, Ed. pp. 275–299. Technomic, Lancaster, PA.

Park, J.B. 1984. *Biomaterials Science and Engineering*, Plenum Press, New York.

Park, J.B. and Kim S.S. 1993. Prevention of mural thrombus in porous inner tube of double-layered tube by saline perfusion. *Bio-Med. Mater. Eng.*, 3: 101–116.

Park, J.B. and Lakes, R. 1992. *Biomaterials: An Introduction*, 2nd ed. pp. 141–168, Plenum Press, New York.

Park, K.D., Okano, T., Nojiri, C., and Kim S.W. 1988. Heparin immobilized onto segmented polyurethane effect of hydrophilic spacers. *J. Biomed. Mater. Res.*, 22: 977–992.

Ratner, B.D., Hoffman, A.S., Schoen, F.J., and Lemons, J.E. 1996. *Biomaterials Science: An Introduction to Materials in Medicine*, Academic Press, New York.

Raurdy, T.G., Moorlag, H.E., Schkenraad, J.M., van der Mei, H.C., and Busscher, H.J. 1997. Detachment of human endothelial under flow from wettability gradient surface with different functional groups, *Cell Mater.*, 7: 123–133.

Sato, K. 1983. Radiation sterilization of medical products. *Radioisotopes*, 32: 431–439.

Shalaby, W.S. 1988. Polymeric materials. In: *Encyclopedia of Med. Dev. Instr.*, J.G. Webster, Ed. pp. 2324–2335, Wiley-Interscience, New York.

Sharma, C.P. and Szycher, M. Eds. 1991. *Blood Compatible Materials and Devices: Perspective Toward the 21st Century*, Technomic Publishing Co. Inc., Lancaster, PA.

van Wachem, P.B., Beugeling, T., Feijen, J., Bantjes, A., Detmers, J.P., and van Aken, W.G. 1985. Interaction of cultured human endothelial cells with polymeric surfaces of different wettabilities, *Biomaterials*, 6: 403–408.

31

Composite Biomaterials

31.1 Structure.. 31-1
31.2 Bounds on Properties.. 31-2
31.3 Anisotropy of Composites... 31-3
31.4 Particulate Composites... 31-4
31.5 Fibrous Composites.. 31-6
31.6 Porous Materials 31-9
31.7 Biocompatibility.. 31-12
31.8 Summary.. 31-13
References... 31-13

Roderic S. Lakes
*University of Wisconsin,
Madison*

Composite materials are solids which contain two or more distinct constituent materials or phases, on a scale larger than the atomic. The term "composite" is usually reserved for those materials in which the distinct phases are separated on a scale larger than the atomic and in which properties such as the elastic modulus are significantly altered in comparison with those of a homogeneous material. Accordingly, reinforced plastics such as fiberglass as well as natural materials such as bone are viewed as composite materials, but alloys such as brass are not. A foam is a composite in which one phase is empty space. Natural biological materials tend to be composites. Natural composites include bone, wood, dentin, cartilage, and skin. Natural foams include lung, cancellous bone, and wood. Natural composites often exhibit hierarchical structures in which particulate, porous, and fibrous structural features are seen on different micro-scales (Katz, 1980; Lakes, 1993). In this chapter, fundamentals of composite materials and their applications in biomaterials (Park and Lakes, 1992) are explored. Composite materials offer a variety of advantages in comparison with homogeneous materials. These include the ability for the scientist or engineer to exercise considerable control over material properties. There is the potential for stiff, strong, lightweight materials as well as for highly resilient and compliant materials. In biomaterials, it is important that each constituent of the composite be biocompatible. Moreover, the interface between constituents should not be degraded by the body environment. Some applications of composites in biomaterials are: (1) dental filling composites, (2) reinforced methylmethacrylate bone cement and ultra-high-molecular-weight polyethylene, and (3) orthopedic implants with porous surfaces.

31.1 Structure

The properties of composite materials depend very much on *structure*. Composites differ from homogeneous materials in that considerable control can be exerted over the larger scale structure and hence over the desired properties. In particular, the properties of a composite material depend on the *shape* of the heterogeneities, on the *volume fraction* occupied by them, and on the *interface* among the constituents. The shape of the heterogeneities in a composite material is classified as follows. The principal inclusion shape categories are: (1) the particle, with no long dimension, (2) the fiber, with one long dimension, and (3) the platelet or lamina, with two long dimensions, as shown in Figure 31.1. The inclusions may

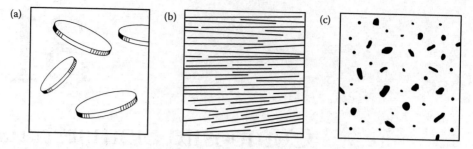

FIGURE 31.1 Morphology of basic composite inclusions: (a) particle, (b) fiber, and (c) platelet.

vary in size and shape within a category. For example, particulate inclusions may be spherical, ellipsoidal, polyhedral, or irregular. If one phase consists of voids, filled with air or liquid, then the material is known as a cellular solid. If the cells are polygonal, then the material is a honeycomb; if the cells are polyhedral, then it is a foam. It is necessary in the context of biomaterials to distinguish the above structural cells from biological cells, which occur only in living organisms. In each composite structure, we may moreover make the distinction between random orientation and preferred orientation.

31.2 Bounds on Properties

Mechanical properties of many composite materials depend on structure in a complex way; however, for some structures, the prediction of properties is relatively simple. The simplest composite structures are the idealized Voigt and Reuss models, shown in Figure 31.2. The dark and light areas in these diagrams represent the two constituent materials in the composite. In contrast to most composite structures, it is easy to calculate the stiffness of materials with the Voigt and Reuss structures, since in the Voigt structure the strain is the same in both constituents; in the Reuss structure, the stress is the same. The Young modulus, E, of the Voigt composite is

$$E = E_i V_i + E_m[1 - V_i] \tag{31.1}$$

where E_i is the Young modulus of the inclusions, V_i is the volume fraction of inclusions, and E_m is the Young modulus of the matrix. The Voigt relation for the stiffness is referred to as the rule of mixtures.

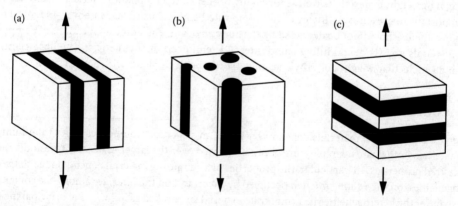

FIGURE 31.2 Voigt (a) laminar; (b) fibrous; and Reuss (c) composite models, subjected to tension force indicated by arrows.

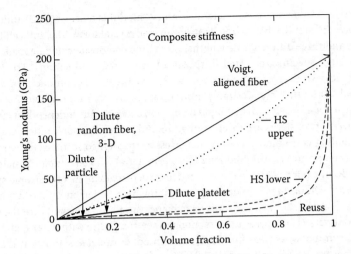

FIGURE 31.3 Stiffness versus volume fraction for Voigt and Reuss models, as well as for dilute isotropic suspensions of platelets, fibers, and spherical particles embedded in a matrix. Phase moduli are 200 and 3 GPa.

The Reuss stiffness E, represented by

$$E = \left[\frac{V_i}{E_i} + \frac{1 - V_i}{E_m} \right]^{-1}$$

(31.2)

is less than that of the Voigt model. The Voigt and Reuss models provide upper and lower bounds, respectively, upon the stiffness of a composite of arbitrary phase geometry (Paul, 1960). The bounds are far apart if, as is common, the phase moduli differ a great deal, as shown in Figure 31.3. For composite materials which are isotropic, the more complex relations of Hashin and Shtrikman (1963) provide tighter bounds upon the moduli (Figure 31.3); both the Young and shear moduli must be known for each constituent to calculate these bounds.

31.3 Anisotropy of Composites

Observe that the Reuss laminate is identical to the Voigt laminate, except for a rotation with respect to the direction of load. Therefore, the stiffness of the laminate is *anisotropic*, that is, dependent on direction (Lekhnitskii, 1963; Nye, 1976; Agarwal and Broutman, 1980). Anisotropy is characteristic of composite materials. The relationship between stress σ_{ij} and strain ε_{kl} in anisotropic materials is given by the tensorial form of Hooke's law as follows:

$$\sigma_{ij} = \sum_{k=1}^{3} \sum_{l=1}^{3} C_{ijkl} \varepsilon_{kl}$$

(31.3)

Here C_{ijkl} is the elastic modulus tensor. It has $3^4 = 81$ elements; however, since the stress and strain are represented by symmetric matrices with six independent elements each, the number of independent modulus tensor elements is reduced to 36. An additional reduction to 21 is achieved by considering elastic materials for which a strain energy function exists. Physically, C_{2323} represents a shear modulus since it couples a shear stress with a shear strain. C_{1111} couples axial stress and strain in the 1 or x-direction, but it is not the same as Young's modulus. The reason is that Young's modulus is measured with the lateral strains free to occur via the Poisson effect, while C_{1111} is the ratio of axial stress to strain when there is only one nonzero strain value; there is no lateral strain. A modulus tensor with 21 independent elements describes a *triclinic* crystal, which is the least symmetric crystal form. The unit cell has three different oblique angles and three different side lengths. A triclinic composite could be made with groups of fibers of three different spacings, oriented in three different oblique directions. Triclinic modulus elements such as C_{2311}, known as cross-coupling constants, have the effect of producing a shear stress in response to a uniaxial strain; this is undesirable in many applications. An *orthorhombic* crystal or an *orthotropic* composite has a unit cell with orthogonal angles. There are nine independent elastic moduli. The associated engineering constants are three Young's moduli, three Poisson's ratios, and three shear moduli; the cross-coupling constants are zero when stresses are aligned to the symmetry directions. An example of such a composite is a unidirectional fibrous material with a rectangular pattern of fibers in the cross-section. Bovine bone, which has a laminated structure, exhibits orthotropic symmetry, as does wood. In a material with *hexagonal* symmetry, out of the nine C elements, there are five independent elastic constants. For directions in the transverse plane, the elastic constants are the same, hence the alternate name transverse isotropy. A unidirectional fiber composite with a hexagonal or random fiber pattern has this symmetry, as does human Haversian bone. In *cubic* symmetry, there are three independent elastic constants: a Young's modulus, E, a shear modulus, G, and an independent Poisson's ratio, v. Cross-weave fabrics have cubic symmetry. Finally, an *isotropic* material has the same material properties in any direction. There are only two independent elastic constants, hence E, G, v, and also the bulk modulus B are related in an isotropic material. Isotropic materials include amorphous solids, polycrystalline metals in which the grains are randomly oriented, and composite materials in which the constituents are randomly oriented.

Anisotropic composites offer superior strength and stiffness in comparison with isotropic ones. Material properties in one direction are gained at the expense of properties in other directions. It is sensible, therefore, to use anisotropic composite materials only if the direction of application of the stress is known in advance.

31.4 Particulate Composites

It is often convenient to stiffen or harden a material, commonly a polymer, by the incorporation of particulate inclusions. The shape of the particles is important (see Christensen, 1979). In isotropic systems, stiff platelet (or flake) inclusions are the most effective in creating a stiff composite, followed by fibers, and the least effective geometry for stiff inclusions is the spherical particle, as shown in Figure 31.3. A dilute concentration of spherical particulate inclusions of stiffness E_i and volume fraction V_i, in a matrix (with Poisson's ratio assumed to be 0.5) denoted by the subscript m, gives rise to a composite with a stiffness E:

$$E = \frac{5(E_i - E_m)V_i}{3 + 2(E_i/E_m)} + E_m \tag{31.4}$$

The stiffness of such a composite is close to the Hashin–Shtrikman lower bound for isotropic composites. Even if the spherical particles are perfectly rigid compared with the matrix, their stiffening effect at low concentrations is modest. Conversely, when the inclusions are more compliant than the matrix, spherical ones reduce the stiffness the least and platelet ones reduce it the most. Indeed, soft platelets are suggestive of crack-like defects. Soft platelets therefore result not only in a compliant composite, but also a weak one. Soft spherical inclusions are used intentionally as crack stoppers to enhance the toughness of polymers such as polystyrene (high-impact polystyrene), with a small sacrifice in stiffness.

Particle reinforcement has been used to improve the properties of bone cement. For example, inclusion of bone particles in polymethyl-methacrylate (PMMA) cement somewhat improves the stiffness and improves the fatigue life considerably (Park et al., 1986). Moreover, the bone particles at the interface with the patient's bone are ultimately resorbed and are replaced by ingrown new bone tissue. This approach is in the experimental stages.

Rubber used in catheters, rubber gloves, and so on is usually reinforced with very fine particles of silica (SiO_2) to make the rubber stronger and tougher.

Teeth with decayed regions have traditionally been restored with metals such as silver amalgam. Metallic restorations are not considered desirable for anterior teeth for cosmetic reasons. Acrylic resins and silicate cements had been used for anterior teeth, but their poor material properties led to short service life and clinical failures. Dental composite resins have virtually replaced these materials and are very commonly used to restore posterior teeth as well as anterior teeth (Cannon, 1988).

The dental composite resins consist of a polymer matrix and stiff inorganic inclusions (Craig, 1981). A representative structure is shown in Figure 31.4. The particles are very angular in shape. The inorganic inclusions confer a relatively high stiffness and high wear resistance on the material. Moreover, since they are translucent and their index of refraction is similar to that of dental enamel, they are cosmetically acceptable. Available dental composite resins use quartz, barium glass, and colloidal silica as fillers. Fillers have particle size from 0.04 to 13 μm, and concentrations from 33% to 78% by weight. In view of the greater density of the inorganic filler phase, a 77 wt% of filler corresponds to about 55 vol%. The matrix consists of a polymer, typically bisphenol A glycidyl methacrylate (BIS-GMA). In restoring a cavity, the dentist mixes several constituents, and then places them in the prepared cavity to polymerize. In order for this procedure to be successful, the viscosity of the mixed paste must be sufficiently low and the polymerization must be controllable. Low-viscosity liquids such as triethylene glycol dimethacrylate are used to lower the viscosity and inhibitors such as butylated trioxytoluene are used to prevent premature polymerization. Polymerization can be initiated by a thermochemical initiator, such as benzoyl peroxide, or by a photochemical initiator (benzoin alkyl ether) which generates free radicals when subjected to ultraviolet light from a lamp used by the dentist.

Dental composites have a Young's modulus in the range 10–16 GPa, and the compressive strength from 170 to 260 MPa (Cannon, 1988). As shown in Table 31.1, these composites are still considerably less stiff than dental enamel, which contains about 99% mineral. Similar high concentrations of mineral particles in synthetic composites cannot easily be achieved, in part because the particles do not pack densely. Moreover, an excessive concentration of particles raises the viscosity of the unpolymerized paste. An excessively high viscosity is problematic since it prevents the dentist from adequately packing the paste into the prepared cavity; the material will then fill in crevices less effectively.

The thermal expansion of dental composites, as with other dental materials, exceeds that of tooth structure. Moreover, there is a contraction during polymerization of 1.2–1.6%. These effects are thought

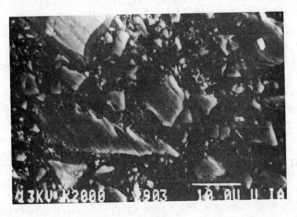

FIGURE 31.4 Microstructure of a dental composite. Miradapt® (Johnson & Johnson) 50% by volume filler: barium glass and colloidal silica. (Adapted from Park, J.B. and Lakes, R.S. 1992. *Biomaterials*, 2nd ed., Plenum Press, New York.)

TABLE 31.1 Properties of Bone, Teeth, and Biomaterials

Material	Young's Modulus E (GPa)	Density ρ (g/cm³)	Strength (MPa)	References
Hard Tissue				
Tooth, bone, human compact bone, longitudinal direction	17	1.8	130 (tension)	Craig and Peyton (1958); Reilly and Burstein (1975); Peters et al. (1983); Park and Lakes (1992)
Tooth dentin	18	2.1	138 (compression)	
Tooth enamel	50	2.9		
Polymers				Park and Lakes (1992)
Polyethylene (UHMW)	1	0.94	30 (tension)	
PMMA	3	1.1	65 (tension)	
PMMA bone cement	2	1.18	30 (tension)	
Metals				Park and Lakes (1992)
316L Stainless steel (wrought)	200	7.9	1000 (tension)	
CoCrMo (cast)	230	8.3	660 (tension)	
CoNiCrMo (wrought)	230	9.2	1800 (tension)	
Ti6A14V	110	4.5	900 (tension)	
Composites				
Graphite-epoxy (unidirectional fibrous, high modulus)	215	1.63	1240 (tension)	Schwartz (1992)
Graphite-epoxy (quasi-isotropic fibrous)	46	1.55	579 (tension)	Schwartz (1992)
Dental composite resins (particulate)	10–16		170–260 (compression)	Cannon (1988)
Foams				Gibson and Ashby (1988)
Polymer foams	10^{-4}–1	0.002–0.8	0.01–1 (tension)	

to contribute to leakage of saliva, bacteria, and so on, at the interface margins. Such leakage in some cases can cause further decay of the tooth.

Use of colloidal silica in the so-called "microfilled" composites allows for these resins to be polished, so that less wear occurs and less plaque accumulates. It is more difficult, however, to make these with a high fraction of filler. All the dental composites exhibit creep. The stiffness changes by a factor of 2.5–4 (depending on the particular material) over a time period from 10 s to 3 h under steady load (Papadogianis et al., 1985). This creep may result in indentation of the restoration, but wear seems to be a greater problem.

Dental composite resins have become established as restorative materials for both anterior and posterior teeth. The use of these materials is likely to increase as improved compositions are developed and in response to concern over long-term toxicity of silver–mercury amalgam fillings.

31.5 Fibrous Composites

Fibers incorporated in a polymer matrix increase the stiffness, strength, fatigue life, and other properties (Agarwal and Broutman, 1980; Schwartz, 1992). Fibers are mechanically more effective in achieving a stiff, strong composite than are particles. Materials can be prepared in fiber form with very few defects which concentrate stress. Fibers such as graphite are stiff (with a Young modulus of 200–800 GPa) and strong (with the tensile strength of 2.7–5.5 GPa). Composites made from these can be as strong as steel but much lighter, as shown in Table 31.1. The stiffness of a composite with aligned fibers, if it is loaded along the fibers, is equivalent to the Voigt upper bound (Equation 31.1). Unidirectional fibrous composites, when loaded along the fibers, can have strengths and stiffnesses comparable to that of steel, but with much less weight (Table 31.1). However, if it is loaded transversely to the fibers, such a composite will be compliant, with a stiffness not much greater than that of the matrix alone. While unidirectional fiber composites can be made very strong in the longitudinal direction, they are weaker than the matrix alone when loaded transversely, as a result of stress concentration around the fibers. If stiffness and strength are needed in all directions, the fibers may be oriented randomly. For such a 3-D isotropic composite, for a low concentration of fibers,

$$E = \frac{E_i V_i}{6} + E_m \qquad (31.5)$$

so the stiffness is reduced by about a factor of 6 in comparison with an aligned composite as illustrated in Figure 31.3. However, if the fibers are aligned randomly in a plane, the reduction in stiffness is only by a factor of 3. The degree of anisotropy in fibrous composites can be very well controlled by forming laminates consisting of layers of fibers embedded in a matrix. Each layer can have fibers oriented in a different direction. One can achieve quasi-isotropic behavior in the laminate plane; such a laminate is not as strong or as stiff as a unidirectional one, as illustrated in Table 31.1. Strength of composites depends on such particulars as the brittleness or ductility of the inclusions and the matrix. In fibrous composites, failure may occur by (1) fiber breakage, buckling, or pullout, (2) matrix cracking, or (3) debonding of fiber from matrix.

Short fiber composites are used in many applications. They are not as stiff or as strong as composites with continuous fibers, but they can be formed economically by injection molding or by *in situ* polymerization. Choice of an optimal fiber length can result in improved toughness, due to the predominance of fiber pullout as a fracture mechanism.

Carbon fibers have been incorporated in the high-density polyethylene used in total knee replacements (Figure 31.5). The standard ultra-high-molecular-weight polyethylene (UHMWPE) used in these implants

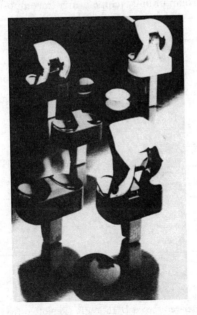

FIGURE 31.5 Knee prostheses with polyethylene tibial components reinforced with carbon fiber.

is considered adequate for most purposes for implantation in older patients. A longer wear-free implant lifetime is desirable for use in younger patients. It is considered desirable to improve the resistance to creep of the polymeric component, since excessive creep results in an indentation of that component after long-term use. Representative properties of carbon-reinforced UHMWPE are shown in Figure 31.6 (Sclippa and Piekarski, 1973). Enhancements of various properties by a factor of 2 are feasible.

PMMA used in bone cement is compliant and weak in comparison with bone. Therefore, several reinforcement methods have been attempted. Metal wires have been used clinically as macroscopic "fibers" to reinforce PMMA cement used in spinal stabilization surgery (Fishbane and Pond, 1977). The wires are made of a biocompatible alloy such as cobalt–chromium alloy or stainless steel. Such wires are not currently used in joint replacements owing to the limited space available. Graphite fibers have been incorporated in bone cement (Knoell et al., 1975) on an experimental basis. Significant improvements in the mechanical properties have been achieved. Moreover, the fibers have an added beneficial effect of reducing the rise in temperature which occurs during the polymerization of the PMMA in the body. Such high temperature can cause problems such as necrosis of a portion of the bone into which it is implanted. Thin, short titanium fibers have been embedded in PMMA cement (Topoleski et al., 1992); a toughness increase of 51% was observed with a 5% volumetric fiber content. Fiber reinforcement of PMMA cement has not found much acceptance since the fibers also increase the viscosity of the unpolymerized material. It is consequently difficult for the surgeon to form and shape the polymerizing cement during the surgical procedure.

Metals are currently used in bone plates for immobilizing fractures and in the femoral component of total hip replacements. A problem with currently used implant metals is that they are much stiffer than bone, so they shield the nearby bone from mechanical stress. Stress shielding results in a kind of disuse atrophy: the bone resorbs (Engh and Bobyn, 1988). Therefore, composite materials have been investigated as alternatives (Bradley et al., 1980; Skinner, 1988). Fibrous composites can deform to higher strains (to about 0.01) than metals (0.001 for a mild steel) without damage. This resilience is an attractive characteristic for more flexible bone plates and femoral stems. Flexible composite bone plates are effective in promoting healing (Jockish et al., 1992). Composite hip replacement prostheses have been made with carbon fibers in a matrix of polysulfone and polyetherether ketone. These prostheses experience heavy load with a static component. Structural metals such as stainless steel and cobalt–chromium alloys do not creep significantly at room or body temperature. In composites which contain a polymer

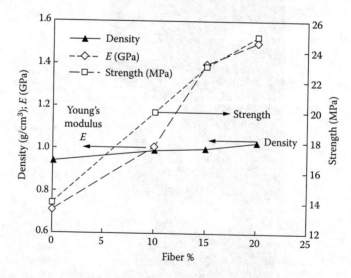

FIGURE 31.6 Properties of carbon fiber-reinforced UHMWPE. (Replotted from Sclippa, E. and Piekarski, K. 1973. *J. Biomed. Mater. Res.*, 7, 59–70. With permission.)

constituent, creep behavior is a matter of concern. The carbon fibers exhibit negligible creep, but polymer constituents tend to creep. Prototype composite femoral components were found to exhibit fiber-dominated creep of small magnitude and are not expected to limit the life of the implant (Maharaj and Jamison, 1993).

Fibrous composites have also been used in external medical devices such as knee braces (Yeaple, 1989), in which biocompatibility is not a concern but light weight is crucial.

31.6 Porous Materials

The presence of voids in porous or cellular solids will reduce the stiffness of the material. For some purposes, that is both acceptable and desirable. Porous solids are used for many purposes: flexible structures such as (1) seat cushions, (2) thermal insulation, (3) filters, (4) cores for stiff and lightweight sandwich panels, (5) flotation devices, and (6) to protect objects from mechanical shock and vibration; and in biomaterials, as coating to encourage tissue ingrowth. Representative cellular solid structures are shown in Figure 31.7.

The stiffness of an open-cell foam is given by (Gibson and Ashby, 1988)

$$E = E_s[V_s]^2 \qquad (31.6)$$

where E_s is the Young modulus and V_s is the volume fraction of the solid phase of the foam; V_s is also called the relative density.

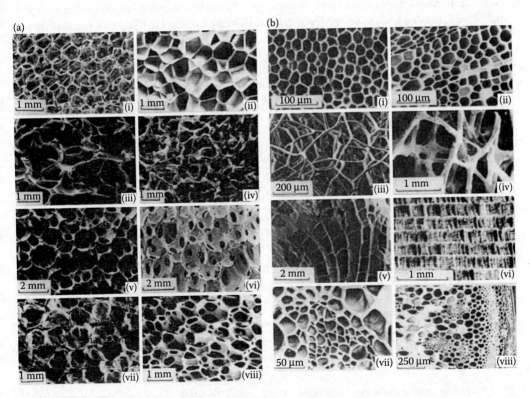

FIGURE 31.7 Cellular solid structures. (a) Synthetic cellular solids: (i) open-cell polyurethane, (ii) closed-cell polyethylene, (iii) foamed nickel, (iv) foamed copper, (v) foamed zirconia, (vi) foamed mullite, (vii) foamed glass, and (viii) polyester foam with both open and closed cells. (b) Natural cellular solids: (i) cork, (ii) balsa wood, (iii) sponge, (iv) cancellous bone, (v) coral, (vi) cuttlefish bone, (vii) iris leaf, and (viii) plant stalk. (After Gibson, L.J. and Ashby, M.F. 1988. *Cellular Solids: Structure and Properties*, Pergamon Press, Oxford.)

The strength for crushing of a brittle foam and the elastic collapse of an elastomeric foam is given, respectively, by

$$\sigma_{crush} = 0.65\sigma_{f,s}[V_s]^{3/2} \tag{31.7}$$

$$\sigma_{coll} = 0.05E_s[V_s]^2 \tag{31.8}$$

Here $\sigma_{f,s}$ is the fracture strength of the solid phase. These strength relations are valid for relatively small density. Their derivation is based on the concept of *bending* of the cell ribs and is presented by Gibson and Ashby (1988). Most man-made closed-cell foams tend to have a concentration of material at the cell edges, so that they behave mechanically as open cell foams. The salient point in the relations for the mechanical properties of cellular solids is that the *relative density* dramatically influences the stiffness and the strength. As for the relationship between stress and strain, a representative stress–strain curve is shown in Figure 31.8. The physical mechanism for the deformation mode beyond the elastic limit depends on the material from which the foam is made. Trabecular bone, for example, is a natural cellular solid, which tends to fail in compression by crushing. Many kinds of trabecular bone appear to behave mechanically as an open cell foam. For trabecular bone of unspecified orientation, the stiffness is proportional to the cube of the density and the strength as the square of the density (Gibson and Ashby, 1988), which indicates behavior dominated by bending of the trabeculae. For bone with oriented trabeculae, both stiffness and strength in the trabecular direction are proportional to the density, a fact which indicates behavior dominated by axial deformation of the trabeculae.

Porous materials have a high surface area to volume ratio. When porous materials are used in biomaterial applications, the demands upon the inertness and biocompatibility are likely to be greater than for a homogeneous material.

Porous materials, when used in implants, allow tissue ingrowth (Spector et al., 1988a,b). The ingrowth is considered desirable in many contexts, since it allows a relatively permanent anchorage of the implant to the surrounding tissues. There are actually two composites to be considered in porous implants: (1) the

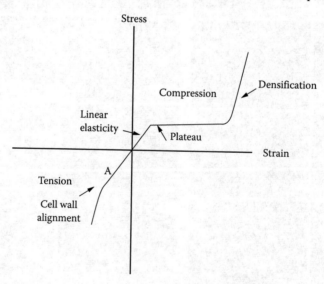

FIGURE 31.8 Representative stress–strain curve for a cellular solid. The plateau region for compression in the case of elastomeric foam (a rubbery polymer) represents elastic buckling; for an elastic–plastic foam (such as metallic foam), it represents plastic yield, and for an elastic-brittle foam (such as ceramic) it represents crushing. On the tension side, point "A" represents the transition between cell wall bending and cell wall alignment. In elastomeric foam, the alignment occurs elastically, in elastic plastic foam it occurs plastically, and an elastic-brittle foam fractures at A.

implant prior to ingrowth, in which the pores are filled with tissue fluid which is ordinarily of no mechanical consequence; and (2) the implant filled with tissue. In the case of the implant prior to ingrowth, it must be recognized that the stiffness and strength of the porous solid are much less than in the case of the solid from which it is derived.

Porous layers are used on bone-compatible implants to encourage bony ingrowth (Galante et al., 1971; Ducheyne, 1984). The pore size of a cellular solid has no influence on its stiffness or strength (though it does influence the toughness); however, pore size can be of considerable biological importance. Specifically, in orthopedic implants with pores larger than about 150 μm, bony ingrowth into the pores occurs and this is useful to anchor the implant. This minimum pore size is on the order of the diameter of osteons in normal Haversian bone. It was found experimentally that pores <75 μm in size did not permit the ingrowth of bone tissue. Moreover, it was difficult to maintain fully viable osteons within pores in the 75–150 μm size range. Representative structure of such a porous surface layer is shown in Figure 31.9. Porous coatings are also under study for application in anchoring the artificial roots of dental implants to the underlying jawbone. Porous hydroxyapatite has been studied for use in repairing large defects in bone (Meffert et al., 1985; Holmes et al., 1986). Hydroxyapatite is the mineral constituent of bone and has the nominal composition $Ca_{10}(PO_4)_6(OH)_2$. Implanted hydroxyapatite is slowly resorbed by the body over several years and replaced by bone. Tricalcium phosphate is resorbed more quickly and has been considered as an implant constituent to speed healing.

When a porous material is implanted in bone, the pores become filled first with blood which clots, then with osteoprogenitor mesenchymal cells, then, after about 4 weeks, bony trabeculae. The ingrown bone then becomes remodeled in response to mechanical stress. The bony ingrowth process depends on the degree of mechanical stability in the early stages of healing. If too much motion occurs, the ingrown tissue will be collagenous scar tissue, not bone.

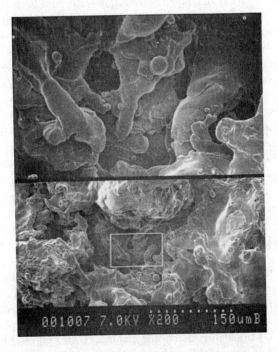

FIGURE 31.9 Irregular pore structure of porous coating in Ti5Al4V alloy for bony ingrowth. The top scanning electron microscopic picture is a ×5 magnification of the rectangular region of the bottom picture (×200). (From Park, J.B. and Lakes, R.S. 1992. *Biomaterials*, 2nd ed., Plenum Press, New York.)

Porous materials used in soft tissue applications include polyurethane, polyamide, and polyester velours used in percutaneous devices. Porous reconstituted collagen has been used in artificial skin, and braided polypropylene has been used in artificial ligaments. As in the case of bone implants, the porosity encourages tissue ingrowth which anchors the device.

Blood vessel replacements are made with porous materials which encourage soft tissue to grow in, eventually forming a new lining, or neointima. The new lining consists of the patient's own cells. It is a natural nonthrombogenic surface resembling the lining of the original blood vessel. This is a further example of the biological role of porous materials as contrasted with the mechanical role.

Ingrowth of tissue into implant pores is not always desirable. For example, sponge (polyvinyl alcohol) implants used in early mammary augmentation surgery underwent ingrowth of fibrous tissue, and contracture and calcification of that tissue, resulting in hardened, calcified breasts. Current mammary implants make use of a balloon-like nonporous silicone rubber layer enclosing silicone oil or gel, or perhaps a saline solution in water. A porous layer of polyester felt or velour attached to the balloon is provided at the back surface of the implant so that limited tissue ingrowth will anchor it to the chest wall and prevent it from migrating.

Foams are also used externally to protect the human body from injury. Examples include knee pads, elbow pads, wrestling mats, and wheelchair cushions. Since these foams are only in contact with skin rather than any internal organs, they are not subject to rigorous biocompatibility requirements. They are therefore designed based on mechanical considerations. Foam used in sports equipment must have the correct compliance to limit impact force without bottoming out. Foam used in wheelchair cushions is intended to prevent pressure sores in people who suffer limited mobility. The properties of cushions are crucial in reducing illness and suffering in people who are confined to wheelchairs or hospital beds for long periods. Prolonged pressure on body parts can obstruct circulation in the capillaries. If this lasts too long, it may cause a sore or ulcer called a pressure sore, also called a bed sore. In its most severe manifestation, a pressure sore can form a deep crater-like ulcer in which underlying muscle or bone is exposed (Dinsdale, 1974). A variety of flexible cushion materials have been tried to minimize the incidence and severity of pressure sores (Garber, 1985). Viscoelastic foam allows the cushion to progressively conform to the body shape. However, progressive densification of the foam due to creep results in a stiffer cushion which must be periodically replaced.

Porous materials are produced in a variety of ways. For example, in the case of bone-compatible surfaces they are formed by sintering of beads or wires. Vascular and soft tissue implants are produced by weaving or braiding fibers as well as by nonwoven "felting" methods. Protective foams for use outside the body are usually produced by the use of a "blowing agent" which is a chemical which evolves gas during the polymerization of the foam. An interesting approach to produce microporous materials is the replication of structures found in biological materials: the *replamineform* process (White et al., 1976). The rationale is that the unique structure of communicating pores is thought to offer advantages in the induction of tissue ingrowth. The skeletal structure of coral or echinoderms (such as sea urchins) is replicated by a casting process in metals and polymers; these have been tried in vascular and tracheal prostheses as well as in bone substitutes.

31.7 Biocompatibility

Carbon itself has been successfully used as a biomaterial. Carbon-based fibers used in composites are known to be inert in aqueous (even seawater) environments; however, they do not have a track record in the biomaterials setting. *In vitro* studies by Kovacs (1993) disclose substantial electrochemical activity of carbon fiber composites in an aqueous environment. If such composites are placed near a metallic implant, galvanic corrosion is a possibility. Composite materials with a polymer matrix absorb water when placed in a hydrated environment such as the body. Moisture acts as a plasticizer of the matrix and shifts the glass transition temperature toward lower values (DeIasi and Whiteside, 1978), hence a reduction in stiffness and an increase in mechanical damping. Water immersion of a graphite epoxy cross-ply composite (Gopalan et al., 1989) for 20 days reduced the strength by 13% and the stiffness by 9%. Moisture absorption by polymer constituents also causes swelling. Such swelling can be beneficial in dental composites since it offsets some of the shrinkage due to polymerization.

Flexible composite bone plates are effective in promoting healing (Jockish et al., 1992), but particulate debris from composite bone plates gives rise to a foreign body reaction similar to that caused by UHMWPE.

31.8 Summary

Composite materials are a relatively recent addition to the class of materials used in structural applications. In the biomaterials field, the ingress of composites has been even more recent. In view of their potential for high performance, composite materials are likely to find increasing use as biomaterials.

References

Agarwal, A.G. and Broutman, L.J. 1980. *Analysis and Performance of Fiber Composites*, Wiley, New York.

Bradley, J.S., Hastings, G.W., and Johnson-Hurse, C. 1980. Carbon fiber reinforced epoxy as a high strength, low modulus material for internal fixation plates, *Biomaterials* 1, 38–40.

Cannon, M.L. 1988. Composite resins, In: *Encyclopedia of Medical Devices and Instrumentation*, J.G. Webster, Ed., Wiley, New York.

Christensen, R.M. 1979. *Mechanics of Composite Materials*, Wiley, New York.

Craig, R. 1981. Chemistry, composition, and properties of composite resins, In: *Dental Clinics of North America*, H. Horn, Ed., W.B. Saunders, Philadelphia, PA.

Craig, R.G. and Peyton, F.A. 1958. Elastic and mechanical properties of human dentin, *J. Dental Res.*, 37, 710–718.

DeIasi, R. and Whiteside, J.B. 1978. *Effect of Moisture on Epoxy Resins and Composites: Advanced Composite Materials—Environmental Effects*, J.R. Vinson, Ed., ASTM Publication STP 658, ASTM, Philadelphia, PA.

Dinsdale, S.M. 1974. Decubitus ulcers: Role of pressure and friction in causation, *Arch. Phys. Med. Rehabil.*, 55, 147–152.

Ducheyne, P. 1984. Biological fixation of implants, In: *Functional Behavior of Orthopaedic Biomaterials*, G.W. Hastings and P. Ducheyne, Eds., CRC Press, Boca Raton, FL.

Engh, C.A. and Bobyn, J.D. 1988. Results of porous coated hip replacement using the AML prosthesis, In: *Non-Cemented Total Hip Arthroplasty*, R. Fitzgerald, Jr Ed., Raven Press, New York.

Fishbane, B.M. and Pond, R.B. 1977. Stainless steel fiber reinforcement of polymethylmethacrylate, *Clin. Orthop.*, 128, 490–498.

Galante, J., Rostoker, W., Lueck, R., and Ray, R.D. 1971. Sintered fiber metal composites as a basis for attachment of implants to bone, *J. Bone Joint Surg.*, 53A, 101–114.

Garber, S.L. 1985. Wheelchair cushions: A historical review, *Am. J. Occup. Ther.*, 39, 453–459.

Gibson, L.J. and Ashby, M.F. 1988. *Cellular Solids: Structure and Properties*, Pergamon Press, Oxford.

Gopalan, R., Somashekar, B.R., and Dattaguru, B. 1989. Environmental effects on fiber–polymer composites, *Polym. Degradat. Stabil.*, 24, 361–371.

Hashin, Z. and Shtrikman, S. 1963. A variational approach to the theory of the elastic behavior of multiphase materials, *J. Mech. Phys. Solids*, 11, 127–140.

Holmes, D.E., Bucholz, R.W., and Mooney, V. 1986. Porous hydroxyapatite as a bone graft substitute in metaphyseal defects, *J. Bone Joint Surg.*, 68, 904–911.

Jockish, K.A., Brown, S.A., Bauer, T.W., and Merritt, K. 1992. Biological response to chopped carbon reinforced PEEK, *J. Biomed. Mater. Res.*, 26, 133–146.

Katz, J.L. 1980. Anisotropy of Young's modulus of bone. *Nature*, 283, 106–107.

Knoell, A., Maxwell, H., and Bechtol, C. 1975. Graphite fiber reinforced bone cement. *Ann. Biomed. Eng.*, 3, 225–229.

Kovacs, P. 1993. *In vitro* studies of the electrochemical behavior of carbon–fiber composites, In: *Composite Materials for Implant Applications in the Human Body: Characterization and Testing, ASTM STP 1178*, R.D. Jamison and L.N. Gilbertson, Eds., ASTM, Philadelphia, PA, pp. 41–52.

Lakes, R.S. 1993. Materials with structural hierarchy, *Nature*, 361, 511–515.

Lekhnitskii, S.G. 1963. *Theory of Elasticity of an Anisotropic Elastic Body*, Holden-Day, San Francisco.

Maharaj, G.R. and Jamison, R.D. 1993. Creep testing of a composite material human hip prosthesis, In: *Composite Materials for Implant Applications in the Human Body: Characterization and Testing, ASTM STP 1178*, R.D. Jamison and L.N. Gilbertson, Eds., ASTM, Philadelphia, PA, pp. 86–97.

Meffert, R.M., Thomas, J.R., Hamilton, K.M., and Brownstein, C.N. 1985. Hydroxyapatite as allopathic graft in the treatment of periodontal osseous defects, *J. Periodontol.*, 56, 63–73.

Nye, J.F. 1976. *Physical Properties of Crystals*, Oxford University Press, Oxford.

Papadogianis, Y., Boyer, D.B., and Lakes, R.S. 1985. Creep of posterior dental composites, *J. Biomed. Mater. Res.*, 19, 85–95.

Park, J.B. and Lakes, R.S. 1992. *Biomaterials*, 2nd ed., Plenum Press, New York.

Park, H.C., Liu, Y.K., and Lakes, R.S. 1986. The material properties of bone–particle impregnated PMMA, *J. Biomech. Eng.*, 108, 141–148.

Paul, B. 1960. Prediction of elastic constants of multiphase materials, *Trans. AIME*, 218, 36–41.

Peters, M.C., Poort, H.W., Farah, J.W., and Graig, R.G. 1983. Stress analysis of a tooth restored with a post and a core, *J. Dental Res.*, 62, 760–763.

Reilly, D.T. and Burstein, A.H. 1975. The elastic and ultimate properties of compact bone tissue, *J. Biomech.*, 8, 393–405.

Schwartz, M.M. 1992. *Composite Materials Handbook*, 2nd ed., McGraw-Hill, New York.

Sclippa, E. and Piekarski, K. 1973. Carbon fiber reinforced polyethylene for possible orthopaedic usage, *J. Biomed. Mater. Res.*, 7, 59–70.

Skinner, H.B. 1988. Composite technology for total hip arthroplasty, *Clin. Orthop. Rel. Res.*, 235, 224–236.

Spector, M., Miller, M., and Beals, N. 1988a. Porous materials, In: *Encyclopedia of Medical Devices and Instrumentation*, J.G. Webster, Ed., Wiley, New York.

Spector, M., Heyligers, I., and Robertson, J.R. 1988b. Porous polymers for biological fixation, *Clin. Orthop. Rel. Res.*, 235, 207–219.

Topoleski, L.D.T., Ducheyne, P., and Cackler, J.M. 1992. The fracture toughness of titanium fiber reinforced bone cement, *J. Biomed. Mater. Res.*, 26, 1599–1617.

White, R.A., Weber, J.N., and White, E.W. 1976. Replamineform: a new process for preparing porous ceramic, metal, and polymer prosthetic materials, *Science*, 176, 922.

Yeaple, F. 1989. Composite knee brace returns stability to joint, *Design News*, 46, 116.

32

Biodegradable Polymeric Biomaterials: An Updated Overview

32.1 Introduction 32-1
32.2 Glycolide/Lactide-Based Biodegradable Linear Aliphatic
Polyesters... 32-4
Glycolide-Based Biodegradable Homopolymer
Polyesters • Glycolide-Based Biodegradable Copolyesters Having
Aliphatic Polyester-Based Co-Monomers • Glycolide-Based
Biodegradable Copolyesters with Nonaliphatic Polyester-Based
Co-Monomers • Glycolide-Derived Biodegradable Polymers
Having Ether Linkage • Lactide Biodegradable Homopolymers and
Copolymers
32.3 Nonglycolide/Lactide-Based Linear Aliphatic Polyesters...... 32-11
32.4 Nonaliphatic Polyester-Type Biodegradable Polymers........... 32-11
Aliphatic and Aromatic Polycarbonates • Poly(alkylene oxalates)
and Copolymers • Amino Acid-Based Poly(ester amide)s and
Copolymers • Poly(carbonate-acetal)s from Dihydroxyacetone
32.5 Biodegradation Properties of Synthetic Biodegradable
Polymers.. 32-21
Theoretical Modeling of Degradation Properties • The Role of Free
Radicals in Degradation Properties
32.6 Role of Linear Aliphatic Biodegradable Polyesters in Tissue
Engineering and Regeneration 32-24
32.7 Supercritical Carbon Dioxide Sterilization 32-27
Defining Terms 32-29
References.. 32-29
Further Information.. 32-37

C. C. Chu
Cornell University

32.1 Introduction

The term biodegradation is loosely associated with biomaterials that could be broken down by nature either through hydrolytic mechanisms without the help of enzymes or through enzyme-catalyzed mechanisms. Terms such as absorbable, erodible, and resorbable have also been used in the literature to indicate biodegradation.

The interests in biodegradable polymeric biomaterials for biomedical engineering use have increased dramatically during the past decades. This is because this class of biomaterials has two major advantages that nonbiodegradable biomaterials do not have. First, they do not elicit permanent chronic foreign-body reactions because they are gradually absorbed by the human body and do not permanently leave any traces of residual in the implantation sites. Second, some of them have recently been found to be able to regenerate tissues, the so-called tissue engineering, through the interaction of their biodegradation with immunologic cells like macrophages. Hence, surgical implants/devices made from biodegradable biomaterials could be used as temporary scaffolds for tissue regeneration. This approach toward the reconstruction of injured, diseased, or aged tissues is one of the most promising fields in the next century.

Although the earliest and most commercially significant biodegradable polymeric biomaterials were originated from linear aliphatic polyesters such as polyglycolide, polylactide, poly(ε-caprolactone), and their copolymers from poly(α-hydroxyacetic acids) family, the subsequent introduction of several new synthetic and natural biodegradable polymeric biomaterials extends the domain beyond this family of simple aliphatic polyesters. These relatively newer, commercially significant biodegradable polymeric biomaterials include poly(orthoesters), polyanhydrides, polysaccharides, poly(ester-amides), tyrosine-based polyarylates or polyiminocarbonates or polycarbonates, poly(D,L-lactide-urethane), poly(β-hydroxybutyrate), poly[bis(carboxylatophenoxy) phosphazene], poly(amino acids), pseudo-poly(amino acids), copolymers derived from amino acids and nonamino acids, and amino acid-based poly(ester amide)s and poly(ester urethane).

All the above biodegradable polymeric biomaterials could be generally divided into nine groups based on their chemical origin: (1) Biodegradable linear aliphatic polyesters [e.g., polyglycolide, polylactide, poly-ε-caprolactone (PCL), poly(hydroxybutyrate)] and their copolymers within the aliphatic polyester family such as poly(glycolide-L-lactide) copolymer and poly(glycolide-ε-caprolactone) copolymer and their melt-blending of glycolide and lactide base (Shalaby, 1994); (2) biodegradable copolymers between linear aliphatic polyesters in (1) and monomers other than linear aliphatic polyesters such as poly(glycolide-trimethylene carbonate) (TMC) copolymer, poly(L-lactic acid-L-lysine) copolymer, tyrosine-based polyarylates or polyiminocarbonates or polycarbonates, poly(D,L-lactide-urethane), and nonamino acid-based poly(ester-amide); (3) polyanhydrides; (4) poly(orthoesters); (5) poly(ester-ethers) such as poly-p-dioxanone (PDS); (6) polysaccharides such as hyaluronic acid, chitin, and chitosan; (7) polyamino acids such as poly-L-glutamic acid and poly-L-lysine; (8) amino acid-based poly(ester amide)s and poly(ester urethane); (9) inorganic biodegradable polymers such as polyphosphazene and poly[bis(carboxylatophenoxy) phosphazene] which have a nitrogen–phosphorus backbone instead of ester linkage.

The earliest, most successful, and frequent biomedical applications of biodegradable polymeric biomaterials have been in wound closure (Chu et al., 1997; Chu, in press). All synthetic absorbable wound closure biomaterials are made from the different combinations of five building blocks: glycolide, L-lactide, ε-caprolactone, trimethylene carbonate (1,3-dioxan-2-one), and p-dioxanone (1,4 dioxane-2-one). Table 32.1 lists the type of building blocks required to fabricate all commercially available absorbable wound closure biomaterials.

This family of absorbable polymeric biomaterials is also the one most studied for their chemical, physical, mechanical, morphological, and biological properties and their changes with degradation time and environment. Some of these absorbable biomaterials such as Vicryl have also been commercially used as surgical meshes for repair of hernia or body wall. Table 32.2 lists the important physical, thermal, and mechanical properties of the most common aliphatic polyesters.

A newcomer to the absorbable suture family is TephaFlex® from Tepha which received FDA approval for marketing in April 2007 (FDA, 2007). TephaFlex is made from a new class of biopolymer that is different from the traditional polyglycolide and polylactide family. TephaFlex is a member of the class of biomaterials known as polyhydroxyalkanoates, particularly poly-4-hydroxybyutrate (P4HB). P4HB is a natural biomaterial produced by numerous microorganisms through a fermentation process based on Tepha-patented recombinant DNA technology. Because of the biological production of P4HB, it does not contain residual metal catalysts and hence very biocompatible (Martin and Williams, 2003). Due to its thermoplastic character, P4HB can be molded by conventional melt-based processes such as melt-spinning, extrusion, and blowing. Table 32.3 shows the effect of 3HB co-monomer on physical and thermal properties of P4HB copolymers. When compared with synthetic absorbable aliphatic polyesters, P4HB shows the most elastomeric character with T_g close to PCL as shown in Table 32.4.

TABLE 32.1 Building Blocks of Commercial Synthetic Absorbable Sutures

	Glycolide	L-Lactide	ε-Caprolactone	Trimethylene Carbonate (1,3-dioxan-2-one)	p-Dioxanone (1,4-dioxane-2-one)
Dexon, Dexon II, Dexon S, Bondek, Safil Surucryl, PolySynFA, Biovek	X				
Vicryl, Vicryl Rapide, Vicryl Plus, Panacryl, Polysorb	X	X			
Maxon	X			X	
Monocryl, Monocryl Plus, Suruglyde	X		X		
PDS, PDSII, PDS Plus, Monodek, MonoPlus, Surusynth					X
Biosyn	X			X	X
Monosyn	X		X	X	
Caprosyn	X	X	X	X	
Orthodek		X			

The next largest biomedical application of biodegradable polymeric biomaterials that are commercially satisfactory is drug control/release devices. Some well-known examples in this application are polyanhydrides and poly(orthoester). Other biodegradable polymeric biomaterials, particularly totally resorbable composites, have also been experimentally used in the field of orthopedics, mainly as components for internal bone fracture fixation such as PDS pins. However, their wide acceptance in other parts of orthopedic implants may be limited due to their inherent mechanical properties and their biodegradation rate. Besides the commercial uses described above, biodegradable polymeric biomaterials have been experimented with as (1) vascular grafts, (2) vascular stents, (3) vascular couplers for vessel anastomosis, (4) nerve growth conduits, (5) augmentation of defected bone, (6) ligament/tendon prostheses, (7) intramedullary plug during total hip replacement, (8) anastomosis ring for intestinal surgery,

TABLE 32.2 Properties of Commercially Important Synthetic Absorbable Polymers

Polymer	Crystallinity	T_m (°C)	T_g (°C)	T_{dec} (°C)	Fiber Strength (MPa)	Modulus (GPa)	Elongation (%)
PGA	High	230	36	260	890	8.4	30
PLLA	High	170	56	240	900	8.5	25
PLA	None	—	57	—	—	—	—
Polyglactin910[a]	High[b]	200	40	250	850	8.6	24
Polydioxanone	High	106	<20	190	490	2.1	35
Polyglyconate[c]	High[b]	213	<20	260	550	2.4	45
Poliglecaprone25[d]	—	<220	−36	~15	91,100[e]	113,000[e]	39

Source: Adapted from Kimura, Y., 1993. *Biomedical Applications of Polymeric Materials*, pp. 164–190. CRC Press, Boca Raton, FL; Chu, C.C., von Fraunhofer, J.A., and Greisler, H.P., 1997. *Wound Closure Biomaterials and Devices*, CRC Press, Boca Raton, FL.

[a] Glycolide per lactide = 9/1.

[b] Depending on the copolymer composition.

[c] Glycolide per TMC = 9/1.

[d] 2/0 size Monocryl (glycolide-ε-caprolactone copolymer).

[e] PSI unit.

TABLE 32.3 Effect of 3HB Co-Monomers on the Properties of Absorbable Elastomeric P4HB Copolymers Incorporating 3HB

Percentage of 4HB Monomer (by ^{1}H NMR)	Durometer Hardness (Shore A scale)	Glass Transition Temperature, T_g (°C)
24	92.5	−10.3
28	82.3	−11.1
31	69.4	−13.2
33	62.2	−14.4
35	59.5	−17.2

Source: Data adapted from Martin, D.P. and Williams, S.F. 2003. *Biochem. Eng. J.*, 16: 97–105.

TABLE 32.4 Comparisons of Properties of P4HB with Other Synthetic Absorbable Aliphatic Polyesters

	Melting Temperature, T_m (°C)	T_g (°C)	Tensile Strength (MPa)	Tensile Modulus (MPa)	Elongation at Break (%)	Absorption Rate
PGA	225	36–45	70	6900	<3	6 weeks
PLLA	175		28–50	1200–2700	6	1.5–5 years
DL-PLA	Amorphous		29–35	1900–2400	6	3 months
PCL	57	−62	16	400	80	2 years
P3HB	180		36	2500	3	2 years
P4HB	60	−51	50	70	1000	8–52 weeks

Source: Data adapted from Martin, D.P. and Williams, S.F. 2003. *Biochem. Eng. J.*, 16: 97–105.
Abbreviations: DL-PLA, copolymer of *p*- and L-Lactide; P3HB, poly-3-hydroxybutyrate; PCL, polycaprolactone.

and (9) drug-eluting stents in treating restenosis of blood vessels and ureteroureterostomies for accurate suture placement.

Owing to space limitation, the emphasis of this chapter will be on the commercially most significant and successful biomedical biodegradable polymers based on (1) linear aliphatic polyesters, (2) some very recent research and development of important classes of synthetic biodegradable polymers, (3) a theoretical approach to modeling the hydrolytic degradation of glycolide/lactide-based biodegradable polymers, (4) the effects of some new extrinsic factors on the degradation of the most commercially significant biodegradable polymers, (5) the new biomedical applications of this class of synthetic biodegradable polymers in tissue engineering and regeneration, (6) the newly developed amino acid-based poly(ester amide)s and their copolymers (pseudo-proteins), and (7) a newly developed sterilization method (supercritical carbon dioxide, or scCO$_2$) for these absorbable biomaterials. The details of the applications of this family and other biodegradable polymeric biomaterials and their chemical, physical, mechanical, biological, and biodegradation properties can be found in other recent reviews (Barrows, 1986; Vert et al., 1992; Kimura, 1993; Park et al., 1993; Shalaby, 1994; Hollinger, 1995; Chu et al., 1997; Ikada et al., 2000; Gunatillake et al., 2006; Nair et al., 2007; Yu et al. 2010; Woodruff and Hutmacher, 2010; Chu, in press).

32.2 Glycolide/Lactide-Based Biodegradable Linear Aliphatic Polyesters

This class of biodegradable polymers is the most successful, important, and commercially widely used biodegradable biomaterials in surgery. It is also the class of biodegradable biomaterials that were most extensively studied in terms of degradation mechanisms and structure–property relationships. Among them, polyglycolide or polyglycolic acid (PGA) is the most important one because most other biodegradable polymers are derived from PGA either through copolymerization, for example, poly(glycolide-L-lactide) copolymer or through modified glycolide monomer, for example, PDS.

32.2.1 Glycolide-Based Biodegradable Homopolymer Polyesters

PGA can be polymerized either directly or indirectly from glycolic acid. The direct polycondensation produces a polymer of M_n less than 10,000 because of the requirement of a very high degree of dehydration (99.28% up) and the absence of monofunctional impurities. For PGA of molecular weight higher than 10,000, it is necessary to proceed through the ring-opening polymerization of the cyclic dimers of glycolic acid. Numerous catalysts are available for this ring-opening polymerization.

They include organometallic compounds and Lewis acids (Chujo et al., 1967a; Wise et al., 1979). For biomedical applications, stannous chloride dihydrate or trialkyl aluminum are preferred. PGA was found to exhibit an orthorhombic unit cell with dimensions $a = 5.22$ Å, $b = 6.19$ Å, and c (fiber axis) = 7.02 Å (Chujo et al., 1967b). The planar zigzag-chain molecules form a sheet structure parallel to the ac-plane and do not have the polyethylene-type arrangement (Chatani et al., 1968). The molecules between two adjacent sheets orient in opposite directions. The tight molecular packing and the close approach of the ester groups might stabilize the crystal lattice and contribute to the high melting point, T_m, of PGA (224–230°C). The glass transition temperature, T_g, ranges from 36 to 40°C. The specific gravities of PGA are 1.707 for a perfect crystal and 1.50 in a completely amorphous state (Chujo et al., 1967a). The heat of fusion of 100% crystallized PGA is reported to be 12 kJ/mol (45.7 cal/g) (Brandrup and Immergut, 1975). A study of injection-molded PGA disks reveals their IR spectroscopic characteristics (Chu et al., 1995). As shown in Figure 32.1, the four bands at 850, 753, 713, and 560 cm⁻¹ are associated with the amorphous regions of the PGA disks and could be used to assess the extends of hydrolysis. Peaks associated with the crystalline phase included those at 972, 901, 806, 627, and 590 cm⁻¹. Two broad, intense peaks at 1142 and 1077 cm⁻¹ can be assigned to C–O stretching modes in the ester and oxymethylene groups, respectively. These two peaks are associated mainly with ester and oxymethylene groups originating in the amorphous domains. Hydrolysis could cause both these C–O stretching modes to substantially decrease in intensity.

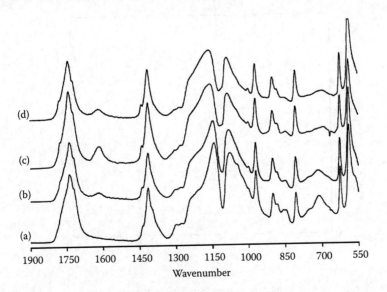

FIGURE 32.1 FTIR spectra of PGA disks as a function of *in vitro* hydrolysis time in phosphate buffer of pH 7.44 at 37°C: (a) 0 day; (b) 55 h; (c) 7 days; (d) 21 days.

32.2.2 Glycolide-Based Biodegradable Copolyesters Having Aliphatic Polyester-Based Co-Monomers

Other commercially successful glycolide-based biodegradable polymeric biomaterials are the copolymers of glycolide with other monomers within linear aliphatic polyesters such as lactides, carbonates, and ε-caprolactone. The glycolide–lactide random copolymers are the most studied and have a wide range of properties and applications, depending on the composition ratio of glycolide to lactide. Figure 32.2 illustrates the dependence of biodegradation rate on the composition of glycolide to lactide in the copolymer. For wound closure purposes, a high concentration of glycolide monomer is required for achieving proper mechanical and degradation properties. Vicryl sutures, sometime called polyglactin 910, contain a 90/10 molar ratio of glycolic to L-lactide and this molar ratio is important for the Vicryl suture to retain crystalline characteristics. For biomedical use, Lewis acid catalysts are preferred for the copolymers (Wise et al., 1979).

Ethicon introduced a similar glycolide-L-lactide copolymer suture in late 1990s, Panacryl®, but basically reversed the molar ratio of Vicryl®, 5/95 molar ratio of glycolide to L-lactide. As a result of predominant L-lactide component in Panacryl suture, its absorption behaves more like PLA than PGA, that is, Panacryl requires at least 1.5 years or longer to be completely absorbed in living tissues. Such a prolonged absorption profile *in vivo* may be associated with some reported postoperation complications (Farnsworth, 2002; Vakili et al., 2004; Goldstein et al., 2007). It is well known that a prolonged *in vivo* degradation period of absorbable sutures could expose patients to the risk of late-stage tissue reactions and hence may cancel out the advantage of slow degradation. For example, Eittenmuller et al. (1989a) reported that 47.7% (9 of 19 patients) treated with PLA plates and screws for ankle fracture had an inflammatory reaction nearly 3 years after operation. Bostman (1991) expressed a similar concern as he reported that late inflammatory reaction encountered in 8% of the patients is a worrisome complication. As a result, Panacryl was withdrawn from the market by Ethicon in mid-2000. Deknatel introduced a 100% PLA absorbable suture (Orthodek®) that is intended for wounds required a prolonged strength support like in orthopedic field. Vicryl sutures are sterilized by ethylene oxide like other synthetic absorbable sutures.

If D,L- instead of L-lactide is used as the co-monomer, the U-shaped relationship between the level of crystallinity and glycolide composition disappears. This is because polylactide from 100% D,L-lactide

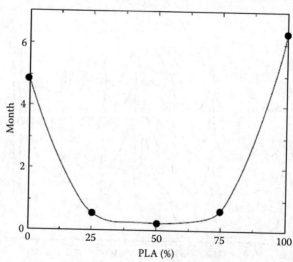

FIGURE 32.2 The effect of poly(L-lactide) composition in polyglycolide on the time required for 50% mass loss implanted under the dorsal skin of rat. (From Miller, R.A., Brady, J.M., and Cutright, D.E., 1977. *J. Biomed. Mater. Res.*, 11: 711. With permission.)

composition is totally amorphous. IR bands associated with Vicryl molecules in the amorphous domains are 560, 710, 850, and 888 cm^{-1}, whereas 590, 626, 808, 900, and 972 cm^{-1} are associated with the crystalline domains (Fredericks et al., 1984). Like PGA, these IR bands could be used to assess the extent of hydrolysis.

A relatively new block copolymer of glycolide and carbonates, such as TMC, has been commercialized. Maxon is made from a block copolymer of glycolide and 1,3-dioxan-2-one (trimethylene carbonate or GTMC) and consists of 32.5 wt% by weight (or 36 mol%) of TMC (Casey and Roby, 1984; Katz et al., 1985). Maxon is a poly(ester-carbonate). The polymerization process of Maxon is divided into two stages. The first stage is the formation of a middle block which is a random copolymer of glycolide and 1,3-dioxan-2-one. Diethylene glycol is used as an initiator and stannous chloride dihydrate (SnCl$_2 \cdot$ 2H$_2$O) serves as the catalyst. The polymerization is conducted at about 180°C. The weight ratio of glycolide to TMC in the middle block is 15:85. After the synthesis of the middle block, the temperature of the reactive bath is raised to about 220°C to prevent the crystallization of the copolymer, and additional glycolide monomers as the end blocks are added into the reaction bath to form the final triblock copolymer.

The latest glycolide-based copolymer that has become commercially successful is Monocryl® suture. It is a segmented block copolymer consisting of both soft and hard segments. The purpose of having soft segments in the copolymer is to provide good handling properties such as pliability, whereas the hard segments are used to provide adequate strength. The generic copolymerization process between glycolic acid and ε-caprolactone was recently reported by Fukuzaki et al. (1989, 1991) in Japan. The resulting copolymers were low-molecular-weight biodegradable copolymers of glycolic acid and various lactones for potential drug delivery purposes. The composition of lactone ranged from as low as 15 to as high as 50 mol% and the weight average for molecular weight ranged from 4510 to 16,500. The glass transition temperature ranged from 18 to −43°C, depending on the copolymer composition and molecular weight.

Monocryl is made from two stages of the polymerization process (Bezwada et al., 1995). In the first stage, soft segments of prepolymer of glycolide and ε-caprolactone are made. This soft segmented prepolymer is further polymerized with glycolides to provide hard segments of polyglycolide. Monocryl has a composition of 75% glycolide and 25% ε-caprolactone and should have a higher molecular weight than those glycolide/ε-caprolactone copolymers reported by Fukuzaki et al., for adequate mechanical properties required by sutures. The most unique aspect of Monocryl monofilament suture is its pliability as claimed by Ethicon (Bezwada et al., 1995). The force required to bend a 2/0 suture is only about 2.8 × 10^4 lb-in.^{2} for Monocryl, while the same sized PDSII® and Maxon® monofilament sutures require about 3.9 and 11.6 × 10^4 lb-in.^{2} force, respectively. This inherent pliability of Monocryl is due to the presence of soft segments and T_g resulting from the ε-caprolactone co-monomer unit. Its T_g is expected to be between 15°C and −36°C.

32.2.3 Glycolide-Based Biodegradable Copolyesters with Nonaliphatic Polyester-Based Co-Monomers

In this category, the most important one is the glycolide copolymer consisting of poly(ethylene 1,4-phenylene-bis-oxyacetate) (PEPBO) (Jamiokowski and Shalaby, 1991). The development of this type of glycolide-based copolymer was initiated because of the adverse effect of γ-irradiation on the mechanical properties of glycolide-based synthetic absorbable sutures. There is a great desire to develop γ-irradiation sterilizable, synthetic, absorbable polymers to take advantage of the highly convenient and reliable method of sterilization.

Shalaby et al. recently reported that incorporation of about 10 mol% of a polymeric radiostabilizer like PEPBO into PGA backbone chains would make the copolymer sterilizable by γ-irradiation without a significant accelerated loss of mechanical properties upon hydrolysis when compared with the unirradiated copolymer control (MPG) (Jamiokowski et al., 1991). The changes in tensile-breaking force of both MPG and PGA sutures implanted intramuscularly and subcutaneously in rats for various periods show the great advantage of such copolymers. MPG fibers γ-irradiated at 2.89 Mrad did not show any loss in tensile-breaking force during the first 14 days postimplantation when compared with unimplanted samples. On the contrary, PGA sutures γ-irradiated at 2.75 Mrad lost 62% of the tensile-breaking force of their unimplanted samples. There was no tensile-breaking force remaining for the irradiated PGA at the end of 21 days, whereas both 2.89 and 5 Mrad irradiated MPG retained 72% and 55% of their corresponding 0 day controls, respectively. The inherent, more hydrolytic resistance of MPG must be attributed to the presence of an aromatic group in the backbone chains. This aromatic polyester component is also responsible for the observed γ-irradiation stability. It is not known at this time that whether the new γ-irradiation-resistant MPG is biocompatible with biologic tissues due to the lack of published histologic data.

Another common co-monomer that has been frequently used to conjugate with aliphatic polyesters is poly(ethylene glycol) (PEG) for the purpose of providing hydrophilicity and possible water solubility to normally hydrophobic and water-insoluble aliphatic polyesters (Kumar et al., 2001; Huh et al., 2003; Lee et al., 2003; Chen et al., 2004, 2005; Ganaha et al., 2004; Jeong et al., 2004; Kwon and Kim, 2004). For example, triblock copolymers of PLGA and PEG are water-soluble for sustained delivery of peptides, and proteins (Choi et al., 2004; Kwon and Kim, 2004; Chen et al., 2005). Other uses of PEG-aliphatic polyester copolymers include gene delivery (Jeong et al., 2004), angiostatin delivery via stent (Ganaha et al., 2004), plasmid TGF-β delivery for promoting diabetic wound healing (Lee et al., 2003). Due to the increasing hydrophilicity, those PEG-aliphatic polyesters hydrolytically degrade at faster rates than unmodified aliphatic polyesters.

In addition to the use of PEG to modify aliphatic polyesters for improved hydrophilicity and water solubility, poly(vinyl alcohol) was also used to modify aliphatic polyesters (Breitenbach and Kissel, 1998; Breitenbach et al., 2000; Jung et al., 2000; Pistel et al., 2001); these PVA-modified aliphatic polyesters show surface erosion degradation mode rather than the bulk mode found in nonmodified aliphatic polyesters. Ionic groups such as sulfobutyl and dimethylamino amine were further incorporated into the PVA-modified aliphatic polyesters to generate either anionic or cationic charges for potential drug delivery (Jung et al., 2000).

32.2.4 Glycolide-Derived Biodegradable Polymers Having Ether Linkage

PDS® is derived from the glycolide family with better flexibility. It is polymerized from ether-containing lactones, 1,4-dioxane-2,5-dione (i.e., *p*-dioxanone) monomers with a hydroxylic initiator and tin catalyst (Shalaby, 1994). The resulting polymer is semi-crystalline with T_m about 106–115°C and T_g about −10–0°C. The improved flexibility of PDS relative to PGA as evidenced in its lower T_g is due to the incorporation of an ether segment in the repeating unit which reduces the density of ester linkages for intermolecular hydrogen bonds. Because of the less dense ester linkages in PDS when compared with PGA or glycolide-L-lactide copolymers, PDS is expected and has been shown to degrade at a slower rate *in vitro* and *in vivo*. PDS having an inherent viscosity of 2.0 dL/g in hexafluoroisopropanol is adequate for making monofilament sutures. Recently, an advanced version of PDS, PDSII, was introduced. PDSII was achieved by subjecting the melt-spun fibers to a high temperature (128°C) for a short period of time. This additional treatment partially melts the outermost surface layer of PDS fibers and leads to a distinctive skin-core morphology. The heat employed also results in larger crystallites in the core of the fiber than the untreated PDS fiber. The tensile strength-loss profile of PDSII sutures is better than that of PDS sutures.

A variety of copolymers having high molar ratios of PDS compared to other monomers within the same linear aliphatic polyester family have been reported for the purpose of improving the mechanical and biodegradation properties (Shalaby, 1994). For example, copolymer of PDS (80%) and PGA (up to 20%) has an absorption profile similar to Dexon® and Vicryl sutures but it has compliance similar to PDS. Copolymer of PDS (85%) and poly-L-lactide (PLLA; up to 15%) results in a more compliant (low modulus) suture than homopolymer PDS but with absorption profiles similar to PDS (Bezwada et al., 1990).

Copolymer fibers made from PDS and monomers other than linear aliphatic polyester such as morpholine2,5-dione (MD) exhibit rather interesting biodegradation properties. This copolymer fiber was absorbed 10–25% earlier than PDS. The copolymer, however, retained a tensile-breaking strength profile similar to PDS with a slightly faster strength loss during the earlier stage, that is, the first 14 days (Shalaby, 1994). This ability to break the inherent fiber structure–property relationship through copolymerization is a major improvement in biodegradation properties of absorbable sutures. It is interesting to recognize that a small percentage (3%) of MD in the copolymer suture is sufficient to result in a faster mass-loss profile without the expense of its tensile strength-loss profile. The ability to achieve this ideal biodegradation property might be attributed to both an increasing hydrophilicity of the copolymer and the disruption of crystalline domains due to MD moiety. As described later, the loss of suture mass is mainly due to the destruction of crystalline domains, whereas the loss of tensile-breaking strength is chiefly due to the scission of tie-chain segments located in the amorphous domains. The question is why MD–PDS copolymeric suture retains its strength-loss similar to PDS. The possible explanation is that the amide functional groups in MD could form stronger intermolecular hydrogen bonds than ester functional groups. This stronger hydrogen bond contributes to the strength retention of the copolymer of PDS and MD during *in vivo* biodegradation. The incorporation of MD moiety into PDS also lowers the unknot and knot strength of unhydrolyzed specimens, but increases elongation at break. This suggests that the copolymer of PDS and MD should have a lower level of crystallinity than PDS which is consistent with its observed faster mass loss *in vivo*.

To improve γ-irradiation stability of PDS, radiostabilizers such as PEPBO have been copolymerized with PDS to form segmented copolymers the same way as PEPBO with glycolide described above (Koelmel et al., 1991; Shalaby, 1994). The incorporation of 5–10% of such stabilizer in PDS has been shown not only to improve γ-irradiation resistance considerably, but to also increase the compliance of the material. For example, PEPBO–PDS copolymer retained 79, 72, and 57% of its original tensile-breaking strength at 2, 3, and 4 weeks in *in vivo* implantation, whereas PDS homopolymer retained only 43, 30, and 25% at the corresponding periods, respectively. It appears that an increasing (CH_2) group between the two ester functional groups of the radiation stabilizers improves the copolymer resistance toward γ-irradiation.

32.2.5 Lactide Biodegradable Homopolymers and Copolymers

Polylactides, particularly PLLA, and copolymers having >50% L- or D,L-lactide have been explored for medical use without much success mainly due to their much slower absorption and difficulty in melt processing. PLLAs are prepared in solid state through ring-opening polymerization due to their thermal instability and should be melt-processed at the lowest possible temperature (Shalaby, 1994). Other methods such as solution spinning, particularly for high molecular weight, and suspension polymerization have been reported as better alternatives. PLLA is a semi-crystalline polymer with $T_m = 170°C$ and $T_g = 56°C$. This high T_g is mainly responsible for the extremely slow biodegradation rate reported in the literature. The molecular weight of lactide-based biodegradable polymers suitable for medical use ranges from 1.5 to 5.0 dL/g inherent viscosity in chloroform. Ultra-high-molecular weight of polylactides have been reported (Tunc, 1983; Leenslag and Pennings, 1984). For example, an intrinsic viscosity as high as 13 dL/g was reported by Leenslag et al. High-strength PLLA fibers from this ultra-high-molecular-weight polylactide was made by hot-drawing fibers from solutions of good solvents. The resulting fibers had tensile-breaking strength close to 1.2 GPa (Gogolewski and Pennings, 1983). Due to a dissymmetric nature of lactic acid, the polymer made from the optically inactive racemic mixture of D and L enantiomers, poly-DL-lactide, however, is an amorphous polymer.

Lactide-based copolymers having a high percentage of lactide have recently been reported, particularly those copolymerized with aliphatic polycarbonates such as TMC or 3,3-dimethyltrimethylene carbonate (DMTMC) (Shieh et al., 1990). The major advantage of incorporating TMC or DMTMC units into lactide is that the degradation products from TMC or DMTMC are largely neutral pH and hence are considered to be advantageous. Both *in vitro* toxicity and *in vivo* nonspecific foreign body reactions like sterile sinuses have been reported in orthopedic implants made from PGA and/or PLLA (Eitenmuller et al., 1989; Bostman et al., 1990; Daniels et al., 1992; Hofmann, 1992; Winet and Hollinger, 1993).

Several investigators indicated that the glycolic or lactic-acid rich-degradation products have the potential to significantly lower the local pH in a closed and less body-fluid buffered regions surrounded by bone (Sugnuma et al., 1992). This is particularly true if the degradation process proceeds with a burst mode (i.e., a sudden and rapid release of degradation products). This acidity tends to cause abnormal bone resorption and/or demineralization. The resulting environment may be cytotoxic (Daniels et al., 1992). Indeed, inflammatory foreign body reactions with a discharging sinus and osteolytic foci visible on x-ray have been encountered in clinical studies (Eitenmuller et al., 1989). Hollinger et al. recently confirmed the problem associated with PGA and/or PLLA orthopedic implants (Winet and Hollinger, 1993). A rapid degradation of a 50:50 ratio of glycolide–lactide copolymer in bone chambers of rabbit tibias has been found to inhibit bone regeneration. However, emphasis has been placed on the fact that extrapolation of *in vitro* toxicity to *in vivo* biocompatibility must consider microcirculatory capacity. The increase in the local acidity due to a faster accumulation of the highly acidic degradation products is also known to lead to an accelerated acid-catalyzed hydrolysis in the immediate vicinity of the biodegradable device. This acceleration in hydrolysis could lead to a faster loss of mechanical property of the device than we expect. This finding suggests the need to use components in totally biodegradable composites so that degradation products with less acidity would be released into the surrounding area. A controlled slow release rather than a burst release of degradation products at a level that the surrounding tissue could timely metabolize them would also be helpful in dealing with the acidity problem. Copolymers of composition ratio of 10DMTMC/90LLA or 10TMC/90LLA appear to be a promising absorbable orthopedic device. Other applications of this type of copolymers include nerve growth conduits, tendon prostheses, and coating materials for biodegradable devices.

Another unique example of l-lactide copolymer is the copolymer of l-lactide and 3-(S)[(alkyloxy-carbonyl) methyl]-1,4-dioxane-2,5-dione, a cyclic diester (Kimura, 1993). The most unique aspect of this new biodegradable copolymer is the carboxyl acid pendant group which obviously would make the new polymer not only more hydrophilic and hence faster biodegradation, but also more reactive toward future chemical modification through the pendant carboxyl group. The availability of these carboxyl-reactive pendant sites could be used to chemically bond antimicrobial agents or other biochemicals like growth factors for making future wound closure biomaterials having new and important biological functions. Unfortunately, there are no reported data to evaluate the performance of this new absorbable polymer for biomedical engineering use up to now.

Block copolymers of PLLA with poly(amino acids) have also been reported as a potential controlled drug-delivery system (Nathan and Kohn, 1994). This class of copolymers consists of both ester and amide linkages in the backbone molecules and is sometimes referred as poly(depsipeptides) or poly(esters-amides). Poly(depsipeptides) could also be synthesized from ring-opening polymerization of morpholine-2,5-dione and its derivatives (Helder et al., 1986). Barrows has also made a series of nonamino acid-based poly(ester-amides) from polyesterification of diols that contain preformed amide linkages, such as amidediols (Barrows, 1994).

The introduction of poly(ethylene oxide) (PEO) into PLLA in order to modulate the hydrophilicity and degradability of PLLA for drug control/release biomaterials has been reported and an example is the triblock copolymer of PLA/PEO/PLA (Li et al., 1998). Biomaterials having an appropriate PLLA and PEO block length were found to have a hydrogel property that could deliver hydrophilic drugs as well as hydrophobic ones such as steroids and hormones. Another unique biodegradable biomaterial consisting of a star-block copolymer of PLLA, PGA, and PEO was also reported for protein drug-delivery devices (Li and Kissel, 1998). This star-shaped copolymer has four or eight arms made of PEO, PLLA, and PGA. The glass transition temperature and the crystallinity of this star-shaped block copolymer were significantly lower than the corresponding linear PLLA and PGA.

Because of the characteristics of very slow biodegradation rate of PLLA and the copolymers having a high composition ratio of PLLA, their biomedical applications have been mainly limited to (1) orthopedic surgery, (2) drug control/release devices, (3) coating materials for suture, (4) vascular grafts, and (5) surgical meshes to facilitate wound healing after dental extraction.

32.3 Nonglycolide/Lactide-Based Linear Aliphatic Polyesters

All glycolide/lactide-based linear aliphatic polyesters are based on poly(α-hydroxy acids). Recently, there are two unique groups of linear aliphatic polyesters based on poly(w-hydroxy acids) and the most famous ones are poly(ϵ-caprolactone) (Kimura, 1993), poly(β-hydroxybutyrate) (PHB), poly(β-hydroxyvalerate) (PHV), and the copolymers of PHB/PHV (Gross, 1994). Poly(ϵ-caprolactone) has been used as a co-monomer with a variety of glycolide/lactide-based linear aliphatic polyesters described earlier. PHB and PHV belong to the family of poly(hydroxyalkanoates) and are mainly produced by prokaryotic types of microorganisms like *Pseudomonas olevorans* or *Alcaligenes eutrophus* through biotechnology. PHB and PHV are the principal energy and carbon storage compounds for these microorganisms and are produced when there are excessive nutrients in the environment. These naturally produced PHB and PHV are stereochemically pure and are isotactic. They could also be synthesized in labs, but the characteristic of stereoregularity is lost.

This family of biodegradable polyesters is considered to be environmentally friendly because they are produced from propionic acid and glucose and could be completely degraded to water, biogas, biomass, and humic materials (Gross, 1994). Their biodegradation requires enzymes. Hence, PHB, PHV, and their copolymers are probably the most important biodegradable polymers for environmental use. However, the biodegradability of this class of linear aliphatic polyesters in human or animal tissues has been questionable. For example, high-molecular-weight PHB or PHB/PHV fibers do not degrade in tissues or simulated environments over periods of up to 6 months (Williams, 1990). The degradability of PHB could be accelerated by γ-irradiation or copolymerization with PHV.

An interesting derivative of PHB, poly(β-malic acid) (PMA), has been synthesized from ϵ-benzyl malolactonate followed by catalytic hydrogenolysis. PMA differs from PHB in that the $-(CH_3)$ substituent is replaced by $-COOH$ (Kimura, 1993). The introduction of pendant carboxylic acid group would make PMA more hydrophilic and easier to be absorbed.

32.4 Nonaliphatic Polyester-Type Biodegradable Polymers

32.4.1 Aliphatic and Aromatic Polycarbonates

The most significant aliphatic polycarbonates are based on DMTMC and TMC. They are made by the same ring-opening polymerization as glycolide-based biodegradable polyesters. The homopolymers are biocompatible with a controllable rate of biodegradation. Pellets of poly(ethylene carbonate) were absorbed completely in 2 weeks in the peritoneal cavity of rats. A slight variation of this polycarbonate, that is, poly(propylene carbonate), however, did not show any sign of absorption after 2 months (Barrows, 1986). Copolymers of DMTMC/ϵ-caprolactone and DMTMC/TMC have been reported to have adequate properties for wound closure, tendon prostheses, and vascular grafts. The most important advantage of aliphatic polycarbonates is the neutral pH of the degradation products.

Poly(BPA-carbonates) made from bisphenol A (BPA) and phosgene is nonbiodegradable, but an analog of poly(BPA-carbonate) like poly(iminocarbonates) have been shown to degrade in about 200 days (Barrows, 1986). In general, this class of aromatic polycarbonates takes an undesirably long period to degrade, presumably due to the presence of an aromatic ring which could protect adjacent ester bonds to be hydrolyzed by water or enzymes. Different types of degradation products of this polymer under different pH environments are produced. At pH >7.0, the degradation products of this polymer are BPA, ammonia, and CO_2, while insoluble poly(BPA-carbonate) oligomers were produced with pH <7.0

(Barrows, 1986). The polymer had good mechanical properties and acceptable tissue biocompatibility. Unfortunately, there is currently no commercial use of this class of polymer in surgery.

32.4.2 Poly(alkylene oxalates) and Copolymers

This class of high-crystalline biodegradable polymers was initially developed (Shalaby, 1994) for absorbable sutures and their coating. They consist of $[-ROOC-COO-]_n$ repeating unit where R is $(CH_2)_x$ with x ranging from 4 to 12. R could also be cyclic (1,4-*trans*-cyclohexanedimethanol) or aromatic (1,4-benzene, 1,3-benzene dimethanol) for achieving higher melting temperature. The biodegradation properties depend on the number of (CH_2) group, x, and the type of R group (i.e., acyclic versus cyclic or aromatic). In general, a higher number of methylene group and/or the incorporation of cyclic or aromatic R group would retard the biodegradation rate and hence make the polymer absorbed slower. For example, there was no mass of the polymer with $x = 4$ remaining *in vivo* (rats) after 28 days, while the polymer with $x = 6$ retained 80% of its mass after 42 days *in vivo*. An isomorphic copolyoxalate consisting of 80% cyclic R group like 1,4-*trans*-cyclohexanedimethanol and 20% with acyclic R group like 1,6-hexanediol retained 56% of its original mass after 180 days *in vivo*. By varying the ratio of cyclic to acyclic monomers, copolymers with a wide range of melting temperatures could be made, for example, copolymer of 95/5 ratio of cyclic (i.e., 1,4-*trans*-cyclohexanedimethanol)/acyclic (i.e., 1,6-hexanediol) monomers had a $T_m = 210°C$, while the copolymer with 5/95 ratio had a $T_m = 69°C$. Poly(alkylene oxalates) with $x = 3$ or 6 had been experimented with drug control/release devices. The tissue reaction to this class of biodegradable polymers has been minimal.

32.4.3 Amino Acid-Based Poly(ester amide)s and Copolymers

The rationale for designing poly(ester amide)s (PEAs) is to combine the predictable hydrolytic-induced degradability and biocompatibility of linear aliphatic polyesters with the high-performance and enzymatically catalyzed biodegradability of polyamides and the potential chemical reactive sites of amide in polyamides into one single entity. Instead of using the block copolymer approach to provide both ester and amide linkages in a polymer backbone, PEAs have both ester and amide linkages within the same repeating unit and different versions of PEAs have been reported.

Two basic types of PEAs exist: nonamino-acid-based PEAs synthesized from polyesterification of amidediol monomers (which contain preformed amide linkages from aliphatic diamines) (Barrows, 1994; Paredes et al. 1998) and amino-acid-based PEAs (AA-PEAs) synthesized from solution polycondensation of amino acids, diols, and dicarboxylic acids (Katsarava et al., 1985, 1999; Chu and Katsarava, 2003; Guo et al., 2005; Guo and Chu, 2007a,b, 2008, 2010; Jokhadze et al., 2007; De Wit et al., 2008; Deng et al., 2009, 2011; Pang et al., 2010; Pang and Chu, 2010a,b; Chkhaidze et al., 2011). PEAs obtained from amidediols (i.e., nonamino-acid based) cannot be considered bioassimilative polymers because the water-soluble amidediols (first product of biodegradation) were extensively excreted without change (i.e., without the liberation of toxic diamine) in the urine.

Katsarava and Chu et al. reported the synthesis of high-molecular-weight amino acid-based poly(ester-amides) (AA-PEAs) of M_w from 24,000 to 167,000 with narrow polydispersity ($M_w/M_n = 1.20-1.81$) via solution polycondensation of di-*p*-toluenesulfonic acid salts of bis-(α-amino acid) α,ω-alkylene diesters and di-*p*-nitrophenyl esters of diacids (Katsarava et al., 1999). These AA-PEAs consist of naturally occurring and nontoxic building blocks and had excellent film and fiber-forming properties. These AA-PEA polymers were mostly amorphous materials with T_g from −7.3 to 109°C. The rationale for making AA-PEAs is to combine the well-known absorbability and biocompatibility of linear aliphatic polyesters with the high performance and the flexibility of potential chemical reactive sites of amide of polyamides. AA-PEAs could be biodegraded either by enzyme and/or nonenzymatic mechanisms. There have been several trials of this new class of AA-PEA copolymers as the coating for drug-eluting stents as well as synthetic vaccines at present.

The approach of using amino acid, diols, and dicarboxylic acid as the three building blocks to form AA-PEAs is a better one because of the biocompatibility of the amino acids used to provide amide linkages. In addition, due to the presence of amino acids with amide linkages, these AA-PEAs have "pseudo-protein" characteristics, that is, exhibiting both protein and nonprotein characteristics simultaneously. Because of the extensive variety and availability of these three core components, AA-PEAs with a wide spectrum of chemical, physical, mechanical, thermal, and biological properties can and has been explored and tailored to suit specific clinical needs. For example, an expansive range of AA-PEA hydrophobicity to hydrophilicity can be engineered. Neutral, cationic, and anionic AA-PEAs have also been developed in the Chu's lab (Katsarava et al., 1999; Chu and Katsarava, 2003; Guo et al., 2005; Guo and Chu, 2007a,b, 2008, 2010; Jokhadze et al., 2007; Deng et al., 2009, 2011; Pang and Chu, 2010a,b; Pang et al., 2010; Chkhaidze et al., 2011; Song and Chu, 2012). The cationic AA-PEAs have been tested for gene delivery (Song, 2007; Yamanouchi et al., 2008; Wu, 2010), whereas the anionic AA-PEAs have been tried as synthetic vaccines like H1N1 (Cawthon et al., 2007).

These amino-acid-based AA-PEAs consisted of naturally occurring and nontoxic building blocks, a generic chemical structure of the repeating unit of AA-PEAs is shown in Figure 32.3. AA-PEAs have excellent film- and fiber-forming properties. AA-PEAs of M_w from 24,000 to 167,000 with narrow polydispersity ($M_w/M_n = 1.20–1.81$) were successfully synthesized via solution polycondensation of di-*p*-toluenesulfonic acid salts of bis(α-amino acid) α,ω-alkylene diesters and di-*p*-nitrophenyl esters of diacids. These AA-PEA polymers are initially semicrystalline polymers from solution polycondensation, but, depending on the type of amino acids, some AA-PEAs, such as L-phenylalanine and L-leucine, become amorphous after first melting and cooling, whereas others like Gly-based PEAs show consistent melting-crystallization upon repeated heating and cooling. For example, the Gly-based PEAs are highly crystalline, and repeated heating and cooling did not change their melting—crystallization property, and their melting temperature decreased with an increase in the methylene chain length in the diacid segment (Paredes et al., 1998). These Gly-based PEAs also showed similar total heat of fusion regardless of whether the polymer was from the polymerization medium or subsequent isothermal crystallization in solution. The lack of crystallization capability from repeated thermal process of Phe and Leu-based PEAs may be attributed to their relatively lower glass transition temperature, T_g, the bulky side group that makes regular chain packing difficult or the extensive inter- and intramolecular hydrogen bond capability from both the amide and the ester linkages in the AA-PEA backbones that retards the chain mobility required for crystallization. The T_g of all reported AA-PEAs ranged from −7.3°C to 109°C.

The first-generation AA-PEAs are of saturated nature (AA-SPEAs): saturated carbon-to-carbon linkages on the backbone, that is, the lack of >C=C< double bond functionality in the AA-PEA backbone. Recently, two new generations of AA-PEAs, unsaturated AA-PEAs (AA-UPEAs), were reported (Guo et al. 2005; Guo and Chu, 2007a,b, 2008; Pang et al. 2010; Pang and Chu, 2010a,b), and Figure 32.4 shows the chemical structure of the repeating unit of these two different types of unsaturated AA-PEAs. The most unique aspect of these AA-UPEAs is that there are >C=C< double bonds built into either the diamide or the diester backbone segments or as a pendant group of the polymer backbones. The effect of >C=C< double bond on the T_g, however, depends on the location of the double bonds. In the case of double bonds in the AA-UPEA backbone, AA-UPEAs would have a much higher T_g and T_m than

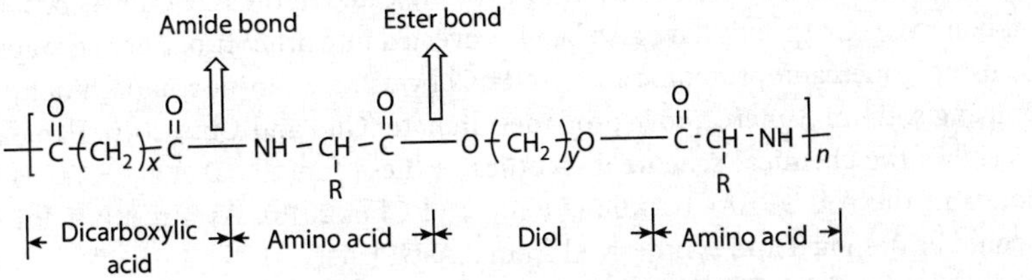

FIGURE 32.3 A generic chemical structure of the repeating unit of amino acid-based poly(ester amide)s.

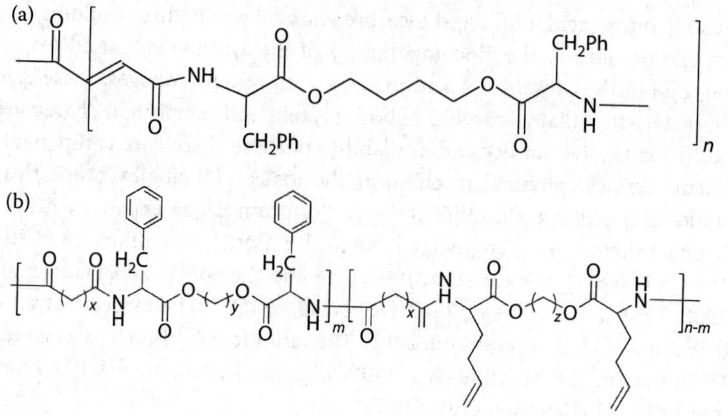

FIGURE 32.4 Chemical structure of the repeating unit of unsaturated poly(ester amide)s (AA-UPEAs). (a) Unsaturated bonds located in the AA-UPEA backbone; (b) unsaturated bonds located as the pendant to the AA-UPEA backbone.

saturated AA-PEAs because of the rigidity of the >C=C< bonds in the backbone. There are two options for the >C=C< bonds to be located in the AA-UPEA backbone: diamide (from diacid) or diester (from diol) segments. The AA-UPEAs based only on fumaryl, FPB, and FPH (i.e., the >C=C< double bond in the diamide segment) had higher T_g than those AA-UPEAs having the same double bond in the diester segment. This is because the >C=C< double bond in the diamide segment could also conjugate with the two carbonyl groups and resulted in a higher rigidity of the polymer backbone, while the >C=C< double bond in the diester segment is isolated by the adjacent methylene group, the lack of conjugation.

Contrary to the unsaturated AA-UPEAs having double bonds in the backbone, those unsaturated AA-UPEAs having pendant >C=C< double bonds (Pang et al., 2010; Pang and Chu, 2010a,b) actually lowers their T_g when compared with the corresponding saturated AA-PEAs. For example, 2-Phe-4 and 8-Phe-4 had T_g of 55°C and 40°C, respectively, while the Phe-based UPEA copolymers with pendant >C=C< double bonds (from 2-allyl glycine) had T_g values ranging from 20°C to 38°C, depending on methylene chain length in diacid, diols, as well as the feed ratio of regular amino acid to 2-allyl glycine. This suggested that the presence of 2-allyl glycine unit in the AA-UPEA backbone could impart additional chain flexibility due to the increasing free volume from pendant double bonds which could act as internal plasticizers, lowered the intermolecular interaction between copolymer chains. Therefore, more allylglycine contents could result in higher chain flexibility and hence lower T_g values as reported (Pang et al., 2010; Pang and Chu, 2010a,b).

These >C=C< double bonds in unsaturated AA-UPEAs also provide potential reactive sites for either synthesizing additional derivatives or attaching biologically active agents to render biological activity to AA-UPEAs. An example of synthesizing additional derivatives from AA-UPEAs is the reported studies of AA-UPEA-based hydrogels via photocrosslinking with PEG diacrylate precursor (Guo and Chu, 2005; Pang and Chu, 2010b). Figure 32.5 illustrates the scanning electron microscopic images of a AA-UPEA-based hydrogel. Figure 32.5a is from AA-UPEAs with pendant >C=C< double bonds, whereas Figure 32.5b is from AA-UPEAs with >C=C< located in the AA-UPEAs backbone. These pendant or backbone >C=C< groups have also been converted into other functional groups like thiol-based –COOH by using 3-mercaptopropionic acid, –NH$_3$Cl by using 2-aminoethanethiol hydrochloride, and –SO$_3$Na by using sodium-3-mercapto-1-propanesulfonate (Guo and Chu, 2010; Pang and Chu, 2010a). Figure 32.6 shows the chemical scheme to synthesize these functional AA-PEAs via the unsaturated >C=C< bonds in the AA-UPEAs backbone (Guo and Chu, 2010). As a result, additional functional AA-PEAs could be designed and synthesized from AA-UPEAs.

Beside the unsaturated AA-UPEA approach to provide additional functionality to AA-PEAs via their unsaturated >C=C< bonds, other efforts could also provide chemical functionality to AA-SPEAs, the

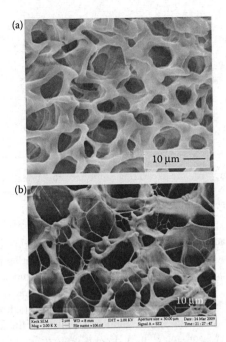

FIGURE 32.5 Scanning electron microscopic images of two representative hybrid hydrogel fabricated from (a) Phe-based unsaturated AA-UPEAs, and poly(ethylene glycol) diacrylate (PEGDA) and (b) Arg-based unsaturated AA-UPEAs and pluronic acid diacrylate.

copolymer approach. Chu et al. recently reported two different copolymer means to provide pendant functional groups via either L-lysine or other amino acid co-monomer (Jokhadze et al., 2007; Deng et al., 2009, 2011). The first copolymer approach led to the AA-PEA copolymers having pendant-free carboxylic acid (located in the Lys block) over a wide range of desirable concentrations (Jokhadze et al., 2007). These free carboxylic acids provide the reactive sites for the attachment of biologically active agents, such as nitric oxide derivative, and the resulting AA-PEA copolymers would have biological activity and intelligence similar to that of nitric oxide (Lee and Chu, 1996, 1998).

The second copolymer approach used a new monomer of ε-(benzyloxycarbonyl)-amino acid-N-carboxyanhydride (Z-amino acid-NCA) and its ring-opening reaction with the regular AA-PEA

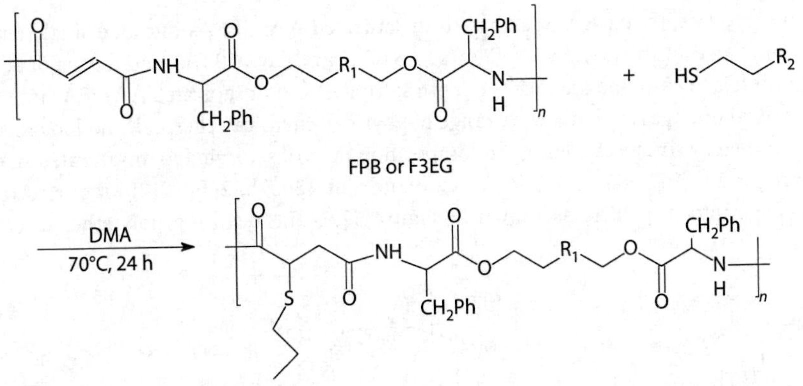

FIGURE 32.6 Chemical scheme to illustrate the synthesis of pendant functional AA-PEAs from the unsaturated >C=C< bonds in the AA-UPEA backbone. (Adapted from Guo, K. and Chu, C.C., 2010. *J. Appl. Polym. Sci.* 117(6): 3386–3394.)

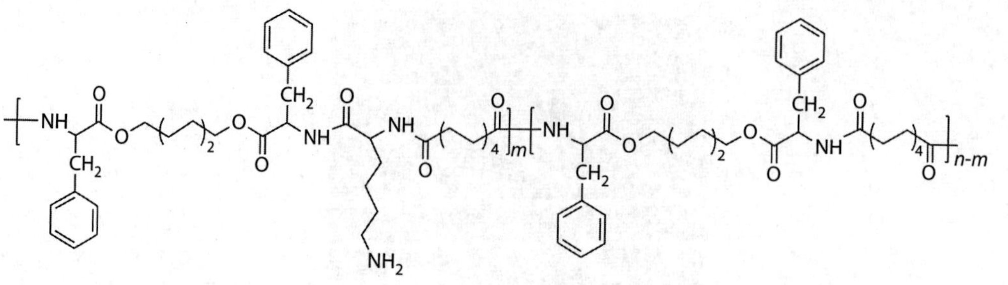

FIGURE 32.7 Chemical structure of the repeating unit of functional AA-PEAs synthesized via ε-(benzyloxycarbonyl)-amino acid-*N*-carboxyanhydride (*Z*-amino acid-NCA) route (the second copolymer approach as described above) (Deng et al., 2010).

monomers (di-*p*-toluenesulfonic acid salts of bis-(α-amino acid) α,ω-alkylene diesters and di-*p*-nitrophenyl esters of diacids). The resulting functional AA-PEAs could have either free pendant –NH₂, –OH or –COOH, depending on the type of the new *Z*-amino acid-NCA monomer (Deng et al., 2009, 2011). For example, if Lys is used (*Z*-Lys-NCA), the resulting AA-PEA copolymer would have pendant –NH₂ functionality. Note the difference in pendant functional group between the first and second copolymer approaches even though the same Lys was used. The chemical structure of the functional AA-PEA copolymers from the second copolymer approach (Figure 32.7) is quite different from the chemical structure of the functional AA-PEAs from the first copolymer approach. In the first copolymer approach (Jokhadze et al., 2007), each of the two amino acids is distinctively located at two different blocks, for example, Phe in one block and Lys in another block. In the second copolymer approach (Deng et al., 2009, 2011), two amino acids are located in the same block and directly connected by a peptide bond, and one of these two amino acids is also located in a separate block. Deng et al. (2009) reported that the pendant –NH₂ group can be attached by a NHS-fluorescein, and the resulting dye-tagged AA-PEAs exhibit fluorescence characteristic.

Glilies et al. also recently reported another method of synthesizing functional AA-PEAs with free pendant amino groups (De Wit et al., 2008). They incorporated bis(L-lysine) R,ω-alkylene diester monomer into the PEA, and the pendant amine group can be recovered after deprotection reaction. However, the chemical structure of Glilies et al.'s functional AA-PEAs differs from that of Deng et al.'s in that the two amino acids within the same block in the Glilies et al.'s study are separated by diacid spacer on the AA-PEA backbone, while the two amino acids in the same block in the Deng et al.'s study are directly connected via a peptide bond.

An effort to integrate saturated AA-SPEAs with unsaturated AA-UPEAs into one single entity was recently reported and an example is shown in Figure 32.8 (Guo and Chu, 2007a), and the major advantage of such an integration is to combine the merits of both saturated and unsaturated AA-PEAs into one single entity via chemical linkages so that a wide range of physical, chemical, thermal, and biological properties could be obtained by simply changing the composition ratio of saturated to unsaturated AA-PEAs.

Beside ester and amide linkages in AA-PEAs, Guo and Chu (2007b, 2008, 2010) reported the addition of ether linkage into AA-PEAs as shown in Figure 32.9. The resulting poly(ether ester amide)

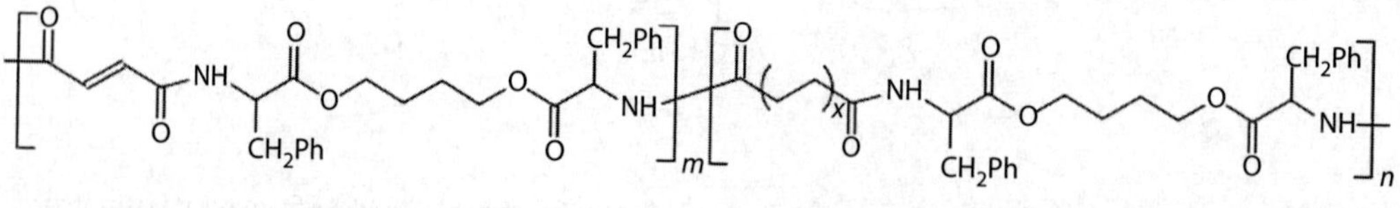

FIGURE 32.8 The chemical structure of the repeating unit of saturated and unsaturated amino acid-based poly(ester amide)s. (Adapted from Guo, K. and Chu, C.C., 2007a. *J. Polym. Sci. Polym. Chem. Ed.*, 45: 1595–1606.)

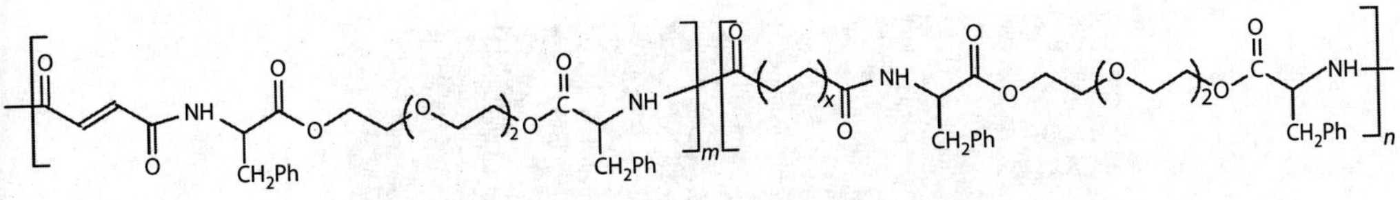

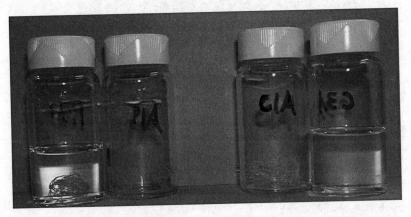

FIGURE 32.9 The chemical structure of the repeating unit of the copolymer of saturated and unsaturated poly(ester ether amide)s. (Adapted from Guo, K. and Chu, C.C., 2007b. *Biomacromolecules*, 8(9): 2851–2861.)

(AA-PEEA) would have three types of linkages: ether, ester, and amide. The ether linkage was introduced by the use of oligo(ethylene glycol). The AA-PEEAs had T_g values lower than that of the AA-PEAs of similar structures due to the incorporation of ether bonds in the backbones. An increase in the number of ether bonds in PEEA resulted in a lower T_g value. The solubility of the PEEA polymers in a wide range of common organic solvents was significantly improved when compared with the corresponding AA-PEAs. Guo et al. (2008) stated that by adjusting monomers feed ratio between saturated AA-SPEEAs and unsaturated AA-UPEEAs, AA-USPEEA copolymers could have controlled chemical, physical, and biodegradation properties.

Both saturated AA-SPEAs and AA-UPEAs were easily biodegraded by enzymes such as lipase or α-chymotrypsin; however, their biodegradability in pure saline buffer is slow as shown in Figure 32.10. The Phe-based AA-PEA fibers were completely biodegraded after 2 days exposure to α-chymotrypsin at 0.1 mg/mL concentration (far right), while these AA-PEA fibers remained intact in phosphate-buffered saline (PBS) at the same duration.

It appears that an increase in the hydrophobicity of AA-PEAs (via longer methylene groups in diols and dicarboxylic acid segments) leads to a faster enzyme-catalyzed biodegradation (Tsitlanadze et al., 2004a,b). In addition to the hydrophobicity factor to interpret this relationship between the length of methylene groups and enzyme-catalyzed biodegradation rate, the lack of intermolecular hydrogen bonds resulting from misalignment of the adjacent AA-PEA macromolecules was also suggested as a possible cause behind such a relationship. The presence of ether linkage in AA-PEEAs accelerates the enzymatic hydrolysis rates (in terms of weight loss) and was found to be much faster than those of AA-PEAs. The zero-order-like biodegradation kinetics and molecular weight data of AA-PEAs and AA-PEEAs also suggested surface erosion biodegradation mechanisms like peeling onions which is very different from the well-known bulk hydrolytic degradation of aliphatic polyesters, that is, degrading throughout the whole biomaterials.

FIGURE 32.10 Enzyme effect on the biodegradation of Phe-based AA-PEA fibers. α-Chymotrypsin concentration at 0.1 mg/mL. The two bottles on the left were treated by PBS, whereas the two bottles on the right were treated by α-chymotrypsin in PBS. The duration of immersion were 24 (inner bottles) and 48 h (outer bottles).

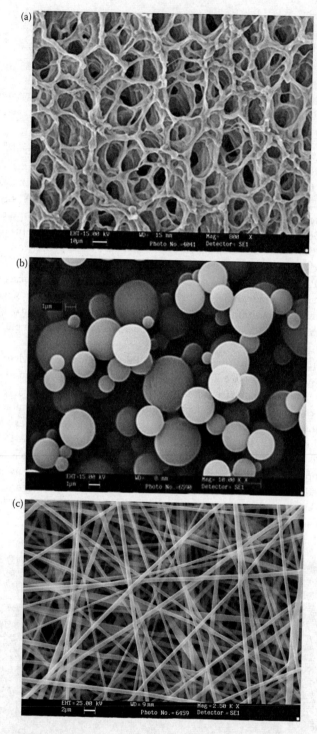

FIGURE 32.11 Variety of physical forms of AA-PEAs engineered. (a) 3D microporous hydrogel; (b) micro/nano-spheres; (c) electrospun fibrous membrane.

A variety of physical forms of AA-PEAs, such as fibers, films, electrospun 3D microporous fibrous membranes, hydrogels, hollow gel tube, and micro/nanospheres have been successfully engineered to meet specific clinical needs and they are shown in Figure 32.11 (Guo and Chu, 2005, 2009; Song, 2007; Chu and Sun, 2008; Li and Chu, 2009; Horwitz et al., 2010; Pang and Chu, 2010; Wu, 2010; Song and Chu, 2012). These physical forms of AA-PEAs have been used to deliver drugs and proteins (e.g., bFGF, IL-12, pactlitaxel, albumin, nitric oxide derivatives, gallium nitrate, antibiotics, biotin) via preloading, postloading, or chemical conjugation modes.

The most unique biological property of these biodegradable amino acid-based poly(ester amide)s is the very low foreign-body inflammatory response that the AA-PEAs can induce as well as their support of more natural wound healing (Lee et al., 2002; Schwartz et al., 2008; DeFife et al., 2009; Horwitz et al., 2010; Wu, 2010). As shown in Figure 32.12, DeFife et al. (2009) reported that human peripheral blood monocytes cultured on AA-PEA films secreted over fivefold less IL-6 proinflammatory cytokine release over 24 h than the classical absorbable aliphatic polyesters like polyglycolide and lactide copolymers (50/50 molar ratio), poly-n-butylmethacrylate (PBMA), and tissue culture-treated polystyrene (TCPS) as IL-6 is known to increase macrophage cytotoxic activity. The very low inflammatory response toward AA-PEA-based biomaterials is further confirmed by examining the IL-1β receptor antagonist secreted by monocytes, and a similar pattern of release of IL-1β, a potent proinflammatory cytokine, on monocyte cultured AA-PEA biomaterials. The amounts of IL-1β released on AA-PEAs were one-quarter to one-half of the FDA-approved absorbable PLGA and nonabsorbable PBMA biomaterials.

The low inflammatory characteristic of AA-PEAs was further confirmed in an *in vivo* porcine coronary artery model of AA-PEA-coated stent (Lee et al., 2002) as well as *in vivo* study of the wound healing performance of Phe-based PEA fibrous membrane for treating second-degree burns in a porcine model (Schwartz et al., 2008). In the porcine coronary artery model, 28 days postimplantation, the AA-PEA copolymer-coated 316L stainless-steel stent (Genic stent) exhibited statistically similar inflammatory score as the bare stent control (1.18 ± 0.38 of AA-PEA-coated stent versus 1.11 ± 0.32 of bare stent control). There was no statistical difference inb% area of stenosis and neointimal hyperplasia between the AA-PEA-coated and bare stents either. These biocompatibility data in an *in vivo* porcine arterial model also suggest that these new biodegradable AA-PEA copolymers induce very low level of inflammatory response.

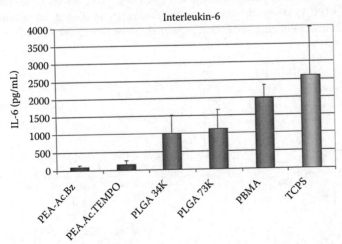

FIGURE 32.12 *In vitro* inflammatory response of Leu–Lys-based AA-PEA copolymers in terms of cytokine IL-6 secretion upon seeding monocytes onto AA-PEA films. PEA-Ac.Bz is a protected AA-PEA copolymer (i.e., the –COOH pendant group in the Lys segment is protected by a benzyl ester). PEA.Ac.TEMPO is a deprotected AA-PEA and its –COOH group was conjugated with a nitroxyl radical, 4-amino-2,2,6,6-tetramethylpiperidine-1-oxy (or 4-amino TEMPO. PLGA is a poly(lactic-*co*-glycolic acid) copolymer with a molecular weight of 36,000 (Resomer RG 502) and 73,000 Da (Resomer RG 504). PBMA is *n*-poly(butyl methacrylate). TCPS is a tissue culture polystyrene plate.

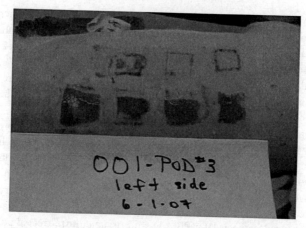

FIGURE 32.13 Drug-eluting AA-PEA fibrous membranes for treating partial thickness wound in a porcine model after 3 days postoperation. Gallium nitrate drug was physically impregnated within AA-PEA fibrous membranes (far right). DuoDerm as the commercial control (far left and third from left). Pure AA-PEA fibrous membrane (second from left) also served as a control.

The *in vivo* porcine burn model study showed that the AA-PEA-based fibrous membranes with or without impregnated drug (gallium nitrate) showed accelerated wound healing with a healing rate of 4–5 days faster than the commercial DuoDerm® control as shown in Figure 32.13 (Schwartz et al., 2008). Therefore, this new family of AA-PEAs appear to support a more natural wound healing process by promoting reendothelialization and lowering foreign-body-induced inflammatory response.

32.4.4 Poly(carbonate-acetal)s from Dihydroxyacetone

The building blocks of all existing synthetic absorbable or biodegradable polymeric biomaterials have largely from the human body metabolic products like PGA, PLA, and PCL. The newly reported poly(carbonate-acetal)s (PCA) are synthesized from dihydroxyacetone (DHA), an intermediate of glucose metabolism (Zelikin and Putnam, 2005; Zawaneha et al., 2005; Henderson et al., 2010). Figure 32.14

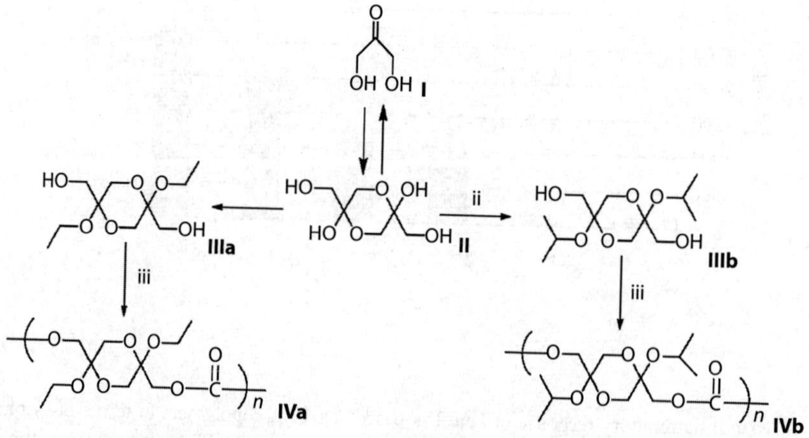

FIGURE 32.14 The chemical scheme to illustrate the synthesis of poly(carbonate-acetal)s from the dimer of dihydroxyacetone. **I**—Dihydroxyacetone; **II**—dimer of dihydroxyacetone; **IIIa**—2,5-diethoxy-1,4-dioxane-2,5-dimethanol; **IIIb**—2,5-diisopropoxy-1,4-dioxane-2,5-dimethanol; **IVa**—poly(carbonate-acetal) from **IIIa**; **IVb**—poly(carbonate-acetal) from **IIIb**. (Adapted from Zelikin, A.N. and Putnam, D., 2005. *Macromolecules*, 38: 5532–5537.)

shows the synthesis scheme of poly(carbonate-acetal)s from the dimer form of DHA with the help of triphosgene. The resulting PCA has yields from 56% to 93% with weight-average molecular weight from 28×10^3 to 48×10^3, and T_g ranging from 42°C to 61°C. The wettability (in terms of water contact angle) of these PCA ranges from 76° to 88°, and is similar to those Phe-based poly(ester amide)s (Horwitz et al., 2010). A preliminary MTT assay and cell proliferation study (NIH/3T3 cell line) indicate that poly(carbonate-acetal)s are not cytotoxic and support cell growth. A PCA derivative from PEGylated DHA diblock copolymer has shown good hemostatic property (Henderson et al., 2010), while this PEGylated DHA physically cross-linked hydrogel can act as a space filler and has been tested for prevention of seroma following ablative and reconstructive surgeries (Zawaneha et al., 2005).

32.5 Biodegradation Properties of Synthetic Biodegradable Polymers

The reported biodegradation studies of a variety of biodegradable polymeric biomaterials have mainly focused on their tissue biocompatibility, the rate of drug release, or loss of strength and mass. Recently, the degradation mechanisms and the effects of intrinsic and extrinsic factors, such as pH (Chu, 1981, 1982), enzymes (Williams and Mort, 1977; Williams and Chu, 1984; Williams, 1979; Chu and Williams, 1983), γ-irradiation (Campbell et al., 1981; Chu and Campbell, 1982; Chu and Williams, 1983; Williams and Chu, 1984; Zhang et al., 1993), electrolytes (Pratt et al., 1993), cell medium (Chu et al., 1992), superoxide (Lee et al., 1999, 2000), annealing treatment (Chu and Browning, 1988), plasma surface treatment (Loh et al., 1992), external stress (Miller and Williams, 1984; Chu, 1985a), and polymer morphology (Chu and Kizil, 1989), and on a chemical means to examine the degradation of PGA fibers (Chu and Louie, 1985) have been systemically examined and the subject has been recently reviewed (Chu, 1985b, 1991, 1995a,b; Hollinger, 1995; Chu et al., 1997). Table 32.5 is an illustration of structural factors of polymers that could control their degradation. Besides these series of experimental studies of a variety of factors that could affect the degradation of biodegradable polymeric biomaterials, there are two new areas that broaden the above traditional study of biodegradation properties of biodegradable polymers into the frontier of science. They are theoretical modeling and the role of free radicals.

32.5.1 Theoretical Modeling of Degradation Properties

The most systematic theoretical modeling study of degradation properties of biodegradable biomaterials was reported by Pratt and Chu who used computational chemistry to theoretically model the effects of a variety of substituents which could exert either steric effect and/or inductive effect on the degradation properties of glycolide/lactide-based biodegradable polymers (Pratt and Chu, 1993, 1994a,b). This

TABLE 32.5　Structural Factors to Control the Polymer Degradability

Factors	Methods of Control
Chemical structure of main chain and side groups	Chemical linkages and functional groups
Aggregation state	Processing, copolymerization
Crystalline state	Polymer blend, copolymerization feed ratio, processing temperature
Hydrophilic/hydrophobic balance	Copolymerization, chemical linkages, introduction of functional groups
Surface area	Micropores, nanotechnology
Shape and morphology	Fiber, film, hydrogels, composite

Source: Adapted from Kimura, Y., 1993. *Biomedical Applications of Polymeric Materials*, pp. 164–190. CRC Press, Boca Raton, FL.

new approach could provide scientists with a better understanding of the relationship between the chemical structure of biodegradable polymers and their degradation behavior at a molecular level. It also could help the future research and development of this class of polymers through the intelligent prediction of structure–property relationships. In those studies, Pratt and Chu examined the affect of various derivatives of linear aliphatic polyester (PGA) and a naturally occurring linear polysaccharide (hyaluronic acid) on their hydrolytic degradation phenomena and mechanisms.

The data showed a decrease in the rate of hydrolysis by about a factor of 106 with isopropyl ct-substituents, but nearly a sixfold increase with t-butyl α-substituents (Pratt and Chu, 1993). The role of electron-donating and electron-withdrawing groups on the rate of hydrolytic degradation of linear aliphatic polyesters was also theoretically modeled by Pratt and Chu (Pratt and Chu, 1994a). Electron-withdrawing substituents to the carbonyl group would be expected to stabilize the tetrahedral intermediate resulting from hydroxide attack, that is, favoring hydroxide attack but disfavoring alkoxide elimination. Electron-releasing groups would be expected to show the opposite effect. Similarly, electronegative substituents on the alkyl portion of the ester would stabilize the forming alkoxide ion and favor the elimination step. Pratt and Chu found that the rate of ester hydrolysis is greatly affected by halogen substituents due primarily to charge delocalization. The data suggest that the magnitude of the inductive effect on the hydrolysis of glycolic esters decreases significantly as the location of the substituent is moved further away from the α-carbon because the inductive effect is very distance-sensitive. In all three locations of substitutions (α and γ), Cl and Br substituents exhibited the largest inductive effect compared to other halogen elements.

Therefore, Pratt and Chu concluded that the rate of ester hydrolysis is greatly affected by both alkyl and halogen substituents due primarily to either steric hindrance or charge delocalization. In the steric effect, alkyl substituents on the glycolic esters cause an increase in activation enthalpies and a corresponding decrease in reaction rate, up to about three carbon sizes, while bulkier alkyl substituents other than isopropyl make the rate-determining elimination step more facile. It appears that aliphatic polyesters containing isopropyl groups, or slightly larger linear alkyl groups, such as *n*-butyl, *n*-pentyl, and so on, would be expected to show a longer strength retention, given the same fiber morphology. In the inductive effect, ct-substituents on the acyl portion of the ester favor the formation of the tetrahedral intermediate through charge delocalization, with the largest effect seen with Cl substitution, but retard the rate-determining alkoxide elimination step by stabilizing the tetrahedral intermediate. The largest degree of stabilization is caused by the very electronegative F substituent.

32.5.2 The Role of Free Radicals in Degradation Properties

Salthouse et al. had demonstrated that the biodegradation of synthetic absorbable sutures is closely related to macrophage activity through the close adhesion of macrophage onto the surface of the absorbable sutures (Matlaga and Salthouse, 1980). It is also known that inflammatory cells, particularly leukocytes and macrophages, are able to produce highly reactive oxygen species such as superoxide ($\cdot O^{2-}$) and hydrogen peroxide during inflammatory reactions toward foreign materials (Badwey and Kamovsky, 1980; Devereux et al., 1991). These highly reactive oxygen species participate in the biochemical reaction, frequently referred to as a respiratory burst, which is characterized by the one electron reduction of O_2 into superoxide via either NADPH or NADH oxidase as shown below. The reduction of O_2 results in an increase in O_2 uptake and the consumption of glucose.

$$2O_2 + NADPH \xrightarrow{\text{(NADPH oxidase)}} 2\cdot O_2^- + NADP^+ + H^+ \tag{32.1}$$

The resulting superoxide radicals are then neutralized to H_2O_2 via cytoplasmic enzyme superoxide dismutase (SOD).

$$2\cdot O^{2-} + 2H^+ \xrightarrow{\text{(SOD)}} H_2O_2 + O_2 \tag{32.2}$$

Williams et al. suggested that these reactive oxygen species may be harmful to polymeric implant surfaces through their production of highly reactive, potent, and harmful hydroxyl radicals $\cdot OH$ in the presence of metals like iron as shown in the following series of redox reactions (Williams and Zhong, 1991; Ali et al., 1993; Zhong et al., 1994).

$$\cdot O_2 + M^{n+} \rightarrow O_2 + M^{(n-1)+} \tag{32.3}$$

$$H_2O_2 + M^{(n-1)+} \rightarrow \cdot OH + HO^- + M^{n+} \tag{32.4}$$

The net reaction will be

$$\cdot O^{2-} + H_2O_2 \rightarrow \cdot OH + HO^- + O_2 \tag{32.5}$$

and is often referred to as the metal-catalyzed Haber–Weiss reaction (Haber and Weiss, 1934).

Although the role of free radicals in the hydrolytic degradation of synthetic biodegradable polymers is largely unknown, a very recent study using absorbable sutures like Vicryl in the presence of an aqueous free radical solution prepared from H_2O_2 and ferrous sulfate, $FeSO_4$, raised the possibility of the role of free radicals in the biodegradation of synthetic absorbable sutures (Williams and Zhong, 1991; Zhong et al., 1994). As shown below, both $\cdot OH$ radicals and OH^- are formed in the process of oxidation of Fe^{2+} by H_2O_2 and could exert some influence on the subsequent hydrolytic degradation of Vicryl sutures.

$$Fe^{2+} + H_2O_2 \rightarrow Fe^{3+} + \cdot OH + OH^-$$

SEM results indicated that Vicryl sutures in the presence of free radical solutions exhibited many irregular surface cracks at both 7 and 14 days *in vitro*, while the same sutures in the two controls (H_2O_2 or $FeSO_4$ solutions) did not have these surface cracks. Surprisingly, the presence of surface cracks of Vicryl sutures treated in the free radical solutions did not accelerate the tensile-breaking strength-loss as would be expected. Thermal properties of Vicryl sutures under the free radical and 3% H_2O_2 media showed the classical well-known maximum pattern of the change of the level of crystallinity with hydrolysis time. The level of crystallinity of Vicryl sutures peaked at 7 days in both media (free radical and 3% H_2O_2). The time for peak appearance in these two media was considerably earlier than Vicryl sutures in conventional physiological buffer media. Based on Chu's suggestion of using the time of the appearance of the crystallinity peak as an indicator of degradation rate, it appears that these two media accelerated the degradation of Vicryl sutures when compared with regular physiological buffer solution. Based on their findings, Williams et al. proposed the possible routes of the role of $\cdot OH$ radicals in the hydrolytic degradation of Vicryl sutures (Zhong et al., 1994). Unfortunately, the possible role of OH^-, one of the byproducts of Fenton reagents ($H_2O_2/FeSO_4$), was not considered in the interpretation of their findings. OH^- species could be more potent than OH toward hydrolytic degradation of synthetic absorbable sutures. This is because hydroxyl anions are the sole species which attack carbonyl carbon of the ester linkages during alkaline hydrolysis. Since an equal amount of $\cdot OH$ and OH^- are generated in Fenton reagents, the observed changes in morphological, mechanical, and thermal properties could be partially attributed to OH^- ions as well as $\cdot OH$ radicals.

Besides hydroxyl radicals, the production of superoxide ions and singlet oxygen during phagocytosis has been well documented (Babior et al., 1973). Although the role of superoxide in simple organic ester hydrolysis has been known since the 1970s (Johnson, 1976; Mango and Bontempeli, 1976; San Fillipo et al., 1976; Forrester and Purushotham, 1984, 1987), its role in the hydrolytic degradation of synthetic biodegradable polyester-based biomaterials has remained largely unknown. Such an understanding of the superoxide ion role during the biodegradation of foreign materials has become increasingly desirable because of the advanced understanding of how the human immune system reacts to foreign materials and the increasing use of synthetic biomaterials for human body repair.

Lee and Chu examined the reactivity of the superoxide ion toward biodegradable biomaterials having an aliphatic polyester structure at different reaction conditions such as temperature, time, and superoxide ion concentration (Lee et al., 1999; Lee and Chu, 2000). Due to the extreme reactivity of the superoxide ion, it has been observed that the effect of superoxide ion-induced hydrolytic degradation of PDLLA and PLLA was significant in terms of changes in molecular weights and thermal properties (Lee et al., 1999). The superoxide ion-induced fragmentation of PDLLA would result in a mixture of various species with different chain lengths. A combined GPC method with a chemical tagging method revealed that the structure of oligomer species formed during the superoxide-induced degradation of PDLLA and PLLA was linear. The significant reduction in molecular weight of PDLLA by superoxide ion was also evident in the change of thermal properties like T_g. The linear low-molecular species (oligomer, trimers, and dimers) in the reaction mixture could act as an internal plasticizer to provide the synergetic effects of lowering T_g by increasing free volume. The effect of the superoxide ion-induced hydrolytic degradation on molecular weight of PLLA was similar to PDLLA but with a much smaller magnitude. The mechanism of simple hydrolysis of ester by superoxide ion proposed by Forrester et al. was subsequently modified to interpret the data obtained from the synthetic biodegradable polymers.

In addition to PDLLA and PLLA, superoxide ions also have a significant adverse effect on the hydrolytic degradation of synthetic absorbable sutures (Lee and Chu, 2000). A significant reduction in molecular weight has been found along with mechanical and thermal properties of these sutures over a wide range of superoxide ion concentrations, particularly during the first few hours of contact with superoxide ions. For example, the PGA suture lost almost all of its mass at the end of 24 h contact with superoxide ions at 25°C, while the same suture would take at least 50 days in an *in vitro* buffer for a complete mass loss. The surface morphology of these sutures was also altered drastically. The exact mechanism, however, is not fully known yet; Lee et al. suggested the possibility of simultaneous occurrence of several main-chain scissions by three different nucleophilic species.

Lee and Chu also reported that the addition of Fenton agent or hydrogen peroxide to the degradation medium would retard the well-known adverse effect of the conventional γ-irradiation sterilization of synthetic absorbable sutures (Lee and Chu, 1996). They found that these γ-irradiated sutures retained better tensile-breaking strength in the Fenton medium than in the regular buffer media. Chu et al. postulated that the γ-irradiation-induced α-carbon radicals in these sutures react with the hydroxyl radicals from the Fenton agent medium and hence neutralize the adverse effect of α-carbon radicals on the backbone chain scission. This mechanism is supported by the observed gradual loss of ESR signal of the sutures in the presence of the Fenton agent in the medium.

Instead of the adverse effect of free radicals on the degradation properties of synthetic biodegradable polyesters, Lee and Chu described an innovative approach of covalent bonding nitroxyl radicals onto these biodegradable polymers so that the nitroxyl radical attached polymers would have biological functions similar to nitric oxide (Lee and Chu, 1996, 1998). The same approach was also used to chemically attach nitroxyl radicals onto the amino acid-based biodegradable poly(ester amide) copolymers (Chu and Katsarava, 2003). A preliminary *in vitro* cell culture study of these new biologically active absorbable aliphatic polyesters indicated that they could retard the proliferation of human smooth muscle cells as native nitric oxides do. The full potential of this new biologically active biodegradable polymers is currently under investigation by Chu for a variety of therapeutic applications like drug-eluting stents and vascular grafts.

32.6 Role of Linear Aliphatic Biodegradable Polyesters in Tissue Engineering and Regeneration

The use of biodegradable polymers as the temporary scaffolds either to grow cells/tissues *in vitro* for tissue engineering applications or to regenerate tissues *in vivo* has very recently become a highly important aspect of research and development that broadens this class of biodegradable polymers beyond their traditional use in wound closure and drug control/release biomaterials. The scaffolds used in either tissue engineering or regeneration are to provide support for cellular attachment and subsequent controlled proliferation into a predefined shape or form. Obviously, a biodegradable scaffold would be preferred because of the elimination of chronic foreign body reaction and the generation of additional volume for regenerated tissues.

Although many other biodegradable polymers of natural origin such as alginate (Atala et al., 1994), hyaluronate (Benedetti et al., 1993; Larsen et al., 1993), collagen (Hirai and Matsuda, 1995), and laminin (Dixit, 1994) have been experimented with for such a purpose, synthetic biodegradable polymers of linear aliphatic polyesters such as PGA, PLA, and their copolymers (Bowald et al., 1979, 1980; Greisler, 1982; Greisler et al., 1985, 1987a,b, 1988a,b,c; Greisler, 1991; Freed et al., 1993; Mikos et al., 1993; Yu and Chu, 1993; Yu et al., 1994; Mooney et al., 1994, 1995, 1996a,b,c; Kim et al., 1998; Kim and Mooney, 1998; Yu et al., 2010) have received more attention because of their consistent sources, reproducible properties, means to tailor their properties, and versatility in manufacturing processes.

Biodegradable polymers must be fabricated into stable textile structures before they can be used as the scaffold for tissue engineering or regeneration. The stability of the scaffold structure is important during tissue engineering and regeneration in order to maintain its proper size, shape, or form upon the shear force imposed by the circulating culture media in a bioreactor, the contractile force imposed by the growing cells on the scaffold surface, and other forces like the compression from surrounding tissues.

Kim et al. reported that, although ordinary nonwoven PGA matrices have very good porosity (to facilitate diffusion of nutrients) with a high surface-to-volume ratio (to promote cell attachment and proliferation) and have been used to engineer dental pulp and smooth muscle tissues having comparable biological contents as the native tissues (Mooney et al., 1996c; Kim et al., 1998), these nonwoven PGA matrices could not maintain their original structure during tissue engineering due to the relatively weak nonwoven textile structure and stronger contractile force exerted by the attached and proliferated cells/tissues (Kim and Mooney, 1998). This led to deformed engineered tissues that may have undesirable properties; for example, the smooth muscle engineered on collagen gels exhibited significant contraction over time (Ziegler and Nerem, 1994; Hirai and Matsuda, 1995).

Because of this shortcoming of the existing nonwoven PGA matrices, Kim and Mooney (1998) very recently reported the use of PLLA to stabilize the PGA matrices. A 5% (w/v) PLLA solution in chloroform was sprayed onto PGA nonwoven matrices (made of 12 µm diameter PGA fibers) of 97% porosity and either 3 or 0.5 mm thickness. The PLLA-impregnated PGA nonwovens could be subjected to additional heat treatment at 195°C to enhance their structural stability further. Figure 32.15 shows the morphology of such a heat-annealed PLLA-impregnated PGA nonwoven matrix (Kim and Mooney, 1998). The PLLA was deposited mainly on the crosspoints of PGA fibers and hence interlocked the possible sliding of PGA fibers upon external force. Depending on the amount of PLLA used and subsequent heat treatment, the resulting PLLA-impregnated PGA nonwoven matrices had an increase in compressive modulus of 10–35-fold when compared with the original PGA non-woven. The PLLA-impregnated PGA nonwoven matrices also retained their initial volume (101 ± 4%) and about same shape as the original during the seven weeks in culture, while the untreated PGA nonwoven exhibited severe distortion in shape and contracted about 5% of its original volume. Since PLLA is well known to degrade at a much slower rate than PGA, its presence on the PGA fiber surface would be expected to make the treated PGA nonwoven matrices degrade at a much slower rate than the untreated PGA nonwoven. For example, the PLLA-treated PGA nonwoven retained about 80% of its initial mass, while the untreated PGA control had only 10% at the end of the 7-week culture.

Linear aliphatic polyesters such as PGA, its lactide copolymer, and PDS have also been fabricated into both woven and knitted forms for the *in vivo* regeneration of blood vessels in animals (Bowald et al., 1979, 1980; Greisler, 1982; Greisler et al., 1985, 1987a, 1988c, 1991; Yu and Chu, 1993; Yu et al., 1994). The published results from a variety of animals like dogs and rabbits indicate that full-wall healing with

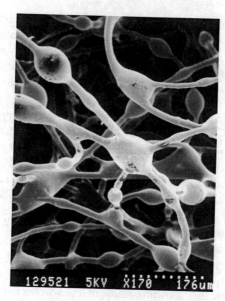

129521   5KV   X170   176um

FIGURE 32.15   Scanning electron micrograph of the exterior of PLLA-impregnated and annealed PGA matrix. (From Kim, B.S. and Mooney, D.J., 1998. *J. Biomed. Mater. Res.*, 41: 322–332. With permission.)

pseudo-endothelial lining was observed. This class of synthetic biodegradable polymers are promising candidates for the regeneration of vascular tissue.

These encouraging findings were believed to be associated with the intense macrophage/biomaterial interactions (Greisler, 1988a; Greisler et al., 1989). This interaction leads to a differential activation of the macrophage which, in turn, yields different macrophage products being released into the microenvironment (Greisler et al., 1991). Greisler et al. (1988b) have documented active stimulatory or inhibitory effects of various bioresorbable and nonresorbable materials on myofibroblast, vascular smooth muscle cell, and endothelial cell regeneration, and has shown a transinterstitial migration to be their source when lactide/glycolide copolymeric prostheses are used. The rate of tissue ingrowth parallels the kinetics of macrophage-mediated prosthetic resorption in all lactide/glycolides studied (Greisler, 1982; Greisler et al., 1985, 1987a, 1988a). Macrophage phagocytosis of the prosthetic material is observed histologically as early as 1 week following implantation of a rapidly resorbed material, such as PGA or polyglactin 910 (PG910), and is followed by an extensive increase in the myofibroblast population and neovascularization of the inner capsules (Greisler, 1982; Greisler et al., 1985, 1986). Autoradiographic analyses using tritiated thymidine demonstrated a significantly increased mitotic index within these inner capsular cells, that mitotic index paralleling the course of prosthetic resorption (Greisler, 1991). Polyglactin 910, for example, resulted in a mitotic index of $20.1 \pm 16.6\%$ three weeks following implantation, progressively decreasing to $1.2 \pm 1.3\%$ after 12 weeks. The more slowly resorbed poly-*p*-dioxanone prostheses demonstrated a persistently elevated mitotic index, $7.1 \pm 3.8\%$, 12 weeks after implantation, a time in which the prosthetic material was still being resorbed. By contrast, Dacron never yielded greater than a $1.2 \pm 1.3\%$ mitotic index (Greisler, 1991). These mitotic indices correlated closely with the slopes of the inner capsule thickening curves, suggesting that myofibroblast proliferation contributed heavily to this tissue deposition.

Therefore, the degradation property of synthetic biodegradable polymers somehow relates to macrophage activation which subsequently leads to the macrophage production of the required growth factors that initiate tissue regeneration. Different degradation properties of synthetic biodegradable polymers would thus be expected to result in different levels of macrophage activation, that is, different degrees of tissue regeneration.

One major obstacle of using those commercially available absorbable polymers like aliphatic polyester-based as scaffolds for tissue engineering is the inherent foreign-body-induced inflammatory response that these FDA-approved biomaterials can induce. This obstacle may be able to be solved by the very recent development of amino acid-based biodegradable poly(ester amide)s (AA-PEAs). Two very recent studies (Horwitz et al., 2010; Jun, 2010) suggest that not only the AA-PEAs themselves exhibit much lower foreign-body inflammatory response than those FDA-approved absorbable polymeric biomaterials, but also can tame the inflammatory response of these FDA biomaterials when coupled with AA-PEAs. The details can be found in Section 32.4.3.

32.7 Supercritical Carbon Dioxide Sterilization

There has been relatively little innovation in the area of medical device sterilization over the past many decades. Ethylene oxide (ETO) and gamma irradiation (γ-irradiation) are the only technologies currently available for medical devices. In particular, medical devices made from absorbable or biodegradable polymers such as absorbable sutures, surgical meshes, bone screws, and plates are sterilized almost exclusively by ETO due to undesirable chemical/thermal degradation from γ-irradiation or autoclave (Shalaby and Jamiolkowski, 1984; Shalaby and Linden, 1996). Although variations on γ-irradiation (namely, radiochemical sterilization pioneered by Shalaby et al., 2003) have been discovered and show promise in reducing absorbable biomaterial degradation, cobalt-60 γ-irradiation is still required and these facilities are generally housed in large industrial or research institutions that contribute to high operating costs associated with this technology.

Thus, ETO sterilization is a standard method used for all absorbable polymer sterilization due to its effectiveness and lack of acceptable alternative means. In addition to the need of a prolonging period of degassing (e.g., 8–48 h depending on the material), the EPA and other government agencies have started to monitor ETO in response to personal and environmental issues because of the concern of both the short- and long-term adverse effects of residual ETO in sterilized products (e.g., cytotoxicity, delayed healing, etc.), and the fact that ETO is a recognized carcinogen and the precautionary measures needed to operate around the toxic and explosive nature of ETO. In an OSHA published web site (http://www.osha.gov/SLTC/ethyleneoxide/), it states: "EtO possesses several physical and health hazards that merit special attention. EtO is both flammable and highly reactive. Acute exposures to EtO gas may result in respiratory irritation and lung injury, headache, nausea, vomiting, diarrhea, shortness of breath, and cyanosis. Chronic exposure has been associated with the occurrence of cancer, reproductive effects, mutagenic changes, neurotoxicity, and sensitization."

The need of a viable alternative can also be illustrated from a practical standpoint. Due to safety concerns and barriers related to high upfront capital investment, medical device manufacturers do not normally have in house ETO or γ-irradiation facilities. The sterilization is done offsite, resulting in loss of product control, increased production time, and significant elevation of costs.

Thus, the development of alternative sterilization processes that are capable of achieving validated sterility assurance levels of 10-6 (SAL6)—the benchmark for medical devices—without the use of dangerous ETO or damaging γ-irradiation is of great importance. NovaSterilis has developed a viable sterilization technology based on supercritical carbon dioxide technology (US patent 7,108,832). This alternative sterilization protocol uses supercritical carbon dioxide ($scCO_2$) to sterilize absorbable biomaterials to a sterility assurance level of 10-6 (SAL6) while maintaining the mechanical properties of the biomaterials.

The NovaSterilis $scCO_2$ sterilization process involves the use of low temperature, low pressure, and a proprietary peracetic acid-based, nontoxic sterilization additive called Novakill. CO_2 has a unique critical point, defined by a pressure ($P_c = 1099$ psi) and a temperature ($T_c = 31.1°C$) at which the liquid and vapor phases become indistinguishable. $scCO_2$ has the density of a liquid, with increased solvating power but no surface tension. The inherent properties of $scCO_2$ such as density, solvency, gas-like viscosity, diffusivity, compressibility, and very low surface tension facilitate penetration to the interior

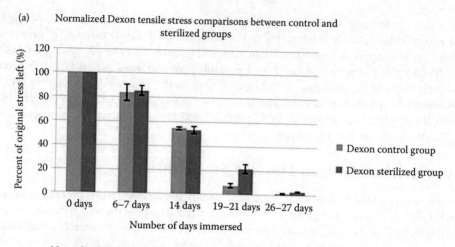

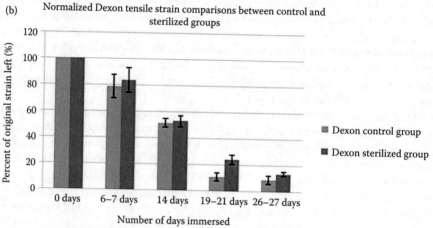

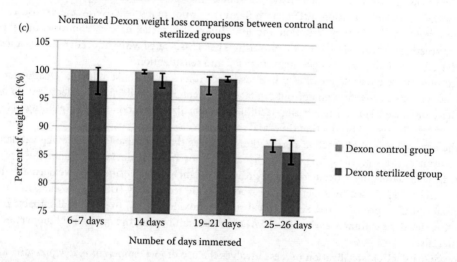

FIGURE 32.16 (a) Comparison of the tensile stresses of the sterilized and control groups of Dexon sutures upon *in vitro* degradation in pH 7.4 buffer over a period of 27 days. (b) Comparison of the tensile strains of sterilized and control groups of Dexon sutures upon *in vitro* degradation in pH 7.4 buffer over a period of 27 days. (c) Comparison of the modulus values of the sterilized and control groups of Dexon sutures upon *in vitro* degradation in pH 7.4 buffer over a period of 27 days.

of bone or soft tissue, thereby allowing inactivation of embedded pathogens. $scCO_2$ retains the diffusive properties of CO_2 gas and thus can rapidly penetrate substrates.

The supercritical form of CO_2 is a more potent biocide than argon, nitrogen, and nitrous oxide used under similar conditions, suggesting that its potency as a sterilant is derived from its chemical nature as well as transformation to the supercritical state. In fact, $scCO_2$ on its own has been used to achieve high levels of disinfection (Dillow et al., 1999), but to attain the sterility assurance level required for medical devices (SAL6), a treatment must reduce the probability of contamination to 1 in one million, when the initial bioburden of an item is ≥106 colony forming units (CFUs) of a bioindicator organism. NovaSterilis developed NovaKill additive, a peracetic acid-based (PAA) entrainer (White et al., 2006). Addition of NovaKill to a sterilization cycle using $scCO_2$ results in a SAL6 reduction in *B. atrophaeus* (standard biological indicator), which meets the definition for sterility. Furthermore, NovaSterilis has shown that $scCO_2$ in the presence of Novakill additive can be used to inactive viruses and a host of organisms including bacteria, molds, and other fungi.

In a recent collaborative preliminary study, Chu et al. have demonstrated that PGA sutures (Dexon) can be sterilized by $scCO_2$ without any adverse effect on their tensile and hydrolytic degradation properties. In addition to achieving SAL6 sterilization on these sutures, we showed that the various tensile properties (e.g., tensile strain, tensile stress, and Young's modulus) were unchanged between experimental (sterilized) and control groups (Figure 32.16). Furthermore, the data in Figure 32.16 also show that the $scCO_2$ sterilization process led to a better retention of Dexon suture mechanical properties than the standard gas sterilization method (as control in Figure 32.16) upon *in vitro* degradation over a period of 27 days. Whether the NovaSterilis $scCO_2$ sterilization technology could be applied to other absorbable polymers, further in-depth study would be required.

Defining Terms

Biodegradation: Materials that could be broken down by nature either through hydrolytic mechanisms without the help of enzymes and/or enzymatic mechanism. It is loosely associated with absorbable, erodable, resorbable.

Tissue Engineering: The ability to regenerate tissue through the help of artificial materials and devices.

References

Ali, S.A.M., Zhong, S.P., Doherty, P.J., and Williams, D.F., 1993. Mechanisms of polymer degradation in implantable devices. I. Poly(caprolactone). *Biomaterials*, 14: 648.

Atala, A., Kim, W., Paige, K.T., Vancanti, C.A., and Retil, A., 1994. Endoscopic treatment of vesicoureterall reflux with a chondrocye-alginate suspension. *J. Urol.*, 152: 641–643.

Babior, B.M., Kipnes R.S., and Cumutte, J.T., 1973. Biological defense mechanisms. The production by leukocytes of superoxide, a potential bactercidal agent. *J. Clin. Invest.*, 52: 741.

Badwey, J.A. and Kamovsky, M.L., 1980. Active oxygen species and the functions of phagocytic leucocytes. *Ann. Rev. Biochem.*, 49: 695.

Barrows, T.H., 1986. Degradable implant materials: A review of synthetic absorbable polymers and their applications. *Clin. Mater.*, 1: 233–257.

Barrows, T.H., 1994. Bioabsorbable poly(ester-amides). In: *Biomedical Polymers: Designed-to-Degrade Systems*, S.W. Shalaby, Ed., New York, Hanser, Chap. 4.

Benedetti, L., Cortivo, R., Berti, T., Berti, A., and Pea, F., 1993. Biocompatibility and biodegradation of different hyaluronan derivatives (Hyaff) implanted in rats. *Biomaterials*, 14: 1154–1160.

Bezwada, R.S., Jamiolkowski, D.D., Lee, I.Y., Agarwal, V., Persivale, J., Trenka-Benthin, S., Erneta, M., Suryadevara, J., Yang, A., and Liu, S., 1995. Monocryl suture: A new ultra-pliable absorbable monofilament suture. *Biomaterials*, 16: 1141–1148.

Bezwada, R.S., Shalaby, S.W., Newman, H.D. Jr., and Kafrawy, A., 1990. Bioabsorbable copolymers of *p*-dioxanone and lactide for surgical devices. *Trans. Soc. for Biomater.*, XIII: 194.

Bostman, O.M., 1991. Absorbable implants for the fixation of fractures. *J. Bone Joint Surg. Am.*, 73: 148.

Bostman, O.M., Hirvensalo, E., Vainionpaa, S. et al., 1990. Degradable polyglycolide rods for the internal fixation of displaced bimalleolar fractures. *Intern. Orthop.* (Germany), 14: 1–8.

Bowald, S., Busch, C., and Eriksson, I., 1979. Arterial regeneration following polyglactin 910 suture mesh grafting. *Surgery*, 86: 722–729.

Bowald, S., Busch, C., and Eriksson, I., 1980. Absorbable material in vascular prosthesis. *Acta Chir. Scand.*, 146: 391–395.

Brandrup, J. and Immergut, E.H., 1975. *Polymer Handbook*, 2nd ed., New York, Wiley.

Breitenbach, A. and Kissel, T. 1998. Biodegradable comb polyesters: Part I. Synthesis, characterisation and structural analysis of poly(lactide) and poly(lactic-co-glycolide) grafted onto water soluble poly(vinyl alcohol) as backbone. *Polymer* 39: 3261–3271.

Breitenbach, A., Pistel, K.F., and Kissel, T. 2000. Biodegradable comb polyesters: Part II. Erosion and release properties of poly(vinyl alcohol)-graft-poly(lactic-co-glycolic acid). *Polymer* 41: 4781–4792.

Campbell, N.D. and Chu, C.C., 1981. The effect of γ-irradiation on the biodegradation of polyglycolic acid synthetic sutures, the Tensile Strength Study. *27th International Symposium on Macromolecules, Abstracts of Communications*, Vol. II, pp. 1348–1352, Strasbourg, France, July 6–9, 1981.

Casey, D.J. and Roby, M.S., 1984. Synthetic copolymer surgical articles and method of manufacturing the same. *US Patent* 4,429,080, American Cyanamid.

Cawthon, A.G., Defife, K.M., Vitiello, A., Charles, C.H., Landis, G., Mendy, J., Parcher, B., Bigger, J.E., and Turnell, W.G., 2007, Novel polymer vaccine protects ferrets against lethal challenge with highly pathogenic avian influenza virus, In: *World Vaccine Congress*, Washington, D.C., Four Seasons Hotel, March 19–22, 2007.

Chatani, Y., Suehiro, K., Okita, Y., Tadokoro, H., and Chujo, K., 1968. Structural studies of polyesters, I. Crystal structure of polyglycolide. *Die Makromol. Chem.*, 113: 215–229.

Chen, S., Pieper, R., Webster, D.C., and Singh, J. 2005. Triblock copolymers: Synthesis, characterization, and delivery of a model protein. *Int. J. Pharm.*, 288: 207–218.

Chkhaidze, E., Tugushi, D., Kharadze1, D., Gomurashvili, Z., Chu, C.C., and Katsarava, R. 2011. New unsaturated biodegradable poly(ester amide)s composed of fumaric acid, leucine and α,ω-alkylene diols. *J. Macromol. Sci. Part A—Pure & Appl. Chem.* 48(7): 544–555.

Choi, S., Kwon, Y.M., and Kim, S.W. 2004. Control of blood glucose by novel GLP-1 delivery using biodegradable triblock copolymer PLGA–PEG–PLGA in type 2 diabetic rats. *Pharm Res.*, 21: 827–831.

Chu, C.C., 1981. The In-vitro degradation of poly(glycolic acid) sutures: Effect of pH. *J. Biomed. Mater. Res.*, 15: 795–804.

Chu, C.C., 1982. The effect of pH on the *in vitro* degradation of poly(glycolide lactide) copolymer absorbable sutures. *J. Biomed. Mater. Res.*, 16: 117–124.

Chu, C.C., 1985a. Strain-accelerated hydrolytic degradation of synthetic absorbable sutures. In: *Surgical Research Recent Development*, ed. C.W. Hall, Pergamon Press, San Antonio, TX.

Chu, C.C., 1985b. The Degradation and biocompatibility of suture materials. In: *CRC Critical Reviews in Biocompatibility*, ed. D.F. Williams, Vol. 1(3), CRC Press, Boca Raton, FL, pp. 261–322.

Chu, C.C., 1991. Recent advancements in suture fibers for wound closure. In: *High-Tech Fibrous Materials: Composites, Biomedical Materials, Protective Clothing, and Geotextiles*, ed. T.L. Vigo and A.F. Turbak, ACS Symposium Series #457, American Chemical Society, Washington, DC, pp. 167–213.

Chu, C.C., 1995a. Biodegradable suture materials: Intrinsic and extrinsic factors affecting biodegradation phenomena. In: *Handbook of Biomaterials and Applications*, ed. D.L. Wise, D.E. Altobelli, E.R. Schwartz, M. Yszemski, J.D. Gresser, and D.J. Trantolo, Marcel Dekker, New York.

Chu, C.C. 1995b. Biodegradable suture materials: Intrinsic and extrinsic factors affecting biodegradation. In: *Encyclopedic Handbook of Biomaterials and Applications, Part A: Materials*, Vol. 1, ed. D.L. Wise, Marcel Dekker, New York, Chap. 17, pp. 543–688.

Chu, C.C., An overview of surgical suture materials, In: *Biotextiles as Medical Implants*, ed. M.W. King and B.S. Gupta, Chap. 16, Woodhead Publisher (In Press).

Chu, C.C. and Browning, A., 1988. The study of thermal and gross morphologic properties of polyglycolic acid upon annealing and degradation treatments. *J. Biomed. Mater. Res.*, 22: 699–712.

Chu, C.C. and Campbell, N.D., 1982. Scanning electron microscope study of the hydrolytic degradation of poly(glycolic acid) suture. *J. Biomed. Mater. Res.*, 16: 417–430.

Chu, C.C., Hsu, A., Appel, M., and Beth, M. 1992. The effect of macrophage cell media on the *in vitro* hydrolytic degradation of synthetic absorbable sutures. *4th World Biomaterials Congress*, April 27–May 1, 1992, Berlin, Germany.

Chu, C.C. and Katsarava, R., 2003. Elastomeric Functional Biodegradable Copolyester Amides and Copolyester Urethanes. US Patent 6,503,538, January 7, 2003.

Chu, C.C. and Kizil, Z., 1989. The effect of polymer morphology on the hydrolytic degradation of synthetic absorbable sutures. *3rd International ITV Conference on Biomaterials—Medical Textiles*, Stuttgart, Germany, June 14–16, 1989.

Chu, C.C. and Louie, M., 1985. A chemical means to study the degradation phenomena of polyglycolic acid absorbable polymer. *J. Appl. Polym. Sci.*, 30: 3133–3141.

Chu, C. C. and Sun, D., 2008. New electrospun synthetic biodegradable poly(ester amide) drug-eluting fibrous membranes for potential wound treatment, *AATCC Symposium Proceeding Medical, Nonwovens, and Technical Textiles*, Oct. 6–7, 2008, Durham, NC, pp. 60–76.

Chu, C.C., von Fraunhofer, J.A., and Greisler, H.P., 1997. *Wound Closure Biomaterials and Devices*, CRC Press, Boca Raton, FL.

Chu, C.C. and Williams, D.F., 1983. The effect of γ-irradiation on the enzymatic degradation of polyglycolic acid absorbable sutures. *J. Biomed. Mater. Res.*, 17: 1029.

Chu, C.C., Zhang, L., and Coyne, L., 1995. Effect of irradiation temperature on hydrolytic degradation properties of synthetic absorbable sutures and polymers. *J. Appl. Polym. Sci.* 56: 1275–1294.

Chujo, K., Kobayashi, H., Suzuki, J., Tokuhara, S., and Tanabe, M., 1967a. Ring-opening polymerization of glycolide. *Die Makromol. Chem.*, 100: 262–266.

Chujo, K., Kobayashi, H., Suzuki, J., and Tokuhara, S., 1967b. Physical and chemical characteristics of polyglycolide. *Die Makromol. Chem.*, 100: 267–270.

Daniels, A.U., Taylor, M.S., Andriano, K.P., and Heller, J., 1992. Toxicity of absorbable polymers proposed for fracture fixation devices. *Trans. 38th Ann. Mtg. Orthop. Res. Soc.*, 17: 88.

DeFife, K.M., Grako, K., Cruz-Aranda, G., Price, S., Chantung, R., Macpherson, K., Khoshabeh, R., Gopalan, S., and Turnell, W., 2009. Poly(ester amide) co-polymers promote blood and tissue compatibility. *J. Biomaterials Sci., Polym. Ed.* 20(11): 1495–1511.

Deng, M.X., Wu, J., Reinhart-King, C., and Chu, C.C., 2009. Synthesis and characterization of biodegradable poly(ester amide)s with pendant amine functional groups and *in vitro* cellular response. *Biomacromolecules*, 10(1): 14–20.

Deng, M.X., Wu, J., Reinhart-King, C.A., and Chu, C.C., 2011. Biodegradable functional poly(ester amide)s with pendant hydroxyl functional groups: Synthesis, characterization, fabrication and *in vitro* cellular response. *Acta Biomater.*, 7: 1504–1515.

Devereux, D.F., O'Connell, S.M., Liesch, J.B., Weinstein, M., and Robertson, F.M., 1991. Induction of leukocyte activation by meshes surgically implanted in the peritoneal cavity. *Am. J. Surg.*, 162: 243.

De Wit, M.A., Wang, Z., Atkins, K.M., Mequanint, K., and Gillies, E.R., 2008. Syntheses, characterization, and functionalization of poly(ester amide)s with pendant amine functional groups. *J. Polym. Sci., Part A: Polym. Chem.*, 46: 6376–6392.

Dillow, A.K., Dehghani, F., Hrkach, J.S., Foster, N.R., and Langer, R., 1999. Bacterial inactivation by using near- and supercritical carbon dioxide. *Proc. Natl Acad. Sci. USA*, 96(18): 10344–10348.

Dixit, V., 1994. Development of a bioartificial liver using isolated hepatocytes. *Artif. Organs*, 18: 371–384.

Eitenmuller, J., David, A. et al. 1989a, 'Die Versorgung von Sprunggelenksfrakturen unter ....' Read at Jahrestagung der Deutschen Gesellschaft fur Unfalheikunde, Berlin, Nov. 22, 1989a.

Eitenmüller, K.L., Schmickal, G.T., and Muhr, G., 1989b. Die versorgung von sprunggelenksfrakturen unter verwendung von platten und schrauben aus resorbierbarem polymer material. Presented at Jahrestagung der Deutschen Gesellschaft für Unfallheilkunde, Berlin, November 1989.

Farnsworth. B.N. 2002. Posterior intravaginal slingplasty (infracoccygeal sacropexy) for severe posthysterectomy vaginal vault prolapse: A preliminary report on efficacy and safety. *Int. Urogynecol. J.,* 13: 4–8.

FDA, 2007. 'FDA clears first of its kind suture made using DNA technology', US Food and Drug Administration, February 12, 2007, US Department of Health and Human Services, http://www.fda.gov/bbs/topics/NEWS/2007/NEW01560.html.

Forrester, A.R. and Purushotham, V., 1984. Mechanism of hydrolysis of esters by superoxide. *J. Chem. Soc., Chem. Commun.*, 1505.

Forrester, A.R. and Purushotham, V., 1987. Reactions of carboxylic acid derivatives with superoxide. *J. Chem. Soc. Perkin Trans.* 1: 945.

Fredericks, R.J., Melveger, A.J., and Dolegiewitz, L.J., 1984. Morphological and structural changes in a copolymer of glycolide and lactide occurring as a result of hydrolysis. *J. Polym. Sci. Phys. Ed.* 22: 57–66.

Freed, L.E., Marquis, J.C., Nohia, A., Emmanual, J., Mikos, A.G. and Langer, R., 1993. Neocartilage formation *in vitro* and *in vivo* using cells cultured on synthetic biodegradable polymers. *J. Biomed. Mater. Res.*, 27: 11–23.

Fukuzaki, H., Yoshida, M., Asano, M., Aiba, Y., and Kumakura, M., 1989. Direct copolymerization of glycolic acid with lactones in the absence of catalysts. *Eur. Polym. J.*, 26: 457–461.

Fukuzaki, H., Yoshida, M., Asano, M., Kumakura, M., Mashimo, T., Yuasa, H., Imai, K., Yamandka, H., Kawaharada, U., and Suzuki, K., 1991. A new biodegradable copolymer of glycolic acid and lactones with relatively low molecular weight prepared by direct copolycondensation in the absence of catalysts. *J. Biomed. Mater. Res.*, 25: 315–328.

Ganaha, F., Kao, E.Y., Wong, H., Elkins, C.J., Lee, J., Modanlou, S., Rhee, C. et al. 2004. Stent-based controlled release of intravascular angiostatin to limit plaque progression and in-stent restenosis. *J Vasc Interv Radiol* 15: 601–608.

Gogolewski, S. and Pennings, A.J., 1983. Resorbable materials of poly(L-lactide). II. Fibres spun from solutions of poly(L-lactide) in good solvents. *J. Appl. Polym. Sci.*, 28: 1045–1061.

Goldstein, H.B., Vakili, B., Franco, N., Echols, K.T., and Chesson, R.R., 2007. The effect of suture material on outcomes of surgery for pelvic organ prolapse. *Pelviperineology,* 26: 174–177.

Greisler, H.P., 1982. Arterial regeneration over absorbable prostheses. *Arch. Surg.*, 117: 1425–1431.

Greisler, H.P., 1988. Macrophage–biomaterial interactions with bioresorbable vascular prostheses. *Trans. ASAIO,* 34: 1051–1059.

Greisler, H.P., 1991. Macrophage activation in bioresorbable vascular grafts. In: *Vascular Endothelium: Physiological Basis of Clinical Problems*. eds. J.D. Catravas, A.D. Callow, C.N. Gillis, and U. Ryan, Plenum Press, New York, NATO Advanced Study Institute, pp. 253–254.

Greisler, H.P., Dennis, J.W., Endean, E.D., Ellinger, J., Friesel, R., and Burgess, W., 1989. Macrophage/biomaterial interactions: The stimulation of endothelialization. *J. Vasc. Surg.*, 9: 588–593.

Greisler, H.P., Dennis, J.W., Endean, E.D., and Kim, D.U., 1988b. Derivation of neointima of vascular grafts. *Circ. Suppl. I*, 78: I6–I12.

Greisler, H.P., Ellinger, J., Schwarcz, T.H., Golan, J., Raymond, R.M., and Kim, D.U., 1987a. Arterial regeneration over polydioxanone prostheses in the rabbit. *Arch. Surg.*, 122: 715–721.

Greisler, H.P., Endean, E.D., Klosak, J.J., Ellinger, J., Dennis, J.W., Buttle, K., and Kim, D.U., 1988c. Polyglactin 910/polydioxanone bicomponent totally resorbable vascular prostheses. *J. Vasc. Surg.*, 7: 697–705.

Greisler, H.P., Kim, D.U., Dennis, J.W., Klosak, J.J., Widerborg, K.A., Endean, E.D., Raymond, R.M., and Ellinger, J., 1987b. Compound polyglactin 910/polypropylene small vessel prostheses. *J. Vasc. Surg.*, 5: 572–583.

Greisler, H.P., Kim, D.U., Price, J.B., and Voorhees, A.B., 1985. Arterial regenerative activity after prosthetic implantation. *Arch. Surg.*, 120: 315–323.

Greisler, H.P., Schwarcz, T.H., Ellinger, J., and Kim, D.U., 1986. Dacron inhibition of arterial regenerative activity. *J. Vasc. Surg.*, 747–756.

Greisler, H.P., Tattersall, C.W., Kloask, J.J. et al., 1991. Partially bioresorbable vascular grafts in dogs. *Surgery*, 110: 645–655.

Gross, R.A., 1994. Bacterial polyesters: Structural variability in microbial synthesis. In: *Biomedical Polymers: Designed-to-Degrade Systems*, ed. S.W. Shalaby, Chap. 7, Hanser, New York.

Gunatillake, P., Mayadunne, R., and Adhikari, R., 2006. Recent developments in biodegradable synthetic polymers. *Biotechnol. Annu. Rev.* 12: 301–347.

Guo, K. and Chu, C.C., 2005. Synthesis, characterization and swelling behaviors of novel biodegradable unsaturated poly(ester-amide)s/poly(ethylene glycol) diacrylate hydrogels. *J. Polym. Sci. Polym. Chem. Ed.*, 43: 3932–3944.

Guo, K. and Chu, C.C., 2007a. Synthesis, characterization and biodegradation of copolymers of unsaturated and saturated poly(ester amide)s. *J. Polym. Sci. Polym. Chem. Ed.*, 45: 1595–1606.

Guo, K. and Chu, C.C., 2007b. Synthesis, characterization and biodegradation of novel poly(ether ester amide)s based on L-phenylalanine and oligoethylene glycol. *Biomacromolecules*, 8(9): 2851–2861.

Guo, K. and Chu, C.C., 2008. Copolymers of unsaturated and saturated poly(ether ester amide)s: Synthesis, characterization and biodegradation. *J. Appl. Polym. Sci.*, 110(3): 1858–1869.

Guo, K. and Chu, C.C., 2009. Biodegradable and injectable Paclitaxel-loaded poly(ester amide)s microspheres: Fabrication and characterization, *J. Biomed. Mater. Res. Part B. Appl. Biomater.*, 89 (2): 491–500.

Guo, K. and Chu, C.C., 2010. Synthesis of biodegradable amino acid-based poly(ester amide) and poly(ether ester amide) with pendant functional groups, *J. Appl. Polym. Sci.* 117(6): 3386–3394.

Guo, K., Chu, C.C., Chkhaidze, E., and Katsarava, R., 2005. Synthesis and characterization of novel biodegradable unsaturated poly(ester-amide)s. *J. Polym. Sci. Polym. Chem. Ed.*, 43: 1463–1477.

Haber, F. and Weiss, J., 1934. The catalytic decomposition of hydrogen peroxide by iron salts. *Proc. R. Soc. Lond.*, A, 147: 332.

Helder, J., Feijen, J., Lee, S.J., and Kim, W., 1986. Copolyemrs of D,L-lactic acid and glycine. *Makromol. Chem. Rapid. Commun.*, 7: 193.

Henderson, P.W., Kadouch, D.J.M., Singh, S.P., Zawaneh, P.N., Weiser, J., Yazdi, S., Weinstein, A., Krotscheck, U., Wechsler, B., Putnam, D., and Spector, J.A., 2010. A rapidly resorbable hemostatic biomaterial based on dihydroxyacetone, *J. Biomed. Mater. Res.*, 93A: 776–782.

Hirai, J. and Matsuda, T., 1995. Self-organized, tubular hybrid vascular tissue composed of vascular cells and collagen for low pressure-loaded venous system, *Cell Transpl.*, 4: 597–608.

Hofmann, G.O., 1992. Biodegradable implants in orthopaedic surgery—A review of the state of the art. *Clin. Mater.*, 10: 75.

Hollinger, J.O., 1995. *Biomedical Applications of Synthetic Biodegradable Polymers*, CRC Press, Boca Raton, FL.

Horwitz, J.A., Shum, K.M., Bodle, J.C., Deng, M.X., Chu, C.C., and Reinhart-King, C.A., 2010. Biological performance of biodegradable amino acid-based poly(ester amide)s: Endothelial cell adhesion and inflammation *in vitro. J. Biomed. Mater. Res. Part A*, 95: 371–380.

Huh, K.M., Cho, Y.W., and Park, K., 2003. PLGA–PEG block copolymers for drug formulations. *Drug Deliv. Technol.*, 3(5): 42, 44–49.

Ikada, Y. and Tsuji, H., 2000. Stereocomplex formation between enantiomeric poly(lactic acid)s. 12. Spherulite growth of low-molecular-weight poly(lactic acid)s from the melt. *Macromol. Rapid Commun.*, 21: 117–132.

Jamiokowski, D.D. and Shalaby, S.W., 1991. A polymeric radiostabilizer for absorbable polyesters. In: *Radiation Effect of Polymers*, ed. R.L. Clough and S.W. Shalaby, Chap. 18, pp. 300–309. ACS Symposium Series # 475, ACS, Washington, DC.

Jeong, J.H., Kim, S.W., and Park, T.G., 2004. Biodegradable triblock copolymer of PLGA–PEG–PLGA enhances gene transfection efficiency. *Pharm. Res.*, 21: 50–54.

Johnson, R.A., 1976. Bis(3-methylbenzoyl)peroxide B-0-031 35 Di-m-ioluoyl peroxide. *Tetrahedron Lett.*, 331.

Jokhadze, G., Machaidze, M., Panosyan, H., Chu, C.C., and Katsarava, R., 2007. Synthesis and characterization of functional elastomeric biodegradable poly(ester amide)s copolymers. *J. Biomater. Sci. Polym. Ed.* 18(4): 411–438.

Jung, T., Breitenbach, A., and Kissel, T., 2000. Sulfobutylated poly(vinyl alcohol)-graft-poly(lactide-co-glycolide)s facilitate the preparation of small negatively charged biodegradable nanospheres. *J. Control Rel.*, 67: 157–169.

Katsarava, R., Beridze, V., Arabuli, N., Kharadze, D., Chu, C.C., and Won, C.Y., 1999. Amino acid based bioanalogous polymers. Synthesis and study of regular poly(ester amide)s based on bis(α-amino acid) α, ω-alkylene diesters and aliphatic dicarboxylic acids. *J. Polym. Sci. Part A: Polym Chem.*, 37: 391–407.

Katsarava, R.D., Kharadze, D.P., Japaridze, N., Avalishvili, L.M., Omiadze, T.N., and Zaalishvili, M.M. 1985. Hetero-chain polymers based on natural amino-acids. Synthesis of polyamides from N-alpha, N-epsilon-bis(trimethylsilyl) lysine alkyl esters. *Makromol. Chem.*, 186: 939–954.

Katz, A., Mukherjee, D.P., Kaganov, A.L., and Gordon, S., 1985. A new synthetic monofilament absorbable suture made from polytrimethylene carbonate. *Surg. Gynecol. Obstet.*, 161: 213–222.

Kim, B.S. and Mooney, D.J., 1998. Engineering smooth muscle tissue with a predefined structure. *J. Biomed. Mater. Res.*, 41: 322–332.

Kim, B.S., Putman, A.J., Kulik, T.J., and Mooney, D.J., 1998. Optimizing seeding and culture methods to engineer smooth muscle tissue on biodegradable polymer matrices. *Biotechnol. Bioeng.*, 57: 64–54.

Kimura, Y., 1993. Biodegradable polymers. In: *Biomedical Applications of Polymeric Materials*, eds. T. Tsuruta, T. Hayashi, K. Kataoka, K. Ishihara, and Y. Kimura, pp. 164–190. CRC Press, Boca Raton, FL.

Koelmel, D.F., Jamiokowski, D.D., Shalaby, S.W., and Bezwada, R.S., 1991. Low modulus radiation sterilizable monofilament sutures. *Polym. Prepr.*, 32: 235–236.

Kumar, N., Ravikumar, M.N.V., and Domb, A.J. 2001. Biodegradable block copolymers. *Adv. Drug Deliv. Rev.*, 53:23–44.

Kwon, Y.M. and Kim, S.W., 2004. Biodegradable triblock copolymer microspheres based on thermosensitive sol–gel transition. *Pharm. Res.*, 21: 339–343.

Larsen, N.E., Pollak, C.T., Reiner, K., Leshchiner, E., and Balazs, E.A., 1993. Hylan gel biomaterial: Dermal and immunologic compatibility. *J. Biomed. Meter. Res.*, 27: 1129–1134.

Lee, K.H. and Chu, C.C., 1996. The role of free radicals in hydrolytic degradation of absorable polymeric biomaterials. *5th World Biomaterials Congress*, Toronto, Canada, May 29–June 2.

Lee, K.H. and Chu, C.C., 1998. Molecular design of biologically active biodegradable polymers for biomedical applications. *Macromol. Symp.*, 130: 71.

Lee, K.H. and Chu, C.C., 2000. The effect of superoxide ions in the degradation of five synthetic absorbable suture materials. *J. Biomed. Mater. Res.*, 49(1): 25–35.

Lee, K.H., Chu, C.C., and Fred, J., 1996. Aminoxyl-containing radical spin in polymers and copolymers. *U.S. Patent 5,516,881*, May 16, 1996.

Lee, K.H., Won, C.Y., and Chu, C.C., 1999. Hydrolysis of biodegradable polymers by superoxide ions. *J. Polym. Sci. Part A, Polym. Chem. Ed.*, 37 (18): 3558–3567.

Lee, P.Y., Li, Z., and Huang, L. 2003. Thermosensitive hydrogel as a TGF-beta gene delivery vehicle enhances diabetic would healing. *Pharm. Res.*, 20: 1995–2000.

Lee, S.H., Szinai, I., Carpenter, K., Katsarava, R., Jokhadze, G., Chu, C.C., Scheerder, I.D., and Hong, M.K., 2002. *In vivo* biocompatibility evaluation of stents coated by a new biodegradable elastomeric and functional polymer. *Coron. Artery Dis.*, 13(4): 237–241.

Leenslag, J.W. and Pennings, A.J., 1984. Synthesis of high-molecular weight poly(L-lactide) initiated with tin 2-ethylhexanoate. *Makromol. Chem.*, 188: 1809–1814.

Li, L. and Chu, C.C., 2009. Nitroxyl radical incorporated lectrospun biodegradable poly(ester amide) nanofibrous membranes. *J. Biomater. Sci. Polym. Ed.*, 20: 341–361.

Li, S., Anjard, S., Tashkov, I., and Vert, M., 1998. Hydrolytic degradation of PLA/PEO/PLA triblock copolymers prepared in the presence of Zn metal or CaH$_2$. *Polymer*, 39: 5421–5430.

Li, Y. and Kissel, T., 1998. Synthesis, characteristics and *in vitro* degradation of star-block copolymers consisting of L-lactide, glycolide and branched multi-arm poly(ethylene oxide). *Polymer*, 39: 4421–4427.

Loh, I.H., Chu, C.C., and Lin, H.L., 1992. Plasma surface modification of synthetic absorbable fibers for wound closure. *J. Appl. Biomater.* 3: 131–146.

Magno, F. and Bontempelli, G., 1976. On the reaction kinetics of electrogenerated superoxide ion with aryl benzoates. *J. Electroanal. Chem.*, 68: 337.

Martin, D.P. and Williams, S.F. 2003. Medical applications of poly-4-hydroxybutyrate: A strong flexible absorbable biomaterial. *Biochem. Eng. J.*, 16: 97–105.

Matlaga, V.F. and Salthouse, T.N., 1980. Electron microscopic observations of polyglactin 910 suture sites, In *First World Biomaterials Congress*, Abstr., Baden, Austria, April 8–12, p. 2.

Mikos, A.G., Sarakinos, G., Leite, S.M., Vacanti, J.P., and Langer, R., 1993. Laminated three-dimensional biodegradable forms for use in tissue engineering. *Biomaterials*, 14: 323–330.

Miller, N.D. and Williams, D.F., 1984. The *in vivo* and *in vitro* degradation of poly(glycolic acid) suture material as a function of applied strain. *Biomaterials*, 5: 365–368.

Miller, R.A., Brady, J.M., and Cutright, D.E., 1977. *J. Biomed. Mater. Res.*, 11: 711.

Mooney, D.J., Baldwin, D.F., Vacanti, J.P. and Langer, R., 1996a. Novel approach to fabricate porous sponges of poly(D,L-lactic-co-glycolic acid) without the use of organic solvents. *Biomaterials*, 17: 1417–1422.

Mooney, D.J., Breuer, C., McNamara, K., Vacanti, J.P., and Langer, R., 1995. Fabricating tubular devices from polymers of lactic and glycolic acid for tissue engineering. *Tissue Eng.*, 1: 107–118.

Mooney, D.J., Mazzoni, C.L., Breuer, K., McNamara, J.P., Vacanti, J.P., and Langer, R., 1996b. Stabilized poly-glycolic acid fibre-based tubes for tissue engineering. *Biomaterials*, 17: 115–124.

Mooney, D.J., Organ, G., Vacanti, J.P., and Langer, R., 1994. Design and fabrication of biodegradable polymer devices to engineer tubular tissue. *Cell Transplant*, 3: 203–210.

Mooney, D.J., Powell, C., Piana, J., and Rutherford, B., 1996c. Engineering dental pulp-like tissue *in vitro*. *Biotechnol. Prog.*, 12: 865–868.

Nair, L.S. and Laurencin, C.T., 2007. Biodegradable polymers as biomaterials. *Prog. Polym. Sci.* 32: 762–798.

Nathan, A. and Kohn, J., 1994. Amino acid derived polymers. In: *Biomedical Polymers: Designed-to-Degrade Systems*, ed. S.W. Shalaby, Chap. 5. Hanser Publishers, New York.

Pang, X. and Chu, C.C., 2010a. Synthesis, characterization and biodegradation of novel poly(ester amide)s and their functionalization. *Biomaterials*, 31(14): 3745–3754.

Pang, X., Wu, J., Reinhart-King, C.A., and Chu, C.C., 2010. Synthesis and characterization of functionalized water soluble cationic poly(ester amide)s. *J. Polym. Sci. Part A: Polym. Chem.*, 48: 3758–3766.

Pang, X. and Chu, C.C., 2010b. Synthesis, characterization and biodegradation of poly(ester amide)s based hydrogels. *Polymer*, 51: 4200–4210.

Paredes, N., Rodriguez-Gala, A., and Puiggali, N.J., 1998. Synthesis and characterization of a family of biodegradable poly(ester amide)s derived from glycine. *J. Polym. Sci. Part A: Polym. Chem.*, 36: 1271–1282.

Park, K., Shalaby, W.S.W., and Park. H., 1993. *Biodegradable Hydrogels for Drug Delivery*, Technomic Publishing, Lancaster, PA.

Pistel, K.F., Breitenbach, A., Zange-Volland, R., and Kissel, T. 2001. Brush-like branched biodegradable polyesters: Part III. Protein release from microspheres of poly(vinyl alcohol)-graft-poly(lactic-co-glycolic acid). *J. Control Rel.*, 73: 7–20.

Pratt, L. and Chu, C.C., 1993. Hydrolytic degradation of α-substituted polyglycolic acid: A semi-empirical computational study. *J. Comput. Chem.*, 14: 809–817.

Pratt, L. and Chu, C.C., 1994. The effect of electron donating and electron withdrawing substituents on the degradation rate of bioabsorbable polymers: A semi-empirical computational study. *J. Mol. Struct.*, 304: 213–226.

Pratt, L. and Chu, C.C., 1994b. A computational study of the hydrolysis of degradable polysaccharide biomaterials: Substituent effects on the hydrolytic mechanism. *J. Comput. Chem.*, 15: 241–248.

Pratt, L., Chu, A., Kim, J., Hsu, A., and Chu, C.C., 1993. The effect of electrolytes on the *in vitro* hydrolytic degradation of synthetic biodegradable polymers: Mechanical properties, thermodynamics and molecular modeling. *J. Polym. Sci. Polym. Chem. Ed.*, 31: 1759–1769.

Puelacher, W.C., Mooney, D., Langer, R., Upton, J., Vacanti, J.P., and Vananti, C.A., 1994. Design of nasoseptal cartilage replacements sunthesized from biodegradable polymers and chondrocytes. *Biomaterials*, 15: 774–778.

San Fillipo, Jr., J., Romano, L.J., Chem, C.I., and Valentine, J.S., 1976. Cleavage of esters by superoxide. *J. Org. Chem.*, 4: 586.

Schwartz, S., Demars, S., Chu, C.C., White, J., Cooper, A, Rothrock, M., Adelman, M., and Yurt, R., 2008. Efficacy of poly(ester amide) dressings on partial thickness wound healing. Paper presented at the *3rd World Union of Wound Healing Societies*, June 4–8, Toronto, Canada.

Shalaby, S.W. and Jamiolkowski, D.D., 1984. Monomer process patent, US Patent, 1984, Ethicon, Inc.

Shalaby, S.W., 1994. *Biomedical Polymers: Designed-to-Degrade Systems*, Hanser Publishers, New York.

Shalaby, S.W. and Linden, C.L.J., 1996, Irradiation of Polmers, In *Irradiation of Poymers*, ed. R.L. Clough and S.W. Shalaby, American Chemical Society, Washington, DC, p. 246.

Shalaby, S.W., Doyle, Y., Anneauxa, B.L., Carpentera, K.A., and Schiretz, F.R., 2003. Radiochemical sterilization and its use for sutures. *Nucl. Instrum. Methods Phys. Res. B*, 208: 110–114.

Shieh, S.J., Zimmerman, M.C., and Parsons, J.R., 1990. Preliminary characterization of bioresorbable and nonresorbable synthetic fibers for the repair of soft tissue injuries. *J. Biomed. Mater. Res.*, 24: 789–808.

Song, H., 2007. L-Arginine-based Biodegradable Poly(ester amide)s, their Synthesis, Characterization, Fabrication, and Application as Drug and Gene Carriers, PhD thesis, Cornell University, May 2007.

Song, H. and Chu, C.C., 2012. Synthesis and characterization of a new family of cationic poly (ester amide) s and their biological properties. *J. Appl. Polym. Sci.* 124(5): 3840–3853.

Sugnuma, J., Alexander, H., Traub, J., and Ricci, J.L., 1992. Biological response of intramedullary bone to poly-L-lactic acid. In: *Tissue-Inducing Biomater*, ed. L.G. Cima and E.S. Ron, Mater. Res. Soc. Symp. Proc., Boston, MA, Material Research Society, 252: 339–343.

Tsitlanadze, G., Machaidze, M., Kviria, T., Djavakhishvili, N., Chu, C.C., and Katsarava, R., 2004b. Biodegradation of amino acid based poly(ester amide)s: *in vitro* weight loss and preliminary *in vivo* study. *J. Biomater. Sci. Polym. Ed.* 15(1): 1–24.

Tsitlanadze, G., Machaidze, M., Kviria, T., Katsarava, R., and Chu, C.C., 2004a. *In vitro* enzymatic biodegradation of amino acid based poly(ester amide)s biomaterials. *J. Mater. Sci.: Mater. Med.*, 15: 185–190.

Tunc, D.C., 1983. A high strength absorbable polymer for internal bone fixation. *Trans. Soc. Biomater.*, 6: 47.

Vert, M., Feijen, J., Albertsson, A., Scott, G., and Chiellini, E., 1992. *Biodegradable Polymers and Plastics*, Royal Society of Chemistry, Cambridge, England, UK.

Villa, M.T., White, L.E., Alam, M., Yoo, S.S., and Walton, R.L. 2008. Barbed sutures: A review of the literature. *Plast. Reconstr. Surg.*, 121(3): 102e–108e.

White, A., Burns, D., and Christiansen, T.W., 2006. Effective terminal sterilization using supercritical carbon dioxide. *J. Biotechnol.*, 123(4): 504–515.

Williams, D.F., 1979. Some observations on the role of cellular enzymes in the *in vivo* degradation of polymers. *ASTM Spec. Tech. Publ.*, 684: 61–75.

Williams, D.F., 1990. Biodegradation of medical polymers. In: *Concise Encyclopedia of Medical and Dental Materials*, ed. D.F. Williams, pp. 69–74. Pergamon Press, New York.

Williams, D.F. and Mort, E., 1977. Enzyme-accelerated hydrolysis of polyglycolic acid. *J. Bioeng.*, 1: 231–238.

Williams, D.F. and Chu, C.C., 1984. The effects of enzymes and gamma irradiation on the tensile strength and morphology of poly(p-dioxanone) fibers. *J. Appl. Polym. Sci.*, 29: 1865–1877.

Williams, D.F. and Zhong, S.P., 1991. Are free radicals involved in the biodegradation of implanted polymers. *Adv. Mater.*, 3: 623.

Winet, H. and Hollinger, J.O., 1993. Incorporation of polylactide–polyglycolide in a cortical defect: Neoosteogenesis in a bone chamber. *J. Biomed. Mater. Res.*, 27: 667–676.

Wise, D.L., Fellmann, T.D., Sanderson, J.E., and Wentworth, R.L., 1979. Lactic/glycolic acid polymers. In: *Drug Carriers in Biology and Medicine*, ed. G. Gregoriadis, pp. 237–270. Academic Press, New York.

Woodruff, M.A. and Hutmacher, D.W., 2010, The return of a forgotten polymer— Polycaprolactone in the 21st century. *Progr. Polym. Sci.*, 35: 1217–1256.

Wu, J., 2010. Arginine and Phenylalanine Based Poly(ester amide)s: Synthesis, Characterization and Applications, PhD thesis, Cornell University, August 2010.

Yamanouchi, D., Wu, J., Lazar, A.N., Kent, K.G., Chu, C.C., and Liu, B., 2008. Biodegradable arginine-based poly(ester-amide)s as non-viral gene delivery reagents. *Biomaterials*, 29(22): 3269–3277.

Yu, N.Y.C., Schindeler, A., Little, D.G., and Ruys, A.J., 2010. Biodegradable poly(a-hydroxy acid) polymer scaffolds for bone tissue engineering. *J. Biomed. Mater. Res. Part B: Appl. Biomater.*, 93B: 285–295.

Yu, T.J. and Chu, C.C., 1993. Bicomponent vascular grafts consisting of synthetic biodegradable fibers. Part I. *In vitro* study. *J. Biomed. Mater. Res.*, 27: 1329–1339.

Yu, T.J., Ho, D.M., and Chu, C.C., 1994. Bicomponent vascular grafts consisting of synthetic biodegradable fibers. Part II. *In vivo* healing response. *J. Investigative Surg.* 7: 195–211.

Zawaneha, P.N., Singh, S.P., Paderac, R.F., Henderson, P.W., Spector, J.A., and Putnama, D. 2005. Design of an injectable synthetic and biodegradable surgical biomaterial. *Proc. Natl Acad. Sci., USA*, 107(24): 11014–11019.

Zelikin, A.N. and Putnam, D., 2005. Poly(carbonate-acetal)s from the dimer form of dihydroxyacetone, *Macromolecules*, 38: 5532–5537.

Zhang, L., Loh, I.H., and Chu, C.C., 1993. A combined γ-irradiation and plasma deposition treatment to achieve the ideal degradation properties of synthetic absorbable polymers. *J. Biomed. Mater. Res.*, 27: 1425–1441.

Zhong, S.P., Doherty, P.J., and Williams, D.F., 1994. A preliminary study on the free radical degradation of glycolic acid/lactic acid copolymer. *Plast., Rubber Composites Process. Appl.*, 21: 89.

Ziegler, T. and Nerem, R.M., 1994. Tissue engineering a blood vessel: Regulation of vascular biology by mechanical stress. *J. Cell. Biochem.*, 56: 204–209.

Further Information

Several recent books have very comprehensive descriptions of a variety of biodegradable polymeric biomaterials, their synthesis, physical, chemical, mechanical, biodegradable, and biological properties.

Barrows, T.H., 1986. Degradable implant materials: A review of synthetic absorbable polymers and their applications. *Clin. Mater.*, 1: 233–257.

Bastioli, C., 2005. *Handbook of Biodegradable Polymers*, UK, Smithers Rapra Press.

Chu, C.C., 1995. Biodegradable suture materials: Intrinsic and extrinsic factors affecting biodegradation phenomena, In: *Handbook of Biomaterials and Applications*, eds. D.L. Wise, D.E. Altobelli, E.R. Schwartz, M. Yszemski, J.D. Gresser, and D.J. Trantolo, Marcel Dekker, New York.

Chu, C.C., von Fraunhofer, J.A., and Greisler, H.P., 1997. *Wound Closure Biomaterials and Devices*, CRC Press, Boca Raton, FL.

Domb, A. and Kumar, N., 2011. *Biodegradable Polymers in Clinical use and Clinical Development*, Wiley, New York.

Hollinger, J.O., Ed., 1995. *Biomedical Applications of Synthetic Biodegradable Polymers*, CRC Press, Boca Raton, FL.

Kimura, Y., 1993. Biodegradable polymers, In: *Biomedical Applications of Polymeric Materials*, T. Tsuruta, T. Hayashi, K. Kataoka, K. Ishihara, and Y. Kimura, Eds., pp. 164–190. CRC Press, Boca Raton, FL.

Mittal, V., 2011. *Nanocomposites with Biodegradable Polymers: Synthesis, Properties, and Future Perspectives*, New York, NY, Oxford University Press.

Park, K., Shalaby, W.S.W., and Park. H., 1993. *Biodegradable Hydrogels for Drug Delivery*, Technomic Publishing, Lancaster, PA.

Shalaby, S.W., 1994. *Biomedical Polymers: Designed-to-Degrade Systems*, Hanser Publishers, New York.

Shalaby, S.W. and Burg, K.J.L., 2003. *Absorbable and Biodegradable Polymers*, Boca Raton, CRC Press.

Vert, M., Feijen, J., Albertsson, A., Scott, G., and Chiellini, E., 1992. *Biodegradable Polymers and Plastics*, Royal Society of Chemistry, Cambridge, England, UK.

33

Biologic Biomaterials: Tissue-Derived Biomaterials (Collagen)

33.1 Structure and Properties of Collagen and Collagen-Rich Tissues 33-1
Structure of Collagen • Properties of Collagen-Rich Tissue
33.2 Biotechnology of Collagen 33-11
Isolation and Purification of Collagen • Matrix Fabrication Technology
33.3 Design of a Resorbable Collagen-Based Medical Implant 33-13
Biocompatibility • Physical Dimension • Apparent Density • Pore Structure • Mechanical Property • Hydrophilicity • Permeability
33.4 Tissue Engineering for Tissue and Organ Regeneration 33-17
Defining Terms 33-18
References.. 33-20

Shu-Tung Li
Collagen Matrix Inc.

33.1 Structure and Properties of Collagen and Collagen-Rich Tissues

33.1.1 Structure of Collagen

Collagen is a multifunctional family of proteins of unique structural characteristics. It is the most abundant and ubiquitous protein in the body; its functions ranging from serving crucial biomechanical functions in bone, skin, tendon, and ligament to controlling cellular gene expressions in development (Nimni and Harkness, 1988). Collagen molecules, like all proteins, are formed *in vivo* by enzymatically regulated step-wise polymerization reaction between amino and carboxyl groups of amino acids, where R is a side group of an amino acid residue:

$$
\begin{array}{c}
\quad\;\; O \;\; H \;\; H \\
\quad\;\; \| \;\;\; | \;\;\; | \\
(-C - N - C-)_n \\
\quad\qquad\quad | \\
\quad\qquad\quad R
\end{array}
\qquad (33.1)
$$

The simplest amino acid is *glycine* (Gly) (R=H), where a hypothetical flat sheet organization of polyglycine molecules can form and be stabilized by intermolecular hydrogen bonds (Figure 33.1a). However, when R is a large group as in most other amino acids, the stereochemical constraints frequently force the

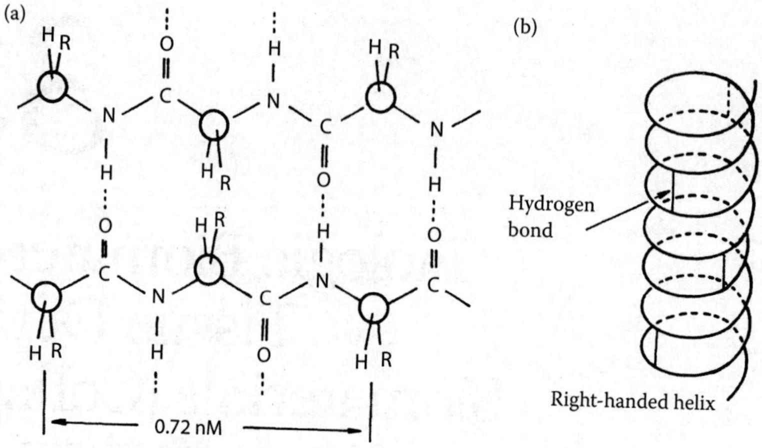

FIGURE 33.1 (a) Hypothetical flat sheet structure of a protein. (b) Helical arrangement of a protein chain.

polypeptide chain to adapt a less constraining conformation by rotating the bulky R groups away from the crowded interactions, forming a helix, where the large R groups are directed toward the surface of the helix (Figure 33.1b). The hydrogen bonds are allowed to form within a helix between the hydrogen attached to nitrogen in one amino acid residue and the oxygen attached to a second amino acid residue. Thus, the final conformation of a protein, which is directly related to its function, is governed primarily by the amino acid sequence of the particular protein.

Collagen is a protein comprised of three polypeptides (α chains), each having a general amino acid sequence of $(-Gly-X-Y-)_n$, where X is any other amino acid and is frequently *proline* (Pro) and Y is any other amino acid and is frequently *hydroxyproline* (Hyp). A typical amino acid composition of collagen is shown in Table 33.1. The application of helical diffraction theory to a high-angle collagen x-ray diffraction pattern (Rich and Crick, 1961) and the stereochemical constraints from the unusual amino acid composition (Eastoe, 1967) led to the initial triple-helical model and subsequent modified triple helix of the collagen molecule. Thus, collagen can be broadly defined as a protein which has a typical triple helix extending over the major part of the molecule. Within the triple helix, glycine must be present as every third amino acid, and proline and hydroxyproline are required to form and stabilize the triple helix.

To date, 19 proteins can be classified as collagen (Fukai et al., 1994). Among the various collagens, type I collagen is the most abundant and is the major constituent of bone, skin, ligament, and

TABLE 33.1 Amino Acid Content of Collagen

Amino Acids	Content, Residues/1000 Residues[a]
Gly	334
Pro	122
Hyp	96
Acid polar (Asp, Glu, Asn)	124
Basic polar (Lys, Arg, His)	91
Other	233

Source: From Eastoe, J.E. 1967. *Treatise on Collagen*, pp. 1–72, Academic Press, New York. With permission.

[a] Reported values are average values of 10 different determinations for tendon tissue.

ndon. Due to the abundance and ready accessibility of these tissues, they have been frequently used s a source for the preparation of collagen. This chapter will not review the details of the structure f the different collagens. The readers are referred to recent reviews for a more in-depth discussion f this subject (Nimni, 1988; van der Rest et al., 1990; Fukai et al., 1994; Brodsky and Ramshaw, 997). It is, however, of particular relevance to review some salient structural features of the type I ollagen in order to facilitate the subsequent discussions of properties and its relation to biomedical pplications.

A type I collagen molecule (also referred to as *tropocollagen*) isolated from various tissues has a nolecular weight of about 283,000 Da. It is comprised of three left-handed helical polypeptide chains Figure 33.2a) which are intertwined forming a right-handed helix around a central molecular axis Figure 33.2b). Two of the polypeptide chains are identical (α_1) having 1056 amino acid residues, and he third polypeptide chain (α_2) has 1029 amino acid residues (Miller, 1984). The triple-helical structure as a rise per residue of 0.286 nm and a unit twist of 108°, with 10 residues in three turns and a *helical pitch* (repeating distance within a single chain) of 30 residues or 8.68 nm (Fraser et al., 1983). More than 95% of the amino acids have the sequence Gly–X–Y. The remaining 5% of the molecules do not have the sequence Gly–X–Y and are, therefore, not triple helical. These nonhelical portions of the molecules are ocated at the N- and C-terminal ends and are referred to as *telopeptides* (9–26 residues) (Miller, 1984). The whole molecule has a length of about 280 nm and a diameter of about 1.5 nm and has a conforma- tion similar to a rigid rod (Figure 33.2c).

The triple-helical structure of a collagen molecule is stabilized by several factors (Figure 33.3): (1) a tight fit of the amino acids within the triple helix—this geometrical stabilization factor can be appreci- ated from a space-filling model constructed from a triple helix with Gly–Pro–Hyp sequence (Figure 33.3); (2) the interchain hydrogen bond formation between the backbone carbonyl and amino hydrogen interactions; and (3) the contribution of water molecules to the interchain hydrogen bond formation.

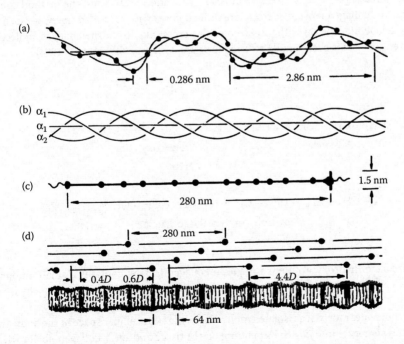

FIGURE 33.2 Formation of collagen, which can be visualized as taking place in several steps: (a) single-chain left-handed helix; (b) three single chains intertwined into a triple stranded helix; (c) a collagen (tropocollagen) molecule; (d) collagen molecules aligned in *D* staggered fashion in a fibril producing overlap and hole regions.

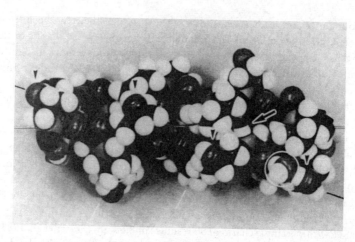

FIGURE 33.3 A space-filling model of the collagen triple helix, showing all the atoms in a 10-residue segment of repeating triplet sequence $(Gly–Pro–Hyp)_n$. The arrow shows an interchain hydrogen bond. The arrowheads identify the hydroxy groups of hydroxyproline in one chain. The circle shows a hydrogen-bonded water molecule. The short white lines identify the ridge of amino acid chains. The short black lines indicate the supercoil of one chain. (Reprinted from *Extracellular Matrix Biochemistry*, In K.A. Piez and A.H. Reddi (Eds.), New York, Piez, K.A., Molecular and aggregate structures of the collagens. p. 5, Copyright 1984, with permission from Elsevier.)

The telopeptides are regions where *intermolecular crosslinks* are formed *in vivo*. A common intermolecular crosslink is formed between an *allysine* (the ε-amino group of *lysine* or hydroxy-lysine has been converted to an aldehyde) of one telopeptide of one molecule and an ε-amino group of a lysine or *hydroxylysine* in the triple helix or a second molecule (Equation 33.2). Thus, the method commonly used to solubilize the collagen molecules from crosslinked *fibrils* with *proteolytic enzymes* such as *pepsin* removes the telopeptides (cleaves the intermolecular crosslinks) from the collagen molecule. The pepsin-solubilized collagen is occasionally referred to as *atelocollagen* (Stenzl et al., 1974).

$$Pr – CH_2 – CH_2 – CH_2 – CHO \quad + \quad H_2N – CH_2 – \overset{\overset{\displaystyle OH}{\displaystyle |}}{CH} – CH_2 – CH_2 – Pr$$

Allysine   Hydroxylysine

$$\to Pr – CH_2 – CH_2 – CH_2 – CH = N – CH_2 – \overset{\overset{\displaystyle OH}{\displaystyle |}}{CH} – CH_2 – CH_2 – Pr$$

Dehydrohydroxylysinonorleucine

(33.2)

Since the presence of hydroxyproline is unique in collagen (*elastin* contains a small amount), the determination of collagen content in a collagen-rich tissue is readily done by assaying the hydroxyproline content.

Collagen does not appear to exist as isolated molecules in the extracellular space in the body. Instead, collagen molecules aggregate into *fibrils*. Depending on the tissue and age, a collagen fibril varies from about 50 to 300 nm in diameter with indeterminate length and can easily be seen under electron microscopy (Figure 33.4). The fibrils are important structural building units for large *fibers* (Figure 33.5). Collagen molecules are arranged in specific orders both longitudinally and in cross-sectionally, and the

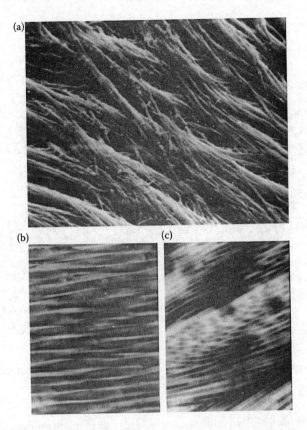

FIGURE 33.4 (a) Scanning electron micrograph of the surface of an adult rabbit bone matrix, showing how the collagen fibrils branch and interconnect in an intricate, woven pattern (×4800). (Adapted from Tiffit, J.T. 1980. *Fundamental and Clinical Bone Physiology*, p. 51, JB Lippincott Co., Philadelphia, PA.) (b) Transmission electron micrographs of (×24,000) parallel collagen fibrils in tendon. (c) Transmission electron micrographs of (×24,000) mesh work of fibrils in skin. ((b) and (c) With kind permission from Springer Science+Business Media: *Biomechanics, Mechanical Properties of Living Tissues*, 2nd ed., 1993, p. 255, New York, Fung, Y.C.)

organization of collagen molecules in a fibril is tissue-specific (Katz and Li, 1972, 1973b). The 2-D structure (the projection of a 3-D structure onto a 2-D plane) of a type I collagen fibril has been unequivocally defined both by an analysis of small-angle x-ray diffraction pattern along the meridian of a collagenous tissue (Bear, 1952) and by examination of the transmission electron micrographs of tissues stained with negative or positive stains (Hodge and Petruska, 1963). In this structure (Figure 33.2d), the collagen molecules are staggered with respect to one another by a distance of D (64–67 nm) or multiple of D, where D is the fundamental repeat distance seen in the small-angle x-ray diffraction pattern, or the repeating distance seen in the electron micrographs. Since a collagen molecule has a length of about $4.4D$, this staggering of collagen molecules creates overlap regions of about $0.4D$ and hole or defect regions of about $0.6D$.

One interesting and important structural aspect of collagen is its approximate equal number of acidic (*aspartic* and *glutamic acids*) and basic (lysines and *arginines*) side groups. Since these groups are charged under physiological conditions, the collagen is essentially electrically neutral (Li and Katz, 1976). The packing of collagen molecules with a D staggering results in clusters of regions where the charged groups are located (Hofmann and Kuhn, 1981). These groups therefore are in close proximity to form intra- and intermolecular hydrogen-bonded *salt-linkages* of the form

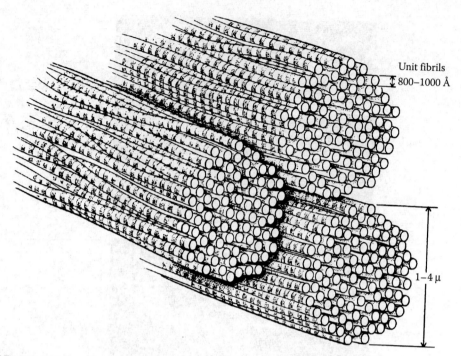

Unit fibrils
800–1000 Å

1–4 μ

FIGURE 33.5 Collagen fibers of the connective tissue in general which are composed of unit collagen fibrils.

(Pr–COO⁻⁺ H₃N–Pr) (Li et al., 1975). In addition, the side groups of many amino acids are nonpolar [alanine (Ala), valine (Val), leucine (Leu), isoleucine (Ile), *proline* (Pro), and *phenolalanine* (Phe)] in character and hence *hydrophobic*; therefore, chains with these amino acids avoid contact with water molecules and seek interactions with the nonpolar chains of amino acids. In fact, the result of molecular packing of collagen in a fibril is such that the nonpolar groups are also clustered, forming hydrophobic regions within collagen fibrils (Hofmann and Kuhn, 1981). Indeed, the packing of the collagen molecules in various tissues is believed to be a result of intermolecular interactions involving both the electrostatic and hydrophobic interactions (Li et al., 1975; Hofmann and Kuhn, 1981; Katz and Li, 1981).

The 3-D organization of type I collagen molecules within a fibril has been the subject of extensive research over the last 40 years (Ramachandran, 1967; Katz and Li, 1972, 1973a,b, 1981; Miller, 1976; Fraser et al., 1983; Yamuchi et al., 1986). Many structural models have been proposed based on an analysis of equatorial and off-equatorial x-ray diffraction patterns of rat-tail-tendon collagen (North et al., 1954; Miller, 1976), *intrafibrillar volume* determination of various collagenous tissues (Katz and Li, 1972, 1973a,b), intermolecular side chain interactions (Hofmann and Kuhn, 1981; Katz and Li, 1981; Li et al., 1981), and intermolecular crosslinking patterns studies (Yamuchi et al., 1986). The general understanding of the 3-D molecular packing in type I collagen fibrils is that the collagen molecules are arranged in hexagonal or near-hexagonal arrays (Katz and Li, 1972, 1981; Miller, 1976). Depending on the tissue, the intermolecular distance varies from about 0.15 nm in rat tail tendon to as large as 0.18 nm in bone and dentin (Katz and Li, 1973b). The axial staggering of the molecules by 1–4D with respect to one another is tissue-specific and has not yet been fully elucidated.

There are very few interspecies differences in the structure of type I collagen molecule. The extensive homology of the structure of type I collagen may explain why this collagen obtained from animal species is acceptable as a material for human implantation.

3.1.2 Properties of Collagen-Rich Tissue

*T*he function of collagenous tissue is related to its structure and properties. This section reviews some important properties of collagen-rich tissues.

3.1.2.1 Physical and Biomechanical Properties

*T*he physical properties of tissues vary according to the amount and structural variations of the collagen fibers. In general, a collagen-rich tissue contains about 75–90% of collagen on a dry weight basis. Table 33.2 is a typical composition of a collagen-rich soft tissue such as skin. Collagen fibers (bundles of collagen fibrils) are arranged in different configurations in different tissues for their respective functions at specific anatomic sites. For example, collagen fibers are arranged in parallel in tendon (Figure 33.4b) and ligament for their high-tensile strength requirements, whereas they are arranged in random arrays in skin (Figure 33.4c) to provide the resiliency of the tissue under stress. Other structure-supporting functions of collagen such as transparency for the lens of the eye and shaping of the ear or tip of the nose can also be provided by the collagen fiber. Thus, an important physical property of collagen is the 3-D organization of the collagen fibers.

The collagen-rich tissues can be thought of as a composite polymeric material in which the highly oriented crystalline collagen fibrils are embedded in the amorphous ground substance of noncollagenous *polysaccharides, glycoproteins,* and elastin. When the tissue is heated, its specific volume increases, exhibiting a glass transition at about 40°C and a melting of the crystalline collagen fibrils at about 56°C. The melting temperature of crystalline collagen fibrils is referred to as the *denaturation temperature* of collagenous tissues.

The stress–strain curves of a collagenous tissue such as tendon exhibit nonlinear behavior (Figure 33.6). This nonlinear behavior of stress–strain of tendon collagen is similar to that observed in synthetic fibers. The initial toe region represents alignment of fibers in the direction of stress. The steep rise in slope represents the majority of fibers stretched along their long axes. The decrease in slope following the steep rise may represent the breaking of individual fibers prior to the final catastrophic failure. Table 33.3 summarizes some mechanical properties of collagen and elastic fibers. The difference in biomechanical properties between collagen and elastin is a good example of the requirements for these proteins to serve their specific functions in the body.

Unlike tendon or ligament, skin consists of collagen fibers randomly arranged in layers or lamellae. Thus skin tissues show mechanical anisotropy (Figure 33.7). Another feature of the stress–strain curve of the skin is its extensibility under small load when compared to tendon. At smaller loads, the fibers are straightened and aligned rather than stretched. Upon further stretching, the fibrous lamellae align with respect to each other and resist further extension. When the skin is highly stretched, the modulus of elasticity approaches that of tendon as expected of the aligned collagen fibers.

Cartilage is another collagen-rich tissue which has two main physiological functions. One is the maintenance of shape (ear, tip of nose, and rings around the trachea) and the other is to provide bearing surfaces at joints. It contains very large and diffuse proteoglycan (protein-polysaccharide)

TABLE 33.2 Composition of Collagen-Rich Soft Tissues

Component	Composition (%)
Collagen	75 (dry), 30 (wet)
Proteoglycans and polysaccharides	20 (dry)
Elastin and glycoproteins	<5 (dry)
Water	60–70

Source: Adapted from Park, J.B. and Lakes, R.S. 1992. *Biomaterials: An Introduction,* 2nd ed., pp. 185–222, Plenum Press, New York.

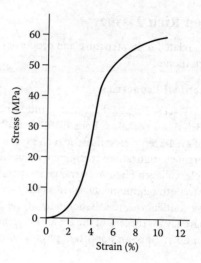

FIGURE 33.6 A typical stress–strain curve for tendon. (Adapted from Rigby, B.J. et al. 1959. *J. Gen. Physiol.* 43:265–283.)

TABLE 33.3 Elastic Properties of Collagen and Elastic Fibers

Fibers	Modulus of Elasticity (MPa)	Tensile Strength (MPa)	Ultimate Elongation (%)
Collagen	1000	50–100	10
Elastin	0.6	1	100

Source: Adapted from Park, J.B. and Lakes, R.S. 1992. *Biomaterials: An Introduction*, 2nd ed., pp. 185–222, Plenum Press, New York.

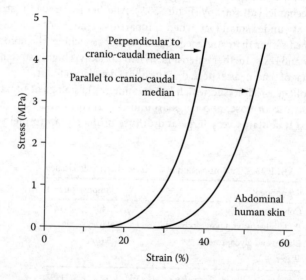

FIGURE 33.7 Stress–strain curves of human abdominal skin. (Adapted from Daly, C.H. 1966. *The Biomechanical Characteristics of Human Skin*. PhD thesis, University of Strathclyde, Scotland.)

TABLE 33.4   Mechanical Properties of Some Nonmineralized Human Tissues

Tissues	Tensile Strength (MPa)	Ultimate Elongation (%)
Skin	7.6	78.0
Tendon	53.0	9.4
Elastic cartilage	3.0	30.0
Heart valves (aortic)		
Radial	0.45	15.3
Circumferential	2.6	10.0
Aorta		
Transverse	1.1	77.0
Longitudinal	0.07	81.0

Source: Adapted from Park, J.B. and Lakes, R.S. 1992. *Biomaterials: An Introduction*, 2nd ed., pp. 185–222, Plenum Press, New York.

molecules which form a gel in which the collagen-rich molecules entangled. They can affect the mechanical properties of the collagen by hindering the movements through the interstices of the collagenous matrix network.

The joint cartilage has a very low coefficient of friction (<0.01). This is largely attributed to the squeeze-film effect between cartilage and synovial fluid. The synovial fluid can be squeezed out through highly fenestrated cartilage upon compressive loading, and the reverse action will take place in tension. The lubricating function is carried out in conjunction with *glycosaminoglycans* (GAG), especially *chondroitin sulfates*. The modulus of elasticity (10.3–20.7 MPa) and tensile strength (3.4 MPa) are quite low. However, wherever high stress is required, the cartilage is replaced by purely collagenous tissue. Mechanical properties of some collagen-rich tissues are given in Table 33.4 as a reference.

33.1.2.2 Physiochemical Properties

33.1.2.2.1 Electrostatic Properties

A collagen molecule has a total of ~240 ε-amino and guanidino groups of lysines, hydroxylysines, and arginines and 230 carboxyl groups of aspartic and glutamic acids. These groups are charged under physiological conditions. In a native fibril, most of these groups interact either intra- or intermolecularly forming salt linkages providing significant stabilization energy to the collagen fibril (Li et al., 1975). Only a small number of charged groups are free. However, the electrostatic state within a collagen fibril can be altered by changing the pH of the environment. Since the pK_a is about 10 for an amino group and about 4 for a carboxyl group, the electrostatic interactions are significantly perturbed at a pH below 4 and above 10. The net result of the pH change is a weakening of the intra- and intermolecular electrostatic interactions, resulting in a swelling of the fibrils. The fibril swelling can be prevented by chemically introducing covalent intermolecular crosslinks. Any bifunctional reagent which reacts with amino, carboxyl, and hydroxyl groups can serve as a crosslinking agent. The introduction of covalent intermolecular crosslinks fixes the physical state of the fibrillar structure and balances the swelling pressures obtained from any pH changes.

Another way of altering the electrostatic state of a collagen fibril is by chemically modifying the electrostatic side groups. For example, the positively charged ε-amino groups of lysine and hydroxylysine can be chemically modified with acetic anhydride, which converts the ε-amino groups to a neutral acetyl group (Green et al., 1953). The result of this modification increases the number of the net negative charges of the fibril. Conversely, the negatively charged carboxyl groups of aspartic and glutamic acid can be chemically modified to a neutral group by methylation (Fraenkel-Conrat and Olcott, 1944). Thus, by adjusting the pH of the solution and applying chemical modification methods, a range of electrostatic properties of collagen can be obtained.

33.1.2.2.2 Ion and Macromolecular Binding Properties

In the native state and under physiological conditions, a collagen molecule has only about 60 free carboxyl groups (Li et al., 1975). These groups have the capability of binding cations such as calcium with a free energy of formation for the protein $-COO-Ca^{2+}$ of about 1.2 kcal/mol. This energy is not large enough to compete for the hydrogen bonded salt-linkage interactions, which have a free energy of formation of about -1.6 kcal/mol. The extent of ion binding, however, can be enhanced in the presence of lyotropic salts such as potassium thiocyanate (KCNS), which breaks the salt linkages, or by shifting the pH away from the *isoelectric point* of collagen. Macromolecules can bind to collagen via covalent bonding, cooperative ionic binding, entrapment, entanglement, and a combination of the above. In addition, binding of charged ions and macromolecules can be significantly increased by modifying the charge profile of collagen as described previously. For example, a complete *N*-acetylation of collagen will eliminate all the positively charged ε-amino groups and, thus, will increase the free negatively charged groups. The resulting acetylated collagen enhances the binding of positively charged ions and macromolecules. On the other hand, methylation of collagen will eliminate the negatively charged carboxyl groups and, thus, will increase the free positively charge moieties. The methylated collagen, therefore, enhances the binding of negatively charged ions and macromolecules (Li and Katz, 1976).

33.1.2.2.3 Fiber-Forming Properties

Native collagen molecules are organized in tissues in specific orders. *Polymorphic* forms of collagen can be reconstituted from the collagen molecules, obtained either from enzymatic digestion of collagenous tissues or by extracting the tissues with salt solutions. The formation of polymorphic aggregates of collagen depends on the environment for reconstitution (Piez, 1984). Native arrangement of the collagen molecules is formed under physiological conditions. Various polymorphic molecular aggregates may be formed by changing the state of intermolecular interactions. For example, when collagen molecules are aggregated under high concentrations of a neutral salt or under nonaqueous conditions, the collagen molecules associate into random arrays having no specific regularities detectable by electron microscopy. The collagen molecules can be induced to aggregate into other polymorphic forms such as the *segment-long-spacing* form where all heads are aligned in parallel and the *fibrous-long-spacing* form where the molecules are randomly aligned in either a head-to-tail, tail-to-tail, or head-to-head orientation.

33.1.2.3 Biologic Properties

33.1.2.3.1 Hemostatic Properties

Native collagen aggregates are intrinsically hemostatic. The mechanism of collagen-induced hemostasis has been the subject of numerous investigations (Wilner et al., 1968; Jaffe and Deykin, 1974; Wang et al., 1978). The general conclusion from these studies is that *platelets* first adhere to a collagen surface. This induces the release of platelet contents, followed by platelet aggregation, leading to the eventual hemostatic plug. The hemostatic activity of collagen is dependent on the size of the collagen aggregate and the native organization of the molecules (Wang et al., 1978). Denatured collagen (*gelatin*) is not effective in inducing hemostasis (Jonas et al., 1988).

33.1.2.3.2 Cell Interaction Properties

Collagen forms the essential framework of the tissues and organs. Many cells, such as epithelial and endothelial cells, are found resting on the collagenous surfaces or within a collagenous matrix such as that of many connective tissue cells. Collagen–cell interactions are essential features during the development stage and during wound healing and tissue remodeling in adults (Kleinman et al., 1981; Lindblad and Kormos, 1991). Studying collagen–cell interactions is useful in developing simulated tissue and organ structures and in investigating cell behavior in the *in vivo* simulated systems. Numerous studies have aimed at developing viable tissues and organs *in vitro* for transplantation applications (Bell et al., 1981; Montesano et al., 1983; Silbermann, 1990; Bellamkonda and Aebischer, 1994; Hubbell, 1995; Moghe et al., 1996; Sittinger et al., 1996).

33.1.2.3.3 Immunologic Properties

Soluble collagen has long been known to be a poor immunogen (Timpl, 1982). A significant level of antibodies cannot be raised without the use of Freund's complete adjuvant (a mixture of mineral oil and heat-killed *mycobacteria*) which augments antibody response. It is known that insoluble collagen is even less immunogenic (Stenzl et al., 1974). Thus, xenogeneic collagenous tissue devices such as porcine and bovine pericardial heart valves are acceptable for long-term implantation in humans. The reasons for the low antibody response against collagen are not known. It may be related to the homology of the collagen structure from different species (low level of foreignness) or to certain structural features associated with collagen (Timpl, 1982).

33.2 Biotechnology of Collagen

33.2.1 Isolation and Purification of Collagen

There are two distinct ways of isolating and purifying collagen material. One is the molecular technology and the other is the fibrillar technology. These two technologies are briefly reviewed here.

33.2.1.1 Isolation and Purification of Soluble Collagen Molecules

The isolation and purification of soluble collagen molecules from a collagenous tissue is achieved by using a proteolytic enzyme such as pepsin to cleave the telopeptides (Miller and Rhodes, 1982). Since telopeptides are the natural crosslinking sites of collagen, the removal of telopeptides renders the collagen molecules and small collagen aggregates soluble in an aqueous solution. The pepsin-solubilized collagen can be purified by repetitive precipitation with a neutral salt. Pepsin-solubilized collagen in monomeric form is generally soluble in a buffer solution at low temperature. The collagen molecules may be reconstituted into fibrils of various *polymorphisms*. However, the reconstitution of the pepsin-solubilized collagen into fibrils of native molecular packing is not as efficient as the intact molecules, since the telopeptides facilitate fibril formation (Comper and Veis, 1977).

33.2.1.2 Isolation and Purification of Fibrillar Collagen

The isolation and purification of collagen fibers relies on the removal of noncollagenous materials from the collagenous tissue. Salt extraction removes the newly synthesized collagen molecules that have not been covalently incorporated into the collagen fibrils. Salt also removes the noncollagenous materials that are soluble in aqueous conditions and are bound to collagen fibrils by nonspecific interactions. *Lipids* are removed by low-molecular-weight organic solvents such as low-molecular-weight ethers and alcohols. Acid extraction facilitates the removal of acidic proteins and GAG due to weakening of the interactions between the acidic proteins and collagen fibrils. Alkaline extraction weakens the interaction between the basic proteins and collagen fibrils and thus facilitates the removal of basic proteins. In addition, various enzymes other than *collagenase* can be used to facilitate the removal of the small amounts of glycoproteins, proteoglycans, and elastins from the tissue. Purified collagen fibers can be obtained through these sequential extractions and enzymatic digestions from the collagen-rich tissues.

33.2.2 Matrix Fabrication Technology

The purified collagen materials obtained from either the molecular technology or from the fibrillar technology are subjected to additional processing to fabricate the materials into useful devices for

TABLE 33.5 Summary of Different Collagen Matrices and Their Medical Applications

Matrix Form	Medical Application
Membrane (film, sheet)	Oral tissue repair; wound dressings; dura repair; patches
Porous (sponge, felt, fibers)	Hemostats; wound dressings; cartilage repair; soft-tissue augmentation
Gel	Drug and biologically active macromolecule delivery; soft- and hard-tissue augmentation
Solution	Soft-tissue augmentation; drug delivery
Filament	Tendon and ligament repair; sutures
Tubular (membrane, sponge) composite	Nerve repair; vascular repair
Collagen/synthetic polymer	Vascular repair; skin repair; wound dressings
Collagen/biological polymer	Soft-tissue augmentation; skin repair
Collagen/ceramic	Hard-tissue repair

specific medical applications. The different matrices and their medical applications are summarized in Table 33.5. The technology in fabricating these matrices are briefly outlined below.

33.2.2.1 Membranous Matrix

Collagen membranes can be produced by drying a collagen solution or a fibrillar collagen dispersion cast on a nonadhesive surface. The thickness of the membrane is governed by the concentration and the initial thickness of the cast solution or dispersion. In general, membrane thickness of up to 0.5 mm can be easily obtained by air-drying a cast collagen material. Additional chemical crosslinking is required to stabilize the membrane from dissolution or dissociation. The membrane produced by casting and air-drying does not permit manipulation of the pore structure. Generally, the structure of a cast membrane is dense and amorphous with minimal *permeability* to macromolecules (Li et al., 1991). Porous membranes may be obtained by freeze-drying a cast solution or dispersion of a predetermined density or by partially compressing a preformed porous matrix to a predetermined density and pore structure.

33.2.2.2 Porous Matrix

Porous collagen matrices are generally obtained by freeze-drying an aqueous volume of collagen solution or dispersion. The freeze-dried porous matrix requires chemical crosslinking to stabilize the structure. A convenient way to stabilize the porous matrix is to crosslink the matrix by vapor using a volatile crosslinking agent such as formaldehyde or glutaraldehyde. The pore structure of the matrix depends, to a large extent, on the concentration of the collagen in the solution or dispersion. Other factors that contribute to the pore structure include the rate of freezing, the size of fibers in the dispersion, and the presence and absence of other macromolecules. *Apparent densities* from 0.05 to 0.3 g matrix per cubic centimeter matrix volume can be obtained. These porous matrices generally have pores from about 50 μm to as large as 1500 μm.

33.2.2.3 Gel Matrix

A *gel matrix* may be defined as a homogeneous phase between a liquid and a solid. As such, a gel may vary from a simple viscous fluid to a highly concentrated putty-like material. Collagen gels may be formed by shifting the pH of a dispersion away from its isoelectric point. Alternatively, the collagen material may be subjected to a chemical modification procedure to change its charge profile to a net positively charged or a net negatively charged protein before hydrating the material to form a gel matrix. For example, native fibers dispersed in water at pH 7 will be in the form of two phases. The dispersed fibers become gel when the pH changes from 7 to 3. Succinylating the primary amino groups of collagen, which converts the positively charged amino groups to negatively charged carboxyl groups, changes the isoelectric point of collagen from about 7 to about 4.5. Such a collagen material swells to a gel at a pH of 7.

3.2.2.4 Solution Matrix

A collagen solution is obtained by dissolving the collagen molecules in an aqueous solution. Collagen molecules are obtained by digesting the insoluble tissue with pepsin to cleave the crosslinking sites of collagen (telopeptides) as previously described. The solubility of collagen depends on the pH, the temperature, the ionic strength of the solution, and the molecular weight. Generally, collagen is more soluble in the cold. Collagen molecules aggregate into fibrils when the temperature of the solution increases to the body temperature. pH plays an important role in solubilizing collagen. Collagen is more soluble at a pH away from the isoelectric point of the protein. Collagen is less soluble at higher ionic strength of a solution. The solubility of collagen decreases with increasing size of molecular aggregates. Thus, collagen becomes increasingly less soluble with increasing extent of crosslinking (Bailey et al., 1970).

33.2.2.5 Filamentous Matrix

Collagen filaments can be produced by extrusion techniques (Schimpf and Rodriquez, 1976; Li and Stone, 1993; Kemp et al., 1995). A collagen solution or dispersion having a concentration in the range 0.5–1.5% (w/v) is first prepared. Collagen is extruded into a coacervation bath containing a high concentration of a salt or into an aqueous solution at a pH of the isoelectric point of the collagen. Tensile strength of 30 MPa has been obtained for the reconstituted filaments.

33.2.2.6 Tubular Matrix

Tubular matrices may be formed either by extrusion through a coaxial cylinder (Stenzl et al., 1974) or by coating collagen onto a mandrel (Li, 1990). Different properties of the tubular membranes can be obtained by controlling the drying properties.

33.2.2.7 Composite Matrix

Collagen can form a variety of homogeneous composites with other water-soluble materials. Ions, peptides, proteins, and polysaccharides can all be uniformly incorporated into a collagen matrix. The methods of homogeneous composite formation include ionic and covalent bonding, entrapment, entanglement, and coprecipitation. A heterogeneous composite can be formed between collagen, ceramics, and synthetic polymers that have distinct properties for medical applications (Li, 1988).

33.3 Design of a Resorbable Collagen-Based Medical Implant

Designing a medical implant for tissue or organ repair requires a thorough understanding of the structure and function of the tissue and organ to be repaired, the structure and properties of the materials used for repair, and the design requirements. There are at present two schools of thought regarding the design of an implant, namely the permanent implant and the *resorbable implant*. The permanent implants intended to permanently replace the damaged tissues or organs are fabricated from various materials including metals and natural or synthetic polymers. For example, most of the weight-bearing orthopedic and oral implants are made of metals or alloys. Nonweight-bearing tissues and organs are generally replaced with implants that are fabricated either from synthetic or natural materials. Implants for blood vessel, heart valve, and most soft tissue repair fall into this class. Permanent implants, particularly those made of synthetic and biological materials, frequently suffer from the long-term effects of material degradation. Material degradation can result from biological processes such as enzymatic degradation or environmentally induced degradation from mechanical, metal-catalyzed oxidation, and from the permeation of body fluids into the polymeric devices (Bruck, 1991). The material degradation is particularly manifested in applications where there is repetitive stress–strain on the implant, such as artificial blood vessels and heart valves.

As a result of the lack of suitable materials for long-term implantation, the concept of using a resorbable template to guide host tissue regeneration (guided tissue regeneration) has received vigorous attention in recent years. This area of research can be categorized into synthetic and biological templates. *Polyglycolic acid* (PGA), *polylactic acid* (PLA), PGA–PLA copolymers, and *polydioxanone* are among the polymers most selected for resorbable medical implant development. Among the biological materials used for resorbable medical implant development, *collagen* has been one of the most popular materials in this category. Collagen-based templates have been developed for skin (Yannas and Burke, 1981), peripheral nerve (Yannas et al., 1985; Li et al., 1990), oral tissue (Blumenthal, 1988; Altman and Li, 1990), and meniscal regeneration (Li et al., 1994; Stone et al., 1997). A variety of other collagen-based templates are being developed for tissue repair and regeneration applications (Goldstein et al., 1989; Ma et al., 1990; Li et al., 1997).

The following discussion is useful in designing a template for tissue repair and regeneration applications. By way of an example, the design parameters listed below are specifically applied to the development of a *resorbable collagen*-based template for guiding meniscal tissue repair and regeneration in the knee joint.

Menisci are semilunar fibrocartilages that are anatomically located between the femoral condyles and tibial plateau, providing stability, weight bearing, shock absorption, and assisting in lubrication of the knee joint. A major portion of the meniscal tissue is avascular except the peripheral rim, which comprises about 10–30% of the total width of the structure and which is nourished by the peripheral vasculature (Arnoczky and Warren, 1982). Collagen is the major matrix material of the *meniscus*, and the fibers are oriented primarily in the circumferential direction in the line of stress for mechanical function. Repair of damaged meniscal tissue in the peripheral vascular rim can be accomplished with sutures. However, in cases where the injured site is in the avascular region, partial or total removal of the meniscal tissue is often indicated. This is primarily due to the inadequacy of the *fibrochondrocytes* alone to self-repair the damaged meniscal tissue. Studies in animals and humans have shown that removal of the meniscus is a prelude to degenerative knees manifested by the development of *osteoarthritis* (Shapiro and Glimcher, 1980; Hede et al., 1992). At present, there is no suitable permanent substitute for meniscal tissue.

33.3.1 Biocompatibility

Biocompatibility of the materials and their degraded products is a prerequisite for resorbable implant development. Purified collagen materials have been used either as implants or have been extensively tested in clinical studies as implants without adverse effects. The meniscus template can be fabricated from purified type I collagen fibers that are further crosslinked chemically to increase the stability and reduce the immunogenicity *in vivo*. In addition, small amounts of noncollagenous materials such as GAG and growth factors can be incorporated into the collagen matrix to improve the osmotic properties as well as the rate of tissue ingrowth.

Since the primary structure of a collagen molecule from bovine is homologous to human collagen (Miller, 1984), the *in vivo* degradation of bovine collagen implant should be similar to the normal host tissue remodeling process during wound healing. For a resorbable collagen template, the matrix is slowly degraded by the host over time. It is known that a number of cell types such as *polymorphonuclear leukocytes*, *fibroblasts*, and *macrophages*, during the wound healing period, are capable of secreting enzyme collagenases which cleave a collagen molecule at 1/4 position from the C-terminal end of the molecule (Woolley, 1984). The enzyme first reduces a collagen molecule to two smaller triple helices which are not stable at body temperature and are subsequently denatured to random coiled polypeptides. These polypeptides are further degraded by proteases into amino acids and short peptides that are metabolized through normal metabolic pathways (Nimni and Harkness, 1988).

Despite the safety record of collagen materials for implantation, during the process of preparing the collagen template, small amounts of unwanted noncollagenous materials could be incorporated into the device such as salts and crosslinking agents. Therefore, a series of biocompatibility testing must be conducted to ensure that the residuals of these materials do not cause any safety issues. The FDA has published a new guideline for biocompatibility testing of implantable devices (Biological Evaluation of Medical Devices, 1995).

33.3.2 Physical Dimension

The physical dimension of a template defines the boundary of regeneration. Thus, the size of the collagen template should match the tissue defect to be repaired. A properly sized meniscal substitute has been found to function better than that which mismatches the physical dimension of the host meniscus (Sommerlath et al., 1991; Li et al., 2002). For a porous, elastic matrix such as the one designed from collagen for meniscal tissue repair, the shape of the meniscus is further defined *in vivo* by the space available between the femoral condyles and tibial plateau within the synovial joint.

33.3.3 Apparent Density

The apparent density is defined as the weight of the dry matrix in a unit volume of matrix. Thus, the apparent density is a direct measure of the empty space which is not occupied by the matrix material per se in the dry state. For example, for a collagen matrix of an apparent density 0.2 g/cm³, the empty space would be 0.86 cm³ for a 1 cm³ total space occupied by the matrix, taking the density of collagen to be 1.41 g/cm³ (Noda, 1972). The apparent density is also directly related to the mechanical strength of a matrix. In weight-bearing applications, the apparent density has to be optimized such that the mechanical properties are not compromised for the intended function of the resorbable implant as described in Section 33.3.5.

33.3.4 Pore Structure

The dimension of a mammalian fibrogenic cell body is on the order of 10–50 μm, depending on the substrate to which the cell adheres (Folkman and Moscona, 1978). In order for cells to infiltrate into the interstitial space of a matrix, the majority of the pores must be significantly larger than the dimension of a cell such that both the cell and its cellular processes can easily enter the interstitial space. In a number of studies using collagen-based matrices for tissue regeneration, it has been found that pore size plays an important role in the effectiveness of the collagen matrix to induce host tissue regeneration (Dagalailis et al., 1980; Chvapil, 1982; Ellis and Yannas, 1996). It was suggested that pore size in the range 100–400 μm was optimal for tissue regeneration. Similar observations were also found to be true for porous metal implants in total hip replacement (Cook et al., 1991). The question of interconnecting pores may not be a critical issue in a collagen template as collagenases are synthesized by most *inflammatory cells* during wound healing and remodeling processes. The interporous membranes which exist in the noninterconnecting pores should be digested as part of resorption and wound healing processes.

33.3.5 Mechanical Property

In designing a resorbable collagen implant for weight-bearing applications, not only the initial mechanical strength is important, but the gradual strength reduction of the partially resorbed template has to be compensated by the strength increase from the regenerated tissue such that at any given time point, the total mechanical properties of the template are maintained. In order to accomplish this goal, one must first be certain that the initial mechanical properties are adequate for supporting the weight-bearing application. For example, compressing the implant with multiple body weights should not cause fraying of the collagen matrix material. It is also of particular importance to design an implant having an adequate and consistent suture pullout strength in order to reduce the incidence of detachment of the implant from the host tissue. The suture pullout strength is also important during surgical procedures as the lack of suture pull strength may result in retrieval and reimplantation of the template. In meniscal tissue repair, the suture pullout strength of 1 kg has been found to be adequate for arthroscopically assisted surgery in simulated placement procedures in human cadaver knees, and this suture pullout strength should be maintained as the minimal strength required for this particular application.

33.3.6 Hydrophilicity

Hydration of an implant facilitates nutrient diffusion. The extent of hydration would also provide information on the space available for tissue ingrowth. The porous collagen matrix is highly hydrophilic and therefore facilitates cellular ingrowth. The biomechanical properties of the hydrophilic collagen matrix such as fluid outflow under stress, fluid inflow in the absence of stress, and the resiliency for shock absorption are the properties also found in the weight-bearing cartilagenous tissues.

33.3.7 Permeability

The permeability of ions and macromolecules is of primary importance in tissues that do not rely on vascular transport of nutrients to the end organs. The diffusion of nutrients into the interstitial space ensures the survival of the cells and their continued ability of growth and synthesis of tissue-specific extracellular matrix. Generally, the permeability of a macromolecule the size of the bovine serum albumin (MW 67,000) can be used as a guideline for probing accessibility of the interstitial space of a collagen template (Li et al., 1994).

33.3.7.1 *In Vivo* Stability

As stated above, the rate of template resorption and the rate of new tissue regeneration have to be balanced so that the adequate mechanical properties are maintained at all times. The rate of *in vivo* resorption of a collagen-based implant can be controlled by controlling the density of the implant and the extent of intermolecular crosslinking. The lower the density, the greater the interstitial space and generally the larger the pores for cell infiltration, leading to a higher rate of matrix degradation. The control of the extent of intermolecular crosslinking can be accomplished by using bifunctional crosslinking agents under conditions that do not denature the collagen. Glutaraldehyde, formaldehyde, adipyl chloride, hexamethylene diisocyanate, and carbodiimides are among the many agents used in crosslinking the collagen-based implants. Crosslinking can also be achieved through vapor phase of a crosslinking agent. The vapor phase crosslinking is effective in crosslinking agents of high vapor pressures such as formaldehyde and glutaraldehyde. The vapor crosslinking is particularly useful for thick implants of vapor-permeable dense fibers where crosslinking in solution produces nonuniform crosslinking. In addition, intermolecular crosslinking can be achieved by heat treatment under high vacuum. This treatment causes the formation of an amide bond between an amino group of one molecule and the carboxyl group of an adjacent molecule and has often been referred to in the literature as dehydrothermal crosslinking.

The shrinkage temperature of the crosslinked matrix has been used as a guide for *in vivo* stability of a collagen implant (Li, 1988). The temperature of shrinkage of collagen fibers measures the transition of the collagen molecules from the triple helix to a random coil conformation. This temperature depends on the number of intermolecular crosslinks formed by chemical means. Generally, the higher the number of intermolecular crosslinks, the higher the thermal shrinkage temperature and more stable the material *in vivo*.

A second method of assessing the *in vivo* stability is to determine the crosslinking density by applying the theory of rubber elasticity to denatured collagen (Wiederhorn and Beardon, 1952). Thus, the *in vivo* stability can be directly correlated with the number of intermolecular crosslinks introduced by a given crosslinking agent.

Another method that has been frequently used in assessing the *in vivo* stability of a collagen-based implant is to conduct an *in vitro* collagenase digestion of a collagen implant. Bacterial collagenase is generally used in this application. The action of bacterial collagenase on collagen is different from that of mammalian collagenase (Woolley, 1984). In addition, the enzymatic activity used in *in vitro* studies is arbitrarily defined. Thus, the data generated from the bacterial collagenase should be viewed with caution. The bacterial collagenase digestion studies, however, are useful in comparing a prototype with a collagen material of known rate of *in vivo* resorption.

Each of the above parameters should be considered in designing a resorbable implant. The interdependency of the parameters must also be balanced for maximal efficacy of the implant.

33.4 Tissue Engineering for Tissue and Organ Regeneration

Biomedical applications of collagen have entered a new era in the last decade. The potential use of collagen materials in medicine has increasingly been appreciated as the science and technology advances.

One major emerging field of biomedical research which has received rigorous attention in recent years is tissue engineering. Tissue engineering is an interdisciplinary science of biochemistry, cell and molecular biology, genetics, materials science, biomedical engineering, and medicine to produce innovative 3-D composites having structure/function properties that can be used either to replace or correct poorly functioning components in humans and animals or to introduce better functional components into these living systems. Thus, the field of tissue engineering requires a close collaboration among various disciplines for success.

Tissue engineering consists primarily of three components: (1) extracellular matrix, (2) cells, and (3) regulatory signals (e.g., tissue-specific growth factors). One of the key elements in tissue engineering is the extracellular matrix which either provides a scaffolding for cells or acts as a delivery vehicle for regulatory signals such as growth factors.

TABLE 33.6 Survey of Collagen-Based Medical Products and Research and Development Activities

Applications	Comments
Hemostasis	Commercial products: sponge, fiber, and felt forms are used in cardiovascular (Abbott and Austin, 1975), neurosurgical (Rybock and Long, 1977), dermatological (Larson, 1988), ob/gyn (Correll et al., 1985), orthopedic (Blanche and Chaux, 1988), and oral surgical applications (Stein et al., 1985)
Dermatology	Commercial products: injectable collagen for soft tissue augmentation (Webster et al., 1984); collagen-based artificial skins (Bell et al., 1981; Yannas and Burke, 1981). Research and Development: collagen-based wound dressings (Armstrong et al., 1986)
Cardiovascular surgery and cardiology	Commercial products: collagen-coated and gelatin-coated vascular grafts (Jonas et al., 1988; Li, 1988), chemically processed human vein graft (Dardik et al., 1974), bovine arterial grafts (Sawyer et al., 1977), porcine heart valves (Angell et al., 1982), bovine pericardial heart valves (Walker et al., 1983), and vascular puncture hole seal device (Merino et al., 1992)
Neurosurgery	Research and development: guiding peripheral nerve regeneration (Archibald et al., 1991; Yannas et al., 1985) and dura replacement material (Collins et al., 1991)
Periodontal and oral surgery	Research and development: collagen membranes for periodontal ligament regeneration (Blumenthal, 1988), resorbable oral tissue wound dressings (Ceravalo and Li, 1988), and collagen/hydroxyapatite for augmentation of alveolar ridge (Gongloff et al., 1985)
Ophthalmology	Commercial products: collagen corneal shield to facilitate epithelial healing (Ruffini et al., 1989). Research and development: collagen shield for drug delivery to the eye (Reidy et al., 1990)
Orthopedic surgery	Commercial products: collagen with hydroxyapatite and autogenous bone marrow for bone repair (Hollinger et al., 1989). Research and development: collagen matrix for meniscus regeneration (Li et al., 1994), collagenous material for replacement and regeneration of Achilles tendon (Kato et al., 1991), and reconstituted collagen template for anterior cruciate ligament (ACL) reconstruction (Li et al., 1997)
Other applications	Research and development: drug delivery support (Sorensen et al., 1990), delivery vehicles for growth factors and bioactive macromolecules (Deatherage and Miller, 1987; Li et al., 1996), and collagenous matrix for delivery of cells for tissue and organ regeneration (Bell et al., 1981)

Type I collagen is the major component of the extracellular matrix and is intimately associated with development, wound healing, and regeneration. The development of the type I collagen-based matrices described in this chapter will greatly facilitate the future development of tissue engineering products for tissue and organ repair and regeneration applications.

To date, collagen-based implants have been attempted for many tissue and organ repair and regeneration applications. A complete historical survey of all potential medical applications of collagen is a formidable task but a selected survey of collagen-based medical products and the research and development activities are summarized in Table 33.6 as a reference.

Defining Terms

Alanine (Ala): One of the amino acids in collagen molecules.

Allysine: The ε-amino group of lysine has been enzymatically modified to an aldehyde group.

Apparent density: Calculated as the weight of the dry collagen matrix per unit volume of matrix.

Arginine (Arg): One of the amino acids in collagen molecules.

Aspartic acid (Asp): One of the amino acids in collagen molecules.

Atelocollagen: A collagen molecule without telopeptides.

Chondroitin sulfate: Sulfated polysaccharide commonly found in cartilages, bone, cornea, tendon, and skin.

Collagen: A family of fibrous insoluble proteins having a triple helical conformation extending over a major part of the molecule. Glycine is present at every third amino acid in the triple helix and proline and hydroxyproline are required in the triple helix.

Collagenase: A proteolytic enzyme that specifically catalyzes the degradation of collagen molecules.

Dehydrohydroxylysinonorleucine (deH-HLNL): A covalently crosslinked product between an allysine and a hydroxylysine residue in collagen fibrils.

D spacing: The repeat distance observed in collagen fibrils by electron microscopic and x-ray diffraction methods.

Elastin: One of the proteins in connective tissue. It is highly stable at high temperatures and in chemicals. It also has rubber-like properties.

Fiber: A bundled group of collagen fibrils.

Fibril: A self-assembled group of collagen molecules.

Fibroblast: Any cell from which connective tissue is developed.

Fibrochondrocyte: Type of cells that are associated with special types of cartilage tissues such as meniscus of the knee and intervertebral disk of the spine.

Fibrous long spacing (FLS): One of the polymorphic forms of collagen where the collagen molecules are randomly aligned in either head-to-tail, tail-to-tail, or head-to-head orientation.

Gelatin: A random coiled form (denatured form) of collagen molecules.

Glutamic acid (Glu): One of the amino acids in collagen molecules.

Glycine (Gly): One of the amino acids in collagen molecules having the simplest structure.

Glycoprotein: A compound consisting of a carbohydrate protein. The carbohydrate is generally hexosamine, an amino sugar.

Glycosaminoglycan (GAG): A polymerized sugar (see polysaccharide) commonly found in various connective tissues.

Helical pitch: Repeating distance within a single polypeptide chain in a collagen molecule.

Hemostat: Device or medicine which arrests the flow of blood.

Hydrophilicity: The tendency to attract and hold water.

Hydrophobicity: The tendency to repel or avoid contact with water. Substances generally are nonpolar in character, such as lipids and nonpolar amino acids.

Hydroxylysine (Hyl): One of the amino acids in collagen molecules.

Hydroxyproline (Hyp): One of the amino acids uniquely present in collagen molecules.

Inflammatory cell: Cells associated with the succession of changes which occur in living tissue when it is injured. These include macrophages, polymorphonuclear leukocytes, and lymphocytes.

Intermolecular crosslink: Covalent bonds formed *in vivo* between a side group of one molecule and a side group of another molecule; covalent bonds formed between a side group of one molecule and one end of a bifunctional agent and between a side group of a second molecule and the other end of a bifunctional agent.

Intrafibrillar volume: The volume of a fibril excluding the volume occupied by the collagen molecule.

In vitro: In glass, as in a test tube. An *in vitro* test is one done in the laboratory, usually involving isolated tissues, organs, or cells.

In vivo: In the living body or organism. A test performed in a living organism.

Isoelectric point: Generally used to refer to a particular pH of a protein solution. At this pH, there is no net electric charge on the molecule.

Isoleucine (Ile): One of the amino acids in collagen molecules.

Leucine (Leu): One of the amino acids in collagen molecules.

Lipid: Any one of a group of fats or fat-like substances, characterized by their insolubility in water and solubility in fat solvents such as alcohol, ether, and chloroform.

Lysine (Lys): One of the amino acids in collagen molecules.

Macrophage: Cells of the reticuloendothelial system having the ability to phagocytose particulate substances and to store vital dyes and other colloidal substances. They are found in loose connective tissues and various organs of the body.

Meniscus: A C-shaped fibrocartilage anatomically located between the femoral condyles and tibial plateau providing stability and shock absorption and assisting in lubrication of the knee joint.

Mycobacterium: A genus of acid-fast organisms belonging to the Mycobacteriaceae which includes the causative organisms of tuberculosis and leprosy. They are slender, nonmotile, Gram-positive rods, and do not produce spores or capsules.

Osteoarthritis: A chronic disease involving the joint, especially those bearing the weight, characterized by destruction of articular cartilage, overgrown of bone with impaired function.

Pepsin: A proteolytic enzyme commonly found in the gastric juice. It is formed by the chief cells of gastric glands and produces maximum activity at a pH of 1.5–2.0.

Permeability: The space within a collagen matrix, excluding the space occupied by collagen molecules, which is accessible to a given size of molecule.

Phenolalanine (Phe): One of the amino acids in collagen molecules.

Platelet: A round or oval disk, 2–4 µm in diameter, found in the blood of vertebrates. Platelets contain no hemoglobin.

Polydioxanone: A synthetic polymer formed from dioxanone monomers which degrades by hydrolysis.

Polyglycolic acid (PGA): A synthetic polymer formed from glycolic acid monomers which degrades by hydrolysis.

Polylactic acid (PLA): A synthetic polymer formed from lactic acid monomers which degrades by hydrolysis.

Polymorphism: Different types of aggregated states of the collagen molecules.

Polymorphonuclear leukocyte: A white blood cell which possesses a nucleus composed of two or more lobes or parts; a granulocyte (neutrophil, eosinophil, basophil).

Polypeptide: Polymerized amino acid molecules formed by enzymatically regulated stepwise polymerization *in vivo* between the carboxyl group of one amino acid and the amino group of a second amino acid.

Polysaccharide: Polymerized sugar molecules found in tissues as lubricant (synovial fluid) or cement (between osteons, tooth root attachment) or complexed with proteins such as glycoproteins or proteoglycans.

Proline (Pro): One of the amino acids commonly occurring in collagen molecules.

Proteolytic enzyme: Enzymes which catalyze the breakdown of native proteins.

Resorbable collagen: Collagen which can be biodegraded *in vivo*.

Salt-linkage: An electrostatic bond formed between a negative charge group and a positive charge group in collagen molecules and fibrils.

Segment-long-spacing (SLS): One of the polymorphic forms of collagen where all heads of collagen molecules are aligned in parallel.

Soluble collagen: Collagen molecules that can be extracted with salts and dilute acids. Soluble collagen molecules contain the telopeptides.

Telopeptide: The two short nontriple helical peptide segments located at the ends of collagen molecules.

Valine (Val): One of the amino acids in collagen molecules.

References

Abbott, W.M. and Austin, W.G. 1975. The effectiveness of mechanism of collagen-induced topical hemostasis. *Surgery* 78:723–729.

Altman, R. and Li, S.T. 1990. Collagen matrix for oral surgical applications. *Int. J. Oral Implantol.* 7:75.

Angell, W.W., Angell, J.D., and Kosek, J.C. 1982. Twelve year experience with glutaraldehyde preserved porcine xenografts. *J. Thorac. Cardiovasc. Surg.* 83:493–502.

Archibald, S.J., Krarup, C., Shefner, J., Li, S.T., and Madison, R. 1991. Collagen-based nerve conduits are as effective as nerve grafts to repair transected peripheral nerves in rodents and non-human primates. *J. Comp. Neurol.* 306:685–696.

Armstrong, R.B., Nichols, J., and Pachance, J. 1986. Punch biopsy wounds treated with Monsel's solution or a collagen matrix. *Arch. Dermatol.* 122:546–549.

Arnoczky, S.P. and Warren, R.F. 1982. Microvasculature of the human meniscus. *Am. J. Sport Med.* 10:90–95.

Bailey, A.J. and Peach, C.M. 1970. Chemistry of the collagen cross-links. Isolation and characterization of two intermediate intermolecular cross-links in collagen. *Biochem. J.* 117(5):819–831.

Bear, R.S. 1952. The structure of collagen fibrils. *Adv. Prot. Chem.* 7:69–160.

Bell, E., Ehrlich, H.P., Buttle, D.J., and Nakatsuji, T. 1981. Living tissue formed *in vitro* and accepted as skin equivalent tissue of full thickness. *Science* 211:1042–1054.

Bellamkonda, R. and Aebischer, P. 1994. Review: Tissue engineering in the nerve system. *Biotechnol. Bioeng.* 43:543–554.

Biological Evaluation and Medical Devices. Use of international standard ISO-10993. Blue Book memorandon G95-1, Rockville, MD, FDA, CDRH, Office of Device Evaluation, May 1, 1995.

Blanche, C. and Chaux, A. 1988. The use of absorbable microfibrillation collagen to control sternal bone marrow bleeding. *Int. Surg.* 73:42–43.

Blumenthal, N.M. 1988. The use of collagen membranes to guide regeneration of new connective tissue attachment in dogs. *J. Periodontol.* 59:830–836.

Brodsky, B. and Ramshaw, J.A. 1997. The collagen triple-helix structure. *Matrix Biol.* 15:545–554.

Bruck, S.D. 1991. Biostability of materials and implants. *J. Long-Term Effects Med. Implants* 1:89–106.

Chvapil, M. 1982. Considerations on manufacturing principles of a synthetic burn dressing: A review. *J. Biomed. Mater. Res.* 16:245–263.

Collins, R.L., Christiansen, D., Zazanis, G.A., and Silver, F.H. 1991. Use of collagen film as a dural substitute: Preliminary animal studies. *J. Biomed. Mater. Res.* 25:267–276.

Comper, W.D. and Veis, A. 1977. Characterization of nuclei *in vitro* collagen fibril formation. *Biopolymers* 16:2133–2142.

Cook, S.D., Thomas, K.A., Dalton, J.E., Volkman, T., and Kay, J.F. 1991. Enhancement of bone ingrowth and fixation strength by hydroxyapatite coating porous implants. *Trans. Orthop. Res. Soc.* 16:550.

Correll, J.T., Prentice, H.R., and Wise, R.C. 1985. Biological investigations of a new absorbable sponge. *Surg. Gynecol. Obstet.* 81:585–589.

Dagalailis, N., Flink, J., Stasikalis, P., Burke, J.F., and Yannas, I.V. 1980. Design of an artificial skin. III. Control of pore structure. *J. Biomed. Mater. Res.* 14:511–528.

Daly, C.H. 1966. *The Biomechanical Characteristics of Human Skin*. Ph.D. thesis, University of Strathclyde, Scotland.

Dardik, H., Veith, F.J., Spreyregen, S., and Dardik I. 1974. Arterial reconstruction with a modified collagen tube. *Ann. Surg.* 180:144–146.

Deatherage, J.R. and Miller, E.J. 1987. Packaging and delivery of bone induction factors in a collagen implant. *Collagen Rel. Res.* 7:225–231.

Eastoe, J.E. 1967. Composition of collagen and allied proteins. In *Treatise on Collagen*, G.N. Ramachandran (Ed.), pp. 1–72, Academic Press, New York.

Ellis, D.L. and Yannas, I.V. 1996. Recent advances in tissue synthesis *in vivo* by use of collagen-glycosaminoglycans copolymers. *Biomaterials* 17:291–299.

Folkman, J. and Moscona, A. 1978. Role of cell shape in growth control. *Nature* 273:345–349.

Fraenkel-Conrat, H. and Olcott, H.S. 1945. Esterification of proteins with alcohols of low molecular weight. *J. Biol. Chem.* 161:259–268.

Fraser, R.D.B., MacRae, T.P., Miller, A., and Suzuki, E. 1983. Molecular conformation and packing in collagen fibrils. *J. Mol. Biol.* 167:497–510.

Fukai, N., Apte, S.S., and Olsen, B.R. 1994. Nonfibrillar collagens. *Meth. Enzymol.* 245:3–28.

Fung, Y.C. 1993. *Biomechanics, Mechanical Properties of Living Tissues*, 2nd ed., p. 255, Springer, New York.

Goldstein, J.D., Tria, A.J., Zawadsky, J.P., Kato, Y.P., Christiansen, D., and Silver, F.H. 1989. Development of a reconstituted collagen tendon prosthesis. A preliminary implantation study. *J. Bone Joint Surg.* 71A: 1183–1191.

Gongloff, R.K., Whitlow, W., and Montgomery, C.K. 1985. Use of collagen tubes for implantation of hydroxyapatite. *J. Oral Maxillofac. Surg.* 43:570–573.

Green, R.W., Ang K.P., and Lam, L.C. 1953. Acetylation of collagen. *Biochem. J.* 54:181–187.

Hede, A., Larson, E., and Sanberg, H. 1992. The long term outcome of open total and partial meniscectomy related to the quantity and site of the meniscus removed. *Int. Orthop.* 16:122–125.

Hodge, A.J. and Petruska, J.A. 1963. Recent studies with the electron microscope on the ordered aggregates of the tropocollagen molecule. In *Aspects of Proteins Structure*, G.N. Ramachandran (Ed.), pp. 289–300, Academic Press, New York.

Hofmann, H. and Kuhn, K. 1981. Statistical analysis of collagen sequences with regard to fibril assembly and evolution. In *Structural Aspects of Recognition and Assembly in Biological Macromolecules*, M. Balaban, J.L. Sussman, W. Traub, and A. Yonath (Eds.), pp. 403–425, Balabann ISS, Rehovot and Philadelphia.

Hollinger, J., Mark, D.E., Bach, D.E., Reddi, A.H., and Seyfer, A.E. 1989. Calvarial bone regeneration using osteogenin. *J. Oral Maxillofac. Surg.* 47:1182–1186.

Hubbell, J.A. 1995. Biomaterials in tissue engineering. *Biotechnology* 13:565–576.

Jaffe, R. and Deykin, D.J. 1974. Evidence for a structural requirement for the aggregation of platelet by collagen. *Clin. Invest.* 53:875–883.

Jonas, R.A., Ziemer, G., Schoen, F.J., Britton, L., and Castaneda, A.R. 1998. A new sealant for knitted dacron prostheses: Minimally cross-linked gelatin. *J. Vasc. Surg.* 7:414–419.

Kato, Y.P., Dunn, M.G., Zawadsky, J.P., Tria, A.J., and Silver, F.H. 1991. Regeneration of Achilles tendon with a collagen tendon prosthesis. *J. Bone Joint Surg.* 73A: 561–574.

Katz, E.P. and Li, S.T. 1972. The molecular organization of collagen in mineralized and nonmineralized tissues. *Biochem. Biophys. Res. Commun.* 3:1368–1373.

Katz, E.P. and Li, S.T. 1973a. The intermolecular space of reconstituted collagen fibrils. *J. Mol. Biol.* 73:351–369.

Katz, E.P. and Li, S.T. 1973b. Structure and function of bone collagen fibrils. *J. Mol. Biol.* 80:1–15.

Katz, E.P. and Li, S.T. 1981. The molecular packing of type I collagen fibrils. In *The Chemistry and Biology of Mineralized Connective Tissues*, A. Veis (Ed.), pp. 101–105, Elsevier, North Holland.

Kemp, P.D., Cavallaro, J.F., and Hastings, D.N. 1995. Effects of carbodiimide crosslinking and load environment on the remodeling of collagen scaffolds. *Tissue Eng.* 1:71–79.

Kleinman, H.K., Klebe, R.J., and Martin, G.R. 1981. Role of collagenous matrices in the adhesion and growth of cells. *J. Cell Biol.* 88:473–485.

Larson, P.O. 1988. Topical hemostatic agents for dermatologic surgery. *J. Dermatol. Surg. Oncol.* (14): 623–632.

Li, S.T. 1988. Collagen and vascular prosthesis. In *Collagen*, Vol. III, M.E. Nimni (Ed.), pp. 253–271, CRC Press, Boca Raton, FL.

Li, S.T. 1990. A multi-layered, semipermeable conduit for nerve regeneration comprised of type I collagen, its method of manufacture and a method of nerve regeneration using said conduit. U.S. Patent 4,963,146.

Li, S.T., Archibald, S.J., Krarup, C., and Madison, R. 1990. Semipermeable collagen nerve conduits for peripheral nerve regeneration. *Polym. Mater. Sci. Eng.* 62:575–582.

Li, S.T., Archibald, S.J., Krarup, C., and Madison, R.D. 1991. The development of collagen nerve guiding conduits that promote peripheral nerve regeneration. In *Biotechnology and Polymers*, C.G. Gebelein (Ed.), pp. 282–293, Plenum Press, New York.

Li, S.T., Bolton, W., Helm, G., Gillies, G., and Frenkel, S. 1996. Collagen as a delivery vehicle for bone morphogenetic protein (BMP). *Trans. Orthop. Res. Soc.* 21:647.

Li, S.T., Golub, E., and Katz, E.P. 1975. On electrostatic side chain complimentarity in collagen fibrils. *J. Mol. Biol.* 98:835–839.

Li, S.T. and Katz, E.P. 1976. An electrostatic model for collagen fibrils: the interaction of reconstituted collagen with Ca^{2+}, Na^+, and Cl^-. *Biopolymers* 15:1439–1460.

Li, S.-T, Rodkey, W.G., Yuen, D., Hansen, P., and Steadman, J.R. 2002. Type I collagen-based template for meniscus regeneration. In *Tissue Engineering and Biodegradable Equivalents. Scientific and Clinical Applications*, K.-U. Lewandrowski, D.L. Wise, D.J. Trantolo, J.D. Gresser, M.J. Yaszemski, and D.E. Altobelli (Eds.), Chapter 13, pp. 237–266, Marcel Dekker, Inc., New York.

Li, S.T. and Stone, K.R. 1993. Prosthetic ligament. U.S. Patent 5,263,984.

Li, S.T., Sullman, S., and Katz, E.P. 1981. Hydrogen bonded salt linkages in collagen. In *The Chemistry and Biology of Mineralized Tissues*, A. Veis (Ed.), pp. 123–127, Elsevier, North Holland.

Li, S.T., Yuen, D., Charoenkul, W., Ulreich, J.B., and Speer, D.P. 1997. A type I collagen ligament for ACL reconstruction. *Trans. Soc. Biomater.* XX:407.

Li, S.T., Yuen, D., Li, P.C., Rodkey, W.G., and Stone, K.R. 1994. Collagen as a biomaterial: an application in knee meniscal fibrocartilage regeneration. *Mater. Res. Soc. Symp. Proc.* 331:25–32.

Lindblad, W.J. and Kormos, A.I. 1991. Collagen: a multifunctional family of proteins. *J. Reconstruct. Microsurg.* 7:37–43.

Ma, S., Chen, G., and Reddi, A.H. 1990. Collaboration between collagenous matrix and osteoginin is required for bone induction. *Ann. NY Acad. Sci.* 580:524–525.

Merino, A., Faulkner, C., Corvalan, A., and Sanborn, T.A. 1992. Percutaneous vascular hemostasis device for interventional procedures. *Catheterizat. Cardiovasc. Diagn.* 26:319–322.

Miller, A. 1976. Molecular packing in collagen fibrils. In *Biochemistry of Collagen*, G.N. Ramachandran and H. Reddi (Eds.), pp. 85–136, Plenum Press, New York.

Miller, E.J. 1984. Chemistry of the collagens and their distribution. In *Extracellular Matrix Biochemistry*, K.A. Piez and A.H. Reddi (Eds.), pp. 41–82, Elsevier, New York.

Miller, E.J. and Rhodes, R.K. 1982. Preparation and characterization of the different types of collagen. *Meth. Enzymol.* 82:33–63.

Moghe, P.V., Berthiaume, F., Ezzell, R.M., Toner, M., Tompkins, R.C., and Yarmush, M.L. 1996. Culture matrix configuration and composition in the maintenance of hepatocyte polarity and function. *Biomaterials* 17:373–385.

Montesano, R., Mouron, P., Amherdt, M., and Orci, L. 1983. Collagen matrix promotes reorganization of pancreatic endocrine cell monolayers into islet-like organoids. *J. Cell Biol.* 97:935–939.

Nimni M.E. (Ed.) 1988. *Collagen*, Vols. I, II, and III. CRC Press, Boca Raton, FL.

Nimni, M.E. and Harkness, R.D. 1988. Molecular structures and functions of collagen. In *Collagen*, Vol. I, M.E. Nimni (Ed.), pp. 1–78, CRC Press, Boca Raton, FL.

Noda, H. 1972. Partial specific volume of collagen. *J. Biochem.* 71:699–703.

North, A.C.T., Cowan, P.M., and Randall, J.T. 1954. Structural units in collagen fibrils. *Nature* 174:1142–1143.

Park, J.B. and Lakes, R.S. 1992. *Biomaterials: An Introduction*, 2nd ed., pp. 185–222, Plenum Press, New York.

Piez, K.A. 1984. Molecular and aggregate structures of the collagens. In *Extracellular Matrix Biochemistry*, K.A. Piez and A.H. Reddi (Eds.), p. 5, Elsevier, New York.

Ramachandran, G.N. 1967. Structure of collagen at the molecular level. In *Treatise on Collagen*, Vol. I, G.N. Ramachandran (Ed.), pp. 103–183, Academic Press, New York, London.

Reidy, J.J., Limberg, M., and Kaufman, H.E. 1990. Delivery of fluorescein to the anterior chamber using the corneal collagen shield. *Ophthalmology* 97:1201–1203.

Rich, A. and Crick, F.H.C. 1961. The molecular structure of collagen. *J. Mol. Biol.* 3:483–505.

Rigby, B.J., Hiraci, N., Spikes, J.D., and Eyring, H. 1959. The mechanical properties of rat tail tendon. *J. Gen. Physiol.* 43:265–283.

Ruffini, J.J., Aquavella, J.V., and LoCascio, J.A. 1989. Effect of collagen shields on corneal epithelialization following penetrating keratoplasty. *Ophthal. Surg.* 20:21–25.

Rybock, J.D. and Long, D.M. 1977. Use of microfibrillar collagen as a topical hemostatic agent in brain tissue. *J. Neurosurg.* 46:501–505.

Sawyer, P.N., Stanczewski, B., and Kirschenbaum, D. 1977. The development of polymeric cardiovascular collagen prosthesis. *Artif. Organs* 1:83–91.

Schimpf, W.C. and Rodriquez F. 1976. Fibers from regenerated collagen. *Ind. Eng. Chem. Prod. Res. Rev.* 16:90–92.

Shapiro, F. and Glimcher, M.J. 1980. Induction of osteoarthrosis in the rabbit knee joint: Histologic changes following meniscectomy and meniscal lesions. *Clin. Orthop.* 147:287–295.

Silbermann, M. 1990. *In vitro* systems for inducers of cartilage and bone development. *Biomaterials* 11:47–49.

Sittinger, J.B., Bugia, J., Rotter, N., Reitzel, D., Minuth, W.W., and Burmester, G.R. 1996. Tissue engineering and autologous transplant formation: Practical approaches with resorbable biomaterials and new cell culture techniques. *Biomaterials* 17:237–242.

Sommerlath, K., Gallino, M., and Gillquist, J. 1991. Biomechanical characteristics of different artificial substitutes for the rabbit medial meniscus and the effect of prosthesis size on cartilage. *Trans. Orthop. Res. Soc.* 16:375.

Sorensen, T.S., Sorensen, A.I., and Merser, S. 1990. Rapid release of gentamicin from collagen sponge. *Acta Orthop. Scand.* 61:353–356.

Stein, M.D., Salkin, L.M., Freedman, A.L., and Glushko, V. 1985. Collagen sponge as a topical hemostatic agent in mucogingival surgery. *J. Periodontol.* 56:35–38.

Stenzl, K.H., Miyata, T., and Rubin, A.L. 1974. Collagen as a biomaterial. *Ann. Rev. Biophys. Bioeng.* 3:231–253.

Stone, K.R., Steadman, J.R., Rodkey, W.R., and Li, S.T. 1997. Regeneration of meniscal cartilage with the use of a collagen scaffold. *J. Bone Joint Surg.* 79A:1770–1777.

Tiffit, J.T. 1980. The organic matrix of bone tissue. In *Fundamental and Clinical Bone Physiology*, M.R. Urist (Ed.), p. 51, JB Lippincott Co., Philadelphia, PA.

Timpl, R. 1982. Antibodies to collagen and procollagen. *Meth. Enzymol.* 82:472–498.

van der Rest, M., Dublet, B., and Champliaud, M.F. 1990. Fibril-associated collagens. *Biomaterials* 11:28–31.

Walker, W.E., Duncan, J.M., Frazier, O.H., Liversay, J.J., Ott, D.A., Reul, G.J., and Cooly, D.A. 1983. Early experience with the Ionescu-Shiley pericardial xenograft valve. *J. Thorac. Cardiovasc. Surg.* 86:570–575.

Wang, C.-L., Miyata, T., Weksler, B., Rubin, A., and Stenzel, K.H. 1978. Collagen-induced platelet aggregation and release: Critical size and structural requirements of collagen. *Biochim. Biophys. Acta* 544:568–577.

Webster, R.C., Kattner, M.D., and Smith, R.C. 1984. Injectable collagen for augmentation of facial areas. *Arch. Otolaryngol.* 110:652–656.

Wiederhorn, N. and Beardon, G.V. 1952. Studies concerned with the structure of collagen: II. Stress–strain behavior of thermally controlled collagen. *J. Polym. Sci.* 9:315–325.

Wilner, G.D., Nossel, H.L., and Leroy, E.C. 1968. Activation of Hageman factor by collagen. *J. Clin. Invest.* 47:2608–2615.

Woolley, D.E. 1984. Mammalian collagenases. In *Extracellular Matrix Biochemistry*, K.A. Piez and A.H. Reddi (Eds.), pp. 119–151, Elsevier, New York.

Yamuchi, M., Katz, E.P., and Mechanic, G.L. 1986. Intermolecular cross-linking and stereospecific molecular packing in type I collagen fibrils of the periodontal ligament. *Biochemistry* 25:4907–4913.

Yannas, I.V. and Burke, J.F. 1981. Design of an artificial skin. I. Basic design principles. *J. Biomed. Mater. Res.* 14:65–80.

Yannas, I.V., Orgill, D.P., Silver, J., Norregaad, T., Ervas, N.N., and Schoene, W.C. 1985. Polymeric template facilitates regeneration of sciatic nerve across a 15 mm gap. *Polym. Mater. Sci. Eng.* 53:216–218.

Biologic Biomaterials: Silk

34.1 Structure and Properties 34-1
34.2 Sources of Silk Proteins 34-2
    Silkworm Silk (*B. mori*) • *B. mori* Silk Fibroin Structure
34.3 Processing Silk Proteins 34-3
34.4 Engineered Silk Matrices for Cell-Based Engineering
    and Drug Delivery 34-4
    Silk Fibroin Micro-/Nanofibrous Nets/Mats/
    Membranes • Regenerated Silk Fibroin Films and
    Coatings • Surface-Decorated Silk Fibroin Films • Silk Fibroin as
    a 3D Scaffold Matrix • Regenerated Silk Fibroin Hydrogels • Silk
    Microspheres
34.5 Applications of Silkworm Silk for Bone and Cartilage
    Tissue Engineering 34-11
    Silk-Based Bone Tissue Engineering • Silk-Based Cartilage Tissue
    Engineering
34.6 Silk Degradation 34-13
34.7 Silk Immunological Responses 34-13
34.8 Conclusions 34-14
Acknowledgments 34-14
References 34-14

Biman Mandal
Tufts University

David L. Kaplan
Tufts University

34.1 Structure and Properties

Silks are naturally produced protein polymers synthesized and processed into fibers by a variety of insects and spiders [1–5]. The functions of silks include web construction and prey capture (spider webs), reproduction (cocoons), and safety lines (dragline) [5–7]. Silks also exhibit a unique combination of material properties including lightweight (1.3 g/cm³), high strength (up to 4.8 GPa as the strongest fiber known in nature), and high toughness with elasticity up to 35% [8]. The toughness of dragline silk is comparable to high-tenacity fibers such as Kevlar 49, while elasticity is 4–7 times higher. In addition, silk as a biopolymer is remarkably stable under thermal conditions (up to ~250°C) allowing processing over a wide range of conditions (Table 34.1) [7].

Silk fibers are composed of a filament core, silk fibroin, and a glue-like coating consisting of a family of sericin proteins. The most widely studied silks are cocoon silk from the mulberry silkworm *Bombyx mori* and the dragline silks from spiders such as *Areneus diadematus* and *Nephila clavipes* [3,8–11]. Structurally, silk fibroins are characterized as natural block (peptide domains) copolymers composed of hydrophobic blocks with highly preserved repetitive sequences consisting of short side-chain amino acids such as glycine and alanine, and smaller hydrophilic blocks with more complex sequence chemistry including some charged amino acids [6,12]. The hydrophobic blocks are responsible for the formation of β-sheets (crystals), formed through hydrogen bonding and hydrophobic interactions, as the basis for the high-tensile strength of silk fibroins [13,14]. These ordered hydrophobic blocks combined with

TABLE 34.1   Mechanical Properties of Silk and Other Biodegradable Polymeric Materials

Source of Biomaterial	Modulus (GPa)	UTS (MPa)	Strain (%) at Break	References
B. mori silk (with sericin)	5–12	500	19	[138]
B. mori silk (without sericin)	15–17	610–690	4–16	[138]
B. mori silk	10	740	20	[139]
N. clavipes silk	11–13	875–972	17–18	[139]
Collagen	0.0018–0.046	0.9–7.4	24–68	[140]
Cross-linked collagen	0.4–0.8	47–72	12–16	[140]
Polylactic acid	1.2–3.0	28–50	2–6	[141]

the less ordered hydrophilic blocks give rise to the combined elasticity and toughness of silk fibroin materials, such as the native fibers [3,10,15].

Mechanistic insight has been developed into how silk fibroin solutions are processed to insoluble fibers by various organisms. The process involves spinning a highly concentrated silk fibroin solution in a non-Newtonian liquid crystalline state, where the silk fibroins are lubricated and stabilized by water through micelle-like structures as a result of phase separation due to silk fibroin's intrinsic hydrophilic–hydrophobic blocks [3,9]. The process is known to be mediated by the content and location of water. The silk fibroin concentration in the gland gradually increases, leading to the formation of micelles and gels [9]. Also, the silk fibroin protein organizes into a metastable state that maintains sufficient water content to avoid premature conversion to insoluble β-sheet structures. Upon spinning via the figure eight head movement of the silkworm or the pulling by the legs of spiders, chain alignment leads to the final assembly of β-sheet crystalline blocks [9]. In the final stages of spinning the fibers in silkworms, hydrophilic proteins, termed sericins, form composite matrices by coating the core fibroin fibers [3,9]. Once formed, silk fibers are insoluble in most organic solvents, water, and dilute acids and bases; hexafluoroisopropanol (HFIP), calcium nitrate, lithium bromide, and lithium thiocyanate can be used to solubilize silk [16,17]. The repetitive peptide domains in the silk fibroin sequence form the core basis for genetically engineered silk-like polymers, in cassette-like approaches, in host systems such as bacteria, yeast, mammalian cells, and plants [11,18,19].

34.2 Sources of Silk Proteins

Many animals produce silk proteins for various different needs [20]; however, silkworm silk proteins are the most extensively studied and abundant due to the 5000 years of domestication known as sericulture for textile-related needs. A wash after harvesting cocoons removes the sericin coating on the silk fibers yielding *B. mori* silk fibroin [21]. Similar processes are applicable to silk fibers produced by wild silkworms (such as *Antheraea pernyi*, *Antheraea mylitta*, or *Samia cynthiaricini* [21]) providing silk proteins with differing amino acid sequences. Spider silk is also widely studied due to its mechanical properties; however, its limited availability from native sources requires biotechnology-generated sources via cloning and expression in a range of heterologous hosts as listed earlier. Although it is possible to harvest milligrams of spider silk from fibers of egg cocoons or webs, or directly from the animal via controlled silking, this is time-consuming and inefficient. For example, a 3.4 m² rug produced from major ampullate silk fibers of *Nephila madagascarenis* spiders took 70 people 4 years to complete, consisted of silk collected from over 1 million spiders, and cost of over half a million US dollars [22]. Unfortunately, attempts to farm spiders on an industrial scale have been unsuccessful due to their cannibalistic nature. Progress in the production of spider silk-like proteins using recombinant DNA technology continues to progress to provide alternative silk options [23]. Recombinant DNA technology has also been used to prepare chimaeric/hybrid silk-like proteins incorporating silkworm silk-like or spider silk-like sequences to enhance protein solubility, improve biomineralization/cell adhesion, and related needs [24].

34.2.1 Silkworm Silk (*B. mori*)

B. mori silkworm farming and use in textiles and in broader studies has facilitated an understanding of the composite protein structure and more recently the broader potential for biomedical applications. Structurally, *B. mori* silk fibroin fibers consist of two proteins: a light chain (~26 kDa) and a heavy chain (~390 kDa) which are present in a 1:1 stoichiometric ratio and linked by a single disulfide bond [25]. These proteins are coated with the family of hydrophilic proteins called sericins (20–310 kDa) [2,25,26]. The disulfide linkage between the Cys-c20 (20th residue from the carboxyl terminus) of the heavy chain and the Cys-172 of the light chain holds the fibroin together and a 25 kDa glycoprotein, named P25, has been reported to be noncovalently linked to these proteins [27]. Silk fibroin can be highly purified from sericins by boiling the silk cocoons in an alkaline solution, sometimes with a surfactant to improve the purification process. Twenty to thirty percent of the silk cocoon mass is sericin, which is removed during this alkali degumming (sericin removal) process.

34.2.2 *B. mori* Silk Fibroin Structure

Silk fibroin from *B. mori* consists primarily of glycine (Gly) (43%), alanine (Ala) (30%), and serine (Ser) (12%) [2]. The heavy chain of the protein consists of 12 domains that form the crystalline (β-sheet) regions in the silk fibers, which are interspersed with nonrepetitive and less-organized domains (noncrystalline) in the proteins. The crystalline domains in the fibers consist of Gly-X repeats, with X being most often Ala, followed by Ser, threonine (Thr), and valine (Val) [28]. The crystalline-forming silk domains have an average of 381 residues (596 in size in the seventh domain to 36 in the 12th domain). Each domain consists of hexapeptide subdomains: GAGAGS, GAGAGY, GAGAGA, or GAGYGA, where G is glycine, A is alanine, S is serine, and Y is tyrosine. These subdomains end with tetrapeptides such as GAAS or GAGS [25,28,29]. The less crystalline regions of the fibroin heavy chain are known as linkers or spacers and are reported to have an identical 25 nonrepetitive amino acid residue sequence, not found in the crystalline regions [28]. The primary sequence for the fibroin results in a hydrophobic protein with a natural coblock polymer design, a design feature found in all silkworm and spider silks [9,12]. A number of silk polymorphs have been reported, including the glandular state prior to crystallization (silk I), the spun silk state which consists of the β-sheet secondary structure (silk II), and an air/water-assembled interfacial silk (silk III, with a helical structure) [2,9,30]. The silk I structure is known to be water-soluble and upon exposure to heat or physical spinning, easily converts into a silk II structure. The silk I structure is also observed *in vitro* in aqueous conditions and converts into a β-sheet structure when exposed to methanol or certain salts [31]. The β-sheet structures are asymmetric with one side occupied with hydrogen side chains from glycine and the other occupied with the methyl side chains from the alanines that populate the hydrophobic domains. The β-sheets are arranged so that the methyl groups and hydrogen groups of opposing sheets interact to form the intersheet stacking in the crystals. Strong hydrogen bonds and van der Waals forces generate a structure that is thermodynamically stable [2], to the point that high pressure and temperature during autoclaving do not significantly impact the structure. The inter- and intra-chain hydrogen bonds form between-amino acids perpendicular to the axis of the chains and the fiber [2]. The silk II structure excludes water and therefore is slow to degrade via hydrolysis or proteolytic activity.

34.3 Processing Silk Proteins

Natural silkworm silk fibers require little processing for use as textile materials (e.g., dyeing [32–34], chemical modification to render them water proof prior [35,36]). However, in order to prepare alternative material morphologies with silk (e.g., films, foams, hydrogels, fibers, spheres) or composite materials,

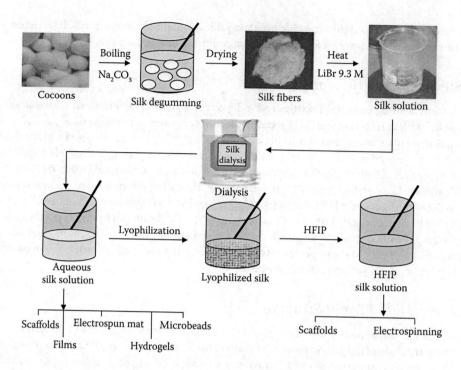

FIGURE 34.1 Processing steps of *B. mori* silk cocoons to form regenerated silk solution.

it is typically necessary to regenerate silk by dissolution in a solvent capable of denaturing the protein (by breaking the strong intermolecular hydrogen bonds—stacks of β-sheets), through the use of concentrated aqueous solutions of inorganic/organic salts, fluorinated solvents, ionic liquids, or strong acids (Figure 34.1) [37–39]. Once dissolved, the regenerated silk protein than can be processed into a variety of different material morphologies (Figure 34.2); for example, silk fibers with micron-scale diameters can be prepared by hand-drawing or dry-/wet-spinning, and silk fibers with nanometer-scale diameters can be prepared by electrospinning. Silk films can be fabricated by casting and dip-/spin-coating; silk hydrogels can be prepared by exposure of aqueous solutions of silk proteins (after dialysis to remove any denaturant) to various stimuli including salt, shear, and sonication. Similarly, silk foams/scaffolds can be prepared by freeze-drying frozen silk and or hydrogels, gas foaming, or salt-leaching; silk spheres can be prepared by electrospraying or precipitation upon addition of solvent to a solution of silk, and silk capsules can be prepared by adsorption of the protein at the interface of a water-in-oil emulsion. These silk materials are often treated with alcohols (typically methanol and or ethanol) or aqueous solutions of salts (such as potassium phosphate) in order to induce β-sheet formation to render them insoluble in water while also changing the mechanical properties [37–39].

34.4 Engineered Silk Matrices for Cell-Based Engineering and Drug Delivery

Over the last decade, numerous studies have explored the potential of native and regenerated silk fibroin-based biomaterials in the context of biomedical applications (Table 34.2). Majority of research activity has been focused on mulberry silk fibroin from *B. mori* due to the availability of this material as outlined earlier.

Biomaterials need to fulfill certain criteria, including physical, chemical, and biological cues to guide cells into functional tissues via cell migration, adhesion, and differentiation. Degradation is also important, particularly for many biomaterial applications and in regeneration needs in medicine, in general. Ideally, biomaterials need to degrade at a rate commensurate with new tissue formation to allow cells

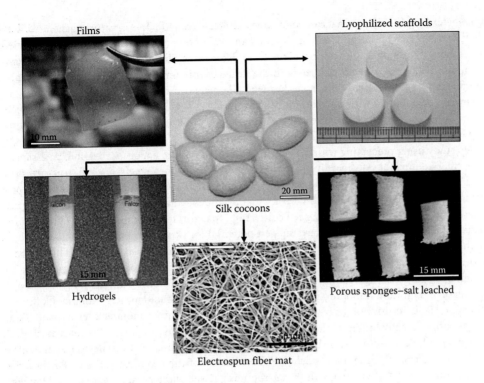

FIGURE 34.2 Various silk fibroin matrix formats prepared using regenerated silk solution.

to deposit new extracellular matrix (ECM) and regenerate functional tissue during the remodeling process. In addition, the biomaterial needs to include provisions for mechanical support appropriate to the level of functional tissue development. In general, biomaterials must be biocompatible and elicit little to no host immune response. Since silk proteins satisfy these criteria, new possibilities to expand silk-based materials for cellular therapeutic applications are being pursued, past the more traditional suture uses for silks.

34.4.1 Silk Fibroin Micro-/Nanofibrous Nets/Mats/Membranes

Scaffolds for tissue engineering can be used to mimic the structure and biological function of the ECM. In native ECMs, collagen fibers are organized in a 3D porous network that forms hierarchical structures

TABLE 34.2 Processing of Regenerated Silk Fibroin and Related Biomedical Applications

Silk Format	Processing Method	Major Applications	References
Film	Casting, layer-by-layer	Coating materials, wound dressings, biosensors, drug delivery	[56–77]
Hydrogel	Sol–gel transition	Bone repair, drug delivery, cartilage engineering	[96–99]
Nonwoven mat/ net/membrane	Fiber deposition, electrospinning	Bone repair, wound dressing, skin tissue engineering	[40–55]
Microspheres	Spray-drying, oil–water emulsion	Drug and growth factor delivery	[112–116]
3D porous sponge	Salt leaching, freeze-drying, gas foaming	Bone and cartilage tissue engineering, drug release	[78–95,117–126]

from nanometer length scales to macroscopic tissue architectures [40]. The structures generated with silks, such as via electrospinning, contain similar nanoscale fibers with micro-scale interconnected pores, resembling the topographic features of the ECM. Nonwoven fibrous silk fibroin nets/mats/membranes can also be fabricated with diameters in the range of micrometers in their native or partially dissolved forms [41–43]. Similarly, finer meshes with diameters in the range of tens to hundreds of nanometers can be obtained with electrospun silk fibroin fibers [44–50]. Nonwoven microfibrous nets support the adhesion, proliferation, and cell–cell interactions of a wide variety of human cell types including epithelial cells, endothelial cells, glial cells, keratinocytes, osteoblasts, and fibroblasts [43]. A follow-up study using precoating with fibronectin supported *in vitro* endothelialization, an essential step for vascularization [42]. After seeding in fibronectin-coated silk fibroin nets, normal structure, proliferative activity, migration, cell–cell interactions, and other phenotypic features were observed in primary human endothelial cells of macro-/microvascular origin. No alteration in the structural integrity of the nonwoven nets was observed during cell cultivation. In addition, cytocompatibility of these nonwoven nets to keratinocytes and osteoblasts suggest potential for skin or bone repair. The biocompatibility of these nonwoven microfibrous meshes composed of partially dissolved native silk fibroin fibers has also been reported [41]. After subcutaneous implant, the nonwoven microfibrous meshes induced a mild foreign body response without fibrosis. Microarray analysis of 23 proinflammatory genes identified an increase in migration inhibitory factor transcript level in implantation sites with the silk fibroin mesh. No appreciable infiltration of lymphocytes was observed within 6 months after implantation, further suggesting biocompatibility. These silk fibroin mesh implants supported the regeneration of vascularized reticular connective tissue based on cytokeratins, vimentin, and Col-I detection, and morphological, histological, and immunohistochemical evaluation of the regenerated tissue. Further, the silk fibroin mesh implants integrated with the surrounding tissue while no apparent degradation was observed within 6 months of implantation. An *in vivo* study [51] further identified silk fibroin-based membranes/meshes as promising materials for skin regeneration. Similar to the above system, micron-diameter fiber mats, nonwoven nanofibrous nets/mats prepared by electrospinning, can be used for similar goals [44,46,47] and support the attachment, spreading, and proliferation of human bone marrow stromal cells, keratinocytes, and fibroblasts *in vitro* [47,48,52]. In an *in vivo* study, the biocompatibility of silk fibroin nonwoven nanofiber membranes/nets and their effect on guided repair of critical-sized calvarial bone defects were assessed in a rabbit model [45]. The nanofiber membranes/nets were formed by electrospinning regenerated silk fibroin solution in 98% formic acid and treated with 50% methanol. The resulting nonwoven nanofibrous membranes contained randomly deposited fibers with diameters ranging from 150 to 300 nm. The membranes supported the *in vitro* attachment, spreading, proliferation, and differentiation of MC3T3-E1 osteoblast-like cells. When evaluated *in vivo* in a rabbit calvarial bone defect model, the silk fibroin nonwoven nanofibrous membranes showed good biocompatibility and structural stability. The membranes enhanced bone formation over 12 weeks with no evidence of inflammatory reactions. This study further suggests that nonwoven silk fibroin nanofibrous nets/mats/membranes have potential for guided regeneration of bones in nonload bearing sites [53–55].

34.4.2 Regenerated Silk Fibroin Films and Coatings

Silk was first evaluated for cellular responses on 2D films in tissue culture wells. The films formed from silkworm fibroin collected from glands of *B. mori* and *A. pernyi* wild silkworms were comparable to collagen films in terms of supporting the attachment, spreading, and proliferation of murine L-929 fibroblasts [56–57] and the growth of human and animal cell lines [58,59]. Cell attachment to positively charged residues like arginine near the C-terminus of the nonrepetitive (hydrophilic) regions of the silk fibroin sequence was identified as an important feature, considering the surface of mammalian cells is predominantly negatively charged [56,58]. Further observations identified stronger cell adhesion on films formed by silk fibroins from *A. pernyi* than those from *B. mori* [56]. The difference in terms of cell attachment was attributed to the presence of the tripeptide Arg(R)-Gly(G)-Asp(D), a recognition site or integrin-mediated cell adhesion [60–62], a sequence found in the silk fibroin sequence from the wild silkworms, but not the domestic silkworms [56].

Regenerated silk fibroin has been used as a coating material for cell culture and tissue engineering [63–67]. Coating poly(D,L-lactic acid) films with regenerated silk fibroin improved interactions between osteoblasts and the polymer films [66,67]. The surface of 2D and 3D polyurethane scaffolds were coated by dipping in 3–4% (w/w) silk fibroin solutions from *B. mori*, resulting in a stable silk fibroin coating with a thickness of 200–600 nm [63]. The effect of silk fibroin coatings on 2D poly(carbonate)-urethane substrates on attachment, proliferation, metabolism, and ECM synthesis of four strains of human fibroblasts was also evaluated [64]. Improved cell attachment, which resulted in a 2.5-fold increase in total cell numbers by day 30 in culture, was found on the silk fibroin films. Concurrently, the silk fibroin coating significantly affected the metabolism of fibroblasts, inducing higher glucose uptake and lower glutamine consumption in the initial stages of cultivation. The coating also enhanced the extracellular assembly of collagen type I (Col-I).

Fibroblasts seeded on silk fibroin-coated substrates did not secrete appreciable levels of cytokines such as IL-1β, TNF-α, or TGF-β1, all of which are implicated in inflammation and tissue repair during wound healing. However, IL-6 secretion, another important cytokine involved in inflammation reactions and wound healing, was enhanced by the silk fibroin coating after 2 weeks. Using similar methodology, the response of human fibroblasts seeded on silk-fibroin-coated 3D polyurethane scaffolds was assessed [65], and cell attachment, proliferation, and cellular metabolism were also found, as above. However, in comparison to the 2D substrates, expression of IL-6 with silk fibroin-coated 3D scaffolds was not significantly affected, nor was the extracellular assembly. These studies provided an experimental basis for silk fibroin as a coating material for tissue-engineering scaffolds. An all-aqueous stepwise (layer-by-layer) deposition technique was used to assemble nanoscale thin-film silk fibroin coatings on a number of substrates, and the response of human bone marrow mesenchymal stem cells (hMSCs) to the coatings was assessed [68]. Mechanistically, the main driving force were hydrophobic interactions and partial electrostatic interactions for the deposition and stabilization of the silk fibroin on the solid substrate surfaces, thus both hydrophilic and hydrophobic materials could be coated. The thickness of the multilayered film coatings was linearly correlated with the number of layers, each of which had a controlled thickness in the range of a few to tens of nanometers depending on the concentration of silk fibroin used in the process and the level of salt. The silk fibroin underwent a structural transition from a mixture of random coil and α-helices (silk I) to organized β-sheets (silk II structure) and supported the attachment, proliferation, and differentiation of the hMSCs. This simple, yet versatile, technique has the potential to be used to generate silk fibroin films with controlled morphological and structural features for clinical applications such as drug delivery and tissue engineering.

For drug delivery, nanolayer coatings of silk fibroin containing model small-molecule drugs and proteins, such as rhodamine B and azoalbumin, were studied in Reference 69, as were heparin, paclitaxel, and clopidogrel for vascular systems [70]. Cell attachment and viability with human aortic endothelial cells and human coronary artery smooth muscle cells on the drug-incorporated silk coatings demonstrated that paclitaxel and clopidogrel inhibited smooth muscle cell proliferation and retarded endothelial cell proliferation [70]. The silk multilayers with heparin promoted human aortic endothelial cell proliferation while inhibiting human coronary artery smooth muscle cell proliferation, which was a desired outcome for the prevention of restenosis [70]. Solid adenosine powder reservoirs coated with silk fibroin were investigated for local and sustained delivery of the anticonvulsant adenosine from the encapsulated reservoirs [71]. These reports demonstrated that silk coatings are effective for drug-eluting coatings.

34.4.3 Surface-Decorated Silk Fibroin Films

Surface modifications with Arg–Gly–Asp (RGD) or specific growth factors/integrin binding sites have also been pursued with silks. RGD coupling, via carbodiimide chemistry, to silk fibroin films and fibers for attachment, spreading, proliferation, and differentiation of human Saos-2 osteoblasts, fibroblasts, and hMSCs were assessed [72,73]. In additional studies, RGD modification of silk fibroin enhanced the adhesion and proliferation of human tenocytes and supported differentiation based on elevated transcript levels for decorin and Col-I [74]. Increased cell density and enhanced differentiation of cells on RGD-coupled silk matrices were shown, mediated by cell–cell interactions [73]. Surface modification with parathyroid hormone, which affects the differentiation of osteoblasts *in vitro* [75] and *in vivo* [76], was used to cell responses on the silk fibroin films [72]. Silk fibroin films decorated with bone morphogenetic protein-2 (BMP-2) via covalent coupling enhanced osteogenic differentiation of hMSCs [77]. Compared to adsorbed BMP-2, covalently coupled BMP-2 was retained on the surface at a significantly higher level for a longer period in culture. Within 1 week, 70% of the adsorbed BMP-2 was released from the film surface. By the end of week 4, only 10% of the adsorbed BMP-2 remained, while 50% of the coupled BMP-2 was still present. More importantly, both covalently coupled and surface-adsorbed BMP-2 remained active and enhanced osteogenic differentiation of the bone marrow stromal cells. The covalently immobilized BMP-2 was more effective than soluble BMP-2 likely due to the slower degradation and higher protein concentration in the local microenvironment. These studies demonstrated that the diversity of amino acid side-chain residues contained in silk fibroin provides useful and accessible options for surface decorations with adhesion ligands and specific growth/morphogen factors where in most cases, biological activity was retained and in some cases improved. These strategies open up further options for selective chemical enhancements of the silk fibroin biomaterial to encode functions related to directing cell and tissue outcomes in a tissue-engineering context.

34.4.4 Silk Fibroin as a 3D Scaffold Matrix

Tissue engineering combines cells and bioactive factors in a defined microenvironment with biomaterial scaffolds that are maintained in bioreactors with controlled environmental stimuli for functional tissue repair and regeneration [78,79]. A key component is the biomaterial scaffold, which acts as a 3D support. Scaffolds should (1) be biocompatible to the host immune system where the engineered tissue will be implanted; (2) support cell attachment, migration, cell–cell interactions, cell proliferation, and differentiation; (3) biodegrade at a controlled rate to match the rate of neotissue growth and facilitate the integration of engineered tissue into the surrounding host tissue; (4) provide structural support for cells and neotissue formed in the scaffold during the initial stages of postimplantation; and (5) be versatile in processing options to alter structure and morphology related to tissue-specific needs (Figure 34.3).

34.4.4.1 Silk Fibroin Porous Sponges

Although silk has been used clinically worldwide as suture material for centuries, only recently has it been exploited as a scaffold biomaterial for cell culture and tissue engineering *in vitro* and *in vivo*. Porous 3D sponge scaffolds are important for tissue engineering for cell attachment, proliferation, and migration, as well as for nutrient and waste transport (Figure 34.3). 3D porous sponges have been formed from regenerated silk fibroin solutions, using both aqueous and solvent approaches and using porogens, gas foaming, and lyophilization [80]. Solvent-based sponges were prepared using salt (e.g., sodium chloride) or sugar as porogen. Solvents such as 1,1,3,3-hexafluoropropanol (HFIP) do not solubilize salt or sugar; therefore, pore sizes in the sponges reflect the size of the porogen used in the process [80]. Similarly, a gradient of pore sizes can be generated by stacking porogens of different sizes within a scaffold. Further, sponges with varying porosity can be controlled by stacking variations of salt/HFIP–silk solutions. Solvent-based porous sponges can also be prepared by addition of a small amount of solvent (ethanol, methanol, DMSO) into the aqueous silk fibroin solution before processing [81]. As with the solvent-based scaffolds, aqueous-based porous silk sponges can be prepared using salt crystals as porogens, with control of pore sizes from 300 to 1000 μm, by manipulating the percent silk solution and the size of the salt crystals. Pore sizes are generally a little smaller than the size of salt crystals utilized in the process due to the limited solubilization of the surface of the crystals during supersaturation of the silk solution prior to solidification [82]. The highly porous scaffolds (porosity up to 99%) prepared by salt

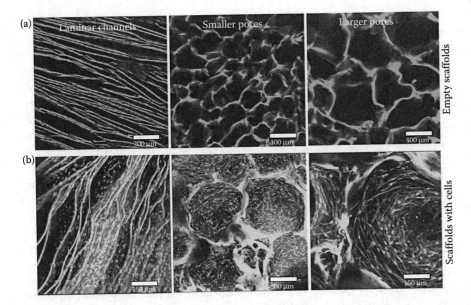

FIGURE 34.3 Silk fibroin scaffolds with various pore sizes prepared using regenerated silk solution. Unseeded silk scaffolds (a) and human bone marrow stem cell-seeded scaffolds (b). Cells are stained with rhodamine-phalloi-din (actin-red) and Hoechst 33342 (nuclei-green false color).

leaching possess a useful combination of high compressive strength and uniform, interconnected pores with controllable pore size and size distribution. In the case of the HFIP-derived scaffolds, a large range of concentrations (6–20%, w/v) can be used that exceed those (4–10%, w/v) for the aqueous-derived scaffolds. Stiffness, compressive strength, and modulus were elevated with an increase in percent silk fibroin solution utilized in the process to form the sponges [82]. Further, enzymatic degradation of aqueous-based sponges was more rapid than for the solvent-based sponges, likely due to higher porosity of the matrices along with less β-sheets [82]. It has also been observed that aqueous-based sponges have rougher surface morphology than solvent-based sponges due to the partial solubilization of the surface of the salt particles. Improved cell attachment was noted for the aqueous silk fibroin sponges in comparison to the solvent-based porous sponges, likely due to these rougher surfaces and high porosity.

Porous 3D silk sponges have been widely utilized in a number of cell studies to generate connective tissues. RGD-coupled silk sponges seeded with hMSCs cultured in osteogenic media resulted in the differentiation of the cells, with deposition of hydroxyapaptite and upregulation of bone markers *in vitro* [83]. Tissue-engineered silk sponges were found useful for healing critical-size femur defects in rats [84]. Further, studies using aqueous porous sponges with large pore sizes (900 μm) were used for bone tissue engineering where structures similar to trabecular bone were observed after 28 days of hMSC differentiation in osteogenic media [85]. Solvent-based silk sponges were cultured with hMSCs in chondrogenic media resulting in the upregulation of collagen type II and glycosaminoglycan transcripts when compared to sponges composed of collagen or cross-linked collagen [86]. The structural integrity of the silk sponges compared with rapidly degrading collagen-based sponges was in part responsible for the differences in gene regulation [86]. Chondrocytes from New Zealand white rabbits were cultured in silk fibroin sponges and proliferated faster and generated a higher content of glycosaminoglycans compared with collagen sponges [87]. Further, porous silk fibroin scaffold sponges seeded with rabbit chondrocytes, in chondrogenic media, yielded a frictional coefficient similar to that of native cartilage after 28 days of culture [88,89]. In skin-related study, sponges formed from a blend of poly(vinyl alcohol) (PVA), chitosan, and silk fibroin showed the best healing of epidermis and dermis of rats when compared to the paired or single polymers [90].

In drug delivery-related studies, silk scaffolds/matrices have been widely used. Horseradish peroxidase (HRP) enzyme gradients were immobilized on silk 3D scaffolds to prepare new functional scaffolds including regional patterning of the gradients to control cell and tissue outcomes [91]. Recently, adenosine release via silk-based implants to the brain of rats have been successfully used for refractory epilepsy treatments [92,93]. Silk-based implants to release adenosine demonstrated therapeutic ability, including the sustained release of adenosine over a period of 2 weeks, with diffusion from the silk, slow degradation of the matrix, biocompatibility, and the delivery of predetermined doses of adenosine [92]. Nerve growth factor (NGF)-loaded silk fibroin nerve conduits have guided the sprouting of axons and to physically protect the axonal cone for peripheral nerve repair [94]. NGF release from the differently prepared silk fibroin nerve conduits was prolonged over 3 weeks, while the total amount of NGF released depended on the procedures used in the preparation of the nerve conduits, such as air-drying or freeze-drying [94]. Silk fibroin scaffolds containing insulin-like growth factor I (IGF-I) were also prepared for controlled IGF-I release in the context of cartilage repair [95].

34.4.5 Regenerated Silk Fibroin Hydrogels

Silk hydrogels can be formed from regenerated fibroin solution by sol–gel transition in the presence of acid, ions, or other additives [96–101]. In addition, temperature, silk fibroin concentration, and pH significantly impact the gelation process. Gelation time decreases with an increase in silk fibroin concentration, temperature, concentration of additives such as Ca^{2+}, glycerol, and poly(ethylene oxide), or a decrease in pH [98,99]. During the gelation process, silk undergoes a structural transition from random coil to β-sheet due to enhanced hydrophobic interactions and hydrogen bond formation [98–100,102,103]. For composites, regenerated silk fibroin can also be blended with other biopolymers such as chitosan and gelatin to form hydrogels [96,104,105] and scaffolds [106]. In addition, genetically engineered silk fibroin-like polymers have been used for hydrogels [107–110]. Silk fibroin hydrogels have been studied for controlled release/delivery of bioactive agents such as plasmid DNA, viruses, and growth factors [17,98].

Silk fibroin hydrogels have been explored for guided tissue repair. The repair of confined, critical-sized cancellous bone defects in a rabbit model using silk fibroin hydrogels was reported [111]. These hydrogels were prepared by adding 1 M citric acid to a 2% (w/v) regenerated silk fibroin aqueous solution until passing the isoelectric point (3.8), and subsequently used for *in vitro* cytotoxicity and cytocompatibility evaluations with a human osteoblast-like cell line (MG63). The silk fibroin hydrogels showed cytocompatibility comparable to poly(D,L-lactide-glycolide), based on cell proliferation, differentiation, and the release of the inflammation-related cytokine IL-6. These silk fibroin hydrogels supported the healing of critical-sized cancellous bone defects *in vivo* in 12 weeks with no obvious inflammatory reactions. Similarly, with further processing, such as freeze-drying, microporous silk fibroin sponges were formed from hydrogels and used for cell culture and tissue engineering [87–89,99]. Microporous silk fibroin sponges were combined with rabbit chondrocytes for cartilage tissue engineering [87–89], and the cells proliferated and maintained differentiated phenotype better than in collagen gels used as controls. The mechanical properties of the regenerated cartilage tissue demonstrated culture time-dependent changes that correspond to the temporal and spatial deposition of cartilage-like ECMs [88,89]. These results suggest the potential of hydrogel-derived silk fibroin sponges as 3D porous scaffolds for chondrocyte-based cartilage regeneration.

34.4.6 Silk Microspheres

Silk spheres were explored for drug delivery applications and in tissue regeneration. These silk microspheres were processed using spray-drying; however, the sizes of the microspheres were above 100 μm, which is suboptimal for drug delivery [112]. Lipid vesicle templating can also be used to efficiently load bioactive molecules for local controlled release [113]. The lipid was subsequently removed by methanol or NaCl, resulting in silk microspheres with β-sheet structure and ~2 μm in diameter [113]. Silk microspheres loaded with HRP demonstrated controlled and sustained release of active enzyme over 10–15 days [113]. Growth factor delivery via silk microspheres in alginate gels was more efficient in delivering BMP-2 than IGFs, probably due to the sustained release of the growth factor [114]. Additionally, growth factors were reported to successfully form linear concentration gradients in scaffolds to control osteogenic and chondrogenic differentiation of hMSCs. A new mode to generate micro- and nanoparticles from silk was reported based on blending with PVA [115]. This method simplifies the overall process compared with lipid templating and provides high yield and good control over feature sizes, from 300 nm to 20 μm, depending on the ratio of PVA/silk used [115]. Silk fibroin microparticles containing BMP-2, BMP-9, and BMP-14 were prepared by dropwise addition of ethanol and exhibited mean diameters of 2.7 ± 0.3 μm, encapsulation efficiencies of 67.9–97.7% depending on the type and amount of BMP loaded, and slow release of BMP over 14 days [116].

34.5 Applications of Silkworm Silk for Bone and Cartilage Tissue Engineering

34.5.1 Silk-Based Bone Tissue Engineering

Bone consists of a highly mineralized ECM, leading to tissue rigidity and strength. The complexity of bone tissues and their morphological, structural, and functional diversity impart difficulties to the repair of critical-sized bone defects. Cortical (compact) bone provides mechanical and protective functions, whereas cancellous (spongy) bone mainly provides metabolic functions [117]. In addition, bone is essential to calcium homeostasis. Despite immune compatibility, bone repair using autologous tissue is often not the best treatment option as it is associated with disadvantages such as limited donor tissue supply, repeated surgery, second site morbidity with additional pain, and long rehabilitation times [78,84]. Silk fibroin scaffolds for the repair of bones have been explored [45,83–85,111,118]. As previously reported, silk fibroin hydrogels [111] and membranes/nets [45] without preseeded cells have been used for guided bone regeneration. In recent years, the technique has evolved to use 3D porous silk fibroin scaffolds and MSCs for the repair of critical-sized bone defects [83–85,118,119].

HFIP- and aqueous-derived 3D porous silk fibroin scaffolds have been used for hMSC-based bone tissue engineering *in vitro* and *in vivo* [83–85,118]. Prior to cell seeding, the hMSCs were characterized for the expression of surface markers and the capacity to differentiate into cells of multiple lineages, with hMSCs staining positive for CD105, CD44, and CD71 and negative for CD34 and CD31 [83–118]. When cultured in BMP-2-containing osteogenic medium under static conditions for 4 weeks, the hMSCs seeded in HFIP-derived porous 3D silk fibroin scaffolds (pore size ~200 mm) showed enhanced osteogenic differentiation over the controls (collagen scaffolds) based on real-time RT-PCR for bone-related gene markers, by immunohistochemistry and microcomputerized tomography for calcium deposition. With RGD modification of the scaffolds, enhanced differentiation of hMSCs was observed, and more organized ECM structures were formed [118]. When cultured under dynamic conditions, the stability of the HFIP-derived silk fibroin scaffolds were found beneficial in terms of maintaining high cell density and promoting the differentiation of hMSCs [83–118]. In spinner flask cultures (5 weeks) at 60 rpm, hMSCs generated trabecular-like bone networks with an ECM similar to that of bone [83]. This engineered bone-like tissue was implanted into critical-sized calvarial bone defects in nude mice and compared with hMSCs freshly seeded on the scaffolds, scaffolds alone and unfilled defects as controls. After 5 weeks of implantation, the engineered bone implants and freshly seeded scaffolds were integrated with the surrounding tissue and stained positive for bone sialoprotein, osteopontin, and osteocalcin, which were absent in the controls (scaffolds alone and unfilled defects). Compared to hMSC freshly seeded implants, the tissue-engineered bone implants showed more substantial bone formation. Within 5 weeks, these tissue-engineered implants started to transform from trabecular-like bone networks to structures similar to the physiological healing process of intra-membraneous bone [83]. Collectively, these observations suggested that a tissue engineering approach combining 3D porous silk fibroin scaffolds and hMSCs offers options for the repair of critical-sized bone defects, where the contribution of host cells is not sufficient for a proper healing. Aqueous-derived silk fibroin scaffolds showed improved bone-tissue engineering outcomes when compared to HFIP-derived silk fibroin scaffolds *in vitro* [85]. This has implications for silk protein processing modes related to biomaterial matrix interactions with stem cells for tissue engineering. New approaches to combine micron-range silk powders with HFIP regenerated silk to fabricate reinforced high-strength reinforced protein–protein composite scaffolds for *in vitro* and *in vivo* applications [120].

34.5.2 Silk-Based Cartilage Tissue Engineering

Adult articular cartilage has limited self-repair capacity due to low cell density, low cell proliferation, slow matrix turnover, and a lack of a vascular supply. Damage in articular cartilage tissue due to developmental abnormalities, trauma, or age-related degeneration such as osteoarthritis often result in extensive chronic pain, gradual loss of mobility, and disability. Current treatment methods are often not sufficient to achieve timely recovery of normal cartilage functions [121]. Most synthetic polymers used in cartilage tissue engineering, especially poly(lactide) (PLA), poly(glycolide) (PGA), or copolymers poly(lactide-*co*-glycolide) (PLGA), can induce inflammation *in vivo* [122,123]. For biomaterials considered for this tissue, collagen suffers from rapid degradation [86] and high swelling [82], while alginate also has limitations including fast degradation, insufficient mechanical properties, inhibitory effects on spontaneous repair, and unfavorable immunological responses [124,125]. The useful combination of high strength, porosity, processability, good biocompatibility, and ability to support cell adhesion, proliferation, and differentiation as described above suggests 3D porous silk fibroin scaffolds as candidates for stem-cell- and chondrocyte-based cartilage tissue engineering [86,126,127]. 3D HFIP-derived silk fibroin scaffolds (pore size ~200 mm) and hMSCs were used for *in vitro* cartilage tissue engineering and outcomes were compared with unmodified and cross-linked collagen scaffolds [86].

Similar to the studies conducted for bone-tissue engineering [83,118], the structurally stable, slow degrading scaffolds (cross-linked collagen scaffolds, silk, and RGD-modified silk scaffolds) were essential to maintain sufficient cell density and to promote the formation of cartilage-like ECMs, based on DNA content and glycosaminoglycan deposition. hMSCs in the porous silk fibroin scaffolds deposited higher amounts of cartilage-specific ECM components (GAGs and Col-II) and expressed higher levels of Col-II mRNA than hMSCs in the collagen-based scaffolds. 3D porous aqueous-derived silk scaffolds (pore size ~550 mm) were also used for *in vitro* cartilage tissue engineering using MSCs and chondrocytes [126,127]. MSCs successfully adhered, proliferated, and differentiated along the chondrogenic lineage in the aqueous-derived silk fibroin scaffolds, based on confocal microscopy, real-time PCR, histology, and immunohistochemistry.

In 3D cultivation with highly porous, aqueous-derived silk fibroin scaffolds, within 3 weeks the majority of MSCs were embedded in lacunae-like spaces and acquired a spherical morphology, which has been found to be essential for the synthesis of ECM components related to cartilage tissue [128]. In the presence of inducers like dexamethasone and TGF-b3, the proliferation of MSCs peaked and switched to a more active differentiating stage. Further, within 3 weeks, the MSCs expressed high levels of cartilage-related ECM transcripts [Col-II, aggrecan (AGC), Col-X, and Col-II/Col-I ratio] and deposited an ECM rich in Col-II protein and sulfated proteoglycans based on immunohistochemistry. No calcium deposition occurred, confirming the absence of osteogenesis. These results supported the presence of chondrogenesis under the cultivation conditions within silk scaffolds. A rather homogeneous cell and ECM distribution was achieved due to the unique features of these aqueous-derived scaffolds, including a rough, hydrophilic surface and high pore interconnectivity [126,127]. The distribution of Col-II protein in the 3D constructs also showed a zonal pattern with more protein deposited in the outer regions, an architecture similar to native articular cartilage tissue. In a follow-up study, combined adult human chondrocytes (hCHs) with aqueous-derived porous silk fibroin scaffolds (pore size ~550 mm) were used for *in vitro* cartilage tissue engineering [126]. After cell seeding, the hCHs attached to, proliferated, and redifferentiated in the scaffolds based on cell morphology, expression of cartilage-related gene transcripts, and the presence of a cartilage-like ECM rich in GAGs and Col- II. Compared to MSCs, the hCHs attached more slowly on the aqueous silk fibroin 3D scaffolds. Cell density was critical for the differentiation of culture-expanded hCHs in the 3D aqueous-derived silk fibroin scaffolds. Significant levels of cartilage-related transcripts (AGC, Col-II, Sox 9, Col-II/Col-I ratio) were upregulated, and uniform deposition of cartilage-specific ECM components (Col-II and GAGs) were observed. The hCH-based constructs were significantly different than those from MSCs with respect to cell morphology and zonal structure. Collectively, these studies demonstrated the potential of porous 3D silk fibroin scaffolds in autologous cell-based cartilage tissue engineering.

34.6 Silk Degradation

The degradation of biomaterials is important related to full regeneration or restoration of full tissue structure and function *in vivo*. Thus, control over the rate of degradation is an important feature in designing functional tissue scaffold biomaterials [129]. Commerical silk fibroin fibers (which are routinely coated with waxes and dyes) retain more than 50% of their mechanical properties after 2 months of implantation *in vivo*; thus, they are defined as a nondegradable biomaterial by the *United States Pharmacopeia* [130]. Other polymers such as PLA, PGA, and PLGA hydrolyze at rates based on the polyester composition, purity, and processing conditions. The degradation of these polymers is usually controlled by varying the ratio of monomers or by altering molecular weight and crystallization [131]. Further, degradation products of polymers like PLA generate low-molecular-weight acids, which can decrease local pH and result in inflammation [132].

Natural polymers like collagen and silks degrade via the action of proteases. Typically, the rate of collagen degradation is altered by cross-linking in order to reduce the rate of enzymatic degradation. Cross-linking of collagen impact cell interactions and may also reduce immunogenicity [133]. The degradation byproducts of collagen are peptides and amino acids. In the case of silks, the rate of fibroin degradation depends on the structure, primarily β-sheet content. Degradation of silk fibroin films and fibers has been explored using several types of proteases, including α-chymotrypsin and collagenases [130,134]. A correlation between *in vitro* and *in vivo* rates of degradation of silk fibroin fibers has also been established [130]. Similarly, the degradation of silk fibers and silk films when exposed to different enzymes has been assessed [134]. Films degraded faster than the fibers based on weight loss. The weight loss was accompanied by a change in average molecular weight of silk from 120 kDa for control silk films to 53 kDa for silk films degraded with α-chymotrypsin over 17 days. Tensile strength properties of silk fibers decreased without a significant change in molecular weight of the silk protein [134]. Silk fibroin porous sponges from regenerated *B. mori* fibers degraded differently with different processing conditions [82]. Aqueous processed 3D sponges, with similar pore sizes, degraded more slowly upon exposure to proteases with an increased percent silk present during the processing. Solvent-processed sponges degraded more slowly than the aqueous-processed systems with similar pore sizes: 65% mass remained after 21 days when compared to aqueous-based sponges, which degraded completely in 4 days upon exposure to proteases. The difference in degradation was likely due to differences in content or distribution of crystallinity [82]. It is generally understood that silk fibroin degradation can be regulated by changing crystallinity [135], pore size, porosity, and molecular weight distribution (MWD). A change in MWD can be achieved by treating the silk fibroin under alkaline conditions and with heat. A decrease in MWD may disrupt ordered structures and reduce cross-links, potentially resulting in faster degradation.

34.7 Silk Immunological Responses

Sutures made from virgin silk (nondegummed silk with sericin) compared with sutures from degummed silk (without sericin) showed differences in hypersensitivity [5]. In early studies, the inflammatory response of degummed silk fibroin *in vitro* was comparable with polystyrene and poly(2-hydroxyethyl methacrylate), with less adhesion of immunocompetent cells [136]. Further, silk films implanted *in vivo* induced lower inflammatory response than collagen films and PLA films [137]. Similarly, silk fibroin nonwoven mats implanted subcutaneously in rats induced a weak foreign body response and no fibrosis. Although there was minor upregulation of inflammatory pathways at the implantation site, there was no invasion by lymphocytes after 6 months *in vivo* [41].

34.8 Conclusions

The range of molecular structures, remarkable mechanical properties, morphology control, versatile processability, and surface modifications suggest that silk fibroin is a useful polymeric biomaterial for design, engineering, and processing into matrices for various medical applications including controlled drug delivery, guided tissue repair, and functional tissue engineering. Different forms of silk matrices with varied surface morphology, useful mechanical features, biocompatibility, slow degradation, and ability to support cell adhesion, proliferation, and differentiation have expanded silk-based biomaterials as promising scaffolds for a wide range of bioengineering needs. To date, the primary impact with silk-based biomaterials has been with the fibroin from *B. mori* silkworm, while other varieties of silkworm silks and spider silks are being actively studied as potential alternatives. As new sources of silk proteins become available, such as from other silkworms and from spiders, as well as via genetic engineering, an expanded range of material properties can be anticipated for biomaterials. Future research toward incorporating cell signaling factors via the aqueous processing modes available during the formation of silk biomaterial matrices, and to induce vascular networks in silks *in vivo*, to further enhance the impact for this family of protein biomaterials will offer novel options to match complex mechanical and biological functions with tissue-specific needs.

Acknowledgments

We thank our many colleagues for their various contributions to the work cited. We also thank the NIH, NSF, and the AFOSR for support of the research.

References

1. Kaplan D, Adams WW, Farmer B, Viney C. Silk—Biology, structure, properties, and genetics. *ACS Symp Ser* 1994;544:2–16.
2. Kaplan DL, Mello CM, Arcidiacono S, Fossey S, Senecal K, Muller W. Silk. In: McGrath K, Kaplan DL, editors. *Protein Based Materials*. Boston, MA: Birkhauser; 1998, pp. 103–31.
3. Vollrath F, Knight DP. Liquid crystalline spinning of spider silk. *Nature* 2001;410:541–48.
4. Vollrath F. Biology of spider silk. *Int J Biol Macromol* 1999;24:81–8.
5. Altman GH, Diaz F, Jakuba C, Calabro T, Horan RL, Chen J et al. Silk-based biomaterials. *Biomaterials* 2003;24:401–16.
6. Winkler S, Kaplan DL. Molecular biology of spider silk. *J Biotechnol* 2000;74:85–93.
7. Wong Po Foo C, Kaplan DL. Genetic engineering of fibrous proteins: Spider dragline silk and collagen. *Adv Drug Deliv Rev* 2002;54:1131–43.
8. Gosline JM, Guerette PA, Ortlepp CS, Savage KN. The mechanical design of spider silks: From fibroin sequence to mechanical function. *J Exp Biol* 1999;202:3295–303.
9. Jin HJ, Kaplan DL. Mechanism of silk processing in insects and spiders. *Nature* 2003;424:1057–61.
10. Vollrath F. Strength and structure of spiders' silks. *J Biotechnol* 2000;74:67–83.
11. Lazaris A, Arcidiacono S, Huang Y, Zhou JF, Duguay F, Chretien N et al. Spider silk fibers spun from soluble recombinant silk produced in mammalian cells. *Science* 2002;295:472–76.
12. Bini E, Knight DP, Kaplan DL. Mapping domain structures in silks from insects and spiders related to protein assembly. *J Mol Biol* 2004;335:27–40.

13. Simmons A, Ray E, Jelinski LW. Solid-state C-13 NMR of *Nephila clavipes* dragline silk establishes structure and identity of crystalline regions. *Macromolecules* 1994;27:5235–7.

14. Simmons AH, Michal CA, Jelinski LW. Molecular orientation and two-component nature of the crystalline fraction of spider dragline silk. *Science* 1996;271:84–7.

15. Vollrath F. Spiders' webs. *Curr Biol* 2005;15:R364–5.

16. Mello CM, Arcidiacono S, Senecal K, Mcgrath K, Beckwitt R, Kaplan DL. Spider silk—Nature's high-performance fiber. *Abstr Pap Am Chem Soc* 1994;207:80-Btec.

17. Haider M, Megeed Z, Ghandehari H. Genetically engineered polymers: Status and prospects for controlled release. *J Control Rel* 2004;95:1–26.

18. Prince JT, McGrath KP, DiGirolamo CM, Kaplan DL. Construction, cloning, and expression of synthetic genes encoding spider dragline silk. *Biochemistry* 1995;34:10879–85.

19. Scheller J, Guhrs KH, Grosse F, Conrad U. Production of spider silk proteins in tobacco and potato. *Nat Biotechnol* 2001;19:573–7.

20. Sutherland TD, Young JH, Weisman S, Hayashi CY, Merritt DJ. Insect silk: One name, many materials. *Ann Rev Entomol* 2010;55:171–88.

21. Kundu SC, Dash BC, Dash R, Kaplan DL. Natural protective glue protein, sericin bioengineered by silkworms: Potential for biomedical and biotechnological applications. *Progr Polym Sci* 2008;33:998–1012.

22. Anonymous. The 50 best inventions of 2009: Spider web silk. Time 2009; http://www.time.com/time/specials/packages/article/0,28804,1934027 1934003 1933990,00.html.

23. Vendrely C, Scheibel T. Biotechnological production of spider-silk proteins enables new applications. *Macromol Biosci* 2007;7:401–9.

24. Hardy JG, Scheibel TR. Silk-inspired polymers and proteins. *Biochem Soc Trans* 2009;37:677–81.

25. Zhou CZ, Confalonieri F, Medina N, Zivanovic Y, Esnault C, Yang T et al. Fine organization of *B. mori* fibroin heavy chain gene. *Nucleic Acids Res* 2000;28:2413–9.

26. Inoue S, Tanaka K, Arisaka F, Kimura S, Ohtomo K, Mizuno S. Silk fibroin of *B. mori* is secreted, assembling a high molecular mass elementary unit consisting of H-chain, L-chain, and P25, with a 6:6:1 molar ratio. *J Biol Chem* 2000;275:40517–28.

27. Tanaka K, Inoue S, Mizuno S. Hydrophobic interaction of P25, containing Asn-linked oligosaccharide chains, with the H–L complex of silk fibroin produced by *B. mori*. *Insect Biochem Mol Biol* 1999;29:269–76.

28. Zhou CZ, Confalonieri F, Jacquet M, Perasso R, Li ZG, Janin J. Silk fibroin: Structural implications of a remarkable amino acid sequence. *Proteins* 2001;44:119–22.

29. Gage LP, Manning RF. Internal structure of the silk fibroin gene of *B. mori*. I. The fibroin gene consists of a homogeneous alternating array of repetitious crystalline and amorphous coding sequences. *J Biol Chem* 1980;255:9444–50.

30. Motta A, Fambri L, Migliaresi C. Regenerated silk fibroin films: Thermal and dynamic mechanical analysis. *Macromol Chem Phys* 2002;203:1658–65.

31. Huemmerich D, Slotta U, Scheibel T. Processing and modification of films made from recombinant spider silk proteins. *Appl Phys A* 2006;82:219–22.

32. Bajaj P. Finishing of textile materials. *J Appl Polym Sci* 2002;83:631–59.

33. Freddi G, Tsukada M, Kato H, Shiozaki H. Dyeability of silk fabrics modified with dibasic acid anhydrides. *J Appl Polym Sci* 1994;52:769–73.

34. Das S. The preparation and processing of tussah silk. *J Soc Dyers Colourists* 1992;108:481–6.

35. Arai T, Freddi G, Innocenti R, Kaplan DL, Tsukada M. Acylation of silk and wool with acid anhydrides and preparation of water-repellent fibers. *J Appl Polym Sci* 2001;82:2832–41.

36. Arai T, Freddi G, Innocenti R, Tsukada M. Preparation of water-repellent silks by a reaction with octadecenylsuccinic anhydride. *J Appl Polym Sci* 2003;89:324–32.

37. Hardy JG, Romer LM, Scheibel TR. Polymeric materials based on silk proteins. *Polymer* 2008;49:4309–27.

38. Hardy JG, Scheibel TR. Production and processing of spider silk proteins. *J Polym Sci Part A Polym Chem* 2009;47:3957–63.

39. Fu C, Shao Z, Vollrath F. Animal silks: Their structures, properties and artificial production. *Chem Commun* 2009;43:6515–29.

40. Kadler KE, Holmes DF, Trotter JA, Chapman JA. Collagen fibril formation. *Biochem J* 1996;316:1–11.

41. Dal Pra I, Freddi G, Minic J, Chiarini A, Armato U. De novo engineering of reticular connective tissue *in vivo* by silk fibroin nonwoven materials. *Biomaterials* 2005;26:1987–99.

42. Unger RE, Peters K, Wolf M, Motta A, Migliaresi C, Kirkpatrick CJ. Endothelialization of a non-woven silk fibroin net for use in tissue engineering: Growth and gene regulation of human endothelial cells. *Biomaterials* 2004;25:5137–46.

43. Unger RE, Wolf M, Peters K, Motta A, Migliaresi C, James Kirkpatrick C. Growth of human cells on a non-woven silk fibroin net: A potential for use in tissue engineering. *Biomaterials* 2004;25:1069–75.

44. Wang M, Jin HJ, Kaplan DL, Rutledge GC. Mechanical properties of electrospun silk fibers. *Macromolecules* 2004;37:6856–64.

45. Kim KH, Jeong L, Park HN, Shin SY, Park WH, Lee SC et al. Biological efficacy of silk fibroin nanofiber membranes for guided bone regeneration. *J Biotechnol* 2005;120:327–39.

46. Jin HJ, Fridrikh SV, Rutledge GC, Kaplan DL. Electrospinning *Bombyx mori* silk with poly(ethylene oxide). *Biomacromolecules* 2002;3:1233–9.

47. Min BM, Jeong L, Nam YS, Kim JM, Kim JY, Park WH. Formation of silk fibroin matrices with different texture and its cellular response to normal human keratinocytes. *Int J Biol Macromol* 2004;34:281–8.

48. Min BM, Lee G, Kim SH, Nam YS, Lee TS, Park WH. Electrospinning of silk fibroin nanofibers and its effect on the adhesion and spreading of normal human keratinocytes and fibroblasts *in vitro*. *Biomaterials* 2004;25:1289–97.

49. Ohgo K, Zhao CH, Kobayashi M, Asakura T. Preparation of nonwoven nanofibers of *Bombyx mori* silk, *Samia cynthiaricini* silk and recombinant hybrid silk with electrospinning method. *Polymer* 2003;44:841–6.

50. Ayutsede J, Gandhi M, Sukigara S, Micklus M, Chen HE, Ko F. Regeneration of *Bombyx mori* silk by electrospinning, Part 3: Characterization of electrospun nonwoven mat. *Polymer* 2005;46:1625–34.

51. Sugihara A, Sugiura K, Morita H, Ninagawa T, Tubouchi K, Tobe R et al. Promotive effects of a silk film on epidermal recovery from full-thickness skin wounds. *Proc Soc Exp Biol Med* 2000;225:58–64.

52. Jin HJ, Chen J, Karageorgiou V, Altman GH, Kaplan DL. Human bone marrow stromal cell responses on electrospun silk fibroin mats. *Biomaterials* 2004;25:1039–47.

53. Puelacher WC, Vacanti JP, Ferraro NF, Schloo B, Vacanti CA. Femoral shaft reconstruction using tissue-engineered growth of bone. *Int J Oral Maxillofac Surg* 1996;25:223–8.

54. Livingston T, Ducheyne P, Garino J. *In vivo* evaluation of a bioactive scaffold for bone tissue engineering. *J Biomed Mater Res* 2002;62:1–13.

55. Zhu L, Liu W, Cui L, Cao Y. Tissue-engineered bone repair of goat femur defects with osteogenically induced bone marrow stromal cells. *Tissue Eng* 2006;12:1369–77.

56. Minoura N, Aiba S, Higuchi M, Gotoh Y, Tsukada M, Imai Y. Attachment and growth of fibroblast cells on silk fibroin. *Biochem Biophys Res Commun* 1995;208:511–6.

57. Minoura N, Aiba S, Gotoh Y, Tsukada M, Imai Y. Attachment and growth of cultured fibroblast cells on silk protein matrices. *J Biomed Mater Res* 1995;29:1215–21.

58. Gotoh Y, Tsukada M, Minoura N. Effect of the chemical modification of the arginyl residue in *Bombyx mori* silk fibroin on the attachment and growth of fibroblast cells. *J Biomed Mater Res* 1998;39:351–7.

59. Inouye K, Kurokawa M, Nishikawa S, Tsukada M. Use of *Bombyx mori* silk fibroin as a substratum for cultivation of animal cells. *J Biochem Biophys Methods* 1998;37:159–64.

60. Pierschbacher MD, Ruoslahti E. Cell attachment activity of fibronectin can be duplicated by small synthetic fragments of the molecule. *Nature* 1984;309:30–3.

61. Pierschbacher MD, Ruoslahti E. Variants of the cell recognition site of fibronectin that retain attachment-promoting activity. *Proc Natl Acad Sci USA* 1984;81:5985–8.

62. Ruoslahti E, Pierschbacher MD. New perspectives in cell adhesion: RGD and integrins. *Science* 1987;238:491–7.

63. Petrini P, Parolari C, Tanzi MC. Silk fibroin-polyurethane scaffolds for tissue engineering. *J Mater Sci Mater Med* 2001;12:849–53.

64. Chiarini A, Petrini P, Bozzini S, Pra ID, Armato U. Silk fibroin/poly(carbonate)-urethane as a substrate for cell growth: *In vitro* interactions with human cells. *Biomaterials* 2003;24:789–99.

65. Dal Pra I, Petrini P, Charini A, Bozzini S, Fare S, Armato U. Silk fibroin-coated three-dimensional polyurethane scaffolds for tissue engineering: Interactions with normal human fibroblasts. *Tissue Eng* 2003;9:1113–21.

66. Cai K, Yao K, Lin S, Yang Z, Li X, Xie H et al. Poly(D,L-lactic acid) surfaces modified by silk fibroin: Effects on the culture of osteoblast *in vitro*. *Biomaterials* 2002;23:1153–60.

67. Cai K, Yao K, Cui Y, Yang Z, Li X, Xie H et al. Influence of different surface modification treatments on poly(D,L-lactic acid) with silk fibroin and their effects on the culture of osteoblast *in vitro*. *Biomaterials* 2002;23:1603–11.

68. Wang X, Kim HJ, Xu P, Matsumoto A, Kaplan DL. Biomaterial coatings by stepwise deposition of silk fibroin. *Langmuir* 2005;21:11335–41.

69. Wang X, Hu X, Daley A, Rabotyagova O, Cebe P, Kaplan DL. Nanolayer biomaterial coatings of silk fibroin for controlled release. *J Control Rel* 2007;121:190–9.

70. Wang X, Zhang X, Castellot J, Herman I, Iafrati M, Kaplan DL. Controlled release from multilayer silk biomaterial coatings to modulate vascular cell responses. *Biomaterials* 2008;29:894–903.

71. Pritchard EM, Szybala C, Boison D, Kaplan DL. Silk fibroin encapsulated powder reservoirs for sustained release of adenosine. *J Control Rel* 2010;144:159–67.

72. Sofia S, McCarthy MB, Gronowicz G, Kaplan DL. Functionalized silk-based biomaterials for bone formation. *J Biomed Mater Res* 2001;54:139–48.

73. Chen J, Altman GH, Karageorgiou V, Horan R, Collette A, Volloch V et al. Human bone marrow stromal cell and ligament fibroblast responses on RGD-modified silk fibers. *J Biomed Mater Res A* 2003;67:559–70.

74. Kardestuncer T, McCarthy MB, Karageorgiou V, Kaplan D, Gronowicz G. RGD-tethered silk substrate stimulates the differentiation of human tendon cells. *Clin Orthop Relat Res* 2006;448:234–9.

75. Ishizuya T, Yokose S, Hori M, Noda T, Suda T, Yoshiki S et al. Parathyroid hormone exerts disparate effects on osteoblast differentiation depending on exposure time in rat osteoblastic cells. *J Clin Invest* 1997;99:2961–70.

76. Uzawa T, Hori M, Ejiri S, Ozawa H. Comparison of the effects of intermittent and continuous administration of human parathyroid hormone (1–34) on rat bone. *Bone* 1995;16:477–84.

77. Karageorgiou V, Meinel L, Hofmann S, Malhotra A, Volloch V, Kaplan D. Bone morphogenetic protein-2 decorated silk fibroin films induce osteogenic differentiation of human bone marrow stromal cells. *J Biomed Mater Res A* 2004;71:528–37.

78. Langer R, Vacanti JP. Tissue engineering. *Science* 1993;260:920–6.

79. Vunjak-Novakovic G, Meinel L, Altman G, Kaplan D. Bioreactor cultivation of osteochondral grafts. *Orthodont Craniofac Res* 2005;8:209–18.

80. Nazarov R, Jin HJ, Kaplan DL. Porous 3-D scaffolds from regenerated silk fibroin. *Biomacromolecules* 2004;5:718–26.

81. Tamada Y. New process to form a silk fibroin porous 3-D structure. *Biomacromolecules* 2005;6:3100–6.

82. Kim UJ, Park J, Kim HJ, Wada M, Kaplan DL. Three dimensional aqueous-derived biomaterial scaffolds from silk fibroin. *Biomaterials* 2005;26:2775–85.

83. Meinel L, Karageorgiou V, Fajardo R, Snyder B, Shinde-Patil V, Zichner L et al. Bone tissue engineering using human mesenchymal stem cells: Effects of scaffold material and medium flow. *Ann Biomed Eng* 2004;32:112–22.

84. Meinel L, Fajardo R, Hofmann S, Langer R, Chen J, Snyder B et al. Silk implants for the healing of critical size bone defects. *Bone* 2005;37:688–98.

85. Kim HJ, Kim UJ, Vunjak-Novakovic G, Min BH, Kaplan DL. Influence of macroporous protein scaffolds on bone tissue engineering from bone marrow stem cells. *Biomaterials* 2005;26:4442–52.

86. Meinel L, Hofmann S, Karageorgiou V, Zichner L, Langer R, Kaplan D et al. Engineering cartilage-like tissue using human mesenchymal stem cells and silk protein scaffolds. *Biotechnol Bioeng* 2004;88:379–9.

87. Aoki H, Tomita N, Morita Y, Hattori K, Harada Y, Sonobe M et al. Culture of chondrocytes in fibroin—Hydrogel sponge. *Biomed Mater Eng* 2003;13:309–16.

88. Morita Y, Tomita N, Aoki H, Wakitani S, Tamada Y, Suguro T et al. Visco-elastic properties of cartilage tissue regenerated with fibroin sponge. *Biomed Mater Eng* 2002;12:291–8.

89. Morita Y, Tomita N, Aoki H, Sonobe M, Wakitani S, Tamada Y et al. Frictional properties of regenerated cartilage *in vitro*. *J Biomech* 2006;39:103–9.

90. Yeo JH, Lee KG, Kim HC, Oh HYL, Kim AJ, Kim SY. The effects of PVA/chitosan/fibroin (PCF)-blended spongy sheets on wound healing in rats. *Biol Pharm Bull* 2000;23:1220–3.

91. Vepari CP, Kaplan DL. Covalently immobilized enzyme gradients within three-dimensional porous scaffolds. *Biotechnol Bioeng* 2006;93:1130–7.

92. Wilz A, Pritchard EM, Li T, Lan JQ, Kaplan DL, Boison D. Silk polymer based denosine release: Therapeutic potential for epilepsy. *Biomaterials* 2008;29:609–16.

93. Li T, Ren G, Kaplan DL, Boison D. Human mesenchymal stem cell grafts engineered to release adenosine reduce chronic seizures in a mouse model of CA3-selective epileptogenesis. *Epilepsy Res.* 2009;84:238–41.

94. Uebersax L, Mattotti M, Papaloizos M, Merkle HP, Gander B, Meinel L. Silk fibroin matrices for the controlled release of nerve growth factor (NGF). *Biomaterials* 2007;28:4449–60.

95. Uebersax L, Merkle HP, Meinel L. Insulin-like growth factor I releasing silk fibroin scaffolds induce chondrogenic differentiation of human mesenchymal stem cells. *J Control Rel* 2008;127:12–21.

96. Chen X, Li WJ, Zhong W, Lu YH, Yu TY. pH sensitivity and ion sensitivity of hydrogels based on complex-forming chitosan/silk fibroin interpenetrating polymer network. *J Appl Polym Sci* 1997;65:2257–62.

97. Ayub ZH, Arai M, Hirabayashi K. Mechanism of the gelation of fibroin solution. *Biosci Biotechnol Biochem* 1993;57:1910–2.

98. Hanawa T, Watanabe A, Tsuchiya T, Ikoma R, Hidaka M, Sugihara M. New oral dosage form for elderly patients: Preparation and characterization of silk fibroin gel. *Chem Pharm Bull (Tokyo)* 1995;43:284–8.

99. Kim UJ, Park J, Li C, Jin HJ, Valluzzi R, Kaplan DL. Structure and properties of silk hydrogels. *Biomacromolecules* 2004;5:786–92.

100. Motta A, Migliaresi C, Faccioni F, Torricelli P, Fini M, Giardino R. Fibroin hydrogels for biomedical applications: Preparation, characterization and *in vitro* cell culture studies. *J Biomater Sci Polym Ed* 2004;15:851–64.

101. Yoo MK, Kweon HY, Lee KG, Lee HC, Cho CS. Preparation of semi-interpenetrating polymer networks composed of silk fibroin and poloxamer macromer. *Int J Biol Macromol* 2004;34:263–70.

102. Ayub ZH, Arai M, Hirabayashi K. Quantitative structural analysis and physical properties of silk fibroin hydrogels. *Polymer* 1994;35:2197–200.

103. Kang GD, Nahm JH, Park JS, Moon JY, Cho CS, Yeo JH. Effects of poloxamer on the gelation of silk fibroin. *Macromol Rapid Commun* 2000;21:788–91.

104. Gil ES, Spontak RJ, Hudson SM. Effect of beta-sheet crystals on the thermal and rheological behavior of protein-based hydrogels derived from gelatin and silk fibroin. *Macromol Biosci* 2005;5:702–9.

105. Gil ES, Frankowski DJ, Spontak RJ, Hudson SM. Swelling behavior and morphological evolution of mixed gelatin/silk fibroin hydrogels. *Biomacromolecules* 2005;6:3079–87.

106. Gobin AS, Froude VE, Mathur AB. Structural and mechanical characteristics of silk fibroin and chitosan blend scaffolds for tissue regeneration. *J Biomed Mater Res A* 2005;74:465–73.

107. Dinerman AA, Cappello J, Ghandehari H, Hoag SW. Swelling behavior of a genetically engineered silk-elastinlike protein polymer hydrogel. *Biomaterials* 2002;23:4203–10.

08. Dinerman AA, Cappello J, Ghandehari H, Hoag SW. Solute diffusion in genetically engineered silk-elastinlike protein polymer hydrogels. *J Control Rel* 2002;82:277–87.

09. Megeed Z, Haider M, Li D, O'Malley Jr. BW, Cappello J, Ghandehari H. *In vitro* and *in vivo* evaluation of recombinant silk-elastinlike hydrogels for cancer gene therapy. *J Control Rel* 2004;94:433–45.

10. Haider M, Leung V, Ferrari F, Crissman J, Powell J, Cappello J et al. Molecular engineering of silk-elastinlike polymers for matrixmediated gene delivery: Biosynthesis and characterization. *Mol Pharm* 2005;2:139–50.

11. Fini M, Motta A, Torricelli P, Giavaresi G, Nicoli Aldini N, Tschon M et al. The healing of confined critical size cancellous defects in the presence of silk fibroin hydrogel. *Biomaterials* 2005;26:3527–36.

112. Hino T, Tanimoto M, Shimabayashi S. Change in secondary structure of silk fibroin during preparation of its microspheres by spray-drying and exposure to humid atmosphere. *J Colloid Interface Sci* 2003;266:68–73.

113. Wang X, Wenk E, Matsumoto A, Meinel L, Li C, Kaplan DL. Silk microspheres for encapsulation and controlled release. *J Control Rel* 2007;117:360–70.

114. Wang X, Wenk E, Zhang X, Meinel L, Vunjak-Novakovic G, Kaplan DL. Growth factor gradients via microsphere delivery in biopolymer scaffolds for osteochondral tissue engineering. *J Control Rel* 2009;134:81–90.

115. Wang X, Yucel T, Lu Q, Hu X, Kaplan DL. Silk nanospheres and microspheres from silk/PVA blend films for drug delivery. *Biomaterials* 2010;31:1025–35.

116. Bessa PC, Balmayor ER, Azevedo HS, Nürnberger S, Casal M, van Griensven M, Reis RL, Redl H. Silk fibroin microparticles as carriers for delivery of human recombinant BMPs, physical characterization and drug release. *J Tissue Eng Regen Med* 2010;4:349–55.

117. Sandy C, Marks J, Odgren PR. Structure and development of the skeleton. In: John PB, Lawrence GR, Gideon AR, editors. *Principles of Bone Biology*. 2nd ed., vol. 1. New York, USA: Academic Press; 2002. pp. 3–15.

118. Meinel L, Karageorgiou V, Hofmann S, Fajardo R, Snyder B, Li C et al. Engineering bone-like tissue *in vitro* using human bone marrow stem cells and silk scaffolds. *J Biomed Mater Res A* 2004;71:25–34.

119. Kim HJ, Kim HS, Matsumoto A, Chin IJ, Jin HJ, Kaplan DL. Processing windows for forming silk fibroin biomaterials into a 3D porous matrix. *Aust J Chem* 2005;58:716–20.

120. Rajkhowa R, Gil ES, Kluge J, Numata K, Wang L, Wang X, Kaplan DL. Reinforcing silk scaffolds with silk particles. *Macromol Biosci* 2010;10:599–611.

121. Tuan RS, Boland G, Tuli R. Adult mesenchymal stem cells and cell based tissue engineering. *Arthritis Res Ther* 2003;5:32–45.

122. Cancedda R, Dozin B, Giannoni P, Quarto R. Tissue engineering and cell therapy of cartilage and bone. *Matrix Biol* 2003;22:81–91.

123. Athanasiou KA, Niederauer GG, Agrawal CM. Sterilization, toxicity, biocompatibility and clinical applications of polylactic acid/polyglycolic acid copolymers. *Biomaterials* 1996;17:93–102.

124. Fragonas E, Valente M, Pozzi-Mucelli M, Toffanin R, Rizzo R, Silvestri F et al. Articular cartilage repair in rabbits by using suspensions of allogenic chondrocytes in alginate. *Biomaterials* 2000;21:795–801.

125. Hunziker EB. Articular cartilage repair: Basic science and clinical progress. A review of the current status and prospects. *Osteoarthritis Cartilage* 2002;10:432–63.

126. Wang Y, Blasioli DJ, Kim HJ, Kim HS, Kaplan DL. Cartilage tissue engineering with silk scaffolds and human articular chondrocytes. *Biomaterials* 2006;27:4434–42.

127. Wang Y, Kim UJ, Blasioli DJ, Kim HJ, Kaplan DL. *In vitro* cartilage tissue engineering with 3D porous aqueous-derived silk scaffolds and mesenchymal stem cells. *Biomaterials* 2005;26:7082–94.

128. von der Mark K, Gauss V, von der Mark H, Muller P. Relationship between cell shape and type of collagen synthesised as chondrocytes lose their cartilage phenotype in culture. *Nature* 1977;267:531–2.

129. Lanza R, Langer R, Vacanti J. *Principles of Tissue Engineering*. San Diego, CA: Academic Press; 2000.

130. Horan RL, Antle K, Collette AL, Wang Y, Huang J, Moreau JE et al. *In vitro* degradation of silk fibroin. *Biomaterials* 2005;26:3385–93.

131. Oh JE, Nam YS, Lee KH, Park TG. Conjugation of drug to poly(D,L-lactic-*co*-glycolic acid) for controlled release from biodegradable microspheres. *J Control Rel* 1999;57:269–80.

132. Solheim E, Sudmann B, Bang G, Sudmann E. Biocompatibility and effect on osteogenesis of poly(ortho ester) compared to poly(D,L-lactic acid). *J Biomed Mater Res* 2000;49:257–63.

133. Basu S, Cunningham LP, Pins GD, Bush KA, Taboada R, Howell AR et al. Multiphoton excited fabrication of collagen matrixes cross-linked by a modified benzophenone dimer: Bioactivity and enzymatic degradation. *Biomacromolecules* 2005;6:1465–7.

134. Arai T, Freddi G, Innocenti R, Tsukada M. Biodegradation of *B. mori* silk fibroin fibers and films. *J Appl Polym Sci* 2004;91:2383–90.

135. Minoura N, Tsukada M, Nagura M. Physico-chemical properties of silk fibroin membrane as a biomaterial. *Biomaterials* 1990;11:430–4.

136. Santin M, Motta A, Freddi G, Cannas M. *In vitro* evaluation of the inflammatory potential of the silk fibroin. *J Biomed Mater Res* 1999;46:382–9.

137. Meinel L, Hofmann S, Karageorgiou V, Kirker-Head C, McCool J, Gronowicz G et al. The inflammatory responses to silk films *in vitro* and *in vivo*. *Biomaterials* 2005;26:147–55.

138. Perez-Rigueiro J, Viney C, Llorca J, Elices M. Mechanical properties of single-brin silkworm silk. *J Appl Polym Sci* 2000;75:1270–7.

139. Cunniff P, Fossey S, Auerbach M, Song J, Kaplan D, Adams WW et al. Mechanical and thermal properties of dragline silk from the spider *N. clavipes*. *Polym Adv Technol* 1994;5:401–10.

140. Pins G, Christiansen D, Patel R, Silver F. Self-assembly of collagen fibers: Influence of fibrillar alignment and Decorin on mechanical properties. *Biophys J* 1997;73:2164–72.

141. Engelberg I, Kohn J. Physicomechanical properties of degradable polymers used in medical applications: A comparative study. *Biomaterials* 1991;12:292–304.

35

Biofunctional Hydrogels

35.1 Introduction 35-1
35.2 Synthetic Hydrogels 35-2
    Common Polymeric Hydrogel Materials • *In Situ* Gelation
35.3 Hydrogel Biofunctionality 35-3
    Engineering Cellular Adhesion • Presentation of Growth Factors
    and Other Signaling Molecules • Cell-Mediated Hydrogel
    Degradation • Incorporating Specific Biofunctionality into
    Hydrogels
35.4 Importance of Physical Properties of Hydrogels 35-8
35.5 Design of Complex Biofunctional Hydrogels 35-9
35.6 Summary 35-10
References 35-11

Melissa K. McHale
Rice University

Jennifer L. West
Rice University

35.1 Introduction

Hydrogels are water-swollen matrices that are generally formed from hydrophilic polymers that have been chemically or physically crosslinked to prevent dissolution. Perhaps the most recognizable hydrogel material is the soft contact lens. Hydrogels are appropriate for this application because they (1) generally exhibit excellent biocompatibility, (2) allow for transport of molecules (in this case primarily gases) needed for tissue function and survival, and (3) possess appropriate mechanical properties for contact with soft tissue. Most synthetic hydrogel materials are relatively bioinert, resisting protein adsorption and cell adhesion. Modification of bioinert hydrogels with bioactive sequences can generate materials with biological functionalities such as biospecific cell adhesion, cell signaling, and enzymatic reactivity.

The prototypical biofunctional hydrogel is the extracellular matrix (ECM) that surrounds the cells of all tissues. This highly functional milieu is comprised of crosslinked proteins and polysaccharides that act to provide cell adhesion and mechanical support to tissues while also guiding various cellular processes. Rational design strategies for many cell- and tissue-interacting materials strive to emulate the functionality of the ECM. In addition, some components of the ECM, such as collagen and hyaluronic acid, have been extensively studied as hydrogel materials for various biomedical applications, including cardiovascular tissue engineering (Masters et al. 2004) and stem-cell differentiation (Chung and Burdick 2009). These naturally derived materials have advantages in that certain aspects of their bioactivity are intrinsic and have evolved over the millennia for optimal cell–material interactions. However, they suffer from difficulties associated with isolation and purification, and control over mechanical properties is limited. Because many recent reviews (Nicodemus and Bryant 2008; Tibbitt and Anseth 2009) and a chapter in this book have provided an extensive look at these natural biomaterials, this chapter will focus primarily on the incorporation of biofunctionality into synthetic hydrogel materials.

35.2 Synthetic Hydrogels

Synthetic polymers serve as foundation elements for hydrogel scaffolds, offering precise control over many of the chemical and physical characteristics of these matrices. This control, or "tuning," is a strong advantage over naturally derived materials, which can suffer from purity issues and batch-to-batch variation. From a bioactivity standpoint, the hydrophilic nature of synthetic hydrogels discourages attachment of proteins and therefore prevents cell interaction with these materials, which are generally not recognized through traditional biological adhesion mechanisms. As such, the polymeric materials act as bioinert platform into which specific bioactivity can be designed. It should be noted, however, that some biofunctionalities are actually based on the inherent inertness of these matrices. Consider, for example, the application of a thin hydrogel to the luminal surface of an injured blood vessel to act as a barrier to thrombosis (Hill-West et al. 1994), or a similar method to prevent the formation of postoperative tissue adhesions in peritoneal sites (Yaacobi et al. 1993). As the field of biomaterials grows, however, strategies to impart specific and complex bioactivities to hydrogel matrices are becoming more common and eagerly pursued.

35.2.1 Common Polymeric Hydrogel Materials

Hydrophilic polymers such as poly(hydroxyethyl methacrylate) (PHEMA), poly(vinyl alcohol) (PVA), poly(N-vinyl-2-pyrrolidone) (PNVP), and poly(ethylene glycol) (PEG) are readily formed into highly hydrated materials whose physical and chemical properties are amenable to interaction with cells and tissues. Table 35.1 shows some recent applications of these frequently used hydrogel materials. It is also common for hydrogels to appear in heterogeneous formulations made up of two or more hydrophilic monomers. This diversity allows for greater control over the properties of hydrogel matrices. For example, PHEMA materials can be made to take in greater amounts of water with the inclusion of methacrylic acid as a comonomer or designed to swell less by incorporating the more hydrophobic methyl methacrylate (Ratner et al. 2004).

PEG is an especially popular biomaterial choice for applications including cell substrates, tissue engineering scaffolds, and drug delivery devices. While the options for formulating PEG hydrogels are extensive, in one specific strategy photoreactive PEG diacrylate mixed with a chemical initiator (2,2-dimethoxy-2-phenyl-acetophenone) is polymerized upon exposure to long-wavelength UV light ($10 \, mW/cm^2$, 365 nm). This rapid polymerization process is amenable to cell encapsulation (Bryant et al. 2000). The low viscosity of PEG precursor solutions means that they are readily formed into various geometries (e.g., tubular structures representative of blood vessels) and that the hydrogels can be

TABLE 35.1 Recent Applications of Common Synthetic, Biofunctional Hydrogel Materials

Material	Abbreviation	Application	References
Poly(ethylene glycol)	PEG	Proangiogenic matrix	Leslie-Barbick et al. (2011); Moon et al. (2010)
		Drug/protein delivery	Zustiak and Leach (2011)
Poly(hydroxyethyl methacrylate)	PHEMA	Stem-cell differentiation	Guvendiren and Burdick (2010)
		Cardiac tissue scaffold[a]	Madden et al. (2010)
		Drug-eluting contact lens	Anderson et al. (2009); Xu et al. (2010)
Poly(N-isopropyl acrylamide)	PNIPAAm	Injectable glucose sensor	Shibata et al. (2010)
Poly(N-vinyl-2-pyrrolidone)	PNVP	Spinal tissue scaffold[a]	Boelen et al. (2007)
Poly(vinyl alcohol)	PVA	Cartilage scaffold	Bichara et al. (2011)
		Drug-eluting sensor coating	Vaddiraju et al. (2009)

[a] Used as a copolymer.

endered as coatings to biomedical devices or body tissues. In addition, this polymer, which is bioinert in its unmodified form, is easily functionalized to allow for an abundance of bioactivity. For this reason, PEG is discussed as an exemplary system in many of the sections that follow.

35.2.2 *In Situ* Gelation

The ability of some hydrogels to be formed *in situ* is a notable advantage since it provides an alternative to invasive biomaterial implantation strategies. In these methods, prepolymer solutions are delivered directly to the site of action (e.g., via syringe and needle) prior to initiation of the polymerization reaction. Many hydrogel synthesis protocols are amenable to *in situ* applications; however, those that require nonbiocompatible chemical activators or that are significantly exothermic are obviously ill-suited for such purposes. Synthetic elastin-mimetic hydrogels were employed in this manner to fill cartilage tissue defects in an osteochondral goat model (Nettles et al. 2008). Injection of the aqueous prepolymer solution proved a facile delivery method, while crosslinking *in situ* is believed to have enhanced tissue integration with the synthetic matrix, leading to increased cell and tissue infiltration. Though this example makes use of a chemically crosslinked polymer, even photoreactive polymerization strategies can thus be undertaken since fiber-optic devices now make delivering light to locations within the body almost trivial.

35.3 Hydrogel Biofunctionality

As mentioned, the hydrophilic nature of synthetic hydrogels results in materials that are resistant to protein adsorption and cell adhesion. This means that if the hydrogel function necessitates the capacity to interact with or respond to cells or tissues, additional modification must be made. For these purposes, the three most common types of engineered biofunctionality are (1) adhesion, (2) protein/growth factor presentation to control cell signaling, and (3) enzymatic degradation.

35.3.1 Engineering Cellular Adhesion

To engineer adhesion into the inert matrices formed by synthetic hydrogels, researchers aim to recapitulate the binding events that occur between cells and the ECM. The majority of cell–ECM interactions are mediated through a class of cell surface receptors called integrins. These transmembrane proteins bind to specific sites on matrix proteins allowing the cell to sense and interact with its environment. In addition, integrin binding can induce intracellular signaling that affects processes including migration, proliferation, and protein synthesis (Mann and West 2002). Though creating a heterogeneous synthetic scaffold that incorporates whole proteins such as collagen or fibronectin would accomplish the goal of creating a cell-adhesive matrix, this methodology is rarely preferred. For one reason, whole proteins would prove unstable in the cellular environment due to their susceptibility to enzymatic digestion. Furthermore, large proteins have many functional domains, only a few of which are needed for cell attachment. The inclusion of superfluous functionality could confound or even hinder the efficacy of synthetic matrices, which are often hailed as materials with "specifically designed" bioactivity.

Seminal work in this area over two decades ago used systematic studies of the amino acid sequences of various ECM proteins to determine that a minimal peptide unit is all that is required for recognition by cell surface receptors (Pierschbacher and Ruoslahti 1984). The most well studied of these peptides is the Arg–Gly–Asp (RGD) sequence which is ubiquitously distributed in proteins, including fibronectin, collagen, laminin, and vitronectin. RGD binds to many members of the integrin family, and as such serves as a ligand for a wide variety of cell surface receptors. The addition of this short peptide sequence has been shown to confer adhesive properties to otherwise inert synthetic hydrogels in a concentration-dependent manner (Figure 35.1).

An even greater level of specificity can be introduced by incorporating adhesion sequences derived from other ECM proteins (Table 35.2). These additional sequences permit the design of materials

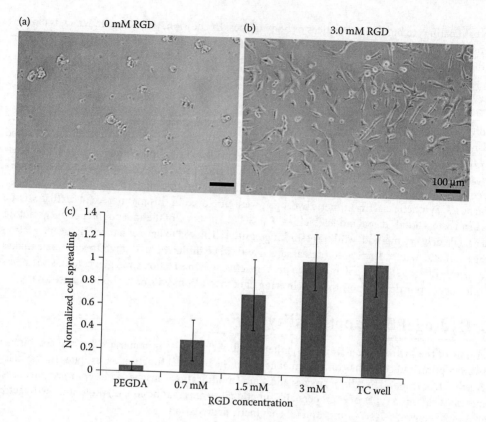

FIGURE 35.1 Engineering cell adhesion. Synthetic hydrogels generally allow very little cellular interaction (a), but can be functionalized with peptides, such as the fibronectin-derived RGD sequence to promote extensive cell adhesion and spreading (b). This effect can be tuned since the degree of cell interaction depends on the concentration of the RGD peptide within the hydrogel (c). PEG-based hydrogels containing 3 mM RGD permit cell spreading that is similar to that seen on tissue culture (TC) wells. (Courtesy of Christy Franco, Rice University.)

that encourage selective cell binding. As an example, consider engineering a vascular substitute that must allow the attachment and spreading of endothelial cells (ECs) and smooth muscle cells (SMCs) while remaining unreactive to circulating blood platelets, which can form dangerous thrombotic structures upon binding. While RGD would be a good peptide of choice for EC and SMC attachment, it will also react with platelets, and therefore is nonideal. There are, however, other short

TABLE 35.2 Cell Adhesion Peptides

Peptide	Source
DELPQLVTLPHPN LHGPEILDVPST[a]	Fibronectin
DGEA	Collagen
IKVAV	Laminin
KQAGDV	Fibrinogen
REDV	Fibronectin
RGD	Fibronectin, collagen, laminin, vitronectin
VAPG	Elastin
YIGSR	Laminin

[a] Commonly referred to as connecting segment 1 (CS1).

equences like YIGSR or IKVAV, which are derived from the basement membrane protein laminin, hat will selectively bind EC and elicit no reactivity from circulating blood cells (Jun and West 2005; 'ittkau et al. 2005). As another example, the VAPG peptide has been shown to bind SMCs but not Cs, fibroblasts, or platelets when covalently attached to a PEG hydrogel (Gobin and West 2003b). MC adhesion was followed by extensive cell spreading, with both factors responding to the ligand n a dose-dependent manner. When combined, these findings have important implications in the reation of a complex vascular graft material that provides selective cell incorporation but is also hrombo-resistant. Furthermore, these basic units of bioactivity are easily applied to applications or a variety of cell and tissue types.

35.3.2 Presentation of Growth Factors and Other Signaling Molecules

The biofunctionality of hydrogel matrices can be extended by including factors known to influence cellular function and tissue development. Growth factors and cytokines are examples of molecules that are generally available to cells in their native environment and have important roles in processes such as proliferation, migration, and protein synthesis. Factors recently incorporated into hydrogel materials include vascular endothelial growth factor (VEGF), platelet-derived growth factor (PDGF), and transforming growth factor-beta (TGF-β).

VEGF and PDGF are known participants in the process of vasculature development and are, therefore, of great interest to individuals attempting to create functional biomaterial constructs for applications in tissue engineering and regenerative medicine. In a recent study, a hydrogel containing VEGF and the adhesive ligand RGD was implanted in the mouse cornea to evaluate its proangiogenic properties (Moon et al. 2010). As shown in Figure 35.2, this bioactive material was infiltrated with functional vessels after only 7 days. A similar response was generated by hydrogels containing PDGF, which acts to promote angiogenesis by upregulating VEGF synthesis among other methods (Saik et al. 2011). These studies indicate that soluble and/or matrix-tethered growth factors have potential to direct the cellular organization and infiltration that lead to the formation of a de novo blood vessel network. Importantly,

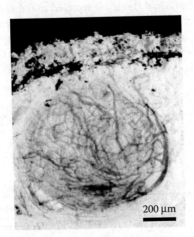

FIGURE 35.2 Proangiogenic growth factor induces functional vessel formation. VEGF incorporated into a degradable PEG-based hydrogel stimulated the formation of blood vessels within the hydrogel material upon implantation in the mouse cornea. These vessels are functional as demonstrated by their perfusion with Dextran-Texas red that was injected intravenously in the mouse. (Reprinted from *Biomaterials*, 31(14), Moon, J.J. et al. Biomimetic hydrogels with pro-angiogenic properties, 3840–7. Copyright 2010, with permission from Elsevier.)

these new vessels are not only pervasive throughout the synthetic hydrogel material, but are also connected to host vasculature as evidenced by perfusion with a small dextran molecule. Incorporation of this proangiogenic functionality into engineered matrices could help maintain the viability of cells within tissue grafts thereby expanding their utility.

TGF-β is another growth factor with important implications for tissue development as it is known to influence the synthesis of ECM proteins. Rat mesenchymal stem cells loaded in hydrogel composites containing TGF-β1 upregulated genes for collagen matrix synthesis over a 14-day period are illustrated in Park et al. (2009). In addition to indicating that the growth factor is a potent stimulator of protein synthesis, the cartilage-specific ECM components (i.e., collagen II and aggrecan) impacted in this study seem to support the hypothesis that TGF-β has also a role in directed stem-cell differentiation.

35.3.3 Cell-Mediated Hydrogel Degradation

Biomaterials intended for use as scaffolds for tissue engineering should be capable of dynamically responding to the events that occur during the process of histogenesis. This means that while serving the functions of physical support and bioactive guide, synthetic hydrogel matrices must also be amenable to cell migration and ECM accumulation. Perhaps the most effective way of achieving this dynamic reorganization is to permit the synthetic material to degrade as new tissue is formed. The timing of these events is critical. A material that dissolves too quickly may fail to provide appropriate protective or physical roles in the short term, whereas scaffolds that are slow to dissipate risk stifling protein synthesis and discouraging cell-mediated reorganization of new tissue. These caveats imply that to be appropriately termed "biofunctional," degradation processes should either be controlled by or in response to cell's natural regeneration cues.

Wound healing is an example of a natural process that involves the active replacement of tissue matrix. Some of the most important factors in this event are the cell-secreted proteolytic enzymes, which work to degrade ECM molecules in a specific manner thereby permitting cell migration and organization of the newly formed tissue. Plasmin is one of these enzymes, as is the family of matrix metalloproteinases (MMPs), that includes collagenases, elastases, and gelatinases (Stamenkovic 2003).

Analysis of the ECM proteins that serve as natural substrates of MMPs has aided the discovery of short peptide sequences that are susceptible to these cell-secreted enzymes (Table 35.3). Incorporation of protease-sensitive segments within synthetic hydrogels creates matrices that are able to adapt to tissue formation. For example, when the elastase-sensitive polyalanine sequence was covalently incorporated as block copolymer with PEG, SMCs in the resulting hydrogel exhibited increased ECM synthesis and up-regulated migratory behavior in comparison to nondegradable controls (Mann et al. 2001). Further, in important steps toward the vascularization of tissue-engineered hydrogels, collagenase-sensitive scaffolds have been shown to encourage tubulogenesis in cocultures of EC and pericyte precursors, while similar, nondegradable materials fail to induce this spontaneous assembly of capillary-like structures (Moon et al. 2010).

TABLE 35.3 Select Enzyme-Degradable Peptide Substrates

Peptide	Cleaved By
AAPV↓RGG	Elastase
L↓GPA	Collagenase
AAAA↓AAAAA	Elastase
GGPQG↓IWGQG	Collagenase
GPS↓G	Cathepsin K
NR↓V	Plasmin

↓ Indicates the site of cleavage.

5.3.4 Incorporating Specific Biofunctionality into Hydrogels

A simplistic approach to incorporating biomolecules in a hydrogel is to physically entrap them during the polymerization process. Of course because there is no covalent attachment to the matrix itself, these methods often mean that hydrogel biofunctionality is transient and thus available only until the active moiety diffuses away or is internalized by resident cells. For the same reason, however, physical entrapment may be adapted to create a controlled delivery device, wherein release is dependent on the size and diffusion profile of the encapsulated agent. While this method is feasible for whole proteins, soluble, untethered adhesion peptides have been shown to be detrimental to cell–material interactions as they can occupy cell surface receptors leaving them unavailable for binding to the substrate.

Longer-acting functionalization can be accomplished by covalently incorporating bioactive molecules using some of the same chemistries employed for polymerization. In the PEG system, the reactive succinimidyl carboxymethyl (SCM) ester group on heterobifunctional acrylate–PEG–SCM readily reacts with free amines on peptides and proteins to create a molecule that is then crosslinked into the hydrogel structure during photopolymerization (Figure 35.3). The number of amines present on the peptide or protein dictates the orientation of the conjugated entity within the polymer matrix. In other words, peptides with only one amine group will conjugate to a single PEG chain and will appear in the hydrogel as a pendant, whereas molecules with multiple amines will be decorated with up to an equal number of PEG chains and thus have several possible points of incorporation. Importantly, growth factors, such as those mentioned in Section 35.3.3, have been covalently immobilized in a PEG scaffold while maintaining appropriate function (Gobin and West 2003a). This is a significant advantage because it means that the biochemical factor does not have to be continuously delivered and instead has prolonged activity, due in part to decreased cellular internalization.

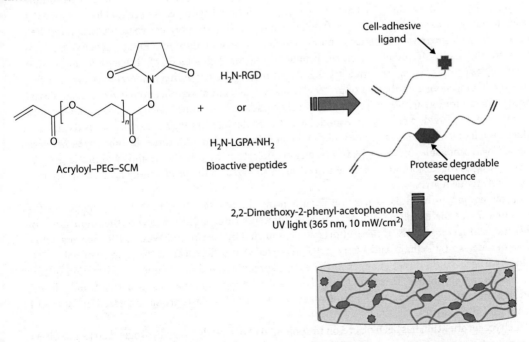

FIGURE 35.3 Biofunctional PEG-based hydrogel. The heterobifunctional acryloyl–PEG–SCM is reacted with bioactive peptides such as the cell-adhesive RGD or protease-degradable leu-gly-pro-ala (LGPA). When these PEG-conjugated molecules are photocrosslinked into a hydrogel using a chemical initiator and long-wave UV light, cells are able to interact with this synthetic matrix.

35.4 Importance of Physical Properties of Hydrogels

Physical properties are also important in the biofunctionality of a synthetic hydrogel used as a cell substrate or tissue replacement. Knowledge of the interplay between these material parameters and the biological response allows for precise tuning of matrices for tissue engineering applications, but also feeds the body of knowledge that helps determine the status and progression of certain disease states (e.g., cancer and atherosclerosis) for which altered tissue mechanics are hallmarks. The important physical properties include strength and elasticity, as well as the hydrogel network characteristics that dictate how molecules move within the polymer mesh. In tissue engineering applications, strength and elasticity must be carefully matched in order for the material to assume the initial structural role when substituted for excised or otherwise damaged tissues. Articular cartilage mimetics, for example, must be both strong and flexible enough to support the mechanical load and shearing forces within a knee joint. Another case in point is the application of a synthetic vascular graft. The compliance mismatch between currently available polymeric materials and the native blood vessel is a leading cause of implant failure. When the synthetic graft displays a stiffness that is significantly greater than that of the adjacent tissue, the stress that results from this disparity induces a protective response from vascular SMCs—forcing them to proliferate and secrete additional matrix. The overproduction of cells and ECM generates a tissue outgrowth, termed intimal hyperplasia, which occludes the lumen of the graft and leads to failure. As hydrogels are adapted for use in vascular applications, particular attention is given to the precise tuning of mechanical properties in order to alleviate the risk for this complication (Hahn et al. 2007; Padavan et al. 2011).

Properties of the hydrogel network, including water content and number average molecular weight between crosslinks (M_c), ultimately determine the network mesh size (ζ) and thereby influence the biofunctional properties of the material. Previous studies have shown the structure of this network to be dependent upon the crosslink density, which is influenced greatly by the molecular weight and volume fraction of the reactive synthetic macromer. In using a PEG-based hydrogel as a scaffold for cartilage tissue engineering, Bryant and Anseth (2002) noted that decreasing the polymer volume fraction resulted in materials with lower water contents and higher compressive moduli, providing a range of physical substrates that had differing effects on the production of cartilaginous ECM. The authors found that chondrocytes produced a maximum level of collagen II in hydrogels with a moderate network density, while the homogenous distribution of proteoglycans was favored at significantly lower levels of crosslinking. To accommodate this difference, hydrogel degradation was tuned such that the initial network was sufficient to provide a compressive modulus in the physiological range of cartilaginous tissues and induce high levels of collagen synthesis, but as the matrix degraded with time, the more open network structure was amenable to proteoglycan dispersion. This study highlights the ability to produce functional hydrogels that accommodate not only cell survival, but also the production and accumulation of appropriate tissue matrix.

A growing body of work is focused on documenting the role of a single substrate property—stiffness—in a multitude of cell behaviors including differentiation. A 2010 review of the importance of synthetic hydrogel materials in these efforts was completed by Nemir and West (2010). Seminal work over a decade ago by Pelham and Wang (1997) reported that differences in the rigidity of polyacrylamide hydrogels could direct changes in the shape, spreading, and focal adhesion formation of epithelial cells and fibroblasts. This initial study has inspired dozens of others using a variety of hydrogel materials and cell types. Some of the results from work with fibroblasts are summarized in Table 35.4 (Nemir and West 2010).

Much recent attention has been placed on the potential of discretely tuned hydrogel matrices to direct stem-cell differentiation down specific lineages. Engler et al. (2006) cultured mesenchymal stem cells on polyacrylamide gels with stiffnesses ranging from 0.1 to 1 kPa. On the softest materials, cells exhibited a neuronal-like morphology, while systematically increasing the hydrogel rigidity led to the appearance of myoblasts and then eventually osteoblasts. This directed differentiation was accomplished in basic

TABLE 35.4 Fibroblast Response to Increasing Substrate Rigidity

Factor	Response
Spread area	↑
Migration speed	↓
Stress fiber formation	↑
Focal adhesion formation	↑
Proliferation	↑
Apoptosis	↓
Adhesion/traction forces	↑
Cell modulus	↑

Source: Adapted from Nemir, S. and J. L. West. 2010. *Ann Biomed Eng* 38(1): 2–20.

↑ Indicates increase and ↓ indicates decrease.

culture media and was measured not only by the morphological appearance of the cells, but also with genetic analysis. The findings have become critical considerations for the design of biofunctional hydrogels for use in the culture of stem cells.

35.5 Design of Complex Biofunctional Hydrogels

Advances in the biomaterials field are providing the means of generating complex and highly specialized 3-D scaffolds for cell culture and tissue regeneration. Many such strategies make use of the tunable chemistries of synthetic hydrogel materials. Especially popular are the photo-reactive polymers, which can be formed into scaffolds using a range of light sources (e.g., mercury lamps and lasers). Photolithographic techniques have been widely employed to pattern hydrogel structures that are used to guide cell–material interactions in both 2-D and 3-D. In addition, studies of biofunctionalized surfaces contribute a wealth of information to the field of cell biology. These artificial matrices present controlled stimuli (e.g., topography, biochemical cues, and mechanical properties) individually or in combination to elucidate cellular behaviors relating to differentiation, proliferation, mechanotransduction, and protein synthesis, among others. In a recent application of photopolymerized PEG hydrogels, investigators were able to control the surface presentation of biomolecules on the nanometer scale and to vary substrate elasticity in the physiological range from 0.6 kPa to 6 MPa (Aydin et al. 2010). This system was used to study the effects of matrix elasticity on fibroblast adhesion and morphology, but is applicable to a wide variety of cell types.

Photolithography is also used to generate 3-D biofunctional materials. For example, Bryant et al. (2007) used a polymer template and photomask to simultaneously create a controlled, microporous architecture and patterned macrostructure within a degradable PHEMA hydrogel. PMMA microspheres served as a space-filling mold around which a PHEMA solution was polymerized, generating a range of pore sizes (62–147 μm) that were dependent on the diameter of the original PMMA spheres. At the same time, a photomask placed in the light path restricted polymerization to only certain areas and effectively patterned channels (360–730 μm) in the material. In this manner, the hydrogel's architecture can be tailored to generate scaffolds amenable to the growth of cells and tissues with varying physiospatial requirements.

Toward the goal of "organ printing," investigators have engineered biofunctional, cell-laden, hydrogel structures with complex architectures. The use of cell-friendly reaction schemes, such as the free-radical initiated and UV-catalyzed photopolymerization of PEG, allows incorporation of cells directly into a hydrogel matrix. This encapsulation process eliminates the need for subsequent seeding protocols and can provide a more homogeneous distribution of cells within the scaffold. As illustration, the Bhatia

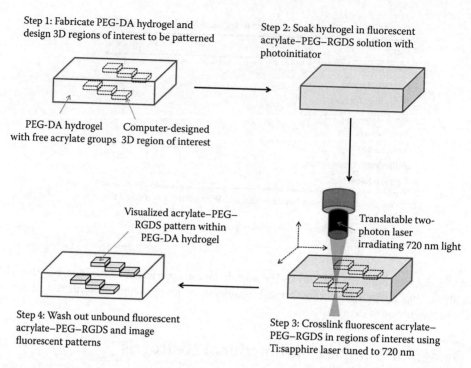

Step 1: Fabricate PEG-DA hydrogel and design 3D regions of interest to be patterned

PEG-DA hydrogel with free acrylate groups   Computer-designed 3D region of interest

Step 2: Soak hydrogel in fluorescent acrylate–PEG–RGDS solution with photoinitiator

Translatable two-photon laser irradiating 720 nm light

Visualized acrylate–PEG–RGDS pattern within PEG-DA hydrogel

Step 4: Wash out unbound fluorescent acrylate–PEG–RGDS and image fluorescent patterns

Step 3: Crosslink fluorescent acrylate–PEG–RGDS in regions of interest using Ti:sapphire laser tuned to 720 nm

FIGURE 35.4 Laser scanning lithography creates complex biofunctional hydrogels. A PEG diacrylate (PEG-DA) hydrogel was fabricated and 3D regions of interest were designed using confocal microscope software. Fluorescent monoacrylate PEG-RGDS solution with photoinitiator was soaked into the PEG-DA hydrogel, and a Ti:sapphire laser tuned to 720 nm was used to crosslink the fluorescent PEG-RGDS moieties in desired free form 3D patterns. (Adapted from Hoffmann, J. C. and J. L. West. 2010. *Soft Matter* 6(20): 5056–63.)

group used a layer-by-layer method to pattern a liver-mimetic structure from a prepolymer solution of PEG diacrylate, RGD adhesion peptides, and hepatocytes (Tsang et al. 2007). The 3-D, photopatterned constructs presented a cell microenvironment designed to recapitulate the hepatocyte ECM, and as such, supported better viability and function than unpatterned hydrogel disks.

Laser-based photomodification of hydrogels is a relatively new technique for generating complex, 3-D microenvironments. In early application of this approach, growth factors and peptides were incorporated into PEG dimethacrylate hydrogels formed using laser-based layer-by-layer stereolithography (Mapili et al. 2005). More recent advancement of a technique called laser scanning lithography (LSL) improves on previous work by employing confocal microscopes and multiphoton lasers to decrease synthesis times and to increase patterning resolution (Miller and West 2008). As shown in Figure 35.4, computer-generated, 3-D regions of interest take the place of a traditional photomask and allow patterning within hydrogels with high resolution and the capacity to generate physiologically relevant features ranging in size from 1 μm to 1 mm. In addition, iterations of the LSL process permit incorporation of multiple biomolecules to aid in the construction of complex cellular microenvironments (Hoffmann and West 2010). These precisely fabricated biofunctional matrices provide opportunities for controlled biological interaction.

35.6 Summary

Biofunctional hydrogels are popular materials for use in applications of tissue engineering, drug delivery, and *in vitro* cell culture. Synthetic polymers such as PEG provide versatile building blocks upon which specific bioactivity (e.g., cell adhesion) can be designed. With tunable mechanical properties, incorporation of signaling molecules, and cell-driven matrix remodeling, these materials serve a variety f purposes and have been shown to modulate cell behaviors including proliferation, migration, pro- ein synthesis, and even differentiation. As technologies for synthesizing and modifying these materials dvance, synthetic hydrogels will prove even more useful for regenerative medicine and drug delivery urposes.

References

Anderson, E. M., M. L. Noble, S. Garty et al. 2009. Sustained release of antibiotic from poly(2-hydroxyethyl methacrylate) to prevent blinding infections after cataract surgery. *Biomaterials* 30(29): 5675–81.

Aydin, D., I. Louban, N. Perschmann et al. 2010. Polymeric substrates with tunable elasticity and nano-scopically controlled biomolecule presentation. *Langmuir* 26(19): 15472–80.

Bichara, D. A., X. Zhao, H. Bodugoz-Senturk et al. 2011. Porous poly(vinyl alcohol)-hydrogel matrix-engineered bio-synthetic cartilage. *Tissue Eng Part A* 17(3–4): 301–9.

Boelen, E. J., L. H. Koole, L. W. van Rhijn, and C. S. van Hooy-Corstjens. 2007. Towards a functional radi-opaque hydrogel for nucleus pulposus replacement. *J Biomed Mater Res B Appl Biomater* 83(2): 440–50.

Bryant, S. J. and K. S. Anseth. 2002. Hydrogel properties influence ECM production by chondrocytes photoencapsulated in poly(ethylene glycol) hydrogels. *J Biomed Mater Res* 59(1): 63–72.

Bryant, S. J., J. L. Cuy, K. D. Hauch, and B. D. Ratner. 2007. Photo-patterning of porous hydrogels for tissue engineering. *Biomaterials* 28(19): 2978–86.

Bryant, S. J., C. R. Nuttelman, and K. S. Anseth. 2000. Cytocompatibility of UV and visible light photo-initiating systems on cultured NIH/3T3 fibroblasts *in vitro*. *J Biomater Sci Polym Ed* 11(5): 439–57.

Chung, C. and J. A. Burdick. 2009. Influence of three-dimensional hyaluronic acid microenvironments on mesenchymal stem cell chondrogenesis. *Tissue Eng Part A* 15(2): 243–54.

Engler, A. J., S. Sen, H. L. Sweeney, and D. E. Discher. 2006. Matrix elasticity directs stem cell lineage speci-fication. *Cell* 126(4): 677–89.

Fittkau, M. H., P. Zilla, D. Bezuidenhout et al. 2005. The selective modulation of endothelial cell mobility on RGD peptide containing surfaces by YIGSR peptides. *Biomaterials* 26(2): 167–74.

Gobin, A. S. and J. L. West. 2003a. Effects of epidermal growth factor on fibroblast migration through bio-mimetic hydrogels. *Biotechnol Prog* 19(6): 1781–5.

Gobin, A. S. and J. L. West. 2003b. Val-ala-pro-gly, an elastin-derived non-integrin ligand: smooth muscle cell adhesion and specificity. *J Biomed Mater Res A* 67(1): 255–9.

Guvendiren, M. and J. A. Burdick. 2010. The control of stem cell morphology and differentiation by hydro-gel surface wrinkles. *Biomaterials* 31(25): 6511–8.

Hahn, M. S., M. K. McHale, E. Wang, R. H. Schmedlen, and J. L. West. 2007. Physiologic pulsatile flow bio-reactor conditioning of poly(ethylene glycol)-based tissue engineered vascular grafts. *Ann Biomed Eng* 35(2): 190–200.

Hill-West, J. L., S. M. Chowdhury, M. J. Slepian, and J. A. Hubbell. 1994. Inhibition of thrombosis and intimal thickening by *in situ* photopolymerization of thin hydrogel barriers. *Proc Natl Acad Sci USA* 91(13): 5967–71.

Hoffmann, J. C. and J. L. West. 2010. Three-dimensional photolithographic patterning of multiple bioactive ligands in poly(ethylene glycol) hydrogels. *Soft Matter* 6(20): 5056–63.

Jun, H. W. and J. L. West. 2005. Modification of polyurethaneurea with PEG and YIGSR peptide to enhance endothelialization without platelet adhesion. *J Biomed Mater Res B Appl Biomater* 72(1): 131–9.

Leslie-Barbick, J. E., C. Shen, C. S. Chen, and J. West. 2011. Micron-scale spatially patterned, covalently immobilized VEGF on hydrogels accelerates endothelial tubulogenesis and increases cellular angio-genic responses. *Tissue Eng Part A* 17(1–2): 221–9.

Madden, L. R., D. J. Mortisen, E. M. Sussman et al. 2010. Proangiogenic scaffolds as functional templates for cardiac tissue engineering. *Proc Natl Acad Sci USA* 107(34): 15211–6.

Mann, B. K., A. S. Gobin, A. T. Tsai, R. H. Schmedlen, and J. L. West. 2001. Smooth muscle cell growth in photopolymerized hydrogels with cell adhesive and proteolytically degradable domains: Synthetic ECM analogs for tissue engineering. *Biomaterials* 22(22): 3045–51.

Mann, B. K. and J. L. West. 2002. Cell adhesion peptides alter smooth muscle cell adhesion, proliferation, migration, and matrix protein synthesis on modified surfaces and in polymer scaffolds. *J Biomed Mater Res* 60(1): 86–93.

Mapili, G., Y. Lu, S. C. Chen, and K. Roy. 2005. Laser-layered microfabrication of spatially patterned functionalized tissue-engineering scaffolds. *J Biomed Mater Res Part B Appl Biomater* 75B(2): 414–24.

Masters, K. S., D. N. Shah, G. Walker, L. A. Leinwand, and K. S. Anseth. 2004. Designing scaffolds for valvular interstitial cells: Cell adhesion and function on naturally derived materials. *J Biomed Mater Res A* 71(1): 172–80.

Miller, J. S. and J. L. West. 2008. Biomimetic hydrogels to support and guide tissue formation. In *Micro and Nanoengineering of the Cell Microenvironment: Technologies and Applications*. A. Khademhosseini, J. Borenstein and M. Toner (eds.). Boston, MA: Artech House Publishers.

Moon, J. J., J. E. Saik, R. A. Poche et al. 2010. Biomimetic hydrogels with pro-angiogenic properties. *Biomaterials* 31(14): 3840–7.

Nemir, S. and J. L. West. 2010. Synthetic materials in the study of cell response to substrate rigidity. *Ann Biomed Eng* 38(1): 2–20.

Nettles, D. L., K. Kitaoka, N. A. Hanson et al. 2008. *In situ* crosslinking elastin-like polypeptide gels for application to articular cartilage repair in a goat osteochondral defect model. *Tissue Eng Part A* 14(7): 1133–40.

Nicodemus, G. D. and S. J. Bryant. 2008. Cell encapsulation in biodegradable hydrogels for tissue engineering applications. *Tissue Eng Part B Rev* 14(2): 149–65.

Padavan, D. T., A. M. Hamilton, L. E. Millon, D. R. Boughner, and W. Wan. 2011. Synthesis, characterization and *in vitro* cell compatibility study of a poly(amic acid) graft/cross-linked poly(vinyl alcohol) hydrogel. *Acta Biomater* 7(1): 258–67.

Park, H., J. S. Temenoff, Y. Tabata et al. 2009. Effect of dual growth factor delivery on chondrogenic differentiation of rabbit marrow mesenchymal stem cells encapsulated in injectable hydrogel composites. *J Biomed Mater Res A* 88(4): 889–97.

Pelham, R. J., Jr. and Y. Wang. 1997. Cell locomotion and focal adhesions are regulated by substrate flexibility. *Proc Natl Acad Sci USA* 94(25): 13661–5.

Peppas, N. A., J. Z. Hilt, A. Khademhosseini, and R. Langer. 2006. Hydrogels in biology and medicine: From molecular principles to bionanotechnology. *Adv Mater* 18(11): 1345–60.

Pierschbacher, M. D. and E. Ruoslahti. 1984. Cell attachment activity of fibronectin can be duplicated by small synthetic fragments of the molecule. *Nature* 309(5963): 30–33.

Ratner, B. D., A. S. Hoffman, F. J. Schoen, and J. E. Lemons. 2004. *Biomaterials science: An introduction to materials in medicine*. London: Elsevier Academic Press.

Saik, J. E., D. J. Gould, E. M. Watkins, M. E. Dickinson, and J. L. West. 2011. Covalently immobilized platelet-derived growth factor-BB promotes angiogenesis in biomimetic poly(ethylene glycol) hydrogels. *Acta Biomater* 7(1): 133–43.

Shibata, H., Y. J. Heo, T. Okitsu et al. 2010. Injectable hydrogel microbeads for fluorescence-based *in vivo* continuous glucose monitoring. *Proc Natl Acad Sci USA* 107(42): 17894–8.

Stamenkovic, I. 2003. Extracellular matrix remodelling: The role of matrix metalloproteinases. *J Pathol* 200(4): 448–64.

Tibbitt, M. W. and K. S. Anseth. 2009. Hydrogels as extracellular matrix mimics for 3D cell culture. *Biotechnol Bioeng* 103(4): 655–63.

Tsang, V. L., A. A. Chen, L. M. Cho et al. 2007. Fabrication of 3D hepatic tissues by additive photopatterning of cellular hydrogels. *FASEB J* 21(3): 790–801.

Vaddiraju, S., H. Singh, D. J. Burgess, F. C. Jain and F. Papadimitrakopoulos. 2009. Enhanced glucose sensor linearity using poly(vinyl alcohol) hydrogels. *J Diabetes Sci Technol* 3(4): 863–74.

Xu, J., X. Li, and F. Sun. 2010. Cyclodextrin-containing hydrogels for contact lenses as a platform for drug incorporation and release. *Acta Biomater* 6(2): 486–93.

Yaacobi, Y., A. A. Israel, and E. P. Goldberg. 1993. Prevention of postoperative abdominal adhesions by tissue precoating with polymer solutions. *J Surg Res* 55(4): 422–6.

Zustiak, S. P. and J. B. Leach. 2011. Characterization of protein release from hydrolytically degradable poly(ethylene glycol) hydrogels. *Biotechnol Bioeng* 108(1): 197–206.

36

Soft Tissue Replacements

36.1 Blood-Interfacing Implants...36-1
   Introduction • Heart Valve Prostheses • TAHs or Ventricular
   Assist Devices • Vascular Prostheses • Conclusions
Defining Terms 36-17
References..36-19
36.2 Nonblood-Interfacing Implants for Soft Tissues....................36-23
   Sutures and Allied Augmentation Devices • Percutaneous
   and Skin Implants • Maxillofacial Implants • Ear and
   Eye Implants • Space-Filling Implants • Fluid Transfer
   Implants • Technologies of Emerging Interest
References..36-33
Further Information..36-35

K. B. Chandran
University of Iowa

K. J. L. Burg
Clemson University

S. W. Shalaby[*]
Poly-Med, Inc.

36.1 Blood-Interfacing Implants

36.1.1 Introduction

Blood comes in contact with foreign materials for a short term in extracorporeal devices such as *dialysers*, *blood oxygenators*, ventricular assist devices, and *catheters*. Long-term vascular implants include heart valve prostheses, *vascular grafts*, and *cardiac pacemakers* among others. In this section, we will be concerned with the development of biomaterials for long-term implants, specifically for heart valve prostheses, total artificial heart (TAH), and vascular grafts. The primary requirements for biomaterials for long-term implants are biocompatibility, nontoxicity, and durability. Furthermore, the material should be nonirritating to the tissue, be resistant to *platelet* and *thrombus* deposition, be nondegradable in the physiological environment, and neither absorb blood constituents nor release foreign substances into the bloodstream (Shim and Lenker, 1988). In addition, design considerations include that the implant should mimic the function of the organ that it replaces without interfering with the surrounding anatomical structures and must be of suitable size and weight. The biomaterials chosen must be easily available, inexpensive, easily machinable, sterilizable, and have a long storage life. The selection of material will also be dictated by the strength requirement for the implant being made. As an example, an artificial heart valve prosthesis is required to open and close on an average once every second. The biomaterial chosen must be such that the valve is durable and will not fail under *fatigue stress* after implantation in a patient. As sophisticated measurement techniques and detailed computational analyses become available with the advent of supercomputers, knowledge on the complex dynamics of the functioning of the implants is increasing. Improvements in design based on such knowledge and improvements in selection and manufacture of biomaterials will minimize problems associated with

---

[*] This chapter is dedicated to the memory of Dr. Shalaby W. Shalaby.

blood-interfacing implants and significantly improve the quality of life for patients with implants. This chapter discusses the development of biomaterials for blood-interfacing implants as well as problems associated with and future directions in the development of such implants.

36.1.2 Heart Valve Prostheses

Attempts at replacing diseased natural human valves with prostheses began about four decades ago. The details of the development of heart valve prostheses, design considerations, *in vitro* functional testing, and durability testing of valve prototypes can be found in several monographs (Shim and Lenker, 1988; Chandran, 1992). The heart valve prostheses can be broadly classified into *mechanical prostheses* (made of nonbiological material) and *bioprostheses* (made of biological tissue). Currently available mechanical and tissue heart valve prostheses in the United States are listed in Table 36.1.

36.1.2.1 Mechanical Heart Valves

Lefrak and Starr (1970) describe the early history of mechanical valve development. The initial designs of mechanical valves were of centrally occluding caged ball or caged disk type. The Starr–Edwards caged ball prostheses, commercially available at present, were successfully implanted in the mitral position in 1961. The caged ball prosthesis is made of a polished Co–Cr alloy (Stellite 21®) cage and a silicone rubber ball (Silastic®), which contains 2 wt% barium sulfate for *radiopacity* (Figure 36.1). The valve *sewing rings* use a silicone rubber insert under a knitted composite polytetrafluoroethylene (PTFE-*Teflon*®) and *polypropylene* cloth. Even though these valves have proven to be durable, the centrally occluding design of the valve results in a larger pressure drop in flow across the valve and higher *turbulent stresses* distal to the valve compared to other designs of mechanical valve prostheses (Yoganathan et al., 1979a,b, 1986; Chandran et al., 1983). The relatively large profile design of caged ball or disk construction also increases the possibility of interference with anatomical structures after implantation. The *tilting disk valves*, with improved hemodynamic characteristics, were introduced in the late 1960s. The initial design consisted of a polyacetal (*Delrin*®) disk with a Teflon sewing ring. Delrin acetal resins are thermoplastic polymers manufactured by the polymerization of *formaldehyde* (Shim and Lenker, 1988). Even though Delrin exhibited excellent wear resistance and mechanical strength with satisfactory performance after more than 20

TABLE 36.1 Heart Valve Prostheses Developed and Currently Available in the United States

Type	Name	Manufacturer
Caged ball	Starr–Edwards	Baxter Health Care, Irvine, CA
Tilting disk	Medtronic-Hall	Medtronic Blood Systems, Minneapolis, MN
	Lillehei–Kaster	Medical, Inc., Inner Grove Heights, MN
	Omni-Science	
Bileaflet	St. Jude Medical	St. Jude Medical, Inc., St. Paul, MN
	Carbomedics	Carbomedics, Austin, TX
	ATS Valve	ATS Medical, St. Paul, MN
	On-X Valve	Medical Carbon Research Inst., Austin, TX
Porcine bioprostheses	Carpentier–Edwards (CE) porcine CE SAV	Edwards Lifesciences, Irvine, CA
	Hancock II Hancock-modified orifice	Medtronic, Santa Ana, CA
	Freestyle	St. Jude Medical, Inc., St. Paul, MN
	Biocor	CarboMedics, Inc., Austin, TX
	Mitroflow	
Pericardial bioprostheses	Carpentier–Edwards CE PERIMOUNT	Edwards Lifesciences, Irvine, CA

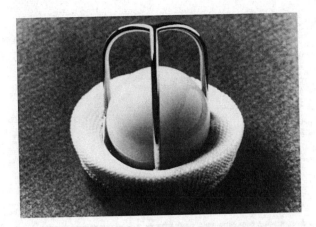

FIGURE 36.1 A caged-ball heart valve prosthesis. (Courtesy of Baxter Health Care, Irvine, CA.)

years of implantation, it was also found to swell when exposed to humid environments such as *autoclaving* and blood contact. To avoid design and manufacturing difficulties due to the swelling phenomenon, the Delrin disk was soon replaced by the *pyrolytic carbon* disk and has become the preferred material for mechanical valve prosthesis occluders to date. Pyrolytic carbons are formed in a fluidized bed by pyrolysis of a gaseous hydrocarbon in the range 1000–2400°C. For biomedical applications, carbon is deposited onto a preformed polycrystalline graphite substrate at temperatures below 1500°C (low-temperature isotropic pyrolytic carbon, *LTI* Pyrolite®). Increase in strength and wear resistance is obtained by codepositing silicone (up to 10 wt%) with carbon in applications for heart valve prostheses. The pyrolytic carbon disks exhibit excellent blood compatibility, as well as wear and fatigue resistance. The guiding *struts* of tilting disk valves are made of *titanium* or Co–Cr alloys (*Haynes 25*® and Stellite 21). The Co–Cr-based alloys, along with pure titanium and its alloy (Ti6A14V), exhibit excellent mechanical properties as well as resistance to corrosion and thrombus deposition. A typical commercially available tilting disk valve with a pyrolytic carbon disk is shown in Figure 36.2a. A tilting disk valve with the leaflet made of *ultra-high-molecular-weight polyethylene* (Chitra valve—Figure 36.2b) is currently marketed in India. The advantages of *leaflets* with relatively more flexibility compared to pyrolytic carbon leaflets are discussed in Chandran et al. (1994a). Another new concept in a tilting disk valve design introduced by Reul et al. (1995) has an S-shaped leaflet with leading and trailing edges being parallel to the direction of blood flow. The housing for the valve is nozzle-shaped to minimize flow separation at the inlet and energy loss in flow across the valve. Results from *in vitro* evaluation and animal implantation have been encouraging.

In the late 1970s, a bileaflet design was introduced for mechanical valve prostheses and several different bileaflet models are being introduced into the market today. The leaflets as well as the housing of the bileaflet valves are made of pyrolytic carbon, and the bileaflet valves show improved hemodynamic characteristics, especially in smaller sizes compared to tilting disk valves. A typical bileaflet valve is shown in Figure 36.3. Design features to improve the hydrodynamic characteristics of the mechanical valves include the opening angle of the leaflets (Baldwin et al., 1997) as well as having an open-pivot design in which the pivot area protrudes into the orifice and is exposed to the washing action of flowing blood (Drogue and Villafana, 1997). Other design modifications to improve the mechanical valve function include the use of double polyester (Dacron®) velour material for the suture ring to encourage rapid and controlled tissue ingrowth, and mounting the cuff on a rotation ring that surrounds the orifice ring to protect the cuff mounting mechanism from deeply placed annulus sutures. A PTFE (Teflon) insert in the cuff provides pliability without excessive drag on the sutures. Tungsten (20 wt%) is incorporated into the leaflet substrate in order to visualize the leaflet motion *in vivo*.

Another attempt to design a mechanical valve that mimics the geometry and function of the trileaflet aortic valve is that of Lapeyre et al. (1994) (Figure 36.4a,b). The geometry of the valve affords true central

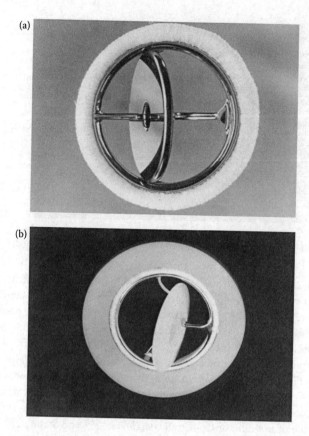

FIGURE 36.2 (a) Photograph of a typical tilting disk valve prosthesis. (Courtesy of Medtronic Heart Valves, Minneapolis, MN.) (b) Chitra tilting disk valve prosthesis with the occluder made of ultra-high-molecular-weight polyethylene. (Courtesy of Sree Chitra Tirunal Institute for Medical Sciences and Technology, India.)

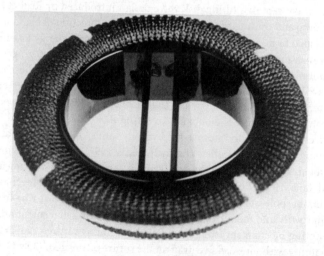

FIGURE 36.3 A CarboMedics bileaflet valve with pyrolytic carbon leaflets and housing. (Courtesy of Sulzer-CarboMedics, Austin, TX.)

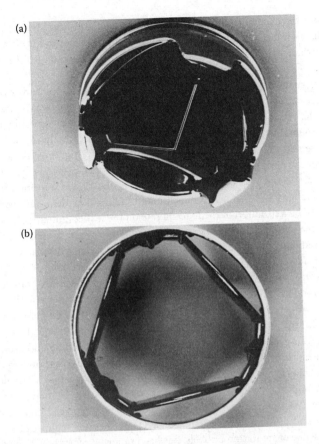

(a)

(b)

FIGURE 36.4 A tri-leaflet heart valve prosthesis under development. (Courtesy of Triflo Medical, Inc., Costa Mesa, CA.)

flow characteristics with reduced backflow. Accelerated fatigue tests have also shown good wear characteristics for this design and the valve is undergoing further evaluation, including animal studies. Other improvements in the mechanical valves that augment performance include machining of the valve housing to fit a disk so as to produce optimal washing and minimal regurgitation (McKenna, 1997); a supra-annular design so that a larger-sized valve can be inserted in the aortic position in the case of patients with small aortic annulus (Bell, 1997); and coating of a titanium alloy ring with a thin, uniform, and strongly adherent film of high-density turbostratic carbon (Carbofilm™) (Bona et al., 1997) in order to integrate the structural stability of the metal alloy to the nonthrombogenecity of pyrolytic carbon. Details of contemporary design efforts in mechanical valve design and potential future biomaterials such as Boralyn® (boron carbide) are discussed in Wieting (1997).

In spite of the desirable characteristics of the biomaterials used in the heart valve prostheses, problems with *thromboembolic complications* are significant with implanted valves, and patients with mechanical valves are under long-term anticoagulant therapy. The mechanical stresses induced by the flow of blood across the valve prostheses have been linked to the lysis and activation of *formed elements of blood* (red blood cells, white blood cells, and platelets) resulting in the deposition of thrombi in regions with relative stasis in the vicinity of the prostheses. Numerous *in vitro* studies with mechanical valves in pulse duplicators simulating physiological flow have been reported in the literature and have been reviewed by Chandran (1988) and Dellsperger and Chandran (1991). Such studies have included measurement of velocity profiles and turbulent stresses distal to the valve due to flow across the valve. The aim of these studies has been the correlation of regions prone to thrombus deposition and tissue overgrowth with explanted valves and the experimentally measured bulk turbulent shear stresses as well as regions of relative stasis. In spite of improvements in the design of the prostheses to afford a centralized flow with minimal flow disturbances and fluid mechanical stresses, the problems with thrombus deposition remain significant.

Reports of strut failure, material *erosion*, and leaflet escapes, as well as *pitting* and erosion of valve leaflets and housing have resulted in numerous investigations of the *closing dynamics* of mechanical valves. The dynamics of the leaflet motion and its impact with the valve housing or seat stop are very complex and a number of experimental and numerical studies have appeared recently in the literature. As the leaflet impacts against the seat stop and comes to rest instantaneously, high positive and negative pressure transients are present on the outflow and inflow side of the occluder, respectively, at the instant when the leaflet impacts against the seat stop or the guiding strut (Leuer, 1986; Chandran et al., 1994a). The *negative pressure transients* have been shown to reach magnitudes below the *liquid vapor pressure* and have been demonstrated to be a function of the loading rate on the leaflet inducing the valve closure. As the magnitudes of negative pressure transients go below the liquid vapor pressure, *cavitation bubbles* are initiated and the subsequent collapse of the cavitation bubbles may also be a factor in the lysis of red blood cells, platelets, and *valvular structures* (Chandran et al., 1994a; Lee et al., 1994). Typical cavitation bubbles visualized in an *in vitro* study with tilting disk and bileaflet valves are shown in Figure 36.5. A correlation is also observed between the region where cavitation bubbles are present, even though for a period of time less than a millisecond after valve closure, and sites of pitting and erosion reported in the pyrolytic carbon material in the valve housing and on the leaflets with explanted valves (Kafesjian, 1994) as well as those used in TAHs (Leuer, 1987). An electron micrograph of pitting and erosion observed in the pyrolytic carbon valve housing of an explanted bileaflet mechanical valve is shown in Figure 36.6. The pressure transients at valve closure are substantially smaller in mechanical valves with a flexible occluder, and leaflets made of ultra-high-molecular-weight polyethylene (Figure 36.2b) may prove to be advantageous based on the closing dynamic analysis (Chandran et al., 1994a). A correlation between the average velocity of the leaflet edge and the negative pressure transients in the same region at the instant of valve closure, as well as the presence of cavitation bubbles, has been reported recently (Chandran et al., 1997).

(a)

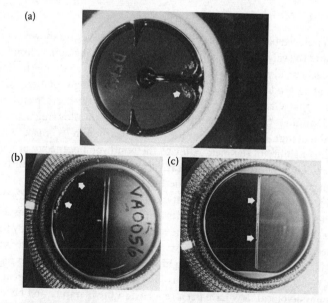

(b)

(c)

FIGURE 36.5 Cavitation bubbles visualized on the inflow side of the valves *in vitro*: (a) Medtronic-Hall tilting disk valve; (b) Edwards–Duromedics bileaflet valve; (c) CarboMedics bileaflet valve. (Adapted from Chandran, K.B., Lee, C.S., and Chen, L.D. 1994a. *J. Heart Valve Dis.* 3(Suppl. 1): S65–S76.)

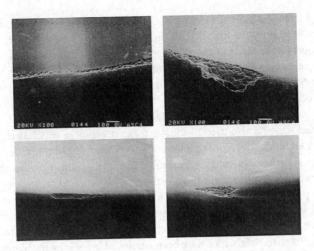

FIGURE 36.6 Photographs showing pitting on pyrolytic carbon surface of a mechanical heart valve. (Courtesy of Baxter Health Care, Irvine, CA.)

This study demonstrated that for the valves of the same geometry (e.g., tilting disk) and size, the leaflet edge velocity as well as the negative pressure transients were similar. However, the presence of cavitation bubbles depended on the local interaction between the leaflet and the seat stop. Hence, it was pointed out that magnitudes of leaflet velocity or presence of pressure transients below the liquid vapor pressure might not necessarily indicate cavitation inception with mechanical valve closure. Chandran et al. (1998) have also demonstrated the presence of negative pressure transients in the atrial chamber with implanted mechanical valves in the mitral position in animals, demonstrating that the potential for cavitation exists with implanted mechanical valves. Similar to the *in vitro* results, the transients were of smaller magnitudes with the Chitra valve made of flexible leaflets, and no pressure transients were observed with tissue valve implanted in the mitral position *in vivo*. The demonstration of the negative pressure transients with mechanical valve closure also shows that this phenomenon is localized and the flow chamber or valve holder rigidity with the *in vitro* experiments will not affect the closing dynamics of the valve.

The pressure distribution on the leaflets and impact forces between the leaflets and guiding struts have also been experimentally measured in order to understand the causes for strut failure (Chandran et al., 1994b). The flow through the clearance between the leaflet and the housing at the instant of valve closure (Lee and Chandran, 1994a,b) and in the fully closed position (Reif, 1991) and the resulting wall shear stresses within the clearance are also being suggested as responsible for clinically significant hemolysis and thrombus initiation. Detailed analysis of the complex closing dynamics of the leaflets may also be exploited in improving the design of the mechanical valves to minimize problems with structural failure (Cheon and Chandran, 1994). Further improvements in the design of the valves based on the closing dynamics as well as improvements in material may result in minimizing thromboembolic complications with implanted mechanical valves.

36.1.2.2 Biological Heart Valves

The first biological valves implanted were *homografts* with valves explanted from cadavers within 48 h after death. Preservation of the valves included various techniques of sterilization, freeze-drying, and immersing in antibiotic solution. The use of homografts is not popular due to problems with long-term durability and due to limited availability except in a few centers (Shim and Lenker, 1988; Lee and Boughner, 1991). Attempts were also made in the early 1960s in the use of *xenografts* (valves made from animal tissue), and porcine bioprostheses became commercially available after the introduction of the glutaraldehyde (rather than formaldehyde, which was initially used) fixation technique. Glutaraldehyde reacts with tissue proteins to form crosslinks and results in improved durability (Carpentier et al., 1969).

The valves are harvested from 7–12-month-old pigs and attached to supporting *stents* and preserved. The stent provided support to preserve the valve in the natural shape and to achieve normal opening and closing. Initial supports were made of metal and subsequently flexible polypropylene stents were introduced. The flexible stents provided the advantage of ease of assembling the valve, and *finite element analyses* have demonstrated reduction in stresses at the juncture between the stent and tissue leaflets resulting in increased durability and increased leaflet coaptation area (Reis et al., 1971; Hamid et al., 1985). A typical porcine bioprosthesis is included in Figure 36.7a.

Fixed bovine pericardial tissue is also used to construct heart valves in which design characteristics such as orifice area, valve height, and degree of coaptation can be specified and controlled. Thus, the geometry and flow dynamics past *pericardial prostheses* mimic those of the natural human aortic valves more closely. Due to the low-profile design of pericardial prostheses and increased orifice area, these valves are less stenotic compared to porcine bioprostheses, especially in smaller sizes (Chandran et al., 1984). In the currently available bioprostheses, the stents are constructed from polypropylene, *Acetol*® homopolymer or copolymer, Elgiloy wire, or titanium. A stainless-steel radiopaque marker is also introduced to visualize the valve *in vivo*. Other biomaterials, which have been employed in making the bioprostheses, include *fascia lata* tissue as well as human *duramater* tissue. The former was prone to deterioration and hence unsuitable for bioprosthetic application, whereas the latter lacked commercial availability.

The advantage with bioprostheses is the freedom from thromboembolism and hence not requiring long-term anticoagulant therapy in general. These prostheses are preferable in patients who do not

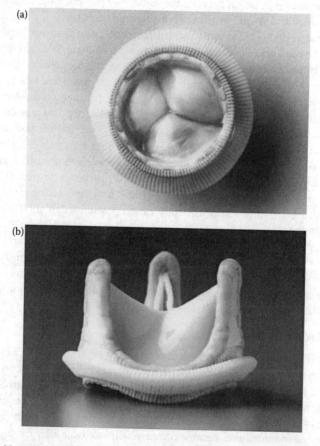

(a)

(b)

FIGURE 36.7 Typical bioprostheses: (a) Hancock porcine bioprosthesis. (Courtesy of Medtronic Heart Valves, Minneapolis, MN.) (b) PhotoFix™ α pericardial prosthesis. (Courtesy of Sulzer-CarboMedics, Inc., Austin, TX.)

lerate anticoagulants. On the other hand, bioprosthetic valves are prone to *calcification* and leaflet tear ith an average lifetime of about 10 years before replacement is necessary, and is generally attributed to he tissue fixation process. Numerous attempts are being made to improve the design as well as fixation n bioprostheses in order to minimize problems with calcification and increase duration of the function f the implant. As an example, a bovine pericardial trileaflet valve (Figure 36.7b) treated with a non-ldehyde fixation resulting in collagen crosslink formation without a new "foreign" chemical process Phillips and Printz, 1997) has been introduced in the European market. A nonaldehyde iodine-based terilization process also sterilizes the valve.

Numerous studies linking the mechanical stresses on the leaflets with calcification, focal thinning, and leaflet failure (Thubrikar et al., 1982a; Sabbah et al., 1985), and design improvements to minimize the stresses on the leaflets (Thubrikar et al., 1982b) have been reported in the literature. Further details on he effects of tissue fixation and mechanical effects of fixation on the leaflets are reported elsewhere (Lee and Boughner, 1991). Improvements in fixation techniques as well as in design of the bioprostheses are continually being made in order to minimize problems with calcification of the leaflets and to improve the durability and functional characteristics of bioprosthetic heart valves (Piwnica and Westaby, 1998). The biomaterials used in commercially available mechanical and bioprosthetic heart valves are included in Table 36.2. Table 36.3 includes a summary of the problems associated with implanted artificial heart valves.

36.1.2.3 Synthetic Heart Valves

Concurrently, efforts have also been made in the development of valve prostheses made of synthetic material. Several attempts to make bileaflet (Braunwald et al., 1960) and trileaflet valves (Roe et al., 1958; Gerring et al., 1974; Ghista and Reul, 1977; Hufnagel, 1977) made of polyurethanes, polyester fabrics,

TABLE 36.2 Biomaterial Used in Heart Valve Prostheses

Type	Component	Biomaterial
Caged ball	Ball/occluder	Silastic
	Cage	Stellite 21/titanium
	Suture ring	Silicone rubber insert under knitted composite Teflon/polypropylene cloth
Tilting disk	Leaflet	Delrin; pyrolytic carbon (carbon deposited on graphite substrate); ultra-high-molecular polyethylene
	Housing/strut	Haynes 25/titanium
	Suture ring	Teflon/Dacron
Bileaflet	Leaflets	Pyrolytic carbon
	Housing	Pyrolytic carbon
	Suture ring	Double velour Dacron tricot knit polyester
Porcine bioprostheses	Leaflets	Porcine aortic valve fixed by stabilized glutaraldehyde
	Stents	Polypropylene stent covered with Dacron; lightweight Elgiloy wire covered with porous knitted Teflon cloth
	Suture ring	Dacron; soft silicone rubber insert covered with porous, seamless Teflon cloth
Porcine bioprostheses	Leaflets	Porcine pericardial tissue fixed by stabilized glutaraldehyde before leaflets are sewn to the valve stents
	Stents	Polypropylene stent covered with Dacron; Elgiloy wire and nylon support band covered with polyester and Teflon cloth
	Suture ring	PTFE fabric over silicone rubber filter

Source: Shim, H.S. and Lenker, J.A.: Heart valve prostheses. *Encyclopedia of Medical Devices and Instrumentation.* 1988. Vol. 3. pp. 1457–1474. Wiley Interscience, New York. Copyright Wiley-VCH Verlag GmbH & Co. KGaA. Reproduced with permission; Dellsperger and Chandran, 1988.

TABLE 36.3   Common Problems with Implanted Prosthetic Heart Valves

I. Mechanical valves
    a. Thromboembolism
    b. Structural failure
    c. Red blood cell and platelet destruction
    d. Tissue overgrowth
    e. Damage to endothelial lining
    f. Paravalvular/perivalvular leakage
    g. Tearing of sutures
    h. Infection
II. Bioprosthetic valves
    a. Tissue calcification
    b. Leaflet rupture
    c. Paravalvular/perivalvular leakage
    d. Infection

Source: Adapted from Yoganathan, A.P., Corcoran, W.H., and Harrison, E.C. 1979a. *J. Biomech.* 12: 135–152; Shim, H.S. and Lenker, J.A.: Heart valve prostheses. *Encyclopedia of Medical Devices and Instrumentation.* 1988. Vol. 3. pp. 1457–1474. Wiley Interscience, New York. Copyright Wiley-VCH Verlag GmbH & Co. KGaA. Reproduced with permission; Chandran, K.B. 1992. *Cardiovascular Biomechanics.* New York University Press, New York.

and silicone rubber were not successful due to problems with durability of relatively thin leaflets made of synthetic material. With the advent of the TAH and *left ventricular assist devices* in the 1980s, an additional impetus on the development of synthetic valves is present. Due to problems with thrombus deposition in the vicinity of the mechanical valves used in the TAH and subsequent stroke episodes in patients with permanent implants, the use of the device is currently restricted as a bridge to transplantation. In such temporary use before a donor heart becomes available (on an average of several weeks), the four mechanical prostheses used in the TAH results in substantial cost. Hence, efforts are being made to replace the mechanical valves with those made with synthetic material. With *vacuum forming* or *solution casting* techniques, synthetic valves can be made at a fraction of the cost of mechanical valves, provided their function in a TAH environment for several weeks will be satisfactory. Implantation of synthetic trileaflet valves (Russel et al., 1980; Harold et al., 1987), even more recently, has resulted in limited success due to leaflet failure and calcification. Hemodynamic comparison of vacuum formed and solution cast trileaflet valves to currently available bioprostheses have produced satisfactory results (Chandran et al., 1989a,b). *Finite element analysis* of synthetic valves can be exploited in design improvements similar to those reported for bioprostheses (Chandran et al., 1991a).

36.1.3 TAHs or Ventricular Assist Devices

Artificial circulatory support can be broadly classified into two categories. The first category is for those patients who undergo open heart surgery to correct *valvular disorders*, ventricular *aneurysm*, or coronary artery disease. In several cases, the heart may not recover sufficiently after surgery to take over the pumping action. In such patients, ventricular assist devices are used as extracorporeal devices to maintain circulation until the heart recovers. Other ventricular assist devices include *intra-aortic balloon pumps* as well as *cardiopulmonary* bypass. Within several days or weeks, when the natural heart recovers, these devices will be removed. In the second category are patients with advanced stages of cardiomyopathy and are subjects for heart transplantation. Due to problems in the availability of suitable donor hearts, not all patients with a failed heart are candidates for heart transplantation. For those patients not selected for transplantation, the concept of replacing the natural heart with a total artificial heart has gained attention in recent years (Akutsu and Kolff, 1958; Jarvick, 1981; DeVries and Joyce, 1983; Unger, 1989; Kambic and Nose, 1991). A number of attempts in the permanent implantation of TAH with pneumatically powered units were made in the 1980s. However, due to neurological complications as a result of thromboembolism, infection, and hematological and renal complications, permanent implantations are currently suspended. If a suitable donor heart is not readily available, TAHs can be used as "bridge to transplantation" for several weeks until a donor heart becomes available. Until recently, most of the circulatory assist devices were pneumatically driven and a typical pneumatic heart is shown in Figure 36.8a. It has two chambers for the left and right ventricles with inlet and outlet valves for each of the chambers. A line coming from the external pneumatic driver passes through the skin and is attached to the diaphragm housing through the connector shown in the photograph. Thus, the patient is tethered to an external pneumatic drive. He can move around for a short period of time by attaching the pneumatic line to a portable driver that he can carry.

Electrically driven blood pumps, which can afford tether-free operation within the body, unlike those of the pneumatically powered pumps, are currently at various stages of development for long-term use (of more than 2 years). The components of such devices include the blood pump in direct contact with

(a)

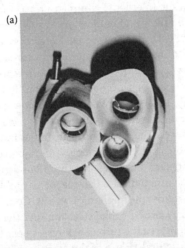

(b)

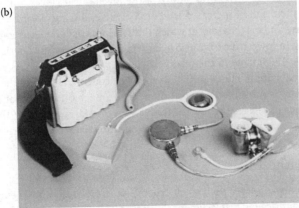

FIGURE 36.8 Typical prototype designs of TAHs: (a) pneumatically powered TAH. The right and left ventricular chambers, inflow and outflow valves, as well as the connector for the pneumatic line are visible in the photograph; (b) electrically powered TAH. Shown are the external battery pack, transcutaneous energy transmission system (TETS) primary and secondary coils, implanted electronics, energy converter and the blood pumps, compliance chamber, and the subcutaneous access port. (Courtesy of G. Rosenberg, Pennsylvania State University.)

blood, energy converter (from electrical to mechanical energy), variable column compensator, implantable batteries, transcutaneous energy transmission system, and external batteries. The blood pump configuration in these devices includes sac, diaphragm, and *pusher plate devices*. Materials used in blood-contacting surfaces in these devices are synthetic polymers (polyurethanes, segmented polyurethanes, *Biomer®*, and others). Segmented polyurethane elastomer used in prosthetic ventricles with a thromboresistant additive modifying the polymeric surface has resulted in improved blood compatibility and reduced thromboembolic risk in animal trials (Farrar et al., 1988). Design considerations include reduction of regions of stagnation of blood within the blood chamber and minimizing the mechanical stresses induced on the formed elements in blood. Apart from the characteristics of these materials to withstand repetitive high mechanical stresses and to minimize failure due to fatigue, surface interaction with blood is also another crucial factor. An electrically powered TAH intended for long-term implantation is shown in Figure 36.8b. The details of the design considerations for the circulatory assist devices are included in Rosenberg (1995) and details of the evaluation of the electrically powered heart are included in Rosenberg et al. (1995).

Due to significant problems with thromboembolic complications and subsequent neurological problems with long-term implantation of TAH in humans, attention has been focused on minimizing factors responsible for thrombus deposition. In order to eliminate crevices formed with the quick connect system, valves sutured in place at the inflow and outflow orifices were offered as an alternative in the Philadelphia Heart (Wurzel et al., 1988). An alternative quick connect system using precision-machined components has been demonstrated to reduce valve- and connector-associated thrombus formation substantially (Holfert et al., 1987). Several *in vitro* studies have been reported in the literature in order to assess the effect of fluid dynamic stresses on thrombus deposition (Phillips et al., 1979; Tarbell et al., 1986; Baldwin et al., 1990; Jarvis et al., 1991). These have included flow visualization and *laser Doppler anemometry* velocity and turbulence measurements within the ventricular chamber as well as in the vicinity of the inflow and outflow orifices. The results of such studies indicate that the flow within the chamber generally has a smooth washout of blood in each pulsatile flow cycle with relatively large turbulent stresses and regions of stasis found near the valves. The thrombus deposition found with implanted TAH in the vicinity of the inflow valves also indicates that the major problem with the working of these devices is still with the flow dynamics across the mechanical valves. Computational flow dynamic analysis within the ventricular chamber may also be exploited to improve the design of the valve chambers and the mechanical valves in order to reduce the turbulent stresses near the vicinity of the inflow and outflow orifices (Kim et al., 1992). Structural failure of the mechanical valves, initially reported with the TAH, may have been the result of increased load on the valves during closure due to the relatively large dp/dt (p is the pressure and t is the time) at which the TAH was operated. Attempts at reducing the dp/dt during closure of the inflow valves have also been reported with modified designs of the artificial heart driver (Wurzel et al., 1988). Due to the relatively large dp/dt at which TAHs are operated, there is increased possibility of cavitation bubble initiation, and subsequent collapse of the bubbles may also be another important reason for thrombus deposition near the mechanical valve at the inflow orifice. Introducing synthetic valves to replace the mechanical valves (Chandran et al., 1991b) may prove to be advantageous with respect to cavitation initiation and may minimize thrombus formation.

36.1.4 Vascular Prostheses

In advanced stages of vascular diseases such as obstructive *atherosclerosis* and aneurysmal dilatation, when other treatment modalities fail, replacement of diseased segments with vascular prostheses is a common practice. Vascular prostheses can be classified as given in Table 36.4.

36.1.4.1 Surgically Implanted Biological Grafts

Arterial homografts, even though initially used in large scale, resulted in aneurysm formation especially in the proximal suture line (Strandness and Sumner, 1975). Still, a viable alternative is to use the

TABLE 36.4 Classification of Vascular Prostheses

Prosthesis	Comments
Surgically implanted biological grafts	
Autograft	Graft transplanted from part of a patient's body to another
	Example: saphenous vein graft for peripheral bypass
Allograft	Homograft. Transplanted vascular graft tissues derived from the same species as recipient. Example: glutaraldehyde-treated umbilical cord vein graft
Xenograft	Heterograft. Surgical graft of vascular tissues derived from one species to a recipient of another species. Example: modified bovine heterograft
Surgically implanted synthetic grafts	
Dacron (polyethylene terephthalate)	Woven, knitted
PTFE (polytetrafluoroethylene)	Expanded, knitted
Other	Nylon, polyurethane

saphenous vein graft from the same patient. Vein grafts have a failure rate of about 20% in 1 year and up to 30% in 5 years after implantation. Vein grafts from the same patients are also unavailable or unsuitable in about 10–30% of the patients (Abbott and Bouchier-Hayes, 1978). Modified *bovine heterograft* and glutaraldehyde-treated *umbilical cord vein grafts* have also been employed as vascular prostheses with less success compared to autologous vein grafts.

36.1.4.2 Surgically Implanted Synthetic Grafts

Prostheses made of synthetic material for vascular replacement have been used for over 40 years. Polymeric materials currently used as implants include *nylon*, polyester, *PTFE*, polypropylene, polyacrylonitrile, and silicone rubber (Park and Lakes, 1992). However, Dacron (polyethylene terephthalate) and PTFE are the more common vascular prosthesis materials currently available. These materials exhibit the essential qualities for implants—they are biocompatible, resilient, flexible, durable, and resistant to sterilization and biodegradation. Detailed discussion on the properties, manufacturing techniques, and testing of Dacron prostheses is included in Guidoin and Couture (1992). Figure 36.9a depicts a Dacron vascular graft having a bifurcated configuration. Figure 36.9b shows expanded PTFE vascular grafts having a variety of configurations and sizes: straight, straight with external reinforcement rings (to resist external compression), and bifurcated.

Synthetic vascular grafts implanted as large-vessel replacements have resulted in reasonable degrees of success. However, in medium- and small-diameter prostheses (less than 6 mm in diameter), loss of *patency* within several months after implantation is more acute. Graft failure due to thrombosis or intimal hyperplasia with thrombosis is primarily responsible in failures within 30 days after implantation, and intimal hyperplasia formation is the reason for failure within 6 months after surgery. Soon after implantation, a layer of *fibrin* and fibrous tissue covers the intimal and outer surface of the prosthesis, respectively. A layer of *fibroblasts* replaces the fibrin and is referred to as *neointima*. In the later stages, *neointimal hyperplasia* formation occurs and ultimately results in the occlusion of the vessels in small-diameter vascular grafts. Attempts are being made currently in suitably modifying the surface characteristics of the prostheses in order to reduce the problems with loss of patency. Studies are also being performed in order to understand the mechanical stresses induced at the anastomotic region, which may result in deposits on the intimal surface and occlusion of the vessels (Chandran and Kim, 1994). The alterations in mechanical stresses with the implantation of vascular prostheses in the arterial circulation may include changes in the deformation and stress concentrations at the anastomotic site. Altered fluid shear stresses at the intimal surface in the vicinity of the anastomosis has also been suggested as important particularly since the loss of patency is present more often at the distal anastomosis.

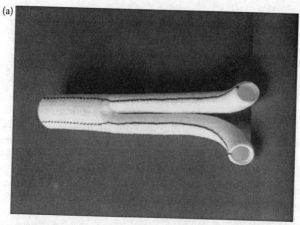

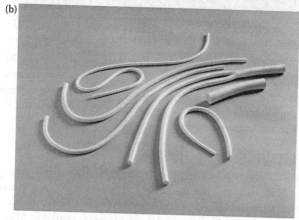

FIGURE 36.9 (a) Photograph of a Dacron vascular graft having a bifurcated configuration. (b) Photograph of expanded PTFE vascular grafts with straight, straight with external reinforcement rings to resist compression, and bifurcated configurations. (Courtesy of W.L. Gore and Associates, Inc., Flagstaff, AZ.)

The vascular prostheses should have the same dynamic response after implantation as the host artery in order to reduce the effect of abnormal mechanical stresses at the junction. For a replacement graft of the same size as the host artery, mismatch in *compliance* may be the most important factor resulting in graft failure (Abbott and Bouchier-Hayes, 1978). In implanting the prostheses, *end-to-end configuration* is common in the reconstruction of peripheral arteries. *End-to-side configuration* is common in coronary artery bypass where blood will flow from the host artery (aorta) to the prosthesis branching out at the anastomotic site. At the other end, the graft is attached distal to the occlusion in the host (coronary) vessel to enable perfusion of the vascular bed downstream from the occlusion. Numerous studies analyzing the abnormal flow dynamics within the anastomotic geometry and stress distribution within the vascular material at the junction to the prostheses have been reported in delineating the causes for intimal hyperplasia formation and loss of patency (Rodgers et al., 1987; Ojha et al., 1990; Keynton et al., 1991; Chandran et al., 1992; Kim and Chandran, 1993; Kim et al., 1993; Rhee and Tarbell, 1994) and a detailed discussion on the mechanical aspects of vascular prostheses can be found in Chandran and Kim (1994). Improvements in the blood–surface interactions are also being attempted in order to improve the functioning capability of vascular grafts. Attempts at seeding the grafts with *endothelial cells* (Hunter et al., 1983), and modifying the graft material properties by removing the *crimping* and heat fusing a coil of bendable and dimensionally stable polypropylene at the outer surface to make it kink-resistant (Guidoin t al., 1983), and employing a compliant and biodegradable graft that will promote regeneration of arterial wall in small caliber vessels (Van der Lei et al., 1985, 1986) are a few examples of such improvements.

36.1.4.3 Transluminally Placed Endovascular Prostheses (Stent-Grafts)

Endoluminal approaches to treating vascular disease involve the insertion of a prosthetic device into the vasculature through a small, often percutaneous, access site created in a remote vessel, followed by the intraluminal delivery and deployment of a prosthesis via transcatheter techniques (Veith et al., 1995). In contrast to conventional surgical therapies for vascular disease, the use of transluminally placed endovascular prostheses are distinguished by their "minimally invasive" nature. Because these techniques do not require extensive surgical intervention, they have the potential to simplify the delivery of vascular therapy, improve procedural outcomes, decrease procedural costs, reduce morbidity, and broaden the patient population that may benefit from treatment. Not surprisingly, endoluminal therapies have generated intense interest within the vascular surgery, interventional radiology, and cardiology communities over recent years.

The feasibility of using transluminally placed endovascular prostheses, or stent-grafts, for the treatment of traumatic vascular injury (Marin et al., 1994), atherosclerotic obstructions (Cragg and Dake, 1993), and aneurysmal vascular disease (Parodi et al., 1991; Dake et al., 1994; Yusuf et al., 1994) has been demonstrated in human beings. Endoluminal stent-grafts continue to evolve to address a number of cardiovascular pathologies at all levels of the arterial tree. Figure 36.10a depicts endoluminal stent-grafts

(a)

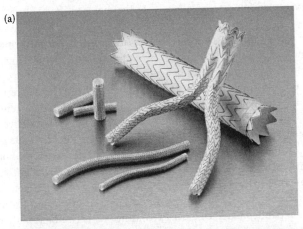

(b)

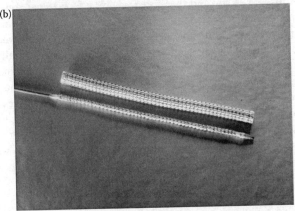

FIGURE 36.10 (a) Endoluminal stent-grafts of straight and bifurcated configurations and sizes currently under clinical investigation. (b) A stent-graft implant consisting of an ePTFE graft that is externally supported by a self-expanding nitinol stent. (Courtesy of W.L. Gore and Associates, Inc., Flagstaff, AZ.)

having a variety of configurations (straight, bifurcated) and functional diameters (peripheral, aortic) that are currently under clinical investigation.

Endoluminal stent-grafts are catheter-deliverable endoluminal prostheses comprised of an intravascular stent component and a biocompatible graft component. The function of these devices is to provide an intraluminal conduit that enables blood flow through pathologic vascular segments without the need for open surgery. The stent component functions as an arterial attachment mechanism and provides structural support to both the graft and the treated vascular segment. By design, stents are delivered to the vasculature in a low-profile, small-diameter delivery configuration and can be elastically or plastically expanded to a secondary, large-diameter configuration upon deployment. Vascular attachment is achieved by the interference fit created when a stent is deployed within the lumen of a vessel having a diameter smaller than that of the stent. The graft component, on the other hand, is generally constructed from a biocompatible material such as expanded polytetrafluoroethylene (ePTFE), woven polyester (Dacron), or polyurethane. The graft component has a number of real and theoretical functions, including segregating potential thromboemboli or atheroemboli from the bloodstream, presenting a physical barrier to mass transport between the bloodstream and arterial wall, and mitigating cellular infiltration and the host inflammatory response. Figure 36.10b shows a stent-graft implant consisting of an ePTFE graft that is externally supported along its entire length by a self-expanding nitinol stent. The implant is radially constrained and attached to the leading end of a dual lumen polyethylene delivery catheter that allows transluminal delivery and deployment. Following introduction into the vascular system, the implant is positioned fluoroscopically within the diseased segment and released from the delivery system.

Mechanical properties play an important role in determining the *in vivo* performance of an endoluminal stent-graft. Since the graft component typically lacks significant structural integrity, the mechanical behavior of the stent-graft predominantly depends upon the mechanical properties of its stent component. The type of mechanism required to induce dilatation from the delivery (small-diameter) configuration to the deployed (large-diameter) configuration typically classifies stents. Self-expanding stents are designed to spontaneously dilate (i.e., elastically recover) from the delivery diameter up to a maximal, predetermined deployed diameter, whereas balloon-expandable stents are designed to be plastically enlarged over a range of values with the use of appropriately sized and pressurized dilatation balloons. Consequently, self-expanding stents exert a continuous, radially outward directed force on periluminal tissues, whereas balloon-expandable stents assume a fixed diameter that resists recoil of the surrounding periluminal tissues. Both types of stents exhibit utilitarian features. For example, in comparison to balloon-expandable devices, self-expanding stents can be rapidly deployed without the use of dilatation balloons, are elastic and therefore less prone to external compression, can radially adapt to postdeployment vascular remodeling, and retain some of the natural compliance of the vascular tissues. In contrast, balloon-expandable stents are much more versatile when it comes to conforming to irregular vascular morphologies because their diameter can be radially adjusted via balloon dilatation. Since the luminal diameter of self-expanding stents cannot be adjusted (i.e., enlarged) to any appreciable degree, accurate sizing of the host vessel is critical. A sizing mismatch resulting in oversizing can cause overcompression of the self-expanding stent and obstructive invagination of the stent into the lumen. Undersizing, in turn, can result in a poor interference fit, inadequate anchoring, device migration, and/or leakage of blood into the abluminal compartment. In either case, the stent provides a scaffold that structurally supports the graft material. Ongoing work in the field of biomedical engineering is directed at optimizing the biomechanical and biological performance of these devices.

36.1.5 Conclusions

In the last four decades, we have observed significant advances in the development of biocompatible materials to be used in blood-interfacing implants. In the case of mechanical heart valve prostheses, pyrolytic carbon has become the material of choice for the occluder and the housing. The pyrolytic carbon is chemically inert and exhibits very little wear even after more than 20 years of use. However, thromboembolic complications still remain significant with mechanical valve implantation. The complex dynamics of valve function and the resulting mechanical stresses on the formed elements of blood appear to be the main cause for initiation of thrombus. More recent reports of structural failure with implanted mechanical valves and pitting and erosion observed on the pyrolytic carbon surfaces have resulted in investigations on cavitation bubble formation during valve closure. Along with further improvements in biomaterials for heart valves, detailed analysis of the closing dynamics and design improvements to minimize the adverse effects of mechanical stresses may be the key to reducing thrombus deposition. Improvements in mechanical heart valves or further developments in durable synthetic leaflet valves may also be vital for the development of TAHs for long-term implantation without neurologic complications.

In the case of vascular grafts, the mismatch of material properties (compliance) between the host artery and the graft, as well as geometric considerations in end-to-side anastomoses, appears to be important for the loss of patency within several months after implantation, particularly with medium- and small-diameter arterial replacement. Most of the vascular grafts are stiffer compared to the host artery and it has been suggested that the mechanical stresses resulting from the discontinuity at the junction is the major cause for neointimal hyperplasia formation and subsequent occlusion of the conduit. Developments with more compliant grafts and in modifying the surface interaction of the graft with blood (endothelialization or other treatment of the graft material) may result in reducing the problems with loss of patency. Recent advances in the use of minimally invasive stent-grafts also show promise in improving the quality of life of patients with vascular disease.

Defining Terms

Acetol: Product of the addition of 2 mol of alcohol to 1 mol of an aldehyde.
Aneurysms: Abnormal bulging or dilatation of a segment of a blood vessel or myocardium.
Artery: Blood vessel transporting blood in a direction away from the heart.
Atherosclerosis: Lipid deposits in the intima of arteries.
ATS valve: A bileaflet mechanical valve made by ATS (Advancing the Standard), Inc.
Autoclaving: Sterilizing by steam under pressure.
Biomer: Segmented polyurethane elastomer.
Bioprostheses: Prosthetic heart valves made of biological tissue.
Blood oxygenators: Extracorporeal devices to oxygenate blood during heart bypass surgery.
Bovine heterograft: Graft material (arterial) transplanted from bovine species.
Calcification: Deposition of insoluble salts of calcium.
Cardiac pacemakers: Prosthesis implanted to stimulate cardiac muscles to contract.
Cardiopulmonary bypass: Connectors bypassing circulation to the heart and the lungs.
Catheters: Hollow cylindrical tubing to be passed through the blood vessels or other canals.
Cavitation bubbles (vapor cavitation): Formation of vapor bubbles due to transient reduction in pressure to below the liquid vapor pressure.
Closing dynamics: Dynamics during the closing phase of heart valves.
Compliance: A measure of ease with which a structure can be deformed; ratio of volumetric strain to increase in unit pressure.
Crimping: Creasing of the synthetic vascular grafts in the longitudinal direction to accommodate the large intermittent flow of blood.
Delrin: Polyacetal made by Union Carbide.
Dialysers: Devices to filter the blood of waste products taking over the function of the kidney.
dp/dt: Slope of the pressure versus time curve of the ventricles.
Duramater: A tough fibrous membrane forming the outer cover of the brain and the spinal cord.

Electrohydraulic blood pump: Blood pumps energized by the conversion of electrical to hydraulic energy.

End-to-end configuration: End of the vascular graft anastamosed to the end of the host artery.

End-to-side configuration: End of the vascular graft anastamosed to the side of the host.

Endothelial cells: A layer of flat cells lining the intimal surface of blood vessels.

Erosion: A state of being worn away.

Fascia lata: A sheet of fibrous tissue enveloping the muscles of the thigh.

Fatigue stress: Level of stress below which the material would not undergo fatigue failure (107 cycles are used as the normal limit).

Fibrin: An elastic filamentous protein derived from fibrinogen in coagulation of the blood.

Fibroblasts: An elongated cell with cytoplasmic processes present in connective tissue capable of forming collagen fibers.

Finite element analysis: Structural analysis with the aid of a computer that divides the structure into finite elements and applies the laws of mechanics on each element.

Formaldehyde: Formic aldehyde, methyl aldehyde, a pungent gas used as antiseptic.

Formed elements in blood: Red blood cells, white blood cells, platelets, and other cells in whole blood.

Haynes 25: Co–Cr alloy.

Homografts: Transplants (heart valves, arterial segments, etc.) from the same species.

Intra-aortic balloon pumps: A balloon catheter inserted in the descending aorta and alternately inflated and deflated timed to the EKG in order to assist the ventricular pumping.

Laser Doppler anemometry: A velocity measurement device using the principle of Doppler shifted frequency of laser light by particles moving with the fluid.

Leaflets: Occluders on valves that open and close to aid blood flow in one direction.

Left ventricular assist devices: Prosthetic devices to assist the left ventricle in pumping blood.

Liquid vapor pressure: Pressure at which liquid vaporizes.

LTI: Low-temperature (below 1500°C) isotropic pyrolytic carbon.

Mechanical prostheses: Prostheses made of nonbiological material.

Negative pressure transients: Reduction in pressure for a short duration.

Neointima: Newly formed intimal surface.

Neointimal hyperplasia: Growth of new intimal surface formed by fibroblasts.

Nylon: Synthetic polymer with condensation polymerization.

Patency: State of being freely open.

Pericardial prostheses: Heart valve prosthesis made with fixed bovine pericardial tissue.

Pitting: Depression or indent on a surface.

Platelet: One of the formed elements of blood responsible for blood coagulation.

Polypropylene: One of the vinyl polymers with good flex life and good environmental stress crack resistance.

Polytetrafluoroethylene (PTFE): A fluorocarbon polymer known as Teflon.

Pusher plate devices: Artificial heart devices working with pusher plates moving the blood.

Pyrolytic carbon: Carbon deposited onto preformed polycrystalline graphite substrate.

Radiopacity: Being opaque to x-ray.

Sewing rings: Rings surrounding the housing of artificial heart valves used to sew the valve to the tissue orifice with suture.

Solution casting: Casting by pouring molten material on dyes to form a structure.

Stellite 21: Co–Cr alloy.

Stent: A device used to maintain the bodily orifice or cavity.

Strut: A projection in the structure such as guiding struts in heart valves used to guide the leaflets during opening and closing.

TAH: Total artificial heart replacing a failed natural heart.

Teflon: See PTFE.

Thromboembolic complications: Complications due to breaking away (emboli) of thrombus blocking the distal blood vessels.

Thrombus: A clot in the blood vessels or in the cavities of the heart formed from the constituents of blood.

Tilting disk valves: Valves with a single leaflet tilting open and shut.

Titanium: Highly reactive metal having low density, good mechanical properties, and biocompatibility due to tenacious oxide layer formation.

Turbulent stresses: Stresses generated in the fluid due to agitated random motion of particles.

Ultra-high-molecular-weight polyethylene: Linear thermoplastics with very high molecular weight ($>2 \times 10^6$ g/mol) used for orthopedic devices such as acetabular cup for hip joint replacement.

Umbilical cord vein grafts: Vascular graft made from umbilical cord veins.

Vacuum forming: A manufacturing technique for thermoplastic polymer in which a sheet is heated and formed over a mold while a vacuum is present under the sheet.

Valvular disorders: Diseased states of valves such as stenosis.

Valvular structures: Components of valves such as leaflets, struts, etc.

Vascular grafts: Grafts to replace segments of diseased vessels.

Xenografts: Grafts obtained from species other than that of the recipient.

References

Abbott, W.M. and Bouchier-Hayes, D.J. 1978. The role of mechanical properties in graft design. In *Graft Materials in Vascular Surgery*, Dardick, H., ed. Year Book Medical Publishers, Chicago, IL, pp. 59–78.

Akutsu, T. and Kolff, W.J. 1958. Permanent substitutes for valves and hearts. *Trans. Am. Soc. Art. Intern. Organs (ASAIO)* 4: 230–235.

Baldwin, J.T., Campbell, A., Luck, C., Ogilvie, W., and Sauter, J. 1997. Hydrodynamics of the CarboMedics® aortic kinetic™ prosthetic heart valve. In *Surgery for Acquired Aortic Valve Disease*. Piwnica, A. and Westaby, S., eds. ISIS Medical Media, Oxford, pp. 365–370.

Baldwin, J.T., Tarbell, J.M., Deutsch, S., Geselowitz, D.B., and Rosenberg, G. 1988. Hot-film wall shear probe measurements inside a ventricular assist device. *Am. Soc. Mech. Eng. (ASME) J. Biomech. Eng.* 110: 326–333.

Bell, R.S. 1997. CarboMedics® supra-annular Top Hat™ aortic valve. In *Surgery for Acquired Aortic Valve Disease*. Piwnica, A. and Westaby, S., eds., ISIS Medical Media, Oxford, pp. 371–375.

Bona, G., Rinaldi, S., and Vallana, F. 1997. Design characteristics of the BICARBON™ bileaflet heart valve prosthesis. In *Surgery for Acquired Aortic Valve Disease*. Piwnica, A. and Westaby, S. eds. ISIS Medical Media, Oxford, pp. 392–396.

Braunwald, N.S., Cooper, T., and Morrow, A.G. 1960. Complete replacement of the mitral valve: Successful application of a flexible polyurethane prosthesis. *J. Thorac. Cardiovasc. Surg.* 40: 1–11.

Carpentier, A., Lamaigre, C.G., Robert, L., Carpentier, S., and Dubost, C. 1969. Biological factors affecting long-term results of valvular heterografts. *J. Thorac. Cardiovasc. Surg.* 58: 467–483.

Chandran, K.B. 1988. Heart valve prostheses: *In vitro* flow dynamics. In *Encyclopedia of Medical Devices and Instrumentation*, Vol. 3. Webster, J.G., Ed., Wiley Interscience, New York, pp. 1475–1483.

Chandran, K.B. 1992. *Cardiovascular Biomechanics*. New York University Press, New York.

Chandran, K.B. and Aluri, S. 1997. Mechanical valve closing dynamics. Relationship between velocity of closing, pressure transients, and cavitation initiation. *Ann. Biomed. Eng.* 25: 926–938.

Chandran, K.B. and Kim, Y.H. 1994. Mechanical aspects of vascular graft-host artery anastomoses. *IEEE Eng. Med. Biol. Mag.* 13: 517–524.

Chandran, K.B., Cabell, G.N., Khalighi, B., and Chen, C.J. 1983. Laser anemometry measurements of pulsatile flow past aortic valve prostheses. *J. Biomech.* 16: 865–873.

Chandran, K.B., Cabell, G.N., Khalighi, B., and Chen, C.J. 1984. Pulsatile flow past aortic valve bioprostheses in a model human aorta. *J. Biomech.* 17: 609–619.

Chandran, K.B., Fatemi, R., Schoephoerster, R., Wurzel, D., Hansen, G., Pantalos, G., Yu, L.-S., and Kolff, W.J. 1989a. *In vitro* comparison of velocity profiles and turbulent shear distal to polyurethane trileaflet and pericardial prosthetic valves. *Artif. Organs* 13: 148–154.

Chandran, K.B., Schoephoerster, R.T., Wurzel, D., Hansen, G., Yu, L.-S., Pantalos, G., and Kolff, W.J. 1989b. Hemodynamic comparison of polyurethane trileaflet and bioprosthetic heart valves. *Trans. Am. Soc. Artif. Intern. Organs (ASAIO)* 35: 132–138.

Chandran, K.B., Kim, S.-H., and Han, G. 1991a. Stress distribution on the cusps of a polyurethane trileaflet heart valve prosthesis in the closed position. *J. Biomech.* 24: 385–395.

Chandran, K.B., Lee, C.S., Shipkowitz, T., Chen, L.D., Yu, L.S. and Wurzel, D. 1991b. *In vitro* hemodynamic analysis of flexible artificial ventricle. *Artif. Organs* 15: 420–426.

Chandran, K.B., Gao, D., Han, G., Baraniewski, H., and Corson, J.D. 1992. Finite element analysis of arterial anastomosis with vein, Dacron® and PTFE grafts. *Med. Biol. Eng. Comp.* 30: 413–418.

Chandran, K.B., Lee, C.S., and Chen, L.D. 1994a. Pressure field in the vicinity of mechanical valve occluders at the instant of valve closure: Correlation with cavitation initiation. *J. Heart Valve Dis.* 3(Suppl. 1): S65–S76.

Chandran, K.B., Lee, C.S., Aluri, S., Dellsperger, K.C., Schreck, S., and Wieting, D.W. 1994b. Pressure distribution near the occluders and impact forces on the outlet struts of Björk–Shiley convexo-concave valves during closing. *J. Heart Valve Dis.* 5: 199–206.

Chandran, K. B., Dexter, E. U., Aluri, S., and Richenbacher, W.E. 1998. Negative pressure transients with mechanical heart-valve closure: Correlation between *in vitro* and *in vivo* results. *Ann. Biomed. Eng.* 26: 546–556.

Cheon, G.J. and Chandran, K.B. 1994. Transient behavior analysis of a mechanical monoleaflet heart valve prosthesis in the closing phase. *Am. Soc. Mech. Eng. J. Biomech. Eng.* 116: 452–459.

Cragg, A.H. and Dake, M.D. 1993. Percutaneous femoropoliteal graft placement. *Radiology* 187: 643–648.

Dake, M.D., Miller, D.C., Semba, C.P. et al. 1994. Transluminal placement of endovascular stent-grafts for the treatment of descending thoracic aortic aneurysms. *N. Engl. J. Med.* 331: 1729–1734.

Dellsperger, K.C. and Chandran, K.B. 1991. Prosthetic heart valves. In *Blood Compatible Materials and Devices. Perspectives towards the 21st Century.* Sharma, C.P. and Szycher, M., eds. Technomic Publishing Company Inc., Lancaster, PA, pp. 153–165.

DeVries, W.C. and Joyce, L.D. 1983. The artificial heart. *CIBA Clin. Symp.*, 35: 1–32.

Drogue, J. and Villafana, M. 1997. ATS Medical open pivot™ valve. In *Surgery for Acquired Aortic Valve Disease.* Piwnica, A. and Westaby, S., eds. ISIS Medical Media, Oxford, pp. 410–416.

Farrar, D.J., Litwak, P., Lawson, J.H., Ward, R.S., White, K.A., Robinson, A.J., Rodvein, R., and Hill, J.D. 1988. *In vivo* evaluations of a new thromboresistant polyurethane for artificial heart blood pumps. *J. Thorac. Cardiovasc. Surg.* 95: 191–200.

Gerring, E.L., Bellhouse, B.J., Bellhouse, F.H., and Haworth, F.H. 1974. Long term animal trials of the Oxford aortic/pulmonary valve prosthesis without anticoagulants. *Trans. ASAIO* 20: 703–708.

Ghista, D.N. and Reul, H. 1977. Optimal prosthetic aortic leaflet valve: Design, parametric and longevity analysis: Development of the avcothane-51 leaflet valve based on the optimal design analysis. *J. Biomech.* 10: 313–324.

Guidoin, R. and Couture, J. 1991. Polyester prostheses: The outlook for the future. In *Blood Compatible Materials and Devices. Perspectives towards the 21st Century.* Sharma, C.P. and Szycher, M., eds. Technomic Publishing Company, Inc., Lancaster, PA, pp. 153–165.

Guidoin, R., Gosselin, C., Martin, L., Marios, M., Laroche, F., King, M., Gunasekara, K., Domurado, D., and Sigot-Luizard, M.F. 1983. Polyester prostheses as substitutes in the thoracic aorta of dogs. I. Evaluation of commercial prostheses. *J. Biomed. Mater. Res.* 17: 1049–1077.

Hamid, M.S., Sabbah, H.N., and Stein, P.D. 1985. Finite element evaluation of stresses on closed leaflets of bioprosthetic heart valves with flexible stents. *Finite Elem. Anal. Des.* 1: 213–225.

Harold, M., Lo, H.B., Reul, H., Muchter, H., Taguchi, K., Gierspien, M., Birkle, G., Hollweg, G., Rau, G., and Messmer, B.J. 1987. The Helmholtz Institute tri-leaflet polyurethane heart valve prosthesis: Design, manufacturing, and first *in vitro* and *in vivo* results. In *Polyurethanes in Biomedical Engineering II.* Planck, H., Syre, I., and Dauner, M., eds., Elsevier, Amsterdam, pp. 321–356.

Holfert, J.W., Reibman, J.B., Dew, P.A., De Paulis, R., Burns, G.L., and Olsen, D.B. 1987. A new connector system for total artificial hearts: Preliminary results. *Trans. ASAIO* 10: 151–156.

Hufnagel, C.A. 1977. Reflections on the development of valvular prostheses. *Med. Instrum.* 11: 74–76.

Hunter, G.C., Schmidt, S.P., Sharp, W.V., and Malindzak, G.S. 1983. Controlled flow studies in 4 mm endothelialized Dacron® grafts. *Trans. ASAIO* 29: 177–182.

Jarvick, R.K. 1981. The total artificial heart. *Sci. Am.* 244: 66–72.

Jarvis, P., Tarbell, J.M., and Frangos, J.A. 1991. An *in vitro* evaluation of an artificial heart. *Trans. ASAIO* 37: 27–32.

Kafesjian, R., Howanec, M., Ward, G.D., Diep, L., Wagstaff, L.S., and Rhee, R. 1994. Cavitation damage of pyrolytic carbon in mechanical heart valves. *J. Heart Valve Dis.* 3 (Suppl. 1): S2–S7.

Kambic, H.E. and Nose, Y. 1991. Biomaterials for blood pumps. In *Blood Compatible Materials and Devices. Perspectives Towards the 21st Century.* Sharma, C.P. and Szycher, M., eds. Technomic Publishing Company, Inc., Lancaster, PA, pp. 141–151.

Keynton, R.S., Rittgers, S.E., and Shu, M.C.S. 1991. The effect of angle and flow rate upon hemodynamics in distal vascular graft anastomoses: An *in vitro* model study. *ASME J. Biomech. Eng.* 113: 458–463.

Kim, S.H., Chandran, K.B., and Chen, C.J. 1992. Numerical simulation of steady flow in a two-dimensional total artificial heart model. *ASME J. Biomech. Eng.* 114: 497–503.

Kim, Y.H. and Chandran, K.B. 1993. Steady flow analysis in the vicinity of an end-to-end anastomosis. *Biorheology* 30: 117–130.

Kim, Y.H., Chandran, K.B., Bower, T.J., and Corson, J.D. 1993. Flow dynamics across end-to-end vascular bypass graft anastomoses. *Ann. Biomed. Eng.* 21: 311–320.

Lapeyre, D.M., Frazier, O.H., and Conger, J.L. 1994. *In vivo* evaluation of a trileaflet mechanical heart valve. *ASAIO J.* 40: M707–M713.

Lee, C.S. and Chandran, K.B. 1994. Instantaneous backflow through peripheral clearance of Medtronic Hall valve at the moment of closure. *Ann. Biomed. Eng.* 22: 371–380.

Lee, C.S. and Chandran, K.B. 1995. Numerical simulation of instantaneous backflow through central clearance of bileaflet mechanical heart valves at the moment of closure: Shear stress and pressure fields within the clearance. *Med. Biol. Eng. Comp.* 33: 257–263.

Lee, C.S., Chandran, K.B., and Chen, L.D. 1994. Cavitation dynamics of mechanical heart valve prostheses. *Artif. Organs* 18: 758–767.

Lee, J.M. and Boughner, D.R. 1991. Bioprosthetic heart valves: Tissue mechanics and implications for design. In *Blood Compatible Materials and Devices. Perspectives Towards the 21st Century.* Sharma, C.P. and Szycher, M., eds. Technomic Publishing Company, Inc., Lancaster, PA, pp. 167–188.

Lefrak, E.A. and Starr, A., Eds. 1970. *Cardiac Valve Prostheses.* Appleton-Century-Crofts, New York.

Leuer, L. 1987. Dynamics of mechanical valves in the artificial heart. *Proc. 40th Ann. Conf. Eng. Med. Biol.* (ACEMB), p. 82.

Marin, M.L., Veith, F.J., Panetta, T.F. et al. 1994. Transluminally placed endovascular stented graft repair for arterial trauma. *J. Vasc. Surg.* 20: 466–473.

McKenna, J. 1997. The Ultracor™ prosthetic heart valve. In *Surgery for Acquired Aortic Valve Disease.* Piwnica, A. and Westaby, S., eds. ISIS Medical Media, Oxford, pp. 337–340.

Ojha, M., Ethier, C.R., Johnston, K.W., and Cobbold, R.S.C. 1990. Steady and pulsatile flow fields in an end-to-side arterial anastomosis model. *J. Vasc. Surg.* 12: 747–753.

Park, J.B. and Lakes, R.S. 1992. *Biomaterials: An Introduction*, 2nd ed. Plenum Press, New York.

Parodi, J.C., Palmaz, J.C., and Barone, H.D. 1991. Transfemoral intraluminal graft implantation for abdominal aortic aneurysms. *Ann. Vasc. Surg.* 5: 491–499.

Phillips, R.E. and Printz, L.K. 1997. PhotoFix™ α: A pericardial aortic prosthesis. In *Surgery for Acquired Aortic Valve Disease.* Piwnica, A. and Westaby, S., eds. ISIS Medical Media, Oxford, pp. 376–381.

Phillips, W.M., Brighton, J.A., and Pierce, W.S. 1979. Laser Doppler anemometer studies in unsteady ventricular flows. *Trans. ASAIO* 25: 56–60.

Piwnica, A. and Westaby, S., Eds. 1997. *Surgery for Acquired Aortic Valve Disease.* ISIS Medical Media, Oxford.

Reif, T.H. 1991. A numerical analysis of the back flow between the leaflets of a St. Jude Medical cardiac valve prosthesis. *J. Biomech.* 24: 733–741.

Reis, R.L., Hancock, W.D., Yarbrough, J.W., Glancy, D.L., and Morrow, A.G. 1971. The flexible stent. *J. Thorac. Cardiovasc. Surg.* 62: 683–691.

Reul, H., Steinseifer, U., Knoch, M., and Rau, G. 1995. Development, manufacturing and validation of a single leaflet mechanical heart valve prosthesis. *J. Heart Valve Dis.* 4: 513–519.

Rhee, K. and Tarbell, J.M. 1994. A study of wall shear rate distribution near the end-to-end anastomosis of a rigid graft and a compliant artery. *J. Biomech.* 27: 329–338.

Rodgers, V.G.J., Teodori, M.F., and Borovetz, H.S. 1987. Experimental determination of mechanical shear stress about an anastomotic junction. *J. Biomech.* 20: 795–803.

Roe, B.B., Owsley, J.W., and Boudoures, P.C. 1958. Experimental results with a prosthetic aortic valve. *J. Thorac. Cardiovasc. Surg.* 36: 563–570.

Rosenberg, G. 1995. Artificial heart and circulatory assist devices. In *The Biomedical Engineering Handbook.* Bronzino, J.D., ed. CRC Press, Boca Raton, FL, pp. 1839–1846.

Rosenberg, G., Snyder, A.J., Weiss, W.J., Sapirstein, J.S., and Pierce, W.S. 1995. *In vivo* testing of a clinical-size totally implantable artificial heart. In *Assisted Circulation 4.* F. Unger, ed. Springer, Berlin, pp. 235–248.

Russel, F.B., Lederman, D.M., Singh, P.I., Cumming, R.D., Levine, F.H., Austen, W.G., and Buckley, M.J. 1980. Development of seamless trileaflet valves. *Trans. ASAIO* 26: 66–70.

Sabbah, H.N., Hamid, M.S., and Stein, P.D. 1985. Estimation of mechanical stresses on closed cusps of porcine bioprosthetic valves: Effect of stiffening, focal calcium and focal thinning. *Am. J. Cardiol.* 55: 1091–1097.

Shim, H.S. and Lenker, J.A. 1988. Heart valve prostheses. In *Encyclopedia of Medical Devices and Instrumentation*, Vol. 3. Webster, J.G., ed. Wiley Interscience, New York, pp. 1457–1474.

Strandness, D.E. and Sumner, D.S. 1975. Grafts and grafting. In *Hemodynamics for Surgeons.* Grune and Stratton, New York, pp. 342–395.

Tarbell, J.M., Gunishan, J.P., Geselowitz, D.B., Rosenberg, G., Shung, K.K., and Pierce, W.S. 1986. Pulsed ultrasonic Doppler velocity measurements inside a left ventricular assist device. *ASME J. Biomech. Eng.* 108: 232–238.

Thubrikar, M.J., Skinner, J.R., and Nolan, S.P. 1982a. Design and stress analysis of bioprosthetic valves *in vivo*. In *Cardiac Bioprostheses.* Cohn, L.H. and Gallucci, V., eds. Yorke Medical Books, New York, pp. 445–455.

Thubrikar, M.J., Skinner, J.R., Eppink, T.R., and Nolan, S.P. 1982b. Stress analysis of porcine bioprosthetic heart valves *in vivo*. *J. Biomed. Mater. Res.* 16: 811–826.

Unger, F. 1989. *Assisted Circulation*, Vol. 3. Springer, Berlin.

Van der Lei, B., Wildevuur, C.R.H., Niewenhuis, P., Blaauw, E.H., Dijk, F., Hulstaert, C.E., and Molenaar, I. 1985. Regeneration of the arterial wall in microporous, compliant, biodegradable vascular grafts after implantation into the rat abdominal aorta. *Cell Tissue Res.* 242: 569–578.

Van der Lei, B., Wildevuur, C.R.H., and Nieuwenhuis, P. 1986. Compliance and biodegradation of vascular grafts stimulate the regeneration of elastic laminae in neoarterial tissue: An experimental study in rats. *Surgery* 99: 45–51.

Veith, F.J., Abbott, W.M., Yao, J.S.T. et al. 1995. Guidelines for development and use of transluminally placed endovascular prosthetic grafts in the arterial system. *J. Vasc. Surg.* 21: 670–685.

Wieting, D.W. 1997. Prosthetic heart valves in the future. In *Surgery for Acquired Aortic Valve Disease.* Piwnica, A. and Westaby, S., eds. ISIS Medical Media, Oxford, pp. 460–478.

Wurzel, D., Kolff, J., Missfeldt, W., Wildevuur, W., Hansen, G., Brownstein, L., Reibman, J., De Paulis, R., and Kolff, W.J. 1988. Development of the Philadelphia heart system. *Artif. Organs* 12: 410–422.

Yoganathan, A.P., Corcoran, W.H., and Harrison, E.C. 1979a. *In vitro* velocity measurements in the vicinity of aortic prostheses. *J. Biomech.* 12: 135–152.

Yoganathan, A.P., Corcoran, W.H., and Harrison, E.C. 1979b. Pressure drops across prosthetic aortic heart valves under steady and pulsatile flow—*In vitro* measurements. *J. Biomech.* 12: 153–164.

Yoganathan, A.P., Woo, Y.R., and Sung, H.W. 1986. Turbulent shear stress measurements in the vicinity of aortic heart valve prostheses. *J. Biomech.* 19: 433–442.

Yusef, S.W., Baker, D.M., Chuter, T.A.M. et al. 1994. Transfemoral endoluminal repair of abdominal aortic aneurysm with bifurcated graft. *Lancet* 344: 650–651.

36.2 Nonblood-Interfacing Implants for Soft Tissues

Most tissues other than bone and cartilage are of the soft category. Soft tissue implants do not generally interface directly with blood; the exceptions are located primarily in the cardiovascular systems. Nonblood-interfacing soft tissue implants are used to augment or replace natural tissues or to redirect specific biological functions. The implants can be transient, that is, of short-term function and thus made of absorbable materials. In contrast, the implants can be long term, that is, of prolonged function and thus made of nonabsorbable materials.

The successful development of a new biomedical device or implant, including those used for soft tissues, encompasses (1) acquiring specific biological and biomechanical data about the implant site and its function, to meet carefully developed product requirements; (2) constructing a prototype and evaluating its physical and biological properties both *in vitro* and *in vivo*, using appropriate benchtop and animal models; and (3) conducting a clinical study following a successful battery of animal safety studies. The extent of the studies associated with any specific milestone can vary considerably and is dependent on intended application and the availability of historical safety and clinical data for the material or design. Several general guidelines are common to all soft tissue implants; specifically, the implant must (1) exhibit physical properties (e.g., flexibility and texture), which are equivalent or comparable to those specified in the product profile; (2) maintain the expected physical properties after implantation for a defined time period; (3) elicit no adverse tissue reaction; (4) display no carcinogenic, toxic, allergenic, and/or immunogenic effects; (5) be readily sterilized without compromising physicochemical properties; and (6) be designed with regard to esthetics. In addition to these criteria, a clinically translatable product is expected to (1) be easily produced in high quantity at a reasonable cost; (2) have acceptable esthetic quality; (3) be enclosed in durable, properly labeled, easy-access packaging; and (4) have adequate shelf stability.

The most common types of soft tissue implants are (1) sutures and allied augmentation devices; (2) percutaneous and cutaneous systems; (3) maxillofacial devices; (4) ear and eye prostheses; (5) space-filling implants; and (6) fluid transfer devices.

36.2.1 Sutures and Allied Augmentation Devices

Sutures and staples are the most common types of augmentation devices. Interest in using tapes and adhesives has increased and will continue to do so, as new, efficacious systems are developed.

36.2.1.1 Sutures and Suture Anchors

Sutures are usually packaged as a thread attached to a metallic needle. Although most needles are made of stainless-steel alloys, the thread component can be made of various materials, and the type used determines the class of the entire suture. In fact, it is common to refer to the thread as the suture. Presently, most needles are drilled (mechanically or by laser) at one end for thread insertion. The thread may be secured in the needle hole by crimping or adhesive attachment. Among the critical physical properties of sutures are their diameter, *in vitro* knot strength, needle-holding strength, needle penetration force, ease of knotting, knot security, and *in vitro* strength retention profile (Postelthwait et al., 1959).

Two types of threads are used in suture manufacturing and are distinguished according to the retention of their properties in the biologic environment, namely whether they are absorbable or nonabsorbable (Shalaby, 1985). Sutures are also categorized according to their chemistry and source, that is, whether they are naturally derived (e.g., catgut, silk, and cotton) or synthetically manufactured (e.g., nylon, polyethylene terephthalate, polypropylene, and polyglycolide and its copolymers) or from a metallic source (e.g., stainless steel and tantalum). Sutures may also be categorized with respect to their configuration, that is, whether they are monofilament, twisted, or braided multifilament (i.e., "braids").

The absorbable catgut, the first known suture, is made primarily of collagen derived from sheep intestinal submucosa and is crosslinked with a chromic salt to increase its *in vivo* strength retention and slow its absorption. This treatment extends the functional performance of a catgut suture from 1 to 2 weeks to about 3 weeks. Catgut sutures are packaged in a specially formulated fluid to prevent drying and maintain necessary compliance for surgical handling and knot formation.

The use of synthetic absorbable sutures has exceeded that of catgut over the past three decades (Shalaby, 1985, 1988). This increase is attributed to many factors specific to the synthetic materials, including (1) higher initial breaking strength and superior handling characteristics; (2) availability of sutures with a broad range of *in vivo* strength retention profiles; (3) considerably milder tissue reactions and no immunogenic response; and (4) reproducible properties and highly predictable *in vivo* performance. Polyglycolide (PG) was the first synthetic absorbable suture to be introduced, approximately five decades ago. Because of the high modulus of oriented fibers, PG is made mostly in the braided form. A typical PG suture braid absorbs in about 4 months and retains partial *in vivo* strength after 3 weeks. Braids made of the 90/10 glycolide/L-lactide copolymer have a comparable or improved strength retention profile and faster absorption rate relative to PG. The copolymeric sutures absorb in about 3 months and have gained wide acceptance by the surgical community.

As with other types of braided sutures, an absorbable coating that improves suture handling and knot formation has been added to the absorbable braids. To minimize the risk of infection and tissue drag that are sometimes associated with braided sutures, four types of monofilament sutures were commercialized. These absorbable monofilaments were designed by combining appropriate materials, such as polydioxanone (PDS) and copolymers of glycolide with caprolactone or trimethylene carbonate, specifically to target the lower modulus, higher compliance of braided, absorbable sutures (Shalaby, 1985, 1988).

Members of the nonabsorbable family of sutures include braided silk (a natural protein), nylon, and polyethylene terephthalate (PET). These braids are used as coated sutures. Although silk sutures have retained wide acceptance by surgeons, nylon and, in particular, PET sutures are used for critical procedures where high strength and predictable long-term performance are required. Meanwhile, the use of cotton sutures has radically decreased because of their low strength and occasional tissue reactivity due to contaminants. Monofilaments are important forms of nonabsorbable sutures and are primarily limited to polypropylene, nylon, and stainless steel. An interesting application of monofilament sutures is illustrated in the use of polypropylene loops (or "haptics," used to anchor the lens) for intraocular lenses (IOLs). The polypropylene sutures exhibit not only the desirable properties of monofilaments, but also the biologic inertness necessary for ocular application; these sutures elicit minimal tissue reactions with use in almost all surgical sites. With the exception of its natural tendency to undergo hydrolytic degradation and, hence, continued loss of mechanical strength postoperatively, nylon monofilament has similar attributes to those of polypropylene monofilaments. Because of their exceptionally high modulus, stainless-steel sutures are not used in soft tissue repair because they can tear these tissues. All sutures can be sterilized by gamma radiation, except those made of synthetic absorbable polymers, polypropylene, or cotton, which are sterilized by ethylene oxide (Shalaby, 1985, 1988).

The tissue suture anchor is related to the suture and is used to attach soft tissue to bone, particularly in shoulder repair. Suture anchors have been used routinely over the past two decades. Sutures are linked to anchors through an eyelet on the anchor. The anchor is embedded into bone and the affixed suture can be used to reattach the soft tissue. Initially, metal anchors were used; however, these implants can cause complications with revision surgeries (Bottoni et al., 2008). Absorbable materials, including polyglycolide, polylactide, and copolymers thereof, have been used clinically as anchors. More recently, blends of tricalcium phosphate and polyglycolide/polylactide have been used to improve anchor osteo-conductivity. Initial concerns regarding early weakening of polyglycolide anchors and subsequent release of acidic degradants, particularly during the crucial tissue healing stage, have lead to the development of slower absorbing lactide/glycolide and lactide anchors.

36.2.1.2 Nonsuture Fibrous and Microporous Implants

Woven PET and polypropylene fabrics are commonly used as surgical meshes for abdominal wall repair and similar surgical procedures where surgical "patching" is required. Recently, absorbable mesh with fast and slow degrading fiber components was introduced into the clinic. This unique construction facilitates a wide range of mechanical, chemical, and physical properties and allows modulation of the mesh absorption profile. Braid forms and similar construction made of multifilament PET yarns have been used for repairing tendons and ligaments. Microporous foams of polytetrafluoroethylene (PTFE) are used as pledgets (to aid in anchoring sutures to soft tissues) and in repair of tendons and ligaments. Microporous collagen and chitosan-based foams are used in wound repair to accelerate healing (Shalaby, 1985).

36.2.1.3 Clips, Staples, and Pins

Ligating clips are most commonly used for temporary or long-term management of the flow in tubular tissues. Titanium clips are among the oldest and versatile types of clips; tantalum and stainless steel have also found use in ligation. Thermoplastic polymers such as nylon can be injection-molded into different forms of ligating clips. These clips are normally designed to have a latch and living hinge. Absorbable polymers made of lactide/glycolide copolymers and PDS have been successfully converted to ligating clips, incorporating different design features for a broad range of applications.

Staples generally provide a less expensive, faster alternative to sutures; however, staples provide less initial wound security and are limited to locations which do not have large tensile loads and do not have inflamed and/or thicker or more sensitive tissue (Tobias, 2007). Metallic staples were introduced about four decades ago as strong competitors to sutures for wound augmentation; their use has grown considerably over the past 20 years for everything from skin closure procedures to a multiplicity of internal surgical applications. Major advantages associated with the use of staples include ease of application and reduction of surgical time, minimized tissue trauma, and reduction in contamination. Metallic staples can be made of tantalum, stainless steel, or titanium–nickel alloys. Staples find use particularly in the closure of large incisions, such as those associated with bowel or gastric surgery. Many interesting applications of small staples have been discovered for ophthalmic and endoscopic use, both of which are fast-growing areas of minimally invasive surgery. Thermoplastic materials based on lactide/glycolide copolymers have been used to produce absorbable staples for skin and internal wound closures (Shall and Cawley, 1994). These staples consist primarily of two interlocking components, a fastener and a receiver. The staples are advantageous in that they provide a quick means of closure with comparable infection resistance. Polyethylene glycol-based gel formed have been developed to serve as suture or staple adjuvants, reducing the number of necessary sutures or staples (Allan et al., 1999a).

Traditional suturing and stapling of skin require puncturing of the epidermis and dermis, increasing the chance of infection and of tearing the wound site; hence, additional focus over the past decade has been on subcuticular closure, where only the dermis is punctured by the fastener. Attempts have been made, with limited success, to commercialize lactide/glycolide subcutaneous pin fasteners that are introduced directly across interdigitated dermal wound edges. Unfortunately, the zigzag-like or serpentine tissue configuration can lead to wound healing issues and an esthetically displeasing result. Accordingly, absorbable pronged clips (similar to bandage clips) and barbed sutures are being investigated as potential subcuticular devices.

36.2.1.4 Surgical Tapes

Surgical tape may be used to adhere skin grafts to a wound site or to close a surgical wound in select cases, particularly low-tension wounds, where sutures are not desired. Tape also offers the obvious surgical advantage of avoiding a needle stick. Previous studies suggest that, when the wound edges are aligned and closely approximated using tape, the wound tensile strength exceeds that of sutured wounds up to approximately 150 days into the healing process (Chen et al., 2001). This difference is attributed to the higher density, ordered packing of collagen at earlier time frames in the taped wound site. Tapes avoid abscesses and/or tissue necrosis that can occur with suturing (Brunius and Ahrén, 1969); tape can also result in a more esthetically pleasing end result (i.e., avoiding cross-hatching scars caused by needle skin puncture), assuming that the wound edges are properly aligned and the tape remains adhered throughout the healing process. Tape may be used to align wound edges of weakened tissues that would not withstand suturing. Tape can be susceptible to peeling, particularly in an infected or a moist wound site; however, careful management in a clinical setting avoids deleterious effects of peeling (Webster and Davis, 1975). A small fraction of patients are allergic to tape adhesive; and application of tape to these individuals can result in tissue swelling and increased healing times. Obese patients may experience greater swelling; tape must be applied accordingly as undue wound tension due to swelling and constriction by tape can cause blistering. Tape removal is faster and less painful than removal of nonabsorbable sutures. Clearly, the wound depth and involved tissues will influence the cosmetic outcome and scar area, where retracted incised subcutaneous muscles will result in a larger scar area.

36.2.1.5 Tissue Adhesives

Tissue adhesives are used to repair exceptionally soft and/or fragile tissues, which cannot be easily repaired with sutures because sutures inflict substantial damage through tissue penetration, knotting, and associated biomechanical stresses. The wide range of soft tissues and related regenerative capacity means that the development of a "one size fits all" tissue adhesive is difficult. Generally, the ultimate tissue adhesive should be easy to apply, painless, and absorbable. Furthermore, this adhesive must wet and bond to tissues and polymerize without causing excessive heat or toxic response. The two most common types of tissue adhesives in clinical use, neither of which satisfy all the criteria, are based on alkyl-*O*-cyanoacrylates and fibrin. The latter is a natural adhesive derived from fibrinogen, which is one of the clotting components of blood. Although fibrin is used in Europe (Lovisetto et al., 2007), its use in the United States has been approved only recently for specific use in cardiovascular surgery; the slow approval was because of the perceived risk of fibrin contamination with hepatitis and/or immune disease viruses. Due to its limited mechanical strength (tensile strength and elastic modulus of 0.1 and 0.15 MPa, respectively), fibrin is used mostly as a sealant and for adjoining delicate tissues, as in nerve anastomoses.

Meanwhile, three members of the cyanoacrylate family of adhesives, *n*-butyl-, *iso*-butyl-, and 2-octyl-cyanoacrylates, are used in a number of countries as sealants and adhesives. Butyl-cyanoacrylates and octyl-cyanoacrylates are considered "blocking agents," as they provide a barrier to microbial invasion. These cyanoacrylates, although not considered absorbable, are generally sloughed from the wound site within 5–10 days following application. In 2006, a U.S. Food and Drug Administration (US FDA) panel unanimously recommended that the tissue adhesive for the topical approximation of skin (i.e., not inclusive of nontopical use, such as tissue adhesive for use in embolization of cerebral arteriovenous malformation or tissue adhesive for ophthalmic use, which still require premarket approval) be reclassified from class III to class II with special controls; a notice announcing the reclassification of this device type was issued shortly thereafter (Mattamal, 2010). The *n*-butyl and 2-octyl-cyanoacrylates were only recently approved for use in the United States; the *iso*-butyl-cyanoacrylate has not yet been approved for use in the United States because of lack of sufficient safety data (Singer et al., 2008). The *n*-butyl-cyanoacrylate is approved in the United States for topical skin approximation as well as for embolization of cerebral arteriovenous malformations prior to surgical removal of malformed vessels. The 2-octyl-cyanoacrylate is also approved for topical skin approximation and is purported to have less toxicity and up to four times the strength of *n*-butyl-cyanoacrylate. Due to a fast rate of polymerization and limited ability to localize the adhesive to the specific surgical site, the *in vivo* performance of cyanoacrylates can be unpredictable. Cyanoacrylates may be used at high-tension wound sites if they are used in conjunction with an allied tissue fastener (e.g., surgical tape or other). Because of their low strength, cyanoacrylates are generally limited to use in traumatized or fragile tissues (such as scalp, face, spleen, liver, and kidney) or after extensive surgery on soft lung tissues. A major safety concern of these alkyl cyanoacrylates is related to their nonabsorbable nature. Hence, a number of investigators have directed their attention to certain alkoxy-alkyl cyanoacrylates, which can be converted to polymeric adhesives with acceptable absorbable profiles and rheological properties. Methoxypropyl cyanoacrylate, for example, has demonstrated both the absorbability and high compliance that is advantageous to soft tissue repair and is currently marketed as a sealant for veterinary use.

36.2.2 Percutaneous and Skin Implants

Percutaneous implants are found in a variety of applications where extracorporeal access, across the skin, to intracorporeal tissues, organs, or devices is required, both for temporary and chronic use. Examples of percutaneous implants include a port that is implanted to allow delivery of medication or nutrients, or a post that is used to connect hearing aids with the bone in the skull. Skin implants serve to minimize fluid loss and infection following loss of skin, usually due to burns. Skin implants have been designed as temporary and as permanent coverings.

36.2.2.1 Percutaneous Devices

Skin is highly proliferative, thus presenting a challenge to the design of a percutaneous implant that must be stable in the long term. Epithelium will rapidly grow to cover a seemingly denuded surface, including that of a smooth percutaneous device. Epithelial growth can result in avulsion or extrusion of a percutaneous implant or in marsupialization, where a pouch is formed around the implant. Of most concern is the invasion of bacteria into the space between the implant and the surrounding tissue (von Recum and Park, 1979). One obvious solution would appear to be to provide a rough surface that allows tissue integration. However, a rough surface is attractive to epithelium but also to bacteria; hence, infection is a large risk. Also, dermal cells rapidly turn over, so the long-term stability of a percutaneous implant is questionable. Several factors that influence the design of percutaneous devices include

1. Target application, or the function the device will serve, that is, transmitting signals (such as pressure, sound waves, temperature), energy (such as electricity, power), fluids (such as blood, spinal fluid), or providing foundational support (as in a dental or auricular post)
2. Engineering design criteria, including material type/constituents (ceramic, glass, metal, polymer, or composite), physical features (such as skirt, surface coating, surface texture), esthetics, and mechanical stresses (soft or hard interface, porous or smooth interface)
3. Host microenvironment, as determined by the species (e.g., cow, human, mouse, rabbit, sheep), and biochemical/biomechanical aspects of the implant location (e.g., abdomen, cranium, oral cavity)
4. Surgical and postsurgical handling and care

Percutaneous devices that are anchored in bone appear to have high rates of success due to a relatively intact interface between the implant and tissue (Reyes et al., 2000). However, devices that are anchored in soft tissue are susceptible to interfacial microtrauma and subsequent infection and failure (Fukano et al., 2006). Attempts have been made to incorporate antibiotics into the implants, but this raises concern that antibiotic resistance may develop with time. Poly(2-hydroxyethyl methacrylate) [poly(HEMA)], a soft material used in contact lenses, has been assessed as a potential material for percutaneous implants. Poly(HEMA) may be surface-treated or processed to include porous components. Preliminary findings suggest that, regardless of surface treatment, poly(HEMA) implants with pores of 40 micron or more allow connective tissue ingrowth and hence enhanced stabilization of the implants (Isenhath et l., 2007). No percutaneous devices are completely satisfactory; nevertheless, some researchers believe that addition of hydroxyapatite may lead to a successful approach. Hydroxyapatite-based percutaneous devices have been associated with less epidermal downgrowth when compared with silicone rubber control specimens in animal dental studies. Diamond-like carbon surface coatings inhibit infection, so a combination of hydroxyapatite and diamond-like coatings may be useful and are currently being investigated (Smith et al., 2006). Indeed, the surface topography has been consistently found to play a large role in tissue integration, where grooved surfaces seem to promote less infection and better tissue ingrowth than either smooth or pitted surfaces (Chehroudi and Brunette, 2002). Researchers have investigated coatings such as laminin-5, which keratinocytes normally produce to enhance migration, adhesion, and ingrowth (El-Ghannam et al., 1998; Uchida et al., 2004). More work will be necessary to pinpoint a simple and effective solution to the long-term maintenance of percutaneous implants.

36.2.2.2 Artificial Skins

A major cause of death for severely burned patients is infection as well as fluid and electrolyte loss. A wide variety of artificial skins have been developed to close burn wounds following excision of necrotic tissue (Jaksic and Burke, 1987). Criteria for artificial skins include good adherence to the wound site, elasticity, durability, bacterial resistance, hemostaticity, antisepticity, ease of application, ease of removal, nontoxicity, biocompatibility, nonantigenicity, durability, and low cost. Artificial skins that are permanent replacements have the added criteria of being esthetically pleasing.

After many early attempts to make artificial skin using tanned collagens, collagen gels, and collagen-impregnated PET mesh, a wound-covering dermis with controlled physicochemical properties was designed using a crosslinked collagen-polysaccharide (chondroitin 6-sulfate) composite membrane (Chvapil, 1982). This particular configuration was specifically constructed to have tunable porosity, flexibility, and moisture flux rate, but required an epidermal autograft. Subsequently, temporary artificial bilayered skin substitutes were developed, where temporary tissue-engineered replacements are particularly useful alternatives for burns requiring larger area coverage. These devices can be similar to a synthetic dressing, incorporating a nylon mesh and a silicone rubber component, but also integrating allogeneic fibroblasts. Of note, in these clinically available devices, the fibroblasts are grown on the construct; subsequently, the cellular construct is frozen for later transport. Hence, the purpose to the temporary covering is to stimulate or to allow fibrovascular growth into the wound bed by providing appropriate cellular products, for example, matrix proteins and growth factors. A related dermal technology was developed as a "permanent" covering, incorporating allogeneic fibroblasts on a degradable mesh. This product is also cryopreserved for shipping. Implantation of allogenic fibroblast/polymer constructs has proved to be useful for providing long-term skin replacement. Human fibroblasts are seeded on the nylon mesh and allowed to proliferate in culture, the concept being that the cells will release necessary growth factors and thus stimulate healing response in the wound. The cellular meshes are frozen, thus killing the cells but retaining the factors in the mesh for release following grafting. This device prevents water evaporation but has not been found to induce fibrovascular growth that may be necessary for preparing the wound bed for a permanent graft or skin substitute.

Epithelial cells derived from a burn patient may be cultured *in vitro* to cover a wound area, potentially a feasible option for superficial or partial thickness wounds. Deep dermal or full thickness skin wounds can be treated with a sheet of keratinocytes that are grown on mouse cell feeder layers. Although the mouse cells are not integrated in the substitute, the device is classified clinically as a xenotransplant. A related type of bilayered, tissue-engineered skin substitute has been developed that includes allogeneic combinations of human fibroblasts in bovine collagen and human epidermal cells (Hu et al., 2006). Research is focused on producing similar substitutes without bovine collagen.

36.2.3 Maxillofacial Implants

Maxillofacial implants may be used to correct defects such as those following head or neck cancer surgery or to correct congenital defects such as cleft palate. Maxillofacial implants are either extraoral, that is, those used to reconstruct defective regions in the maxilla, mandible, and face, or intraoral, those used to repair maxilla, mandibular, and facial bone defects. Polymeric implants used in extraoral repair should (1) be mechanically and chemically stable, (2) be easy to fabricate, (3) match color, texture, and features of the native tissue, and (4) easily attach to the native tissue. Polyvinyl chloride, polymethylmethacrylate, silicone, and polyurethane are used in the manufacture of these implants, with silicone being the most commonly used material due to its versatility. Rapid prototyping provides a means of building patient-customized molds with which silicone implants may be cast. Material requirements for the intraoral implants are similar to those of the extraoral implants, but lead largely to metals such as tantalum, titanium, and cobalt chromium alloys, although silicones and polymethylmethacrylate are used for gum and chin augmentation.

36.2.4 Ear and Eye Implants

Biomaterials have been commonly used in contact lens and IOL fabrication for the eye as well as to provide cochlear implants and middle ear repair. Ear implants are useful in correcting hearing loss due to middle ear hereditary defects such as otosclerosis or diseases such as chronic otitis media. A wide range of biomaterials have been investigated for middle and inner ear reconstruction, including bioglass, polymethylmethacrylate, polytetrafluoroethylene, polyethylene, silicone rubber, stainless steel, and tantalum for middle ear application and polytetrafluoroethylene–carbon composites, porous polyethylene, and pyrolytic carbon for cochlear, or inner ear, implants.

Design criteria for middle ear replacement include maintenance of shape, size, and acoustic transmission over decades. The implant is placed in a diseased environment and therefore must be extrusion- and resorption-resistant. The ends of middle ear ossicular implants must integrate well with bone (e.g., the stapes) or to soft tissue (e.g., the tympanic membrane) (Hoffmann et al., 2003). Ear implants have most recently been fashioned from porous high-molecular-weight polyethylene, hydroxyapatite, bioglass, or autograft from bone or cartilage. High-molecular-weight polyethylene implants can elicit a chronic foreign body response and are often subject to degradation over time. Bioglass can easily be broken into small fragments through the foreign body response and partially absorbed with time, while hydroxyapatite seems to elicit a more favorable response although resulting in encapsulation with connective tissue and epithelium. Cartilage autografts tend to resorb quickly, whereas bone autografts do not. Certainly tissue ingrowth and encapsulation with time can diminish sound conduction.

Cochlear, or inner ear, implants have undergone rapid advances over the past decade, particularly with respect to size. The implant is surgically placed under the skin behind the ear. An external microphone collects the sound, while a speech processor filters the sound to select audible speech and sends the sound signals to a transmitter (located behind the outer ear), and subsequently transmits power and the processed sound signals to the internal implant, consisting of a receiver and a stimulator secured in bone beneath the skin, which converts the signals into electric impulses, sending them through an internal cable to electrodes in the cochlea, which send the impulses to the nerves in the scala tympani and then to the brain (Gantz, 1987; White, 1982). The platinum (or other conducting metal) electrodes are mounted on silicone rubber and are connected to the internal receiver on one end and inserted into the cochlea deeper in the skull. Some individuals had have tissue necrosis of the skin flaps surrounding the implants, symptomatic of a percutaneous implant; hence, combination approaches may be used to minimize this reaction, for example, using hydroxyapatite-anchored bone implants.

Orbital repair materials are generally selected according to the size of the orbital defect. PDS, titanium meshes, bone, bone plus PDS/titanium mesh are used accordingly, where the absorbable PDS is reserved for small defects, while the combination products are used in large defect repair (Jaquiéry et al., 2007). Vision is directly correlated with many everyday simple activities, such as driving, reading, recognizing, recreating, and writing. The deterioration of eyesight has given rise to a great need for and the design of ocular implants. An IOL is an implant that is designed to correct vision by replacing a cloudy natural lens. The original IOLs were made of polymethylmethacrylate, a material which was found to be biocompatible in the eye, but which limited surgeries to larger incisions due to its rigidity. Early IOLs also allowed passage of light from the entire electromagnetic spectrum, with subsequent designs providing filtering of ultraviolet. Accordingly, soft materials such as silicone and acrylic were introduced, which could be folded for insertion through a smaller incision. An IOL includes an optics part, which is connected to the haptics, which one the appendages or struts that take various forms and are used to anchor the lens in place. Depending on the implant, the haptics may or may not be made of the same material as the lens. The shape of the lens plays an important role in determining not only the refractive index, but also the local tissue response, for example, the migration of lens epithelial cells onto the posterior capsule. For example, preliminary studies suggest that lenses with sharp corners can inhibit posterior capsule opacification, caused by cellular migration (Nishi et al., 2000). Foldable IOLs are more susceptive to discoloration/opacification and slight changes in refractive index, the latter perhaps attributable to the folding during surgical implantation. Preliminary studies have also focused on the development of light-adjustable IOLs that can be adjusted to tune refractive index postoperatively (Packer et al., 2004). IOLs have been developed that allow both distance vision and near vision.

Many blinding diseases of the eye have no implant solution or even therapy. With the progression of tissue engineering, one approach being investigated toward the treatment of adult onset blindness is the transplantation of retinal pigmented epithelium, either in sheets or spheroids. A major challenge in transplanting cellular sheets is the development of readily detachable (e.g., thermoresponsive) or absorbable materials on which to culture sheets of these or precursor cells. Both polyester-based absorbable materials and gelatin scaffolds have been tested as cell carriers in small-animal studies and have provided platforms on which cells could be delivered in more organized fashion. Nonetheless, the surgical handling of monolayer cellular sheets is challenging and the clinical feasibility of culturing cells on scaffolds for extended times preoperatively is low.

36.2.5 Space-Filling Implants

Pectoral, penile, testicular, and vaginal implants are silicone-based; implantation of these devices is considered elective surgery rather than surgery to improve physical health. Breast implants, the most common space-filling implants, have been an ongoing topic of regulatory interest. Early attempts to augment breast tissue were conducted with silicone or paraffin injections; with no means of containment, these liquids could not maintain shape or form and were more susceptible to infection, causing patient pain and complications. Subsequently, sponges made of polyvinyl alcohol were applied; however, these nonabsorbable, porous materials were infiltrated by soft tissue and calcified with time. Silicone or saline-filled silicone shell implants were developed for total breast reconstruction. Once implanted, these devices would naturally induce a foreign body response; the formation of collagen around the implants would in some instances become so tightly packed due to capsular contraction that a "marble" breast resulted. Additionally, some implants were susceptible to leakage and questions ensued, particularly with respect to silicone leakage. These implants were in use in the 1960s, before the US FDA had regulatory oversight of these devices. Accordingly, the US FDA did not initially approve silicone-filled implants for use; however, they approved a compassionate need exemption policy in 1992, which allowed silicone-filled implants to remain available, primarily to reconstruction patients and women who already had breast implants needing replacement. Saline-filled implants, however, were approved for use in 2000, and in late 2006, the US FDA approved specific silicone gel-filled breast implants with a number of postapproval conditions, including continued studies and rigorous patient-tracking requirements. The silicone breast implant envelope can be smooth or textured, where the debate continues as to whether the textured implants are more likely to leak and/or induce a greater capsular contraction. The development of tissue-engineered breast is ongoing, where fat or normal breast tissue may be derived from the patient and combined with an absorbable scaffold for transplantation (Holder et al., 1998). Composite injectables, comprised of cells loaded on absorbable beads and delivered in a degradable gel from a syringe, are of high interest as they conform to irregular defects, may be implanted in a minimally invasive manner, and may be readily modulated to serve a particular patient, or a particular application (Gomillion and Burg, 2006). A wide array of absorbable and/or degradable materials may be used in these composite systems, thus facilitating a wide range of application needs.

36.2.6 Fluid Transfer Implants

Fluid transfer implants, or shunts, are implemented to relieve fluid-affiliated problems related to conditions such as chronic ear infection, glaucoma, hydrocephalus, and urinary incontinence. Chronic ear infection, such as acute otitis media, results in inflammation of the middle ear and fluid accumulation. Drainage tubes, that is, tympanostomy tubes, are inserted into the ear drum to ventilate the middle ear, reduce fluid accumulation, and allow pressure equalization between the middle and outer ear, before being intentionally extruded or surgically removed. These tubes are temporary implants and have been made from polyethylene, PTFE, silicone, stainless steel, or titanium, where PTFE and silicone are the most frequently used materials. Problems with the implants can include premature extrusion, lack of timely extrusion, blockages, or the stimulation of fibrotic tissue that affects long-term hearing. The tube surface energy, microtopography, and chemistry affect biofilm formation following implantation. Ionized silicone tubes are more resistant to biofilm formation when compared with untreated silicone tubes; the ionized tubes have increased surface tension and decreased adhesion. The propensity for the development of tube blockages decreases with decreased biofilm formation. Phosphorylcholine, a zwitterionic phospholipid, has been used as a PTFE tubing coating; however, while preclinical studies have suggested a coating-induced decrease in biofilm formation, clinical studies have not shown significant differences in outcome when compared with other materials.

Glaucoma is a disease in which the optic nerve is damaged, causing loss of vision and possible increased pressure of the fluid in the eye. To treat glaucoma-related fluid pressure increase, a tube can be implanted to decrease the high intraocular fluid pressure caused by the aqueous humor, the fluid between the cornea and the lens of the eye (Hong et al., 2005). The tube serves as a conduit, directing fluid from the anterior eye chamber to the external subconjunctival space. Tubes may include a pressure-sensitive, unidirectional valve that provides resistance to the aqueous flow and prevents early, postoperative abnormally low pressure in the eye, while allowing later release of fluid once higher pressures are realized. The tube is attached to an endplate which is used to anchor the implant appropriately and to allow greater surface area for fluid release and distribution. If not designed carefully with respect to material and shape, the end plates can be particularly attractive to protein and plasma, which can lead to tissue inflammation, fibrosis, and obstruction of the tube. Additionally, the endplates are susceptible to micromotion, stemming from ocular movement. Endplates with opening/holes (fenestrations) can reduce micromotion by allowing integration of tissue to anchor the plates. Tubes and plates are typically made of silicone or polypropylene, where the stiffer polypropylene material may stimulate greater tissue reactions and become obstructed by cellular activities related to wound healing; consequently, researchers are investigating combining this device with an absorbable drug delivery plug to regulate fluid flow as well as the wound healing process.

Hydrocephalus, commonly known as "water on the brain," is a state where excess cerebrospinal fluid accumulates in the brain, causing abnormally increased intracranial pressure. Without treatment, this condition is potentially life-threatening. Hydrocephalus can be treated by draining the fluid through a shunt to a place such as the peritoneal cavity. A shunt consists of a perforated ventricular catheter, which allows collection of fluid from the cerebral ventricular spaces and flow through a valve that connects to a second catheter that is subcutaneously implanted to release fluid into the peritoneal cavity. These shunts, like other fluid transfer devices, are susceptible to failure by obstruction and infection. The largest reason for failure is blockage of the shunt, often caused by tissue ingrowth into the ventricular catheter. Valves have been developed that allow adjustment postsurgical implantation. Some implants have slits at the discharge end, which open above a critical fluid pressure. Recent focus has been on the impregnation of antimicrobials into the silicone in order to reduce the potential for infection (Zhong and Bellamkonda, 2008).

The urinary system presents an interesting biomaterials challenge of moving fluid in the correct direction as well as providing a fluid-tight seal. Urinary incontinence, the involuntary loss of bladder control, is difficult to treat with implants, because of the balance required in sealing liquid while not allowing salt or other urine-derived products to deposit and form blockages. Additionally, these conditions are difficult to control for infection. Urethral plugs have been used to simply prevent urine release; these devices are inserted/removed by the individual with each urination and promote higher rates of infection. Urethral slings can be placed around the urethra and attached to the abdominal wall, to treat urinary incontinence by repositioning the urethra and applying pressure to retain urine. Slings can be autograft or xenograft tissues, typically fascia or dermis, or synthetic polymers. A wide range of synthetic materials, including polyethylene, polyethyleneterephthalate, polypropylene, and PTFE, have been used in fabricating slings and have had limited long-term success as they are nonabsorbable materials and will eventually succumb to or cause mesh erosion, infection, pain, or fistula formation. Urethral injection therapy has been used, with moderate success, in building up the urethral sphincter valve, using biomaterials such as PTFE, glutaraldehyde cross-linked collagen, and autologous fat (Tsai et al., 2005). PTFE, although promising for the intended bulking application, is suspected to leach particles that can migrate throughout the body, potentially causing complications; products with this material have not acquired US FDA regulatory approval for use at this time. Type I collagen materials were the first US FDA approved implants for injectable application to urinary incontinence; they are bovine derived and can cause an allergic response in a small percentage of patients, as well as cause; a large inflammatory response in the majority of patients. Additionally, collagen resorbs with time; thus, a patient requires repeated injections with time. Similarly, injected fat resorbs with time. Pyrolytic carbon-coated zirconium oxide beads suspended in a water-based carrier gel containing beta-glucan are approved for United States use at this time. This injectable implant has short-term clinical results similar to collagen, but requires a large gauge needle for injection due to the large bead size (approximately 500 microns, on average), thereby increasing the chance for infection. It is thought that the high-modulus metal beads induce an acute inflammatory response, causing a granulomatous reaction and acute urine retention postinjection. Hyaluronic acid/dextranomer bead composites have also found application and are superior in their handling, as the beads are sufficiently small (approximately 100 microns, on average) to allow the use of small gauge needles. Although this injectable has distinct handling advantages and avoids issues related to migration, it does not promote tissue regeneration and is not perceived as superior to collagen alternatives. To improve the current state of the art, injectable implants are needed that are biocompatible, that stimulate regeneration of tissue, that do not migrate, and that absorb accordingly after promoting tissue growth.

Tissue-engineered devices also have applications in urinary repair; for example, an alginate-chondrocyte system was tested clinically to treat vesicoureteral reflux, a condition in which urine flows in reverse, from the bladder into the ureters or kidneys. The cellular material was endoscopically injected about the ureters to provide a "bulking" effect and prevent backflow of liquid. Preliminary results suggested that, in select patients, by transplanting the hydrogel system as a bulking agent below a refluxing ureter, neocartilage gradually developed to correct the reflux. Barring consistent clinical outcomes, other approaches are being developed, for example, injection of nonurologic autologous cells or injection of stem cells at different stages of differentiation. Uroepithelial cells, combined with porous, absorbable polyester matrices, for example, show promise in the replacement of urologic tissues.

36.2.7 Technologies of Emerging Interest

Implant fixation continues to be an ongoing area of new developments across all applications. Polyetherether ketone (PEEK) dental healing caps, that is, temporary caps used to protect exposed implants while a dental crown is being manufactured, already find clinical use. However, a process for uniaxial solid-state orientation, using a range of compressive forces and temperatures, has been developed to produce stock sheets of PEEK for machining dental implants, resulting in substantial increases in strength and modulus (Deng et al., 1999a; Clupper et al., 2004). Surface treatment of materials influences surface charge, topography, and conductivity. Surface treatment has obvious effects on cell adhesion and integration of traditional implants with surrounding tissues, and it has a profound effect on the success or failure of a tissue-engineered device. Research is ongoing to introduce cementless, polymeric

ndosteal dental implants for anchoring artificial teeth and bridging natural ones. For example, stud-
es addressing the use of surface phosphonylation to create hydroxyapatite-like substrates show that
1) surface-microtextured polypropylene and polyethylene transcortical implants in goat tibia having
phosphonate functionalities (with or without immobilized calcium ions) do induce bone ingrowth
nd (2) microtexture and surface-phosphonylated (with and without immobilized calcium ions) rods
nade of PEEK and similarly treated rods of carbon fiber-reinforced PEEK induce bone ingrowth when
mplanted in the toothless region of the lower jaw of goats (Allan et al., 1999b, 2000; Anneaux et al.,
2004). The use of surface-phosphonylated and posttreated (with a bridging agent) ultra-high-molecular-
weight polyethylene fibers and fabric produce high strength and modulus composites at exceptionally
ow filler loading (Deng et al., 1999b). Among these composites are those based on methyl methacrylate
matrices, similar to those used in bone cement.

The development of new biomaterials will continue to allow the bounds of medical possibilities to
be pushed forward. One common limiting factor across all nonblood-contacting applications is lack
of ideal biomaterials. Recent wound repair research, for example, has focused on the development of
p-dioxanone-based polyaxial polyesters and polyether-esters and their conversion into monofilament
sutures with modulated strength retention profiles and greater range of breaking strength retention
(Baum et al., 2010). The emergence of materials with new profiles into the clinical setting will allow
greater selection and better match of a biomaterial to a particular application. As another example,
researchers are continually introducing new bioinspired materials to human medicine. Gecko-inspired
adhesives, for example, are being assessed, the design of which emulate the microscopic hairs on a
gecko's foot, which adhere to surfaces through van der Waals forces (Autumn et al., 2000). The aggregate output of these seemingly weak forces is an enormously powerful adhesive, one that can potentially
form the basis for an adhesive tape that could be used again and again.

As new materials and processing of new materials evolve, so too will methods of assessing the devices.
Tissue test systems, or 3D-engineered tissues fabricated from cellular materials, will be increasingly useful in the design process (Burg and Boland, 2003). Test systems/organ culture may be used to test select
cellular responses to materials, for example, organ cultures have already been successfully developed to
assess epidermal response to percutaneous implants (Fukano et al., 2006; Fleckman and Olerud, 2008).
As the logistical hurdles of rapid prototyping of cellular materials are removed, complex tissues can be
built that better simulate the complexities and interactions in native tissue, thereby facilitating the development of enhanced biologically based diagnostics that will radically increase the speed of the implant
design and evaluation process and allow the development of personalized implants (Burg et al., 2010).

References

Allan, J.M., Kline, J.D., Wrana, J.S., Flagle, J.A., Corbett, J.T., and Shalaby, S.W. 1999a. Absorbable gel-
forming sealant/adhesives as a staple adjuvant in wound repair. *Trans. Soc. Biomater.* 22:374.

Allan, J.M., Wrana, J.S., Dooley, R.L., Budsberg, S., and Shalaby, S.W. 1999b. Bone ingrowth into surface-
phosphonylated polyethylene and polypropylene. *Trans. Soc. Biomat.* 22:468.

Allan, J.M., Wrana, J.S., Linden, D.E., Faris, H., Budsberg, S., Dooley, R.L., and Shalaby, S.W. 2000. Bone
formation into surface phosphonylated polymeric implants. *Crit. Rev. Biomed. Eng.* 28:377.

Anneaux, B.L., Hollinger, J.O., Budsburg, S.C., Fulton, L.K., and Shalaby, S.W. 2004. Surface activated
PEEK-based endosteal implants. 7th World Biomaterials Congress. *Trans. Soc. Biomater.* 27:967.

Autumn, K., Yiching, A., Liang, S., Hsieh T., Zesch, W., Chan, W.P., Kenny, T.W., Fearing, R., and Full, R.J.
2000. Adhesive force of a single gecko foot-hair. *Nature* 405:681.

Baum, B.P., Ingram, D.R., Linden, D.E., Taylor, M.S., Burg, K.J.L., and Shalaby, S.W. 2010. Modulation of
the properties of p-dioxanone copolymeric monofilament sutures. *Trans. Soc. Biomater.* 32(2):778.

Bottoni, C.R., Brooks, D.E., DeBerardino, T.M., Owens B.D., Judson, K.L., Eggers J.S., Mays M.Z., Brunius
U., and Ahrén C. 2008. A comparison of bioabsorbable and metallic suture anchors in a dynamically
loaded, intra-articular caprine model. *Orthopedics* 31(11):1106.

Brunius, U. and Ahrén, C. 1969. Healing impairment in skin incisions closed with silk sutures. A tensiometric and histologic study in the rat. *Acta Chir. Scand.* 135(5):369.

Burg, K.J.L. and Boland, T. 2003. Bioengineered devices: Minimally invasive tissue engineering composites and cell printing. *IEEE Eng. Med. Biol.* 22(5):84.

Burg, T.C., Parzel, C.A., Groff, R.E., Pepper, M., and Burg, K.J.L. 2010. Building off-the-shelf tissue engineered composites. *Philos. Trans. Royal Soc. A.* 368:1839–1862.

Chehroudi, B. and Brunette, D.M. 2002. Subcutaneous microfabricated surfaces inhibit epithelial recession and promote long-term survival of percutaneous implants. *Biomaterials* 23(1):229.

Chen, H.-H., Tsai, W.-S., Yeh, C.-Y., Wang, J.-Y., and Tang, R. 2001. Prospective study comparing wounds closed with tape with sutured wounds in colorectal surgery. *Arch. Surg.* 136:802.

Chvapil, M. 1982. Considerations on manufacturing principles of a synthetic burn dressing: A review. *J. Biomed. Mater. Res.* 16:245.

Clupper, D.C., Carpenter, K.A., Anneaux, B.L., and Shalaby, S.W. 2004. Orthogonal solid state orientation of absorbable polymers for orthopedic devices. 7th World Biomaterials Congress. *Trans. Soc. Biomater.* 27:458.

Deng, M., Wrana, J.S., Allan, J.M., and Shalaby, S.W. 1999a. Tailoring mechanical properties of polyetherether ketone for implants using solid-state orientation. *Trans. Soc. Biomater.* 22:477.

Deng, M., Allan, J.M., Lake, R.A., Gerdes, G.A., and Shalaby, S.W. 1999b. Effect of phosphonylation on UHMW-PE fabric-reinforced composites. *Trans. Soc. Biomater.* 22:470.

El-Ghannam, A., Starr, L., and Jones, J. 1998. Laminin-5 coating enhances epithelial cell attachment, spreading, and hemidesmosome assembly on Ti–6Al–4V implant material *in vitro*. *J. Biomed. Mater. Res.* 41:30.

Fleckman, P. and Olerud, J.E. 2008. Models for the histologic study of the skin interface with percutaneous biomaterials. *Biomed. Mater.* 3(3):1.

Fukano, Y., Knowles, N.G., Usui, M.L., Underwood, R.A., Hauch, K.D., Marshall, A.J., Ratner, B.D. et al., 2006. Characterization of an *in vitro* model for evaluating the interface between skin and percutaneous biomaterials. *Wound Rep Reg.* 14:484.

Gantz, B.J. 1987. Cochlear implants: An overview. *Acta Otolaryng. Head Neck Surg.* 1:171.

Gomillion, C. and Burg, K.J.L. 2006. Stem cells and soft tissue engineering. *Biomaterials* 27(36):6052.

Hoffmann, K.K., Kuhn, J.J., and Strasnick, B. 2003. Bone cements as adjuvant techniques for ossicular chain reconstruction. *Otol. Neurotol.* 24(1):24.

Holder, W.D., Jr., Gruber, H.E., Moore, A.L., Culberson, C.R., Anderson, W., Burg, K.J.L., and Mooney, D.J. 1998. Cellular ingrowth and thickness changes in poly-L-lactide and polyglycolide matrices implanted subcutaneously in the rat. *J. Biomed. Mater. Res.* 41:412–421.

Hong, C.-H., Arosemena, A., Zurakowski, D., and Ayyala, R.S. 2005. Glaucoma drainage devices: A systematic literature review and current controversies. *Surv. Ophthal.* 50(1):48–60.

Hu, S., Kirsner, R.S., Falanga, V., Phillips, T., and Eaglstein, W.H. 2006. Evaluation of Apligrafs persistence and basement membrane restoration in donor site wounds: A pilot study. *Wound Rep. Reg.* 14:427.

Isenhath, S.N., Fukano, Y., Usui, M.L., Underwood, R.A., Irvin, C.A., Marshall, A.J., Hauch, K.D., Ratner, B.D., Fleckman, P., and Olerud, J.E. 2007. A mouse model to evaluate the interface between skin and a percutaneous device. *J. Biomed. Mater. Res. A.* 83A(4):915.

Jaksic, T. and Burke, J.F. 1987. The use of "artificial skin" for burns. *Ann. Rev. Med.* 38:107.

Jaquiéry, C., Aeppli, C., Cornelius, P., Palmowsky, A., Kunz, C., and Hammer, B. 2007. Reconstruction of orbital wall defects: Critical review of 72 patients. *Int. J. Oral Maxillofac. Surg.* 36(3):193.

Lovisetto, F., Zonta, S., Rota, E., Mazzilli, M., Bardone M., Bottero, L., Faillace, G., and Longoni, M. 2007. Use of human fibrin glue (tissucol) versus staples for mesh fixation in laparoscopic transabdominal preperitoneal hernioplasty. A prospective, randomized study. *Ann. Surg.* 245(2):222.

Mattamal, G.J. 2010. Recent US FDA reclassification on the regulation of tissue adhesives for skin approximation in clinical applications. *Mat. Sci. Forum.* 638:624.

Nishi, O., Nishi, K., and Wickström, K. 2000. Preventing lens epithelial cell migration using intraocular lenses with sharp rectangular edges. *J. Cataract. Refract. Surg.* 26(10):1543.

Packer, M., Fine, I.H., Hoffman, R.S., and Piers, A. 2004. Improved functional vision with a modified prolate intraocular lens. *J. Cataract. Refract. Surg.* 30:986.

Postelthwait, R.W., Schauble, J.F., Dillan, M.L., and Morgan, J. 1959. An evaluation of surgical suture material. *Surg. Gyn. Obstet.* 108:555.

Reyes, R.A., Tjellström, G., and Granström, E. 2000. Evaluation of implant losses and skin reactions around extraoral bone-anchored implants: A 0- to 8-year follow-up. *Otolaryngol. Head Neck Surg.* 122(2):272.

Shalaby, S.W. 1985. Fibrous materials for biomedical applications. In *High Technology Fibers: Part A*. Lewin, M. and Preston, J., eds. Marcel Dekker, New York.

Shalaby, S.W. 1988. Bioabsorbable polymers. In *Encyclopedia of Pharmaceutical Technology*, Vol. 1. Boylan, J.C. and Swarbrick, J., eds. Marcel Dekker, New York.

Shall, L.M. and Cawley, P.W. 1994. Soft tissue reconstruction in the shoulder. Comparison of suture anchors, absorbable staples, and absorbable tacks. *Am. J. Sports Med.* 22:715.

Singer, A.J., Quinn, J.V., and Hollander, J.E. 2008. The cyanoacrylate topical skin adhesives. *Am. J. Emerg. Med.* 26(4):490.

Smith, T.J., Galm, A., Chatterjee, S., Wells, R., Pedersen, S., Parizi, A.M., Goodship, A.E., and Blunn, G.W. 2006. Modulation of the soft tissue reactions to percutaneous orthopaedic implants. *J. Orthop. Res.* 24(7):1377.

Tobias, K.M. 2007. Surgical stapling devices in veterinary medicine: A review. *Vet. Surg.* 36(4):341.

Tsai, C.-C., Lin, V., and Tang, L. 2005. Injectable biomaterials for incontinence and vesico-ureteral reflux: Current status and future promise. *J. Biomed. Mater. Res. B Appl. Biomater.* 77(1):171.

Uchida, M., Oyane, A., Kim, H.-M., Kokubo, T., and Ito, A. 2004. Biomimetic coating of laminin-apatite composite on titanium metal and its excellent cell-adhesive properties. *Adv. Mater.* 16(13):1071.

von Recum, A.G. and Park, J.B. 1979. Percutaneous devices. *Crit. Rev. Bioeng.* 5:37.

Webster, D. J. T. and Davis, P. W. 1975. Closure of abdominal wounds by adhesive strips: A clinical trial. *Brit. Med. J.* 3(5985):696–698.

White, R.L. 1982. Review of current status of cochlear prostheses. *IEEE Trans. Biomed. Eng.* 29(4):233.

Zhong, Y. and Bellamkonda, R.V. 2008. Biomaterials for the central nervous system. *J. R. Soc. Interface* 5:957.

Further Information

Lanza, R.P., Langer, R., and Chick, W.L., Eds. 1997. *Principles of Tissue Engineering*. Academic Press, San Diego, CA.

Lynch, W. 1982. *Implants: Reconstructing the Human Body*. Van Nostrand Reinhold, New York.

Mattamal, G.J. 2008. US FDA perspective on the regulations of medical-grade polymers: Cyanoacrylate polymer medical device tissue adhesives. *Expert Rev. Med. Dev.* 5(1):41.

Park, J.B. and Lakes, R.S. 1992. *Biomaterials Science and Engineering*, 2nd ed. Plenum Press, New York.

Shalaby, S.W., Ed. 1994. *Biomedical Polymers Designed to Degrade Systems*. Hanser, New York.

Yannas, I.V. and Burke, I.F. 1980. Design of an artificial skin: 1. Basic design principles. *J. Biomed. Mater. Res.* 14:107.

37

Hard Tissue Replacements

Sang-Hyun Park
Orthopedic Hospital
University of California,
Los Angeles

Adolfo Llinás
Fundacion Cosme and
Damian
Universidad de los Andes

Vijay K. Goel
University of Toledo

37.1 Long Bone Repair 37-1
  Wires and Cables • Pins • Screws • Plates • Intramedullary Nails
37.2 Joint Replacements 37-8
  Implant Fixation Methods
37.3 Total Joint Replacements 37-12
  Hip Joint Replacement • Knee Joint Replacement • Ankle
  Joint Replacement • Shoulder Joint Replacement • Elbow Joint
  Replacement • Finger Joint Replacement (Metacarpophalangeal
  and Interphalangeal Joints) • Prosthetic Intervertebral
  Disk • Prostheses for Limb Salvage
Defining Terms 37-19
References 37-19

The use of biomaterials to restore the function of traumatized or degenerated connective tissues and thus to improve the quality of life of a patient has become widespread. In the past, implants were designed with insufficient cognizance of biomechanics. Accordingly, the clinical results were not very encouraging. An upsurge of research activities into the mechanics of joints and biomaterials has resulted in better designs with better *in vivo* performance. The improving long-term success of total joint replacements for the lower limb is testimony to this. As a result, researchers and surgeons have developed and used fixation devices for the joints, including artificial spine disks. A large number of devices are also available for the repair of the bone tissue. This chapter provides an overview of the contemporary scientific work related to the use of biomaterials for the repair of bone (e.g., fracture) and joint replacements ranging from a hip joint to a spine.

37.1 Long Bone Repair

The principal functions of the skeleton are to provide a frame to support the organ systems and to determine the direction and range of body movements. Bone provides an anchoring point (insertion), for most skeletal muscles and ligaments. When the muscles contract, long bones act as levers, with the joints functioning as pivots, to cause body movement.

Bone is the only tissue able to undergo spontaneous regeneration and to remodel its micro- and macrostructure. This is accomplished through a delicate balance between *osteogenic* (bone-forming) and *osteoclastic* (bone-removing) processes (Brighton 1984; Kakar and Einhorn 2009). Bone can adapt to a new mechanical environment by changing the equilibrium between osteogenesis and osteoclasis. These processes will respond to changes in the static and dynamic stress applied to bone; that is, if more stress than the physiological is applied, then the equilibrium tilts toward more osteogenic activity. Conversely, if less stress is applied, then the equilibrium tilts toward osteoclastic activity (it is known as the Wolff's law of bone remodeling) (Wolff 1986).

Nature provides different types of mechanisms to repair fractures in order to be able to cope with different mechanical environments about a fracture (Hulth 1989; Giannoudis et al. 2007; Einhorn et al. 2008; Kakar and Einhorn 2009). For example, incomplete fractures (fissures), which only allow micromotion between the fracture fragments, heal with a small amount of fracture-line *callus*, known as *primary healing*. In contrast, complete fractures which are unstable and, therefore, generate macromotion heal with a voluminous callus stemming from the sides of the bone, known as *secondary healing* (Brighton 1984; Hulth 1989; Einhorn et al. 2008; Kakar and Einhorn 2009).

The goals of fracture treatment are to obtain rapid healing, to restore function, and to preserve anatomic shape, without general or local complications. Implicit to the selection of the treatment method is the need to avoid potentially deleterious conditions, for example, the presence of excessive motion between bone fragments which may delay or prevent fracture healing (Brighton 1984; Brand and Rubin 1987; Einhorn et al. 2008).

Each fracture pattern and location results in a unique combination of characteristics ("fracture personality") that require specific treatment methods. The treatments can be nonsurgical or surgical. Examples of nonsurgical treatments are immobilization with casting (plaster or resin) and bracing with plastic apparatus. The surgical treatments are divided into external fracture fixation, which does not require opening the fracture site, and internal fracture fixation, which requires opening the fracture.

With external fracture fixation, the bone fragments are held in alignment by pins placed through the skin onto the skeleton, structurally supported by external bars. With internal fracture fixation, the bone fragments are held by wires, screws, plates, and/or intramedullary devices (Figure 37.1). All the internal fixation devices should meet the general requirement of biomaterials, that is, biocompatibility, sufficient strength within dimensional constrains, and corrosion resistance. In addition, the device should also provide a suitable mechanical environment for fracture healing. From this perspective, stainless steel, cobalt–chrome alloys, and titanium alloys are most suitable for internal fixation. Detailed mechanical properties of the metallic alloys are discussed in the chapter on metallic biomaterials. Most internal fixation devices persist in the body after the fracture has healed, often causing discomfort and requiring removal. Recently, biodegradable polymers, for example, polylactic acid (PLA) and polyglycolic acid (PGA), have been used to treat minimally loaded fractures, thereby eliminating the need for a second surgery for implant removal. A summary of the basic application of biomaterials in internal fixation is presented in Table 37.1. A description of the principal failure modes of internal fixation devices is presented in Table 37.2.

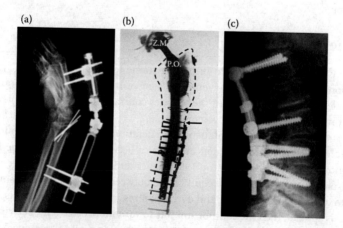

FIGURE 37.1 Radiographs of (a) an internal and external fixation of the wrist shows the entire fixation apparatus; (b) a total hip joint replacement in a patient who sustained a femoral fracture and was treated with double bone plates, screws, and surgical wire (arrows); (c) application of screws (pedicle screw) and rods in spine fusion.

TABLE 37.1 Biomaterials Applications in Internal Fixation

Materials	Properties	Application
Stainless steel	Low cost, easy fabrication	Surgical wire (annealed)
		Pin, plate, screw
		IM nail
Ti alloy	High cost	Surgical wire
	Low density and modulus	Plate, screws, IM nails
	Excellent bony contact	
Co–Cr alloys	High cost	Surgical wire
(wrought)	High density and modulus	IM nails
	Difficult fabrication	
PLA	Resorbable	Pin, screw
PGA	Weak strength	
Nylon	Nonresorbable plastic	Cerclage band

TABLE 37.2 Failure Modes of Internal Fixation Devices

Failure Mode	Failure Location	Reasons of Failure
Overload	Bone fracture site	Small size implant
	Implant screw hole	Unstable reduction
	Screw thread	Early weight bearing
Fatigue	Bone fracture site	Early weight bearing
	Implant screw hole	Small size implant
	Screw thread	Unstable reduction
		Fracture nonunion
Corrosion	Screw head-plate hole	Different alloy implants
	Bent area	Overtightening screw
		Missalignment of screw
		Overbent
Loosening	Screw	Motion
		Wrong choice of screw type
		Osteoporotic bone

37.1.1 Wires and Cables

Surgical wires and cables are used to reattach large fragments of bone, like the greater trochanter, which is often detached during total hip replacement. They are also used to provide additional stability in long-oblique or spiral fractures of long bones which have already been stabilized by other means (Figure 37.1b). Similar approaches based on the use of wires have been employed to restore stability in the lower cervical spine region and in the lumbar segment as well.

Twisting and knotting is unavoidable when fastening wires to bone; however, by doing so, the strength of the wire can be reduced by 25% or more, due to stress concentration (Tencer et al. 1993). This can be partially overcome by using a thicker wire, since its strength increases in direct proportional to its diameter. The deformed regions of the wire are more prone to corrosion than the undeformed, because of the higher strain energy. To decrease this problem and ease handling, most wires are annealed to increase the ductility.

Braided multistrain (multifilament) wire is an attractive alternative because it has a similar tensile strength than a monofilament wire of equal diameter, but has more flexibility and higher fatigue strength. However, bone often grows into the grooves of the braided multistrain wire, making it exceedingly difficult to remove, since it prevents the wire from sliding when pulled. When a wire is used with other metallic implants, the metal alloys should be matched to prevent galvanic corrosion (Park and Lakes 2007).

37.1.2 Pins

Straight wires are called Steinmann pins; however, if the pin diameter is <2.38 mm, then it is called Kirschner wire. They are widely used, primarily, to hold fragments of bones together provisionally or permanently and to guide large screws during insertion. To facilitate implantation, the pins have different tip designs which have been optimized for different types of bone (Figure 37.2). The trochar tip is the most efficient in cutting; hence it is often used for cortical bone.

The holding power of the pin comes from elastic deformation of surrounding bone. In order to increase the holding power to bone, threaded pins are used. Most pins are made of 316L stainless steel; however, recently, biodegradable pins made of PLA or PGA have been employed for the treatment of minimally loaded fractures.

The pins can be used as part of elaborate frames designed for external fracture fixation (Figure 37.1a). In this application, several pins are placed above and below the fracture, but away from it. After the fracture fragments are manually approximated (reduced) to resemble the intact bone, the pins are attached to various bars, which upon assembly will provide stability to the fracture.

37.1.3 Screws

Screws are the most widely used devices for fixation of bone fragments. There are two types of bone screws: (1) cortical bone screws, which have small threads, and (2) cancellous screws, which have large threads to get more thread-to-bone contact. They may have either V or buttress threads (Figure 37.3). The cortical screws are subclassified further according to their ability to penetrate into self-tapping and nonself-tapping (Figure 37.3). The self-tapping screws have cutting flutes which thread the pilot drill-hole during insertion; in contrast, the nonself-tapping screws require a tapped pilot drill-hole for insertion.

The holding power of screws can be affected by the size of the pilot drill-hole, the depth of screw engagement, the outside diameter of the screw, and quality of the bone (Cochran 1982; DeCoster et al. 1990; Ricci et al. 2010). Therefore, the selection of the screw type should be based on the assessment of the quality of the bone at the time of insertion. Under identical conditions, self-tapping screws provide a slightly greater holding power than nonself-tapping screws (Tencer et al. 1993).

Screw pullout strength varies with time after insertion *in vivo*, and it depends on the growth of bone into the screw threads and/or resorption of the surrounding bone (Wermelin et al. 2008; Ricci et al. 2010). The bone immediately adjacent to the screw often undergoes *necrosis* initially, but if the screw

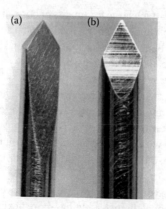

FIGURE 37.2 Types of metallic pin tip: (a) trocher end and (b) diamond end.

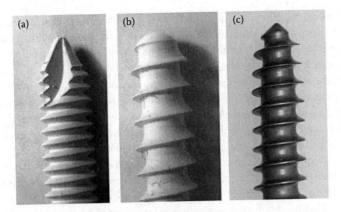

FIGURE 37.3 Bone screws: (a) a self-tapping V-threaded screw (has a cutting flute), (b) a nonself-tapping and buttress threaded screw, and (c) a nonself-tapping cancellous screw (pedicle screw).

is firmly fixed, when the bone revascularizes, permanent secure fixation may be achieved. This is particularly true for titanium alloy screws or screws with a roughened thread surface, with which bone ongrowth results in an increase in removal torque (Hutzschenreuter and Brümmer 1980). When the screw is subject to micro- or macromovement, the contacting bone is replaced by a membrane of fibrous tissue, the purchase is diminished, and the screw loosens.

The two principal applications of bone screws are: (1) as interfragmentary fixation devices to "lag" or fasten bone fragments together and (2) to attach a metallic or plastic bone plate to bone (Mazzocca et al. 2009). Interfragmentary fixation is used in most fractures involving cancellous bone, and in those oblique fractures in cortical bone. In order to lag the fracture fragments, the head of the screw must engage the cortex on the side of insertion without gripping the bone, while the threads engage cancellous bone and/or the cortex on the opposing side. When screws are employed for bone plate fixation, the bone screw threads must engage both cortices. In order to minimize bone damage due to trial and error during drilling, when placing screws in a broad area of cancellous bone, preliminary pins may be placed initially, and when optimal placement is obtained, cannulated drills and screws may be used to obtain maximal purchase and a perfect location. Screws are also used for a fixation of spine fractures (for plate fixation or compression of bone fragment) and for a spine fusion (Figure 37.1c).

37.1.4 Plates

Plates are available in a wide variety of shapes and are intended to facilitate fixation of bone fragments. They range from the very rigid, intended to produce primary bone healing, to the relatively flexible, intended to facilitate physiological loading of bone (Mazzocca et al. 2009).

The rigidity and strength of a plate in bending depends on the cross-sectional shape (mostly thickness) and material from which it is made. Consequently, the weakest region in the plate is the screw hole, especially if the screw hole is left empty, due to a reduction of the cross-sectional area in this region. The effect of the material on the rigidity of the plate is defined by the elastic modulus of the material for bending and by the shear modulus for twisting (Cochran 1982). Thus, given the same dimensions, a titanium alloy plate will be less rigid than a stainless steel plate, since the elastic modulus of these alloys is 110 and 200 GPa, respectively.

Stiff plates often shield the underlying bone from the physiological loads necessary for its healthful existence (O'Sullivan et al. 1989; Perren 2002). Similarly, flat plates closely applied to the bone prevent blood vessels from nourishing the outer layers of the bone (Perren 1989). For these reasons, the current clinical trend is to use more flexible plates (titanium alloy) to allow micromotion, and low-contact plates (only small surface of the plate contacts to bone), to allow restoration of vascularity to the bone (Uhthoff and Finnegan 1984; Claes 1989). The underlying goals of this philosophical change are to increase the fracture healing rate, to decrease the loss of bone mass in the region shielded by the plate, and, consequently, to decrease the incidence of refracture which occurs following plate removal.

The interaction between bone and the plate is extremely important, since the two are combined into a composite structure. The stability of the plate–bone composite and the service life of the plate depend on accurate fracture reduction. The plate is most resistant in tension; therefore, in fractures of long bones, the plate is placed along the side of the bone which is typically loaded in tension. Having excellent apposition of the bone fragments, as well as developing adequate compression between them, is critical in maintaining the stability of the fixation and preventing the plate from repetitive bending and fatigue failure. Interfragmentary compression also creates friction at the fracture surface, increasing resistance to torsional loads (Tencer et al. 1993; Parren 2002). On the contrary, too much compression causes microfractures and necrosis of contacting bone due to the collapse of vesicular canals. Good mechanical stability of the plate fixation requires strong compression between bone and the plate. However, it disturbs periosteal blood supply to the cortical bone. In order to minimize contact between bone and the plate, low-contact bone plate designs have been used to promote cortical perfusion (Uhthoff et al. 2006; Mazzocca et al. 2009).

Compression between the fracture fragments can be achieved with a special type of plate called a *dynamic compression plate* (DCP). The DCP has elliptic-shaped screw holes with its long axis oriented parallel to that of the plate. The screw hole has a sliding ramp to the long axis of the plate. Figure 37.4 explains the principle of the DCP. Bone plates are often contoured in the operating room, in order to conform to an irregular bone shape, to achieve maximum contact of the fracture fragments and anatomic reduction of bone fragments. However, excessive bending decreases the service life of the plate. The most common failure modes of a bone plate-screw fixation are screw loosening and plate failure. The latter typically occurs through a screw hole, due to fatigue and/or crevice corrosion (Uhthoff et al. 2006). The locking compression plate is another type of plate system where the plate and screw can be locked onto the plate. In locking compression plate (LCP), screw holes in a plate and head of screw are threaded for interlocking (Figure 37.5h). Advantages of the locking compression plate are: no compression of the plate onto the bone is required; anatomic reduction of bone fragments can be achieved easily during surgery; and postoperative screw loosening can be reduced (Perren 2002; Wagner and Frigg 2009). Additionally, fracture and plate stability can be achieved without direct contact of the plate to the bone, and in some constructs, the plate–screw unit can behave mechanically as an internal fixator (Wagner 2003).

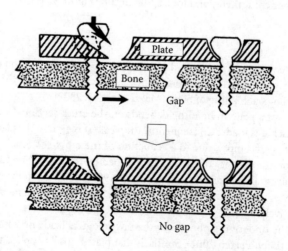

FIGURE 37.4 Principle of a DCP for fracture fixation. During tightening a screw, the screw head slides down on a ramp in a plate screw hole result in pushing the plate away from a fracture end and compressing the bone fragments together.

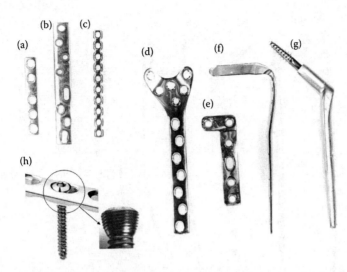

FIGURE 37.5 Bone plates: (a) DCP, (b) hybrid compression plate (lower part has dynamic compression screw holes), (c) reconstruction bone plate (easy contouring), (d) buttress bone plate, (e) L-shaped buttress plate, (f) nail plate (for condylar fracture), (g) dynamic compression hip screw, and (h) locking plate and screw head (circle).

In the vicinity of the joints, where the diameter of long bones is wider, the cortex thinner, and cancellous bone abundant, plates are often used as a buttress or retaining wall. A buttress plate applies force to the bone perpendicular to the surface of the plate and prevents shearing or sliding at the fracture site. Buttress plates are designed to fit specific anatomic locations and often incorporate other methods of fixation besides cortical or cancellous screws, for example, a large lag screw or an I-beam. For the fusion of vertebral bodies following diskectomy, spinal plates are used along with bone grafts. These plates are secured to the vertebral bodies using screws. Similar approaches have been employed to restore stability in the thoracolumbar and cervical spine region as well. Figure 37.5 illustrates various types of bone plates.

37.1.5 Intramedullary Nails

Intramedullary devices (IM nails) are used as internal struts, to stabilize long bone fractures. IM nails are also used for fixation of femoral neck or intertrochanteric bone fractures; however, this application requires the addition of long screws. A gamut of designs are available, going from solid to cylindrical, with shapes such as cloverleaf, diamond, and "C" (slotted cylinders). Figure 37.6 shows variety of intramedullary devices.

Compared to plates, IM nails are better positioned to resist multidirectional bending than a plate or an external fixator, since they are located in the center of the bone. However, their torsional resistance is less than that of the plate (Mazzocca et al. 2009). Therefore, when designing or selecting an IM nail, a high polar moment of inertia is desirable to improve torsional rigidity and strength. The torsional rigidity is proportional to the elastic modulus and the moment of inertia. For nails with a circular cross-section, torsional stiffness is proportional to the fourth power of the radius of the nail. The wall thickness of the nail also affects the stiffness. A slotted, open-section nail is more flexible in torsion and bending and allows easy insertion into a curved medullary canal, for example, that of the femur (Tencer et al. 1993). However, in bending, a slot is asymmetrical with respect to rigidity and strength. For example, a slotted nail is strongest when bending is applied so that the slot is near the neutral plane; the nail is weakest when oriented so that the slot is under tension.

In addition to the need to resist bending and torsion, it is vital for an IM nail to have a large contact area with the internal cortex of the bone to permit torsional loads to be transmitted and resisted by shear

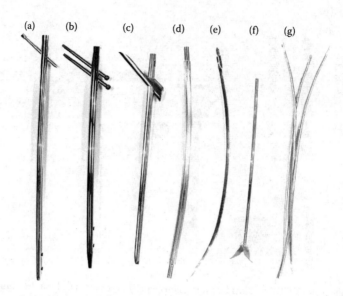

FIGURE 37.6 Intramedullary devices: (a) Gross–Kempf (slotted), (b) Uniflex (Ti alloy, slotted), (c) Kuntscher, (d) Samson, (e) Harris, (f) Brooker–Wills distal locking pin, and (g) Enders pins.

stress. Two different concepts are used to develop shear stress: (1) a three-point, high-pressure contact, achieved with the insertion of curved pins and (2) a positive interlocking between the nail and intramedullary canal, to produce a unified structure. Positive interlocking can be enhanced by reaming the intramedullary canal. Reaming permits a larger, longer, nail–bone contact area and allows the use of a larger nail, with increased rigidity and strength (Kessler et al. 1986; Mazzocca et al. 2009).

The addition of screws through the bone and nail, proximal and distal to the fracture, known as *interlocking*, increases torsional stability and prevents shortening of the bone, especially in unstable fractures (Perren 1989). The IM nail, which has not been interlocked, allows interfragmentary compressive force, due to its low resistance to axial load. Another advantage of the IM nails is that they do not require opening the fracture site, since they can be inserted through a small skin incision, typically located in one extreme of the bone. The insertion of an IM nail, especially those that require reaming of the medullary canal, destroys the intramedullary vessels which supply two-thirds of the cortex. However, this is not of clinical significance because revascularization occurs rapidly (Kessler et al. 1986; O'Sullivan et al. 1989).

37.2 Joint Replacements

Our ability to replace damaged joints with prosthetic implants has brought relief to millions of patients, who would otherwise have been severely limited in their most basic activities and doomed to a life in pain. It is estimated that about 16 million people in the United States are affected by osteoarthritis, one of the various conditions that may cause joint degeneration and may lead a patient to a total joint replacement.

Joint degeneration is the end stage of a process of destruction of the articular cartilage, which results in severe pain, loss of motion, and, occasionally, in angular deformity of the extremity (Buckwalter et al. 1993). Unlike bone, cartilage has a very limited capacity for repair (Safran and Seiber 2010). Therefore, when exposed to a severe mechanical, chemical, or metabolic injury, the damage is permanent and often progressive.

Under normal conditions, the functions of cartilage are to provide a congruent articulation between bones, to transmit load across the joint, and to allow low-friction movements between opposing joint surfaces. The sophisticated manner in which these functions are performed become evident from some of the mechanical characteristics of normal cartilage. For example, due to the leverage geometry of the muscles and the dynamic nature of human activity, the cartilage of the hip is exposed to about eight times body weight fast walking (Paul 1976). Over a period of 10 years, an active person may subject the cartilage of the hip to more than 10 million weight bearing cycles (Schmalzried and Huk 2004). From the point of view of the optimal lubrication provided by synovial fluid, cartilage's extremely low frictional resistance makes it 15 times easier to move opposing joint surfaces than to move an ice-skate on ice (Mow and Hayes 1991).

Cartilage functions as a unit with subchondral bone, which contributes to shock absorption by undergoing viscoelastic deformation of its fine trabecular structure. Although some joints, like the hip, are intrinsically stable by virtue of their shape, the majority require an elaborate combination of ligaments, meniscus, tendons, and muscles for stability. Because of the large multidirectional forces that travel through the joint, its stability is a dynamic process. Receptors within the ligaments fire, when stretched during motion, producing an integrated muscular contraction that provides stability for that specific displacement. Therefore, the ligaments are not passive joint restraints as once believed. The extreme complexity and high level of performance of biologic joints determine the standard to be met by artificial implants.

Total joint replacements are permanent implants, unlike those used to treat fractures, and the extensive bone and cartilage removed during implantation makes this procedure irreversible. Therefore, when faced with prosthesis failure and the impossibility to reimplant, the patient will face severe shortening of the extremity, instability or total rigidity of the joint, difficulty in ambulation, and often will be wheel chair-ridden.

The design of an implant for joint replacement should be based on the kinematics and dynamic load transfer characteristic of the joint. The material properties, shapes, and methods used for fixation of the implant to the patient determine the load transfer characteristics. This is one of the most important elements that determine long-term survival of the implant, since bone responds to changes in load transfer with remodeling process, mentioned earlier as Wolff's law. Overloading the implant–bone interface or shielding it from load transfer may result in bone resorption and subsequent loosening of the implant (Sarmiento et al. 1990). The articulating surfaces of the joint should function with minimum friction and produce the least amount of wear products (Charnley 1979). The implant should be securely fixed to the body as early as possible (ideally immediately after implantation); however, removal of the implant should not require destruction of large amount of surrounding tissues. Loss of tissue, especially of bone, makes reimplantation difficult and often shortens the life span of the second joint replacement (Dupont and Charnley 1972).

Decades of basic and clinical experimentation have resulted in a vast number of prosthetic designs and material combinations (Tables 37.3 and 37.4) (Griss 1984). In the following section, the most relevant achievements in fixation methods and prosthetic design for different joints will be discussed at a conceptual level. Most joints can undergo partial replacement (hemiarthroplasty), that is, reconstruction of only one side of the joint while retaining the other. This is indicated in selected conditions when global joint degeneration has not taken place. This section will focus on total joint replacement, since this allows for a broader discussion of the biomaterials used.

37.2.1 Implant Fixation Methods

The development of a permanent fixation mechanism of implants to bone has been one of the most formidable challenges in the evolution of joint replacement. There are three types of methods of fixation: first, by means of mechanical interlock, which is achieved by press-fitting the implant (Cameron 1994a), by using polymethylmethacrylate (PMMA), which is called bone cement, as a grouting agent (Charnley 1979), or by using threaded components (Albrektsson et al. 1994); second, by means of biological fixation, which is achieved by using textured or porous surfaces, which allow bone to grow into the interstices (Cameron 1994b); and finally, by means of direct chemical bonding between the implant

TABLE 37.3 Biomaterials for Total Joint Replacements

Materials	Applications	Properties
Co–Cr alloy	Stem, head (ball)	Heavy, hard, stiff
(casted or wrought)	Cup, porous coating	High wear resistance
	Metal backing	
Ti alloy	Stem, porous coating	Low stiffness
	Metal backing	Low wear resistance
Pure titanium	Porous coating	Excellent osseous integration
Tantalum	Porous structure	Excellent osseous integration
		Good mechanical strength
Alumina	Ball, cup	Hard, brittle
		High wear resistance
Zirconia	Ball	Heavy and high toughness
		High wear resistance
UHMWPE	Cup	Low friction, wear debris
		Low creep resistance
PMMA	Bone cement fixation	Brittle, weak in tension
		Low fatigue strength

Notes: Stem, femoral hip stem/chondylar knee stem; Head, femoral head of the hip stem; Cup, acetabular cup of the hip.

and bone, for example, by coating the implant with calcium hydroxyapatite, which has a similar mineral composition to bone (Morscher 1992). Each of the fixation mechanisms has an idiosyncratic behavior, and their load transfer characteristics as well as the failure mechanisms are different. Further complexity arises from prosthesis which combine two or more of the fixation mechanisms in different regions of the implant. Multiple mechanisms of fixation are used in an effort to customize load transfer to requirements of different regions of bone, in an effort to preserve bone mass. Loosening, unlocking, or debonding between the implant and bone constitute some of the most important mechanisms of prosthetic failure.

37.2.1.1 Bone Cement Fixation

Fixation of implants with polymethylmethacrylate (PMMA) bone cement provides immediate stability, allowing the patients to bare all of their weight on the extremity at once. In contrast, implants which depend on bone ingrowth require the patient to wait about 12 weeks to bear full weight.

Bone cement functions as a grouting material; consequently, its anchoring power depends on its ability to penetrate between bone trabeculae during the insertion of the prosthesis (Charnley 1979). Being a

TABLE 37.4 Types of Total Joint Replacements

Joint	Types
Hip	Ball and socket, surface replacement
Knee	Hinged, semiconstrained, surface replacement
	Unicompartment or bicompartment
Shoulder	Ball and socket, surface replacement
Ankle	Surface replacement
Elbow	Hinged, semiconstrained
Wrist	Ball and socket, space filler
Finger	Hinged, space filler
Spine	Ball and socket, surface replacement

iscoelastic polymer, it has the ability to function as a shock absorber. It allows loads to be transmitted niformly between the implant and bone, reducing localized high-contact stress.

Fixation with bone cement creates bone–cement and cement–implant interfaces, and loosening may ccur at either one. The mechanisms to enhance the stability of the metal–cement interface constitute an rea of controversy in joint replacement. Some investigators have focused their efforts on increasing the ond between the metal and cement by roughening the implant, or precoating it with PMMA to prevent inking of the prosthesis within the cement mantle, and circulation of debris within the interface (Park t al. 1978; Barb et al. 1982; Harris and Davies 1988). In contrast, others polish the implant surfaces and avor wedge-shaped designs which encourage sinking of the prosthesis within the cement, to profit from he viscoelastic deformation of the mantle by loading the cement in compression (Ling 1992).

The problems with bone–cement interface may arise from intrinsic factors, such as the properties of the PMMA and bone, as well as extrinsic factors such as the cementing technique. Refinements in the cementing technique, such as pulsatile lavage of the medullary canal, optimal hemostasis of the cancellous bone, as well as drying of medullary canal and pressurized insertion of the prosthesis, can result in a cement–bone interface free of gaps, with maximal interdigitation with cancellous bone (Harris and Davies 1988). Despite optimal cementing technique, a thin fibrous membrane may appear in various regions of the interface, due to various factors, for example, to the toxic effect of free methylmethacrylate monomer, to necrosis of the bone resulting from high polymerization temperatures, or to devascularization during preparation of the canal (Little et al. 2008). Although a fibrous membrane in the bone–cement interface may be present in a well-functioning implant, it may also increase in width over time (most probably as a result of the accumulation of polyethylene wear debris from the bearing couple) and may result in macromotion, bone loss, and eventual loosening (Ebramzadeh et al. 1994). Finally, the cement strength itself may be improved by removing air bubbles with mixing monomer and polymer under vacuum and/or centrifuging it (Harris and Davies 1988). During implantation, various devices are used to guarantee uniform thickness of the mantle to minimize risk of fatigue failure of the cement (Oh et al. 1978).

37.2.1.2 Porous Ingrowth Fixation

Bone ingrowth can occur with inert implants that provide pores larger than 25 microns in diameter, which is the size required to accommodate an osteon. For the best ingrowth, pore size should be ranged in clinical practice from 100 to 350 microns and pores should be interconnected to one another with a similar size of opening (Cameron 1994b). Implant motion inhibits bony ingrowth and large bone–metal gap prolongs or prevents the osseointegration time (Curtis et al. 1992). Therefore, precise surgical implantation and prevention of postoperative weight bearing for about 12 weeks are required for implant fixation.

The porous-coated implants require active participation of the bone in the fixation of the implant, in contrast to cementation where the bone has a passive role. Therefore, porous-coated implants are best indicated in conditions where the bone mass is near-normal. The implant design should allow the ingrown bone to be subjected to continuous loading within a physiologic range in order to prevent loss of bone mass due to stress shielding. Porous ingrowth prosthesis are notoriously difficult to remove, and substantial bone damage often results from the removal process. For this reason, they should be optimized to provide predictable ingrowth with a minimal area of surgically accessible porous-coated surface.

Commercially pure titanium, titanium alloy, tantalum, and calcium hydroxyapatite (HA) are currently used as porous coating materials. With pure titanium, three different types of porosity can be achieved: plasma spray coating (1), and sintering of wire (2) or beads (3) on a implant surface (Figure 37.7) (Morscher 1992). Thermal processing of the porous coating may weaken the underlying metal (implant). Additional problems may result from flaking of the porous coating materials, since loosened metal particles may cause severe wear, when they migrate into the articulation (bearing couple) (Agins et al. 1988). A thin calcium hydroxyapatite coating over the porous titanium surface has been used in an effort to enhance osseointegration; however, it improves only early-stage interfacial strength (Friedman 1992; Capello and Bauer 1994). The long-term degradation and/or resorption of hydroxyapatite are still under investigation.

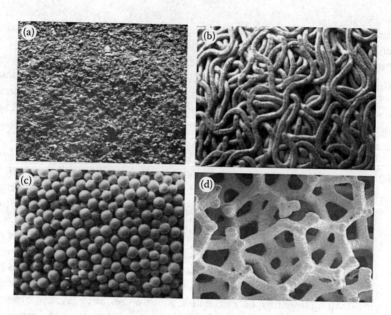

FIGURE 37.7 Scanning electron micrographs of four different types of porous structure: (a) plasma-sprayed coating, (b) sintered wire mesh coating, (c) sintered beads coating, and (d) Hedrocel® porous tantalum.

Recently, a cellular, structural biomaterial comprised of 15–25% tantalum (75–85% porous) has been developed. The average pore size is about 550 µm, and the pores are fully interconnected (Figure 37.7d). The porous tantalum is a bulk material (i.e., not a coating) and is fabricated via a proprietary chemical vapor infiltration process in which pure tantalum is uniformly precipitated onto a reticulated vitreous carbon skeleton. The porous tantalum possesses sufficient compressive strength for most physiological loads, and tantalum exhibits excellent biocompatibility (Black 1994). However, unlike traditional porous coatings, this porous tantalum is not a coating, but rather can be mechanically attached or diffusion bonded to substrate materials such as Ti alloy. Current commercial applications included polyethylene-porous tantalum acetabular components for total hip joint replacement and repair of defects in areas of cancellous bone, such as the acetabulum, femoral condyles, and tibial metaphysis.

37.3 Total Joint Replacements

37.3.1 Hip Joint Replacement

The prosthesis for total hip replacement consists of a femoral component and an acetabular component (Figure 37.8a and b). The femoral stem is divided into head, neck, and shaft. The femoral stem is made of Ti alloy or Co–Cr alloy (316L stainless steel was used earlier) and is fixed into a reamed medullary canal by cementation or press-fitting. Femoral head is made of Co–Cr alloy, alumina, or zirconia. Although Ti alloy heads function well under clean articulating conditions, they have fallen into disuse because of their low wear resistance to third bodies, for example, bone or cement particles. Acetabular component is generally made of ultra-high-molecular-weight polyethylene (UHMWPE).

The prostheses can be monolithic when they consist of one part, or modular when they consist of two or more parts and require assembly during surgery. Monolithic components are often less expensive and less prone to corrosion or disassembly. However, modular components allow customization of the implant intraoperatively, and during future revision surgeries, for example, modifying the length of an extremity by using a different femoral neck length after the stem has been cemented in place, or exchanging a worn polyethylene-bearing surface for a new one without removing the well-functioning part of the prosthesis from the bone. In modular implants (Figure 37.8a), the femoral head is fitted to

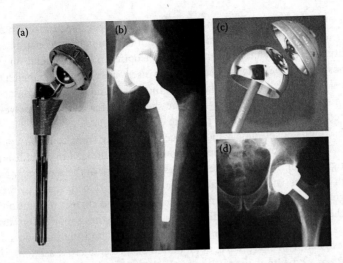

FIGURE 37.8 (a) Modular total hip system: head, femoral stem, porous-coated proximal wedge, porous-coated metal backing for cup UHMWPE cup, (b) radiograph of bone cement fixed hip joint (monolithic femoral and acetabular component), (c) hip surface replacement system (metal on metal), and (d) radiograph of surface-replaced hip joint.

the femoral neck with a Morse taper, which allows changes in head material, size, and neck length. Table 37.5 illustrates the most frequently used combinations of material in total hip replacement.

When the acetabular component is monolithic, it is made UHMWPE; when it is modular, it consists of a metallic shell and an UHMWPE insert. The metallic shell seeks to decrease the microdeformation of the UHMWPE and to provide a porous surface for fixation of the cup (Skinner 1992). The metallic

TABLE 37.5 Possible Combination of Total Hip Replacements

Femoral Component			Acetabular Component		
Fixation	Stem	Ball	Cup	Backing	Fixation
PMMA		Co–Cr alloy	Co–Cr alloy		PMMA
	Co–Cr alloy	Alumina	UHMWPE	Metal	Screw, or press-fitting
Bone ingrowth					
Press-fitting	Ti alloy	Zirconia	Alumina	None	Bone ingrowth

shell allows worn polyethylene liners to be exchanged. In cases of repetitive dislocation of the hip after surgery, the metallic shell allows for replacement of the old liner with a more constrained one, to provide additional stability. Great effort has been placed on developing an effective retaining system for the insert, as well as on maximizing the congruity between the insert and the metallic shell. Dislodgment of the insert results in dislocation of the hip and damage of the femoral head, since it contacts the metallic shell directly. Micromotion between the insert and the shell produces additional polyethylene debris which can eventually contribute to bone loss (Friedman et al. 1994).

The hip joint is a ball-and-socket joint, which derives its stability from congruity of the implants, pelvic muscles, and capsules. The prosthetic hip components are optimized to provide a wide range of motion without impingement of the neck of the prosthesis on the rim of the acetabular cup, to prevent dislocation. The design characteristics must enable implants to support loads that may reach more than eight times body weight (Paul 1976). Proper femoral neck length and correct restoration of the center of motion and femoral offset decrease the bending stress on the prosthesis–bone interface. High stress concentration or stress shielding may result in bone resorption around the implant. For example, if the femoral stem is designed with sharp corners (diamond-shaped in a cross-section), then the bone in contact with the corners of the implant may necrose and resorb (Glyn-Jones et al. 2005). In order to preserve femoral bone, hip resurfacing is also available. In the hip resurfacing, only part of the femoral head is removed and replaced with a metallic shell, thus preserving the neck, intertrochanteric region, and proximal femur intact for future revisions (Amstutz and Le Duff 2009) (Figure 37.8c and d). While preserving bone is an attractive concept, achieving consistent long-term fixation without utilizing the proximal femur for fixation remains a challenge (Malviya et al. 2010).

Load bearing and motion of the prosthesis produce wear debris from the articulating surface, and from the interfaces where there is micromotion, for example, stem–cement interface. Bone chip, cement chip, or broken porous coating are often entrapped in the articulating space and cause severe polyethylene wear (third-body wear). The principal source of wear under normal conditions is the UHMWPE bearing surface in the cup. Approximately 150,000 particles are generated with each step and a large proportion of these particles are smaller than 1 micron (McKellop et al. 1995). Cells from the immune system of the host, for example, *macrophages*, are able to identify the polyethylene particles as foreign and initiate a complex inflammatory response. This response may lead to rapid focal bone loss (*osteolysis*), bone resorption, loosening, and/or fracture of the bone. Recently, low-wear UHMWPE has been developed using a crosslinking of polyethylene molecular chains. There are several effective methods of crosslinking polyethylene, including irradiation of crosslinking, peroxide crosslinking, and silane crosslinking (Shen et al. 1998; McKellop et al. 1999). Gamma-radiated crosslinked polyethylene has been clinically tested and shows very low wear rate (Garcia-Rey et al. 2008; Manley and Sutton 2008; Rajadhyaksha et al. 2009). Numerous efforts are underway to modify the material properties of articulating materials to harden and improve the surface finish of the femoral head (Friedman et al. 1994). Currently, metal–metal and ceramic–ceramic hip prostheses are used widely due to their low wear rate (Lang et al. 2008; Tateiwa et al. 2008; Durr 2009). However, nano-sized particles from the metal–metal prosthesis may cause complex biological responses (Papageorgiou et al. 2007; Callaghan et al. 2008; Endres et al. 2008; Manley and Sutton 2008; Mehmood et al. 2008; Hallab and Jacobs 2009; Kanaji et al. 2009). This biological reaction can take place around the joint, in the form of a large sterile effusion, microscopic tissue necrosis, or metallosis, and are collectively referred to as ARMD (adverse reaction to metal debris) (Langton et al. 2010). More specifically, Willert et al. (2005) described a local tissue reaction with an aseptic lymphocyte-dominated vasculitis-associated lesion, having histologic features that include diffuse perivascular infiltrates of T and B lymphocytes and plasma cells, high endothelial venules, massive fibrin exudation, accumulation of macrophages with drop-like inclusions, and infiltrates of eosinophilic granulocytes and necrosis. There are a few reports of squeaking noises from a ceramic–ceramic hip system during patient walking. However, the cause of the noise is unknown (Ranawat and Ranawat 2007).

37.3.2 Knee Joint Replacement

The prosthesis for total knee joint replacement consists of a femoral, a tibial, and/or a patellar components. Compared to the hip joint, knee joint has a more complicated geometry and movement biomechanics and is not intrinsically stable. In a normal knee, the center of movement is controlled by the geometry of the ligaments. As the knee moves, the ligaments rotate on their bony attachments and the center of movement also moves. The eccentric movement of the knee helps distribute the load throughout the entire joint surface (Mündermann et al. 2008).

The prostheses for total knee replacement (Figure 37.9) can be divided according to the extent they rely on the ligaments for stability: (1) Constrained: these implants have a hinge articulation, with a fixed axis of rotation, and are indicated when all of the ligaments are absent, for example, in reconstructive procedures for tumor surgery. (2) Semiconstrained prosthesis: these implants control posterior displacement of the tibia on the femur and media-lateral angulation of the knee, but rely on remaining ligaments and joint capsule to provide the rest of the constraint. Semiconstrained prosthesis is often used in patients with severe angular deformities of the extremities, or in those that require revision surgery, when moderate ligamentous instability has developed. (3) Nonconstrained: these implants provide minimal or no constraint. The prosthesis that provides minimal constrain requires resection of the posterior cruciate ligament during implantation, and the prosthetic constrain reproduces that normally provided by this ligament. The ones that provide no constrain spare the posterior cruciate ligament. These implants are indicated in patients who have joint degeneration with minimal or no ligamentous instability. As the degree of constraint increases with knee replacements, the need to use of femoral and tibial intramedullary extensions of the prosthesis is greater, since the loads normally shared with the ligaments are then transferred to the prosthesis–bone interface.

Total knee replacements can be implanted with cement or without cement, the latter relying on porous coating for fixation. The femoral components are typically made of Co–Cr alloy and the monolithic tibial components are made of UHMWPE. In modular components, the tibial polyethylene component assembles onto a titanium alloy tibial tray. The patellar component is made of UHMWPE, and a titanium alloy back is added to components designed for uncemented use. The relatively small size of the patellar component compared to the forces that travel through the extensor mechanism and the small area of bone available for anchorage of the prosthesis make the patella vulnerable.

The wear characteristic of the surface of tibial polyethylene is different from that of acetabular components. The point contact stress and sliding motion of the components result in delamination and fatigue wear of the UHMWPE (Walker 2000). Presumably, because of the relatively larger particle

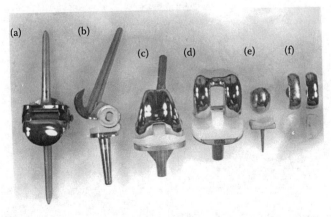

FIGURE 37.9 Various types of knee joints: (a) metal hinged, (b) hinged with plastic liner, (c) intramedullary fixed semiconstrained, (d) surface replacement, (e) unicompartmental replacement, and (f) bicompartmental replacement.

size of polyethylene debris, osteolysis around a total knee joint is less frequent than in a total hip replacement.

37.3.3 Ankle Joint Replacement

Total ankle replacements had not met with as much success as total hip and knee replacements, and typically loosened within a few years of service (Claridge et al. 1991; Guyer and Richardson 2008; Durr 2009; Coetzee and Deorio 2010). This was due, presumably, to the high load transfer demand over the relatively small ankle surface area and the need to replace three articulating surfaces (tibial, talar, and fibular). The joint configurations that have been used are cylindrical, reverse cylindrical, and spherical. The materials used to construct ankle joints are usually Co–Cr alloy and UHMWPE. Degeneration of the ankle joint is currently treated with fusion of the joint, since prosthesis for total ankle replacement is considered to be in intermediate stages of development. The current outcomes have improved and the trend suggests that they will approach, in the future, those of total hip and knee replacement (Fevang et al. 2007). Figure 37.10a shows ankle and other total joint replacements.

37.3.4 Shoulder Joint Replacement

The prosthesis for total shoulder replacement consists of a humeral and a glenoid component (Figure 37.10b). Like the femoral stem, the humeral component can be divided into head, neck, and shaft. Variations in the length of the neck result in change in the length of the extremity. Even though the patient's perception of length of the upper extremity is not as accurate as that of the lower extremity, varying lengths of the neck are used to fine-tune the tension of the soft tissues to obtain maximal stability and range of motion (Wiater and Fabing 2009).

The shoulder has the largest range of motion in a body, which results from a shallow ball-and-socket joint, which allows for a combination of rotation and sliding motions between the joint surfaces. To compensate for the compromise in congruity, the shoulder has an elaborate capsular and ligamentous structure, which provides the basic stabilization. In addition, the muscle girdle of the shoulder provides additional dynamic stability. A decrease in the radius of curvature of the implant to compensate for soft tissue instability will result in a decrease in the range of motion (Neer 1990).

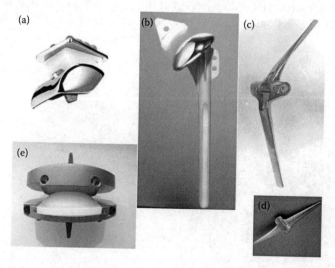

FIGURE 37.10 Miscellaneous examples of prostheses for total joint replacement: (a) ankle, (b) socket-ball shoulder joint, (c) hinged elbow joint, (d) elastomer finger joint, and (e) spine disk.

37.3.5 Elbow Joint Replacement

The elbow joint is a hinge-type joint allowing mostly flexion and extension but having a polycentric motion (Goel et al. 1989). The elbow joint implants are hinged (Figure 37.10c), semiconstrained, or unconstrained. These implants, like those of the ankle, have a high failure rate and are not used commonly. The high loosening rate is the result of high rotational moments, limited bone stock for fixation, and minimal ligamentous support (Morrey 1993; Chalidis et al. 2009). In contrast to fusions of the ankle which function well, fusions of the elbow result in a moderate degree of incapacitation.

37.3.6 Finger Joint Replacement (Metacarpophalangeal and Interphalangeal Joints)

Finger joint replacements are divided into three types: (1) hinge, (2) polycentric, and (c) space-filler (Murray 2003, 2006; Joyce 2004). The most widely used are the space-filler type (Figure 37.10d). These are made of high-performance silicone rubber (polydimethylsiloxane) and are stabilized with a passive fixation method. This method depends on the development of a thin, fibrous membrane between the implant and bone, which allows pistoning of the prosthesis. This fixation can provide only minimal rigidity of the joint (O'Donovan et al. 1991). Implant wear and cold flow associated with erosive cystic changes of adjacent bone have been reported with the silicone implant (Carter et al. 1986; Maistrelli 1994).

37.3.7 Prosthetic Intervertebral Disk

Spinal fusion has become a very popular surgical procedure indicated for chronic disabling back pain caused by degenerative disk disorders during the past 20 years. However, surgeons and patients are somewhat frustrated with the results of spinal fusion because of (1) no significant improvement of the clinical success rate of spinal fusion in spite of many new surgical techniques and instruments, (2) difficulty in obtaining a consistently high rate of solid fusion, (3) morbidities of spinal fusion, (4) accelerated adjacent level degeneration, (5) a long postoperative recuperation period, and (6) increasing cost of spinal fusion (Glassman et al. 2009). Alternative approaches to spinal fusion have been sought out and many in the past conceived the idea of disk replacement. Several designs have undergone clinical trials in human, mostly in Europe and recently in the United States (Figure 37.10e). Some other designs are in various stages of development (Hedman et al. 1991; Bono and Garfin 2004). These designs range from flexible polymer inserts to ball-and-socket of hinge-type designs. Surgical treatment of degenerative disorders of the spine is about to repeat the successful revolution of joint arthroplasty of the hip and knee. An ideal design for total disk prosthesis is to provide a proper range of motion (quantity), proper patterns of motion (quality), proper stiffness in compression, bending and torsion, and stability. In general, the center of rotation moves posterior on flexion and anterior on extension. Excessive amount of motion or abnormal patterns of motion will produce changes in stress flow through the facet joints and adjacent levels. Total disk prosthesis with an adequate amount of motion but with abnormal patterns of motion may be as deleterious as lack of motion to the surrounding structures.

37.3.8 Prostheses for Limb Salvage

Prosthetic implant technology has brought new life style to thousands of patients who would lose their limbs due to bone cancer. The treatment for primary malignant bone cancer of the extremities was amputation. Significant advances in the bone tumor treatment have taken place in the last two decades. The major treatment methods for limb reconstruction following bone tumor resection are resection arthrodesis (fusion of two bones), allograft-endoprosthetic composite, and endoprosthetic reconstruction. Endoprosthetic reconstruction is an extension of a total joint replacement(s) component to the resected bone area and is most popular option due to an advantage of fast postoperative recovery

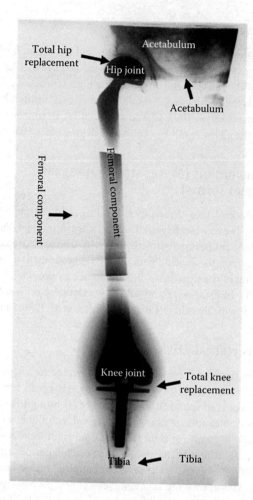

FIGURE 37.11 Radiographic appearance (montage) of a modular endoprosthetic replacement. Entire femur, hip joint, and knee joint of the bone tumor patient were replaced with prostheses for limb salvage.

(Figure 37.11). Therefore, material and fixation method for limb salvage endoprostheses are exactly the same for total joint replacements. Femur, tibia, humerus, pelvis, and scapular are often resected and replaced endoprostheses. Similar to total joint replacements, disadvantages of the endoprosthetic reconstruction are prosthesis loosening due to polyethylene wear and cement failure, and mechanical failure of the prostheses.

Most of the endoprostheses for the limb salvage are expandable type (Ward et al. 1996). Expandable endoprostheses are required for children who have a potential of skeletal growth. Several expandable prostheses require an open surgical procedure to be lengthened, whereas others have been developed that can be lengthened by servomechanisms within the endoprosthesis. Modular segmental system is a new option for expandable endoprosthesis. They can easily be revised to longer modular components to gain length over time. Modular segmental system has several advantages over the mechanically expandable one. The use of the modular system allows for intraoperative customization of the endoprosthesis during the surgery. It minimizes discrepancy between the custom implant and actual skeletal defect due to the radiographic magnification and uncertainty of margin of tumor resection. It allows the surgeon to assemble the prosthesis intraoperatively. The cost of the modular system is less than the cost of an expandable custom endoprosthesis. The modular system allows for simpler and ess expensive revision when failures occur, obviating the need for an entirely new prosthesis when only one part needs to be replaced. On the other hand, modular system has a high chance of corrosion failure at the Morse tapers and dislodgment at the Morse taper fittings. It can be lengthened only in certain increments. Modular component system has additional applications: metastatic bone disease, failure of internal fixation, severe acute fractures with poor bone quality, and failure of total joints with insufficient bone stock.

Defining Terms

Bone resorption: A type of bone loss due to the greater osteoclastic activity than the osteogenic activity.

Callus: Unorganized meshwork of woven bone which is formed following fracture of bone to achieve an early stability of the fracture.

Fibrous membrane: Thin layer of soft tissue which covers an implant to isolate from the body.

Necrosis: Cell death caused by enzymes or heat.

Osseointegration: Direct contact of bone tissues to an implant surface without fibrous membrane.

Osteolysis: Dissolution of bone mineral from the bone matrix.

Primary healing: Bone healing in which union occurs directly without forming callus.

Secondary healing: Bone union with a callus formation.

Stress shielding: Bone is protected from stress by the stiff implant.

Wolff's law: Bone develops or adapts the structure most suited to resist the forces acting upon it.

References

Agins, H. J., Alcock, N. W., Bansal, M. et al. 1988. Metallic wear in failed titanium-alloy total hip replacements. A histological and quantitative analysis. *J Bone Joint Surg Am* 70(3): 347–356.

Albrektsson, T., Carlsson, L. V., Morberg, P. et al. 1994. Directly bone-anchored implants. In *Bone Implant Interface*, ed. R. Hurley, pp. 97–120. St. Louis: Mosby.

Amstutz, H. C. and Le Duff, M. J. 2009. Current status of hemi-resurfacing arthroplasty for osteonecrosis of the hip: A 27-year experience. *Orthop Clin North Am* 40(2): 275–282.

Barb, W., Park, J. B., Kenner, G. H., and Von Recum, A. F. 1982. Intramedullary fixation of artificial hip joints with bone cement-precoated implants. I. Interfacial strengths. *J Biomed Mater Res* 16(4): 447–458.

Black, J. 1994. Biological performance of tantalum. *Clin Mater* 16(3): 167–173.

Bono, C. M. and Garfin, S. R. 2004. History and evolution of disc replacement. *Spine J* 4(Suppl 6): 145S–150S.

Brand, R. A. and Rubin, C. T. 1987. Fracture healing. In *Scientific Basics of Orthopaedics*, 2nd ed. eds. J. Albert and R. Brand, pp. 325–340. Norwalk: Appleton & Lange.

Brighton, C. T. 1984. The biology of fracture repair. *Instr Course Lect* 33:60–82.

Buckwalter, J. A., Woo, S. L., Goldberg, V. M. et al. 1993. Soft-tissue aging and musculoskeletal function. *J Bone Joint Surg Am* 75(10): 1533–1548.

Callaghan, J. J., Cuckler, J. M., Huddleston, J. I., and Galante, J. O. 2008. How have alternative bearings (such as metal-on-metal, highly cross-linked polyethylene, and ceramic-on-ceramic) affected the prevention and treatment of osteolysis? *J Am Acad Orthop Surg* 16(Suppl 1): S33–S38.

Cameron, H. U. 1994a. Smooth metal–bone interface. In *Bone Implant Interface*, ed. R. Hurley, pp. 121–144. St. Louis: Mosby.

Cameron, H. U. 1994b. The implant–bone interface: Porous metals. In *Bone Implant Interface*, ed. R. Hurley, pp. 121–144. St. Louis: Mosby.

Capello, W. N. and Bauer, T. W. 1994. Hydroxyapatite in orthopaedic surgery. In *Bone Implant Interface*, ed. R. Hurley, pp. 121–144. St. Louis: Mosby.

Carter, P. R., Benton, L. J., and Dysert, P. A. 1986. Silicone rubber carpal implants: A study of the incidence of late osseous complications. *J Hand Surg Am* 11(5): 639–644.

Chalidis, B., Dimitriou, C., Papadopoulos, P., Petsatodis, G., and Giannoudis, P. V. 2009. Total elbow arthroplasty for the treatment of insufficient distal humeral fractures. A retrospective clinical study and review of the literature. *Injury* 40(6): 582–590.

Charnley, J. 1979. *Low Friction Arthroplasty of the Hip.* Berlin: Springer.

Claes, L. 1989. The mechanical and morphological properties of bone beneath internal fixation plates of differing rigidity. *J Orthop Res* 7(2): 170–177.

Claridge, R. J., Hart, M. B., Jones, R. A. et al. 1991. Replacement arthroplasties of the ankle and foot. In *Disorder of the Foot & Ankle,* 2nd Ed. ed. M. Jahss, pp. 2647–2664. Philadelphia, PA: Saunders.

Cochran, G. V. B. 1982. Biomechanics of orthopaedic structures. In *A Primer in Orthopaedic Biomechanics,* ed. G.V.B. Cochran, pp. 143–215. New York: Churchill Livingstone.

Coetzee, J. C. and Deorio, J. K. 2010. Total ankle replacement systems available in the United States. *Instr Course Lect* 59: 367–374.

Curtis, M. J., Jinnah, R. H., Wilson, V. D., and Hungerford, D. S. 1992. The initial stability of uncemented acetabular components. *J Bone Joint Surg Br* 74(3): 372–376.

Decoster, T. A., Heetderks, D. B., Downey, D. J., Ferries, J. S., and Jones, W. 1990. Optimizing bone screw pullout force. *J Orthop Trauma* 4(2): 169–174.

Dupont, J. A. and Charnley, J. 1972. Low-friction arthroplasty of the hip for the failures of previous operations. *J Bone Joint Surg Br* 54(1): 77–87.

Durr, H. R. 2009. The problem of fractures of ceramic heads. What should be done? *Orthopade* 38(8): 698–703.

Ebramzadeh, E., Sarmiento, A., McKellop, H. A., Llinas, A., and Gogan, W. 1994. The cement mantle in total hip arthroplasty. Analysis of long-term radiographic results. *J Bone Joint Surg Am* 76(1): 77–87.

Einhorn, T. A., Laurencin, C. T., and Lyons, K. 2008. An AAOS-NIH symposium. Fracture repair: Challenges, opportunities, and directions for future research. *J Bone Joint Surg Am* 90(2): 438–442.

Endres, S., Bartsch, I., Sturz, S., Kratz, M., and Wilke, A. 2008. Polyethylene and cobalt–chromium molybdenum particles elicit a different immune response *in vitro. J Mater Sci Mater Med* 19(3): 1209–1214.

Fevang, B. T., Lie, S. A., Havelin, L. I. et al. 2007. 257 ankle arthroplasties performed in Norway between 1994 and 2005. *Acta Orthop* 78(5): 575–583.

Friedman, R. J. 1992. Advances in biomaterials and factors affecting implant fixation. *Instr Course Lect* 41: 127–136.

Friedman, R. J., Black, J., Galante, J. O., Jacobs, J. J., and Skinner, H. B. 1994. Current concepts in orthopaedic biomaterials and implant fixation. *Instr Course Lect* 43: 233–255.

Garcia-Rey, E., Garcia-Cimbrelo, E., Cruz-Pardos, A., and Ortega-Chamarro, J. 2008. New polyethylenes in total hip replacement: A prospective, comparative clinical study of two types of liner. *J Bone Joint Surg Br* 90(2): 149–153.

Giannoudis, P. V., Einhorn, T. A., and Marsh, D. 2007. Fracture healing: The diamond concept. *Injury* 38(Suppl 4): S3–S6.

Glassman, S. D., Polly, D. W., Bono, C. M., Burkus, K., and Dimar, J. R. 2009. Outcome of lumbar arthrodesis in patients sixty-five years of age or older. *J Bone Joint Surg Am* 91(4): 783–790.

Glyn-Jones, S., Gill, H. S., Beard, D. J., McLardy-Smith, P., and Murray, D. W. 2005. Influence of stem geometry on the stability of polished tapered cemented femoral stems. *J Bone Joint Surg Br* 87(7): 921–927.

Goel, V. K., Lee, I. K., and Blair, W. F. 1989. Stress distribution in the ulna following a hinged elbow arthroplasty. A finite element analysis. *J Arthroplasty* 4(2): 163–171.

Griss, P. 1984. Assessment of clinical status of total joint replacement. In *Functional Behavior of Orthopaedic Biomaterials,* eds. P. Ducheyne and G. W. Hastings, pp. 21–48. Boca Raton, FL: CRC Press.

Guyer, A. J. and Richardson, G. 2008. Current concepts review: Total ankle arthroplasty. *Foot Ankle Int* 29(2): 256–264.

Hallab, N. J. and Jacobs, J. J. 2009. Biologic effects of implant debris. *Bull NYU Hosp Jt Dis* 67(2): 182–188.

Harris, W. H. and Davies, J. P. 1988. Modern use of modern cement for total hip replacement. *Orthop Clin North Am* 19(3): 581–589.

Hedman, T. P., Kostuik, J. P., Fernie, G. R., and Hellier, W. G. 1991. Design of an intervertebral disc prosthesis. *Spine (Phila Pa 1976)* 16(Suppl 6): S256–S260.

Hulth, A. 1989. Current concepts of fracture healing. *Clin Orthop Relat Res* 249: 265–284.

Hutzschenreuter, P. and Brümmer, H. 1980. Screw design and stability. In *Current Concepts of Internal Fixation*, ed. H. Uhthoff, pp. 244–250. Berlin: Springer.

Joyce, T. J. 2004. Currently available metacarpophalangeal prostheses: Their designs and prospective considerations. *Expert Rev Med Devices* 1(2): 193–204.

Kakar, S. and Einhorn, T. A. 2009. Biology and enhancement of skeletal repair. In *Skeletal Trauma-Basic Science, Management, and Reconstruction*, 4th ed. eds. B. D. Browner, A. M. Levine, J. B. Jupiter, P. G. Trafton, and C. Krettek, pp. 33–50. Philadelphia, PA: Saunders.

Kanaji, A., Caicedo, M. S., Virdi, A. S. et al. 2009. Co–Cr–Mo alloy particles induce tumor necrosis factor alpha production in MLO-Y4 osteocytes: A role for osteocytes in particle-induced inflammation. *Bone* 45(3): 528–533.

Kessler, S. B., Hallfeldt, K. K., Perren, S. M., and Schweiberer, L. 1986. The effects of reaming and intramedullary nailing on fracture healing. *Clin Orthop Relat Res* 212: 18–25.

Lang, J. E., Whiddon, D. R., Smith, E. L., and Salyapongse, A. K. 2008. Use of ceramics in total hip replacement. *J Surg Orthop Adv* 17(1): 51–57.

Langton, D. J., Jameson, S. S., Joyce, T. J. et al. 2010. Early failure of metal-on-metal bearings in hip resurfacing and large-diameter total hip replacement: A consequence of excess wear. *J Bone Joint Surg Br* 92(1): 38–46.

Ling, R. S. 1992. The use of a collar and precoating on cemented femoral stems is unnecessary and detrimental. *Clin Orthop Relat Res* 285: 73–83.

Little, J. P., Gray, H. A., Murray, D. W., Beard, D. J., and Gill, H. S. 2008. Thermal effects of cement mantle thickness for hip resurfacing. *J Arthroplasty* 23(3): 454–458.

Maistrelli, G. L. 1994. Polymer in orthopaedic surgery. In *Bone Implant Interface*, ed. R. Hurley, pp. 169–190. St. Louis: Mosby.

Malviya, A., Ramaskandhan, J., Holland, J. P., and Lingard, E. A. 2010. Metal-on-metal total hip arthroplasty. *J Bone Joint Surg Am* 92(7): 1675–1683.

Manley, M. T. and Sutton, K. 2008. Bearings of the future for total hip arthroplasty. *J Arthroplasty* 23 (Suppl 7): 47–50.

Mazzocca, A. D., DeAngelelis, J. P., Caputo, A. E. et al. 2009. Principles of internal fixation. In *Skeletal Trauma—Basic Science, Management, and Reconstruction*, 4th ed. eds. B. D. Browner, A. M. Levine, J. B. Jupiter, P. G. Trafton, and C. Krettek, pp. 83–142. Philadelphia, PA: Saunders.

McKellop, H., Shen, F. W., Lu, B., Campbell, P., and Salovey, R. 1999. Development of an extremely wear-resistant ultra high molecular weight polyethylene for total hip replacements. *J Orthop Res* 17(2): 157–167.

McKellop, H. A., Campbell, P., Park, S. H. et al. 1995. The origin of submicron polyethylene wear debris in total hip arthroplasty. *Clin Orthop Relat Res* 311: 3–20.

Mehmood, S., Jinnah, R. H., and Pandit, H. 2008. Review on ceramic-on-ceramic total hip arthroplasty. *J Surg Orthop Adv* 17(1): 45–50.

Morrey, B. F. 1993. *The Elbow and its Disorders,* 2nd ed. Philadelphia, PA: Saunders.

Morscher, E. W. 1992. Current status of acetabular fixation in primary total hip arthroplasty. *Clin Orthop Relat Res* 274: 172–193.

Mow, V. C. and Hayes, W. C. 1991. *Basic Orthopaedic Biomechanics*. New York: Raven Press.

Mündermann, A., Dyrby, C. O., D'Lima, D. D., Colwell, C. W., Jr., and Andriacchi, T. P. 2008. *In vivo* knee loading characteristics during activities of daily living as measured by an instrumented total knee replacement. *J Orthop Res* 26(9): 1167–1172.

Murray, P. M. 2003. New-generation implant arthroplasties of the finger joints. *J Am Acad Orthop Surg* 11(5): 295–301.

Murray, P. M. 2006. Prosthetic replacement of the proximal interphalangeal joint. *Hand Clin* 22(2): 201–206.

Neer, C. S. 1990. *Shoulder Reconstruction*. Philadelphia, PA: Saunders.

O'Donovan, T. M., Terrono, A. L., and Millender, L. H. 1991. Silicone rubber arthroplasty of the wrist. *Semin Arthroplasty* 2(2): 85–90.

Oh, I., Carlson, C. E., Tomford, W. W., and Harris, W. H. 1978. Improved fixation of the femoral component after total hip replacement using a methacrylate intramedullary plug. *J Bone Joint Surg Am* 60(5): 608–613.

O'Sullivan, M. E., Chao, E. Y., and Kelly, P. J. 1989. The effects of fixation on fracture-healing. *J Bone Joint Surg Am* 71(2): 306–310.

Papageorgiou, I., Brown, C., Schins, R. et al. 2007. The effect of nano- and micron-sized particles of cobalt–chromium alloy on human fibroblasts *in vitro*. *Biomaterials* 28(19): 2946–2958.

Park, J. B. and Lakes, R. S. 2007. *Biomaterials: An Introduction*, 3rd ed. New York: Springer.

Park, J. B., Malstrom, C. S., and Von Recum, A. F. 1978. Intramedullary fixation of implants pre-coated with bone cement: A preliminary study. *Biomater Med Devices Artif Organs* 6(4): 361–373.

Paul, J. P. 1976. Loading on normal hip and knee joints and joint replacement. In *Advances in Hip and Knee Joint Technology*, eds. M. Schaldach and D. Hohmann, pp. 53–77. Berlin: Springer.

Perren, S. M. 1989. The biomechanics and biology of internal fixation using plates and nails. *Orthopedics* 12(1): 21–34.

Perren, S. M. 2002. Evolution of the internal fixation of long bone fractures. The scientific basis of biological internal fixation: Choosing a new balance between stability and biology. *J Bone Joint Surg Br* 84(8): 1093–1110.

Rajadhyaksha, A. D., Brotea, C., Cheung, Y. et al. 2009. Five-year comparative study of highly cross-linked (crossfire) and traditional polyethylene. *J Arthroplasty* 24(2): 161–167.

Ranawat, A. S. and Ranawat, C. S. 2007. The squeaking hip: A cause for concern-agrees. *Orthopedics* 30(9): 738, 743.

Ricci, W. M., Tornetta, P., III, Petteys, T. et al. 2010. A comparison of screw insertion torque and pullout strength. *J Orthop Trauma* 24(6): 374–378.

Safran, M. R. and Seiber, K. 2010. The evidence for surgical repair of articular cartilage in the knee. *J Am Acad Orthop Surg* 18(5): 259–266.

Sarmiento, A., Ebramzadeh, E., Gogan, W. J., and McKellop, H. A. 1990. Cup containment and orientation in cemented total hip arthroplasties. *J Bone Joint Surg Br* 72(6): 996–1002.

Schmalzried, T. P. and Huk, O. L. 2004. Patient factors and wear in total hip arthroplasty. *Clin Orthop Relat Res* (418): 94–97.

Shen, F. W., McKellop, H. A., and Salovey, R. 1998. Morphology of chemically crosslinked ultrahigh molecular weight polyethylene. *J Biomed Mater Res* 41(1): 71–78.

Skinner, H. B. 1992. Current biomaterial problems in implants. *Instr Course Lect* 41: 137–144.

Tateiwa, T., Clarke, I. C., Williams, P. A. et al. 2008. Ceramic total hip arthroplasty in the United States: Safety and risk issues revisited. *Am J Orthop (Belle Mead NJ)* 37(2): E26–E31.

Tencer, A. F., Johnson, K. D., Kyle, R. F., and Fu, F. H. 1993. Biomechanics of fractures and fracture fixation. *Instr Course Lect* 42: 19–55.

Uhthoff, H. K. and Finnegan, M. A. 1984. The role of rigidity in fracture fixation. An overview. *Arch Orthop Trauma Surg* 102(3): 163–166.

Uhthoff, H. K., Poitras, P., and Backman, D. S. 2006. Internal plate fixation of fractures: Short history and recent developments. *J Orthop Sci* 11(2): 118–126.

Wagner, M. 2003. General principles for the clinical use of the LCP. *Injury* 34(Suppl 2): B31–B42.

Wagner, M.A. and Frigg, R. 2009. Locking plates: Development, biomechanics, and clinical application. In *Skeletal Trauma—Basic Science, Management, and Reconstruction*, 4th ed. eds. B. D. Browner, A. M. Levine, J. B. Jupiter, P. G. Trafton, and C. Krettek, pp. 143–176. Philadelphia, PA: Saunders.

Walker, P. S. 2000. Design criteria for total knee. In *Surgery of the Knee*. 3rd ed. Vol. 1, eds. J. Insall and W. Scott, pp. 284–314. New York: Churchill Livingstone.

Ward, W. G., Yang, R. S., and Eckardt, J. J. 1996. Endoprosthetic bone reconstruction following malignant tumor resection in skeletally immature patients. *Orthop Clin North Am* 27(3): 493–502.

Wermelin, K., Suska, F., Tengvall, P., Thomsen, P., and Aspenberg, P. 2008. Stainless steel screws coated with bisphosphonates gave stronger fixation and more surrounding bone. Histomorphometry in rats. *Bone* 42(2): 365–371.

Wiater, J. M. and Fabing, M. H. 2009. Shoulder arthroplasty: Prosthetic options and indications. *J Am Acad Orthop Surg* 17(7): 415–425.

Willert, H. G., Buchhorn, G. H., Fayyazi, A. et al. 2005. Metal-on-metal bearings and hypersensitivity in patients with artificial hip joints. A clinical and histomorphological study. *J Bone Joint Surg Am* 87(1): 28–36.

Wolff J. 1986. *The Law of Bone Remodeling*, R Maquet, R Furlong (trans), Berlin: Springer.

IV

Bioelectric Phenomena

Roger C. Barr
Duke University

38 Basic Electrophysiology *Roger C. Barr* **38**-1
Galvani and the Beginning of Scientific Electrophysiology • The Electrical Structure of
Active Membrane • Energy and the Resting Potential • Membrane Stimulation • Action
Potentials and Membrane Currents in a Patch • Action Potential Wave Forms
following Patch Stimulation • Propagation • Field Stimulation • Galvani in
Hindsight • Magnetics • Failures • Linkages • References

39 Volume Conductor Theory *Robert Plonsey* **39**-1
Basic Relations in the Idealized Homogeneous Volume Conductor • Monopole and
Dipole Fields in the Uniform Volume of Infinite Extent • Volume Conductor Properties
of Passive Tissue • Effects of Volume Conductor Inhomogeneities: Secondary Sources
and Images • References

40 Electrical Conductivity of Tissues *Bradley J. Roth* **40**-1
Introduction • Cell Suspensions • Fiber Suspensions • Syncytia •
Defining Terms • Acknowledgments • References • Further Information

41 Cardiac Microimpedances *Andrew E. Pollard* **41**-1
Introduction • Microimpedances Derived from Literature-Based Data • Impact of
Microimpedance Measurement Availability • Multisite Stimulation for Microimpedance
Measurements • Acknowledgments • References

42 Membrane Models *Anthony Varghese* **42**-1
Introduction • The Action Potential • Patch-Clamp Data • General Formulations of
Membrane Currents • Nerve Cells • Skeletal Muscle Cells • Endocrine Cells • Cardiac
Cells • Epithelial Cells • Smooth Muscle • Plant Cells • Simplified Models • Defining
Terms • For Further Information • References

**43 Computational Methods and Software for Bioelectric Field
Problems** *Christopher R. Johnson* **43**-1
Introduction • Problem Formulation • Model Construction and Mesh
Generation • Numerical Methods • Adaptive Methods • Software for Bioelectric Field
Problems • Acknowledgments • References

44 The Potential Fields of Triangular Boundary Elements *A. van Oosterom* **44**-1
Introduction • Preliminaries • Potential Field of a Uniform Double
Layer • Potential Field of a Uniform Monolayer • Potential Field of a
Linearly Distributed Double Layer • Potential Field of a Linearly Distributed
Monolayer • Analysis • Discussion • References

45 Principles of Electrocardiography *Edward J. Berbari* **45**-1
Introduction • Physiology • Instrumentation • Conclusions • References • Further
Information

46 Electrodiagnostic Studies *Sanjeev D. Nandedkar* **46**-1
Introduction • Anatomy • Physiology • EMG and Force
Generation • Pathology • Instrumentation • EDX Study • Motor Nerve
Conduction • Sensory Nerve Conduction • Needle EMG • Single Fiber and Macro
EMG • Evoked Potentials • Somatosensory Evoked Potential • Brainstem Auditory
Evoked Response • Visual Evoked Potential • Engineering in EDX • References

47 Principles of Electroencephalography *Joseph D. Bronzino* **47**-1
Historical Perspective • EEG Recording Techniques • Use of Amplitude Histographs
to Quantify the EEG • Frequency Analysis of the EEG • Nonlinear Analysis of the
EEG • Defining Terms • References • Further Information

48 Biomagnetism *Jaakko Malmivuo* **48**-1
Theoretical Background • Sensitivity Distribution of Dipolar Electric and Magnetic
Leads • Magnetocardiography • Magnetoencephalography • References

49 Electrical Stimulation of Excitable Tissue *Dominique M. Durand* **49**-1
Introduction • Fundamental Principles of Electrical Stimulation • Membrane-
Electric Field Interaction • Electrode–Tissue Interface • Stimulation of Excitable
Tissue • Conclusion • Acknowledgment • References

38

Basic Electrophysiology

38.1 Galvani and the Beginning of Scientific Electrophysiology 38-1
38.2 The Electrical Structure of Active Membrane............................38-3
Patches • A Mathematical Model of the Patch
38.3 Energy and the Resting Potential...38-6
38.4 Membrane Stimulation...38-7
38.5 Action Potentials and Membrane Currents in a Patch.............38-9
Resting Phase • Stimulation Phase • Excitation Phase • Recovery
Phase
38.6 Action Potential Wave Forms following Patch
Stimulation 38-11
Resting Phase • Stimulation Phase • Excitation Phase • Recovery
Phase • End Repolarization
38.7 Propagation...38-13
Comparative Transmembrane Potentials • Propagation Cartoon •
Equivalent Circuit • Intracellular Current Flow • Membrane
Current • Extracellular Path • Propagation Velocity • Two and
Three Dimensions
38.8 Field Stimulation...38-17
38.9 Galvani in Hindsight...38-19
38.10 Magnetics..38-19
38.11 Failures 38-20
38.12 Linkages 38-20
References..38-21

Roger C. Barr
Duke University

38.1 Galvani and the Beginning of Scientific Electrophysiology

In the late 1700s, Luigi Galvani, a faculty member of the Italian University of Bologna, discovered that an electric shock caused frog legs to contract (Figure 38.1) (Galvani, 1791). In so doing, Galvani refuted earlier thinking that the flow of information along nerves was caused by particles moving down the hollow interior of each nerve and showed that nerves functioned electrically. He went on to show that the electrical energy initiating nerve function came from the nerve itself, rather than being provided by a battery or any other source connected to the nerve.

Benjamin Franklin (Franklin, 1784) pointed out the boundless possibilities for error allowed by human imagination. Because of the inability of anyone (then or now) to directly see electrical currents there has been ample opportunity in bioelectricity to demonstrate the truth of Franklin's observation. Indeed Galvani was wrong on some major points. For example, "animal electricity" is not fundamentally different from physical electricity as studied by Volta, now considered classical electromagnetism (e.g., Panofsky and Phillips, 1962). Galvani was nonetheless correct in his most important conclusions—that the underlying mechanism of the transmission of information by nerves is electrical rather than mechanical, and that the sources of the required electrical energy lie within the tissue itself. Thus his

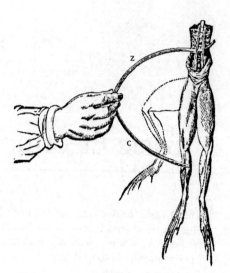

FIGURE 38.1 Galvani experiment. This historical drawing shows a probe touching a frog. The leg, originally extended, contracts (lighter sketch) due to the electrical shock.

field, originally called *Galvanism,* grew to be called *electrophysiology* and now often *bioelectricity* (the latter term embracing both the tissue and human systems that interact with it).

A sketch (Figure 38.2) portraying a view of Galvani's experiment gives more details of what happens as seen from the present day. When a probe (Figure 38.2a) injects a stimulus current into the conducting solution around the nerve, the current initiates a series of *action potentials.* These action potentials are pulse-like changes of the transmembrane potential, the voltage difference across the nerve membrane (defined as potential inside minus the potential outside). In nerves, action potentials involve a voltage change of about 100 mV for a duration of about 3 ms. The energy required to produce each action potential comes mostly from energy stored across the membrane at that site. The succession of action potentials down the nerve fiber occurs because the action potential in each

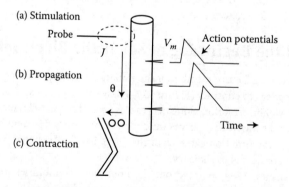

FIGURE 38.2 A modern Galvani-like experiment. An experiment similar to that of Galvani is sketched, shows a probe (a) that creates current density *J* around the tip. The current causes action potentials (b) to occur in the nerve. The action potentials are drawn with stylized triangular waveforms, offset horizontally to suggest the time delay arising from action potentials propagating along the nerve. Symbol θ represents the conduction velocity, usually 1 m/s or more. (θ is used in electrophysiology to be different from voltage *V.*) Neurotransmitters (indicated by small circles at (c) allow the neural excitatory signal to cross into the muscle. Action potentials in the muscle release calcium ions, which leads to muscle contraction.

egment of the nerve stimulates adjacent portions of the membrane. Thus there is a chain reaction of action potentials, loosely analogous to a wall of fire advancing through a forest. At the distal end of the nerve, there is a release of neurotransmitters leading, in the case of the Galvani experiment, to action potentials in the muscle, the release of calcium ions, and the mechanical contraction of the leg (Figure 38.2c).

38.2 The Electrical Structure of Active Membrane

What is it about nerve membrane that allows it to create signals and transmit information? It has taken two centuries of theory and experimental progress to give a good picture of the electrically important structures of the nerve membrane. The most important of these are sketched in Figure 38.3.

38.2.1 Patches

Electrically active membrane often is segmented into patches. The segmentation is sometimes experimental, sometimes numerical, or sometimes conceptual. The core idea is that the elements in a patch are a functional unit. In Figure 38.3, a patch is drawn as the surface area of a cylinder 50 μm in length and 20 μm in diameter. The membrane is a lipid bilayer. The membrane is thin, nominally 50 μm in thickness. Core structures critical to the electrophysiological function are properties of or embedded within the membrane and serve to transport ions back and forth from the outside to the inside, or vice versa (Byrne and Schultz, 1988). Each is itself a complex entity (Hille, 2001) and has properties that justify some discussion. From an electrical perspective, nerve function is accomplished through changes in the transmembrane voltage, so the discussion of each membrane element focuses especially on how that element affects V_m.

Here *patch* is a term of art. Its use implies that the membrane surface area of the patch is large enough that a large number of channels (described later) are present (and thus their properties can be averaged) within the patch, but the patch area is small enough that the patch functions, electrically, without significant spatial variation in the transmembrane voltage. Unless the properties of channels are being

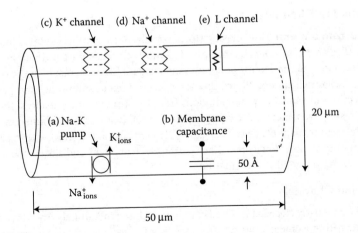

FIGURE 38.3 Electrical structure of a patch of nerve membrane. The membrane is a lipid bilayer. Though the membrane is thin, nominally 50 μm in electrical thickness. Core structures critical to electrophysiological function are portrayed: (a) sodium–potassium pump, (b) membrane capacitance, (c) potassium ion channels, (d) sodium ion channels, and (e) leakage channels.

studied as such, membrane properties (conductivities) are determined for patches of membrane, rather than for individual channels. That is, channels are important to function because of their properties *on the average.*

38.2.1.1 Sodium–Potassium Pump

The Na–K pump consumes energy and actively moves sodium and potassium ions against the gradients of their concentrations, thereby requiring and storing energy. The pump moves Na ions outside and brings K ions inside. The pump carrier is an ATPase. The energy used by the pump, derived ultimately from food, is in effect stored in the form of concentration differences inside versus outside of the membrane, with higher potassium concentration inside as compared with the outside and higher sodium concentrations outside as compared with the inside. From an electrical perspective, the concentration differences result in a highly charged membrane capacitance. For a long time, most investigators thought that there was no net current associated with the sodium–potassium pump, as positive ions are moved in both directions. In the 1950s, however, the Danish scientist Jens Christian Skou showed the pump's existence and that the *stoichiometry* of the pump is unbalanced, with 3 sodium ions moving outward for each 2 of potassium ions brought inside. As a corollary, the original numerical models of membrane electrical function (such as the Hodgkin–Huxley model (Hodgkin and Huxley, 1952)) include no pump current, but more recent models (such as the DiFrancesco–Noble model of the cardiac conduction system (Noble et al., 1994; Cabo and Barr, 1992), the Luo–Rudy model of cardiac ventricular membrane (Noble and Rudy, 2001)) include pump currents. One may think of the Na–K pump as producing major effects by steadily producing small changes over a longer time period, similar by analogy to a refrigerator compressor motor.

38.2.1.2 Membrane Capacitance

Membrane capacitance is approximately 1 $\mu F/cm^2$ of the cell surface area. This area that is capacitive is the whole area of the membrane surface. A high value of specific capacitance occurs because the membrane is very thin, electrically only about 50 μm, and the membrane's dielectric constant is large, about 3. High membrane capacitance is important to membrane electrical function because energy is stored across the membrane when the membrane capacitance is charged, which is most of the time. Membrane capacitance also determines the temporal rate of response of the transmembrane voltage to membrane or axial currents.

38.2.1.3 Potassium Ion Channels

These channels are dynamic, opening and closing stochastically. Each channel contains four gating elements, historically called *particles*. When open, which is more likely when the transmembrane potential is more positive, potassium channels allow potassium ions to pass from the inside to the outside of the membrane. Potassium channels do not allow other ion species, such as sodium ions to pass, except to a minor degree. Selective movement of potassium ions from the inside to the outside of the membrane creates the negative resting transmembrane voltage when the cell is at rest, as explained in detail in the following section. Potassium channels have four gating elements (called *n* gates) within each channel. All have to be open for the channel to be open. Each gating element opens and closes stochastically and apparently independently, to a good approximation.

38.2.1.4 Sodium Ion Channels

Sodium ion channels are mostly closed at rest and can remain closed indefinitely. Sodium channels also are composed of four gating elements, but not the same kind of elements as in a potassium channel. There are three gating elements of one kind (called *m* gates) and one of another kind (called an *h* gate). As with potassium channels, it is the average number of sodium ion channels open or closed at a particular moment that determines sodium conductivity. In contrast to potassium ion channels, sodium ion channels are sensitive to how long they have been open as well as to the transmembrane voltage, and the probability of a sodium channel remaining open decreases with time, even if the transmembrane potential remains elevated. The probability of a sodium channel being open diminishes with time, allowing the return of the membrane to its resting transmembrane voltage.

38.2.1.5 Leakage Channels

Leakage channels are relatively small (i.e., have low conductivity) but allow small numbers of any small ion species to pass from the inside to the outside, or vice versa. In models of nerve fibers, leakage channels often are associated with movement across the membrane of chloride ions. Numerical models show that leakage channels are important to membrane dynamics as well as transmembrane voltages, serving to keep transmembrane voltage changes stable with temporally smooth changes.

Hille has estimated that the maximum number of pores that might fit into a square micron of membrane surface area could be as high as 40,000. In contrast, the actual number of sodium and potassium ion channels appears to be much smaller, on the order of 100–1000. Useful tables have been provided by Hille (Hille, 2001, Table 12.2) and Plonsey (Plonsey and Barr, 2007, Table 4.1). For squid axon the latter gives 330 potassium and 30 sodium channels per square micron. That is, only a small fraction of the membrane surface is occupied by channels.

38.2.2 A Mathematical Model of the Patch

Given the electrical structure of Figure 38.3 one can construct a mathematical model of key relationships in the patch. In particular, one can write

$$I_m = I_C + I_P + I_K + I_{Na} + I_L \tag{38.1}$$

In this equation I_m is the total membrane current, I_C is the capacitive current, I_P is the pump current, and the set of values, I_K, I_{Na}, and I_L are the currents through the potassium, sodium, and leakage channels, respectively. The equation is not for a cell as a whole but rather for each patch within it, as any of these values may vary from patch to patch.

The suggestive form of the equation notwithstanding, it is better to think of the total current I_m as a value imposed on the patch by its external environment, rather than thinking of it as the sum of the components on the right. One might say that a patch is given a certain amount of current and has to figure out what to do with it. To this end, using the standard properties of currents and voltages across a capacitor, one can substitute

$$I_C = C_m \frac{\partial V_m}{\partial t} \tag{38.2}$$

into the equation for I_m and rearrange, giving

$$\frac{\partial V_m}{\partial t} = \frac{1}{C_m}(I_m - I_{ion}) \tag{38.3}$$

where

$$I_{ion} = I_P + I_K + I_{Na} + I_L \tag{38.4}$$

From these equations one sees that the time rate of change of the transmembrane voltage is controlled by the total membrane current required by the patch's environment, I_m, minus the total amount of current flowing through the collection of membrane pumps and channels, I_{ion}.

38.3 Energy and the Resting Potential

A remarkable aspect of electrically active cells is that the voltage of the inside with respect to the outside is significantly negative when the cell is at rest. Left alone, the cell will inevitably return to that rest condition. The resting potential (portrayed in Figure 38.4) is notably different from zero and comes about because of the concentration differences established by the Na–K pump together with the small (but nonzero) ionic conductances at rest, especially the residual conductance of potassium ions.

Qualitatively, the resting potential is generated when potassium ions pass from the intracellular into the extracellular volume, carrying positive charge and thus leaving the interior relatively negative. This process continues until the electric field, exerting an inward force on the potassium ions, is large enough to counterbalance the outward flow due to diffusion down the concentration gradient. (The process is more complicated than this simple explanation, because Cl ions simultaneously pass through the leakage channel.) If there is nonzero conductance for potassium ions only, then equilibrium is achieved at the Nernst potential E_K where

$$E_K = \frac{RT}{F}\ln\frac{[K]_e}{[K]_i} \tag{38.5}$$

In Equation 38.5, R is the gas constant, F is Faraday's constant, and T is the absolute temperature (Kelvin scale). The value of RT/F is approximately 25 mV. From Equation 38.5 E_K then is −74.7 mV. That is, at rest one would have $V_m = E_K$ in a potassium-only system, and that is a good first-order approximation of V_m when the membrane is at rest.

But there are more ions and channels, so a more comprehensive system of equations is required to get a better equation for the resting value of V_m. To this end, suppose one recalls from before that the equation for the time rate of change of the transmembrane potential is

$$\frac{\partial V_m}{\partial t} = \frac{1}{C_m}(I_m - I_{\text{ion}}) \tag{38.6}$$

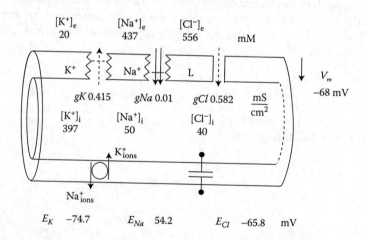

FIGURE 38.4 Origin of the resting potential. The resting potential indicates that electrical energy is stored in the cell. Bracketed quantities are concentrations of each ion species, conductivities gK, gNa, and gL are for each type of channel. Nernst potentials are E_K, E_{Na}, and E_L. The transmembrane potential is V_m, which at the moment −68 mV. The membrane capacitance C_m is charged at rest. At rest there is no capacitive current, by definition, because "at rest" means that V_m is constant.

By definition, at rest the time rate of change of V_m is zero. Thus if the total membrane current is also zero (i.e., if the patch is not being stimulated), one has

$$I_{ion} = I_P + I_K + I_{Na} + I_L = 0 \qquad (38.7)$$

If one follows the Hodgkin–Huxley model, then $I_P = 0$ and the equation becomes

$$g_K(V_m - E_K) + g_{Na}(V_m - E_{Na}) + g_L(V_m - E_L) = 0 \qquad (38.8)$$

where, for example, $I_K = g_K(V_m - E_K)$ and similarly for I_{Na} and I_L. In each case, the equation postulates that the current can be found by multiplying a conductance value (such as g_K) and the difference of the transmembrane potential from the ions' Nernst potential, such as $(V_m - E_K)$.

Solving Equation 38.8 for V_m one finds its value at rest

$$V_m = \frac{g_K E_K + g_{Na} E_{Na} + g_L E_L}{g_K + g_{Na} + g_L} \qquad (38.9)$$

Substituting into the equation the numerical values shown in Figure 38.4, one gets

$$V_m = \frac{-31.0 + 0.542 - 38.296}{1.007} = -68.276 \, \text{mV} \qquad (38.10)$$

which is the result for the resting potential shown in the figure. Comparing this value with the estimate made earlier using the potassium Nernst potential (−74.7 mV), one sees that this value remains negative, but it has a slightly smaller magnitude, reflecting the small sodium and leakage currents.

From the preceding discussion, one sees that nerve membrane in its normal state, left alone, charges itself up to about −65 mV. Such an action is the opposite of what one normally expects—batteries and other objects, left alone, gradually discharge. Electrically excitable membrane is different.

38.4 Membrane Stimulation

Galvani observed the consequences of nerve stimulation but had no way to observe or detect it directly. Since the time of his work, a great deal has been accomplished both experimentally and theoretically, so that the properties of many excitable membranes now can be replicated in detail by numerical models with all key findings confirmed by (or based on) experimental data (Noble and Rudy, 2001).

The most amazing property of excitable membrane is shown in Figure 38.5. In the experiment shown, conducted *in silico*, stimuli of varying amplitudes are applied to the same cylindrical nerve fiber. Stimuli are applied at the left end. Observations of the transmembrane potential versus time are shown for two sites, one at the end (where the stimulus is located), and a second site 2 mm away.

The bottom set of panels show what happens if the stimulus current is directed from the outside to the inside of the fiber. (Such stimuli are considered to have a negative sign, in that positive membrane current is by convention current flowing from the inside to the outside). With negative stimuli of increasing magnitudes of −15, −25, and −40 μA, there is a negative response of the transmembrane potential of increasing magnitude, at the site of the stimulus. The response is most visible during the time of the stimulus but dies off quickly thereafter, so that after a millisecond the fiber has returned to rest. At the second site 2 mm further down the fiber, any effect of the stimuli is barely visible, either during the stimulus or thereafter. That is, nothing much happens.

For comparison, panels a through c show what happens if the stimulus current is directed from the inside to the outside of the membrane. Looking first at panel c, one observes responses that are virtually

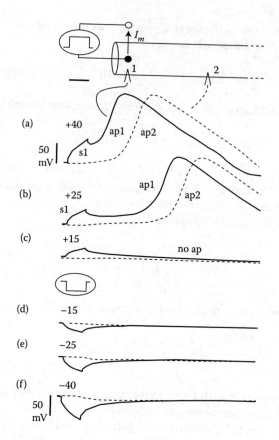

FIGURE 38.5 Stimulation and the membrane response. A cylindrical fiber, sketched at the top, is stimulated by a pair of electrodes placed at one end. For positive stimuli (panels a through c) the source electrode is the solid circle and the sink electrode is the open circle, while for negative stimuli (panels d through f) the source electrode is the open circle and the sink is the positive circle. All stimuli are 400 μs in duration. Stimulus amplitudes vary as given for individual plots. The upward going rectangular stimulus symbol above panels a through c signifies outward (positive) stimulus current, and the downward symbol in the ellipse above panels d through f signifies inward (negative). There are two sets of transmembrane electrodes along the fiber, located at sites 1 and 2. Site 1 is at the left end, and site 2 is 2 mm further down the fiber. The transmembrane voltages at each of these two sites are graphed with a solid line (1) or a dashed line (2). The response of the fiber to stimulation was computed according to the equations of the Hodgkin–Huxley model. Panels a through c show positive stimuli of decreasing magnitude, while panels d through f show negative stimuli of increasing magnitude. Responses to stimulation are discussed in the text. The response at b is marked by an exclamation point, as the response is dramatically different than for panels c through f. The voltage calibration at the bottom applies to all panels.

identical to panel d. That is, the stimulus polarity changed sign, and so did the response, but still little happened in the fiber as a whole.

A dramatically different result is seen in panel b. The stimulus magnitude is increased by less than a factor of 2, and the response *during the time of the stimulus* increases in proportion. But the response no longer dies off after the stimulus is over. Rather, a much bigger and longer response occurs (about 3 times the size and 10 times the duration). This response is called an *action potential*. The ability to generate action potentials (by means discussed later) is perhaps the key characteristic of the excitable tissue. In panel b, another amazing result is seen. Another action potential is observed at site 2, at a later time than the one at site 1. Looking carefully at the action potential at 2, one sees that it is not quite the same as at site 1, in that the response to the external stimulus that is evident at site 1 (identified on the figure as s1) s not present at site 2. It also is notable that the action potential at site 2 does not have a lower amplitude or duration, as compared to the action potential at site 1. That is, the response at site 2 is not a decayed version of the response at site 1 but *another event*, triggered in some fashion by the events at site 1, but a new and distinct response.

Panel a shows the response of the membrane to stimulation if the stimulus amplitude is further increased, as compared to panel b. Again the response is startling. One might expect that the response to the stimulus *itself* would be bigger, and it is. However, the resulting action potentials at both sites 1 and 2 are not bigger—they are virtually the same size. The startling part is that the time relationship of the stimulus to the resulting action potentials is dramatically different, and in particular the action potentials arise much more quickly with the larger stimulus. But again of interest, the time displacement between the action potential at sites 1 and 2 is about the same, roughly half a millisecond.

Suppose one imagines a similar sequence of stimuli being applied to an everyday object such as a paper drinking straw. It is illuminating to thinking about where the response would be of the same type in the straw as in the fiber, and where different. The responses in panels c through f would likely be about the same. The responses to the stimulus itself in panels a and b would be about the same. These are called *passive* responses. But the follow-up action potentials seen after the stimulus in a and b would have no corollary in the straw. These action potentials are called *active* responses.

It also is interesting to think about the responses observed in the fiber in terms of how these responses would be characterized in engineering systems analysis. In such analysis, linear and time-independent systems, the ones most frequently analyzed, are those where the output is proportional to the input, and where a time displacement in the stimulus corresponds to a time displacement in the response. In the fiber system shown in the figure, both conditions are violated. That is, the nerve fiber system's response is neither linear nor is it time independent. That makes its analysis much harder.

38.5 Action Potentials and Membrane Currents in a Patch

In terms of the structure of the membrane and the ionic concentrations within and the outside, how can the events of an action potential be explained? A somewhat simplified portrayal of the major phases is given in terms of dominant effects (Figure 38.6), as follows.

38.5.1 Resting Phase

The resting phase (Figure 38.6a) has already been discussed extensively earlier. Figure 38.5a shows a cartoon with potassium ions moving into the cell from the pump and out through the potassium channels, a small fraction of which are open. Such a process can continue indefinitely. Also, though not drawn, some current flows through all channels, as the resting potential is not the equilibrium potential of any ion species, and all of the channels retain at least minimal conductivity. That is, the membrane has a dynamic equilibrium, but not a Donnan equilibrium (all ions are in equilibrium individually).

38.5.2 Stimulation Phase

Stimulation occurs when current arising from another patch or from an external source passes from the inside to the outside of the membrane (Figure 38.6b). In Figure 38.5b, such a current is shown arising from an unknown location to the left. Though the stimulus current does not immediately change any ionic conductivities, there is a positive change in the transmembrane potential. Recall from Equation 38.6 that

$$\frac{\partial V_m}{\partial t} = \frac{1}{C_m}(I_m - I_{ion}) \tag{38.11}$$

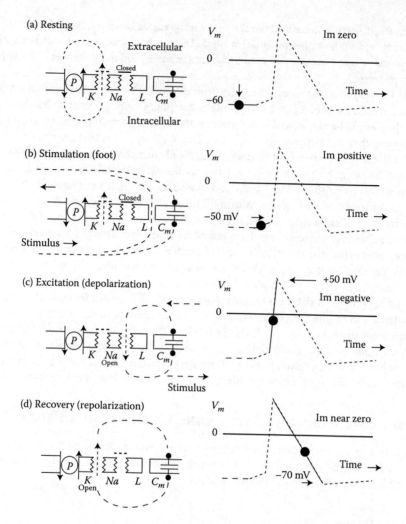

FIGURE 38.6 Patch action potential, cartoon explanation. In each panel a major phase of the action potential is identified, and the major events occurring in that phase are drawn in schematic form. The solid bars are the time period named, and the solid dot is the particular moment discussed in the text. Panels (a) resting phase. In this phase there are small currents of all ions, the most important being potassium. (b) Stimulation, the foot of the action potential. The current paths are indicated by the dotted lines entering the panel (lower line) and leaving the panel (upper) from the left. From the perspective of this patch, these are external stimulus current. (c) Excitation events, the depolarization phase. All ionic paths are active, but the intense inward current driven by sodium ions moving down their concentration gradient is primary. Some current to and from the segment on the right serves to stimulate that segment. (d) Recovery events, the repolarization phase. Potentials fall slightly below and then return to resting values, primarily because of (outward) potassium ion currents, much larger in recovery than at rest.

Even though I_{ion} is zero (when stimulation begins), $\partial V_m/\partial t$ is positive when I_m is positive. For $C_m = 1$ $\mu F/cm^2$ and $I_m = 1007\ \mu A/cm^2$ one has

$$\frac{\partial V_m}{\partial t} = \frac{1}{1}(100 - 0)\frac{A}{F} = 100\frac{C/s}{C/V} = 100\frac{V}{s} = 100\frac{mV}{ms} \tag{38.12}$$

A stimulus of this magnitude and 0.4 ms duration would raise the transmembrane potential by 40 mV. (i.e., it would do so if I_{ion} remained zero throughout the interval of the stimulus, which is only approximately the case.)

38.5.3 Excitation Phase

When there is a rise in the transmembrane potential (toward a less negative value) as the result of an external stimulus, and when the change is of sufficient magnitude and duration, the change in transmembrane potential leads to the *triggering* of sodium channels (Figure 38.6c). Triggering occurs when the probability of a sodium channel being open rises rapidly. The opening of sodium channels produces a rush of sodium ions from the outside to the inside of the membrane. As each sodium ion is positively charged, the inward rush of sodium ions brings along with it a rapid rise in the transmembrane potential.

The numbers of channels of each kind that are open depend on the probability of opening for each one. That probability rises as V_m rises (becomes less negative). This triggering mechanism is built into the structure of each kind of channel. Thereby, when the stimulus increases the transmembrane voltage, it markedly increases the number of sodium channels that are open. Higher V_m also increases somewhat the number of potassium channels that are open. The result is a tremendous influx of sodium ions, driven both by the concentration gradient and by the electric field, offset somewhat by the outward movement of potassium ions. The dominant sodium influx, carrying positively charged ions, in turn causes a further rise in the transmembrane potential, a positive feedback loop that continues until the transmembrane potential approaches the equilibrium potential for sodium ions.

For example, suppose the stimulus opens the sodium channels by increasing the transmembrane voltage, so that $g_{Na} = 10$ mS/cm^2 and $g_K = 5$ mS/cm^2. (Recall that mS is milliSiemens, a unit of conductivity, the inverse of resistivity). If $V_m = -10$ mV the rate of rise of transmembrane potential will be about 285 mV/ms (computed by using Equations 38.3 and 38.4 once again). That extremely rapid rate of rise is enough to cause a shift in V_m of 100 mV or more in less than 1 ms, which is what occurs.

Because the upstroke occurs very rapidly, there is a spatial gradient in V_m. That is, consecutive patches will not have the same transmembrane voltage. The consequence is some current flowing from one patch to the next. In Figure 38.6c, that current is indicated by the current flow path that goes to the right. This current stimulates the next patch along the fiber, as will be discussed in more detail in a subsequent section.

38.5.4 Recovery Phase

The probability of potassium channels being open remains high so long as V_m remains elevated from its resting value. Sodium channels function differently, however, with their probability of being open diminishing with time even if V_m remains well above the baseline. Consequently, sodium channels close while potassium channels continue to be open. The result is that as time goes by I_{ion} comes to be dominated by potassium ions moving outward. Because potassium ions carry positive charges outward, the membrane repolarizes to its resting value (Figure 38.6d). As it returns to the resting value, most of the potassium channels close. The membrane returns to its resting state.

The current loop drawn in Figure 38.6d shows a current loop through the potassium channel, recharging the membrane capacitance. This effect is dominant, although of course, there are nonzero currents through all the channels.

38.6 Action Potential Wave Forms following Patch Stimulation

Having in mind the major phases of the action potential as described earlier, we now examine an action potential in a different way fashion by looking at temporal wave forms (Figure 38.7). These wave forms show the changes with time for the total membrane current I_m, the transmembrane action potential V_m, the current I_K through the potassium ion channel, and the current I_{Na} through the sodium ion channel. In the figure, vertical lines a through e identify for discussion particular moments in each phase of the action potential.

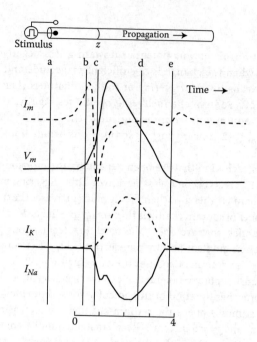

FIGURE 38.7 Patch transmembrane potentials, membrane current, and ionic currents. At the top there is a sketch of a fiber, stimulated at the left end. The wave forms show temporal events at position z, marked along the fiber axis based on a numerical simulation with the Hodgkin–Huxley membrane. All wave forms are plotted for several milliseconds (time calibration at bottom). The wave forms are the total transmembrane current I_m (dashed line), the transmembrane potential V_m (plotted as a solid line), the potassium channel current I_K (dashed line below), and sodium channel current (solid line). Vertical lines a–e identify particular moments for discussion in the text. (Moments a–d correspond to panels a through d in the cartoon of the preceding figure.)

The waveforms of Figure 38.7 (and subsequent figures) are not experimental (indeed, it remains virtually impossible to measure all these kinds of waveforms simultaneously), but rather are computed with a numerical model of the kind first used by Hodgkin and Huxley in their seminal work (Hodgkin and Huxley, 1952). (Detailed information about such simulations is given by Plonsey and Barr (Plonsey, 2007)). Though coming directly from a numerical model, the wave forms shown are firmly based in experimental results, however, as the underlying equations for the model come from matching the experimental data. Moreover, although computed for the unmyelinated giant axon of the squid, the resulting computed wave forms are remarkably similar in important respects to wave forms arising from other kinds of tissue, as shown by Spach for cardiac Purkinje strands (Spach et al., 1973).

38.6.1 Resting Phase

In Figure 38.7, the vertical line (a) crosses each of the four curves at the baseline, during which nothing is changing. Total current I_m is zero and the transmembrane potential V_m is unchanging. Currents I_K and I_{Na} are nonzero, but their magnitudes are too small to be visible on the scale of the graph.

38.6.2 Stimulation Phase

At the time when vertical line (b) intersects with each of the curves in Figure 38.7, one sees the first inklings of the series of events that are required for major shifts. In particular, the total current I_m is sharply above its baseline, indicating a strong stimulus current coming into the patch. Transmembrane potential V_m has increased slightly from the baseline. Owing to that small increase, the potassium conductivity and resulting potassium ion current I_K have become slightly more positive, but the sodium conductivity and resulting sodium ion current I_{Na} have not yet shifted off the baseline. If the stimulus were to end at moment (B), V_m would simply return to the baseline.

38.6.3 Excitation Phase

As the stimulus continues, the amplitude of the sodium current I_{Na} becomes notably negative, so that by moment C, current I_{Na} is negative. Comparing I_{Na} with I_K one sees that the magnitude of I_{Na} is greater (see Figure 38.7). (A dominant sodium current is consistent with the cartoon shown in Figure 38.6c of the previous section.) The consequence is that V_m is moving up sharply at this time. That is, the membrane is rapidly *depolarizing*. Additionally, I_m is sharply negative at this time; that is, there is a significant stimulus current to adjoining patches downstream.

38.6.4 Recovery Phase

Ultimately the magnitude of I_K rises enough to match that of I_{Na} and V_m reaches a peak. Then, as the magnitude of I_K exceeds that of I_{Na}, V_m declines (see Figure 38.7). By time D transmembrane potential V_m is again negative and continuing to decline toward its resting potential. Note that both I_{Na} and I_K remain substantial currents at this time, but quantitatively I_K is dominant (as earlier portrayed in the cartoon in Figure 38.6d.) Current I_m is near zero at time D, indicating that this membrane patch is neither receiving nor providing much stimulus current to adjacent membrane patches at this time.

38.6.5 End Repolarization

As repolarization ends (Figure 38.7), ionic currents are small, but current I_K is sufficiently nonzero to drive the transmembrane potential V_m below its baseline value. The small variations in the total current I_m serve to maintain uniformity of repolarization among adjacent membrane patches.

Looking at instants a through e as a group, one sees that the V_m curve is deceptively simple. Though it seems to be a simple undulation in the transmembrane potential, in fact, the V_m wave shape reflects a complex interaction between currents external to and within the individual membrane patch.

38.7 Propagation

Now understanding the basis for action potentials in one patch, we move on to consider how the action potential propagates down the fiber.

It is important to keep in mind that action potential propagation involves one patch initiating excitation at adjacent sites, in the fashion of a forest fire spreading. (Conversely, a bad analogy is an electric pulse in a cable, where energy moves spatially—nerve action potentials are not like that.) In the nerve, how does the action potential spread?

Here it is useful to first examine wave forms from two closeby sites along a cylindrical fiber (Figure 38.8). Examining first the set of wave forms as a whole (panels b through d), one sees that the second set of wave forms (the dashed lines) are virtually identical to the first set (solid lines), but displaced in time by a fraction of a millisecond. Looking carefully, one also sees that the dashed set is not diminished in amplitude as compared to the first set; that is, the wave forms are not being degraded as they propagate.

Now looking at specific individual features of the waveforms, the first relative to the second, one sees the following points of note: Along the vertical line drawn at time t the intersection of the vertical line with the I_m curves (at points b1 and b2) shows that at time t site 1 (d1) has negative total membrane current. Therefore, at time t site 1 is sending current to other sites (such as site 2). In comparison, the

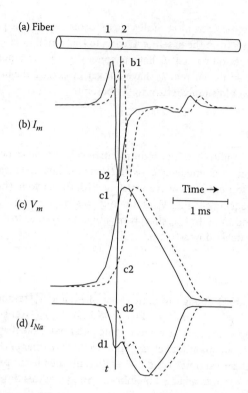

FIGURE 38.8 Propagation: Action potentials and currents from two sites. A cylindrical fiber is sketched at the top (a), with two sites separated by 2 mm axially identified by number 1 (solid) and 2 (dashed). Temporal wave forms obtained by the numerical simulation arising from each of these two sites are shown. Panel (b) total membrane current I_m, (c) transmembrane potential V_m, (d) current through the sodium ion channel I_{Na}. The time calibration bar applies to all wave forms.

vertical line crosses the I_m curve for site 2 at point d2. The elevation of d2 above the baseline shows that this site has positive total membrane current; that is, this site is receiving stimulation from adjacent sites (such as site 1).

Again comparing sites in detail, we see that at time t site 1 has a high magnitude and inward sodium current I_{Na} (point d1 on the figure) and at action potential nearing its peak (c1). In contrast, at site 2, there is still little sodium channel current (point d2 still near baseline), and the action potential of site 2 is only starting to enter the depolarization phase (point c2, small rise from the baseline).

Putting together the picture of propagation in cartoon fashion (Figure 38.9), one sees that what is happening at sites 1 and 2 is distinct but tightly linked.

38.7.1 Comparative Transmembrane Potentials

In Figure 38.9, the panels show spatial wave forms and a cartoon explanation of what is happening during propagation. Panel a identifies two sites along a cylindrical fiber, site 1 (solid) and site 2 (dashed). Panel b shows curves of $I_m(Z)$ and $V_m(Z)$. The former shows that total current at site 1 is negative ("losing current") while total current at site 2 is positive ("gaining current") at this moment. The site being stimulated, site 2, has relatively low V_m while the site providing stimulation has relatively high V_m.

38.7.2 Propagation Cartoon

A qualitative explanation is given in panel c. At time t the high probability of sodium channels being open (left) allows strong current flow inward, and current along the fiber axis from site 1 toward site 2,

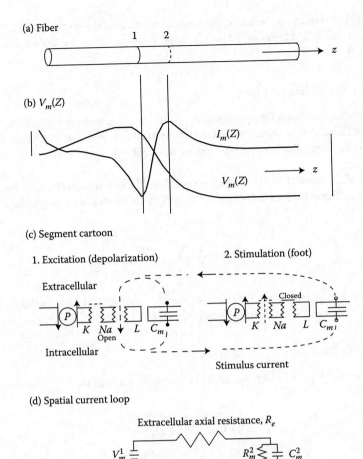

FIGURE 38.9 Propagation of spatial relationships. The panels show spatial wave forms and a cartoon explanation of what is happening during propagation. (a) Two sites along a cylindrical fiber, site 1 (solid) and site 2 (dashed). (b) At a certain time t, curves of $I_m(Z)$ and $V_m(Z)$ are shown. These curves plot *spatial* changes, in contrast to earlier figures that plotted *temporal* changes. The vertical bars mark the positions of these two sites on the graphs, which extend from one end of the fiber to the other, for the time shown. (c) Cartoon showing strong current flow through sodium channels at site 1 leading to charging currents at site 2. Intracellular and extracellular axial currents allow this linkage. (d) An equivalent electrical circuit for this moment. Longitudinal paths are identified by their specific resistivities R_i and R_e (units of Ω m) and must be converted to resistances in ohm based on the cross-sections of the paths, for example, fiber radius.

intracellular. The current's return path is extracellular. The current along the fiber axis produces changes at site 2, that is, site 2 is being stimulated.

38.7.3 Equivalent Circuit

Panel d is an electrical "equivalent" electrical circuit for this moment. It sometimes is called the *local current loop*. The equivalent circuit shows a battery replacing the membrane patch at site 1, axial resistors for the intracellular and extracellular pathways inside and outside of the fiber, and, in parallel, resistance membrane resistance and capacitance replacing site 2. That is, at this moment the battery (at site 1) is charging the capacitance at site 2, with some current also flowing through site 2's passive membrane resistance. One might think of the process of propagation as having the whole local current loop move along the fiber.

38.7.4 Intracellular Current Flow

A critical aspect of the explanation of propagation, as shown in the cartoon, is the flow of current longitudinally along the fiber, both in the intracellular and extracellular volumes. The resistances formed by the spaces thus determine whether enough current flows for propagation to occur, and how fast propagation may occur.

Each of the paths of the equivalent circuit may be described in mathematical form, thus making it possible to construct mathematical models of propagation. On the intracellular longitudinal path, currents are Ohmic, so

$$I_i = -\frac{1}{r_i}\frac{\partial \phi_i}{\partial z} \tag{38.13}$$

where ϕ_i is the intracellular potential (in Volts), z is the axial coordinate (in m), r_i is the resistance per length for the fiber (Ω/m), and I_i is the resulting axial current (A).

38.7.5 Membrane Current

The membrane current is the spatial derivative of the intracellular current, so

$$I_m = \frac{1}{2\pi a}\frac{\partial I_i}{\partial z} = \frac{1}{2\pi a}\frac{1}{r_i}\frac{\partial^2 \phi_i}{\partial z^2} \tag{38.14}$$

In situations when a large conducting volume surrounds the fiber, $\phi_i \approx V_m$, the membrane current goes as the second spatial derivative of the transmembrane potential. Also, the expression can be written more simply using the substation $r_i = R_i/\pi a^2$ where R_i is the specific resistance (in Ω m), so that one has

$$I_m = \frac{a}{2R_i}\frac{\partial^2 V_m}{\partial z^2} \tag{38.15}$$

Often numerical simulations proceed by using this equation to find I_m and then Equation 38.3 to find the change in V_m, for each site along a fiber. It is conventional to compute all membrane currents in units of current per area, for example, A/m². A detailed discussion of the steps in a numerical simulation is given by Plonsey and Barr (Plonsey, 2007, Section 5.4).

38.7.6 Extracellular Path

Current on the extracellular path of the loop can be written in a form analogous to Equation 38.13. However, that is rarely done. More commonly the cross-sectional area of the extracellular space is considered large, and therefore the voltage drops along the extracellular path are considered to be virtually zero *insofar as determining the axial or membrane currents*.

Extracellular voltages (on out to the body surface), though often small in magnitude as compared to transmembrane voltages, are nonetheless extremely important because it is such extracellular voltages that are observed in most clinical measurements. Computation of the extracellular field may be complex but has been accomplished successfully, both in principle and in practice, by solving Poisson's equation n the outside volume. A good review has been provided in the text by Gulrajani (1998) and in this Handbook in the chapters by Johnson and Van Oosterom.

38.7.7 Propagation Velocity

Propagation velocity is markedly affected by membrane properties such as sodium conductance, by the rate at which channels open, and by the resistance of intracellular and extracellular connections from one patch to the adjoining patches. There is no simple closed-form mathematical expression for the propagation velocity, in general. There is, however, a very useful expression for changes in propagation velocity, which is

$$\theta = \sqrt{\frac{Ka}{2R_i}} \qquad (38.16)$$

In this equation, θ is the conduction velocity, K is an unknown constant, the radius is a, and R_i is the specific resistance of the intracellular medium, in Ω cm. It is assumed that the fiber is cylindrical and that propagation is away from the ends. Constant K has to be determined experimentally (or numerically). That is done by finding values for all variables in one experiment and choosing K to make the equation hold. Then the value can be used to estimate changes in velocity for other fibers or other values of resistivity. Usually K will be constant so long as the membrane is of the same kind (e.g., nerve, cardiac, skeletal muscle) and, importantly, the temperature remains constant.

For a particular kind of membrane and the same temperature, the equation shows that velocity goes as the square root of the radius, or as the square root of the intracellular conductivity. Thus, for squid axon at 18.3°C Hodgkin and Huxley estimated the velocity, in m/s, to be approximately

$$\theta = \sqrt{2a} \qquad (38.17)$$

38.7.8 Two and Three Dimensions

The preceding example of propagation was structured geometrically as a one-dimensional cylindrical fiber, as that geometry is relatively simple. Of course, many electrically excitable organs (such as the heart and brain) function in three dimensions. In a corresponding way, analysis of stimulation (e.g., Barr, 2003), evaluation of cell structure (e.g., Spach et al., 2004), and experimental mapping (e.g., Taccardi and Punske, 2002) also can be done in two or three dimensions, though the latter is computer intensive, and one finds it hard to display results unambiguously.

38.8 Field Stimulation

The preceding figures have discussed the stimulation phase based on drawings and graphs arising from transmembrane stimulation. In these cases the stimulus current has come from a source inside the fiber, such as the intracellular volume of an adjacent patch.

With artificial stimulation, common for the treatment of disease, and in Galvani's experiments, both source and sink stimulus electrodes are outside the fiber, that is, there is *field stimulation*. One might ask how such stimulation comes about. To this end, a visual picture of the current flow pattern (Figure 38.10) is helpful.

The cartoon of current flow patterns along extracellular and intracellular pathways (Figure 38.10a) shows the stimulus electrodes, both source (solid square) and sink (open square) electrodes are "in the field." That is, both are outside the fiber. The sink electrode is closer to the fiber's membrane.

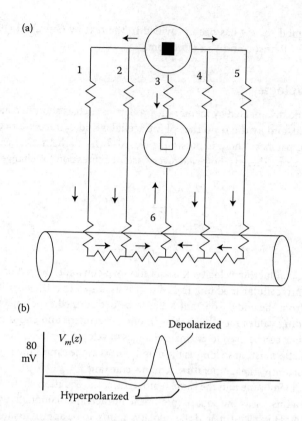

FIGURE 38.10 Field stimulation. (a) Cartoon of current flow patterns along extracellular and intracellular pathways. Here the stimulus electrodes, both source (solid square) and sink (open square), are "in the field," that is, outside the fiber. The plot is spatial, extending along the fiber, for a particular instant. Note that the transmembrane currents are outward (depolarizing) directly under the source but inward (hyperpolarizing) on both the left and right sides. (b) Plot of change in the transmembrane potential created by a field stimulus. The electrode arrangement shown in (a) is used. For stimulation. The plot of the result is spatial, that is, V_m as a function of axial coordinate z. The plot is drawn for a time near the end of the short stimulus.

The resulting current flow pattern, drawn qualitatively in panel a, shows five current flow lines originating from the stimulus source. The center flow line, line 3, flows directly to the sink. Other flow lines, which have a smaller intensity, take more circuitous routes. For example, line 1 flows well to the left, then down and into the fiber, then along the fiber's axis, and then back out of the fiber along pathway 6. Other lines (2, 4, 5) also are drawn with circuitous routes. In the cartoon, they combine to flow out of the fiber and to the sink along pathway 6.

The differing directions of transmembrane current along the different pathways is important. Pathways 1, 2 on the left and pathways 4, 5 on the right hyperpolarize the membrane, because current flow is inward. However, as charge moves outward directly under the source, it is depolarizing. This depolarizing current, if it has sufficient magnitude and duration, will stimulate the fiber's membrane along pathway 6. That is, the membrane is stimulated most strongly directly under the sink electrode. (At first it seems counter-intuitive that the sink electrode rather than the source is associated with the depolarized region, but it becomes logical when current paths are drawn and one sees that arrangement produces outward transmembrane current flow, i.e., forces membrane depolarization.)

For comparison to the qualitative cartoon of Figure 38.10a, a quantitative plot (Figure 38.10b) gives a more precise picture of how transmembrane potential changes underneath a field stimulus. The wave form is shown at the end of a short stimulus (duration 0.4 ms) and thus has a wave shape similar to that of the *activation function* (Rattay, 1990; Plonsey, 2007). Note that the graph is spatial, that is, a function of distance along the fiber, and is drawn for a time near the end of the stimulus. The electrode arrangement shown in (a) is used. Immediately underneath the sink electrode the membrane is depolarized. The depolarized region extends away from the point of maximum depolarization for a distance roughly equal to the distance of the sink from the fiber's axis. On the wings the stimulus hyperpolarizes the membrane. Consequently, with this, the stimulus excitation will begin at the center and propagate outward.

If the stimulus polarity is inverted (source closer, sink further away), the graph of Figure 38.10b will be turned upside down, and the regions on the wings will be depolarized. If the stimulus is large enough and long enough, excitation then will be initiated on both sides of the site of the stimulus electrodes. Note that a stimulus of minimal magnitude may need to have increased magnitude when the stimulus polarity is inverted.

38.9 Galvani in Hindsight

If one now reviews Galvani's experiment with present-day information, one sees that what Galvani did can be explained as follows:

1. Even though invisible to Galvani, the frog's nerves, prior to stimulation, were energized and waiting for stimulation, with cells having stored energy in the form of charged membrane capacitance, reflected in a substantial resting potential.
2. Galvani's electrodes initiated action potentials in the nerves by means of field stimulation.
3. Action potentials produced in membrane patches below the stimulus propagated along the nerve until they reach the junction of the nerve with the muscles of the frog's legs, then across that junction and along the muscle fibers.
4. The action potentials in the muscles (ultimately) caused the release of calcium ions in muscle cells, and these ions caused the frog's muscles to contract.
5. The frog's legs strongly contracted, and this movement was obvious to Galvani or his assistants.

As the intermediate steps could not be observed by Galvani, it is amazing that he and his assistants were able to deduce as much as they did of the mechanisms that are required. Perhaps just as amazing are the limitations that have remained until quite recently or even through the present day—limitations in the direct measurement of currents, especially those of individual ions, limitations of size so that the structure of the individual pumps and channels is only now being unfolded, and limitations of knowledge of the electrical conductivities of cell-to-cell junctions, as well as their surrounding volumes. In each case, bioelectric knowledge has advanced by a slow process of piecing together the results of different kinds of experiments, made at different times, often integrated by the use of mathematical and numerical models of increasing sophistication.

38.10 Magnetics

As one knows from the fundamentals of electromagnetism (Panofsky, 1962), electric currents produce magnetic fields, and changing magnetic fields produce electric currents. The magnetic fields are difficult to measure because they are small in comparison to the earth's magnetic field. Nonetheless, that measurement has been accomplished by Wikswo and van Egeraat (1991), Roth and Passer (1990), Malmivuo and Plonsey (1995), and others (Gulrajani, 1998). Moreover, though not stimulated directly by magnetic fields, electrically active tissue can be stimulated by the electric currents produced by changing magnetic fields. Such magnetic stimulation has important advantages for brain stimulation in that the stimulus is not impeded by regions of poor conductance, such as the bone of the skull (Peterchev et al., 2008).

38.11 Failures

It is the failure of electrophysiological systems to operate normally that give rise to a multitude of human diseases, ranging from leprosy to heart failure. Failure can occur because of changes in the membrane itself, because of improper ionic balance outside the membrane, and because of changes in electrical resistances between cells, especially in organs such as the heart and brain that have many small but coupled cells. As might be expected, a great deal of time and energy has been and is being used to better understand such failures. Remarkable excitation sequences showing initial reentry of cardiac excitation have been presented by Spach et al. (2007). Additionally, understanding has been greatly aided by the understanding of molecular structure, for example, Watson et al. (2007) and Marban (1999).

Therapeutic devices for medical stimulation have now come into routine use over long periods of time, for example, cardiac pacemakers. Large currents ("shocks") of artificial origin also are used to terminate action potentials in some cases, for example, cardiac defibrillators. The transmembrane potential changes induced by such shocks now have been measured in considerable detail (e.g., Zhou et al., 1996, Ideker et al., 2000).

38.12 Linkages

An understanding of the basic electrophysiology of nerve action potentials and propagation and the basic ideas of stimulation provides a conceptual backbone for the other chapters in this section, as well as a starting point for understanding many other electrophysiological events.

In this section of the handbook, some of the relationships with other chapters are as follows: Electrically active membrane exists within a volume conductor, described by Plonsey, that follows the standard laws of electromagnetism but that mathematically is best described in a form with current sources, rather than static charges, and with biological media characterized by the conductivities, rather than by their dielectric constant. Both propagation and observation depend on the electrical conductivity of tissues (Chapter 40), and propagation depends strongly on microimpedances, that is, the resistivities within and immediately around the active tissue (Chapter 41). In this chapter on basic electrophysiology, explanations have used the Hodgkin–Huxley membrane model, but as discussed by Varghese, that is but the simplest of present-day membrane models, which encompass a much broader range of organs and tissues.

A major part of electrophysiology involves the flow of currents into the volume conductor around the active tissues and out on to the body surface, and the voltages these currents produce. Such voltages are relatively easy to measure, for example, the ECG. As a consequence, the science and art of understanding and interpretation of extracellular voltages is highly developed. The chapter by Johnson shows the sophistication of modern models, and the chapter by Van Oosterom provides the mathematical basis for the core of such calculations (which in some fashion, divide volumes into surfaces, and subdivide surfaces into triangles). The major fields of interpretation of waveforms include electrocardiography (for the heart, Chapter 45), for the brain (Chapter 47), and for muscles (Chapter 46). In all systems electrical stimulation is critical to human-engineered intervention by stimulation into the electrophysiological events (Chapter 49). Finally, while the major focus here is on electrical stimulation and measurement, there are systematic corollaries with magnetic stimulation and magnetic fields (Chapter 48).

Outside of this section of the handbook, there are many other linkages. For example, strong linkages exist to the sections on neuroengineering and rehabilitation engineering, for which bioelectricity is the means to the desired end. Galvani would be amazed.

References

Barr RC, Plonsey R. 2003. Field stimulation of 2-D sheets of excitable tissue. *IEEE T Bio-Med Eng* 51:539–40.

Byrne JH, Schultz SG. 1988. *An Introduction to Membrane Transport and Bioelectricity*. Raven Press, New York.

Cabo C, Barr RC. 1992. Propagation model using the DiFrancesco–Nobel equations. *Med Biol Eng Comput* 30:292.

Franklin B. 1784. Report of Dr. Benjamin Franklin, and Other Commissioners, Charged by the King of France, with the Examination of the Animal Magnetism, as Now Practiced in Paris. See also Kathryn Schultz, *Being Wrong*, Harper Collins Publishers, 2010, p. vix.

Galvani L. 1791. *Commentary on the Effect of Electricity on Muscular Motion. Proceedings of the Institute of Sciences at Bologna*. De viribus electricitatis, 1791. The International Centre for the History of Universities and Science (CIS), Università di Bologna. See also http://en.wikipedia.org/wiki/Galvani Wikipedia (Galvani), 2010,

Gulrajani R. 1998. *Bioelectricity and Biomagnetism*. John Wiley and Sons, New York. pp. 525–610.

Hille B. 2001. *Ion Channels of Excitable Membranes*. 3rd Edition. Sinauer Associates, Sunderland, MA.

Hodgkin AL, Huxley AF. 1952. A quantitative description of membrane current and its application to conduction and excitation in nerve. *J Physiol* 117:500–544.

Ideker RE, Chattipakorn TN, Gray RA. 2000. Defibrillation mechanisms: The parable of the blind men and the elephant. *J Cardiovasc Electrophysiol* 11:1008–1013.

Malmivuo J, Plonsey R. 1995. *Bioelectromagnetism: Principles and Applications of Bioelectric and Biomagnetic Fields*. Oxford University Press, New York.

Marban E. 1999. Molecular approaches to arrhythmogenesis. In *Molecular Basis of Cardiovascular Disease*, KR Chien, Ed. Philadelphia, W. B. Saunders, Chapter 14, pp. 313–328.

Noble D, DiFrancesco D, Noble S. 1994. *Oxsoft Heart Program Manual*. Wellesley Hills, MA, NB Datyner.

Noble D, Rudy Y. 2001. Models of cardiac ventricular action potentials: Iterative interaction between experiment and simulation. *Philos Trans R Soc Lond A* 359(1783):1127–1142.

Panofsky WKH, Phillips M. 1962. *Classical Electricity and Magnetism*, 2nd edition. Addison-Wesley, New York.

Peterchev AV, Murphy DL, Lisanby SH. 2008. Repetitive transcranial magnetic stimulator with controllable pulse parameters (cTMS). *IEEE Transactions on Biomedical Engng* 55:257–266.

Plonsey R, Barr RC. 2007. *Bioelectricity: A Quantitative Approach*, 3rd edition. Springer Science + Business Media, New York. ISBN 978-0-387-48864-6.

Rattay F. 1990. *Electrical Nerve Stimulation*. Springer-Verlag, Wien, New York.

Roth BJ, Passer PJ. 1990. A model of the stimulation of a nerve fiber by electromagnetic stimulating. *IEEE Trans BME* 37:588–597.

Spach MS, Barr RC, Johnson EA, Kootsey JM. 1973. Cardiac extracellular potentials: Analysis of complex waveforms about the Purkinje network in dogs. *Circ Res* 31:465.

Spach MS, Heidlage JF, Barr RC, Dolber PC. 2004. Cell size and communication: Role in structural and electrical development and remodeling of the heart. *Heart Rhythm* 1:235–251.

Spach MS, Heidlage JF, Dolber PC, Barr RC. 2007. Mechanism of origin of conduction disturbances in aging human atrial bundles: Experimental and model study. *Heart Rhythm* 4:175–185.

Taccardi B, Punske BB. 2002. Body surface and epicardial mapping: State of the art and future perspectives. *IJBEM* 4:91–94.

Watson JD, Myers RM, Caudy AA, Witkowski JA. 2007. *Recombinant DNA: Genes and Genomes*. 3rd edition. Scientific American Books, New York.

Wikswo JP Jr, van Egeraat JM. 1991. Cellular magnetic fields: Fundamental and applied measurements on nerve axons, peripheral nerve bundles, and skeletal muscle. *J Clin Neurophysiol* 8(2):170.

Zhou XH, Smith WM, Rollins DL, Ideker RE. 1996. Trans-membrane potential changes caused by shocks in guinea pig papillary muscle. *Am J Physiol* 271:H2536–H2546.

39

Volume Conductor Theory

39.1 Basic Relations in the Idealized Homogeneous Volume
Conductor 39-1
39.2 Monopole and Dipole Fields in the Uniform Volume of
Infinite Extent 39-3
39.3 Volume Conductor Properties of Passive Tissue 39-4
39.4 Effects of Volume Conductor Inhomogeneities: Secondary
Sources and Images 39-5
References 39-8

Robert Plonsey
Duke University

This chapter considers the properties of the volume conductor as it pertains to the evaluation of electric and magnetic fields arising therein. The sources of the aforementioned fields are described by $\bar{J}^i$, a function of position and time, which has the dimensions of current per unit area *or* dipole moment per unit volume. Such sources may arise from active endogenous electrophysiologic processes such as propagating action potentials, generator potentials, synaptic potentials, and so on. Sources may also be established exogenously, as exemplified by electric or magnetic field stimulation. Details on how one may quantitatively evaluate a source function from an electrophysiologic process are found in other chapters. For our purposes here, we assume that such a source function $\bar{J}^i$ is known and, furthermore, that it has well-behaved mathematical properties. Given such a source, we focus our attention here on a description of the volume conductor as it affects the electric and magnetic fields that are established in it. As a loose definition, we consider the *volume conductor* to be the contiguous passive conducting medium that surrounds the region occupied by the source $\bar{J}^i$. (This may include a portion of the excitable tissue itself that is sufficiently far from $\bar{J}^i$ to be described passively.)

39.1 Basic Relations in the Idealized Homogeneous Volume Conductor

Excitable tissue, when activated, will be found to generate currents both within itself and also in all surrounding conducting media. The latter passive region is characterized as a *volume conductor*. The adjective *volume* emphasizes that current flow is three-dimensional, in contrast to the confined one-dimensional flow within insulated wires. The volume conductor is usually assumed to be a monodomain (whose meaning will be amplified later), isotropic, resistive, and (frequently) homogeneous. These are simply assumptions, as will be discussed subsequently. The permeability of biologic tissues is important when examining magnetic fields and is usually assumed to be that of free space. The permittivity is a more complicated property, but outside cell membranes (which have a high lipid content), it is also usually considered to be that of free space.

A general, mathematical description of a current source is specified by a function $\bar{J}^i(x, y, z, t)$, namely, a vector field of current density in say milliamperes per square centimeter that varies in both space and time. A study of sources of physiologic origin shows that their temporal behavior lies in a low-frequency range. For example, currents generated by the heart have a power density spectrum that lies mainly under 1 kHz (in fact, clinical ECG instruments have upper frequency limits of 100 Hz), while most other electrophysiologic sources of interest (i.e., those underlying the EEG, EMG, EOG, etc.) are of even lower frequency. Examination of electromagnetic fields in regions with typical physiologic conductivities, with dimensions of under 1 m and frequencies less than 1 kHz, shows that *quasi-static* conditions apply. That is, at a given instant in time, source–field relationships correspond to those found under static conditions.[*] Thus, in effect, we are examining direct current (dc) flow in physiologic volume conductors, and these can be maintained only by the presence of a supply of energy (a "battery"). In fact, we may expect that wherever a physiologic current source $\bar{J}^i$ arises, we also can identify a (normally nonelectrical) energy source that generates this current. In electrophysiologic processes, the immediate repository of energy is the potential energy associated with the varying chemical compositions encountered (extracellular ionic concentrations that differ greatly from intracellular concentrations), but the long-term energy source is the adenosine triphosphate (ATP) that drives various pumps that create and maintain the aforementioned concentration gradients.

On the basis of the aforementioned assumptions, we consider a uniformly conducting medium of conductivity σ and of infinite extent within which a current source $\bar{J}^i$ lies. This, in turn, establishes an electric field $\bar{E}$ and, based on Ohm's law, a conduction current density $\sigma\bar{E}$. The total current density $\bar{J}$ is the sum of the aforementioned currents, namely

$$\bar{J} = \sigma\bar{E} + \bar{J}^i \tag{39.1}$$

Now, by virtue of the quasi-static conditions, the electric field may be derived from a scalar potential Φ (Plonsey and Heppner, 1967) so that

$$\bar{E} = -\nabla\Phi \tag{39.2}$$

Since quasi-steady-state conditions apply, $\bar{J}$ must be solenoidal, and consequently, substituting Equation 39.2 into Equation 39.1 and then setting the divergence of Equation 39.1 to zero show that Φ must satisfy Poisson's equation, namely

$$\nabla^2\Phi = \left(\frac{1}{\sigma}\right)\nabla \cdot \bar{J}^i \tag{39.3}$$

An integral solution to Equation 39.3 is (Plonsey and Collin, 1961)

$$\Phi_p(x', y', z') = -\frac{1}{4\pi\sigma}\int_v \frac{\nabla \cdot \bar{J}^i}{r}\, dv \tag{39.4}$$

where r in Equation 39.4 is the distance from a field point $P(x', y', z')$ to an element of source at $dv(x, y, z)$, that is

$$r = \sqrt{(x - x')^2 + (y - y')^2 + (z - z')^2} \tag{39.5}$$

---

[*] Note that while, in effect, we consider relationships arising when $\partial/\partial t = 0$, all fields are actually assumed to vary in time synchronously with $\bar{J}^i$. Furthermore, for the special case of magnetic field stimulation, the source of the primary electric field, $\partial\bar{A}/\partial t$, where $\bar{A}$ is the magnetic vector potential, must be retained.

Equation 39.4 may be transformed to an alternate form by employing the vector identity

$$\nabla \cdot \left[\left(\frac{1}{r} \right) \bar{J}^i \right] \equiv \left(\frac{1}{r} \right) \nabla \cdot \bar{J}^i + \nabla \left(\frac{1}{r} \right) \cdot \bar{J}^i \tag{39.6}$$

On the basis of Equation 39.6, we may substitute for the integrand in Equation 39.4 the sum $\nabla \cdot [(1/r)\bar{J}^i] - \nabla(1/r) \cdot \bar{J}^i$, giving the following:

$$\Phi_p(x', y', z') = -\frac{1}{4\pi\sigma} \left\{ \int_v \nabla \cdot \left[\left(\frac{1}{r} \right) \bar{J}^i \right] dv - \int_v \nabla \left(\frac{1}{r} \right) \bar{J}^i dv \right\} \tag{39.7}$$

The first term on the right-hand side may be transformed using the divergence theorem as follows:

$$\int_v \nabla \cdot \left[\left(\frac{1}{r} \right) \bar{J}^i \right] dv = \int_s \left(\frac{1}{r} \right) \bar{J}^i \cdot d\bar{S} = 0 \tag{39.8}$$

The volume integral in Equations 39.4 and 39.8 is defined simply to include all sources. Consequently, in Equation 39.8, the surface S, which bounds V, necessarily lies away from $\bar{J}^i$. Since $\bar{J}^i$ thus is equal to zero on S, the expression in Equation 39.8 must likewise equal zero. The result is that Equation 39.4 may also be written as

$$\Phi_p(x', y', z') = -\frac{1}{4\pi\sigma} \int_v \frac{\nabla \cdot \bar{J}^i}{r} dv = \frac{1}{4\pi\sigma} \int_v \bar{J}^i \cdot \nabla \left(\frac{1}{r} \right) dv \tag{39.9}$$

We will derive the mathematical expressions for monopole and dipole fields in the next section, but based on those results, we can give a physical interpretation of the source terms in each of the integrals on the right-hand side of Equation 39.9. In the first, we note that $-\nabla \cdot \bar{J}^i$ is a volume source density, akin to charge density in electrostatics. In the second integral of Equation 39.9, $\bar{J}^i$ behaves with the dimensions of dipole moment per unit volume. This confirms an assertion, above, that $\bar{J}^i$ has a dual interpretation as a current density, as originally defined in Equation 39.1, or a volume dipole density, as can be inferred from Equation 39.9; in either case, its dimension is $mA/cm^2 = mA \cdot cm/cm^3$.

39.2 Monopole and Dipole Fields in the Uniform Volume of Infinite Extent

The monopole and dipole constitute the basic source elements in electrophysiology. We examine the fields produced by each in this section.

If one imagines an infinitely thin wire insulated over its extent except at its tip to be introducing a current into a uniform volume conductor of infinite extent, then we illustrate an idealized point source. Assuming the total applied current to be I_0 and located at the coordinate origin, then, by symmetry, the current density at a radius r must be given by the total current I_0 divided by the area of the spherical surface, or

$$\bar{J} = \frac{I_0}{4\pi r^2} \bar{a}_r \tag{39.10}$$

and $\vec{a}_r$ is a unit vector in the radial direction. This current source can be described by the nomenclature of the previous section as

$$\nabla \cdot \vec{J}^i = -I_0 \delta(r) \tag{39.11}$$

where δ denotes a volume delta function.

One can apply Ohm's law to Equation 39.10 and obtain an expression for the electric field, and if Equation 39.2 is also applied, we get

$$\vec{E} = -\nabla \Phi = \frac{I_0}{4\pi\sigma r^2} \vec{a}_r \tag{39.12}$$

where σ is the conductivity of the volume conductor. Since the right-hand side of Equation 39.12 is a function of r only, we can integrate to find Φ, which is

$$\Phi = \frac{I_0}{4\pi\sigma r} \tag{39.13}$$

In obtaining Equation 39.13, the constant of integration was set equal to zero so that the point at infinity has the usually chosen zero potential.

The dipole source consists of two monopoles of equal magnitude and opposite sign whose spacing approaches zero and whose magnitude during the limiting process increases such that the product of spacing and magnitude is constant. If we start out with both component monopoles at the origin, then the total source and field are zero. However, if we now displace the positive source in an arbitrary direction $\vec{d}$, then cancellation is no longer complete, and at a field point P, we simply see the change in monopole field resulting from the displacement. For a very small displacement, this amounts to (i.e., we retain only the linear term in a Taylor series expansion)

$$\Phi_p = \frac{\partial}{\partial d}\left(\frac{I_0}{4\pi\sigma r}\right) d \tag{39.14}$$

The partial derivative in Equation 39.14 is called the *directional derivative*, and this can be evaluated by taking the dot product of the gradient of the expression enclosed in parentheses with the direction of d (i.e., $\nabla() \cdot \vec{a}_d$, where $\vec{a}_d$ is a unit vector in the $\vec{d}$ direction). The result is

$$\Phi_p = \frac{I_0 d}{4\pi\sigma} \vec{a}_d \cdot \nabla\left(\frac{1}{r}\right) \tag{39.15}$$

By definition, the dipole moment $\vec{m} = I_0 \vec{d}$ in the limits as $d \to 0$; as noted, m remains finite. Thus, finally, the dipole field is given by (Plonsey, 1969)

$$\Phi_p = \frac{1}{4\pi\sigma} \vec{m} \cdot \nabla\left(\frac{1}{r}\right) \tag{39.16}$$

39.3 Volume Conductor Properties of Passive Tissue

If one were considering an active single isolated fiber lying in an extensive volume conductor (e.g., an *in vitro* preparation in a Ringer's bath), then there is a clear separation between the excitable tissue and the surrounding volume conductor. However, consider in contrast the activation proceeding in the *in vivo* heart. In this case, the source currents lie in only a portion of the heart (nominally where $\nabla V_m \neq 0$). The

TABLE 39.1 Conductivity Values for Cardiac Bidomain

S/mm	Clerc (1976)	Roberts and Scher (1982)
g_{ix}	1.74×10^4	3.44×10^{-4}
g_{iy}	1.93×10^{-5}	5.96×10^{-5}
g_{ax}	6.25×10^{-4}	1.17×10^{-4}
g_{ay}	2.36×10^{-4}	8.02×10^{-5}

volume conductor now includes the remaining (passive) cardiac fibers along with an inhomogeneous torso containing a number of contiguous organs (internal to the heart are blood-filled cavities, while external are pericardium, lungs, skeletal muscle, bone, fat, skin, air, etc.).

The treatment of the surrounding multicellular cardiac tissue poses certain difficulties. A recently used and reasonable approximation is that the intracellular space, in view of the many intercellular junctions, can be represented as a continuum. A similar treatment can be extended to the interstitial space. This results in two domains that can be regarded as occupying the same physical space; each domain is separated from the other by the membrane. This view underlies the *bidomain* model (Plonsey, 1989). To reflect the underlying fiber geometry, each domain is necessarily anisotropic, with the high conductivity axes defined by the fiber direction and with an approximate cross-fiber isotropy. A further simplification may be possible in a uniform tissue region that is sufficiently far from the sources, since beyond a few space constants, transmembrane currents may become quite small and the tissue would therefore behave as a single domain (a *monodomain*). Such a tissue would also be substantially resistive. On the other hand, if the membranes behave passively and there is some degree of transmembrane current flow, then the tissue may still be approximated as a uniform monodomain, but it may be necessary to include some of the reactive properties introduced via the highly capacitive cell membranes. A classic study by Schwan and Kay (1957) of the macroscopic (averaged) properties of many tissues showed that the displacement current was normally negligible compared with the conduction current.

It is not always clear whether a bidomain model is appropriate to a particular tissue, and experimental measurements found in the literature are not always able to resolve this question. The problem is that if the experimenter believes the tissue under consideration to be, say, an isotropic monodomain, measurements are set up and interpreted that are consistent with this idea; the inherent inconsistencies may never come to light (Plonsey and Barr, 1986). Thus, one may find impedance data tabulated in the literature for a number of organs, but if the tissue is truly, say, an anisotropic bidomain, then the impedance tensor requires six numbers, and anything less is necessarily inadequate to some degree. For cardiac tissue, it is usually assumed that the impedance in the direction transverse to the fiber axis is isotropic. Consequently, only four numbers are needed. These values are given in Table 39.1 as obtained from, essentially, the only two experiments for which bidomain values were sought.

39.4 Effects of Volume Conductor Inhomogeneities: Secondary Sources and Images

In the preceding sections, we have assumed that the volume conductor is homogeneous, and the evaluation of fields from the current sources given in Equation 39.9 is based on this assumption. Consider what would happen if the volume conductor in which $\bar{J}^i$ lies is bounded by air, and the source is suddenly introduced. Equation 39.9 predicts an initial current flow into the boundary, but no current can escape into the nonconducting surrounding region. We must, consequently, have a transient during which charge piles up at the boundary, a process that continues until the field from the accumulating charges brings the net normal component of electric field to zero at the boundary. To characterize a steady-state condition with no further increase in charge requires satisfaction of the boundary condition that $\partial \Phi / \partial n = 0$ at the surface (within the tissue). The source that develops at the bounding surface is secondary to the initiation of the primary field; it is referred to as a *secondary source*. While the secondary source is essential for the satisfaction of boundary conditions, it contributes to the total field everywhere else.

The preceding illustration is for a region bounded by air, but the same phenomena would arise if the region were simply bounded by one of different conductivity. In this case, when the source is first "turned on," since the primary electric field $\vec{E}_a$ is continuous across the interface between regions of different conductivity, the current flowing into such a boundary (e.g., $\sigma_1\vec{E}_a$) is unequal to the current flowing away from that boundary (e.g., $\sigma_2\vec{E}_a$). Again, this necessarily results in an accumulation of charge, and a secondary source will grow until the applied plus secondary field satisfies the required continuity of current density, namely

$$-\sigma_1\partial\frac{\Phi_1}{\partial_n} = -\sigma_2\partial\frac{\Phi_2}{\partial_n} = J_n \tag{39.17}$$

where the surface normal n is directed from region 1 to region 2. The accumulated single source density can be shown to be equal to the discontinuity of $\partial\Phi/\partial_n$ in Equation 39.17 (Plonsey, 1974), in particular

$$K_s = J_n\left(\frac{1}{\sigma_1} - \frac{1}{\sigma_2}\right)\sigma$$

The magnitude of the steady-state secondary source can also be described as an *equivalent double layer*, the magnitude of which is (Plonsey, 1974)

$$\vec{K}_k^i = \Phi_k(\sigma_k'' - \sigma_k')\vec{n} \tag{39.18}$$

where the condition at the kth interface is described. In Equation 39.18, the two abutting regions are designated with prime and double-prime superscripts, and $\vec{n}$ is directed from the primed to the double-primed region. Actually, Equation 39.18 evaluates the double-layer source for the scalar function $\Psi = \Phi\sigma$, its strength being given by the discontinuity in Ψ at the interface (Plonsey, 1974) (the potential is necessarily continuous at the interface with the value Φ_k called for in Equation 39.18). The (secondary) potential field generated by $\vec{K}_k^i$, since it constitutes a source for Ψ with respect to which the medium is uniform and infinite in extent, can be found from Equation 39.9 as

$$\Psi_P^S = \sigma_P\Phi_P^S = \frac{1}{4\pi}\sum_k\int_k\Phi_k(\sigma_k'' - \sigma_k')\vec{n}\cdot\nabla\left(\frac{1}{r}\right)ds \tag{39.19}$$

where the superscript S denotes the secondary source/field component (alone). Solving Equation 39.19 for Φ, we get

$$\Phi_P^S = \frac{1}{4\pi\sigma_P}\sum_k\int_k\Phi_k(\sigma_k'' - \sigma_k')\vec{n}\cdot\nabla\left(\frac{1}{r}\right)ds \tag{39.20}$$

where σ_P in Equations 39.19 and 39.20 takes on the conductivity at the field point. The total field is obtained from Equation 39.20 by adding the primary field. Assuming that all applied currents lie in a region with conductivity σ_a, we then have

$$\Phi_P^S = \frac{1}{4\pi\sigma_a}\int\vec{J}^i\cdot\nabla\left(\frac{1}{r}\right)dv + \frac{1}{4\pi\sigma_P}\sum_k\int_k\Phi_k(\sigma_k'' - \sigma_k')\vec{n}\cdot\nabla\left(\frac{1}{r}\right)ds \tag{39.21}$$

(If the primary currents lie in several conductivity compartments, then each will yield a term similar to the first integral in Equation 39.21.) Note that in Equations 39.20 and 39.21, the secondary source field is similar in form to the field in a homogeneous medium of infinite extent, except that σ_p is piecewise constant and consequently introduces interfacial discontinuities. With regard to the potential, these just cancel the discontinuity introduced by the double layer itself so that Φ_k is appropriately continuous across each passive interface.

The primary and secondary source currents that generate the electrical potential in Equation 39.21 also set up a magnetic field. The primary source, for example, is the forcing function in the Poisson equation for the vector potential $\vec{A}$ (Plonsey, 1981), namely

$$\nabla^2 \vec{A} = -\vec{J}^i \tag{39.22}$$

From this, it is not difficult to show that, due to Equation 39.21 for Φ, we have the following expression for the magnetic field $\vec{H}$ (Plonsey, 1981):

$$\vec{H} = \frac{1}{4\pi} \int \vec{J}^i \times \nabla\left(\frac{1}{r}\right) dv + \frac{1}{4\pi} \sum_k \int \Phi_k (\sigma_k'' - \sigma_k') \vec{n} \times \nabla\left(\frac{1}{r}\right) dS \tag{39.23}$$

A simple illustration of these ideas is found in the case of two semi-infinite regions of different conductivity, 1 and 2, with a unit point current source located in region 1 a distance h from the interface. Region 1, which we may think of as on the "left," has the conductivity σ_1, while region 2, on the "right," is at conductivity σ_2. The field in region 1 is that which arises from the actual point current source plus an image point source of magnitude $(\rho_2 - \rho_1)/(\rho_2 + \rho_1)$ located in region 2 at the mirror-image point (Schwan and Kay, 1957). The field in region 2 arises from an equivalent point source located at the actual source point but of strength $[1 + (\rho_2 - \rho_1)/(\rho_2 + \rho_1)]$. One can confirm this by noting that all fields satisfy Poisson's equation and that at the interface, Φ is continuous while the normal component of current density is also continuous (i.e., $\sigma_1 \partial \Phi_1/\partial n = \sigma_2 \partial \Phi_2/\partial n$).

The potential on the interface is constant along a circular path whose origin is the foot of the perpendicular from the point source. Calling this radius r and applying Equation 39.13, we have for the surface potential Φ_S

$$\Phi_S = \frac{\rho_1}{4\pi\sqrt{h^2 + r^2}} \left(1 + \frac{\rho_2 - \rho_1}{\rho_2 + \rho_1}\right) \tag{39.24}$$

and consequently a secondary double-layer source $\vec{K}_S$ is, according to Equation 39.18

$$\vec{K}_S = \frac{\rho_1}{4\pi\sqrt{h^2 + r^2}} \left(1 + \frac{\rho_2 - \rho_1}{\rho_2 + \rho_1}\right) (\sigma_2 - \sigma_1) \vec{n} \tag{39.25}$$

where $\vec{n}$ is directed from region 1 to region 2. The field from $\vec{K}_S$ in region 1 is exactly equal to that from a point source of strength $(\rho_2 - \rho_1)/(\rho_2 + \rho_1)$ at the mirror-image point, which can be verified by evaluating and showing the equality of the following:

$$\Phi_P = \frac{1}{4\pi\sigma_1} \int \vec{K}_S \cdot \nabla\left(\frac{1}{r}\right) dS = \frac{(\rho_2 - \rho_1)/(\rho_2 - \rho_1)}{4\pi\sigma_1 R} \tag{39.26}$$

where R in Equation 39.26 is the distance from the mirror-image point to the field point P, and r in Equation 39.26 is the distance from the surface integration point to the field point.

References

Clerc, L. 1976. Directional differences of impulse spread in trabecular muscle from mammalian heart. *J. Physiol. (Lond.)* 255: 335.

Plonsey, R. 1969. *Bioelectric Phenomena*. New York, McGraw-Hill.

Plonsey, R. 1974. The formulation of bioelectric source–field relationship in terms of surface discontinuities. *J. Frank Inst.* 297: 317.

Plonsey, R. 1981. Generation of magnetic fields by the human body (theory). In S.-N. Erné, H.-D. Hahlbohm, and H. Lübbig (Eds.), *Biomagnetism*, pp. 177–205. Berlin, W de Gruyter.

Plonsey, R. 1989. The use of the bidomain model for the study of excitable media. *Lect. Math. Life Sci.* 21: 123.

Plonsey, R. and Barr, R.C. 1986. A critique of impedance measurements in cardiac tissue. *Ann. Biomed. Eng.* 14: 307.

Plonsey, R. and Collin, R.E. 1961. *Principles and Applications of Electromagnetic Fields*. New York, McGraw-Hill.

Plonsey, R. and Heppner, D. 1967. Consideration of quasi-stationarity in electrophysiological systems. *Bull. Math. Biophys.* 29: 657.

Roberts, D. and Scher, A.M. 1982. Effect of tissue anisotropy on extracellular potential fields in canine myocardium *in situ*. *Circ. Res.* 50: 342.

Schwan, H.P. and Kay, C.F. 1957. The conductivity of living tissues. *NY Acad. Sci.* 65: 1007.

40

Electrical Conductivity of Tissues

40.1 Introduction 40-1
40.2 Cell Suspensions 40-2
40.3 Fiber Suspensions 40-4
40.4 Syncytia 40-8
Defining Terms 40-11
Acknowledgments 40-11
References 40-11
Further Information 40-12

Bradley J. Roth
Oakland University

40.1 Introduction

One of the most important problems in bioelectric theory is the calculation of the electrical potential, Φ (V), throughout a *volume conductor*. The calculation of Φ is important in impedance imaging, cardiac pacing and defibrillation, electrocardiogram and electroencephalogram analysis, and functional electrical stimulation. In bioelectric problems, Φ often changes slowly enough that we can assume it is *quasistatic* (Plonsey, 1969); we ignore capacitive and inductive effects and the finite speed of propagation of electromagnetic radiation. (Usually for bioelectric phenomena, this assumption is valid for frequencies below about 100 kHz.) Under the quasistatic approximation, the continuity equation states that the divergence, $\nabla\cdot$, of the current density, J (A/m²), is equal to the applied or endogenous source of electrical current, S (A/m³):

$$\nabla \cdot J = S. \tag{40.1}$$

In regions of tissue where there are no sources, S is zero. In these cases, the divergenceless of J is equivalent to the law of *conservation of current* that is often invoked when analyzing electrical circuits. Another property of a volume conductor is that the current density and the electric field, E (V/m), are related linearly by *Ohm's law*

$$J = gE, \tag{40.2}$$

where g is the electrical *conductivity* (S/m). Finally, the relationship between the electric field and the gradient, ∇, of the potential is

$$E = -\nabla\Phi. \tag{40.3}$$

The purpose of this chapter is to characterize the electrical conductivity. This task is not easy, because g is generally a macroscopic parameter (an "effective conductivity") that represents the electrical properties of the tissue averaged over many cells. The effective conductivity can vary with direction, can be complex (contain real and imaginary parts), and can depend on the temporal and spatial frequencies.

Before discussing the conductivity of tissue, consider one of the simplest and most easily understood volume conductors: saline. The electrical conductivity of saline arises from the motion of free ions in response to a steady electric field, and is on the order of 1 S/m. Besides conductivity, another property of saline is its electrical *permittivity*, ε (S s/m). This property is related to the dielectric constant, κ (dimensionless), by $\varepsilon = \kappa\varepsilon_0$, where ε_0 is the permittivity of free space, 8.854×10^{-12} S s/m. Dielectric properties arise from bound charge that is displaced by the electric field, creating a dipole. They can also arise if the applied electric field aligns molecular dipoles (such as the dipole moments of water molecules) that normally are oriented randomly. The DC (direct current) dielectric constant of saline is similar to that of water (about $\kappa = 80$).

The movement of free charge produces conductivity, whereas stationary dipoles produce permittivity. In steady state, the distinction between the two is clear, but at higher frequencies, the concepts merge. In such a case, we can combine the electrical properties into a complex conductivity, g':

$$g' = g + i\omega\varepsilon, \tag{40.4}$$

where ω (rad/s) is the angular frequency ($\omega = 2\pi f$, where f is the frequency in Hz) and i is $\sqrt{-1}$. The real part of g' accounts for the movement of charge in phase with the electric field; the imaginary part accounts for out-of-phase motion. Both the real and the imaginary parts of the complex conductivity may depend on the frequency. For many bioelectric phenomena, the first term in Equation 40.4 is much larger than the second, so the tissue can be represented as purely conductive (Plonsey, 1969). (The imaginary part of the complex conductivity represents a capacitive effect, and therefore technically violates our assumption of quasistationarity. This violation is the only exception we will make to our general rule of a quasistatic potential.)

40.2 Cell Suspensions

The earliest and simplest model describing the electrical conductivity of a biological tissue is a suspension of cells in a saline solution (Cole, 1968; Peters et al., 2001). Let us consider a suspension of spherical cells, each of radius a (Figure 40.1a). The saline surrounding the cells constitutes the *interstitial* space

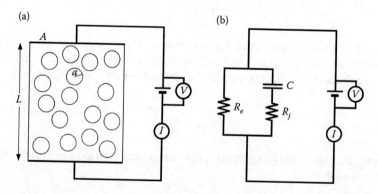

FIGURE 40.1 (a) A schematic diagram of a suspension of spherical cells; the effective conductivity of this suspension is IL/VA. (b) An electric circuit equivalent of the effective conductivity of this suspension.

conductivity σ_e), while the conducting fluid inside the cells constitutes the *intracellular* space (conductivity σ_i). (We shall follow Henriquez (1993) in denoting macroscopic effective conductivities by g and microscopic conductivities by σ.) The cell membrane separates the two spaces: a thin layer having conductivity per unit area G_m (S/m²) and capacitance per unit area C_m (F/m²). One additional parameter—the intracellular volume fraction, f (dimensionless)—indicates how tightly the cells are packed together. The volume fraction can range from nearly zero (a dilute solution) to almost 1. (Spherical cells cannot approach a volume fraction of 1, but tightly packed, nonspherical cells can.) For irregularly shaped cells, the "radius" is difficult to define. In these cases, it is easier to specify the surface-to-volume ratio of the tissue (the ratio of the membrane surface area to tissue volume). For spherical cells, the surface-to-volume ratio is $3f/a$.

We can define operationally the effective conductivity, g, of a cell suspension by the following process (Figure 40.1a): Place the suspension in a cylindrical tube of length L and cross-sectional area A (be sure that L and A are large enough so the volume contains many cells). Apply a DC potential difference V across the two ends of the cylinder (so that the electric field has strength V/L) and measure the total current, I, passing through the suspension. The effective conductivity is IL/VA.

Deriving an expression for the effective conductivity of a suspension of spheres in terms of microscopic parameters is an old and interesting problem in electromagnetic theory (Cole, 1968). For DC fields, the effective conductivity, g, of a suspension of insulating spheres placed in a solution of conductivity σ_e is

$$g = \frac{2(1-f)}{2+f}\sigma_e. \tag{40.5}$$

For most cells, G_m is small enough so the membrane behaves as an insulator; thus, the assumption of insulating spheres is applicable. The net effect of the cells is to decrease the conductivity of the solution (the decrease can be substantial for tightly packed cells).

The cell membrane has a capacitance of about 0.01 F/m² (or, in traditional units, 1 μF/cm²), which causes the electrical conductivity to depend on frequency. The electrical circuit in Figure 40.1b represents the suspension of cells: R_e is the effective resistance to current passing entirely through the interstitial space; R_i is the effective resistance to current passing into the intracellular space; and C is the effective membrane capacitance. (The membrane conductance is usually small enough so that it has little effect, regardless of the frequency.) At low frequencies, all of the current is restricted to the interstitial space, and the electrical conductivity is given approximately by Equation 40.5 above. At large frequencies, C shunts current across the membrane, so that the effective conductivity of the tissue is

$$g = \frac{2(1-f)\sigma_e + (1+2f)\sigma_i}{(2+f)\sigma_e + (1-f)\sigma_i}\sigma_e. \tag{40.6}$$

At intermediate frequencies, the effective conductivity has both real and imaginary parts because the membrane capacitance contributes significantly to the effective conductivity. In these cases, Equation 40.6 still holds if σ_i is replaced by σ_i^*, where

$$\sigma_i^* = \frac{\sigma_i Y_m a}{\sigma_i + Y_m a}, \quad \text{with } Y_m = G_m + i\omega C_m. \tag{40.7}$$

Figure 40.2 shows the effective conductivity (magnitude and phase) as a function of frequency for a typical tissue. The increase in the phase at about 300 kHz is sometimes called the "beta dispersion."

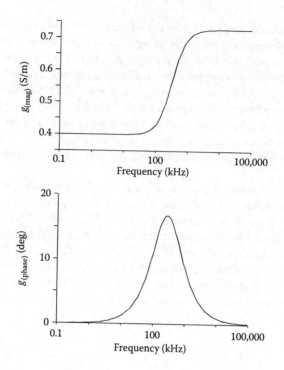

FIGURE 40.2 The magnitude and phase of the effective conductivity as a function of frequency, for a suspension of spherical cells: $f = 0.5$; $a = 20$ μm; $\sigma_e = 1$ S/m; $\sigma_i = 0.5$ S/m; $G_m = 0$; and $C_m = 0.01$ F/m².

40.3 Fiber Suspensions

Many of the most interesting electrically active tissues, such as nerve and skeletal muscle, are better approximated as a suspension of cylinders rather than a suspension of spheres. This difference has profound implications because it introduces *anisotropy*: the effective electrical conductivity depends on direction. Henceforth, we must speak of the longitudinal effective conductivity parallel to the cylindrical fibers, g_L, and the transverse effective conductivity perpendicular to the fibers, g_T. (In theory, the conductivity could be different in three directions; however, the electrical properties in the two directions perpendicular to the fibers are often the same.) In general, the conductivity is no longer a scalar quantity, but is a tensor instead, and must be represented by a 3×3 symmetric matrix. If our coordinate axes lie along the principal directions of this matrix (invariably, the directions parallel to and perpendicular to the fibers), then the off-diagonal terms of the matrix are zero. If, however, we choose our coordinate axes differently, or if the fibers curve so that the direction parallel to the fibers varies over space, we have to deal with tensor properties, including off-diagonal components.

When the electric field is applied perpendicular to the fiber direction, a suspension of fibers is similar to the suspension of cells described above (in Figure 40.1a, we must now imagine that the circles represent cross sections of cylindrical fibers, rather than spherical cells). The expression for the effective transverse conductivity of a suspension of cylindrical cells, of radius a and intracellular conductivity σ_i, placed in a solution of conductivity σ_e, with intracellular volume fraction f, is (Cole, 1968)

$$g_T = \frac{(1-f)\sigma_e + (1+f)\sigma_i^*}{(1+f)\sigma_e + (1-f)\sigma_i^*}\sigma_e,$$

(40.8)

where Equation 40.7 defines σ_i^*. At DC, and for $G_m = 0$, Equation 40.8 reduces to

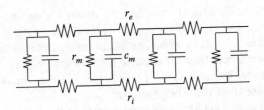

FIGURE 40.3 An electrical circuit representing a one-dimensional nerve or muscle fiber: r_i and r_e are the intra-cellular and extracellular resistances per unit length (Ω/m); r_m is the membrane resistance times unit length (Ω m); and c_m is the membrane capacitance per unit length (F/m).

$$g_T = \frac{1-f}{1+f}\sigma_e. \tag{40.9}$$

When an electric field is applied parallel to the fiber direction, a new behavior arises that is fundamentally different from that observed for a suspension of spherical cells. Return for a moment to our operational definition of the effective conductivity. Surprisingly, the effective longitudinal conductivity of a suspension of fibers depends on the length L of the tissue sample used for the measurement. To understand this dependence, we must consider one-dimensional *cable theory* (Plonsey, 1969). The circuit in Figure 40.3 approximates a single nerve or muscle fiber. Adopting the traditional electrophysiology nomenclature, we denote the intracellular and extracellular resistances per unit length along the fiber by r_i and r_e (Ω/m), the membrane resistance times unit length by r_m (Ω m), and the capacitance per unit length by c_m (F/m). The cable equation governs the transmembrane potential, V_m:

$$\lambda^2 \frac{\partial^2 V_m}{\partial x^2} = \tau \frac{\partial V_m}{\partial t} + V_m, \tag{40.10}$$

where τ is the time constant, $r_m c_m$, and λ is the length constant, $\sqrt{r_m/(r_i + r_e)}$. For a truncated fiber of length L (m) with sealed ends, and with a steady-state current I (A) injected into the extracellular space at one end and removed at the other, the solution to the cable equation is

$$V_m = I r_e \lambda \frac{\sinh(x/\lambda)}{\cosh(L/2\lambda)}, \tag{40.11}$$

where the origin of the x-axis is at the midpoint between the electrodes. The extracellular potential, V_e, consists of two terms: one is proportional to x, and the other is $r_e/(r_i + r_e)$ times V_m. We can evaluate V_e at the two ends of the fiber to obtain the voltage drop between the electrodes, ΔV_e

$$\Delta V_e = \frac{r_i r_e}{r_i + r_e} I \left[L + \frac{r_e}{r_i} 2\lambda \tanh\left(\frac{L}{2\lambda}\right) \right]. \tag{40.12}$$

If L is very large compared to λ, the extracellular voltage drop reduces to

$$\Delta V_e = \frac{r_i r_e}{r_i + r_e} L I \quad L \gg \lambda. \tag{40.13}$$

The leading factor is the parallel combination of the intracellular and extracellular resistances. However, if L is very small compared to λ, the extracellular voltage drop becomes

$$\Delta V_e = r_e L I \quad L \ll \lambda. \tag{40.14}$$

In this case, the leading factor is simply the extracellular resistance alone. Physically, there is a redistribution of current into the intracellular space that occurs over a distance on the order of a length constant. If the tissue length is much longer than a length constant, the current is redistributed completely between the intracellular and extracellular spaces. If the tissue length is much smaller than a length constant, the current does not enter the fiber, but is instead restricted to the extracellular space. If either of these two conditions is met, then the effective conductivity ($IL/A\Delta V_e$, where A is the cross-sectional area of the tissue strand) is independent of L. However, if L is comparable to λ, the effective conductivity depends on the size of the tissue being studied.

Roth et al. (1988) recast the expression for the effective longitudinal conductivity in terms of *spatial frequency*, k (rad/m). This approach has two advantages. First, the temporal and spatial behaviors are both described using frequency analysis. Second, a parameter describing the size of a specific piece of tissue is not necessary: the spatial frequency dependence becomes a property of the tissue, not the measurement. The expression for the DC effective longitudinal conductivity is

$$g_L = \frac{(1-f)\sigma_e + f\sigma_i}{1 + \dfrac{f\sigma_i}{(1-f)\sigma_e} \dfrac{1}{1 + \left(\dfrac{1}{\lambda k}\right)^2}}. \tag{40.15}$$

To relate the effective longitudinal conductivity to Equations 40.13 and 40.14 above, note that $1/k$ plays the same role as L. If $k\lambda \ll 1$, g_L reduces to $(1-f)\sigma_e + f\sigma_i$, which is equivalent to the parallel combination

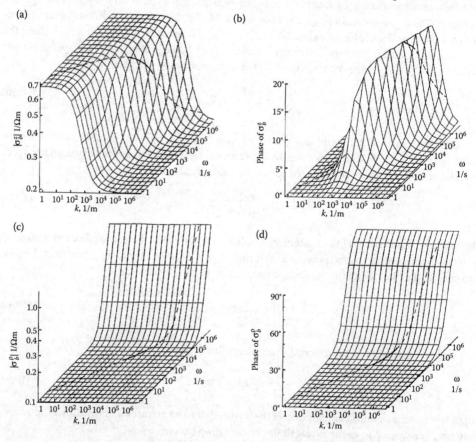

FIGURE 40.4 The magnitude (a, c) and phase (b, d) of the effective longitudinal (a, b) and transverse (c, d) effective conductivities, calculated using the spatial, k, and temporal, ω, frequency model. The parameters used in this calculation are $G_m = 1$ S/m²; $C_m = 0.01$ F/m²; $f = 0.9$; $a = 20$ μm; $\sigma_i = 0.55$ S/m; and $\sigma_e = 2$ S/m. (From Roth, B.J., Gielen, F.L.H., and Wikswo, J.P., Jr. 1988. *Math. Biosci.*, 88:159–189. With permission.)

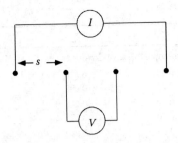

FIGURE 40.5 A schematic diagram of the four-electrode technique for measuring tissue conductivities. Current, I, is passed through the outer two electrodes, and the potential, V, is measured between the inner two. The inter-electrode distance is s.

of resistances in Equation 40.13. If $k\lambda \gg 1$, g_L becomes $(1 - f)\sigma_e$, implying that the current is restricted to the interstitial space, as in Equation 40.14. Equation 40.15 can be generalized to all temporal frequencies by defining λ in terms of Y_m instead of G_m (Roth et al., 1988). Figure 40.4 shows the magnitude and phase of the longitudinal and transverse effective conductivities as functions of the temporal and spatial frequencies.

The measurement of effective conductivities is complicated by the traditionally used electrode geometry. Typically, one uses a four-electrode technique (Steendijk et al., 1993), in which two electrodes inject current and two others measure the potential (Figure 40.5). Gielen et al. (1984) used this method to measure the electrical properties of skeletal muscle and found that the effective conductivity depended on the interelectrode distance. Roth (1989) reanalyzed Gielen et al.'s data using the spatial frequency-dependent model and found agreement with some of the more unexpected features or their data (Figure 40.6). Table 40.1 contains typical values of skeletal muscle effective conductivities and microscopic tissue parameters. Table 40.2 lists nerve effective conductivities.

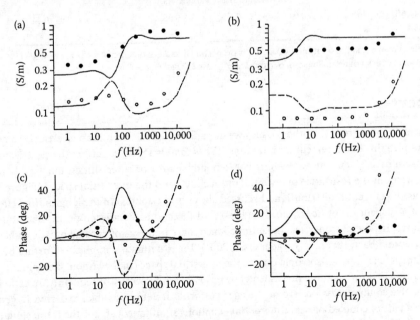

FIGURE 40.6 The calculated (a) amplitude and (b) phase of g_L (solid) and g_T (dashed) as a function of frequency, for an interelectrode distance of 0.5 mm; (c) and (d) show the quantities for an interelectrode distance of 3.0 mm. Circles represent experimental data; g_L (filled), g_T (open). (From Roth, B.J. 1989. *Med. Biol. Eng. Comput.*, 27:491–495. With permission.)

TABLE 40.1 Skeletal Muscle

Reference	g_L	g_T	Note
	Macroscopic Effective Conductivities (S/m)		
Gielen et al.,	0.35	0.086	10 Hz, IED = 3 mm
MBEC, 22:569	0.20	0.092	10 Hz, IED = 0.5 mm
Epstein & Foster,	0.52	0.076	20 Hz, IED = 17 mm
MBEC, 21:51	0.70	0.32	100 kHz, IED = 17 mm
Rush et al., *Circ*	0.67	0.040	0.1 s pulse
Res, 12:40			

Reference	σ_i (S/m)	σ_e (S/m)	f	C_m (F/m^2)	G_m (S/m^2)
	Microscopic Tissue Parameters				
Gielen et al.,	0.55	2.4	0.9	0.01	1.0
MBEC, 24:34					

Note: IED = interelectrode distance; *MBEC = Med & Biol Eng & Comput.*

TABLE 40.2 Nerve

Reference	g_L	g_T	Note
	Macroscopic Effective Conductivities (S/m)		
Tasaki, *J Neurophysiol*,	0.41	0.01	Toad sciatic nerve
27:1199			
Ranck & BeMent, *Exp*	0.57	0.083	Cat dorsal column, 10 Hz
Neurol, 11:451			

Reference	σ_i (S/m)	σ_e (S/m)	f	C_m (F/m^2)	G_m (S/m^2)
	Microscopic Tissue Parameters				
Roth & Altman, *MBEC*,	0.64	1.54	0.35	1	0.44
30:103					

Note: Volume fraction of myelin = 0.27. G_m is proportional to the axon diameter; the above value is for an axon with an outer diameter of 6.5 μm. *MBEC = Med & Biol Eng & Comput.*

40.4 Syncytia

Cardiac tissue is different from the other tissues we have discussed in that it is an electrical *syncytium*: the cells are coupled through intercellular junctions. The *bidomain* model describes the electrical properties of cardiac muscle (Henriquez, 1993). It is essentially a two- or three-dimensional cable model that takes into account the resistance of both the intracellular and the interstitial spaces (Figure 40.7). Thus, the concept of current redistribution, discussed above in the context of the longitudinal effective conductivity of a suspension of fibers, now applies in all directions. Furthermore, cardiac muscle is markedly anisotropic. These properties make impedance measurements of cardiac muscle difficult to interpret (Plonsey and Barr, 1986; Le Guyader et al., 2001). The situation is complicated further because the intracellular space is more anisotropic than is the interstitial space (in the jargon of bidomain modeling, this condition is known as "unequal anisotropy ratios") (Roth, 1997). Consequently, an expression for a single effective conductivity for cardiac muscle is difficult, if not impossible, to derive. In general, one must solve a pair of coupled partial differential equations simultaneously for the intracellular and interstitial potentials.

The bidomain model characterizes the electrical properties of the tissue by four effective conductivities: g_{iL}, g_{iT}, g_{eL}, and g_{eT}, where i and e denote the intracellular and interstitial spaces, and L and T denote the directions parallel to and perpendicular to the myocardial fibers. We can relate these parameters

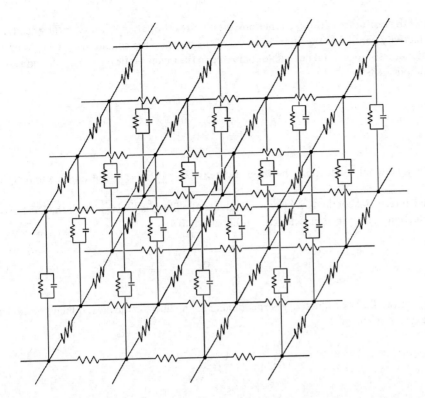

FIGURE 40.7 A circuit representing a two-dimensional syncytium (i.e., a bidomain). The lower array of resistors represents the intracellular space, the upper array represents the extracellular space, and the parallel resistors and capacitors represent the membrane.

to the microscopic tissue properties by using an operational definition of an effective bidomain conductivity, similar to the operational definition given earlier. To determine the interstitial conductivity, first dissect a cylindrical tube of tissue of length L and cross-sectional area A (one must be sure that L and A are large enough so the volume contains many cells, and that the dissection does not damage the tissue). Next, apply a drug to the tissue that makes the membrane essentially insulating (i.e., the length constant is much longer than L). Finally, apply a DC potential difference, V, across the two ends of the cylinder and measure the total current, I. The effective interstitial conductivity is IL/VA. This procedure must be performed twice, once with the fibers parallel to the axis of the cylinder, and once with the fibers perpendicular to it. To determine the effective intracellular conductivities, follow the above procedure but apply the voltage difference to the intracellular space instead of the interstitial space. Although the procedure would be extraordinarily difficult in practice, we can imagine two arrays of microelectrodes that impale the cells at both ends of the cylinder and maintain a constant potential at each end.

Expressions have been derived for the effective bidomain conductivities in terms of the microscopic tissue parameters (Roth, 1988; Henriquez, 1993; Neu and Krassowska, 1993). The effective conductivities in the direction parallel to the fibers are simplest. Imagine that the tissue is composed of long, straight fibers (like skeletal muscle) and that the intracellular space of these fibers occupies a fraction f of the tissue cross-sectional area. If the conductivity of the interstitial fluid is σ_e, then the effective interstitial conductivity parallel to the fibers, g_{eL}, is simply

$$g_{eL} = (1-f)\sigma_e. \tag{40.16}$$

If we neglect the resistance of the gap junctions, we obtain a similar expression for the effective intracellular conductivity parallel to the fibers in terms of the myoplasmic conductivity, σ_i: $g_{iL} = f\sigma_i$. When the gap junctional resistance is not negligible compared to the myoplasmic resistance, the expression for g_{iL} is more complicated:

$$g_{iL} = \frac{1}{1 + \frac{\pi a^2 \sigma_i}{bG}} f\sigma_i,$$

(40.17)

where G is the junctional conductance between two cells (S), b is the cell length (m), and a is the cell radius (m).

The effective interstitial conductivity perpendicular to the fibers is identical with the DC transverse effective conductivity for skeletal muscle given in Equation 40.9

$$g_{eT} = \frac{1-f}{1+f}\sigma_e.$$

(40.18)

The effective intracellular conductivity perpendicular to the fibers is the most difficult to model, but a reasonable expression for g_{iT} is

$$g_{iT} = \frac{1}{1 + \frac{b\sigma_i}{G}}\sigma_i.$$

(40.19)

Table 40.3 contains measured values of the bidomain conductivities (see also Roth (1997)). Typical values of the microscopic tissue parameters are also given in Table 40.3, although some are quite uncertain (particularly G).

In the last 5 years, several research groups examined a variety of techniques to determine bidomain conductivities. Stinstra et al. (2005) used a detailed microscopic model of cardiac tissue to estimate macroscopic electrical parameters, and Hand et al. (2009) derived these conductivities using homogenization. Pollard and Barr (2006) measured conductivities using multisite interstitial stimulation, and extracted anisotropic bidomain conductivities from this data. Sadleir and Henriquez (2006) performed a similar numerical simulation to obtain the bidomain parameters using a Newton–Raphson reconstruction method. Johnston et al. (2006) used a two-step process, getting the interstitial conductivities from closely spaced electrodes and then obtaining the intracellular conductivities from widely spaced

TABLE 40.3 Cardiac Muscle

Reference	g_{iL}	g_{iT}	g_{eL}	g_{eT}
Macroscopic Effective Conductivities (Ventricular Muscle) (S/m)				
Clerc, *J Physiol*, 255:335	0.17	0.019	0.62	0.24
Roberts et al., *Circ Res*, 44:701	0.28	0.026	0.22	0.13
Roberts & Scher, *Circ Res*, 50:342	0.34	0.060	0.12	0.080

Reference	σ_i (S/m)	σ_e (S/m)	f	a (μm)	b (μm)	G (μS)
Microscopic Tissue Parameters						
Roth, *Ann Biomed Eng*, 16:609	1	1	0.7	100	10	3
Neu & Krassowska, *Crit Rev Biomed Eng*, 21:137	0.4	2	0.85	100	7.5	0.05

lectrodes. Finally, Hooks and Trew (2008) analyzed data from plunge electrodes that could be used to determine if the intracellular and extracellular spaces have different conductivities in three directions, that is, the two directions perpendicular to the fiber axis are not equivalent.

Defining Terms

Anisotropy: Having different properties in different directions.

Bidomain: A two- or three-dimensional cable model that takes into account the resistance of both the intracellular and the extracellular spaces (see http://www.scholarpedia.org/article/ The_bidomain_model).

Cable theory: Representation of a cylindrical fiber as two parallel rows of resistors (one each for the intracellular and extracellular spaces) connected in a ladder network by a parallel combination of resistors and capacitors (the cell membrane).

Conductivity: A parameter (g) that measures how well a substance conducts electricity. The coefficient of proportionality between the electric field and the current density. The units of conductivity are siemens per meter (S/m). A siemens is an inverse ohm, sometimes called a "mho" in the older literature.

Conservation of current: A fundamental law of electrostatics, stating that there is no *net* current entering or leaving at any point in a volume conductor.

Interstitial space: The extracellular space between cells in a tissue.

Ohm's law: A linear relation between the electric field and current density vectors.

Permittivity: A parameter (ε) that measures the size of the dipole moment induced in a substance by an electric field. The units of permittivity are siemens second per meter (S s/m), or farads per meter (F/m).

Quasistatic: A potential distribution that changes slowly enough that we can accurately describe it by the equations of electrostatics (capacitive, inductive, and propagation effects are ignored).

Spatial frequency: A parameter governing how rapidly a function changes in space; $k = 1/(2\pi s)$, where s is the wavelength of a sinusoidally varying function.

Syncytium (pl., syncytia): A tissue in which the intracellular spaces of adjacent cells are coupled through intercellular channels so that the current can pass between any two intracellular points without crossing the cell membrane.

Volume conductor: A three-dimensional region of space containing a material that passively conducts electrical current.

Acknowledgments

I thank Dr. Craig Henriquez for several suggestions and corrections, and Barry Bowman for carefully editing the manuscript.

References

Cole, K.S. 1968. *Membranes, Ions, and Impulses*, University of California Press, Berkeley, CA.

Gielen, F.L.H., Wallinga-de Jonge, W., and Boon, K.L. 1984. Electrical conductivity of skeletal muscle tissue: Experimental results from different muscles *in vivo*. *Med. Biol. Eng. Comput.*, 22:569–577.

Hand, P.E., Griffith, B.E., and Peskin, C.S. 2009. Deriving macroscopic myocardial conductivities by homogenization of microscopic models. *Bull. Math. Biol.*, 71:1707–1726.

Henriquez, C.S. 1993. Simulating the electrical behavior of cardiac tissue using the bidomain model. *Crit. Rev. Biomed. Eng.*, 21:1–77.

Hooks, D.A. and Trew, M.L. 2008. Construction and validation of a plunge electrode array for three-dimensional determination of conductivity in the heart. *IEEE Trans. Biomed. Eng.*, 55:626–635.

Johnston, B.M., Johnston, P.R., and Kilpatrick, D. 2006. Analysis of electrode configurations for measuring cardiac tissue conductivities and fibre rotation. *Ann. Biomed. Eng.*, 34:986–996.

Le Guyader, P., Trelles, F., and Savard, P. 2001. Extracellular measurement of anisotropic bidomain myocardial conductivities. I. Theoretical analysis. *Ann. Biomed. Eng.*, 29:862–877.

Neu, J.C. and Krassowska, W. 1993. Homogenization of syncytial tissues. *Crit. Rev. Biomed. Eng.*, 21:137–199.

Peters, M.J., Hendriks, M., and Stinstra, J. G. 2001. The passive DC conductivity of human tissues described by cells in solution. *Bioelectrochemistry*, 53:155–160.

Plonsey, R. 1969. *Bioelectric Phenomena*, McGraw-Hill, New York.

Plonsey, R. and Barr, R.C. 1986. A critique of impedance measurements in cardiac tissue. *Ann. Biomed. Eng.*, 14:307–322.

Pollard, A.E. and Barr, R.C. 2006. Cardiac microimpedance measurement in two-dimensional models using multisite interstitial stimulation. *Am. J. Physiol.*, 290:H1976–H1987.

Roth, B.J. 1988. The electrical potential produced by a strand of cardiac muscle: A bidomain analysis. *Ann. Biomed. Eng.*, 16:609–637.

Roth, B.J. 1989. Interpretation of skeletal muscle four-electrode impedance measurements using spatial and temporal frequency-dependent conductivities. *Med. Biol. Eng. Comput.*, 27:491–495.

Roth, B.J. 1997. Electrical conductivity values used with the bidomain model of cardiac tissue. *IEEE Trans. Biomed. Eng.*, 44:326–328.

Roth, B.J., Gielen, F.L.H., and Wikswo, J.P. Jr. 1988. Spatial and temporal frequency-dependent conductivities in volume-conduction for skeletal muscle. *Math. Biosci.*, 88: 159–189.

Sadleir, R. and Henriquez, C. 2006. Estimation of cardiac bidomain parameters from extracellular measurement: Two dimensional study. *Ann. Biomed. Eng.*, 34:1289–1303.

Steendijk, P., Mur, G., van der Velde, E.T., and Baan, J. 1993. The four-electrode resistivity technique in anisotropic media: Theoretical analysis and application on myocardial tissue *in vivo*. *IEEE Trans. Biomed. Eng.*, 40:1138–1148.

Stinstra, J.G., Hopenfeld, B., and MacLeod, R.S. 2005. On the passive cardiac conductivity. *Ann. Biomed. Eng.*, 33:1743–1751.

Further Information

Mathematics and Physics

Hobbie, R.K. and Roth, B.J. *Intermediate Physics for Medicine and Biology*, 4th Ed., Springer, New York, 2007. (*Contains many examples of the application of physics to medicine, including several chapters about bioelectric and biomagnetic phenomena*).

Jackson, J.D. *Classical Electrodynamics*, 3rd Ed., John Wiley & Sons, New York, 1999 (*The classic graduate level physics text*).

Purcell, E.M. *Electricity and Magnetism*, Berkeley Physics Course, Vol. 2, McGraw-Hill Book Co., New York, 1963. (*A wonderfully written undergraduate physics text full of physical insight*).

Schey, H.M. *Div, Grad, Curl and All That*, 3rd Ed., Norton, New York, 1997. (*An accessible and useful introduction to vector calculus*).

Bioelectric Phenomena and Tissue Models

The texts by Cole and Plonsey, cited above, are classics in the field.

Gabriel, C., Gabriel, S., and Corthout, E. 1996. The dielectric properties of biological tissues: I. Literature survey. *Phys. Med. Biol.*, 41:2231–2249.

Geddes, L.A. and Baker, L.E. 1967. The specific resistance of biologic material—A compendium of data for the biomedical engineer and physiologist. *Med. Biol. Eng. Comput.*, 5:271–293. *(Measured conductivity values for a wide variety of tissues.)*

Plonsey, R. and Barr, R.C. *Bioelectricity, A Quantitative Approach*, 3rd Ed., Springer, New York, 2007. *(An updated version of Plonsey's "Bioelectric Phenomena," and a standard textbook for bioelectricity courses).*

Polk, C. and Postow, E. (Eds.) *CRC Handbook of Biological Effects of Electromagnetic Fields*, CRC Press, Boca Raton, FL, 1986.

Journals: *IEEE Transactions on Biomedical Engineering, Medical & Biological Engineering & Computing, Annals of Biomedical Engineering.*

Cardiac Microimpedances

41.1 Introduction 41-1
41.2 Microimpedances Derived from Literature-Based Data 41-2
41.3 Impact of Microimpedance Measurement Availability 41-4
41.4 Multisite Stimulation for Microimpedance Measurements 41-5
Acknowledgments 41-7
References 41-8

Andrew E. Pollard
University of Alabama at
Birmingham

41.1 Introduction

For many problems in bioelectric theory, investigators analyze the transmembrane (V_m) and interstitial (ϕ_o) potential distributions that arise from models that include prescribed tissue conductivities and ionic currents flowing through membrane channels. These entities dictate the local circuit currents formed during propagation and are usually treated as a continuum for the cardiac muscle along the lines presented by Roth in an earlier chapter:

$$\beta \left(C_m \frac{dV_m}{dt} + I_{\text{ion}} \right) = -\nabla \cdot (\sigma_o \nabla \phi_o) = -\nabla \cdot (\sigma_i \nabla (V_m + \phi_o)) \tag{41.1}$$

where σ_o and σ_i are macroscopic interstitial and intracellular conductivity tensors, respectively, β is a ratio of membrane surface to myocyte volume, C_m is a specific membrane capacitance, and I_{ion} is the total current resulting from ion channels, pumps, and exchangers when the membrane is considered active. An alternate formulation

$$\beta \left(\frac{V_m}{Z_m} \right) = -\nabla \cdot (\sigma_o \nabla \phi_o) = -\nabla \cdot (\sigma_i \nabla (V_m + \phi_o)) \tag{41.2}$$

is available with Z_m, an effective membrane impedance that depends upon the parallel combination of resistive and reactive components when the membrane is considered passive. The quantitative detail for many parameters in Equations 41.1 and 41.2 is extensive. For example, contemporary membrane equations for I_{ion} integrate single-cell data for guinea pig [1], canine [2], rat [3], mouse [4], and rabbit [5] ventricular myocytes. The experimental literature for isolated myocytes provides a wide range of species-, disease-, and region-specific β and Z_m values, with Z_m dictated by the myocyte's input resistance at low frequencies and Z_m reducing as cell capacitance contributes at a higher frequency.

The contemporary data for σ_o and σ_i are more challenging to identify. This important limitation is further complicated by the focus of the available data on macroscopic descriptions of the tissue's electrical properties. The local alterations of intercellular coupling suggested by the structural arrangement of gap junctions and of the collagen network in the cardiac tissue are commonly cited as contributors to arrhythmia development [6]. While altered coupling is accepted as an arrhythmia mechanism, the actual magnitudes for the intrinsic electrical impedances on the cellular size scale, that is, the micro-impedances, remain largely unknown. Because conduction velocities for action potential propagation differ with direction, microimpedances along myocyte axes are assumed to differ from those across myocyte axes and transmural to myocyte layers. In addition, distributions of gap junctions and the arrangement of the extracellular matrix are likely to establish microimpedances for the interstitial (Rox,Roy,Roz) and intracellular (Rix,Riy,Riz) compartments that are distinct from one another, that is (Rox/Rix is not equal to Roy/Riy, Rox/Rix is not equal to Roz/Riz). Therefore, the analytic descriptions arising from core-conductor assumptions are unavailable at the microscopic size scale.

This chapter examines the likely values for (Rox,Roy,Roz) and (Rix,Riy,Riz) as derived from the available data for tissue and cellular electrical properties in the ventricular myocardium. It then considers the impact a rapid and routine measurement strategy would have on an improved understanding of arrhythmia substrate development. Finally, it presents an initial progress achieved toward (Rox,Roy,Roz) and (Rix,Riy,Riz) measurement as a standard component of electrophysiological studies, assuming that closely spaced electrodes are available for stimulation and recording.

41.2 Microimpedances Derived from Literature-Based Data

To derive the likely microimpedances for the cardiac muscle, one may first consider the data available for rabbit ventricular myocytes and tissue preparations. The rationale for focusing on this species and tissue type is practical. First, rabbit ventricular myocytes are widely used in cellular electrophysiology studies and there has been an impressive maturation in the quantitative descriptions of the components for this cell type. Second, the perfused rabbit papillary muscle preparation has been used extensively in studies documenting the time course for core-conductor impedance changes during ischemia and reperfusion; so, the cable-like properties identified in the rabbit ventricle provide a rich source for considering the likely intracellular and interstitial microimpedances along myocyte axes. This chapter focuses attention on building blocks that measure $12.5 \times 12.5 \times 12.5 \ \mu m^3$, as shown schematically in Figure 41.1a. The 12.5 μm edge is below the length of a typical ventricular myocyte (~100 μm) and comparable with reported dimensions for the short axes of individual myocytes (~10–20 μm); so, the resolution of current flowing within a block may be considered as being on a cellular to subcellular size scale. Within each block, intracellular and interstitial compartments are coupled via the membrane. Because Giles and Imaizumi [7] measured the mean total cell capacitance of 72.5 pF in isolated rabbit ventricular myocyte experiments, a $12.5 \times 12.5 \times 12.5 \ \mu m^3$ block of 8.85 pF can be assumed. Here, the building block capacitance is 8.2-fold lower to represent a volume reduction from the reported value of 16,021 to 1875 μm^3. Similarly, the volume reduction supports a direct current (DC) or low frequency membrane impedance for each block of 276 MΩ based on an average cell input resistance of 33.7 MΩ [7].

Consistent with Equations 41.1 and 41.2, orthogonal connections between points located intracellularly and interstitially in adjacent blocks are considered as shown schematically in Figure 41.1b.

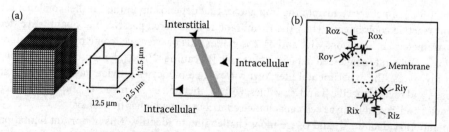

FIGURE 41.1 (a) Schematic of a three-dimensional or tissue model made from blocks in which (b) microimpedances (Rox,Roy,Roz) make interstitial connections to neighbors and microimpedances (Rix,Riy,Riz) make intracellular connections to neighbors. The intracellular and interstitial compartments are coupled by the membrane.

nterstitial coupling is via (Rox,Roy,Roz). Intracellular coupling is via (Rix,Riy,Riz). A standard approach to assess such parameters in an electrically conductive material is to supply current between two stimulating electrodes, record two intermediate voltages, and interpret the composite impedance (CI) as the voltage-to-current ratio with an appropriate structural model. The measured "4-electrode" CIs in heart preparations have been used to identify time intervals over which intercellular uncoupling occurs in animal models of ischemia and infarction [8,9]. However, because those CIs have not been interpreted within frameworks that allow segmentation between interstitial and intracellular compartments, relative contributions from the individual compartments are assumed but not measured.

Traditionally, segmentation has required intracellular access, which involves making sequential recordings with fragile glass microelectrodes in superfused preparations. To interpret those recordings with a continuous one-dimensional core-conductor framework, the flow of supplied current is typically restricted to the myocyte axis by embedding the preparation in oil. Weidmann [10] measured core-conductor impedances in superfused calf trabeculae in this way. More recent investigators have used a related voltage ratio method [11,12] with perfused papillary muscles. Assuming that myocytes align with the x axis in networks assembled from our building blocks, Kleber and Rieger's [11] specific intracellular conductivity for perfused rabbit papillary muscles (6.02 mS/cm) suggests a possible Rix value of 133 kΩ because the block faces through which current flows are separated by only 12.5 μm (1/((6.02 mS/cm) × (0.00125 cm)) = 133). With only 80% of the tissue volume being intracellular [13], however, Rix is likely higher at 166 kΩ. Similarly, using Kleber and Rieger's [11] specific extracellular conductivity (15.85 mS/cm) and assuming that 20% of each block is interstitial, we derive an Rox of 255 kΩ.

Because conduction velocities for action potentials propagating along and across macroscopic fiber axes in the ventricular myocardium differ from one another by a factor of approximately 3 to 1, one would expect values for Roy and Riy to exceed values for Rox and Rix. The macroscopic impedance data to support this expectation are limited. Clerc [14] identified core-conductor impedances along and across fibers by moving superfused calf trabeculae between different experimental chambers to supply current in orthogonal directions that allowed the interpretation of sequential measurements in a manner analogous to that of Weidmann [10]. The special preparations and apparatus required, however, have led most investigators to simply use the 30+-year-old Clerc measurements as if they remained valid for all other species and disease states despite the fact that virtually no present-day investigators use the calf preparation that Clerc studied. Those investigators found interstitial and intracellular conductivities across myocyte axes that were 2.7- and 9.4-fold lower, respectively, than conductivities along myocyte axes. Values for our building blocks were therefore set to Roy = 680 kΩ and Riy = 1560 kΩ. Here, the reader is cautioned on these specific quantities, as considerable variation seems likely and further supports the need for new measurement strategies that will allow microimpedance measurements to be made *in vivo* and *in vitro*.

The identification of microimpedances transmural to the myocyte layers is similarly complicated by the difficulty of segmenting the total tissue impedance into its intracellular and interstitial components. While values for Riz and Roz are likely to be closer to Riy and Roy than to Rix and Rox, recent experimental reports suggest that there may be differences. Hooks et al. [15] measured potential distributions with plunge-needle electrode systems in pig ventricle and found unique directional tissue impedances along fibers, across fibers, and intramurally. Those investigators hypothesized that the total tissue impedance differences were primarily a consequence of reduced gap junction availability, which they attributed to the presence of laminar sheets embedded between myocyte layers. While it is likely that the demonstration by Pope et al. [16] that perimysial collagen surrounding myolaminae formed a mesh with a wide range of sizes and orientations that were typically oblique to myocyte axes in rat ventricle suggests that an improved understanding of any interstitial contribution to the Hooks et al. [15] observation is also important. Because the extent to which cleavage planes between the myolaminae that form at separations of approximately four myocytes will impact Roz and Riz is not known, Roz = Roy and Riz = Riy represent attractive starting points for analyses.

41.3 Impact of Microimpedance Measurement Availability

One intriguing aspect of considering intracellular current flow on a cellular to subcellular size scale as *in vivo* (Rix,Riy,Riz) measurements is the potential for improved understanding of how gap junctions influence arrhythmia substrate development. One-dimensional modeling with explicitly characterized gap junction and cytoplasmic contributions showed propagation with normal gap junction coupling that differed little from propagation in the continuous core-conductor model [1]. However, with moderate uncoupling, the gap junctions caused discontinuous propagation in which large differences and long conduction latencies were maintained between adjacent myocytes. More severe uncoupling caused propagation failure, but only at extremely low propagation velocities. In the ventricular myocardium, Cx43 hemichannels form most gap junctions [17]. Cx43 turnover is rapid with a channel half-life of approximately 1–2 h [18]. The assembly requires a combination of individual connexons into hemichannels that are transported to the membrane where they locate preferentially at myocyte ends and dock to hemichannels from neighboring myocytes to form gap junctions under normal conditions [17]. The steps in the assembly are tightly regulated by binding partners (c-Src, ZO-1), adhesion junction proteins (cadherin, N-cadherin), and trafficking mediators (tubulin, caveolin) [19]. Once assembled, channel conductance then depends upon hemichannel type, phosphorylation state, and cytosolic levels of protons, calcium, and lipid metabolites [20–22]. Channel degradation occurs via lysosomal and proteosomal pathways [17]. Therefore, the intracellular microimpedances are likely to depend upon channel assembly/degradation and upon channel conductance. An ability to document (Rix,Riy,Riz) changes from those derived earlier in the chapter using the available macroscopic electrical data would allow more quantitative definition of these competing influences.

Similarly, an improved understanding of interstitial current flow resulting from (Rox,Roy,Roz) measurements is needed because this critical part of the local circuit current loop alters the action potential propagation on the size scale where propagation fails. Interstitial currents flow through intervening cleft spaces between myocytes and may also flow through the connexons between subjacent fibroblasts that reside with the perimysial collagen matrix [16,23]. The impedances in this part of the loop are likely comparable in magnitude to those in the intracellular part because interstitial potentials recorded during propagation have amplitudes approximately 1/2 of the action potential upstroke's amplitude [24]. However, quantitative data on the interstitium's electrical properties are limited. Fleischauer et al. [25] showed the sensitivity of core-conductor interstitial impedance to interstitial compartment size changes in perfused rabbit papillary muscles. During compartment expansion, they measured core-conductor interstitial impedance reduction. With compartment contraction, that impedance rose. The modulation of the electrical properties of the microvasculature had no effect. Compartment collapse has been proposed as the main mechanism for the rapid rise in core-conductor interstitial impedance [26] that occurs within approximately 1 min of loss of perfusion. Compartment expansion during reperfusion may also be important, as Cascio et al. [12] found that interstitial core-conductor impedance fell below its preischemic value 10 min after reperfusion. An ability to document (Rox,Roy,Roz) changes from those derived earlier in the chapter using the available macroscopic data would allow more quantitative correlations between tissue electrical properties and structural remodeling of the extracellular matrix.

Where microimpedance data are available, those data have been obtained, for the most part, using the highly successful cell pair method (see Metzger and Weingart [27]). With cell pairs, the structural framework is relatively simple and takes advantage of the high membrane resistance for an isolated myocyte. This preparation allows changes in transmembrane potentials recorded in adjacent cells during intracellular stimulation to be considered in terms of a junctional resistance (or conductance) that accounts for myoplasm and gap junction contributions. Cell pairs with myocyte–myocyte connections that are predominantly end to end are assumed to reflect *in vivo* intracellular coupling along myocyte axes [28]. Pairs with more side-to-side connections provide descriptions across myocyte axes and are transmural to myocyte layers. The values reported for junctional resistance vary widely between species, tissue types, and experimental conditions. While junctional resistance values vary widely, it is nteresting to note that Metzger and Weingart [27] measured junctional resistances of approximately 2 MΩ in their rat ventricular myocyte pairs, which primarily included side-to-side connections. That magnitude is close to the Riy and Riz we derived from the available macroscopic electrical properties.

41.4 Multisite Stimulation for Microimpedance Measurements

While the cell pair method provides a unique opportunity to quantify some intracellular electrical properties on the microscopic size scale, the method has limitations. The extracellular matrix must necessarily be digested to provide the pairs. Therefore, (Rox,Roy,Roz) measurements cannot be made with this method. Fragile glass microelectrodes must be attached to adjacent cells for intracellular stimulation and recording. Such intracellular access is technically challenging and complicates data acquisition. The focus on pairs also limits the identification of possible differences between intracellular microimpedances along myocyte axes, and across myocyte axes and transmural to myocyte layers. In a series of recent reports, the author has proposed using very small and closely spaced electrodes for interstitial stimulation and recording as an alternative strategy to provide intracellular and interstitial microimpedance measurements. The main benefits envisioned with this strategy include (i) elimination of the need for intracellular penetration, which is problematic for multicellular preparations where vigorous contractions complicate the ability of investigators to maintain impalements, (ii) rapid implementation under experimental conditions, as the process of stimulation with different electrode combinations to acquire a set of voltage recordings is relatively straightforward in electrophysiological studies, and (iii) its microscopic focus, which distinguishes the approach from studies that use traditional systems that are more typical for macroscopic cardiac mapping.

The approach relies on electrode systems fabricated using microelectrical mechanical systems (MEMS) technology [29]. In practice, complete arrays are positioned well inside tissue space constants and cover myocardial regions that are generally covered by individual electrodes in traditional studies. The importance of achieving this change in scale is evident when considering the tissue microstructure. Figure 41.2a shows a schematic (left) of a set of electrodes with center-to-center separations of 2 mm in a 2 × 2 cm² region. This scale is typical for traditional cardiac electrical mapping. Figure 41.2a (right) shows the same schematic photographed on top of an Hematoxylin and Eosin (H&E) stained section from rabbit left ventricle. The arrows in the center of both panels mark an MEMS array. Figure 41.2b shows a magnified image from Figure 41.2a (right). A black rectangle connects four traditional electrodes. A schematic of an MEMS array is drawn to scale and is bounded by a dashed box in the center of the image. The electrodes separated on a cellular to subcellular size scale are more likely to provide information on (Rox,Roy,Roz) and (Rix,Riy,Riz) than traditional arrangements, including more macroscopic separations.

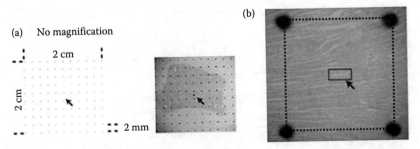

FIGURE 41.2 (a) Schematic of a traditional electrode array used for cardiac mapping beside an H&E stained section from rabbit ventricular epicardium that includes the schematic (no magnification). (b) Image with magnification to include a linear set of electrodes from the schematic in the right part of (a). The central region highlights the size scale for stimulation and recording to measure microimpedances. The central box surrounds electrodes in a linear MEMS array. The arrows in (a) and (b) mark the MEMS array size.

With MEMS arrays, it is practical to record microscopic potential differences (uPDs) and to measure microscopic composite impedances (uCIs) under conditions where the electrode separations are known with precision (25 mm center to center) and are on a size scale comparable to separations available in cell pair experiments. Under these conditions, the high membrane impedance limits redistribution of the supplied current to the intracellular compartment, which allows uCIs measured during stimulation with different electrode combinations near the uPD recording pair to be interpreted primarily based on interstitial current flow. On theoretical grounds [30], positioning a four-electrode arrangement inside a space constant limits the ability of the supplied current to cross the membrane. Stimulating with more widely separated electrodes [31,32] or with higher frequencies [33] then modulates the flow of supplied current to the intracellular compartment to an extent that depends upon electrode separation relative to the space constant.

To assess the feasibility of stimulation and recording strategies based solely on interstitial access with the electrodes, the one-dimensional fiber shown in Figure 41.3a was studied first. The building blocks were laid end to end to represent the structural arrangement along myocyte axes. An electrode pair (open circles) separated by 25 μm recorded uPDs. Multiple stimulating electrodes (filled circles) positioned at 25 μm intervals over the central five myocytes in the model (fine region) and at 400 mm intervals (wide region) outside the fine region supplied the current. Rox and Rix values were prescribed for membrane equation simulations with I_{ion} in Equation 41.1. In each simulation, the activation sequence initiation at one end of the fiber (square wave) was followed by a premature DC stimulus (S2) applied approximately 10 ms after action potentials propagated past the uPD recording pair with interstitial current supplied between two stimulating electrodes located on opposite sides of that pair.

Figure 41.3b shows uPD amplitudes from recordings during stimulation with electrodes separated between 75 μm and 4.5 mm. The supplied current was held constant for all stimuli. Using electrodes in the fine region, relatively large uPDs were recorded, consistent with the concept that the supplied current remained interstitial. Using electrodes in the wide region, relatively small uPDs were recorded, consistent with the redistribution of supplied current to the intracellular compartment. The inspection of the uPD amplitudes resulting from stimulation with the different electrode combinations showed an

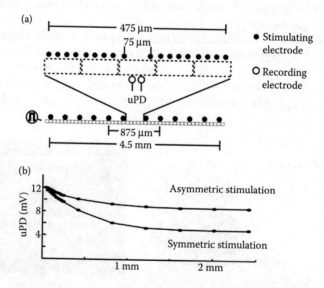

FIGURE 41.3 (a) Arrangement of recording (open circles) and stimulating (filled circles) sites in the fine (top) and wide (bottom) spacing regions. The interstitial current was fixed for simulations with fine or wide spacing. (b) uPDs during symmetric and asymmetric arrangement of the stimulating electrodes. For symmetric arrangements, the horizontal axis denotes the positions for p and q. For asymmetric arrangements, the horizontal axis denotes the positions for q only because p was fixed at a central location.

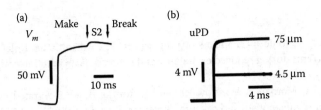

FIGURE 41.4 (a) Initial protocol used to obtain uPDs in the linear electrode array. A constant current S2 pulse of 10 ms duration applied in the action potential plateau caused a modest transmembrane potential change. (b) Unique uPDs were recorded during stimulation of the one-dimensional myocyte network using electrodes separated by 75 μm and 4.5 mm.

exponential decline when separations were relatively fine and an asymptotic response when separations were relatively wide. The separation by one space constant is marked with the dashed vertical line. To interpret the uPDs, an analytic solution resulting from the core-conductor equations was available as

$$\text{uPD} = \frac{\text{uPD}_0}{1 + k_x}\left(\frac{e^{-p/\lambda} + e^{-q/\lambda}}{2} + k_x\right) \qquad (41.3)$$

where p and q were separations of the stimulating electrodes from the central point in the uPD pair, λ was the space constant, uPD_0 was the uPD as p and q approached zero, and k_x was an intracellular to interstitial microimpedance ratio, that is, Rix/Rox. For a given set of uPDs, uPD_0, k_x and λ were determined by nonlinear least-squares analysis given a set of (p,q) values. The direct comparisons between prescribed and measured microimpedances documented (Rox,Rix) accuracies within 1%. Highly accurate microimpedance measurements were also obtained in simulations in which myoplasmic and gap junctional components were treated as discrete entities. That accuracy was maintained over a 10-fold range of junctional resistances. Therefore, the measurement procedure was effective under conditions where the action potential propagation appeared continuous, and as that propagation became discontinuous.

An important aspect of the overall procedure as it is implemented now is that low-magnitude (10–100 nA) supplied currents establish uPDs of approximately 1 mV amplitude. That amplitude is sufficient to ensure straightforward resolution at high signal-to-noise ratios under experimental conditions, while simultaneously causing minimal alteration to V_m. The main advantage of this arrangement is that it causes no change to the intrinsic activation sequence. Figure 41.4a shows the V_m time course during stimulation with electrodes separated by 75 μm. The voltage change between the make and break of the S2 pulse was considerably smaller than the action potential upstroke. Figure 41.4b shows uPDs recorded during multisite stimulation with closely (75 μm) and widely (4.5 mm) separated electrodes. End pulse uPDs were large enough to suggest straightforward resolution in experiments.

While it is tempting to simply adapt this approach for measurements in the y and z directions, the reader is cautioned to recognize the framework for the interpretation of uPD recordings in the one-dimensional fiber, which is the core-conductor model. It is complicated to adapt that model to two- and three-dimensional arrangements of building blocks unless assumptions such as Rix/Riy = Rox/Roy are made. The interested reader is encouraged to review alternate strategies for sheet [32] and tissue [34] arrangements developed by the author and colleagues in which more complete structural frameworks for the interpretation of recorded voltages are presented.

Acknowledgments

This work was supported by National Heart, Lung and Blood Institute Award HL092049 and National Science Foundation Award CBET-0756078.

References

1. Shaw RM and Rudy Y. Ionic mechanisms of propagation in cardiac tissue. Roles of sodium and L-type calcium currents during reduced excitability and decreased gap junction coupling. *Circ. Res.*, 81:727–741, 1997.

2. Cortassa S, Aon MA, Marban E, Winslow RL, and O'Rourke B. An integrated model of cardiac mitochondrial energy metabolism and calcium dynamics. *Biophys. J.*, 84:2734–2755, 2003.

3. Pandit SV, Clark RB, Giles WR, and Demir SS. A mathematical model of action potential heterogeneity in adult rat left ventricular myocytes. *Biophys. J.*, 81:3029–3051, 2001.

4. Bondarenko VE, Szigeti GP, Bett GC, Kim SJ, and Rasmusson RL. Computer model of action potential of mouse ventricular myocytes. *Am. J. Physiol. Heart Circ. Physiol.*, 287:H1378–H1403, 2004.

5. Puglisi JL and Bers DM. LabHEART: An interactive computer model of rabbit ventricular myocyte ion channels and Ca transport. *Am. J. Physiol. Cell Physiol.*, 281:C2049–C2060, 2001.

6. Kleber AG and Rudy Y. Basic mechanisms of cardiac impulse propagation and associated arrhythmias. *Physiol. Rev.*, 84:431–488, 2004.

7. Giles WR and Imaizumi Y. Comparison of potassium currents in rabbit atrial and ventricular cells. *J. Physiol. (London)*, 405:123–145, 1988.

8. Fallert MA, Mirotznik MS, Downing SW, Savage EB, Foster KR, Josephson ME, and Bogen DK. Myocardial electrical impedance mapping of ischemic sheep hearts and healing aneurysms. *Circulation*, 87:199–207, 1993.

9. Coronel R, Wilms-Schopman FJG, and deGroot JR. Origin of ischemia-induced phase 1b ventricular arrhythmias in pig hearts. *J. Am. Coll. Cardiol.*, 39:166–176, 2002.

10. Weidmann S. Electrical constants of trabecular muscle from mammalian heart. *J. Physiol.*, 210:1041–1054, 1970.

11. Kleber AG and Rieger CB. Electrical constants of arterially perfused rabbit papillary muscle. *J. Physiol. (London)*, 385:307–324, 1987.

12. Cascio WE, Yang H, Johnson TA, Muller-Borer BJ, and Lemasters JJ. Electrical properties and conduction in reperfused papillary muscle. *Circ. Res.*, 89:807–814, 2001.

13. Polimeni PI, Williams S, and Weisman H. Application of automatic electrotonic image analyzer to the measurement of myocardial extracellular space. *Comp. Biomed. Res.*, 16:522, 1983.

14. Clerc L. Directional differences of impulse spread in trabecular muscle from mammalian heart. *J. Physiol. (London)*, 255:335–346, 1976.

15. Hooks DA, Trew ML, Caldwell BJ, Sands GB, LeGrice IJ, and Smaill BH. Laminar arrangement of ventricular myocytes influences electrical behavior of the heart. *Circ. Res.*, 101:e103–e112, 2007.

16. Pope AJ, Sands GB, Smaill BH, and LeGrice IJ. Three-dimensional transmural organization of perimysial collagen in the heart. *Am. J. Physiol. Heart Circ. Physiol.*, 295:H1243–H1252, 2008.

17. Saffitz JE, Laing JG, and Yamada KA. Connexin expression and turnover. Implications for cardiac excitability. *Circ. Res.*, 86:723–728, 2000.

18. Musil LS and Goodenough DA. Biochemical analysis of connexin43 intracellular transport, phosphorylation, and assembly into gap junctional plaques. *J. Cell Biol.*, 115:1357–1374, 1991.

19. Hunter AW, Barker RJ, Zhu C, and Gourdie RG. Zonula occludens-1 alters connexin43 gap junction size and organization by influencing channel accretion. *Mol. Biol. Cell*, 16:5686–5698, 2005.

20. Yamada KA, McHowat J, Yan G-X, Donahue K, Peirick J, Kleber AG, and Corr PB. Cellular uncoupling induced by accumulation of long-chain acylcarnitine during ischemia. *Circ. Res.*, 74(1):83–95, 1994.

21. Carmeliet E. Cardiac ionic currents and acute ischemia: From channels to arrhythmias. *Physiol. Rev.*, 79:917–1017, 1999.

22. Duffy HS, Fort AG, and Spray DC. Cardiac connexins: Genes to nexus. *Adv. Cardiol.*, 42:1–17, 2006.

23. Kohl P and Camelliti P. Cardiac myocyte–nonmyocyte electronic coupling: Implications for ventricular arrhythmogenesis. *Heart Rhythm*, 4(2):233–235, 2007.

24. Roberts DE, Hersh LT, and Scher AM. Influence of cardiac fiber orientation on wavefront voltage conduction velocity and tissue resistivity in the dog. *Circ. Res.*, 44:701–712, 1979.

25. Fleischauer J, Lehmann L, and Kleber AG. Electrical resistances of interstitial and microvascular space as determinants of the extracellular electrical field and velocity of propagation in ventricular myocardium. *Circulation*, 92:587–594, 1995.

26. Kleber AG, Rieger CB, and Janse MJ. Electrical uncoupling and increase of extracellular resistance after induction of ischemia in isolated arterially perfused rabbit papillary muscle. *Circ. Res.*, 61:271–279, 1987.

27. Metzger P and Weingart R. Electrical current flow in cell pairs isolated from adult rat hearts. *J. Physiol.*, 366:177–195, 1985.

28. Cabo C, Yao JA, Boyden PA, Chen W, Hussain W, Duffy HS, Ciaccio EJ, Peters NS, and Wit AL. Heterogeneous gap junction remodeling in reentrant circuits in the epicardial border zone of the healing canine infarct. *Cardiovasc. Res.*, 72:241–249, 2006.

29. Pollard AE, Ellis CD, and Smith WM. Linear electrode arrays for stimulation and recording within cardiac tissue space constants. *IEEE Trans. Biomed. Eng.*, 55:1408–1414, 2008.

30. Plonsey RC and Barr RC. A critique of impedance measurements in cardiac tissue. *Ann. Biomed. Eng.*, 14:307–322, 1986.

31. Pollard AE, Smith WM, and Barr RC. Feasibility of cardiac microimpedance measurement using multisite interstitial stimulation. *Am. J. Physiol. Heart Circ. Physiol.*, 287:H2402–H2411, 2004.

32. Pollard AE and Barr RC. Cardiac microimpedance measurement in two-dimensional models using multisite interstitial stimulation. *Am. J. Physiol. Heart Circ. Physiol.*, 290:H1976–H1987, 2006.

33. Barr RC, Nolte LW, and Pollard AE. Bayesian analysis of fiber impedance measurements. *Conf. Proc. IEEE Eng. Med. Biol. Soc.*, 1:423–429, 2007.

34. Pollard AE and Barr RC. A biophysical model for cardiac microimpedance measurements. *Am. J. Physiol. Heart Circ. Physiol.*, 298:H1699–H1709, 2010.

42

Membrane Models

42.1	Introduction	42-1
42.2	The Action Potential	42-2
42.3	Patch-Clamp Data	42-3
42.4	General Formulations of Membrane Currents	42-5

Nernst–Planck Equations • Hodgkin–Huxley Resistor Battery Model • Goldman–Hodgkin–Katz Constant Field Formulation • GHK with Correction for Fixed Surface Charge • Eyring Rate Theory Models of Ionic Currents • Ion Pump • Ion Exchangers • Synapses • Calcium as a Second Messenger

42.5	Nerve Cells	42-9

Sensory Neurons • Efferent Neurons

42.6	Skeletal Muscle Cells	42-14

Frog Sartorius Muscle Cell • Barnacle Muscle

42.7	Endocrine Cells	42-16

Pancreatic β-Cells • Chromaffin Cells • Pituitary Gonadotrophs and Corticotrophs

42.8	Cardiac Cells	42-16

Purkinje Fiber • Sinoatrial Node • Atrial Muscle • Atrioventricular Node • Ventricular Muscle • Amphibian Sinus Venosus and Atrial Cells

42.9	Epithelial Cells	42-19
42.10	Smooth Muscle	42-19
42.11	Plant Cells	42-19
42.12	Simplified Models	42-19

Hill • FitzHugh–Nagumo • Hindmarsh–Rose Models

Defining Terms	42-21
For Further Information	42-21
References	42-22

Anthony Varghese
University of Wisconsin, River Falls

42.1 Introduction

The models discussed in this chapter involve the time behavior of electrochemical activity in excitable cells. These models are systems of ordinary differential equations where the independent variable is time. While a good understanding of linear circuit theory is useful to understand the models presented in this chapter, most of the phenomena of interest involve nonlinear circuits with time-varying components.

Electrical activity in plant and animal cells are caused by two main factors: first, there are differences in the concentrations of ions inside and outside the cell; and second, there are molecules embedded in the cell membrane that allow these ions to be transported across the membrane. The ion concentration differences and the presence of large membrane-impermeant anions inside the cell result in the existence of a polarity: the potential inside a cell is typically 30–100 mV lower than that in the external solution. It is important to note that almost all of this potential difference occurs across the membrane itself. The bulk solutions both inside and outside the cell are, for the most part, at a uniform potential. This *transmembrane potential difference* is in turn sensed by molecules in the membrane that control the flow of ions.

The lipid bilayer, which constitutes the majority of the cell membrane, acts as a capacitor with a specific capacitance that is typically 1 μF/cm^2. The rest of the membrane comprises large protein molecules that act as (1) ion *channels*, (2) ion *pumps*, or (3) ion *exchangers*. The flow of ions across the membrane causes changes in the transmembrane potential, which is typically the main observable quantity in experiments.

42.2 The Action Potential

The main behavior that will be examined in this chapter is the *action potential*. This is a term used to denote a temporal phenomenon exhibited by every electrically excitable cell. A schematic representation of an action potential is shown in Figure 42.1. The transmembrane potential difference of most excitable cells usually stays at some negative potential called the *resting potential*. External current or voltage inputs can cause the potential of the cell to deviate in the positive direction and if the input is large enough, the result is an action potential. An action potential is characterized by a *depolarization*, which typically results in an *overshoot* beyond the 0 mV level (see Figure 42.1) followed by *repolarization*. Some cells may actually *hyperpolarize* before returning to the resting potential.

A key concept in the modeling of excitable cells is the idea of *ion channel selectivity*. A particular type of ion channel will only allow certain ionic species to pass through; most types of ion channels are modeled as being permeant to a single ionic species. In most excitable cells at rest, the membrane is most permeable to potassium. This is because only potassium channels (i.e., channels selective to potassium) are open at the resting potential. For a given stimulus to result in action potential the cell has to be brought to *threshold*, that is, the stimulus has to be larger than some critical size; smaller sub-threshold stimuli will result in an exponential decay to the resting potential. The upstroke, or fast initial depolarization, of the action potential is caused by a large influx of sodium ions as sodium channels open (in some cells, entry of calcium ions through calcium channels is responsible for the upstroke) in response to a stimulus. This is followed by repolarization as potassium ions start flowing out of the cell in response to the new potential gradient. While responses of most cells to subthreshold inputs are usually linear and passive, the suprathreshold response—the action potential—is a nonlinear phenomenon. Unlike

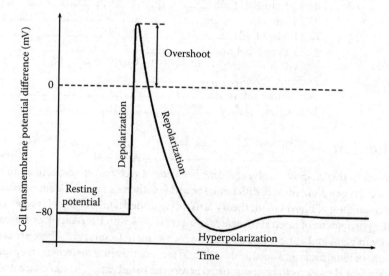

FIGURE 42.1 Schematic representation of an action potential in an excitable cell. The abscissa represents time and the ordinate represents the transmembrane potential.

linear circuits where the principle of superposition holds, the nonlinear processes in cell membranes do not allow responses of two stimuli to be added. If an initial stimulus results in an action potential, a subsequent stimulus administered at the peak voltage will not produce an even larger action potential; instead, it may have no effect at all. Following an action potential, most cells have a *refractory period*, during which they are unable to respond to stimuli. Nonlinear features such as these make modeling of excitable cells a nontrivial task. In addition, the molecular behavior of ion channels includes a stochastic component and, therefore, it is not feasible to construct membrane models from first principles. The models in this chapter were all constructed using empirical data.

In 1952, Alan Hodgkin and Andrew Huxley published a paper showing how a nonlinear empirical model of the membrane processes could be constructed (Hodgkin and Huxley 1952). In the five decades since their work, the Hodgkin–Huxley (abbreviated HH) paradigm of modeling cell membranes has been enormously successful. While the concept of ion channels was not established when they performed their work, one of their main contributions was the idea that ion-selective processes existed in the membrane. It is now known that most of the passive transport of ions across cell membranes is accomplished by ion-selective channels. In addition to constructing a nonlinear model, they also established a method to incorporate experimental data into a nonlinear mathematical membrane model.

42.3 Patch-Clamp Data

The main source of experimental data used to construct models of cell electrophysiology is the *patch clamp* method (Hamill et al. 1981). In the whole-cell patch-clamp configuration, a glass pipette with a very fine tip, typically 1 μm in diameter, containing a solution that is close in ionic composition to the intracellular fluid is brought to the external surface of the cell. A small amount of suction is applied to form a tight seal between the tip of the glass pipette and the membrane and by applying additional suction, the cell membrane under the tip can be ruptured and the fluid in the electrode is allowed to come in physical contact with the internal fluid of the cell. With electrical contact thus established between the fluid of the glass pipette and the interior of the cell, it becomes possible to monitor as well as control cell electrical activity using electronic instruments.

The components of cellular electrophysiology can be summarized schematically in Figure 42.2a. Cell membranes may contain ion channels that allow ions to flow down their electrochemical gradient and ion pumps that move ions against their gradients. The various cell membrane channel, pump, and exchanger currents are summed in $I_{ion} = I_{ion}(V_m, \bar{y})$, which is a nonlinear function of V_m and $\bar{y}$, a vector representing the kinetics of the various channels. The capacitance of the membrane, C_m, responds to changes in the cell transmembrane potential difference, V_m, with a capacitive current, $I_C = C_m(dV_m/dt)$. Using Kirchoff's current law from electrical circuit theory,

$$I_C + I_{ion} = 0 \tag{42.1}$$

which yields the basic differential equation for the cell transmembrane potential difference, V_m:

$$C_m \frac{dV_m}{dt} = -I_{ion}(V_m \cdot \bar{y}) \tag{42.2}$$

The kinetics of $\bar{y}$ is usually defined by a system of equations of the form:

$$\frac{d\bar{y}}{dt} = F(V_m, \bar{y}) \tag{42.3}$$

Cell patch clamping allows experimenters to either inject a current while observing the response in V_m, (current-clamp mode, Figure 42.2b) or impose a waveform, $V_{clamp}(t)$, on the cell transmembrane

A cell membrane model and circuit equivalent

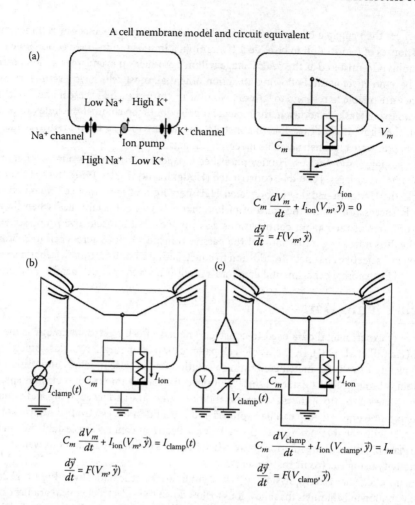

$$C_m \frac{dV_m}{dt} + I_{ion}(V_m, \vec{y}) = 0$$

$$\frac{d\vec{y}}{dt} = F(V_m, \vec{y})$$

$$C_m \frac{dV_m}{dt} + I_{ion}(V_m, \vec{y}) = I_{clamp}(t)$$

$$\frac{d\vec{y}}{dt} = F(V_m, \vec{y})$$

$$C_m \frac{dV_{clamp}}{dt} + I_{ion}(V_{clamp}, \vec{y}) = I_m$$

$$\frac{d\vec{y}}{dt} = F(V_{clamp}, \vec{y})$$

FIGURE 42.2 Schematic view of membrane currents and patch-clamp techniques. (a) Most cells have a low internal concentration of sodium (Na+) and a high internal concentration of potassium (K+) ions while the external concentrations are reversed. Sodium and potassium channels allow these ions to run down their electrochemical gradients while ion pumps can pump these ions against their respective electrochemical gradients. This electrical activity can be represented by an equivalent circuit shown on the left. The cell membrane capacitance is represented by the capacitor C_m and the various ionic currents are added together into a single nonlinear element through which the current I_{ion} passes. Thus, the equation of circuit equivalent is: $C_m/(dV_m/dt) + I_{ion}(V_m, \vec{y}) = 0$ and the time-dependent properties of the nonlinearities of I_{ion} are described by the vector equation $d\vec{y}/dt = F(V_m, \vec{y})$. (b) In the *Current Clamp* mode of the whole cell patch-clamp configuration, one electrode is used to inject a known current $I_{clamp}(t)$ while the other electrode is used to sense the potential inside the cell. (c) In *Voltage Clamp* mode the potential inside the cell is compared to a known voltage supplied by the experimenter and an amplifier is used to supply whatever current is required to keep the cell potential at the specified voltage $V_{clamp}(t)$. The resulting circuit equations are indicated below the circuit diagrams.

potential and observe membrane current, I_m (voltage-clamp mode, Figure 42.2). By choosing appropriate voltage-clamp waveforms, $V_{clamp}(t)$, experimenters can make deductions about the structure of the nonlinear function $F(V_m, \vec{y})$ in Equation 42.3. The membrane current measured during voltage-clamp experiments, $I_m(t) = C_m \, dV_{clamp}/dt + I_{ion}(V_{clamp}, \vec{y})$ is then painstakingly dissected into its essential components due to the various ion channels, pumps, and exchangers by established protocols as well as by trial and error. Using cloned channels overexpressed in cultured cells or *Xenopus* oocytes, a relatively pure current can be studied in isolation.

42.4 General Formulations of Membrane Currents

In this section, we examine the various components common to membrane models. We start with the Nernst–Planck formulation of ion flow across a membrane. Although it is seldom used now, this equation is needed to derive other, more practical models such as the resistor-battery model or the Goldman–Hodgkin–Katz current model. Some preliminary remarks are in order before examining these models. At dilute concentrations, ions in aqueous solutions behave like gas molecules. This is why the *gas constant, R,* is ubiquitous in models of ion flow in cells. Similarly, the phenomenon of chemisorption of gas molecules is used as an analog to study the binding of ions (and drug molecules) to receptors in the cell membrane. In chemisorption under equilibrium conditions, the fraction of gas molecules bound to fixed reaction sites is given by an expression of the form: $[C]^n/(k + [C]^n)$ where $[C]$ is the concentration of gas, k is a constant and n is typically a small positive number. This expression is also derived from Michaelis–Menten-type kinetic schemes. Similar terms arise in many membrane models cited in this chapter and they indicate that some fraction of an ionic species, C, is binding to the receptor molecules on the cell surface.

42.4.1 Nernst–Planck Equations

One of the most general descriptions of ion flow across a membrane is given by the Nernst–Planck equations. This is a partial differential equation where the independent variables represent space (x) and time (t). The main dependent variable is the concentration of the ion $(c(x,t))$. The potential $(u(x,t))$ is usually a fixed function but can be made a dependent variable in which case an additional equation is required. The Nernst–Planck equations can be written as

$$\frac{\partial c(x,t)}{\partial t} = \frac{\partial}{\partial x}\frac{\mu(x,t)}{|z|}\left[\frac{RT}{F}\frac{\partial c(x,t)}{\partial x} + zc(x,t)\frac{\partial u}{\partial x}(x,t)\right] \tag{42.4}$$

where the symbols are defined thus:

Variable	Description	Dimensions
R	Gas constant	8314.41 mJ/(mol K)
T	Temperature	310 K
F	Faraday's constant	96,485 C/mol
u	Potential	mV
c	Ion concentration	Mol L
z	Valence of the ion	
E	Electric field force	mV m^{-1}
μ	Ion mobility	m^2 mV^{-1} s^{-1}

Note that μ can vary with both space and time depending on the type of ion channel or pump and its gating properties. Owing to the complexity of this formulation, it is of limited use when examining behavior at the cellular level but it can be used to derive simpler formulations under certain assumptions as shown below.

42.4.2 Hodgkin–Huxley Resistor Battery Model

This model is the one that is most frequently employed to look at ions flowing through channels and is shown in terms of its circuit equivalent in Figure 42.3. This models the passive flow of ions due to a transmembrane potential gradient, V_m, and a concentration gradient (represented in the battery, E_i)

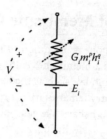

FIGURE 42.3 Circuit representation of membrane current. The conductance can be nonlinear as indicated by the powers p and q on the state variables m_i and h_i, respectively. These state variables are typically time-varying functions of the transmembrane potential difference, V. The battery, E_i represents the electrochemical gradient of the ionic species responsible for the current.

through a nonlinear membrane conductance. From the structure of the circuit, we see that the equation for the current for ionic species i has the form:

$$I_i = G_i m_i^p h_i^q (V_m - E_i) \tag{42.5}$$

where G_i represents the maximum value of the conductance of the membrane, and m_i and h_i are gating variables that vary in time and take values between 0 and 1. p and q are integers that depend on the kinetic characteristics of the membrane channel. For example, in the formulation of the sodium current in the Hodgkin and Huxley (HH, see below) equations, the conductance is $G_{Na} m^3 h$, that is, p is 3 and q is 1, and these values were found to result in the best fit with experimental data.

The above expression can be derived from the Nernst–Planck equations with the assumption that concentration does not vary with time. In addition, the space dimension of Equation 42.4 is reduced to a two-compartment cell interior and exterior model. Thus, the steady state of Equation 42.4 tells us that when there is no net current flow, the transmembrane potential will equal a quantity called the "Nernst" potential: $E_i = RT/z_i F \ln ([C]_o/[C]_i)$. z_i is the valence of the ion, $[C_i]_o$ is the concentration of the ion on the outside and $[C_i]_i$ is the concentration on the inside. Quantities such as ion mobility are effectively lumped into a nonlinear time-varying conductance ($G_i m_i^p h_i^q$).

First-order differential equations are used to model the time behavior of m_i and h_i. For example, the equation for m_i will have the form:

$$\frac{dm_i}{dt} = \alpha_m (1 - m_i) - \beta_m m_i \tag{42.6}$$

where the α_m and β_m are empirically determined functions of the membrane potential. This equation is also written as: $dm_i/dt = (m_i \infty - m_i)/\tau_i$ where $m_i \infty = \alpha_m/(\alpha_m + \beta_m)$ and $\tau_i = 1/(\alpha_m + \alpha_m)$. Voltage-clamp protocols are used by experimenters to characterize $m_i \infty$ and τ_i empirically as functions of V_m for a given cell. As a result, there is no unique derivation for the differential equations describing the time behavior of the gating variables. $m_i \infty$ and τ_i are usually nonlinear functions of voltage. This nonlinear dependence on V_m makes the coupled system of Equations 42.2 and 42.3 a nonlinear system of ordinary differential equations. Selectivity is implicitly modeled by assuming that only one ionic species flows through a current branch. A number of current branches, one for each type of ion channel, are connected in parallel to model the interaction of the various ion currents.

Gating variables, ion channel kinetics, and Markov-state models: Gating variables like m_i and h_i above model the kinetic behavior of ion channels. For example, in the HH equations (see below), the variable "m" is used to model the process of *activation* of the sodium current. At polarized potentials, the sodium current is turned off: m is close to 0 and therefore the sodium current conductance, $G_{Na} m^3 h$, is close to

). As the cell depolarizes (V_m increases, see Figure 42.1), the sodium current turns on (activates) and this is modeled as an increase in the value of m until it approaches 1. Concomitant with this activation is a process that desensitizes (inactivates) the sodium current thus guaranteeing that the sodium current is transient. This is modeled using the inactivation variable h, which goes from a resting value of 1 to a value closer to 0 as V_m increases. This decrease in h causes the sodium conductance, $G_{Na}m^3h$, to decrease even though m may be close to 1. In an excitable cell such as a nerve, skeletal, or cardiac cell, activation of the sodium current causes inward flow of sodium ions resulting in depolarization of the cell; this depolarization further activates the sodium current and a regenerative activation process continues until inactivation desensitizes the current. In the absence of other currents, the cell will stay depolarized but most excitable cells will have an outward potassium current which activates much more slowly than the fast inward sodium current. This outward potassium current causes potassium ions to leave the cell and repolarizes the cell, that is, it brings the transmembrane potential closer to the reversal potential for potassium. The sodium current is affected by repolarization in two ways: it turns off (deactivates) and it becomes resensitized (recovers from inactivation). The deactivation is modeled as a return of the m variable to values close to 0 and the recovery from inactivation is modeled as a return of h to a value closer to 1. These four processes: activation, inactivation, deactivation, and recovery from inactivation are present in many ion channels. Investigations of these processes in squid axons, native mammalian cells, and in cloned channels revealed that the HH formulation of these four processes were deficient in at least three ways. First, inactivation was often found to be coupled to activation rather than being independently voltage dependent as in the Hodgkin–Huxley model. Second, multiple steps were involved each of the four processes and these steps could not be adequately modeled using different values for the exponents (p and q above). Third, unlike the HH model, the speed of activation, for instance, is in some cases decoupled from the speed of deactivation. These observations resulted in the need for a more general framework for kinetics and the most commonly used one is Markov-state models (see Hills 2001, pp. 583–602).

42.4.3 Goldman–Hodgkin–Katz Constant Field Formulation

From Equation 42.4, assuming that potential varies linearly across the membrane and that the ion flux is constant, we obtain an expression for current flow of the form (Goldman 1943):

$$I_i = P_i d_i^p f_i^q \frac{V_m/(RT/zF)}{1 - e^{-\frac{V_m}{RT/zF}}} \left[[C_i]_i - [C_i]_o e^{-\frac{V_m}{RT/zF}} \right] \tag{42.7}$$

where P_i is the maximum permeability of the membrane and d and f are gating variables like m and h in Equation 42.5. This equation is frequently used when large concentration gradients are present.

42.4.4 GHK with Correction for Fixed Surface Charge

When surface charge is present on the inside or outside of the cell membrane, the effective potential gradient sensed by the channel is modified by a correction factor, $V_{surface}$, and the current then has the form (Frankenhaeuser 1960):

$$I_i = P_i d_i^p f_i^q \frac{V_m - V_{surface}/(RT/zF)}{1 - e^{\frac{V_m - V_{surface}}{RT/zF}}} \left[[C_i]_i - [C_i]_o e^{-\frac{V_m - V_{surface}}{RT/zF}} \right] \tag{42.8}$$

42.4.5 Eyring Rate Theory Models of Ionic Currents

An alternative to the Nernst–Planck models of charge diffusion is the rate-theory model which views ion permeation through a channel or pump from a statistical thermodynamics perspective. In this approach, one or more energy barriers are assumed to exist at fixed points in the channel and ions permeate the channel when the energy of the ions overcomes the energy barrier. The case of one barrier is shown schematically in Figure 42.4. The forward and backward ion flux rates can be described using Boltzmann equations as shown below.

$$k_1 = v e^{-(G_b - G_o) - z\delta \frac{V_m}{RT/F}} \tag{42.9}$$

$$k_{-1} = v e^{-(G_b - G_i) + z(1-\delta)\frac{V_m}{RT/F}} \tag{42.10}$$

where k_1 is the forward flux rate from the outside to the inside, and k_{-1} is the flux rate in the other direction; v is some nominal flux; G_o and G_i are the energies at the external and internal surfaces of the cell membrane; G_b is the height of the energy barrier; z is the valence of the permeating ion; δ is the location of the membrane barrier as measured from the external side of the membrane; V_m is the transmembrane potential difference and is implicitly assumed to vary linearly through the thickness of the membrane; and R, T, and F are as defined earlier. Given these flux rates, we can write the flux equations as

$$\text{influx} = [C]_o k_1 \tag{42.11}$$

$$\text{efflux} = [C]_i k_{-1} \tag{42.12}$$

If the net current is then assumed to be the difference between the efflux and the influx, it can be written as

$$I_i = v \left([C]_i e^{-(G_b - G_i) + z(1-\delta)\frac{V_m}{RT/F}} - [C]_o e^{-(G_b - G_o) - z\delta \frac{V_m}{RT/F}} \right) \tag{42.13}$$

The equations for the case of multiple barriers can be derived in a similar way but are much more tedious to work through.

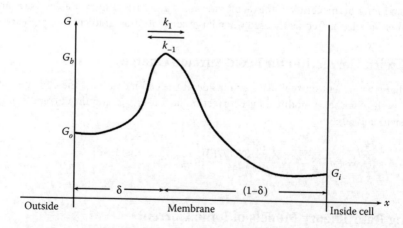

FIGURE 42.4 Schematic representation of energy barrier in a rate theory model of ionic current. A single energy barrier of height G_b located at a fraction δ of the membrane thickness is assumed in this example.

42.4.6 Ion Pump

Ion pumps are membrane molecules that, unlike channels, require energy to function. While the workings of ion pumps can get quite complex especially if the source of energy for these pumps needs to be modeled, most models in use assume a simplied form using Michaelis–Menten terms such as

$$I_p = I_{pmax} \frac{[X]_i}{[X]_i + k_x} \frac{[Y]_o}{[Y]_o + k_y} \tag{42.14}$$

In the above equation, I_{pmax} is the maximum pump current, $[X]_i$ is the concentration of the ionic species on the inside being pumped out and $[Y]_o$ is the concentration of the ionic species on the outside being pumped in. k_x and k_y represent sensitivities of the pump to these ion concentrations.

42.4.7 Ion Exchangers

Ion exchangers are similar to ion pumps but do not require energy directly. Instead, exchangers use the energy stored in a concentration gradient of ion X to transport ion Y in the opposite direction. An example of an exchanger current is the cardiac Na–Ca exhanger, which uses the concentration gradient of sodium (high outside, low inside) to pump one calcium ion out of the cell for every three sodium ions allowed into the cell. An additional difference between exchangers and pumps is that exchangers are more voltage sensitive and are thus more readily operated in the reverse direction under physiological conditions.

42.4.8 Synapses

Yamada and Zucker (1992) have tested various kinetic mechanisms to model calcium control of pre-synaptic release of transmitters. The classic model of postsynaptic response to a synaptic input is the so-called *alpha* function due to Rall (1967) and has the form:

$$G(t) = \frac{t - t_0}{t_{peak}} e^{\frac{t - t_0}{t_{peak}}} \tag{42.15}$$

where G is usually a conductance in a resistor-battery-type branch circuit. Although the alpha function is the one that is most commonly used, more detailed schemes have been constructed using kinetic models (Destexhe et al. 1994).

42.4.9 Calcium as a Second Messenger

Calcium entry into a cell frequently has a number of secondary effects such as initiation of contraction, release of neurotransmitters, and modulation of membrane ion channels. This is usually accomplished by the binding of calcium ions to calcium receptors inside the cell. Michaelis–Menten kinetic schemes with steady-state assumptions are used to model this binding and therefore expressions of the form $f = [Ca^{++}]_i^n / ([Ca^{++}]_i^n + k)$ are frequently employed. Here, f is the fraction of calcium that is bound to the receptor and K is the dissociation constant for the reaction, and n is the number of calcium ions that bind to each receptor molecule.

42.5 Nerve Cells

Nerve cells typically have complex geometries with axons, branching dendrites, spines, and synapses. While it was thought for a long time that dendrites could be modeled using linear resistor–capacitor circuits, it is becoming increasingly clear that nonlinear ionic currents are present in many dendritic trees. Owing to technical difficulties in measuring currents in dendrites and synapses directly, most neuronal models in this chapter describe ionic currents of cell soma or axons. Since the Hodgkin–Huxley equations constitute the basis for membrane modeling, the reader should be familiar with this model before examining the others.

Squid Axon: Hodgkin and Huxley Most models of excitable cells are descendants of this model. The basic circuit equivalent of this model comprises a linear capacitance in parallel with three resistor-battery sub-circuits (one each for sodium, potassium and a nonspecific leakage channel). The HH equations in their original form were

$$C_m \frac{dV}{dt} = -G_{Na}m^3h(V - E_{Na}) - G_K n^4(V - E_K) - G_l(V - E_l)$$

$$\frac{dm}{dt} = \alpha_m(1 - m) - \beta_m m$$

$$\frac{dh}{dt} = \alpha_h(1 - h) - \beta_h h \tag{42.16}$$

$$\frac{dn}{dt} = \alpha_n(1 - n) - \beta_n n$$

The rate constants were given originally as

$$\alpha_m = \frac{(V + 25)/10}{e^{(V+25)/10} - 1} \tag{42.17}$$

$$\beta_m = 4e^{V/18} \tag{42.18}$$

$$\alpha_h = 0.07e^{V/20} \tag{42.19}$$

$$\beta_h = \frac{1}{e^{(V+30)/10} + 1} \tag{42.20}$$

$$\alpha_n = \frac{1}{10} \frac{(V + 10)/10}{e^{(V+10)/10} - 1} \tag{42.21}$$

$$\beta_n = \frac{e(V/80)}{8} \tag{42.22}$$

The physical constants used in these equations are: $G_{Na} = 120$ mS/cm^2, $G_K = 36$ mS/cm^2, $G_l = 0.3$ mS/cm^2, $C_m = 1$ µF/cm^2, $E_{Na} = -115$ mV, $E_K = 12$ mV, and $E_l = -10.613$. The original equations as listed by Hodgkin and Huxley (1952), unfortunately, used a sign convention that has not been followed since. They assumed a resting level of 0 mV for V and that depolarization resulted in negative values for V. Using the sign convention of today for the transmembrane potential, the rate constants can be rewritten by replacing all occurrences of V in the "HH" equations above with $-(V_m + 60)$ with a similar transformation for E_K, E_{Na}, and E_l.

The successes of this model include the ability to predict the velocity of action potential propagation when the spatial aspect is included, the continuous nature of the threshold of the nerve, and the repetitive firing behavior seen under the influence of a constant current. A number of remarks should be made regarding this model that hold for other models as well. First, L'Hopital's Rule allows us to compute the value of expressions of the form $x/(e^x - 1)$ as in Equation 42.17 at the point $x = 0$. Second, for temperatures other than 6.3°C, an acceptable correction is the Q_{10} scaling: multiply each α and β by $\phi = 3^{(T-6.3)/10}$ where the 3 indicates that for each 10°C change in temperature, the speed of the reaction increases threefold (T is in °Celsius). It has been found that the ratio of 3.33 for $G_{Na} : G_K$ in this model achieves a balance between a quick repolarization and continued excitability.

Toad Myelinated Neuron   Frankenhaeuser and Huxley (1964) modified the HH model to describe the fast sodium and delayed rectifier potassium currents with the GHK model rather than the resistor–battery formulation used by Hodgkin and Huxley. In addition, they added a small nonspecific current to account for inward currents late in action potentials of myelinated neurons of the toad *Xenopus laevis*.

Gastropod Neuron   The model of Connor and Stevens (1971) used a HH-type system of differential equations to model repetitive firing in isolated gastropod neurons. This was the first model to include an inactivating potassium current (the A-type current) that has since been used in a number of other cells.

Aplysia Abdominal Ganglion R15 Cell   The bursting behavior of *Aplysia* neurons have been extensively studied. The first model was that of Plant (1976) who extended the HH equations to include an inactivating potassium current, a slow potassium current and a constant hyperpolarizing current due to the Na/K pump. Bertram (1993) modeled bursting in these cells by augmenting an HH model with a calcium current, a second delayed rectifier-type potassium current, and serotonin-activated inward-rectifying potassium current and a negative slope region calcium current. A detailed model including a fast inward sodium current, fast and slow calcium currents, a delayed rectifier and an inward rectifier potassium currents, a sodium–potassium pump, a sodium–calcium exchanger, a calcium pump, and a leakage current is described in Butera et al. (1995).

CA3 Hippocampal Pyramidal Neurons   Traub et al. (1991) have constructed a multicompartment—soma and dendrites—model of hippocampal neurons with upto six membrane currents in each compartment: (i) a fast sodium current, (ii) a calcium current, (iii) a delayed rectifier potassium current, (iv) an inactivating (A-type) potassium current, (v) a long-duration calcium-activated potassium current, and (vi) a short-duration calcium-activated potassium current. Furthermore, calcium concentration changes in a restricted space beneath the membrane is modeled using a simplified linear buffering scheme. Good and Murphy (1996) modified this model to include N-, L-, and T-type calcium currents along with an AMPA-activated current and the effects of β-amyloid block of the A-type current. A branching dendritic version of the Traub et al. (1991) model with synaptic input is described in Traub and Miles (1995).

CA1 Hippocampal Pyramidal Neurons   A model that accurately predicts accomodation in CA1 neurons was constructed by Warman et al. (1994). Using the previous work of Traub et al. (1991) and taking experimental data into consideration, they constructed a 16-compartment model with the following membrane currents: (i) a fast sodium current, (ii) a calcium current, (iii) a delayed rectifier potassium current, (iv) an inactivating (A-type) potassium current, (v) a long-duration calcium-dependent potassium current, (vi) a short-duration calcium and voltage-activated potassium current, (vii) a persistent muscarinic potassium current, and (viii) a leakage current. Unlike the Traub model separate pools of calcium were used to modulate the potassium currents. A linear buffering scheme was assumed for both internal calcium pools but the decay times were assumed to be different in each pool.

Stomatogastric Ganglion Neurons   Epstein and Marder (1990) constructed a HH-type model of the lobster stomatogastric ganglion neuron with a fast sodium current, a delayed rectifier potassium current a voltage-dependent calcium current, a calcium-dependent potassium current, and a linear leakage current to study the mechanism of bursting oscillations in these cells.

Chopper Units in the Anteroventral Cochlear Nucleus   Banks and Sachs (1991) constructed an equivalent cylinder model of chopper units in the anteroventral cochlear nucleus. The model of the soma membrane included a fast sodium current, a delayed rectifier current a linear leakage current and inhibitory and excitatory synaptic currents using the Rall α-wave model.

Lamprey CNS Neurons   The model of Brodin et al. (1991) consisted of voltage-gated sodium, potassium and calcium currents, a calcium-activated potassium current, and a NMDA N-Methyl-D-aspartatae receptor channel. The voltage-dependent block by magnesium of the NMDA was also modeled in this paper. Two compartments were used to model calcium concentration changes inside the cells.

Thalamocortical Cells Neurons in the thalamocortical systems show various kinds of oscillatory behavior during sleep and wake cycles. It has been shown over the last decade that these neurons interact to produce a wide range of oscillatory activity. Huguenard and McCormick (1992) constructed a model of thalamic relay neurons with: (i) a low-threshold transient calcium current, (ii) an inactivating (A-type) potassium current, (iii) a slowly inactivating potassium current, and (iv) a hyperpolarization activated nonspecific current. McCormick and Huguenard (1992) extended the above model to simulate the behavior of thalamocortical relay neurons by adding: (i) a fast sodium current, (ii) a persistent sodium current, (iii) a high-threshold calcium current, (iv) a calcium activated potassium current, and (v) linear leakage currents. Destexhe et al. (1993b) and Destexhe et al. (1993a) have examined similar models as well.

Human Node of Ranvier Schwartz et al. (1995) measured action potentials and separated membrane currents in nodes of Ranvier in human nerve trunks. Their model comprises a fast sodium current, fast and slow potassium currents, and a leakage current.

Dopaminergic Neurons A minimal model of the soma with a fast sodium current and a delayed rectifier potassium current and a dendritic compartment with a sodium–potassium pump, NMDA-activated current, and leakage current was augmented with an L-type calcium current in the dendritic compartment and an A-type potassium current, T-type calcium current, and a calcium-sensitive potassium current in the soma by Li et al. (1996). An improved model with an additional N-type calcium current and another high-voltage-activated calcium current, a sodium–calcium exchanger, a calcium pump, a hyperpolarization activated cation current and cytosolic calcium buffering was constructed by Amini e al. (1999) and a model focusing on the GABA- and NMDA-mediated currents was published by Komendantov et al. (2004).

Cerebellar Granule Cells A model of the soma with three sodium currents (a fast, a persistent, and a resurgent current), a high-threshold calcium current and five potassium currents (fast and slow delayed rectifier currents, an A-type, an inward rectifier, and a calcium-activated potassium current) was constructed by DAngelo et al. (2001).

Prefrontal Cortex Neurons Neurons in the prefrontal cortex show persistent firing activity in the absence of stimuli or neuromodulators. To reconstruct this kind of activity, Winograd and Desexhe (2008) set up a model of the soma with a fast sodium current, an L-type calcium current, two potassium currents (delayed rectifier and slow M-type currents), a leak current, and a hyperpolarization-activated cationic current that is sensitive to cytosolic calcium.

42.5.1 Sensory Neurons

Rabbit Sciatic Nerve Axons A fast sodium current and a leak current was found to be sufficient to model single action potentials in the nodes of Ranvier of axons from rabbit sciatic nerve by Chiu et al. (1979). It is likely that this model should be augmented to include potassium currents in order to model trains of action potentials accurately.

Myelinated Auditory-Nerve Neuron A detailed model of the morphology of myelination and ion channel distribution was formulated by Colombo and Parkins (1987) using the Frankenhaeuser–Huxley model as a base: it includes a fast sodium current, fast potassium current, a leakage current, and a slow sodium current.

Retinal Ganglion Cells Fohlmeister et al. (1990) modeled the retinal ganglion cells using a fast inactivating sodium current, a calcium current, a noninactivating (delayed-rectifier) potassium current, an inactivating potassium current, and a calcium-activated potassium current. An important feature in this model is that it models the calcium concentration inside the cell using a simplified buffering scheme and in this way they are able to model the modulation of potassium currents by calcium. A model with separate L- and N-type calcium currents was constructed by Benison et al. (2001).

Retinal Horizontal Cells The model of Winslow and Knapp (1991) consisted of a fast sodium current, an inactivating (A-type) potassium current, a noninactivating potassium current, an anomalous rectifier potassium current, a calcium-inactivated calcium current, and a linear leakage current. In addition, calcium concentration changes in a restricted region beneath the membrane was also modeled.

Rat Nodose Neurons Schild et al. (1994) built a model comprising fast and slow sodium currents, an A-type potassium current, a delayed rectifier potassium current, T- and L-type calcium currents, a calcium-activated potassium current, a slowly inactivating potassium current, a sodium–calcium exchanger, a sodium–potassium pump, a calcium pump current, and background currents. This model was enhanced with descriptions of vesicular storage and release in Schild et al. (1995) and further tuned to fit myelinated and nonmyelinated neurons in Schild and Kunze (1997).

Muscle Spindle Primary Endings Otten et al. (1995) extended the Frankenhaeuser–Huxley model with modifications to reproduce repetitive firing in sensory endings: in addition to the fast sodium current, fast potassium current, and leakage currents of the FH model, a slowly activating delayed rectifier current was required.

Vertebrate Retinal Cone Photoreceptors A model of vertebrate photoreceptor cells that includes a light-sensitive current, an L-type calcium current, a delayed rectifier potassium current, calcium-sensitive potassium and chloride currents, a hyperpolarization-activated current, a sodium–potassium pump, and a leak current in addition to the response of the cell to a channel blocker was published by Usui et al. (1996).

Primary and Secondary Sensory Neurons of the Enteric Nervous System A model of primary and secondary afferents with a fast sodium current, an N-type calcium current, a delayed rectifier potassium current, a calcium-sensitive potassium current, and a chloride current was set up by Miftakhov and Wingate (1996).

Invertebrate Photoreceptor Neurons The membrane properties of nerve terminals, axons, soma, and microvilli of Type-B photoreceptors of the invertebrate *Hermissenda* were modeled using a fast sodium current, an A-type potassium current, a calcium-dependent potassium current, a delayed rectifier potassium current, a noninactivating calcium current, light-induced sodium and calcium currents, and a leakage current by Fost and Clark (1996).

Fly Optic Lobe Tangential Cells Three families of tangential cells of the blowfly were modeled by Haag et al. (1997). The centrifugal–horizontal cell has an inward calcium current and outward potassium currents. The other cells have a fast sodium current, a delayed rectifier potassium current, and a sodium-dependent potassium current.

Rat Mesencephalic Trigeminal Neurons Negro and Chandler (1997) have constructed a model of sensory neurons involved in brain stem control of jaw musculature. This model of the trigeminal neurons includes a fast sodium current, N- and T-type calcium currents, two A-type potassium currents, a sustained potassium current, a delayed rectifier potassium current, a calcium-dependent potassium current, a hyperpolarization-activated current, and a leakage current.

Primary Afferents and Related Efferents A model comprising a fast sodium current, a delayed rectifier potassium current, a calcium current, and a calcium-dependent potassium current was used to model primary afferents as well as interneurons and efferent neurons connected to the afferents by Saxena et al. (1997). A modification of the HH model was used in Amir et al. (2002) to model A-type dorsal root ganglion neuron cell bodies.

Myelinated Ia Primary Afferent Neurons The intraspinal collateral of a myelinated primary afferent neuron was modeled with a myelination morphology by D'Incamps et al. (1998) and included a fast sodium current, a delayed rectifier potassium current, and a Rall synaptic current at a particular node of Ranvier in the network.

42.5.2 Efferent Neurons

Sympathetic Neurons of the Superior Cervical Ganglia Superior cervical ganglion neurons were modeled by Belluzzi and Sacchi (1991) using the following membrane currents: (i) sodium currents with fast and slow components, (ii) a GHK-type calcium current, (iii) a delayed rectifier potassium current, (iv) an inactivating (A-type) potassium current, and (v) a calcium-activated potassium current. One drawback of this model is that the calcium activation of the potassium channels was modeled using a fixed time delay rather than by allowing the internal calcium concentration to change.

Small Intestine Cholinergic and Adrenergic Neurons   Miftakhov and Wingate (1994a) used the HH equations (fast sodium current, delayed rectifier potassium current, and a leak current attributed to chloride channels) and added a system of equations to model the release of the neurotransmitter acetylcholine by the presynaptic terminal. Similarly a model of release of noradrenaline was modeled in Miftakhov and Wingate (1994b).

Pyloric Constrictor Neurons of the Lobster   Models of the crab lateral pyloric neuron were modified to include a fast sodium current, an A-type potassium current, a delayed rectifier potassium current, a calcium current, a calcium-dependent potassium current, and a leak current by Harris-Warrick et al. (1995a) to examine the effect of the neurotransmitter dopamine on the A-type current. This model was augmented by Harris-Warrick et al. (1995b) to include a hyperpolarization activated current.

Mammalian Spinal Motoneuron   Halter et al. (1995) set up a detailed model of myelinated motoneurons with myelination morphology and ionic currents including: a fast sodium current, fast and slow delayed rectifier potassium currents, and a leak current.

Leech Heartbeat Oscillator Interneuron   Interneurons controlling the leech heartbeat were modeled using: a fast sodium current, an A-type potassium current, an inward rectifier current, fast and slowly inactivating calcium currents, a persistent sodium current, a hyperpolarization activated current, slowly inactivating and persistent potassium currents, and synaptic chloride currents (Nadim et al. 1995).

Snail RPa1 Bursting Neuron   A model including a fast sodium current, a delayed rectifier potassium current, a voltage-dependent calcium current, a voltage- and calcium-dependent calcium current, and a leak current was constructed by Berezetskaya et al. (1996) to investigate the bursting behavior of pacemaker cells of *Helix pomatia*.

Vertebrate Motoneuron   Data from motoneurons from various species were put together to construct a generic model of vertebrate motoneurons by Booth et al. (1997). This model contains a fast sodium current, a delayed rectifier potassium current, L- and N-type calcium currents, and a calcium-dependent potassium current.

Xenopus Central Pattern Generator Neuron   A model of *Xenopus* embryo swimming central pattern generator neurons with HH currents was modified by Tabak and Moore (1998) to include a voltage- and magnesium-sensitive NMDA channel current and a Rall alpha-wave mechanism for non-NMDA postsynaptic currents.

Interstitial Cells of Cajal   Interstitial cells of Cajal are pacemaking cells in the gastrointestinal tract. The model of Youm et al. (2006) includes voltage-dependent sodium, potassium, and calcium currents, an Na–K pump, an Na–Ca exchanger, and a plasmalemmal calcium pump; it also has equations for cytosolic calcium changes. A newer model by Faville et al. (2009) includes a T-type calcium current as well as mitochondrial calcium handling and ER calcium release.

42.6 Skeletal Muscle Cells

42.6.1 Frog Sartorius Muscle Cell

Skeletal muscle cells have a significant amount of current flowing through the cell membrane in the T-tubules of the cells. For this reason, it becomes imperative to model the currents in the T-tubules along with the rest of the cell membrane. The Adrian and Peachey (1973) equations are a system of coupled HH-type circuits and thus have a significant spatial component. The equations describing the velocity field have the same structure as the Hodgkin–Huxley equations. Two models were suggested in the paper: if sodium and potassium channels are assumed to exist in the T-tubules, the usual HH formulation of the corresponding currents are used; otherwise, only a linear leakage current appears in the voltage equation.

42.6.2 Barnacle Muscle

Morris and Lecar (1981) sought to model the oscillatory activity in current-clamped barnacle muscle fibers using just two noninactivating currents: a fast calcium current and a potassium current. It should be kept in mind that their model does not take into account the presence of a calcium chelator (EGTA) inside the cells used to obtain experimental results. Their equations have the same general structure as the HH equations:

$$C_m \frac{dV}{dt} = -G_L(V - E_L) - G_{Ca}m(V - E_{Ca}) - G_K^n(V - E_K) \tag{42.23}$$

$$\frac{dm}{dt} = \lambda_m(m_\infty - m) \tag{42.24}$$

$$\frac{dn}{dt} = \lambda_n(n_\infty - n) \tag{42.25}$$

where

$$m_\infty = \frac{1}{2}\left(1 + \tanh\frac{V - v_1}{v_2}\right) \tag{42.26}$$

$$\lambda_\infty = \lambda_m \cosh\frac{V - v_1}{2v_2} \tag{42.27}$$

$$n_\infty = \frac{1}{2}\left(1 + \tanh\frac{V - v_3}{v_4}\right) \tag{42.28}$$

$$\lambda_n = \lambda_n \cosh\frac{V - v_3}{2v_4} \tag{42.29}$$

Typical values of the parameters are: $C_m = 20\ \mu F/cm^2$, $G_L = 2\ mS/cm^2$, $G_K = 8\ mS/cm^2$, $G_{Ca} = 4mS/cm^2$, $E_L = -50\ mV$, $E_K = -70\ mV$, $E_{Ca} = 100\ mV$, $v_1 = 10\ mV$, $v_2 = 15\ mV$, $v_3 = 10\ mV$, $v_4 = 14.5\ mV$, $\lambda_m = 0.1$, and $\lambda_n = 1/15$. An alternative model of the calcium current was also proposed. Instead of the HH resistor-battery-type formulation, a GHK formulation was suggested:

$$I_{Ca} = G_{Ca}m\frac{V/12.5}{1 - e^{V/12.5}}\left[1 - \frac{[Ca^{-+}]_i}{[Ca^{-+}]_o}e^{V/12.5}\right] \tag{42.30}$$

where typical values of $[Ca^{-+}]_i$ and $[Ca^{-+}]_o$ were 0.001 and 100 mM, respectively.

42.7 Endocrine Cells

42.7.1 Pancreatic β-Cells

An interesting electrophysiological phenomenon occurs in the Islet of Langerhans of the pancreas: the release of insulin is controlled in these islets by trains of action potentials occurring in rapid bursts followed by periods of quiescence. This "bursting" behavior occurs only in intact islets: single cells do not display such bursting activity. Chay and Keizer (1983) was the first attempt to model this phenomenon quantitatively. Sherman et al. (1988) sought to explain the absence of bursting in single β-cells using the idea of "channel-sharing." Keizer (1988) modified this model by substituting an ATP and ADP-dependent K channel instead of the Ca-dependent K channel. This model was then further improved by Keizer and Magnus (1989). Sherman et al. (1990) constructed a domain model to examine the effect of Ca on Ca channel inactivation. Further refinements have been made by Keizer and Young (1993). A new slowly activating calcium-dependent potassium current and a calcium subspace model was added in Goforth et al. (2002) and Zhang et al. (2003). The model of Fridlyand et al. (2003) incorporates a detailed model of calcium uptake and release and sodium, IP_3, and ATP signalling. Bertram and Sherman (1993) use the "phantom burster" model to reconstruct a wide range of burst frequencies.

42.7.2 Chromaffin Cells

The model of Warashina and Ogura (2004) uses voltage-dependent sodium, potassium and calcium currents, a Ca-activated K current, cytosolic calcium handling, and exocytosis to model stimulation–secretion coupling in chromaffin cells of the rat adrenal medulla.

42.7.3 Pituitary Gonadotrophs and Corticotrophs

Li et al. (1995) have constructed a model of membrane fluxes and calcium release from the endoplasmic reticulum of rat pituitary gonadotrophs. The membrane currents modeled include an L- and T-type calcium currents, delayed rectifier and calcium-sensitive potassium currents, and a leak current. A modification of this model was used by LeBeau et al. (1997) to model pituitary corticotroph cells. Shorten and Wall (2000) use voltage-dependent potassium currents, L- and T-type calcium currents, and Ca-activated K currents interacting with a cytosolic calcium subsystem to model bursting behavior in pituitary corticotrophs.

42.8 Cardiac Cells

42.8.1 Purkinje Fiber

Older models of the Purkinje fiber (Noble 1960, 1962; Noble and Tsien 1969; McAllister et al. 1975) failed to model the pacemaking currents correctly. Furthermore, external and internal concentration changes were not modeled until the work of DiFrancesco and Noble (1985) (The original paper contained a number of errors and a corrected listing of the model equations can be found in Varghese and Winslow 1993). Despite the fact that the magnitude of the changes in calcium concentrations is at odds with recent experimental observations, this model has been very influential in directing modeling efforts. Many cardiac models constructed now use the general DiFrancesco–Noble structure. The canine Purkinje fiber cell model (Aslanidi et al. 2009b) is a single-cell model based on an earlier canine endocardial cell model and includes L- and T-type calcium currents and fast and slow delayed rectifier currents along with the currents found in the DiFrancesco–Noble equations. Sampson et al. (2010) constructed a human Purkinje fiber cell model including Markov-state models for many of the ion channel currents.

42.8.2 Sinoatrial Node

As was the case with Purkinje fibers, the pacemaking mechanism was not modeled correctly in earlier models (Bristow and Clark 1982; Yanagihara et al. 1980) and it was only after the Purkinje fiber model of DiFrancesco and Noble (1985) that accurate models of the sinoatrial node models could be constructed. An excellent summary of these modeling efforts can be found in Wilders et al. (1991) complete with listings of the equations. The most detailed model of sinoatrial node cells to date is that of Demir et al. (1994); this model includes a biophysically accurate description of internal calcium buffering and varying extracellular concentrations. A model similar to the ones in Wilders et al. (1991) was augmented to model the effects of acetylcholine changes outside sinoatrial node cells by Dokos et al. (1996). Zhang et al. (2000) set up a pair of sinoatrial models to reconstruct different action potential shapes found in cells from two areas—the center and the periphery—of the rabbit sinoatrial node. Kurata et al. (2002) included a sustained inward current, improved formulation of L-type calcium current and the delayed rectifier current, and cytosolic calcium changes for a rabbit central sinoatrial node cell. Sarai et al. (2003) reconstructed sinoatrial node cell action potential changes due to external calcium and potassium using the same general structure as the ventricular cell model of Matsuoka et al. (2003). Lovell et al. (2004) used Markov-state models of currents to simulate various regions of the rabbit sinoatrial node.

42.8.3 Atrial Muscle

The first detailed model of the excitation–contraction coupling mechanism in cardiac cells was constructed by Hilgemann and Noble (1987) and a single cell model was completed by Earm and Noble (1990). A similarly detailed model of rabbit atrial cells was constructed by Lindblad et al. (1996) and modified to fit the data from human atrial cells by Nygren et al. (1998). Another model of human atrial cells based on the ventricular cell model of Luo and Rudy (1994) but with improved calcium-handling equations was formulated by Courtemanche et al. (1998). The main differences between the Nygren and Courtemanche models are that the latter uses a steady-state approximation for the calcium buffers and that the relative sizes of the rapid and slow components of the delayed rectifier are reversed. The first model of a canine atrial cell was constructed by Ramirez et al. (2000) by tuning the Courtemanche model to data from canine atrial cell experiments; this model reconstructed action potentials from different regions of the canine right atria. Kneller et al. (2002) improved on the Ramirez model to include a Na–Cl transporter and a background chloride current to stabilize concentrations in long time-duration pacing simulations. The rabbit atrial cell model of Aslanidi et al. (2009a) is a modification of the Lindblad model to reproduce action potential characteristics of anatomically distinct areas of the rabbit atria.

42.8.4 Atrioventricular Node

Inada et al. (2009) have developed models of three areas of the rabbit atrioventricular node: the quiescent atrio-nodal and nodal-His cells and the pacemaking Nodal cells. Ten ionic currents were used to construct the models, including voltage-dependent Na, K, and Ca currents, a hyperpolarization activated cationic current, a Na–Ca exchanger and a Na–K pump.

42.8.5 Ventricular Muscle

The first model of ventricular cells (Beeler and Reuter 1977) consisted of (i) a fast inward sodium current, (ii) a slow inward calcium current, (iii) an inward-rectifying potassium current, and (iv) a voltage-dependent potassium current. A simple linear model of calcium buffering was also included. Drouhard and Roberge (1987) improved the Beeler–Reuter model by varying parameters and the equations for the rate constants for sodium activation and inactivation to match the experimental results. Noble et al. (1991) constructed a model of the guinea-pig ventricular cell by varying parameters in equations for the atrial cell model of Earm and Noble (1990). Further refinements including better handling of the fast and slow components of the delayed rectifier current and feedback of length and tension changes on the electrophysiology was incorporated in Noble et al. (1998). Nordin (1993) modified the DiFrancesco and Noble (1985) equations to model ventricular cells. His model included membrane calcium and potassium pumps and subcompartments inside the cell for sodium and calcium concentrations. Luo and Rudy (1991) brought further improvements by including a plateau potassium current and updating all the current characteristics to match the data from whole cell and patch-clamp experiments. A more detailed model with more accurate descriptions of internal calcium concentration changes has also been constructed (Luo and Rudy 1994). The main disadvantage of this effort is the formulation of the calcium release current: it depends on the time of the maximum rate of depolarization and activates with a time delay. This was remedied by the model of Jafri et al. (1998) and also by Priebe and Beuckelmann (1998) for human ventricular cells. A model incorporating a Markov-state model of the transient outward current along with the other ionic currents in Jafri et al. (1998) was described in Greenstein et al. (2000) and a significantly more detailed model comprising a number of stochastically activated calcium release units and a Markov-state model formulation of L-type calcium currents was constructed by Greenstein and Winslow (2002). The adult rat ventricular cell model of Pandit et al. (2003) (also see Pandit et al. 2001) includes the regulatory effects of type-1 diabetes on action potential characteristics. The human ventricular cell model of Bernus et al. (2002) is a simplified (six differential equations) version of the Priebe model but is capable of reproducing a range of behaviors of human ventricular cells. Matsuoka et al. (2003) used newer Na and Ca channel models and include kinetic information in models of the inward rectifier current and Na–K pump and also coupled a muscle contraction component as well. The model of Bondarenko et al. (2004) is notable in that it is a mouse ventricular cell model and incorporates a number of Markov-state models. The canine epicardial ventricular cell model of Hund and Rudy (2004) recreates rate-dependent changes in action potential shape and include the regulatory effects of a CaM kinase. Iyer et al. (2004) model of human left-ventricular epicardial myocytes used Markov state models to construct one of the more complex models (a set of 66 differential equations). Shannon et al. (2004) have set up a model of rabbit ventricular myocytes with a focus on the calcium-handling equations. The human ventricular cell models of ten Tusscher et al. (2004) and ten Tusscher and Panfilov (2006) have been used by a number of groups to compute epicardial, midmyocardial, and endocardial cell action potentials. Livshitz and Rudy (2007) reproduced alternans in calcium transients and the effects of CaM-kinaseII activation in their canine ventricular cell model. Canine endocardial, midmyocardial, and epicardial cell action potentials were modelled by Benson et al. (2008) by modifying the Hund–Rudy model. Mahajan et al. (2008) rabbit ventricular cell model includes detailed Markov-state models of L-type calcium currents to model calcium transients during high pacing rates. Decker et al. (2009) canine epicardial cell model refines the Livschitz model and uses Markov-state models for the L-type Ca current and the slow component of the delayed rectifier to model rate-dependent action potential changes. Gauthier et al. (2012) incorporate metabolism, isometric force production and excitation–contraction coupling along with a membrane model of guinea-pig ventricular myocytes.

42.8.6 Amphibian Sinus Venosus and Atrial Cells

Rasmussion et al. (1990) have constructed a detailed model of the bullfrog sinus venosus pacemaker cells that includes: (i) a delayed rectifier potassium current, (ii) a GHK-type calcium current, linear background (iii) sodium and (iv) calcium currents, (v) a Na–K pump current, (vi) a Na–Ca exchanger current, and (vii) a calcium pump current. Calcium binding to troponin, troponin-Mg, and calmodulin was also included in the model. Furthermore, internal and external sodium, calcium, and potassium were also modeled as time-varying quantities. In addition to the features of the sinus venosus cell, the bullfrog atrial cell (Rasmusson et al. 1990) includes a fast sodium current and an inward rectifying potassium current.

42.9 Epithelial Cells

A detailed model of the slow processes in principal cells of the cortical collecting tubule of the mammalian kidney was built by Tang and Othmer (1996) and includes sodium, potassium, and chloride channels, a sodium–potassium pump, a calcium pump, a sodium–potassium-chloride cotransporter, and a sodium–calcium exchanger.

42.10 Smooth Muscle

Smooth muscle cells like many other kinds of cells have significant current carried by pumps and exchangers. A simple model of smooth muscle cell membrane electrical activity was constructed by Gonzalez-Fernandez and Ermentrout (1994). This model has the same structure as the Morris–Lecar model of barnacle muscle fibers. Besides model parameter differences, the gating variable m was set to its steady-state value of m_∞ and the internal calcium was modeled as a time-varying quantity with a simple linear model of internal buffering. A detailed model of electrical activity in the smooth muscle of the small bowel with L- and T-type calcium currents, a calcium-dependent potassium current, a delayed rectifier potassium current, and a background chloride current has been published by Miftakhov et al. (1992).

42.11 Plant Cells

The electrophysiology of a number of plant cells have been studied and characterized. A plasmalemmal proton pump, a hydrogen-chloride symporter, inward and outward rectifying K^+ currents, and a chloride channel were modeled in the equations representing electrical activity in *Egeria densa* Planchon by Buschmann et al. (1996).

42.12 Simplified Models

A large number of papers have investigated the dynamics of cell electrophysiology by using simplifications of models listed above. A good reason to use simplified models is that mathematical analysis of such models is tractable.

42.12.1 Hill

The model constructed by Hill (1936) was one of the earliest differential equation models of nerve electrical activity. While the behavior of this model was compared with experimental observations in animal preparations, the model is a phenomenological one that only reproduced subthreshold responses. Hill's focus was the modeling of accomodation and he used a time-varying "threshold," U.

The basic model is a linear differential equation with time being the independent variable and voltage, V, and threshold voltage, U, being the dependent variables:

$$\dot{V} = \frac{-1}{k}(V - V_o) + I(t)$$

$$\dot{U} = \frac{-1}{\lambda}(U - U_o) + \frac{1}{\beta}(V - V_o)$$

(42.31)

where V_o and U_o are some steady-state values of voltage and the threshold function and k, λ, and β are relaxation time constants (k is a few milliseconds and λ and β are a few hundred milliseconds) and $I(t)$ is some time-varying current source. The above equations can be solved using the variation of constants method and Hill documented the responses of the model to various functions, $I(t)$, and various parameter values. Such a model is only of use if one is not interested in supra-threshold behavior.

42.12.2 FitzHugh–Nagumo

The FitzHugh–Nagumo equations are also called the Bonhoeffer–Van der Pol equations and have been used as a generic system that shows excitability and oscillatory activity. FitzHugh (1969) showed that much of the behavior of the Hodgkin–Huxley equations can be reproduced by a system of two differential equations:

$$\dot{V} = V - \frac{V^3}{3} - U + I(t)$$
$$\dot{U} = \phi(V - bU + a)$$

(42.32)

where a, b, and ϕ are positive constants (typical values are: $a = 0.7$, $b = 0.8$, and $\phi = 0.08$). With no input current ($I = 0$) the system has a stable resting state and at $I = 0.4$ the system exhibits oscillatory activity. This model reproduces excitability, threshold phenomena, and repetitive firing.

42.12.3 Hindmarsh–Rose Models

The first model of Hindmarsh and Rose (1982a) was an attempt to improve on the FitzHugh–Nagumo model without increasing the number of state variables. In most neurons undergoing repetitive firing, the time between action potentials is usually much greater than the duration of action potentials; however, the FHN model has an action potential duration that is roughly the same order of magnitude as the inter-spike interval. In addition, FHN does not yield a linear current–frequency relationship. These inadequacies were addressed by Hindmarsh and Rose and in their model the action potential duration and the inter-spike interval are closer to experimental recordings. Their model can be written as

$$\dot{V} = -a(f(V) - y - I)$$
$$\dot{y} = b(g(V) - y)$$

(42.33)

where the nonlinearities are defined to be: $f(V) = cV^3 + dV^2 + eV + h$ and $g(V) = f(V) - qe^{rV} + s$. The constants used to model action potentials in snail visceral ganglion neurons were: $a = 5400$ M Ω/s, $b = 30$ s^{-1}, $c = 0.00017$, $d = 0.001$, $e = 0.01$, $h = 0.1$, $q = 0.024$, $r = 0.088$, and $s = 0.046$.

A second model (Hindmarsh and Rose 1982b) sought to include the phenomenon of bursting by adding a third variable. The model had the following form:

$$\dot{V} = -aV^3 + bV^2 + y - z + I$$
$$\dot{y} = c - dV^2 - y$$
$$\dot{z} = r(s(V - V_1) - z)$$

(42.34)

where $a = 1$, $b = 3$, $c = 1$, $d = 5$, $r = 0.001$, $s = 1$, and setting $I = 1$ for a short period triggers the bursting response.

Defining Terms

Action potential: A phenomenon involving temporal changes in the transmembrane potential. An action potential is typically characterized by a fast depolarization followed by a slower repolarization and sometimes hyperpolarization as well.

Depolarization: Depolarization is a process that is said to occur whenever the transmembrane potential becomes more positive than some "resting" potential.

Hyperpolarization: A deviation of the transmembrane potential in the negative direction from a "resting" state is called hyperpolarization.

Ion channel: An ion channel is a protein molecule embedded in the cell membrane. It is thought to have the structure of a pipe with obstructions that gate the flow of ions into and out of the cell.

Ion exchanger: An ion exchanger molecule uses the potential energy in the electrochemical gradients to pump one ionic species into the cell and another species out.

Ion pump: An ion pump molecule uses energy (in the form of ATP molecules) to pump ions against their electrochemical gradients.

Refractory period: A period of time after an action potential during which the cell is unable to undergo another action potential in response to a second stimulus.

Repolarization: Repolarization is a process that usually follows depolarization and causes the transmembrane potential to return to a polarized state.

Selectivity: This is a property of ion channels where a certain type of channel only allows a specific ionic species to pass through it. Some channels are less specific than others and may allow more than one ionic species to pass through it.

Threshold: There is no satisfactory definition nor a quantitative description of threshold that will work for all conditions. A working definition of threshold would be *the state the cell has to reach in order to produce an action potential*. It is usually characterized by the strength of an external stimulus required to bring the cell from some initial state to the threshold state. The problem with this definition is that the threshold stimulus will vary considerably depending on the initial state of the cell: the cell may be in a resting state or it may be undergoing repolarization or depolarization.

Transmembrane potential difference: The potential difference between the inside and the outside of a cell manifests itself very close to the membrane. In many cases, the potential of the external fluid is taken to be the reference or ground potential and the transmembrane potential difference is the same as the cell potential, otherwise also called the membrane potential.

Voltage clamp: This refers to the experimental procedure of using active electronic circuits to hold the transmembrane potential difference at a fixed value by pumping current into the cell.

For Further Information

The best introduction to ion channels and excitable behavior in cells can be found in *Ion Channels of Excitable Membranes*, 3rd ed. by Bertil Hille (Sunderland, MA: Sinauer Associates; 2001).

In the case of neurons, *Principles of Neural Science* by Kandel, Schwartz and Jessell (McGraw-Hill, 2000) is the bible. Detailed discussions of cardiovascular cell membrane phenomena can be found in *Cardiac Electrophysiology*, 5th ed. edited by Zipes and Jalife (Philadelphia, PA; WB Saunders; 2009).

Mathematical analysis of cell models can be found in Guckenheimer et al. (1997), Bertram et al. (1995), and Koch et al. (1995).

Numerical Methods

Most of the models presented in this chapter are systems of first-order nonlinear ordinary differential equations. While the solution of linear ordinary differential equations can be written down explicitly, this is usually impossible for nonlinear systems. The only option to investigate the behavior of these solutions is to compute approximate solutions using numerical time integration. There are a number of numerical methods with varying degrees of accuracy and they fall into two main classes: explicit and implicit methods. The advantage of explicit methods is that they are simpler to implement whereas implicit methods require the use of a nonlinear solver, which can be extremely complicated. The disadvantage of explicit methods is that the errors of these methods are very sensitive to the time step used and generally very small time steps are required to ensure accuracy; implicit methods generally allow much larger time steps. A general guideline would be to try a variable-step explicit method such as a Runge–Kutta method with tight tolerances to control the error; if this proves to be too slow, an implicit method such as the backward difference formula. A good source of integration packages is http://www.netlib.org.

Databases

A number of databases of membrane models have been constructed. The CellML project (Wimalaratne et al. 2009) makes mathematical models like those mentioned in this chapter freely available on the Internet. These models are available at: http://www.cellml.org along with tools to compute numerical solutions for the models, which are also available as XML files. At the time of this writing, the site was regularly being updated and new models were being added when published. This collection of models is curated and annotated.

Models of neuronal cells can also be found at http://senselab.med.yale.edu/ModelDB/ and http://www.cnsorg.org/model-database along with programs and tools for numerical solutions.

References

Adrian, R. H. and L. D. Peachey 1973. Reconstruction of the action potential of frog sartorius muscle. *Journal of Physiology (London) 235*, 103–131.

Amini, B., J. W. Clark, and C. C. Canavier 1999. Calcium dynamics underlying pacemaker-like and burst firing oscillations in midbrain dopaminergic neurons: A computational study. *Journal of Neurophysiology 82*, 2249–2261.

Amir, R., M. Michaelis, and M. Devor 2002. Burst discharge in primary sensory neurons: Triggered by subthreshold oscillations, maintained by depolarizing afterpotentials. *The Journal of Neuroscience 22*(3), 1187–1198.

Aslanidi, O. V., P. Stewart, M. R. Boyett, and H. Zhang 2009a. Mechanisms of transition from normal to reentrant electrical activity in a model of rabbit atrial tissue: Interaction of tissue heterogeneity and anisotropy. *Biophysical Journal 96*, 798–817.

Aslanidi, O. V., P. Stewart, M. R. Boyett, and H. Zhang 2009b. Optimal velocity and safety of discontinuous conduction through the heterogeneous Purkinje-ventricular junction. *Biophysical Journal 97*, 20–39.

Banks, M. I. and M. B. Sachs 1991. Regularity analysis in a compartmental model of chopper units in the anteroventral cochlear nucleus. *Journal of Neurophysiology 65*(3), 606–629.

Beeler, G. W. and H. Reuter 1977. Reconstruction of the action potential of ventricular myocardial fibres. *Journal of Physiology (London) 268*, 177–210.

Belluzzi, O. and O. Sacchi 1991. A five-conductance model of the action potential in the rat sympathetic neurone. *Progress in Biophysics and Molecular Biology 55*, 1–30.

Benison, G., J. Keizer, L. M. Chalupa, and D. W. Robinson 2001. Modeling temporal behavior of postnatal cat retinal ganglion cells. *Journal of Theoretical Biology 210*, 187–199.

Benson, A. P., O. V. Aslanidi, H. Zhang, and A. V. Holden 2008. The canine virtual ventricular wall: A platform for dissecting pharmacological effects on propagation and arrhythmogenesis. *Progress in Biophysics and Molecular Biology 96*, 187–208.

Berezetskaya, N. M., V. N. Kharkyanen, and N. I. Kononenko 1996. Mathematical model of pacemaker activity in bursting neurons of snail, *Helix pomatia*. *Journal of Theoretical Biology 183*, 207–218.

Bernus, O., R. Wilders, C. W. Zemlin, H. Verschelde, and A. V. Panfilov 2002. A computationally efficient electrophysiological model of human ventricular cells. *American Journal of Physiology 282*, H2296–H2308.

Bertram, R. 1993. A computational study of the effects of serotonin on a molluscan burster neuron. *Biological Cybernetics 69*, 257–267.

Bertram, R., M. J. Butte, T. Kiemel, and A. Sherman 1995. Topological and phenomenological classification of bursting oscillations. *Bulletin of Mathematical Biology 57*(3), 413–439.

Bertram, R. and A. Sherman 1993. A calcium-based phantom bursting model for pancreatic islets. *Biological Cybernetics 69*, 257–267.

Bondarenko, V. E., G. P. Szigeti, G. C. Bett, S. J. Kim, and R. L. Rasmusson 2004. Computer model of action potential of mouse ventricular myocytes. *American Journal of Physiology 287*, H1378–1403.

Booth, V., J. Rinzel, and O. Kiehn 1997. Compartmental model of vertebrate motoneurons for Ca^{2+}-dependent spiking and plateau potentials under pharmacological treatment. *Journal of Neurophysiology 78*, 3371–3385.

Bristow, D. G. and J. W. Clark 1982. A mathematical model of primary pacemaking cell in SA node of the heart. *American Journal of Physiology 243*, H207–H218.

Brodin, L., H. G. C. Traven, A. Lansner, P. Wallen, O. Ekeberg, and S. Grillner 1991. Computer simulations of n-methyl-D-aspartate receptor-induced membrane properties in a neuron model. *Journal of Neurophysiology 66*(2), 473–484.

Buschmann, P., H. Sack, A. E. Kohler, and I. Dahnse 1996. Modeling plasmalemmal ion transport of the aquatic plant *Egeriadensa*. *Journal of Membrane Biology 154*, 109–118.

Butera, R. J., J. W. Clark, C. C. Canavier, D. A. Baxter, and J. H. Byrne 1995. Analysis of the effects of modulatory agents on a modeled bursting neuron: Dynamic interactions between voltage and calcium dependent stores. *Journal of Computational Neuroscience 2*, 19–44.

Chay, T. R. and J. Keizer 1983. Minimal model for membrane oscillations in the pancreatic β-cell. *Biophysical Journal 42*, 181–190.

Chiu, S. Y., J. M. Ritchie, R. B. Rogart, and D. Stagg 1979. A quantitative description of membrane currents in rabbit myelinated nerve. *Journal of Physiology (London) 292*, 149–166.

Colombo, J. and C. W. Parkins 1987. A model of electrical excitation of the mammalian auditory-nerve neuron. *Hearing Research 31*, 287–312.

Connor, J. A. and C. F. Stevens 1971. Prediction of repetitive firing behaviour from voltage clamp data on an isolated neurone soma. *Journal of Physiology (London) 213*, 31–53.

Courtemanche, M., R. J. Ramirez, and S. Nattel 1998. Ionic mechanisms underlying human atrial action potential properties: Insights from a mathematical model. *American Journal of Physiology 275*, H301–H321.

D'Angelo, E., T. Nieus, A. Maffei, S. A. P. Rossi, V. Taglietti, A. Fontana, and G. Naldi 2001. Theta-frequency bursting and resonance in cerebellar granule cells: Experimental evidence and modeling of a slow k+-dependent mechanism. *The Journal of Neuroscience 21*(3), 759–770.

Decker, K. F., J. Heijman, J. R. Silva, T. J. Hund, and Y. Rudy 2009. Properties and ionic mechanisms of action potential adaptation, restitution, and accommodation in canine epicardium. *American Journal of Physiology 296*, H1017–H1026.

Demir, S. S., J. W. Clark, C. R. Murphey, and W. R. Giles 1994. A mathematical model of a rabbit sinoatrial node cell. *American Journal of Physiology 266*, C832–C852.

Destexhe, A., A. Babloyantz, and T. J. Sejnowski 1993a. Ionic mechanisms for intrinsic slow oscillations in thalamic relay neurons. *Biophysical Journal 65*(4), 1538–1552.

Destexhe, A., Z. F. Mainen, and T. J. Sejnowski 1994. An efficient method for computing synaptic conductances based on a kinetic model of receptor binding. *Neural Computation 6*, 14–18.

Destexhe, A., D. A. McCormick, and T. J. Sejnowski 1993b. A model for 8–10 Hz spindling in interconnected thalamic relay and reticularis neurons. *Biophysical Journal 65*(6), 2473–2477.

DiFrancesco, D. and D. Noble 1985. A model of cardiac electrical activity incorporating ionic pumps and concentration changes. *Philosophical Transactions of the Royal Society of London B. 307*, 353–398.

D'Incamps, B. L., C. Meunier, M.-L. Monnet, L. Jami, and D. Zytnicki 1998. Reduction of presynaptic action potentials by pad: Model and experimental study. *Journal of Computational Neuroscience 5*, 141–156.

Dokos, S., B. G. Celler, and N. H. Lovell 1996. Vagal control of sinoatrial node rhythm: A mathematical model. *Journal of Theoretical Biology 182*, 21–44.

Drouhard, J.-P. and F. A. Roberge 1987. Revised formulation of the Hodgkin–Huxley representation of the sodium current in cardiac cells. *Computers and Biomedical Research 20*, 333–350.

Earm, Y. E. and D. Noble 1990. A model of the single atrial cell: Relation between calcium current and calcium release. *Proceedings of the Royal Society, London, series B 240*, 83–96.

Epstein, I. R. and E. Marder 1990. Multiple modes of a conditional neural oscillator. *Biological Cybernetics 63*, 25–34.

Faville, R. A., A. J. Pullan, K. M. Sanders, S. D. Koh, C. M. Lloyd, and N. P. Smith 2009. Biophysically based mathematical modeling of interstitial cells of Cajal slow wave activity generated from a discrete unitary potential basis. *Biophysical Journal 96*, 4834–4852.

FitzHugh, R. 1969. Mathematical models of excitation and propagation in nerve. In H. P. Schwan (Ed.), *Biological Engineering*, Chapter 1, pp. 1–85. New York: McGraw-Hill Book Co. Inc.

Fohlmeister, J. F., P. A. Coleman, and R. F. Miller 1990. Modeling the repetitive firing of retinal ganglion cells. *Brain Research 510*, 343–345.

Fost, J. W. and G. A. Clark 1996. Modeling *Hermissenda*: I. Differential contributions of IA and IC to type-B cell plasticity. *Journal of Computational Neuroscience 3*, 137–153.

Frankenhaeuser, B. 1960. Sodium permeability in toad nerve and in squid nerve. *Journal of Physiology (London) 152*, 159–166.

Frankenhaeuser, B. and A. F. Huxley 1964. The action potential in the myelinated nerve fibre of *Xenopus laevis* as computed on the basis of voltage clamp data. *Journal of Physiology (London) 171*, 302–315.

Fridlyand, L. E., N. Tamarina, and L. H. Philipson 2003. Modeling of Ca^{2+} flux in pancreatic β-cells: Role of the plasma membrane and intracellular stores. *American Journal of Physiology 285*, E138–E154.

Gauthier, L. D., J. L. Greenstein, and R. L. Winslow 2012. Toward an integrative computational model of guinea pig cardiac myocyte. *Frontiers in Physiology 3*, 244.

Goforth, P. B., R. Bertram, F. A. Khan, M. Zhang, A. Sherman, and L. S. Satin 2002. Calcium-activated K^+ channels of mouse β-cells are controlled by both store and cytoplasmic Ca^{2+}: Experimental and theoretical studies. *Journal of General Physiology 120*, 307–322.

Goldman, D. E. 1943. Potential, impedence, and rectification in membranes. *Journal of General Physiology 27*, 37–60.

Gonzalez-Fernandez, J. M. and B. Ermentrout 1994. On the origin and dynamics of the vasomotion of small arteries. *Mathematical Biosciences 119*, 127–167.

Good, T. A. and R. M. Murphy 1996. Effect of β-amyloid block of the fast-inactivating K^+ channel on intracellular Ca^{2+} and excitability in a modeled neuron. *Proceedings of the National Academy of Sciences, USA 93*, 15130–15135.

Greenstein, J. L. and R. L. Winslow 2002. An integrative model of the cardiac ventricular myocyte incorporating local control of Ca^{2+} release. *Biophysical Journal 83*, 2918–2945.

Greenstein, J. L., R. Wu, S. Po, G. F. Tomaselli, and R. L. Winslow 2000. Role of the calcium-independent transient outward current $i_{to}1$ in shaping action potential morphology and duration. *Circulation Research 87*, 1026–1033.

Guckenheimer, J., R. Harris-Warrick, J. Peck, and A. Willms 1997. Bifurcation, bursting, and spike frequency adaptation. *Journal of Computational Neuroscience 4*, 257–277.

Haag, J., F. Theunissen, and A. Borst 1997. The intrinsic electrophysiological characteristics of fly lobula plate tangential cells: Ii. Active membrane properties. *Journal of Computational Neuroscience 4*, 349–369.

Halter, J. A., J. S. Carp, and J. R. Wolpaw 1995. Operantly conditioned motoneuron plasticity: Possible role of sodium channels. *Journal of Neurophysiology 73*(2), 867–871.

Hamill, O. P., A. Marty, E. Neher, B. Sakmann, and F. J. Sigworth 1981. Improved patch-clamp techniques for high resolution current recording from cells and cell-free membrane patches. *Pflugers Arch. Ges. Physiol. 391*, 85–100.

Harris-Warrick, R. M., L. Coniglio, N. Barazangi, J. Guckenheimer, and S. Gueron 1995a. Dopamine modulation of transient potassium current evokes phase shifts in a central pattern generator network. *The Journal of Neuroscience 15*(1), 342–358.

Harris-Warrick, R. M., L. Coniglio, R. M. Levini, S. Gueron, and J. Guckenheimer 1995b. Dopamine modulation of two subthreshold currents produces phase shifts in activity of an identified motoneuron. *Journal of Neurophysiology 74*(4), 1404–1420.

Hilgemann, D. W. and D. Noble 1987. Excitation–contraction coupling and extracellular calcium transients in rabbit atrium: Reconstruction of basic cellular mechanisms. *Proceedings of the Royal Society, London, Series B 230*, 163–205.

Hill, A. V. 1936. Excitation and accomodation in nerve. *Proceedings of the Royal Society, Series B 119*, 305–355.

Hille, B. 2001. *Ion Channels of Excitable Membranes* (Third ed.). Sunderland, MA: Sinauer Associates.

Hindmarsh, J. L. and R. M. Rose 1982a. A model of the nerve impulse using two first-order differential equations. *Nature 296*, 162–164.

Hindmarsh, J. L. and R. M. Rose 1982b. A model of the neuronal bursting using three coupled first order differential equations. *Proceedings of the Royal Society, Series B 221*, 87–102.

Hodgkin, A. L. and A. F. Huxley 1952. A quantitative description of membrane current and its application to conduction and excitation in nerve. *Journal of Physiology (London) 117*, 500–544.

Huguenard, J. R. and D. A. McCormick 1992. Simulation of the currents involved in rhythmic oscillations in thalamic relay neurons. *Journal of Neurophysiology 68*(4), 1373–1383.

Hund, T. J. and Y. Rudy 2004. Rate dependence and regulation of action potential and calcium transient in a canine cardiac ventricular cell model. *Circulation 110*, 3168–3174.

Inada, S., J. C. Hancox, H. Zhang, and M. R. Boyett 2009. One-dimensional mathematical model of the atrioventricular node including atrio-nodal, nodal, and nodal-his cells. *Biophysical Journal 97*, 2117–2127.

Iyer, V., R. Mazhari, and R. L. Winslow 2004. A computational model of the human left-ventricular epicardial myocyte. *Biophysical Journal 87*, 1507–1525.

Jafri, M. S., J. J. Rice, and R. L. Winslow 1998. Cardiac Ca^{2+} dynamics: The roles of ryanodine receptor adaptation and sarcoplasmic reticulum load. *Biophysical Journal 74*, 1149–1168.

Keizer, J. 1988. Electrical activity and insulin release in pancreatic beta cells. *Mathematical Biosciences 90*, 127–138.

Keizer, J. and G. Magnus 1989. ATP-sensitive potassium channel and bursting in the pancreatic beta cell. A theoretical study. *Biophysical Journal 89*, 229–242.

Keizer, J. and G. W. D. Young 1993. Effect of voltage-gated plasma membrane Ca^{2+} fluxes on IP_3-linked Ca^{2+} oscillations. *Cell Calcium 14*, 397–410.

Kneller, J., R. J. Ramirez, D. Chartier, M. Courtemanche, and S. Nattel 2002. Time-dependent transients in an ionically based mathematical model of the canine atrial action potential. *American Journal of Physiology 282*, H1437–H1451.

Koch, C., O. Bernander, and R. J. Douglas 1995. Do neurons have a voltage or a current threshold for action potential initiation? *Journal of Computational Neuroscience 2*, 63–82.

Komendantov, A. O., O. G. Komendantova, S. W. Johnson, and C. C. Canavier 2004. A modeling study suggests complementary roles for GABA$_a$ and NMDA receptors and the SK channel in regulating the firing pattern in midbrain dopamine neurons. *Journal of Neurophysiology 91*, 346–357.

Kurata, Y., I. Hisatome, S. Imanishi, and T. Shibamoto 2002. Dynamical description of sinoatrial node pacemaking: Improved mathematical model for primary pacemaker cell. *American Journal of Physiology 283*, H2074–H2101.

LeBeau, A. P., A. B. Robson, A. E. McKinnon, R. A. Donald, and J. Sneyd 1997. Generation of action potentials in a mathematical model of corticotrophs. *Biophysical Journal 73*, 1263–1275.

Li, Y.-X., R. Bertram, and J. Rinzel 1996. Modeling *n*-methyl-D-aspartate-induced bursting in dopamine neurons. *Neuroscience 71*(2), 397–410.

Li, Y.-X., J. Rinzel, L. Vergara, and S. S. Stojilkovic 1995. Spontaneous electrical and calcium oscillations in unstimulated pituitary gonadotrophs. *Biophysical Journal 69*, 785–795.

Lindblad, D. S., C. R. Murphey, J. W. Clark, and W. R. Giles 1996. A model of the action potential and underlying membrane currents in a rabbit atrial cell. *American Journal of Physiology 271*, H1666–H1696.

Livshitz, L. M. and Y. Rudy 2007. Regulation of Ca^{2+} and electrical alternans in cardiac myocytes: Role of CAMKII and repolarizing currents. *American Journal of Physiology 292*, H2854–2866.

Lovell, N. H., S. L. Cloherty, B. G. Celler, and S. Dokos 2004. A gradient model of cardiac pacemaker myocytes. *Progress in Biophysics and Molecular Biology 85*, 301–323.

Luo, C. and Y. Rudy 1991. A model of the ventricular cardiac action potential. *Circulation Research 68*, 1501–1526.

Luo, C. and Y. Rudy 1994. A dynamic model of the cardiac ventricular action potential: I. Simulations of ionic currents and concentration changes. *Circulation Research 74*, 1071–1096.

Mahajan, A., Y. S. Y, D. Sato, A. Baher, R. O. R, L. H. Xie, M. J. Yang, P. S. Chen, J. G. Restrepo, A. Karma, A. Garfinkel, Z. Qu, and J. N. Weiss 2008. A rabbit ventricular action potential model replicating cardiac dynamics at rapid heart rates. *Biophysical Journal 94*, 392–410.

Matsuoka, S., N. Sarai, S. Kuratomi, K. Ono, and A. Noma 2003. Role of individual ionic current systems in ventricular cells hypothesized by a model study. *Japanese Journal of Physiology 53*, 105–123.

McAllister, R. E., D. Noble, and R. W. Tsien 1975. Reconstruction of the electrical activity of cardiac Purkinje fibres. *Journal of Physiology (London) 251*, 1–59.

McCormick, D. A. and J. R. Huguenard 1992. A model of the electrophysiological properties of thalamo-cortical relay neurons. *Journal of Neurophysiology 68*(4), 1373–1383.

Miftakhov, R. N., G. R. Abdusheva, and D. L. Wingate 1996. Model predictions of myoelectrical activity of the small bowel. *Biological Cybernetics 74*, 167–179.

Miftakhov, R. N. and D. L. Wingate 1994a. Mathematical modelling of the enteric nervous network 1: Cholinergic neuron. *Med. Eng. Phys. 16*, 67–73.

Miftakhov, R. N. and D. L. Wingate 1994b. Mathematical modelling of the enteric nervous network 3: Adrenergic neuron. *Med. Eng. Phys. 16*, 451–457.

Miftakhov, R. N. and D. L. Wingate 1996. Electrical activity of the sensory afferent pathway in the enteric nervous system. *Biological Cybernetics 75*, 471–483.

Morris, C. and H. Lecar 1981. Voltage oscillations in the barnacle giant muscle fiber. *Biophysical Journal 35*, 193–213.

Nadim, F., O. H. Olsen, E. DeSchutter, and R. L. Calabrese 1995. Modeling the leech heartbeat elemental oscillator I. Interactions of intrinsic and synaptic currents. *Journal of Computational Neuroscience 2*, 215–235.

Negro, C. A. D. and S. H. Chandler 1997. Physiological and theoretical analysis of K^+ currents controlling discharge in neonatal rat mesencephalic trigeminal neurons. *Journal of Neurophysiology 77*, 537–553.

Noble, D. 1960. A description of cardiac pacemaker potentials based on the Hodgkin–Huxley equations. *Journal of Physiology (London) 154*, 64P–65P.

Noble, D. 1962. A modification of the Hodgkin–Huxley equations applicable to Purkinje fibre action and pace-maker potentials. *Journal of Physiology (London) 160*, 317–352.

Noble, D., S. J. Noble, G. C. L. Bett, Y. E. Earm, W. K. Ho, and I. K. So 1991. The role of sodium–calcium exchange during the cardiac action potential. *Annals of the New York Academy of Sciences 639*, 334–353. Sodium–calcium exchange. *Proceedings of the Second International Conference*, April 1991, Baltimore, MD.

Noble, D. and R. W. Tsien 1969. Reconstruction of the repolarization process in cardiac Purkinje fibres based on voltage clamp measurements of membrane current. *Journal of Physiology (London) 200*, 205–231.

Noble, D., A. Varghese, P. Kohl, and P. Noble 1998. Improved guinea-pig ventricular cell model incorporating a diadic space, i_{Kr} and i_{Ks}, and length- and tension-dependent processes. *Canadian Journal of Cardiology 14*(1), 123–134.

Nordin, C. 1993. Computer model of membrane current and intracellular Ca^{2+} flux in the isolated guinea-pig ventricular myocyte. *American Journal of Physiology 265*, H2117–H2136.

Nygren, A., C. Fiset, L. Firek, J. W. Clark, D. S. L. R. B. Clark, and W. R. Giles 1998. Mathematical model of an adult human atrial cell. The role of K^+ currents in repolarization. *Circulation Research 82*, 63–81.

Otten, E., M. Hulliger, and K. A. Scheepstra 1995. A model study on the influence of a slowly activating potassium conductance on repetitive firing patterns of muscle spindle primary endings. *Journal of Theoretical Biology 173*, 67–78.

Pandit, S. V., R. B. Clark, W. R. Giles, and S. S. Demir 2001. A mathematical model of action potential heterogeneity in adult rat left ventricular myocytes. *Biophysical Journal 81*, 3029–3051.

Pandit, S. V., W. R. Giles, and S. S. Demir 2003. A mathematical model of the electrophysiological alterations in rat ventricular myocytes in type-I diabetes. *Biophysical Journal 84*, 832–841.

Plant, R. E. 1976. Mathematical description of a bursting pacemaker neuron by a modification of the Hodgkin–Huxley equations. *Biophysical Journal 16*, 227–244.

Priebe, L. and D. J. Beuckelmann 1998. Simulation study of cellular electric properties in heart failure. *Circulation Research 82*, 1206–1223.

Rall, W. 1967. Distinguishing theoretical synaptic potentials computed for different soma-dendritic distributions of synaptic input. *Journal of Neurophysiology 30*, 1138–1168.

Ramirez, R. J., S. Nattel, and M. Courtemanche 2000. Mathematical analysis of canine atrial action potentials: Rate, regional factors, and electrical remodeling. *American Journal of Physiology 279*, H1767–H1785.

Rasmusson, R. L., J. W. Clark, W. R. Giles, K. Robinson, R. B. Clark, E. F. Shibata, and D. L. Campbell 1990. A mathematical model of electrophysiological activity in a bullfrog atrial cell. *American Journal of Physiology 259*, H370–H389.

Rasmusson, R. L., J. W. Clark, W. R. Giles, E. F. Shibata, and D. L. Campbell 1990. A mathematical model of a bullfrog cardiac pacemaker cell. *American Journal of Physiology 259*, H352–H369.

Sampson, K. J., V. Iyer, A. R. Marks, and R. S. Kass 2010. A computational model of Purkinje fibre single cell electrophysiology: Implications for the long QT syndrome. *Journal of Physiology (London) 588*, 2643–2655.

Sarai, N., S. Matsuoka, S. Kuratomi, K. Ono, and A. Noma 2003. Role of individual ionic current systems in the SA node hypothesized by a model study. *Japanese Journal of Physiology 53*, 125–134.

Saxena, P., R. Goldstein, and L. Isaac 1997. Computer simulation of neuronal toxicity in the spinal cord. *Neurological Research 19*, 340–349.

Schild, J. H., J. W. Clark, C. C. Canavier, D. L. Kunze, and M. C. Andresen 1995. Afferent synaptic drive of rat medial nucleus tractus solitarius neurons: Dynamic simulation of graded vesicular mobilization, release, and non-NMDA receptor kinetics. *Journal of Neurophysiology 74* (4), 1529–1548.

Schild, J. H., J. W. Clark, M. Hay, D. Mendelowitz, M. C. Andresen, and D. L. Kunze 1994. A- and C-type rat nodose sensory neurons: Model interpretations of dynamic discharge characteristics. *Journal of Neurophysiology 71*(6), 2338–2358.

Schild, J. H. and D. L. Kunze 1997. Experimental and modeling study of Na⁺ current heterogeneity in rat nodose neurons and it impact on neuronal discharge. *Journal of Neurophysiology 78*, 3198–3209.

Schwartz, J. R., G. Reid, and H. Bostock 1995. Action potentials and membrane currents in the human node of Ranvier. *Pflugers Archiv 430*, 283–292.

Shannon, T. R., F. Wang, J. Puglisi, C. Weber, and D. M. Bers 2004. A mathematical treatment of integrated CA dynamics within the ventricular myocyte. *Biophysical Journal 87*, 3351–3371.

Sherman, A., J. Keizer, and J. Rinzel 1990. Domain model for Ca²⁺-inactivation of Ca²⁺ channels at low channel density. *Biophysical Journal 58*, 985–995.

Sherman, A., J. Rinzel, and J. Keizer 1988. Emergence of organized bursting in clusters of pancreatic β-cells by channel sharing. *Biophysical Journal 54*, 411–425.

Shorten, P. R. and D. J. Wall 2000. A Hodgkin–Huxley model exhibiting bursting oscillations. *Bulletin of Mathematical Biology 62*, 695–715.

Tabak, J. and L. E. Moore 1998. Simulation and parameter estimation study of a simple neuronal model of rhythm generation: Role of NMDA and non-NMDA receptors. *Journal of Computational Neuroscience 5*, 209–235.

Tang, Y. and H. G. Othmer 1996. Calcium dynamics and homeostasis in a mathematical model of the principal cell of the cortical collecting tubule. *Journal of General Physiology 107*, 207–230.

ten Tusscher, K. H., D. Noble, P. J. Noble, and A. V. Panfilov 2004. A model for human ventricular tissue. *American Journal of Physiology 286*, H1573–H1589.

ten Tusscher, K. H. and A. V. Panfilov 2006. Alternans and spiral breakup in a human ventricular tissue model. *American Journal of Physiology 291*, H1088–H1100.

Traub, R. D. and R. Miles 1995. Pyramidal cell-to-inhibitory cell spike transduction explicable by active dendritic conductances in inhibitory cell. *Journal of Computational Neuroscience 2*, 291–298.

Traub, R. D., R. K. S. Wong, R. Miles, and H. Michelson 1991. A model of a Ca³ hippocampal pyramidal neuron incorporating voltage-clamp data on intrinsic conductances. *Journal of Neurophysiology 66*(2), 635–650.

Usui, S., Y. Kamiyama, T. Ogura, I. Kodama, and J. Toyama 1996. Effects of zatebradine (ul-fs 49) on the vertebrate retina. In J. Toyama, M. Hiraoka, and I. Kodama (Eds.), *Recent Progress in Electropharmacology of the Heart*, Chapter 4, pp. 37–46. Boca Raton, FL: CRC Press.

Varghese, A. and R. L. Winslow 1993. Dynamics of the calcium subsystem in cardiac Purkinje fibers. *Physica D: Nonlinear Phenomena 68*, 364–386.

Warashina, A. and T. Ogura 2004. Modeling of stimulation-secretion coupling in a chromaffin cell. *Pflügers Archiv 448*(2), 161–174.

Warman, E. N., D. M. Durand, and G. L. F. Yuen 1994. Reconstruction of hippocampal Ca1 pyramidal cell electrophysiology by computer simulation. *Journal of Neurophysiology 71*(6), 2033–2045.

Wilders, R., H. J. Jongsma, and A. C. G. van Ginneken 1991. Pacemaker activity of the rabbit sinoatrial node: A comparison of mathematical models. *Biophysical Journal 60*, 1202–1216.

Wimalaratne, S. M., M. D. Halstead, C. M. Lloyd, E. J. Crampin, and P. F. Nielsen 2009. Biophysical annotation and representation of cellMl models. *Bioinformatics 25*(17), 2263–2270.

Winograd, M. and M. V. S.-V. A Destexhe 2008. Hyperpolarization-activated graded persistent activity in the prefrontal cortex. *Proceedings of the National Academy of Sciences, USA 105*, 7298–7303.

Winslow, R. L. and A. G. Knapp 1991. Dynamic models of the retinal horizontal cell network. *Progress in Biophysics and Molecular Biology 56*, 107–133.

Yamada, W. M. and R. S. Zucker 1992. Time course of transmitter release calculated from simulations of a calcium diffusion model. *Biophysical Journal 61*, 671–682.

Yanagihara, K., A. Noma, and H. Irisawa 1980. Reconstruction of sino-atrial node pacemaker potential based on the voltage clamp experiments. *Japanese Journal of Physiology 30*, 841–857.

Youm, J. B., N. Kim, J. Han, E. Kim, H. Joo, G. G. C. H. Leem, A. Noma, and Y. E. Earm 2006. A mathematical model of pacemaker activity recorded from mouse small intestine. *Philosophical Transactions Series A Mathematical Physical and Engineering Sciences 364*, 1135–1154.

Zhang, H., A. V. Holden, I. Kodama, H. Honjo, M. Lei, T. Varghese, and M. R. Boyett 2000. Mathematical models of action potentials in the periphery and center of the rabbit sinoatrial node. *American Journal of Physiology 279*, H397–H421.

Zhang, M., P. Goforth, R. Bertram, A. Sherman, and L. Satin 2003. The Ca^{2+} dynamics of isolated mouse β-cells and islets: Implications for mathematical models. *Biophysical Journal 84*, 2852–2870.

43

Computational Methods and Software for Bioelectric Field Problems

43.1 Introduction 43-1
43.2 Problem Formulation 43-2
    Example: Simulation of Focal Current Sources in the
    Brain • Example: Simulation of Implantable Cardiac Defibrillators
43.3 Model Construction and Mesh Generation 43-5
    Example: Modeling of Focal Current Sources in the Brain
43.4 Numerical Methods 43-7
    Approximation Techniques: The Galerkin Method • Finite
    Difference Method • Finite Element Method • Boundary
    Element Method • Solution Methods and Computational
    Considerations • Comparison of Methods
43.5 Adaptive Methods 43-15
    Convergence of a Sequence of Approximate Solutions • Energy
    Norms
43.6 Software for Bioelectric Field Problems 43-18
    SCIRun • BioPSE • PowerApps
Acknowledgments 43-24
References 43-24

Christopher R.
Johnson
University of Utah

43.1 Introduction

Computer modeling and simulation continue to become more important in the field of bioengineering. The reasons for this growing importance are manyfold. First, mathematical modeling has been shown to be a substantial tool for the investigation of complex biophysical phenomena. Second, since the level of complexity one can model parallels the existing hardware configurations, advances in computer architecture have made it feasible to apply the computational paradigm to complex biophysical systems. Hence, while biological complexity continues to outstrip the capabilities of even the largest computational systems, the computational methodology has taken hold in bioengineering and has been used successfully to suggest physiologically and clinically important scenarios and results.

This chapter provides an overview of numerical techniques that can be applied to a class of bioelectric field problems. Bioelectric field problems are found in a wide variety of biomedical applications, which range from single cells [59], to organs [62], up to models that incorporate partial to full human structures [44,45,50]. We describe some general modeling techniques that will be applicable, in part, to all the aforementioned applications. We focus our study on a class of bioelectric volume conductor problems that arise in electrocardiography (ECG) and electroencephalography (EEG).

We begin by stating the mathematical formulation for a bioelectric volume conductor, continue by describing the model construction process, and follow with sections on numerical solutions and computational considerations. We continue with a section on error analysis coupled with a brief introduction to adaptive methods. We conclude with a section on software.

43.2 Problem Formulation

As noted in Chapter 39, most bioelectric field problems can be formulated in terms of either the Poisson or the Laplace equation for electrical conduction. Since the Laplace equation is the homogeneous counterpart of the Poisson equation, we will develop the treatment for a general three-dimensional (3D) Poisson problem and discuss simplifications and special cases when necessary.

A *typical* bioelectric volume conductor can be posed as the following boundary value problem:

$$\nabla \cdot \sigma \nabla \Phi = -I_V \quad \text{in } \Omega, \tag{43.1}$$

where Φ is the electrostatic potential, σ is the electrical conductivity tensor, and I_V is the current per unit volume defined within the solution domain, Ω. The associated boundary conditions depend on what type of problem one wishes to solve. There are generally considered to be two different types of conductor problems: direct and inverse volume.

One type of problem deals with the interplay between the description of the bioelectric volume source currents and the resulting volume currents and volume and surface voltages. Here, the problem statement would be to solve Equation 43.1 for Φ with a known description of I_V and the Neumann boundary condition:

$$\sigma \nabla \Phi \cdot \mathbf{n} = 0 \quad \text{on } \Gamma_T, \tag{43.2}$$

which says that the normal component of the electric field is zero on the surface interfacing with air (here denoted by Γ_T). This problem can be used to solve two well-known problems in medicine, the direct EEG and the ECG volume conductor problems. In the direct EEG problem, one usually discretizes the brain and surrounding tissue and skull. One then assumes a description of the bioelectric current source within the brain (this usually takes the form of dipoles or multipoles) and calculates the field within the brain and on the surface of the scalp.

43.2.1 Example: Simulation of Focal Current Sources in the Brain

Figure 43.1 shows the simulation results from a patient-specific model of the head carried out with NeuroFEM (for source simulation) and SCIRun (for mesh generation and visualization). The mesh was composed of 179,643 nodes and 1,067,541 tetrahedral elements and the preliminary simulation was carried out with a dipole source in the right posterior region.

Similarly, in one version of the direct ECG problem, one utilizes descriptions of the current sources in the heart (either dipoles or membrane current source models such as the FitzHugh Nagumo and Beeler Reuter, among others) or defibrillation sources and calculates the currents and voltages within the heart and volume conductor of the chest and voltages on the surface of the torso.

43.2.2 Example: Simulation of Implantable Cardiac Defibrillators

The goal of these simulations was to calculate the electric potentials in the body, and especially in the fibrillating heart, that arise during a shock from an implantable cardiac defibrillator (ICD), over 90,000 of which are implanted annually in the United States alone. Of special interest was the use of such

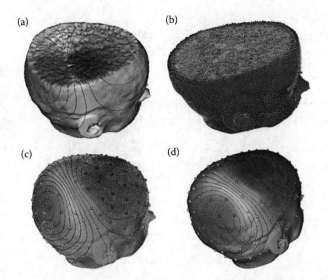

FIGURE 43.1 Illustration of the simulation of the electromagnetic field propagation in a patient-specific brain model. The figure shows a finite element method discretization of the Poisson equation with a patient-specific, five-compartment, geometrical model derived from a segmentation of brain MRI. The solid lines in the simulation images indicate isopotentials and the small white lines are electrical current streamlines.

devices in children, who are both much smaller in size than adults and almost uniformly have some form of anatomical abnormality that makes patient-specific modeling essential.

We have developed a complete pipeline for the patient-specific simulation of defibrillation fields from ICDs, starting from computed tomography (CT) or magnetic resonance imaging (MRI) image volumes and creating hexahedral meshes of the entire torso with heterogeneous mesh density to achieve acceptable computation times [48]. In these simulations, there was effectively a second modeling pipeline that executed each time the user selected a candidate set of locations for the device and the associated shock electrodes. For each such configuration, there was a customized version of the volume mesh that had to be generated and prepared for computation.

Figure 43.2 shows the steps required to implement the customized mesh for each new set of device and electrode locations. The user manipulated an interactive program implemented in SCIRun that allowed very flexible design and placement of the components of the device, an image of which is shown in the leftmost panel of the figure. Modules in SCIRun then carried out a refinement of the underlying hexahedral mesh so that the potentials applied by the device and electrodes were transferred with suitable spatial fidelity to the torso volume conductor (second panel). Then, additional modules in SCIRun computed the resulting electric field throughout the torso and visualized the results, also showing the details of the potentials at the heart and deriving from the simulations a defibrillation threshold value (last two panels of the figure). We have also carried out the initial validation of the complete system by comparing computed to measured defibrillation thresholds and obtained encouraging results [48].

The inverse problems associated with these direct problems involve estimating the current sources I_V within the volume conductor from measurements of voltages on the surface of either the head or the body. Thus, one would solve Equation 43.1 with the boundary conditions:

$$\Phi = \Phi_0 \quad \text{on } \Sigma \subseteq \Gamma_T \tag{43.3}$$

$$\sigma \nabla \Phi \cdot \mathbf{n} = 0 \quad \text{on } \Gamma_T. \tag{43.4}$$

The first is the Dirichlet condition, which says that one has a set of discrete measurements of the voltage of a subset of the outer surface. The second is the natural Neumann condition. While it does not look

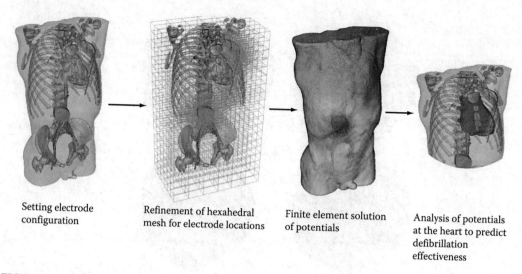

Setting electrode configuration

Refinement of hexahedral mesh for electrode locations

Finite element solution of potentials

Analysis of potentials at the heart to predict defibrillation effectiveness

FIGURE 43.2 Pipeline for computing defibrillation potentials in children. The figures show the steps from the left to the right required to place electrodes and then compute and visualize the resulting cardiac potentials.

much different than the formulation of the direct problem, the inverse formulations are ill-posed. The bioelectric inverse problem in terms of primary current sources does not have a unique solution, and the solution does not depend continuously on the data. Thus, to obtain *useful* solutions, one must try to restrict the solution domain (i.e., number of physiologically plausible solutions) [29] for the former case, and apply the so-called *regularization* techniques to attempt to restore the continuity of the solution on the data in the latter case.

Another bioelectric direct/inverse formulation poses both the problems in terms of scalar values at the surfaces. For the EEG problem, one would take the surface of the brain (cortex) as one bounded surface and the surface of the scalp as the other surface. The direct problem would involve making measurements of voltage of the surface of the cortex at discrete locations and then calculating the voltages on the surface of the scalp. Similarly, for the ECG problem, voltages could be measured on the surface of the heart and used to calculate the voltages at the surface of the torso, as well as within the volume conductor of the thorax. To formulate the inverse problems, one uses measurements on the surface of the scalp (torso) to calculate the voltages on the surface of the cortex (heart). Here, we solve the Laplace equation instead of the Poisson equation because we are interested in the distributions of voltages on a surface instead of current sources within a volume. This leads to the following boundary value problem:

$$\nabla \cdot \sigma \nabla \Phi = 0 \quad \text{in } \Omega \tag{43.5}$$

$$\Phi = \Phi_0 \quad \text{on } \Sigma \subseteq \Gamma_T \tag{43.6}$$

$$\sigma \nabla \Phi \cdot \mathbf{n} = 0 \quad \text{on } \Gamma_T. \tag{43.7}$$

For this formulation, the solution to the inverse problem is unique [87]; however, there still exists the problem of continuity of the solution on the data. The linear algebra counterpart to the elliptic boundary value problem is often useful in discussing this problem of noncontinuity. The numerical solution to all elliptic boundary value problems (such as the Poisson and Laplace problems) can be formulated

In terms of a set of linear equations, $\mathbf{A\Phi} = \mathbf{b}$. For the solution of the Laplace equation, the system can be reformulated as

$$A\Phi_{in} = \Phi_{out}, \tag{43.8}$$

where Φ_{in} is the vector of the data on the inner surface bounding the solution domain (e.g., the electrostatic potentials on the scalp or heart), Φ_{out} is the vector of data that bounds the outer surface (e.g., the subset of voltage values on the surface of the cortex or torso), and A is the *transfer matrix* between Φ_{out} and Φ_{in}, which usually contains the geometry and physical properties (conductivities, dielectric constants, etc.) of the volume conductor. The direct problem is then simply (well) posed as solving Equation 43.8 for Φ_{out} given Φ_{in}. Likewise, the inverse problem is to determine Φ_{in} given Φ_{out}.

A characteristic of A for ill-posed problems is that it has a very large condition number. In other words, the ill-conditioned matrix A is very near to being singular. Briefly, the condition number is defined as $\kappa(A) = \|A\| \cdot \|A^{-1}\|$ or the ratio of maximum to minimum singular values measured in the L_2 norm. The ideal problem conditioning occurs for orthogonal matrices that have $\kappa(A) \approx 1$, while an ill-conditioned matrix will have $\kappa(A) \gg 1$. When one inverts a matrix that has a very large condition number, the inversion process is unstable and is highly susceptible to errors. The condition of a matrix is relative. It is related to the precision level of computations and is a function of the size of the problem. For example, if the condition number exceeds a linear growth rate with respect to the size of the problem, the problem will become increasingly ill-conditioned. See Reference 27 for more about the condition number of matrices.

A number of techniques have arisen to deal with ill-posed inverse problems. These techniques include truncated singular value decomposition (TSVD), generalized singular value decomposition (GSVD), maximum entropy, and a number of generalized least squares schemes, including Twomey and Tikhonov regularization methods. Since this section is concerned more with the numerical techniques for approximating bioelectric field problems, the reader is referred to References 26, 32, 81, and 82 to further investigate the regularization of ill-posed problems. A particularly useful reference for discrete ill-posed problems is the MATLAB® package developed by Per Christian Hansen, which is available via his website [31].

43.3 Model Construction and Mesh Generation

Once we have stated or derived the mathematical equations that define the physics of the system, we must figure out how to solve these equations for the particular domain we are interested in. Most numerical methods for solving boundary value problems require that the continuous domain be broken up into discrete elements, the so-called *mesh* or *grid*, which one can use to approximate the governing equation(s) using the particular numerical technique (finite element, boundary element, finite difference, or multigrid) best suited to the problem.

Because of the complex geometries often associated with bioelectric field problems, the construction of the polygonal mesh can become one of the most time-consuming aspects of the modeling process. After deciding upon the particular approximation method to use (and the most appropriate type of element), we need to construct a mesh of the solution domain, which matches the number of degrees of freedom (DOF) of our fundamental element. For the sake of simplicity, we will assume that we will use linear elements, either tetrahedrons, which are usually used for modeling irregular 3D domains, or hexahedrons used for modeling regular, uniform domains.

There are several different strategies for discretizing the geometry into fundamental elements. For bioelectric field problems, two approaches to mesh generation have become standard: the *divide-and-conquer* (or subsequent subdivision) strategy and the so-called *Delaunay triangulation* strategy.

In using the divide-and-conquer strategy, one starts with a set of points that define the bounding surface(s) in three dimensions (contours in two dimensions). The volume (surface) is repeatedly divided into smaller regions until a satisfactory discretization level has been achieved. Usually, the domain is broken up into eight-node cubic elements, which can then be subdivided into five (minimally) or six tetrahedral elements if so desired. This methodology has the advantage of being fairly easy to program; furthermore, commercial mesh generators exist for the divide-and-conquer method. For use in solving bioelectric field problems, its main disadvantage is that it allows elements to overlap interior boundaries. A single element may span two different conductive regions, for example, when part of an element represents muscle tissue (which could be anisotropic) and the other part of the element falls into a region representing fat tissue. It then becomes very difficult to assign unique conductivity parameters to each element and at the same time accurately represent the geometry.

A second method of mesh generation is the Delaunay triangulation strategy. Given a 3D set of points that define the boundaries and interior regions of the domain to be modeled, one tessellates the point cloud into an optimal mesh of tetrahedra. For bioelectric field problems, the advantages and disadvantages tend to be exactly contrary to those arising from the divide-and-conquer strategy. The primary advantage is that one can create the mesh to fit any predefined geometry, including subsurfaces, by starting with points that define all the necessary surfaces and subsurfaces and then adding additional interior points to minimize the aspect ratio. For tetrahedra, the aspect ratio can be defined as $4\sqrt{(3/2)}(\rho_k/h_k)$, where ρ_k denotes the diameter of the sphere circumscribed about the tetrahedron, and h_k is the maximum distance between two vertices. These formulations yield a value of 1 for an equilateral tetrahedron and a value of 0 for a degenerate (flat) element [7]. The closer to the value of 1, the better. The Delaunay criterion is a method for minimizing the occurrence of obtuse angles in the mesh, yielding elements that have aspect ratios as close to 1 as possible, given the available point set. While the ideas behind Delaunay triangulation are straightforward, the programming is nontrivial and is the primary drawback to this method. Fortunately, there exist several public domain software packages for two- and three-dimensional mesh generation (see Equation 43.6). For more information on mesh generation and various aspects of biomedical modeling, see References 4, 12, 15, 16, 19, 25, 36, 53–55, 57, 58, 66, 71, 75, 76, 79, and 80.

43.3.1 Example: Modeling of Focal Current Sources in the Brain

Figure 43.3 contains the geometric model results from a 15-year-old pediatric patient suffering from epileptic seizures. The segmentations came from a semiautomated tissue classification algorithm developed by Warfield et al. [86], followed by extensive manual inspection and hand editing of mislabeled pixels using Seg3D. The meshing component of the pipeline was implemented in BioMesh3D, a new program that incorporates separate surface fitting and mesh generation programs (e.g., TetGen) in a scripting environment [15,76]. The triangle mesh quality in Panel (a) is excellent, a result of the distributed particle method we have developed [57,58].

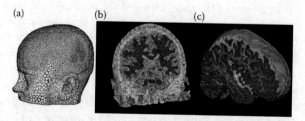

(a)   (b)   (c)

FIGURE 43.3 Example of meshing of the head in a pediatric epilepsy patient. Panel (a) shows the particle distribution over the head surface, and highlights through the variation in particle size the adaptivity of the particles over the skin. Panel (b) shows the associated tetrahedral mesh and panel (c) shows another, higher-resolution view of the mesh, highlighting the cortex and the cerebrospinal fluid.

43.4 Numerical Methods

Because of the geometrical complexity of, and numerous inhomogeneities inherent in, anatomical structures in physiological models, solutions of bioelectric field problems are usually tractable (except in the most simplified of models) only when one employs a numerical approximation method such as the finite difference (FD), the finite element (FE), boundary element (BE), or the multigrid (MG) method to solve the governing field equation(s).

43.4.1 Approximation Techniques: The Galerkin Method

The problem posed in Equation 43.1 can be solved using any of the aforementioned approximation schemes. One technique that addresses three of the previously mentioned techniques (FD, FE, and BE) can be derived by the Galerkin method. The Galerkin method is one of the most widely used methods for discretizing elliptic boundary value problems such as Equation 43.1 and for treating the spatial portion of time-dependent parabolic problems, which are common in models of cardiac wave propagation. While the Galerkin technique is not essential to the application of any of the techniques, it provides for a unifying bridge between the various numerical methods. To express our problem in a Galerkin form, we begin by rewriting Equation 43.1 as

$$A\Phi = -I_v, \tag{43.9}$$

where A is the differential operator, $A = \nabla \cdot (\sigma\nabla)$. An equivalent statement of Equation 43.9 is, find Φ such that $(A\Phi + I_v, \bar{\Phi}) = 0$. Here, $\bar{\Phi}$ is an arbitrary *test function*, which can be thought of physically as a virtual potential field, and the notation $(\phi_1, \phi_2) \equiv \int_\Omega \phi_1 \phi_2 \, d\Omega$ denotes the inner product in $L_2(\Omega)$. Applying Green's theorem, we can equivalently write

$$(\sigma\nabla\Phi, \nabla\bar{\Phi}) - \left\langle \frac{\partial\Phi}{\partial n}, \bar{\Phi} \right\rangle = -(I_v, \bar{\Phi}), \tag{43.10}$$

where the notation $\langle \phi_1, \phi_2 \rangle \equiv \int_S \phi_1 \phi_2 \, dS$ denotes the inner product on the boundary S. When the Dirichlet, $\Phi = \Phi_0$, and Neumann, $\sigma\nabla\Phi \cdot \mathbf{n} = 0$, boundary conditions are specified on S, we obtain the *weak form* of Equation 43.1:

$$(\sigma\nabla\Phi, \nabla\bar{\Phi}) = -(I_v, \bar{\Phi}). \tag{43.11}$$

It is understood that this equation must hold for all test functions, $\bar{\Phi}$, which must vanish at the boundaries where $\Phi = \Phi_0$. The Galerkin approximation ϕ to the weak form solution Φ in Equation 43.11 can be expressed as

$$\phi(\mathbf{x}) = \sum_{i=0}^{N} \phi_i \, \psi_i(\mathbf{x}). \tag{43.12}$$

The trial functions ψ_i, $i = 0,1,\ldots, N$ form a basis for an $N+1$-dimensional space S. We define the *Galerkin approximation* to be that element $\phi \in S$, which satisfies

$$(\sigma\nabla\phi, \nabla\psi_j) = -(I_v, \psi_j) \quad (\forall \, \psi_j \in S). \tag{43.13}$$

Since our differential operator A is positive definite and self-adjoint (i.e., $(A\Phi, \Phi) \geq \alpha \, (\Phi, \Phi) > 0$ for some nonzero positive constant α and $(A\Phi, \bar{\Phi}) = (\Phi, A\bar{\Phi})$, respectively), then we can define a space E

with an inner product defined as $(\Phi, \bar{\Phi})_E = (A\Phi, \bar{\Phi}) \equiv a(\Phi, \bar{\Phi})$ and norm (the so-called energy norm) equal to

$$(\Phi, \bar{\Phi})_E = \left\{ \int_\Omega (\nabla \Phi)^2 d\Omega \right\}^{1/2} = (\Phi, \Phi)_E^{1/2}. \tag{43.14}$$

The solution Φ of Equation 43.9 satisfies

$$(A\Phi, \psi_i) = -(I_v, \psi_i) \quad (\forall\, \psi_i \in S) \tag{43.15}$$

and the approximate Galerkin solution obtained by solving Equation 43.13 satisfies

$$(A\phi, \psi_i) = -(I_v, \psi_i) \quad (\forall\, \psi_i \in S). \tag{43.16}$$

Subtracting Equation 43.15 from Equation 43.16 yields

$$(A(\phi - \Phi), \psi_i) = (\phi - \Phi, \psi_i)_E = 0 \quad (\forall\, \psi_i \in S). \tag{43.17}$$

The difference $\phi - \Phi$ denotes the error between the solution in the infinite dimensional space V and the $N + 1$-dimensional space S. Equation 43.17 states that the error is orthogonal to all basis functions spanning the space of possible Galerkin solutions. Consequently, the error is orthogonal to all elements in S and must therefore be the minimum error. Thus, the Galerkin approximation is an orthogonal projection of the true solution Φ onto the given finite dimensional space of possible approximate solutions. Therefore, the Galerkin approximation is the best approximation in the energy space E. Since the operator is positive definite, the approximate solution is unique. Assume for a moment there are two solutions, ϕ_1 and ϕ_2, satisfying

$$(A\phi_1, \psi_i) = -(I_v, \psi_i) \; (A\phi_2, \psi_i) = -(I_v, \psi_i) \quad (\forall\, \psi_i \in S), \tag{43.18}$$

respectively. Then, the difference yields

$$(A(\phi_1 - \phi_2), \psi_i) = 0 \quad (\forall\, \psi_i \in S). \tag{43.19}$$

The function arising from subtracting one member from another member in S also belongs in S; hence, the difference function can be expressed by the set of A orthogonal basis functions spanning S:

$$\sum_{j=0}^{N} \Delta\phi_j (A(\psi_j, \psi_i)) = 0 \quad (\forall\, \psi_i \in). \tag{43.20}$$

When $i \neq j$, the terms vanish due to the basis functions being orthogonal with respect to A. Since A is positive definite:

$$(A\Phi_i, \Phi_i) > 0 \quad i = 0, \dots, N. \tag{43.21}$$

Thus, $\Delta\phi_i = 0$, $i = 0, \dots, N$, and by virtue of Equation 43.20, $\delta\phi = 0$, such that $\phi_1 = \phi_2$. The identity contradicts the assumption of two distinct Galerkin solutions. This proves the solution is unique [33].

43.4.2 Finite Difference Method

Perhaps the most traditional way to solve Equation 43.1 utilizes the FD approach by discretizing the solution domain Ω using a grid of uniform hexahedral elements. The coordinates of a typical grid point are $x = lh$, $y = mh$, $z = nh$ (l, m, n = integers), and the value of $\Phi(x, y, z)$ at a grid point is denoted by $\Phi_{l,m,n}$. Taylor's theorem can then be utilized to provide the difference equations. For example

$$\Phi_{l+1,m,n} = \left(\Phi + h\frac{\partial \Phi}{\partial x} + \frac{1}{2}h^2\frac{\partial^2 \Phi}{\partial x^2} + \frac{1}{6}h^3\frac{\partial^3 \Phi}{\partial x^3} + \cdots \right)_{l,m,n} \tag{43.22}$$

with similar equations for $\Phi_{l-1,m,n}$, $\Phi_{l,m+1,n}$, $\Phi_{l,m-1,n}$,.... The FD representation of Equation 43.1 is

$$\frac{\Phi_{l+1,m,n} - 2\Phi_{l,m,n} + \Phi_{l-1,m,n}}{h^2} + \frac{\Phi_{l,m+1,n} - 2\Phi_{l,m,n} + \Phi_{l,m-1,n}}{h^2}$$

$$+ \frac{\Phi_{l,m,n+1} - 2\Phi_{l,m,n} + \Phi_{l,m,n-1}}{h^2} = -I_{l,m,n}(v) \tag{43.23}$$

or, equivalently

$$\Phi_{l+1,m,n} + \Phi_{l-1,m,n} + \Phi_{l,m+1,n} + \Phi_{l,m-1,n} + \Phi_{l,m,n+1} + \Phi_{l,m,n-1} - 6\Phi_{l,m,n} = -h^2\,I_{l,m,n}(v). \tag{43.24}$$

If we define the vector $\boldsymbol{\Phi}$ to be $[\Phi_{1,1,1}\ldots\Phi_{1,1,N-1};\ldots\Phi_{1,N-1},1\ldots\Phi_{N-1,N-1,N-1}]^T$ to designate the $(N-1)^3$ unknown grid values, and pull out all the known information from Equation 43.24, we can reformulate Equation 43.1 by its FD approximation in the form of the matrix equation $A\boldsymbol{\Phi} = \mathbf{b}$, where $\mathbf{b}$ is a vector that contains the sources and modifications due to the Dirichlet boundary condition.

Unlike the traditional Taylor's series expansion method, the Galerkin approach utilizes basis functions, such as linear piecewise polynomials, to approximate the true solution. For example, the Galerkin approximation to the sample problem Equation 43.1 would require evaluating Equation 43.13 for the specific grid formation and specific choice of basis function:

$$\int_\Omega \left(\sigma_x \frac{\partial \phi}{\partial x}\frac{\partial \psi_i}{\partial x} + \sigma_y \frac{\partial \phi}{\partial y}\frac{\partial \psi_i}{\partial y} + \sigma_z \frac{\partial \phi}{\partial z}\frac{\partial \psi_i}{\partial z} \right) d\Omega = -\int_\Omega I_v \psi_i\, d\Omega. \tag{43.25}$$

Difference quotients are then used to approximate the derivatives in Equation 43.25. We note that if linear basis functions are utilized in Equation 43.25, one obtains a formulation that corresponds exactly with the standard FD operator. Regardless of the difference scheme or order of basis function, the approximation results in a linear system of equations of the form $A\boldsymbol{\Phi} = \mathbf{b}$, subject to the appropriate boundary conditions.

43.4.3 Finite Element Method

As we have seen above, in the classical numerical treatment for partial differential equations—the FD method—the solution domain is approximated by a grid of uniformly spaced nodes. At each node, the governing differential equation is approximated by an algebraic expression that references adjacent grid points. A system of equations is obtained by evaluating the previous algebraic approximations for each node in the domain. Finally, the system is solved for each value of the dependent variable at each node. In the FE method, the solution domain can be discretized into a number of uniform or nonuniform FEs that are connected via nodes. The change of the dependent variable with regard to location is approximated within each element by an interpolation function. The interpolation function is defined relative to the values of the variable at the nodes associated with each element. The original boundary value problem is then replaced with an equivalent integral formulation (such as Equation 43.13). The interpolation functions are then substituted into the integral equation, integrated, and combined with the results from all other elements in the solution domain. The results of this procedure can be reformulated into a matrix equation of the form $A\Phi = \mathbf{b}$, which is subsequently solved for the unknown variable [3,36].

The formulation of the FE approximation starts with the Galerkin approximation, $(\sigma\nabla\Phi, \nabla\bar{\Phi}) = -(I_v, \bar{\Phi})$, where $\bar{\Phi}$ is our test function. We now use the FE method to turn the continuous problems into a discrete formulation. First, we discretize the solution domain, $\Omega = \cup_{e=1}^{E}\Omega_e$, and define a finite dimensional subspace, $V_h \subset V = \{\bar{\Phi}: \bar{\Phi}$ is continuous on Ω, $\nabla\bar{\Phi}$ is piecewise continuous on $\Omega\}$. One usually defines parameters of the function $\bar{\Phi} \in V_h$ at node points $\alpha_i = \bar{\Phi}(x_i)$, $i = 0,1,\ldots,N$. If we now define the basis functions, $\psi_i \in V_h$, as linear continuous piecewise functions that take the value 1 at node points and zero at other node points, then we can represent the function $\bar{\Phi} \in V_h$ as

$$\bar{\Phi}(x) = \sum_{i=0}^{N} \alpha_i \Psi_i(x), \tag{43.26}$$

such that each $\bar{\Phi} \in V_h$ can be written in a unique way as a linear combination of the basis functions $\Psi_i \in V_h$. Now, the FE approximation of the original boundary value problem can be stated as

$$\text{Find } \Phi_h \in V_h \quad \text{such that } (\sigma\nabla\Phi_h, \nabla\bar{\Phi}) = -(I_v, \bar{\Phi}). \tag{43.27}$$

Furthermore, if $\Phi_h \in V_h$ satisfies Equation 43.27, then we have $(\sigma\nabla\Phi_h, \nabla\Psi_i) = -(I_v, \Psi_i)$ [42,47]. Finally, since Φ_h itself can be expressed as the linear combination

$$\Phi_h = \sum_{i=0}^{N} \xi_i \Psi_i(x) \quad \xi_i = \Phi_h(x_i), \tag{43.28}$$

we can then write Equation 43.27 as

$$\sum_{i=0}^{N} \xi_i (\sigma_{ij}\nabla\Psi_i, \nabla\Psi_j) = -(I_v, \Psi_j) \quad j = 0,\ldots,N, \tag{43.29}$$

subject to the Dirichlet boundary condition. Then the FE approximation of Equation 43.1 can equivalently be expressed as a system of N equations with N unknowns $\xi_i,\ldots,\xi_N$ (e.g., the electrostatic potentials). In matrix form, the above system can be written as $A\xi = b$, where $A = (a_{ij})$ is called the global stiffness matrix and has elements $(a_{ij}) = (\sigma_{ij}\nabla\Psi_i, \nabla\Psi_j)$, while $b_i = -(I_v, \Psi_i)$ and is usually termed the load vector.

For volume conductor problems, A contains all the geometry and conductivity information of the model. The matrix A is symmetric and positive definite; thus, it is nonsingular and has a unique solution. Because the basis function differs from zero for only a few intervals, A is sparse (only a few of its entries are nonzero).

43.4.3.1 Application of the FE Method for 3D Domains

We now illustrate the concepts of the FE method by considering the solution of Equation 43.1 using linear 3D elements. We start with a 3D domain Ω that represents the geometry of our volume conductor and break it up into discrete elements to form a finite dimensional subspace, Ω_h. For 3D domains, we have the choice of representing our function as either tetrahedra

$$\tilde{\Phi} = \alpha_1 + \alpha_2 x + \alpha_3 y + \alpha_4 z, \tag{43.30}$$

or hexahedra

$$\tilde{\Phi} = \alpha_1 + \alpha_2 x + \alpha_3 y + \alpha_4 z + \alpha_5 xy + \alpha_6 yz + \alpha_7 xz + \alpha_8 xyz. \tag{43.31}$$

Because of space limitations, we restrict our development to tetrahedra, knowing that it is easy to modify our formulae for hexahedra. We take out a specific tetrahedra from our finite dimensional subspace and apply the previous formulations for the four vertices

$$\begin{pmatrix} \tilde{\Phi}_1 \\ \tilde{\Phi}_2 \\ \tilde{\Phi}_3 \\ \tilde{\Phi}_4 \end{pmatrix} = \begin{pmatrix} 1 & x_1 & y_1 & z_1 \\ 1 & x_2 & y_2 & z_2 \\ 1 & x_3 & y_3 & z_3 \\ 1 & x_4 & y_4 & z_4 \end{pmatrix} \begin{pmatrix} \alpha_1 \\ \alpha_2 \\ \alpha_3 \\ \alpha_4 \end{pmatrix}, \tag{43.32}$$

or

$$\tilde{\Phi}_i = C\alpha, \tag{43.33}$$

which define the coordinate vertices, and

$$\alpha = C^{-1}\tilde{\Phi}_i, \tag{43.34}$$

which defines the coefficients. From Equations 43.30 and 43.34, we can express $\tilde{\Phi}$ at any point within the tetrahedra

$$\tilde{\Phi} = [1, x, y, z]\alpha = S\alpha = SC^{-1}\tilde{\Phi}_i \tag{43.35}$$

or, most succinctly

$$\tilde{\Phi} = \sum_i N_i \tilde{\Phi}_i. \tag{43.36}$$

$\tilde{\Phi}_i$ is the solution value at node i, and $N = SC^{-1}$ is the local *shape function* or *basis function*. This can be expressed in a variety of ways in the literature (depending, usually, on whether you are reading engineering or mathematical treatments of FE analysis):

$$\Phi_j(N_i) = N_i(x, y, z) = f_i(x, y, z) \equiv \frac{a_i + b_i x + c_i y + d_i z}{6V}, \tag{43.37}$$

where

$$6V = \begin{vmatrix} 1 & x_1 & y_1 & z_1 \\ 1 & x_2 & y_2 & z_2 \\ 1 & x_3 & y_3 & z_3 \\ 1 & x_3 & y_3 & z_4 \end{vmatrix} \tag{43.38}$$

defines the volume of the tetrahedra, V.

Now that we have a suitable set of basis functions, we can find the FE approximation to our 3D problem. Our original problem can be formulated as

$$a(u, v) = (I_v, v) \quad \forall\, v \in \Omega,$$
(43.39)

where

$$a(u,v) = \int_{\Omega} \nabla u \cdot \nabla v \, d\Omega$$
(43.40)

and

$$(I_v,v) = \int_{\Omega} I_v \cdot v \, d\Omega.$$
(43.41)

The FE approximation to the original boundary value problem is

$$a(u_h, v) = (I_v, v) \quad \forall\, v \in \Omega_h,$$
(43.42)

which has the equivalent form

$$\sum_{i=1}^{N} \xi_i a(\Phi_i, \Phi_j) = (I_v, \Phi_j),$$
(43.43)

where

$$a(\Phi_i, \Phi_j) = a(\Phi_i(N_j), \Phi_j(N_i)),$$
(43.44)

which can be expressed by the matrix and vector elements

$$a_{ij} = \int_{\Omega_E} \left(\frac{\partial N_i}{\partial x} \frac{\partial N_j}{\partial x} + \frac{\partial N_i}{\partial y} \frac{\partial N_j}{\partial y} + \frac{\partial N_i}{\partial z} \frac{\partial N_j}{\partial z} \right) d\Omega$$
(43.45)

and

$$I_i = \int_{\Omega_E} N_i I_v \, d\Omega.$$
(43.46)

Fortunately, the above quantities are easy to evaluate for linear tetrahedra. As a matter of fact, there are closed form solutions for the matrix elements (a_{ij}):

$$\int_{\Omega_h} N_1^a N_2^b N_3^c N_4^d \, d\Omega = 6V \frac{a!b!c!d!}{(a+b+c+d+3)!}.$$
(43.47)

Therefore

$$a_{ij} = \int_{\Omega_E} \frac{b_i b_j + c_i c_j + d_i d_j}{6V^2} \, d\Omega = \frac{b_i b_j + c_i c_j + d_i d_j}{6V},$$
(43.48)

and, for the right-hand side (RHS), we have, assuming constant sources,

$$I_i = \int_{\Omega_E} \frac{a_i + b_i x + c_i y + d_i z}{6V} I_v \, d\Omega = \frac{V I_v}{4}.$$
(43.49)

which have the compact forms

$$a_{ij}^{(n)} = \frac{1}{6V}(b_i^{(n)}b_j^{(n)} + c_i^{(n)}c_j^{(n)} + d_i^{(n)}d_j^{(n)})$$

(43.50)

and

$$I_i^{(n)} = \frac{VI_v}{4} \quad \text{for constant sources.}$$

(43.51)

Now, we add up all the contributions from each element into a global matrix and global vector.

$$\sum_{n=1}^{Nel}(a_{ij}^{(n)})(\xi_i) = (I_i^{(n)}),$$

(43.52)

where Nel is equal to the total number of elements in the discretized solution domain and i represents the node numbers (vertices). This yields a linear system of equations of the form $\mathbf{A\Phi} = \mathbf{b}$, where $\mathbf{\Phi}$ is our solution vector of voltages, $\mathbf{A}$ represents the geometry and conductivity of our volume conductor, and $\mathbf{b}$ represents the contributions from the current sources and boundary conditions.

For the FD method, it turns out that the Dirichlet boundary condition is easy to apply while the Neumann condition takes a little extra effort. For the FE method, it is just the opposite. The Neumann boundary condition

$$\nabla\Phi \cdot \mathbf{n} = 0$$

(43.53)

is satisfied automatically within the Galerkin and variational formulations. This can be seen by using Green's divergence theorem

$$\int_\Omega \nabla \cdot \mathbf{A}\,dx = \int_\Gamma \mathbf{A} \cdot \mathbf{n}\,dS,$$

(43.54)

and applying it to the left-hand side of the Galerkin FE formulation:

$$\int_\Omega \nabla v \cdot \nabla w\,d\Omega \equiv \int_\Omega \left[\frac{\partial v}{\partial x_1}\frac{\partial w}{\partial x_1} + \frac{\partial v}{\partial x_2}\frac{\partial w}{\partial x_2}\right]d\Omega$$

$$= \int_\Gamma \left[v\frac{\partial w}{\partial x_1}n_1 + v\frac{\partial w}{\partial x_2}n_2\right]dS - \int_\Omega v\left[\frac{\partial^2 w}{\partial x_1^2} + \frac{\partial^2 w}{\partial x_2^2}\right]d\Omega$$

$$= \int_\Gamma v\frac{\partial w}{\partial n}\,dS - \int_\Omega v\nabla^2 w\,d\Omega.$$

(43.55)

If we multiply our original differential equation, $\nabla^2\Phi = -I_v$, by an arbitrary test function and integrate, we obtain

$$(I_v, v) = -\int_\Omega (\nabla^2\Phi)v\,d\Omega = -\int_\Gamma \frac{\partial\Phi}{\partial n}\,v\,dS + \int_\Omega \nabla\Phi \cdot \nabla v\,d\Omega = a(\Phi, v),$$

(43.56)

where the boundary integral term, $\partial\Phi/\partial n$ vanishes and we obtain the standard Galerkin FE formulation.

To apply the Dirichlet condition, we have to work a bit harder. To apply the Dirichlet boundary condition directly, one usually modifies the (a_{ij}) matrix and b_i vector such that one can use standard linear system solvers. This is accomplished by implementing the following steps.

Assuming we know the ith value of u_i

1. Subtract from the ith member of the RHS the product of a_{ij} and the known value of Φ_i (call it $\bar{\Phi}_i$); this yields the new RHS, $\hat{b}_i = b_i - a_{ij}\bar{\Phi}_j$.
2. Zero the ith row and column of A: $\hat{a}_{ij} = \hat{a}_{ji} = 0$.
3. Assign $\hat{a}_{ii} = 1$.
4. Set the jth member of the RHS equal to $\bar{\Phi}_i$.
5. Continue for each Dirichlet condition.
6. Solve the augmented system, $\hat{A}\Phi = \hat{b}_v$.

43.4.4 Boundary Element Method

For bioelectric field problems with isotropic domains (and few inhomogeneities), another technique, called the BE method, may be utilized. This technique utilizes information only upon the boundaries of interest, and thus reduces the dimension of any field problem by one. For differential operators, the response at any given point to sources and boundary conditions depends only on the response at neighboring points. The FD and FE methods approximate differential operators defined on subregions (volume elements) in the domain; hence, direct mutual influence (connectivity) exists only between neighboring elements, and the coefficient matrices generated by these methods have relatively few nonzero coefficients in any given matrix row. As is demonstrated by Maxwell's laws [39], equations in differential forms can often be replaced by equations in integral forms, for example, the potential distribution in a domain is uniquely defined by the volume sources and the potential and current density on the boundary. The BE method utilizes this fact by transforming the differential operator defined in the domain to integral operators defined on the boundary. In the BE method [6,13,40], only the boundary is discretized; hence, the mesh generation is considerably simpler for this method than for the volume methods. Boundary solutions are obtained directly by solving the set of linear equations; however, potentials and gradients in the domain can be evaluated only after the boundary solutions have been obtained. As this method has a rich history in bioelectric field problems, the reader is referred to some of the classic references for further information regarding the application of the BE method to bioelectric field problems [5,30,67,69].

43.4.5 Solution Methods and Computational Considerations

The application of each of the previous approximation methods to Equation 43.1 yields a system of linear equations of the form $\mathbf{A}\Phi = \mathbf{b}$, which must be solved to obtain the final solution. There are a plethora of available techniques for the solutions of such systems. The solution techniques can be broadly categorized as *direct* and *iterative* solvers. Direct solvers include Gaussian elimination and lower-upper (LU) decomposition, while iterative methods include Jacobi, Gauss–Seidel, successive overrelaxation (SOR), and conjugate gradient (CG) methods, among others. The choice of the particular solution method is highly dependent upon the approximation technique employed to obtain the linear system, upon the size of the resulting system, and upon accessible computational resources. For example, the linear system resulting from the application of the FD or FE method will yield a matrix $\mathbf{A}$ that is symmetric, positive definite, and sparse. The matrix resulting from the FD method will have a specific band-diagonal structure that is dependent on the order of difference equations one uses to approximate the governing equation. The matrix resulting from the FE method will be exceedingly sparse so that only a few of the off diagonal elements will be nonzero. The application of the BE method, on the other hand, will yield a matrix $\mathbf{A}$ that is dense and nonsymmetric and thus requires a different choice of solver.

The choice of the optimal solver is further complicated by the size of the system versus access to computational resources. Sequential direct methods are usually confined to single workstations and thus the size of the system should fit in memory for optimal performance. Sequential iterative methods can be employed when the size of the system exceeds the memory of the machine; however, one pays a price in terms of performance as direct methods are usually much faster than iterative methods. In many cases, the size of the system exceeds the computational capability of a single workstation and one must resort to the use of clusters of workstations and/or parallel computers.

While new and improved methods continue to appear in the numerical analysis literature, the author's studies comparing various solution techniques for direct and inverse bioelectric field problems have resulted in the conclusion that the preconditioned CG methods and MG methods are the best overall performers for volume conductor problems computed on single workstations. Specifically, the incomplete Choleski conjugate gradient (ICCG) method works well for the FE method* and the preconditioned biconjugate gradient (BCG) methods are often utilized for BE methods. When clusters of workstations and/or parallel architectures are considered, the choice is less clear. For use with some high-performance architectures that contain large amounts of memory, parallel direct methods such as LU decomposition become attractive; however, preconditioned CG methods still perform well.

A discussion of parallel computing methods for the solution of biomedical field problems could fill an entire text. Thus, the reader is directed to the following references on parallel scientific computing [18,23,28].

43.4.6 Comparison of Methods

Since we do not have space to provide a detailed, quantitative description of each of the previously mentioned methods, we give an abbreviated summary of the applicability of each method in solving different types of bioelectric field problems.

As outlined above, the FD, FE, and BE methods can all be used to approximate the boundary value problems that arise in biomedical research problems. The choice depends on the nature of the problem. The FE and FD methods are similar in that the entire solution domain must be discretized, while with the BE method, only the bounding surfaces must be discretized. For regular domains, the FD method is generally the easiest method to code and implement, but the FD method usually requires special modifications to define irregular boundaries, abrupt changes in material properties, and complex boundary conditions. While typically more difficult to implement, the BE and FE methods are preferred for problems with irregular, inhomogeneous domains and mixed boundary conditions. The FE method is superior to the BE method for representing nonlinearity and true anisotropy, while the BE method is superior to the FE method for problems where only the boundary solution is of interest or where solutions are wanted in a set of highly irregularly spaced points in the domain. Because the computational mesh is simpler for the BE method than for the FE method, the BE program requires less bookkeeping than an FE program. For this reason, BE programs are often considered easier to develop than FE programs; however, the difficulties associated with singular integrals in the BE method are often highly underestimated. In general, the FE method is preferred for problems where the domain is highly heterogeneous, whereas the BE method is preferred for highly homogeneous domains.

43.5 Adaptive Methods

Thus far, we have discussed how one formulates the problem, discretizes the geometry, and finds an approximate solution. We are now faced with answering the difficult question pertaining to the accuracy

---

* This is specifically for the FE method applied to elliptic problems. Such problems yield a matrix that is symmetric and positive definite. The Choleski decomposition only exists for symmetric, positive-definite matrices.

of our solution. Without reference to experimental data, how can we judge the validity of our solutions? To give yourself an intuitive feel for the problem (and possible solution), consider the approximation of a two-dimensional region discretized into triangular elements. We will apply the FE method to solve the Laplace equation in the region.

First, consider the approximation of the potential field $\Phi(x, y)$ by a two-dimensional Taylor's series expansion about a point (x, y):

$$\Phi(x + h, y + k) = \Phi(x, y) + \left[h \frac{\partial \Phi(x, y)}{\partial x} + k \frac{\partial \Phi(x, y)}{\partial y} \right]$$
$$+ \frac{1}{2!} \left[h^2 \frac{\partial^2 \Phi(x, y)}{\partial^2 x} + 2hk \frac{\partial^2 \Phi(x, y)}{\partial x \partial y} + k^2 \frac{\partial^2 \Phi(x, y)}{\partial^2 y} \right] + \cdots \tag{43.57}$$

where h and k are the maximum x and y distances within an element. Using the first two terms (up to first-order terms) in the above Taylor's expansion, we can obtain the standard linear interpolation function for a triangle:

$$\frac{\partial \Phi(x_i, y_i)}{\partial x} = \frac{1}{2A} [\Phi_i (y_j - y_m) + \Phi_m (y_i - y_j) + \Phi_j (y_m - y_i)], \tag{43.58}$$

where A is the area of the triangle. Likewise, one could calculate the interpolant for the other two nodes and discover that

$$\frac{\partial \Phi(x_i, y_i)}{\partial x} = \frac{\partial \Phi(x_j, y_j)}{\partial x} = \frac{\partial \Phi(x_m, y_m)}{\partial x} \tag{43.59}$$

is constant over the triangle (and thus so is the gradient in y as well). Thus, we can derive the standard linear interpolation formulas on a triangle that represent the first two terms of the Taylor's series expansion. This means that the error due to discretization (from using linear elements) is proportional to the third term of the Taylor's expansion:

$$\epsilon \approx \frac{1}{2!} \left[h^2 \frac{\partial^2 \Phi(x, y)}{\partial^2 x} + 2hk \frac{\partial^2 \Phi(x, y)}{\partial x \partial y} + k^2 \frac{\partial^2 \Phi(x, y)}{\partial^2 y} \right], \tag{43.60}$$

where Φ is the exact solution. We can conjecture, then, that the error due to discretization for first-order linear elements is proportional to the second derivative. If Φ is a linear function over the element, then the first derivative is a constant and the second derivative is zero and there is no error due to discretization. This implies that the gradient must be constant over each element. If the function is not linear, or the gradient is not constant over an element, the second derivative will not be zero and is proportional to the error incurred due to "improper" discretization. Examining Equation 43.60, we can easily see that one way to decrease the error is to decrease the size of h and k. As h and k go to zero, the error tends to zero as well. Thus, decreasing the mesh size in places of high errors due to high gradients decreases the error. As an aside, we note that if one divides Equation 43.9 by hk, one can also express the error in terms of the elemental aspect ratio h/k, which is a measure of the relative shape of the element. It is easy to see that one must be careful to maintain an aspect ratio as close to unity as possible.

The problem with the preceding heuristic argument is that one has to know the exact solution *a priori* before one can estimate the error. This is certainly a drawback considering we are trying to accurately approximate Φ.

43.5.1 Convergence of a Sequence of Approximate Solutions

Let us try to quantify our error a bit further. When we consider the preceding example, it seems to make sense that if we increase the number of DOF we used to approximate our function, the accuracy must approach the true solution. That is, we would hope that the sequence of approximate solutions will *converge* to the exact solution as the number of DOF increases indefinitely:

$$\Phi(x) - \tilde{\Phi}_n(x) \to 0 \quad \text{as } N \to \infty. \tag{43.61}$$

This is a statement of *pointwise convergence*. It describes the approximate solution as approaching arbitrarily close to the exact solution at each point in the domain as the number of DOF increases.

Measures of convergence often depend on how the *closeness* of measuring the distance between functions is defined. Another common description of measuring convergence is *uniform convergence*, which requires that the maximum value of $\Phi(x) - \tilde{\Phi}_n(x)$ in the domain vanish as $N \to \infty$. This is stronger than pointwise convergence as it requires a uniform rate of convergence at every point in the domain. Two other commonly used measures are *convergence in energy* and *convergence in mean*, which involve measuring an *average* of a function of the pointwise error over the domain [14].

In general, proving pointwise convergence is very difficult except in the simplest cases, while proving the convergence of an averaged value, such as energy, is often easier. Of course, scientists and engineers are often much more interested in assuring that their answers are accurate in a pointwise sense than in an energy sense because they typically want to know values of the solution $\Phi(x)$ and gradients $\nabla\Phi(x)$ at specific places.

One intermediate form of convergence is called the *Cauchy convergence*. Here, we require the sequences of two different approximate solutions to approach arbitrarily close to each other:

$$\Phi_m(x) - \tilde{\Phi}_n(x) \to 0 \quad \text{as } M, N \to \infty. \tag{43.62}$$

While the pointwise convergence expression would imply the previous equation, it is important to note that the Cauchy convergence does not imply pointwise convergence, as the functions could converge to an answer other than the true solution.

While we cannot be assured of pointwise convergence of these functions for all but of the simplest cases, there do exist theorems that ensure that a sequence of approximate solutions must converge to the exact solution (assuming no computational errors) if the basis functions satisfy certain conditions. The theorems can only ensure convergence in an average sense over the entire domain but it is usually the case that if the solution converges in an average sense (energy, etc.), then it will converge in the pointwise sense as well.

43.5.2 Energy Norms

The error in energy, measured by the *energy norm*, is defined in general as [88–90]

$$e = \left(\int_\Omega e^T L e \, d\Omega \right)^{1/2}, \tag{43.63}$$

where $e = \Phi(x) - \tilde{\Phi}_n(x)$ and L is the differential operator for the governing differential equation (i.e., it contains the derivatives operating on $\Phi(x)$ and any function multiplying $\Phi(x)$). For physical problems, this is often associated with the energy density.

Another common measure of convergence utilizes the L_2 norm. This can be termed the average error and can be associated with errors in any quantity. The L_2 norm is defined as

$$(e)_{L_2} = \left(\int_\Omega e^T e \, d\Omega \right)^{1/2}. \tag{43.64}$$

While the norms given above are defined on the whole domain, one can note that the square of each can be obtained by summing element contributions

$$(e)^2 = \sum_{i=1}^{M} (e)_i^2, \tag{43.65}$$

where i represents an element contribution and m the total element number. Often for an *optimal* FE mesh, one tries to make the contributions to this square of the norm equal for all elements.

While the absolute values given by the energy or L_2 norms have little value, one can construct a relative percentage error that can be more readily interpreted:

$$\eta = \frac{(e)}{(\Phi)} \times 100. \tag{43.66}$$

This quantity, in effect, represents a weighted RMS error. The analysis can be determined for the whole domain or for element subdomains. One can use it in an adaptive algorithm by checking element errors against some predefined tolerance, η_0, and increasing the DOF only of those areas above the predefined tolerance.

Two other methods, the p and the hp methods, have been found, in most cases, to converge faster than the h method. The p method of refinement requires that one increase the order of the basis function that was used to represent the interpolation (i.e., linear to quadratic to cubic, etc.). The hp method is a combination of the h and p methods and has recently been shown to converge the fastest of the three methods (but, as you might imagine, it is the hardest to implement). To find out more about adaptive refinement methods, see References 2, 14, 22, 43, 47, 71, and 88.

43.6 Software for Bioelectric Field Problems

In the past few years, there have been a number of research software systems that have been created for the computational study of biomedical problems, including bioelectric field problems. Below, I have listed several open source software that are useful for computational bioelectric field problems. The list is meant to be representative and not comprehensive and I apologize for inevitable omissions.

- *SCIRun* (software.sci.utah.edu/scirun) is our own example of a general-purpose, problem-solving environment that has found extremely broad application both within biomedicine [34,46,48,77,85] and in areas as diverse as nuclear physics [49,70] and combustion [63]. An overview of SCIRun will be presented below.
- *CMISS* (www.cmiss.org) also has a very broad technical scope and application domain [9] and is the basis of many simulation studies in bioelectric fields and biomechanics of the heart and other organs [24,35,60], respiratory physiology [78], and bioelectric fields in the gastrointestinal system [68].
- *Simbios* (simbios.stanford.edu) is a newly emerging software system from the NIH-funded "Center for Physics-Based Simulation of Biological Structures" [72]. The biological coverage of Simbios is very broad, with the goal to help biomedical researchers understand biological

form and function as they create novel drugs, synthetic tissues, medical devices, and surgical interventions [8,10,11,20].

- *3D Slicer* (www.slicer.org) is a multiplatform, open source set of tools for visualization and image computing. It is also from an NIH NCBC Center, the "National Alliance for Medical Image Computing" (NA-MIC) (www.na-mic.org) [65]. Slicer includes a wide variety of image processing and visualization capabilities, including segmentation, registration, and analysis [52,56].
- *Seg3D* (www.seg3d.org) is a lightweight 3D segmentation program, which includes interactive volume visualization capabilities [91].
- *Brainstorm* (neuroimage.usc.edu/brainstorm) is an integrated toolkit dedicated to visualization and processing of data recorded from magnetoencephalography (MEG) and EEG. Brainstorm provides a comprehensive set of tools for researchers interested in MEG/EEG [41,61,74].
- *SimBio* and *NeuroFEM* (www.simbio.de and www.neurofem.com) is a combination of programs directed at source localization in the brain using patient-specific FE models with multiple conductivities and even anisotropic conductivity [85].
- *Continuity* (www.continuity.ucsd.edu) is a problem-solving environment for multiscale modeling in bioengineering and physiology with special emphasis on cardiac biomechanics, transport, and electrophysiology.
- *PCEnv* (www.cellml.org/downloads/pcenv) is the Physiome CellML Environment, an integrated software that provides an interface to the cell simulation models of the CellML project.
- *Virtual Cell* (www.nrcam.uchc.edu) is a software system for a wide range of scientists, from experimental cell biologists to theoretical biophysicists, who wish to create models of cellular structure and chemical, electrical, or mechanical function.
- *Neuron* (www.neuron.yale.edu/neuron) is a simulation environment for modeling individual neurons and networks of neurons, which is especially well suited to comparisons with experimental data. It has a very user-friendly interface that provides tools for building, managing, and using models in a way that is numerically sound and computationally efficient.
- *Genesis* (www.genesis-sim.org) has a very similar application domain as Neuron as a general-purpose simulation platform to simulate neural systems ranging from subcellular organelles and biochemical reactions to complex models of single neurons, large networks, and systems-level models.
- *TetGen* (tetgen.berlios.de) creates tetrahedral volume meshes from volume data made from triangulated surfaces for solving partial differential equations by FE or finite volume methods.
- *BioMesh3D* (www.sci.utah.edu/software) is a 3D tetrahedral and hexahedral mesh generator [92].
- *ITK* (www.itk.org), the Insight ToolKit, is a comprehensive set of software functions to perform image processing or analysis. ITK is the basis of many other tools (e.g., SCIRun and Seg3D) as they lack a graphical user interface (UI) and exist only as a C++ class library [37].
- *VTK* (www.vtk.org), the Visualization ToolKit, consists of an extensive library for visualization functions that is a component in many larger systems, for example, 3D slicer [73].
- *ImageVis3D* (www.sci.utah.edu/software) is a volume visualization program that allows for large-scale interactive visualization of scalar field datasets using isosurface extraction and volume rendering. ImageVis3D [93] works on multiple platforms, including desktops and laptops, the iPhone and iPad, and large distributed high-performance computers via the *VisIT* software system.
- *VisIT* (www.vacet.org) is a scalable, parallel software system for visualizing results of large-scale computational simulations. *VisIT* was created as part of the DOE ASCI and SciDAC programs. Research and development of *VisIT* continues as part of the DOE Visualization and Analytics Center for Enabling Technologies (VACET).
- *ECGSim* (www.ecgsim.org) is a program that computes the body surface potentials from the heart and allows the user to make changes in the electrical characteristics of the cells in any region of the heart. Its goal is to provide an educational tool but also a way to study the relationship between

the electric activity of the ventricular myocardium and the resulting potentials on the thorax under both normal and pathological conditions.

- *LabHeart* (www.labheart.org) is primarily a teaching tool that simulates the cardiac action potential, including the individual ionic currents and the fluctuations in intracellular calcium concentration.
- *iCell* is an Internet-based simulation program that allows the user to generate action potentials from a wide range of cell types [21].

43.6.1 SCIRun

This section provides a brief overview of the SCIRun and BioPSE problem-solving environments and presents examples of their use for the solution of bioelectric field problems.

The SCIRun[*] software system is an integrated, extensible, visualization-driven, open source, problem-solving environment that has been developed at the University of Utah's Scientific Computing and Imaging Institute [38].

For an application developer, SCIRun provides a software platform, upon which other applications can be rapidly constructed. SCIRun provides native support for interprocess communication, resource management (e.g., thread migration, memory management), and parallel computing. These operating system type services enable the dataflow aspects of the system. In addition to these low-level services, SCIRun also provides a number of built-in libraries and data structures that developers can use and can build upon. And at the highest level, SCIRun provides a rich set of algorithms for modeling, simulation, and visualization. All these levels of functionality can be leveraged by the developer when constructing new algorithms or applications in SCIRun [46,64,84].

The application program interface (API) to SCIRun is the visual dataflow environment called the network editor. Within the network editor, programs can be visually assembled from the library of available algorithms. The dataflow network for a sample bioelectric field simulation is shown in Figure 43.4.

The boxes in the network are called *modules*, and the lines connecting them are called *datapipes*. The point of attachment, where a datapipe attaches to a module, is called a *dataport*; the dataports on the tops of the modules are input ports, and the ports on the bottoms of the modules are output ports. In SCIRun, the dataports are color-coded to indicate the type of the data. For example, the blue datapipes are for matrices, and the yellow datapipes are for fields. Fields are used to represent 3D geometry as well as the data values that are defined over that geometry. Taken as a whole, the collection of modules and datapipes in a dataflow application is called a *network*, or *net*. Each module can have an optional UI button on its module; if the user presses the UI button, a separate window appears, with controls for viewing and modifying the state of the module's parameters.

43.6.2 BioPSE

SCIRun comes with a set of general-purpose modules that are not specific to any particular application. Modules can also be generated for a specific application, or for adding a set of optional functionality (such as raster data processing), in which case they are organized into a *package*. The package that has been primarily used and extended in this work is called BioPSE [17]. BioPSE stands for biomedical problem-solving environment, and contains all the functionality that is specific to bioelectric field problems.

The example network in Figure 43.4 is solving a bioelectric field problem for a dipolar source in a volume conductor model of a head. The domain is discretized with linear tetrahedral FEs, with five

---

[*] SCIRun is pronounced "ski-run" and derives its name from the Scientific Computing and Imaging (SCI) Institute, which is pronounced "ski" as in "Ski Utah."

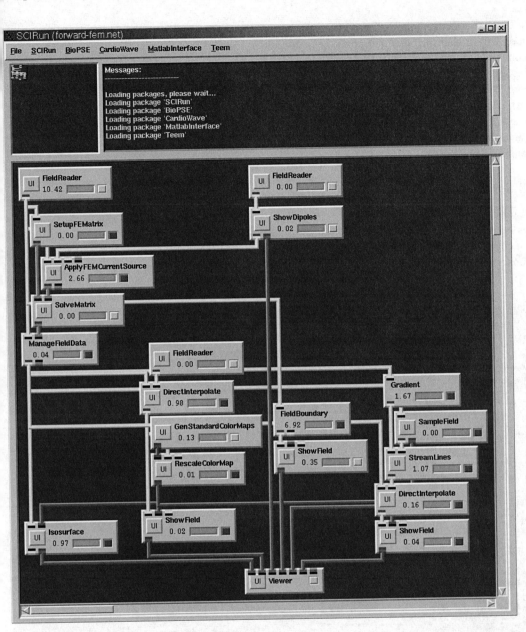

FIGURE 43.4   BioPSE dataflow network for modeling, simulating, and visualizing the bioelectric field generated in a realistic head model due to a single dipole source.

different conductivity types assigned through the volume. The problem is numerically approximated with a linear system, and is solved using the CG method. A set of virtual electrode points are rendered as pseudocolored spheres, to visualize the potentials at those locations on the scalp, and an isopotential surface and several pseudocolored electric field streamlines are also shown.

The BioPSE network implements this simulation and visualization with a collection of interconnected modules. The tetrahedral FE mesh with conductivity values is read in with one of the FieldReaders. That Field is then passed into the SetupFEMatrix module, which produces a stiffness matrix, **A**, as output. The RHS of the linear system, **b**, is generated by the ApplyFEMCurrentSource module, which applies the dipole source as a boundary condition. The linear system $\mathbf{A\Phi} = \mathbf{b}$ is then solved by the SolveMatrix module to recover the potentials at all the nodes in the domain. This solution is then attached to the geometry with the ManageFieldData module, and the results are visualized. A complete description of this application is available in the tutorial section of the SCIRun User's Guide, and can be downloaded from the SCI Institute's website [1].

In addition to the BioPSE modules that appear in the above net, BioPSE also contains modules for generating and using FE lead fields, for constructing separating surfaces from segmented volumes or planar contours, for running boundary element method (BEM) simulations, and for visualizing lead potentials over time.

43.6.3 PowerApps

Historically, one of the major hurdles to SCIRun becoming a tool for the scientist as well as the engineer has been SCIRun's dataflow interface. While visual programming is natural for computer scientists and engineers, who are accustomed to writing software and building algorithmic pipelines, it is overly cumbersome for application scientists. Even when a dataflow network implements a specific application

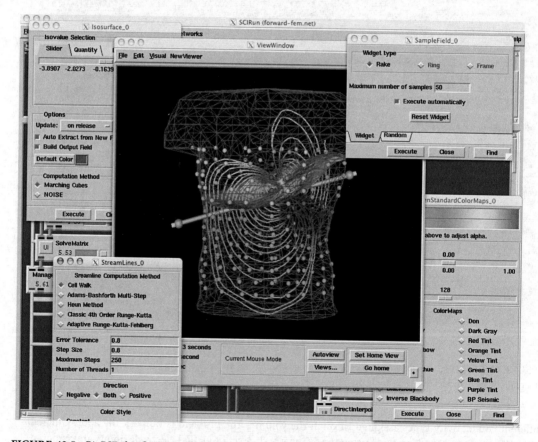

FIGURE 43.5 BioPSE dataflow interface to the forward bioelectric field application. The underlying dataflow network implements the application with modular interconnected components called modules. Data are passed between the modules as input and output parameters to the algorithms. While this is a useful interface for prototyping, it is nonintuitive for end-users; it is confusing to have a separate user interface window to control the settings for each module. Moreover, the entries in the user interface windows fail to provide a semantic context for their settings. For example, the text-entry field on the SampleField user interface that is labeled "Maximum number of samples" is controlling the number of electric field streamlines that are produced for the visualization.

such as the forward bioelectric field simulation network provided with BioPSE and detailed in the BioPSE tutorial), the UI components of the network are presented to the user in separate UI windows, without any semantic context for their settings. For example, SCIRun provides file browser UIs for reading in data. However, on the dataflow network, all the file browsers have the same generic presentation. Historically, there has not been a way to present the filename entries in their semantic context, for example, to indicate that one entry should identify the electrodes input file and another should identify the FE mesh file.

While this interface shortcoming has long been identified, it has only recently been addressed. With the 1.20 release of BioPSE/SCIRun (in October 2003), we introduced *PowerApps*. A PowerApp is a customized interface built atop a dataflow application network. The dataflow network controls the execution and synchronization of the modules that comprise the application, but the generic UI windows are replaced with entries that are placed in the context of a single application-specific interface window.

With the 1.20 release of BioPSE, we released a PowerApp called BioFEM. BioFEM has been built atop the dataflow network shown in Figure 43.4, and provides a useful example for demonstrating the differences between the dataflow and PowerApp views of the same functionality. In Figure 43.5, the dataflow version of the application is shown: the user has separate interface windows for controlling different aspects of the simulation and visualization. In contrast, the PowerApp version is shown in Figure 43.6; here, the application has been wrapped up into a single interface window, with logically arranged and semantically labeled UI elements composed within panels and notetabs.

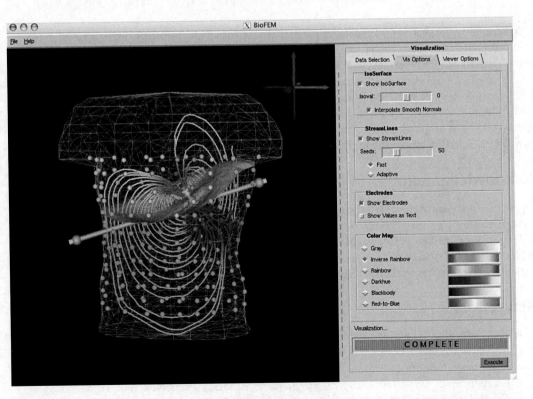

FIGURE 43.6 The BioFEM custom interface. Though the application is functionality equivalent to the dataflow version shown in Figures 43.4 and 43.5, this PowerApp version provides an easier-to-use custom interface. Everything is contained within a single window; the user is led through the steps of loading and visualizing the data with the tabs on the right; the generic control settings have been replaced with contextually appropriate labels; and application-specific tooltips (not shown) appear when the user places the cursor over any user interface element.

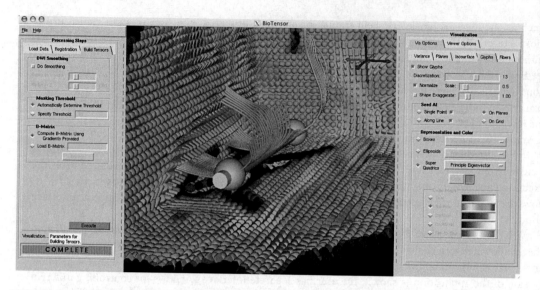

FIGURE 43.7 The BioTensor PowerApp. Just as with BioFEM, we have wrapped up a complicated dataflow network into a custom application. In the left panel, the user is guided through the stages of loading the data, co-registering the diffusion-weighted images, and constructing diffusion tensors. On the right panel, the user has controls for setting the visualization options. In the rendering window in the middle, the user can render and interact with the dataset.

In addition to bioelectric field problems, the BioPSE system can also be used to investigate other biomedical applications. For example, we have wrapped the tensor and raster data processing functionality of the Teem toolkit into the Teem package of BioPSE, and we have used that increased functionality to develop the BioTensor PowerApp, as seen in Figure 43.7. BioTensor presents a customized interface to a 140-module dataflow network. With BioTensor, the user can visualize diffusion-weighted imaging (DWI) datasets to investigate the anisotropic structure of biological tissues. The application supports the import of DICOM and Analyze datasets, and implements the latest diffusion tensor visualization techniques, including superquadric glyphs [51] and tensorlines [83] (both shown).

Acknowledgments

Support for this research comes largely from the NIH Center for Integrative Biomedical Computing (www.sci.utah.edu/cibc), funded by grants from the National Center for Research Resources (5P41RR012553-14) and the National Institute of General Medical Sciences (8 P41 GM103545-14) from the National Institutes of Health. I thank David Weinstein, Jeroen Stinstra, and Rob MacLeod for their contribution to the illustrative examples and the section on software.

References

1. 2010. Scientific Computing and Imaging Institute (SCI), University of Utah, www.sci.utah.edu.
2. A. Ainsworth and J.T. Oden. *A Posteriori Error Estimation in Finite Element Analysis.* Wiley-Interscience, New York, 2000.
3. J.E. Akin. *Finite Element Analysis for Undergraduates.* Academic Press, New York, 1986.
4. Th. Apel, M. Berzins, P.K. Jimack, G. Kunert, A. Plaks, I. Tsukerman, and M. Walkley. Mesh shape and anistropic elements: Theory and practice. *The Mathematics of Finite Elements and Applications X*, p. 367–376, 2000.
5. R.C. Barr, T.C. Pilkington, J.P. Boineau, and M.S. Spach. Determining surface potentials from current dipoles, with application to electrocardiography. *IEEE Trans Biomed Eng*, 13:88–92, 1966.

6. G. Beer and J.O. Watson. *Introduction to Finite and Boundary Element Methods for Engineers*. Wiley, New York, 1992.

7. O. Bertrand. 3D finite element method in brain electrical activity studies. In J. Nenonen, H.M. Rajala, and T. Katila, editors, *Biomagnetic Localization and 3D Modeling*, p. 154–171. Helsinki University of Technology, Helsinki, 1991.

8. T.F. Besier, G.E. Gold, S.L. Delp, M. Fredericson, and G.S. Beaupre. The influence of femoral internal and external rotation on cartilage stresses within the patellofemoral joint. *J Orthop Res*, 26(12):1627–1635, 2008.

9. S. Blackett, D. Bullivant, C. Stevens, and P. Hunter. Open source software infrastructure for computational biology and visualization. *Conf Proc IEEE Eng Med Biol Soc*, 6:6079–6080, 2005.

10. S.S. Blemker, D.S. Asakawa, G.E. Gold, and S.L. Delp. Image-based musculoskeletal modeling: Applications, advances, and future opportunities. *J Magn Reson Imaging*, 25(2):441–451, 2007.

11. G.R. Bowman, X. Huang, Y. Yao, J. Sun, G. Carlsson, L.J. Guibas, and V.S. Pande. Structural insight into RNA hairpin folding intermediates. *J Am Chem Soc*, 130(30):9676–9678, 2008.

12. A. Bowyer. Computing Dirichlet tesselations. *Comput J*, 24:162–166, 1981.

13. C.A. Brebbia and J. Dominguez. *Boundary Elements: An Introductory Course*. McGraw-Hill, Boston, 1989.

14. D.S. Burnett. *Finite Element Method*. Addison Wesley, Reading, MA, 1988.

15. M. Callahan, M.J. Cole, J.F. Shepherd, J.G. Stinstra, and C.R. Johnson. A meshing pipeline for biomedical computing. *Eng Comput*, 25(1):115–130, 2009.

16. C.D. Carbonera and J.F. Shepherd. A constructive approach to constrained hexahedral mesh generation. In *Proceedings of the 15th International Meshing Roundtable*, September 2006.

17. CIBC, 2009. BioPSE: Problem solving environment for modeling, simulation, image processing, and visualization for biomedical computing applications. Scientific Computing and Imaging Institute (SCI), Download from: http://www.scirun.org.

18. E.F. Van de Velde. *Concurrent Scientific Computing*. Springer-Verlag, New York, 1994.

19. C. Deitrich, C.E. Scheidegger, J. Schreiner, J. Comba, L.P. Nedel, and C.T. Silva. Edge transformations for improving mesh quality of marching cubes. *IEEE Trans Vis Comput Graphics*, 15(1):150–159, 2009.

20. S.L. Delp, F.C. Anderson, A.S. Arnold, P. Loan, A. Habib, C.T. John, E. Guendelman, and D.G. Thelen. Opensim: Open-source software to create and analyze dynamic simulations of movement. *IEEE Trans Biomed Eng*, 54(11):1940–1950, 2007.

21. S.S. Demir. Interactive cell modeling web-resource, iCell, as a simulation-based teaching and learning tool to supplement electrophysiology education. *Ann Biomed Eng*, 34:1077–1087, 2006.

22. J.E. Flaherty. *Adaptive Methods for Partial Differential Equations*. SIAM, Philadelphia, 1989.

23. T.L. Freeman and C. Phillips. *Parallel Numerical Algorithms*. Prentice Hall, New York, 1992.

24. A. Garny, P. Kohl, P.J. Hunter, M.R. Boyett, and D. Noble. One-dimensional rabbit sinoatrial node models: Benefits and limitations. *J Cardiovasc Electrophysiol*, 14(10 Suppl):S121–S132, 2003.

25. P.L. George. *Automatic Mesh Generation*. Wiley, New York, 1991.

26. V.B. Glasko. *Inverse Problems of Mathematical Physics*. American Institute of Physics, New York, 1984.

27. G.H. Golub and C.F. Van Loan. *Matrix Computations*. Johns Hopkins, Baltimore, 1989.

28. G.H. Golub and J.M. Ortega. *Scientific Computing: An Introduction with Parallel Computing*. Academic Press, Boston, 1993.

29. F. Greensite, G. Huiskamp, and A. van Oosterom. New quantitative and qualitative approaches to the inverse problem of electrocardiology: Their theoretical relationship and experimental consistency. *Med Phys*, 17(3):369–379, 1990.

30. R.M. Gulrajani, F.A. Roberge, and G.E. Mailloux. The forward problem of electrocardiography. In P.W. Macfarlane and T.D. Veitch Lawrie, editors, *Comprehensive Electrocardiology*, p. 197–236. Pergamon Press, Oxford, England, 1989.

31. P.C. Hansen. Regularization tools: A MATLAB package for analysis and solution of discrete ill-posed problems. Technical report, Technical University of Denmark, 1992. Available via netlib in the library numeralgo/no4.

32. P.C. Hansen. Analysis of discrete ill-posed problems by means of the L-curve. *SIAM Rev*, 34(4):561–580, 1992.

33. C.S. Henriquez, C.R. Johnson, K.A. Henneberg, L.J. Leon, and A.E. Pollard. Large scale biomedical modeling and simulation: From concept to results. In N. Thakor, editor, *Frontiers in Biomedical Computing*. IEEE Press, Philadelphia, 1995.

34. C.S. Henriquez, J.V. Tranquillo, D.M. Weinstein, E.W. Hsu, and C.R. Johnson. Three-dimensional propagation in mathematic models: Integrative model of the mouse heart. In D.P. Zipes and J. Jalife, editors, *Cardiac Electrophysiology: From Cell to Bedside*, Chapter 30, p. 273–281. Saunders, Philadelphia, PA, 4th edition, 2004.

35. D.A. Hooks, K.A. Tomlinson, S.G. Marsden, I.J. LeGrice, B.H. Smaill, A.J. Pullan, and P.J. Hunter. Cardiac microstructure: Implications for electrical propagation and defibrillation in the heart. *Circ Res*, 91(4):331–338, 2002.

36. S.R.H. Hoole. *Computer-Aided Analysis and Design of Electromagnetic Devices*. Elsevier, New York, 1989.

37. L. Ibanez and W. Schroeder. *The ITK Software Guide 2.4*. Kitware, 2005.

38. SCI Institute, 2010. SCIRun: A scientific computing problem solving environment, Scientific Computing and Imaging Institute (SCI), Download from: http://www.scirun.org.

39. J.D. Jackson. *Classical Electrodynamics*. John Wiley & Sons, New York, 1975.

40. M.A. Jawson and G.T. Symm. *Integral Equation Methods in Potential Theory and Elastostatics*. Academic Press, London, 1977.

41. K. Jerbi, J.P. Lachaux, K. N'Diaye, D. Pantazis, R.M. Leahy, L. Garnero, and S. Baillet. Coherent neural representation of hand speed in humans revealed by MEG imaging. *Proc Natl Acad Sci USA*, 104(18):7676–7681, 2007.

42. C.R. Johnson and R.S. MacLeod. Computer models for calculating electric and potential fields in the human thorax. *Ann Biomed Eng*, 19:620, 1991. In *Proceedings of the 1991 Annual Fall Meeting of the Biomedical Engineering Society*.

43. C.R. Johnson and R.S. MacLeod. Expedition in das herz (in German). *GEO*, 1993.

44. C.R. Johnson, R.S. MacLeod, and P.R. Ershler. A computer model for the study of electrical current flow in the human thorax. *Comput Biol Med*, 22(3):305–323, 1992.

45. C.R. Johnson, R.S. MacLeod, and M.A. Matheson. Computer simulations reveal complexity of electrical activity in the human thorax. *Comput Phys*, 6(3):230–237, 1992.

46. C.R. Johnson, S.G. Parker, D. Weinstein, and S. Heffernan. Component-based problem solving environments for large-scale scientific computing. *J Conc Comp Prac Exper*, 14:1337–1349, 2002.

47. C.R. Johnson and A.E. Pollard. Electrical activation of the heart: Computational studies of the forward and inverse problems in electrocardiography. In *Computer Assisted Analysis and Modeling*, p. 583–628. MIT Press, Cambridge, MA, 1990.

48. M. Jolley, J. Stinstra, S. Pieper, R.S. MacLeod, D.H. Brooks, F. Cecchin, and J.K. Triedman. A computer modeling tool for comparing novel ICD electrode orientations in children and adults. *Heart Rhythm J*, 5(4):565–572, 2008.

49. C. Jones, K.-L. Ma, A.R. Sanderson, and L. Myers. Visual interrogation of gyrokinetic particle simulations. *J Phys*, 78:012033 (6pp), 2007.

50. Y. Kim, J.B. Fahy, and B.J. Tupper. Optimal electrode designs for electrosurgery. *IEEE Trans Biomed Eng*, 33:845–853, 1986.

51. G. Kindlmann. Superquadric tensor glyphs. In *Proceedings of the IEEE TVCG/EG Symposium on Visualization 2004*, p. 147–154, May 2004.

52. S. Lankton and A. Tannenbaum. Localizing region-based active contours. *IEEE Trans Imag Proc*, pp. 2029–2039, 11 2008.

53. M. Lizier, J.F. Shepherd, L.G. Nonato, J. Comba, and C.T. Silva. Comparing techniques for tetrahedral mesh generation. In *Proceedings of the Inaugural International Conference of the Engineering Mechanics Institute (EM 2008)*, pp. 1–8, 2008.

54. R.S. MacLeod, C.R. Johnson, and M.A. Matheson. Visualization of cardiac bioelectricity—A case study. In *Proceedings of the IEEE Visualization 92*, p. 411–418. IEEE CS Press, 1992.

55. R.S. MacLeod, C.R. Johnson, and M.A. Matheson. Visualization tools for computational electrocardiography. In *Visualization in Biomedical Computing*, p. 433–444. Bellingham, WA, 1992. Proceedings of the SPIE #1808.

56. M. Maddah, W. Grimson, S. Warfield, and W. Wells. A unified framework for clustering and quantitative analysis of white matter fiber tracts. *Med Image Anal*, pp. 191–202, 04 2008.

57. M. Meyer, P. Georgel, and R.T. Whitaker. Robust particle systems for curvature dependent sampling of implicit surfaces. In *Proceedings of the International Conference on Shape Modeling and Applications (SMI)*, p. 124–133, June 2005.

58. M. Meyer, B. Nelson, R.M. Kirby, and R.T. Whitaker. Particle systems for efficient and accurate finite element visualization. *IEEE Trans Vis Comput Graphics* 13(5): 1015–1026, 2007.

59. C.E. Miller and C.S. Henriquez. Finite element analysis of bioelectric phenomena. *Crit Rev Biomed Eng*, 18:181–205, 1990.

60. A.J. Pullan M.P. Nash. Challenges facing validation of noninvasive electrical imaging of the heart. *Ann Noninvasive Electrocardiol*, 10(1):73–82, 2005.

61. K. N'Diaye, R. Ragot, L. Garnero, and V. Pouthas. What is common to brain activity evoked by the perception of visual and auditory filled durations? a study with MEG and EEG co-recordings. *Brain Res Cogn Brain Res*, 21(2):250–268, 2004.

62. J. Nenonen, H.M. Rajala, and T. Katilia. *Biomagnetic Localization and 3D Modelling*. Helsinki University of Technology, Espoo, Finland, 1992. Report TKK-F-A689.

63. S.G. Parker. Component-based multi-physics simulations of fires and explosions. In *Proceedings of the 12th SIAM Conference on Parallel Processing for Scientific Computing*, 2006. Presented at the Minisymposium on Parallel Dynamic Data Management Infrastructures for Scientific & Engineering Applications.

64. S.G. Parker, D.M. Weinstein, and C.R. Johnson. The SCIRun computational steering software system. In E. Arge, A.M. Bruaset, and H.P. Langtangen, editors, *Modern Software Tools in Scientific Computing*, p. 1–40. Birkhauser Press, Boston, 1997.

65. S. Pieper, B. Lorensen, W. Schroeder, and R. Kikinis. The NA-MIC kit: ITK, VTK, Pipelines, Grids and 3D Slicer as an open platform for the medical image computing community. In *Proceedings of the IEEE International Symposium on Biomedical Imaging*, 4 2006.

66. T.C. Pilkington, B. Loftis, J.F. Thompson, S. L-Y. Woo, T.C. Palmer, and T.F. Budinger. *High-Performance Computing in Biomedical Research*. CRC Press, Boca Raton, FL, 1993.

67. R. Plonsey. *Bioelectric Phenomena*. McGraw-Hill, New York, 1969.

68. A. Pullan, L. Cheng, R. Yassi, and M. Buist. Modelling gastrointestinal bioelectric activity. *Prog Biophys Mol Biol*, 85(2–3):523–550, 2004.

69. Y. Rudy and B.J. Messinger-Rapport. The inverse solution in electrocardiography: Solutions in terms of epicardial potentials. *Crit Rev Biomed Eng*, 16:215–268, 1988.

70. A.R. Sanderson, C.R. Johnson, and R.M. Kirby. Display of vector fields using a reaction diffusion model. In *Proceedings of IEEE Visualization 2004*, p. 115–122, 2004.

71. J.A. Schmidt, C.R. Johnson, J.C. Eason, and R.S. MacLeod. Applications of automatic mesh generation and adaptive methods in computational medicine. In I. Babuska, J.E. Flaherty, W.D. Henshaw, J.E. Hopcroft, J.E. Oliger, and T. Tezduyar, editors, *Modeling, Mesh Generation, and Adaptive Methods for Partial Differential Equations*, p. 367–390. Springer-Verlag, 1995.

72. J.P. Schmidt, S.L. Delp, M.A. Sherman, C.A. Taylor, V.S. Pande, and R.B. Altman. The Simbios national center: Systems biology in motion. *Proc IEEE*, 96(8):1266–1280, 2008.

73. W. Schroeder, K. Martin, and B. Lorensen. *Visualization Toolkit: An Object-Oriented Approach to 3D Graphics, 4th Edition*. Kitware, Clifton Park, NY, 2006.

74. C. Sergent, S. Baillet, and S. Dehaene. Timing of the brain events underlying access to consciousness during the attentional blink. *Nat Neurosci*, 8(10):1391–1400, 2005.

75. J.F. Shepherd. *Topologic and Geometric Constraint-Based Hexahedral Mesh Generation*. PhD thesis, School of Computing, University of Utah, May 2007.

76. J.F. Shepherd and C.R. Johnson. Hexahedral mesh generation constraints. *J Eng Comput*, 24(3):195–213, 2008.

77. J.G. Stinstra, S. Shome, B. Hopenfeld, and R.S. MacLeod. Modeling the passive cardiac electrical conductivity during ischemia. *Med Biol Eng Comput*, 43(6):776–782, 2005.

78. M.H. Tawhai, A.J. Pullan, and P.J. Hunter. Generation of an anatomically based three-dimensional model of the conducting airways. *Annal Biomed Eng*, 28(7):793–802, 2000.

79. J. Thompson, Z. Warsi, and C. Mastin. *Numerical Grid Generation Foundations and Applications*. North Holland, New York, 1985.

80. J. Thompson and N.P. Weatherill. Structed and unstructed grid generation. In T.C. Pilkington, B. Loftis, J.F. Thompson, S. L-Y. Woo, T.C. Palmer, and T.F. Budinger, editors, *High-Performance Computing in Biomedical Research*, p. 63–112. CRC Press, Boca Raton, FL, 1993.

81. A. Tikhonov and V. Arsenin. *Solution of Ill-Posed Problems*. Winston, Washington, DC, 1977.

82. A.N. Tikhonov and A.V. Goncharsky. *Ill-Posed Problems in the Natural Sciences*. MIR Publishers, Moscow, 1987.

83. D. Weinstein, G. Kindlmann, and E. Lundberg. Tensorlines: Advection-diffusion based propagation through diffusion tensor fields. In *Proceedings of IEEE Visualization 1999*, p. 249–253, 1999.

84. D.M. Weinstein, S.G. Parker, J. Simpson, K. Zimmerman, and G.M. Jones. Visualization in the scirun problem-solving environment. In C.D. Hansen and C.R. Johnson, editors, *The Visualization Handbook*, p. 615–632. Elsevier, Burlington, MA, 2005.

85. C.H. Wolters, A. Anwander, X. Tricoche, D.M. Weinstein, M.A. Koch, and R.S. Macleod. Influence of tissue conductivity anisotropy on EEG/MEG field and return current computation in a realistic head model: A simulation and visualization study using high-resolution finite element modeling. *Neuroimage*, 30(3):813–826, 2006.

86. Y. Wu, S.K. Warfield, I.L. Tan, W.M. Wells, D.S. Meier, R.A. van Schijndel, F. Barkhof, and C.R. Guttmann. Automated segmentation of multiple sclerosis lesion subtypes with multichannel MRI. *Neuroimage*, 32(3):1205–1215, 2006.

87. Y. Yamashita. Theoretical studies on the inverse problem in electrocardiography and the uniqueness of the solution. *IEEE Trans Biomed Eng*, 29:719–725, 1982.

88. O.C. Zienkiewicz. *The Finite Element Method in Engineering Science*. McGraw-Hill, New York, 1971.

89. O.C. Zienkiewicz and J.Z. Zhu. A simple error estimate and adaptive procedure for practical engineering analysis. *Int J Num Meth Eng*, 24:337–357, 1987.

90. O.C. Zienkiewicz and J.Z. Zhu. Adaptivity and mesh generation. *Int J Num Meth Eng*, 32:783–810, 1991.

91. CIBC, 2013. Volumetric image segmentation and visualization. Scientific Computing and Imaging Institute (SCI), Download from: http://www.seg3d.org.

92. SCI Institute, 2013. BioMesh3D: Quality mesh generator for biomedical applications. Scientific Computing and Imaging Institute (SCI). Download from http://www.biomesh3d.org.

93. CIBC, 2013. ImageVis3D: A SCIRun Power App for interactive visualization of vary large image volumes. Scientific Computing and Imaging Institute (SCI), Download from: http://www.imagevis3d.org.

44

The Potential Fields of Triangular Boundary Elements

44.1 Introduction 44-1
44.2 Preliminaries 44-2
    Notation • Field Produced by a Line Source • Integral of $r(\lambda)$
44.3 Potential Field of a Uniform Double Layer 44-4
    Properties of Ω_Δ • Autosolid Angle
44.4 Potential Field of a Uniform Monolayer 44-6
44.5 Potential Field of a Linearly Distributed Double Layer 44-9
44.6 Potential Field of a Linearly Distributed Monolayer 44-11
44.7 Analysis 44-12
    Numerical Aspects • Examples
44.8 Discussion 44-17
References 44-18

A. van Oosterom
Radboud University
Nijmegen

44.1 Introduction

The boundary element method (BEM) is a well-known method for computing the (quasi-static) potential in field points on the boundaries of piecewise homogeneous media, as well as inside these, arising from applied forces. The principles of the method for two-dimensional (2D) applications can be found in Reference 1, while three-dimensional (3D) applications to bioelectricity are described, for example, in Reference 2.

As described in Chapter 20, in bioelectricity, the applied forces are impressed electric currents and the medium is a volume conductor configuration comprising a set of nonintersecting surfaces nested inside the body surface. The surfaces considered are the interfaces between any two regions having a different electric conductivity. In the latter case, the surfaces are taken to carry the so-called secondary sources. These are virtual sources that are placed in a virtual, homogeneous, and isotropic medium having an infinite extent. In the BEM, the strengths of the secondary sources are computed such that the continuity conditions of the electric volume conduction theory at these interfaces are satisfied [3].

The requisite basic computations involved in the BEM are those of the potential fields generated by monolayer and/or double-layer sources distributed over the surfaces. On the basis of the superposition theorem, which applies to quasi-static linear media, the potential at each field point is computed as the sum of the contributions of the primary sources and the secondary current sources on all the small triangles considered (Chapter 20).

Initially, in its application to electrocardiography, the BEM was worked out by introducing virtual monolayer current source density at the interfaces [4] and their local strength was expressed in A/m².

Soon after, dipole layer source densities were introduced [5]. These so-called double-layer sources that may be viewed as an infinite number of current dipoles oriented along the local surface normal of the interface, with their total local strength expressed in $Am/m^2 = A/m$.

Another application of the BEM in bioelectricity aims at linking the potential field on a closed internal surface that encompasses all primary sources to the potential field on the surface bounding the conductive medium. An example of this application is the one in which the internal surface is taken to be a surface closely encompassing the heart and the bounding surface is that of the thorax [6–11]. The solving of this type of mixed boundary value problem (Cauchy problem) involves both double layers and monolayers.

The interfaces that are relevant in the field of bioelectricity usually have a complex shape. This necessitates a numerical handling of the computation of the fields generated by sources distributed over the surfaces involved. To this end, the surfaces are subdivided into numerous, small planar elements. By choosing a triangular shape for these elements, an optimal fit of the mesh to interfaces is reached. If the primary source involved is distributed over a surface, the same numerical handling can be used for finding the potential field that it generates.

In early applications of the BEM, the vertices of each triangular element were placed on the surface to be represented; the local source strength was taken to be uniform over the triangle and the field points considered were the centers of gravity of the triangles. For a single surface bounding a volume conductor represented by N_V vertices, this results in $N_t = 2N_V - 4$ triangles. Solving the potential field on the body surface as generated by an internal primary source then demands the solution of a linear system of N_t equations in the N_t unknown field point potentials.

In later applications, the field points were taken to be the vertices of the triangular elements; thus, the field points directly coincide with feasible measurement locations such as the electrodes placed on the body surface as used in electrocardiography. The source strength over a triangle was taken to be proportional to the mean value of the field potentials at its vertices [8]. For a single interface, this reduced the size of the linear system to N_V equations in N_V field point potentials. In such applications, the fields produced by virtual sources on the "elementary" boundary elements, the triangles, need to be computed in the virtual homogeneous volume conductor.

In this chapter, an overview is presented of analytical expressions for the fields produced by a uniform monolayer and a uniform dipole-layer distribution on a triangle, as well as for their variants in which the source strength is linearly distributed over the triangle. Particular attention is given to the computation of the value of the potential generated at the triangle's vertices. The derivations for each of the cases are included. Some of these derivations follow those reported in the literature, while including some more intermediate steps; others are more original. The order in which these topics are presented here is aimed at facilitating the subsequent derivations in this chapter.

44.2 Preliminaries

44.2.1 Notation

Throughout, vectors in 3D space are denoted by lower-case variables with an overhead arrow, for example, $\vec{r}$, and their lengths are denoted by dropping the arrow. The vector product of vectors $\vec{a}$ and $\vec{b}$ is denoted by $\vec{a} \times \vec{b}$ (cross product) and their scalar vector product is denoted as $\vec{a} \cdot \vec{b}$ (dot product). The source triangle is denoted by Δ its normal $\vec{n}$ is found from the cross product of two of its edges. The norm of $\vec{n}$, denoted by n, is twice the area of the source triangle. The normalized version of $\vec{n}$ is denoted by $\vec{n}_n$.

The variables expressed in the domain of linear algebra are denoted as follows: vectors are denoted in lower-case bold, their norms are denoted using regular font, matrices are denoted in upper-case bold, row vectors are denoted as primed, and column vectors are denoted as unprimed. The transpose of a matrix **M** is primed: **M'**. The column vectors having only unit elements are denoted by **u**.

44.2.2 Field Produced by a Line Source

As is evident in the following sections, the expressions for the fields produced by some of the source distributions over a triangle contain terms that can be interpreted as the fields resulting from a line source. This problem is discussed here in some detail to provide a correct physical interpretation of such terms.

The problem to be solved is illustrated in Figure 44.1. A current line density τ (unit: A/m) is impressed in a conductive infinite medium surrounding a line segment with length c having endpoints $\vec{a}$ and $\vec{b}$ relative to the field point depicted as the origin. The potential at the origin, Φ, is found by integration (superposition) of the contributions of point current sources at positions $\vec{r}$ along the line source segment, with strength $I(\vec{r}) = \tau(\vec{r}) c \, d\lambda$, in which λ is a dimensionless integration variable. Accordingly, we have

$$\Phi = \frac{1}{4\pi\sigma} \int_0^1 \frac{\tau(\vec{r})c}{r(\lambda)} \, d\lambda \tag{44.1}$$

with σ denoting the electric conductivity of the medium (unit: S/m), and the potential at infinity taken to be zero is the reference potential. For ease of notation, the factor preceding the integral is dropped. In the sequel, a uniform line source density is assumed with unit strength, that is, $\tau(\vec{r}) = 1\,\text{A/m}$. This leaves the following integral to be determined:

$$I_0 = \int_0^1 \frac{c}{r(\lambda)} \, d\lambda \tag{44.2}$$

Note that this expression is invariant to an overall scaling of the geometry (Figure 44.1).

The distance function $r(\lambda)$ is the length of $\vec{r} = (1 - \lambda)\vec{a} + \lambda\vec{b}$, which can be expressed as $r(\lambda) = \sqrt{c^2\lambda^2 + Q\lambda + a^2}$, in which Q denotes a combination of squared edge lengths: $Q = b^2 - a^2 - c^2$.

The integral is a standard one. By using Dwight (380.001) listed in Reference 12, we have

$$I_0 = \ln(2c^2\lambda + Q + c\,r(\lambda))\big|_{\lambda=0}^{\lambda=1} = \ln\frac{bc + \vec{b}\cdot\vec{c}}{ac + \vec{a}\cdot\vec{c}} = \ln\frac{(b+c)^2 - a^2}{b^2 - (a-c)^2} \tag{44.3}$$

On the basis of the triangle inequalities applied to the triangle with edges (a, b, c), both the numerator and the denominator in the fractions appearing in Equation 44.3 are nonnegative. Moreover, with the

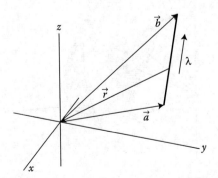

FIGURE 44.1 Diagram introducing the computation of the potential at the origin generated by a line source density along a line segment with endpoints $\vec{a}$ and $\vec{b}$. Here, the vector $\vec{r}$ is drawn from a source point of the line source to the field point, depicted at the origin.

zero reference potential at infinity, the integral must be positive. Hence, the fractions forming the arguments of the logarithms are greater than one. Equation 44.3 holds true throughout the 3D space; at field points coinciding with the line source, its value is infinite.

44.2.3 Integral of $r(\lambda)$

In one of the field problems to be discussed (Section 44.6), the integral over a line segment of $r(\lambda)$ appears rather than that of its reciprocal value appearing in Equation 44.2. By using the result listed as Dwight (380.201) [12] and employing the same notation, the result is

$$I_1 = \left(2bc^2 + (b-a)Q - \frac{D}{2c}I_0 \right)/(4c) \tag{44.4}$$

with $D = Q^2 - 4a^2c^2$, the discriminant of the parabolic expression in $r(\lambda)$.

44.3 Potential Field of a Uniform Double Layer

The first of the fields produced by the sources on the basic, triangular BEM element Δ to be discussed is the one generated by a double layer that is uniformly distributed over Δ. The geometrical configuration involved is depicted in Figure 44.2. The triangle vertices are labeled (k,l,m) in a clockwise order when viewed from the origin. The elementary current dipoles constituting the double layer are lined up in parallel to the triangle normal, pointing into the forward direction of a right-hand cork screw rotated in the order of the vertices $k \rightarrow l \rightarrow m$. Without loss of generality, the field point is taken to be the origin. The potential at $t\,\vec{r}$ follows from taking the integral of the contributions to the potential of elementary current dipoles (Equation 44.16) dipole strength $\vec{d}\,dS$

$$\Phi(\vec{r}) = \frac{1}{4\pi\sigma} \int_{\Delta} \frac{\vec{r} \cdot \vec{d}}{r^3}\, dS \tag{44.5}$$

with $\vec{d}$ as the current dipole surface density (unit: Am/m^2) taken to be uniform over Δ. Note that, as for the line source, the potential is invariant to an overall scaling of the geometry, the tetrahedron formed

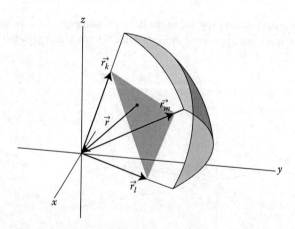

FIGURE 44.2 Diagram introducing the computation of the potential at the origin generated by a uniform current dipole surface source density over a triangle. The nearby curved patch represents the central projection of all elements of the source triangle onto a sphere with unit radius. Here, the vector $\vec{r}$ points from a source location on the triangle to the field point, depicted as the origin.

by the vertex indices of Δ and the field point. The term $\vec{r} \cdot \vec{d}\, dS$ is the component of the local dipole strength $\vec{d}\, dS$ along the vector specifying the source location. Combined with the preceding note, this means that the contribution to the field potential of the elementary sources $\vec{d}\, dS$ is equal to a virtual dipole source at the central projection of dS onto a sphere with unit radius surrounding the field point, now pointing radial, having the same strength as $\vec{d}$. This means that the solution of Equation 44.5 is

$$\Phi(\vec{r}) = \frac{d}{4\pi\sigma} \int_\Delta dS = \frac{d}{4\pi\sigma} \Omega_\Delta \tag{44.6}$$

with Ω_Δ denoting the solid angle subtended by the triangle at the field point of interest [13]. A numerically efficient and accurate expression for Ω_Δ, dating from 1983 [14], reads

$$\Omega_\Delta = 2\arctan \frac{[\vec{r}_k\,\vec{r}_l\,\vec{r}_m]}{r_k\,r_l\,r_m + r_k(\vec{r}_l \cdot \vec{r}_m) + r_l(\vec{r}_m \cdot \vec{r}_k) + r_m(\vec{r}_k \cdot \vec{r}_l)} \tag{44.7}$$

with $[\vec{r}_k\,\vec{r}_l\,\vec{r}_m]$ the triple vector product of the vectors specifying the triangle vertices relative to the field point. In the sequel, this triple vector product is denoted by T. Its numerical value is denoted by T; it equals that of the determinant of the matrix of size 3×3 whose elements are the vertex coordinates of the source triangle relative to the field point; it represents 6 times the volume of the tetrahedron.

44.3.1 Properties of Ω_Δ

As mentioned above, the potential is invariant to an overall scaling of the geometry as seen from the field point, which is also evident from Equation 44.7. The potential profile along a line crossing the source triangle exhibits a discontinuous jump. This corresponds to the discontinuity in the solid angle observed close to the triangle, which jumps from $\Omega_\Delta = -2\pi$ at one side to $\Omega_\Delta = 2\pi$ at the other side, with a positive sign at the side of the semispace into which the elementary dipoles are pointing. Applied to Equation 44.6, we see that a voltage jump of $V_d = d/\sigma$ is observed when crossing the double layer, a value that, in a uniform medium with known conductivity, may be used to specify the double-layer strength.

Expression 44.7 produces the correct sign of the solid angle in this application provided the arctan function produces angles in the range $-\pi$ to π and thus accounts for the signs of the numerator and the denominator (e.g., MATLAB®'s atan2 function).

When moving away from the source triangle, the potential profile rapidly approaches the profile produced by a single dipole placed at the center of gravity of Δ, with strength $D = dS_\Delta$ with S_Δ the area of Δ, directed along its normal

$$\Phi(\vec{r}) = \frac{1}{4\pi\sigma} \frac{\vec{r} \cdot d\vec{S}_\Delta}{r^3} \tag{44.8}$$

which indicates that at increasingly larger distances from Δ, the potential decays as $1/r^2$.

44.3.2 Autosolid Angle

In the early application of the BEM, the field points considered were the centers of gravity of the triangles forming a closed interface. The discontinuity when crossing a double-layer source was treated by using the limit of the solid angle ($\Omega_j \to -2\pi$) while approaching any triangle j from the interior part of the interface along its local normal.

In later applications, the field points were taken to be the vertices of the triangles [15]. In this situation, the BEM requires the specification of the potentials generated by all individual source triangles at all field points, *including those at its own vertices*. However, the solid angle subtended by a triangle at any of its vertices remains to be defined. The singularity needs to be treated with care since their values have a major impact on the accuracy of the entire computed potential field. In the application of the BEM to a closed interface, the total solid angle subtended by the interface at any interior point is -4π. This has led to the practice of assigning a value of

$$\Omega_i = -4\pi - \sum_{j|i \notin \Delta_j} \Omega_{\Delta_j}$$

(44.9)

to any node i (field point), involving the summation over the solid angles subtended by all triangles on the interface carrying node i, but excluding those having node i as a vertex. The solid angle defined in this manner is referred to as the autosolid angle [16]. For a node at an approximately planar patch of the interface, the value of Ω_i is close to -2π; for a locally convex patch, it is more negative, and at a concave patch, it is less negative. An improved handling of this complexity results from the application of the results for the linearly distributed double-layer strength (Section 44.5 and Reference 17).

44.4 Potential Field of a Uniform Monolayer

Figure 44.3 depicts the basic configuration involved in solving the potential field generated by a uniform monolayer on a triangle, with vertices as defined previously, and edges $\vec{e}_k = \vec{r}_l - \vec{r}_k$, $\vec{e}_l = \vec{r}_m - \vec{r}_l$, and $\vec{e}_m = \vec{r}_k - \vec{r}_m$.

At each infinitesimally small part dS of the triangle, an electric current $J dS$ (unit: A) is impressed in the surrounding medium, with J the impressed current surface density (unit: A/m²). The problem to be solved is the computation of the potential at an arbitrary field point. There are a multitude of papers dealing with this problem, or the linearly distributed variant, each exhibiting a different approach to solving the involved surface integrals, and the detail in which the results, or their derivations, are documented [18–23]. The solution presented here, but not the solution method, corresponds to the analytical, closed-form solution described in Reference 24.

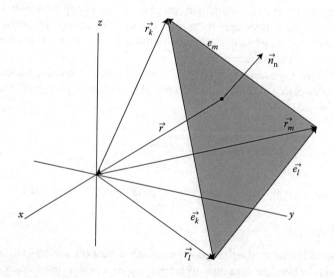

FIGURE 44.3 Diagram introducing some of the variables involved in the computation of the potential at the origin generated by a uniform current surface source density over a triangle. Here, the vector $\vec{r}$ points from a source location on the triangle to the field point, depicted as the origin. The unit normal, $\vec{n}_n$ of the triangle is drawn starting from an arbitrary source location.

The problem to be tackled is the computation of

$$\Phi(\vec{r}) = \frac{1}{4\pi\sigma} \int_{\Delta} \frac{J(\vec{r})}{r} \, dS = \frac{J_{\Delta}}{4\pi\sigma} \int_{\Delta} \frac{1}{r} \, dS \tag{44.10}$$

which is similar to the situation treated in Section 44.2.2, but now involves a surface integral. J_{Δ} is the uniform surface source density over Δ, scaling the potential. In the derivation, its value is set at $J_{\Delta} = 1\,\text{A/m}^2$. Another difference is that the integral, and, hence, the potential, depends linearly on an overall scaling, say, by a factor α. This property is the key to the solution method described here.

In Figure 44.4, the triangle nearest to the field point is the source triangle. Its potential at the field point is denoted by Φ_1, the potential required to be computed. The other triangle has vertices that are obtained by scaling the source triangle vertices by a factor $\alpha \geq 1$. Point $\vec{p}$ is the orthogonal projection of the field point onto the plane of the source triangle; its length h is the height of the tetrahedron as seen from the source triangle. From this point, line segments are drawn orthogonal to the lines carrying the edges of the source triangle; their lengths are denoted by h_k, h_l, and h_m, respectively. In addition, orthogonal projections of the vertex points of the source triangle onto the second triangle are included, outlined by means of their connections shown in white line segments that delineate a triangle having the same size as Δ. In addition, small line segments are shown that connect these projections to the nearby vertices of the source triangle. The latter line segments are parallel to the line connecting the field point and its projection $\vec{p}$ on the plane of Δ. On the basis of the overall scaling of the two tetrahedrons, their length is $l = (\alpha - 1)h$. Note that in this particular example, the projection of the edge $\vec{e}_k$ runs outside the second triangle, which relates to the fact that $\vec{p}$ lies outside the source triangle.

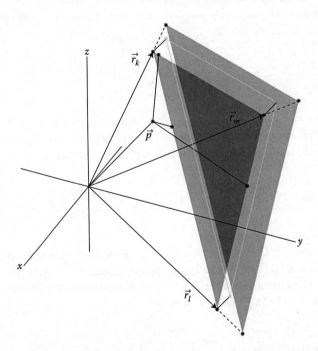

FIGURE 44.4 Diagram introducing the configuration involved in the method for computing the potential at an arbitrary field generated by a uniform current surface source density over a triangle. The triangle closest to the field point (at the origin) is the source triangle, the second triangle has vertices that are scaled versions of those of the source triangle. The vector $\vec{p}$ is the projection of the field point on the plane of the source triangle. Further details are as described in the text.

The second triangle is taken to represent a virtual monolayer source with uniform density and unit strength. The potential Φ_2 generated at the field point is, as discussed above, $\Phi_2 = \alpha\Phi_1$. When the polarity of the sources at the second triangle is reversed, turning its sources into sinks, the potential Φ at the field point generated by the "imperfect sandwich" formed in this manner is

$$\Phi = (1 - \alpha)\Phi_1 \tag{44.11}$$

We now consider taking the limit $\alpha \to 1$, which reduces the distance between the two triangles.

For small values of $l = (\alpha - 1)h$, the combination of the uniform source density on the source triangle and the uniformly distributed sinks over its scaled version has the character of a double layer with strength $d = J(\alpha - 1)h$. For $J = 1$, this produces a potential Φ_{DL} at the field point equal to

$$\Phi_{DL} = \frac{d}{4\pi\sigma}\Omega_\Delta = -\frac{(\alpha - 1)h}{4\pi\sigma}\Omega_\Delta \tag{44.12}$$

(compare Equation 44.6).

By looking at Figure 44.4, we note that there are sinks on two strips on the scaled version of Δ that are not represented in the double-layer activity. In contrast, the contribution of the strip parallel to edge $\vec{e}_k$ is overrepresented in Φ_{DL}. For values of α close to one, the length of these strips tends to the lengths of the longest edges bounding them and their widths can be seen to be $(\alpha - 1)h_j$, $j = (k,l,m)$. The areas that these strips have in common shrink as $(\alpha - 1)^2$ and the contributions of sources on these areas may be neglected for $\alpha \to 1$.

The contributions of each of these strips can be approximated by those of a weighted uniform line source with density $w_j = (\alpha - 1)h_j$. For a strip parallel to any edge j, the approximate contribution to the potential at the field point is (Section 44.2.2)

$$\Phi_j = \frac{1}{4\pi\sigma}w_j\gamma_j = \frac{1}{4\pi\sigma}(\alpha - 1)h_j\gamma_j \tag{44.13}$$

with γ_j the value of the line integral I_0 as in Equation 44.3, here pertaining to edge j. By using an appropriately signed version of the h_j distances, the contributions will be positive or negative as required.

By combining the results shown in Equations 44.11 through 44.13, we see that

$$\Phi = (1 - \alpha)\Phi_1 = \frac{(1 - \alpha)h}{4\pi\sigma}\Omega_\Delta + \frac{1}{4\pi\sigma}(1 - \alpha)\sum_{j=[k,l,m]} h_j\gamma_j \tag{44.14}$$

The required signed distances h_j are found from $h_k = [\vec{r}_k\ \vec{r}_l\ \vec{n}_n]/e_k$, the other two follow by cyclic permutations of the vertex indices (k, l, m). The height of the tetrahedron is $h = [\vec{r}_k\ \vec{r}_l\ \vec{r}_m]/n$.

For $\alpha \to 1$, all approximations mentioned tend to be more realistic and after dividing by $\alpha - 1 > 0$, we find the solution to Equation 44.10 for a uniform density J

$$\Phi(\vec{r}) = \frac{J_\Delta}{4\pi\sigma}\left(h\Omega_\Delta + \sum_{j=[k,l,m]} h_j\gamma_j\right) = \frac{J_\Delta\Gamma_\Delta}{4\pi\sigma} = \frac{J_\Delta}{4\pi\sigma}(h\Omega_\Delta + \mathbf{h}'\gamma) \tag{44.15}$$

in which Γ_Δ represents the value of the right integral in Equation 44.10; the expression on the right includes the numerical vector representations of h_j and γ_j.

44.5 Potential Field of a Linearly Distributed Double Layer

In its application to the BEM, the strength of the double layer, a virtual source in infinite space, is proportional to the local potential of the actual physical problem addressed. For the vertex approach, generally having different potential values at each of the vertices of a triangular element, the uniform double-layer strength over the individual triangles needs to be specified in terms of its vertex values. In the early application of the BEM to bioelectric field problems, Barr et al. [15] took the uniform source strength on a triangle to be proportional to the mean value of its vertex potentials.

Assuming the source strength to be uniform over each triangle implies that the potential over the triangle is constant. Generally, this would imply a discontinuity of the potential across edges shared by neighboring triangles, which is unrealistic. This problem was solved by de Munck [25], who derived a closed-form analytical expression for the field generated by a double layer having a strength that varies linearly between the vertex values. This extended the zero-order approximation of the source distribution as used in the solid-angle formulation to a first-order approximation, rendering the source strength across an edge shared by neighboring triangles to be continuous.

The method used by de Munck for deriving this expression is not always easy to grasp from his paper. Here, a reconstruction is presented of the derivation of this highly significant expression, cast in the notation used in this chapter. Some notations in Reference 25 that easily lead to confusion have been adapted.

The nonuniform variant of Equation 44.5 reads

$$\Phi(\vec{r}) = \frac{1}{4\pi\sigma} \int_{\Delta} d(\vec{r}) \frac{\vec{r} \cdot \vec{n}_{\mathrm{n}}}{r^3} \, dS \tag{44.16}$$

with $d(\vec{r})$ as a scalar function specifying the double-layer strength over the triangle. On the basis of the values at its vertices, $d(\vec{r}_k)$, $d(\vec{r}_l)$, and $d(\vec{r}_m)$, a linear distribution of $d(\vec{r})$ over the triangle can be described as

$$d(\vec{r}) = d(\vec{r}_k)w_k(\vec{r}) + d(\vec{r}_l)w_l(\vec{r}) + d(\vec{r}_m)w_m(\vec{r}) \tag{44.17}$$

in which any of the weighting functions $w_j(\vec{r})$, $j \in (k,l,m)$, has a value one at vertex j, zero values at the remaining two vertices, and a linear course along any straight line passing through vertex j. For vertex k, such a dimensionless weighting function is

$$w_k(\vec{r}) = [\vec{r}, \vec{r}_l, \vec{r}_m]/T = (\vec{r}_l \times \vec{r}_m \cdot \vec{r})/(\vec{r}_l \times \vec{r}_m \cdot \vec{r}_k) = (\vec{r}_l \times \vec{r}_m \cdot \vec{r})/T \tag{44.18}$$

a function that is linear in $\vec{r}$ and satisfies the required values at the vertices of the source triangle. Recall that T is the value of the triple vector product.

By inserting Equation 44.17 in Equation 44.16, the integral can be split up into three integrals of the same type. The one involving $w_k(\vec{r})$ is worked out in detail and the other two are found from a cyclic permutation of the vertex indices. The integral involving $w_k(\vec{r})$, after moving the constant $d(\vec{r}_k)$ in front of it, is

$$\Omega_k = \frac{1}{T} \int_{\Delta} \frac{(\vec{r}_l \times \vec{r}_m \cdot \vec{r})\vec{r} \cdot \vec{n}_{\mathrm{n}}}{r^3} \, dS \tag{44.19}$$

For any $\vec{r}$ starting from the source, viz the source triangle, and ending at the remaining node of the tetrahedron, we have $\vec{r} \cdot \vec{n}_{\mathrm{n}} n = \vec{r} \cdot \vec{n} = \vec{r} \cdot \vec{e}_l \times \vec{e}_m = T$. This leads to the following integral to be evaluated:

$$\Omega_k = \frac{1}{n} \int_{\Delta} \vec{r}_l \times \vec{r}_m \cdot \frac{\vec{r}}{r^3} \, dS = \frac{1}{n} \int_{\Delta} \frac{\vec{z}_k \cdot \vec{r}}{r^3} \, dS \tag{44.20}$$

in which $\vec{z}_k$ is the shorthand for $\vec{r}_l \times \vec{r}_m$ as used in de Munck's paper, with variants for $\vec{z}_l$ and $\vec{z}_m$ defined through a cyclic permutation of the indices (k, l, m). These vectors are normals to those faces of the tetrahedrons that do not have a vertex corresponding to their label; their vector sum equals $\vec{n}$.

The integral in Equation 44.19 can be seen to represent a weighted solid angle. To be valid for a uniform density, the weights should satisfy

$$\Omega_k + \Omega_l + \Omega_m = \Omega_\Delta \tag{44.21}$$

While solving the integral on the right-hand side in Equation 44.20, de Munck introduced a similar type of integral:

$$\vec{H} = \int_\Delta \frac{\vec{r}}{r^3} \times d\vec{S} = \int_\Delta \nabla \frac{1}{r} \times d\vec{S} = \oint \frac{1}{r} d\vec{c} \tag{44.22}$$

Note that this integral is dimensionless.

With the scalar vector product replaced by a cross product, the application of Stoke's law yields the contour integral on the right, the contour being formed by the edges of the source triangle. By using γ_j as the value of the line integral I_0 as in Equation 44.3 pertaining to edge j, we find

$$\vec{H} = \oint \frac{1}{r} d\vec{c} = \sum_{j=k,l,m} \int_0^1 \frac{1}{r(\lambda)} \vec{e}_j \, d\lambda = \sum_{j=k,l,m} \frac{\vec{e}_j}{e_j} \int_0^1 \frac{e_j}{r(\lambda)} \, d\lambda = \sum_{j=k,l,m} \frac{\vec{e}_j}{e_j} \gamma_j \tag{44.23}$$

An alternative expression for $\vec{H}$ results from introducing the representation of the vector $\vec{r}$ as the sum of its components along vectors $\vec{r}_j$: $\vec{r} = (1/T)\sum_{j=k,l,m}(\vec{z}_j \cdot \vec{r})\vec{r}_j$ into the integral on the left-hand side of Equation 44.22. This yields

$$\vec{H} = \frac{1}{T} \int_\Delta \sum_{j=k,l,m} \frac{(\vec{z}_j \cdot \vec{r})\vec{r}_j}{r^3} \times \vec{n}_n dS = \frac{n \, \vec{n}_n}{T} \times \sum_{j=k,l,m} \vec{r}_j \frac{1}{n} \int_\Delta \frac{(\vec{z}_j \cdot \vec{r})}{r^3} \, dS = \frac{\vec{n}}{T} \times \sum_{j=k,l,m} \vec{r}_j \Omega_j \tag{44.24}$$

The most right-hand part of this expression stems from identifying the final part of the preceding expression with the definition of Ω_k in Equation 44.20.

By storing the vectors $(\vec{n}/T) \times \vec{r}_j$ as columns of a matrix **B**, the expression on the right-hand side of Equation 44.24 reads **Bω**, with ω a column vector with elements Ω_j. Equations 44.23 and 44.24 both express $\vec{H}$, with the right-hand side of Equation 44.23 being a vector $\mathbf{y} = \mathbf{E}_n \mathbf{y}$, in which $\mathbf{E}_n$ is a matrix comprising the normalized edges (k,l,m) as its columns. Combining Equations 44.23 and 44.24 leads to the linear system

$$\mathbf{B}\omega = \mathbf{y} \tag{44.25}$$

A straightforward solution of the desired vector ω is impossible since **B** is underdetermined; **n′** is a left eigenvector with zero eigenvalue: $\mathbf{n'B} = [0\ 0\ 0]$, as follows from the fact that for any vertex index j, the vector $\vec{n} \times \vec{r}_j$ lies in the plane of the source triangle and, hence, $\vec{n} \cdot \vec{n} \times \vec{r}_j = 0$. Note that this complication is due to the nature of **B** rather than the nature of **y** as suggested in Reference 25. The complication is removed by adding Condition 44.21 as a row to the system in Equation 44.25. Finally, ω is found as the least-squares solution to the 4×3 linear system

$$\begin{bmatrix} \mathbf{B} \\ \mathbf{u'} \end{bmatrix} \omega = \begin{bmatrix} \mathbf{y} \\ \Omega_\Delta \end{bmatrix} \tag{44.26}$$

The solution, Equation 44.19 of de Munck's paper cast in the notation of this chapter, is

$$\omega = \frac{1}{n^2}(\mathbf{Z'n}\Omega_\Delta - \mathbf{E'_c E_n}\gamma T) \tag{44.27}$$

with Ec a matrix whose columns are the edges of the source matrix stored after one step of cyclic rotation, $[e_l, e_m, e_k]$, and Z a matrix in which the columns are the vectors of $\vec{z}_j$; recall Ω_Δ as found from Equation 44.7.

44.6 Potential Field of a Linearly Distributed Monolayer

We now turn to the final topic, the handling of the refinement of Section 44.4, determining the field of a monolayer, the strength of which is linearly distributed over the triangle. This problem is addressed in a manner similar to the one described in detail in the previous section for the double layer. To this end, the monolayer strength is written as $J(\vec{r}) = J(\vec{r}_k)w_k(\vec{r}) + J(\vec{r}_l)w_l(\vec{r}) + J(\vec{r}_m)w_m(\vec{r})$ (compare Equation 44.17) and after its introduction in Equation 44.10, we have

$$\Phi(\vec{r}) = \frac{1}{4\pi\sigma}\int_\Delta \frac{J(\vec{r})}{r}\,dS = \frac{J_k}{4\pi\sigma}\int_\Delta \frac{w_k(\vec{r})}{r}\,dS + \frac{J_l}{4\pi\sigma}\int_\Delta \frac{w_l(\vec{r})}{r}\,dS + \frac{J_m}{4\pi\sigma}\int_\Delta \frac{w_m(\vec{r})}{r}\,dS, \tag{44.28}$$

with the integral broken up into three subintegrals of the same type.

In the following equation, the integral for the index $j \in (k, l, m)$ is denoted by Γ_j.

$$\Gamma_j = \int_\Delta \frac{w_j(\vec{r})}{r}\,dS = \frac{1}{T}\vec{z}_j \cdot \int_\Delta \frac{\vec{r}}{r}\,dS = \frac{1}{T}\vec{z}_j \cdot \int_\Delta \nabla r\,dS \tag{44.29}$$

with the linear weighting function as in Equation 44.18, (dimension: m). Similar to Condition 44.21, the terms Γ_j should add up to the value of the integral for the uniform distribution:

$$\Gamma_k + \Gamma_l + \Gamma_\Delta. \tag{44.30}$$

Next, an auxiliary vector $\vec{G}$ introduced, similar to the vector $\vec{F}$ in the previous section

$$\vec{G} = \int_\Delta \frac{\vec{r}}{r} \times d\vec{S} = \int_\Delta \nabla r \times d\vec{S} = \oint r\,d\vec{c} \tag{44.31}$$

with the second equality resulting from the application of Stoke's law (dimension: m²). The value of the contour integral is

$$\vec{G} = \oint r\,d\vec{c} = \sum_{j=k,l,m}\int_0^1 r(\lambda)\,\vec{e}_j\,d\lambda = \sum_{j=k,l,m}\frac{\vec{e}_j}{e_j}\int_0^1 r(\lambda)e_j\,d\lambda = \sum_{j=k,l,m}\frac{\vec{e}_j}{e_j}I_{1,j} \tag{44.32}$$

with $I_{1,j}$ the value of the line integral I_1 (Equation 44.4) pertaining to edge j.

Similar to the procedure in the previous section, the synthesis $\vec{r} = (1/T)\sum_{j=k,l,m}(\vec{z}_j \cdot \vec{r})\vec{r}_j$ is inserted in the left integral in Equation 44.31, yielding an alternative for $\vec{G}$

$$\vec{G} = \frac{1}{T}\int_\Delta \sum_{j=k,l,m}\frac{(\vec{z}_j \cdot \vec{r})\vec{r}_j}{r} \times \vec{n}_n\,dS = \vec{n}_n \times \sum_{j=k,l,m}\vec{r}_j\frac{1}{T}\int_\Delta \frac{(\vec{z}_j \cdot \vec{r})}{r}\,dS = \frac{\vec{n}}{n} \times \sum_{j=k,l,m}\vec{r}_j\Gamma_j \tag{44.33}$$

The vectors $(\bar{n}/n) \times \bar{r}$ are stored as columns of a matrix $\mathbf{N}$, which can be seen to be a scaled version of matrix $\mathbf{B}$ introduced in the previous section and hence, like $\mathbf{B}$, is underdetermined. After introducing $\mathbf{y} = \sum_{j=k,l,m} (\bar{e}_j/e_j) I_{1,j}$ and applying Constraint 44.30, this leads to the following 4×3 linear system, to be solved for the monolayer of the source distribution

$$\begin{bmatrix} \mathbf{N} \\ \mathbf{u}' \end{bmatrix} \Gamma = \begin{bmatrix} \mathbf{y} \\ \Gamma_\Delta \end{bmatrix} \tag{44.34}$$

The least-squares solution of this system produces a numerical column vector Γ, the three elements of which are the three integrals in Equation 44.28, thus yielding the final solution

$$\Gamma = (\mathbf{Z}' \, \mathbf{n} \Gamma_\Delta - \mathbf{E}'_c \mathbf{E}_n \mathbf{I}_1)/n \tag{44.35}$$

with matrices $\mathbf{E}_c$ and $\mathbf{E}_n$ as in Equation 44.27, n and $\mathbf{I}_1$ representing column vectors, and the scalar Γ_Δ as found from Equation 44.15.

44.7 Analysis

44.7.1 Numerical Aspects

The basic results discussed in this chapter are Expressions 44.27 and 44.35. These are closed-form analytical expressions for computing the potential fields produced by current sources that are linearly distributed over a triangle of the double-layer type in Equation 44.27 and the monolayer type in Equation 44.35. In turn, these build on the expressions for the corresponding uniform distributions, Equations 44.7 and 44.15. As a consequence, the implementation of these expressions is less forbidding than may appear at first glance. In fact, the results of several of the intermediate and basic computations involved can be used at different points in large-scale implementations as carried out in the BEM. A careful implementation in any code is essential in such applications.

The results in Equations 44.7, 44.15, 44.27, and 44.35 have been tested exhaustively and were found to be accurate. Their values were finite at all points of 3D space as were expected to be from the physical nature of the problem. As discussed in Section 44.3.1, the potential field produced by the double layer on the source triangle itself remains to be defined.

All monolayer potentials in Equations 44.15 and 44.35 resulting from a positive monolayer source strength were positive, as required. For field points in the plane of the source triangle as well as for field points very close to it, the results proved to be accurate within machine precision. To ensure this property, when computing factors γ_j, the absolute value of the denominator in Equation 44.3 was used, after which the machine epsilon was added to the numerator as well as to the denominator. This efficiently suppresses any arguments of the logarithm less than one that may arise due to the rounding-off steps in the numerical handling of the numbers involved in the computation of these essentially positive entities.

44.7.2 Examples

In the following section, some examples are presented of potential fields generated by the expressions discussed in the chapter, also aimed at demonstrating the major properties of these fields. In all these examples, unit values are assigned to the source densities d_Δ and J_Δ as well as to the conductivity σ of the medium.

44.7.2.1 Double Layer

The left panel of Figure 44.5 illustrates the potential field in the plane $z = 0$ of a uniform *double layer* in the plane $z = 0.01$ with its normal directed along the z-axis, computed from Equations 44.6 and 44.7. Lying close to the double-layer source, the potential inside the triangle is almost uniform, with its

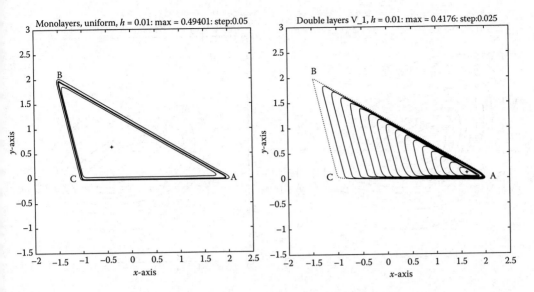

FIGURE 44.5 Left panel: Potential field in the plane $z = 0.01$ generated by a triangularly shaped uniform *double layer* in the plane $z = 0$, having vertices A, B, and C at [2 0 0], [−1.5 2 0], and [−1 0 0], respectively. Right panel: Corresponding result, now for a linearly distributed source strength, with unit value at vertex A and zero values at the other two vertices. Note the different step sizes between the contours used in both panels.

maximum (0.494; position indicated by the asterisks) close to the theoretical limit of 0.5 and with values outside the triangle close to zero. As a consequence, the isopotential lines, drawn at 0.05 V intervals, concentrate along the edges of the triangle. On the right panel, the corresponding field is shown, now generated by a linearly distributed source strength, with its unit value at one of the three vertices ([2 0 0]) and zero at the other two vertices. This field was computed from Equation 44.27. Note that, at this closeness to the double-layer source, the pattern of the potential field closely follows the distribution of the source strength; its maximum is somewhat smaller (0.418) than the limit value of 0.5. Moving away from the source, the potential field exhibits a more diffuse image of the edges of the source, as illustrated in Figure 44.6 for the plane $z = 0.5$, with the maxima of both cases clearly reduced and the maximum observed for the nonuniform case closer to that of the uniform case. When moving further away from Δ, these effects are amplified.

44.7.2.2 Monolayer

The field generated by sources on the same triangle as in the previous example, now generated by a monolayer, is illustrated in Figure 44.7. The field potential generated by a monolayer is defined throughout space, and hence, the illustration (based on Equation 44.15 for the uniform case and on Equation 44.35 for the linearly distributed case) could be produced at the plane of observation coinciding with that of the source triangle. Interestingly, the field shown in the right panel, which is directly at the source plane, has its extreme at a location that lies more than a unit away from the position of the maximal source strength. As for the double layer, the field gets more blurred, with reduced voltages, the further one moves away from the source plane, as is illustrated in Figure 44.8. The potentials at the vertices of the source triangle for all three basic linear source configurations, as well as for the uniform case, are listed in Table 44.1.

Another view on this basic phenomenon is presented in Figure 44.9. It depicts some potential profiles along a line parallel to the z-axis, and thus directed along the normal of the source triangle, and passing through its center of gravity, generated by uniform densities over the triangle. The solid discontinuous line is the profile of the double layer. Including the applied scaling by 4π (Section 44.3.1), the

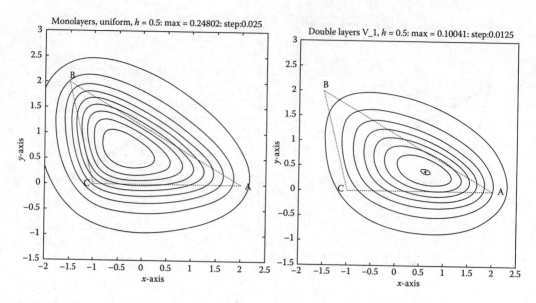

FIGURE 44.6   As in Figure 44.5, with the plane of observation here at $z = 0.5$.

discontinuity has magnitude one (-0.5 to 0.5). The solid continuous line is generated by the monolayer. Here, the characteristic feature is the discontinuity in the slope, changing abruptly from 0.5 to -0.5 while crossing the source in the positive z-direction. This corresponds to the symmetric outflow of the current density from both sides of the monolayer. These curves form the quantification for the triangle of the general profiles of these two fundamental source types as discussed in the major textbooks on potential theory (e.g., Figures 1 through 7 in Panofski and Phillips [13]).

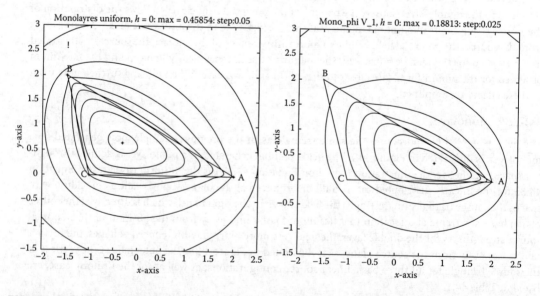

FIGURE 44.7   Left panel: Potential field in the plane $z = 0$, the source plane, generated by a triangularly shaped uniform *monolayer* in the plane $z = 0$, as in Figure 44.5. Right panel: Corresponding result, now for a linearly distributed source strength, with unit value at vertex A and zero values at the other two vertices. Note the different step sizes between contours used in both panels.

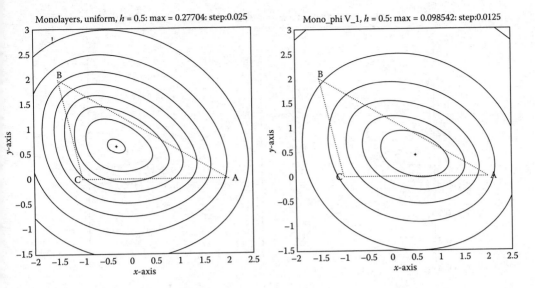

FIGURE 44.8 As in Figure 44.7, here, with the plane of observation at $z = 0.5$.

The solid lines are accompanied by dotted lines representing the potential profiles generated by a single, equivalent single dipole with strength dS_Δ placed at the center of gravity, as well as that of a single, equivalent monopole current source with strength JS_Δ. These curves illustrate that the fields that generated the distributed sources at sufficiently large distances may be approximated by these point sources, the current dipole (decay of the potential as $1/r^2$) and the current monopole (decay of the potential field as $1/r$). Close to the position of such equivalent sources, the correspondence with the fields generated by the surface sources is extremely poor, tending toward infinite values while moving closer to the source location. As a rule of thumb, fields further away than, say, 3 times the size of the triangle expressed, for example, by the radius of the circumscribed circle, may permit field computations based on such equivalent sources. For the computation of the most significant terms in the BEM transfer matrix, the diagonal terms, such approximations are inadequate, as can be seen in Figure 44.9.

44.7.2.3 Singularities

As discussed in Section 44.1, the BEM requires the field potentials generated by sources on a triangle to be known at its own vertices. The handling of this problem for the double layer is discussed in Section 44.3.1, with a special reference to the handling of the autosolid angle as described in Reference 16.

For the monolayer, on the basis of the expressions presented in Section 44.6, it is seen that the field generated in the plane of the source triangle is continuous and finite, including field points on the

TABLE 44.1 Potentials at Vertices A, B, and C of the Triangle Specified in Figure 44.5

	A	B	C
[1 0 0]	0.06996	0.03794	0.05942
[0 1 0]	0.03323	0.08582	0.06954
[0 0 1]	0.03676	0.04788	0.12896
[1 1 1]	0.13992	0.17164	0.25791

Note: First three rows: linearly distributed monolayer current source distributions, with vertex source strengths as specified in the row labels, for example, [1 0 0]: a unit strength at vertex A and zero values at vertices B and C. The lower row represents the uniform case, with potential values seen to be equal to the sum of the other column entries, as required.

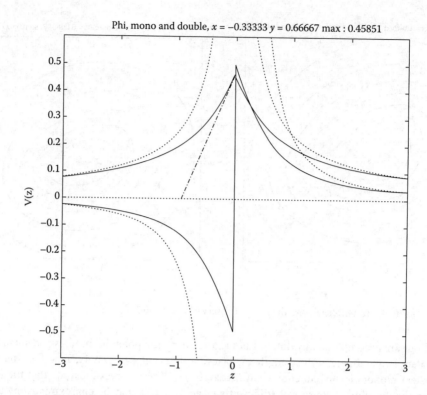

Phi, mono and double, $x = -0.33333$ $y = 0.66667$ max : 0.45851

FIGURE 44.9 Potential profiles along a line parallel to the z-axis, passing through the center of gravity of the triangle, generated by *uniform* source distributions. Solid discontinuous line: double-layer sources; solid continuous line: monolayer sources. Dotted lines: fields generated by a single, equivalent single dipole with strength dS_Δ placed at the center of gravity as well as that of a single, equivalent monopole current source with strength JS_Δ. The dash–dot line represents one of the two tangents to the potential profile of the monolayer at $z \to 0$; its slope is 0.5.

edges, as well as at the vertices. The potentials at the vertices of a monolayer distribution on the source triangle follow from Equation 44.35. Figure 44.7 illustrates that the handling by the expression of these so-called weak singularities is adequate and that the singularity relates to the gradient of the field only at these locations. This can be explained as follows. The term on the left of this expression includes Γ_Δ as computed for the uniform case in Equation 44.15. In its computation, the first term in Equation 44.15 is eradicated by the zero value of the solid angle of the triangle subtended by the observation point in the plane of the triangle and moreover, the factor h is also zero in this case. From the interpretation of the factors h_j in Equation 44.15, it can be seen that these are nonzero only for the edge opposite the vertex of interest, yielding positive contributions $h_j\gamma_j$ for this edge only, while wiping out the singularities in the logarithms γ_j pertaining to the two edges carrying the node of interest. This also justifies the inclusion of the machine epsilon in the logarithm as described above.

A useful set for checking the accuracy of the values found from Equation 44.35 at the critical field points, in the plane of the source triangle, and in particular, those at its vertices, is presented in Table 44.2. Its rows list the values of the vector Γ at the vertices of a rectangular triangle as generated by each of the separate linear distributions. The source triangle is taken to have vertex labels A, B, and C. Its edges form a right angle at vertex C. The lengths of the edges opposite vertices A, B, and C are labeled a, b, and c, respectively.

The right angle in this example facilitates the computation of such results by means of direct integration, using, for example, the results Dw.200.01, Dw.610.1, and Dw.635 [12]. The values for more general triangles, as well as at arbitrary field points in the plane of the source triangle, can be found by forming

TABLE 44.2 Values of Γ at the Vertices A, B, and C of a Rectangular Triangle (Right Angle at C) Generated by Linear Monolayer Source Distributions, with Source Strengths Specified in the Leading Column

	A	B	C
[1 0 0]	$\dfrac{b}{2}\ln\dfrac{a+c}{b}$	$\dfrac{a(c-a)}{2b}$	$\dfrac{ab(a-b)}{2c^2}+\dfrac{ab^3}{2c^3}\ln\dfrac{(a+c)(b+c)}{ab}$
[0 1 0]	$\dfrac{b(c-b)}{2a}$	$\dfrac{a}{2}\ln\dfrac{b+c}{a}$	$\dfrac{ab(b-a)}{2c^2}+\dfrac{a^3b}{2c^3}\ln\dfrac{(a+c)(b+c)}{ab}$
[0 0 1]	$\dfrac{b(b-c)}{2a}+\dfrac{b}{2}\ln\dfrac{a+c}{b}$	$\dfrac{a(a-c)}{2b}+\dfrac{a}{2}\ln\dfrac{b+c}{a}$	$\dfrac{ab}{2c}\ln\dfrac{(a+c)(b+c)}{ab}$
[1 1 1]	$b\ln\dfrac{a+c}{b}$	$a\ln\dfrac{b+c}{a}$	$\dfrac{ab}{c}\ln\dfrac{(a+c)(b+c)}{ab}$

Note: The variables a, b, and c denote the edge lengths, opposite to vertices A, B, and C, respectively. The lower row represents the uniform case, seen to be equal to the sum of the other three elements of the same column, as required.

triangles between the field point and the edges of the source triangle. The subsequent application of the superposition theorem, forming an appropriately weighted sum of the individual results, yields the desired solution.

Note: Table 44.2 has two terms in which the logarithm is absent; also note that, for this rectangular triangle, $\Gamma([111],A) = 2\Gamma([100]A)$ and $\Gamma([111],B) = 2\Gamma([010],B)$.

44.8 Discussion

In this chapter, analytical expressions are described for computing the potential field generated by either a double layer or a monolayer current distribution on a triangle. The pertinent expressions are Equations 44.7, 44.15, 44.27, and 44.35, which remain to be scaled by source strength and $1/4\pi\sigma$.

Next to an application to the computation of the potential field, the BEM can be used in the computation of the magnetic fields outside the body generated by internal electric sources. The virtual, secondary electric sources at the interface may serve for the computation of the effect of inhomogeneities in the electric tissue conductivities on the magnetic field [26]. The numerical handling of the computation of the magnetic fields on the basis of the virtual current source strengths at the triangular elements can be found in Reference 24.

In the vertex approach to the BEM, the expressions pertaining to linearly distributed sources can be used, by which the discontinuities of the source strength across the edges are avoided. The proper handling of the contributions of the current sources on the triangles to their vertex potentials is essential. Equation 44.35 is the proper expression for treating this situation. For the double layer, the concept of the autosolid angle as introduced in Reference 16 can be used.

The computation of the fields for the linearly distributed cases includes factors that are the endpoints of the uniform cases. For sufficiently distal field points, the fields produced by the uniform distributions may be considered as an approximation to the linearly distributed cases.

The suggestions for using higher-order shape functions have been reported in the literature, for example, in Reference 21. When considering their application on any given triangular mesh, one may be well advised to contrast this to a straightforward refinement of the triangulation in which all additional nodes are projections of the triangle refinement onto the actual, generally nonplanar, geometry treated [27].

The interest in the use of the method of fundamental solutions (MFS) appears to be on the increase [28]. This method uses sets of virtual *monopolar* sources, for which the infinite medium potential field is simple. However, by their nature, these sources have an essential singularity at their locus (Figure 44.9), which necessitates the inclusion of an extremely dense set of nodes in the computation of boundary value problems. The claims seen in the literature that the MFS would obviate the complete meshing of the involved surfaces conceal the fact that imaging the results demands the construction of such meshes.

This chapter offers a physical interpretation of the dominant role of the solid angle appearing in all of the expressions for the four major analytical expressions treated in Sections 44.3 through 44.6 and of their properties. This insight has led to the full set of these results, also previously published, in more a condensed report [29].

References

1. Brebbia, C.A., *The Boundary Element Method for Engineers*. 1984, London: Pentech Press.
2. Gulrajani, R.M., *Bioelectricity and Biomagnetism*. 1998, New York: John Wiley & Sons.
3. Smythe, W.R., *Static and Dynamic Electricity*. 1968, New York: McGraw-Hill.
4. Gelernter, H.L. and J.C. Swihart, A mathematical–physical model of the genesis of the electrocardiogram. *Biophys. J.*, 1964. **4**: 285–301.
5. Lynn, M.S. and W.P. Timlake, The numerical solution of singular equations of potential theory. *Numer. Math.*, 1968. **11**: 77–98.
6. Gulrajani, R.M., The forward problem in electrocardiography, in *Bioelectricity and Biomagnetism*. 1998, New York: John Wiley & Sons. pp. 348–380.
7. Martin, R.O., *Inverse Electrocardiography*. 1970, Duke University: Duke, NC, USA.
8. Barr, R.C., M. Ramsey, and M.S. Spach, Relating epicardial to body surface potentials by means of transfer coefficients based on geometry measurements. *IEEE Trans. Biomed. Eng.*, 1977. **BME-24**: 1–11.
9. Colli-Franzone, P. et al., Inverse epicardial mapping in the human case. In *Proceedings of the Symposium on Electrophysiology of the Heart*. 1980, New York: Plenum.
10. Rudy, Y. and J.E. Burns, Noninvasive electrocardiographic imaging. *Ann. Noninv. Electrocardiol.*, 1999. **4**: 340–359.
11. van Oosterom, A. and T.F. Oostendorp, On computing pericardial potentials and current densities. *J Electrocardiol.*, 1992. **25**: 102–106.
12. Dwight, B.H., *Tables of Integrals and Other Mathematical Data*. 1961, New York: Macmillan.
13. Panofski, W.K.H. and M. Phillips, *Classical Electricity and Magnetism*. 1962, London: Addison-Wesley.
14. van Oosterom, A. and J. Strackee, The solid angle of a plane triangle. *IEEE Trans. Biomed. Eng.*, 1983. **BME-30**: 125–126.
15. Barr, R.C. et al., Determining surface potentials from current dipoles with application to electrocardiography. *IEEE Trans. Biomed. Eng.*, 1966. **BME-13**: 88–92.
16. Meijs, J.W.H. et al., On the numerical accuracy of the boundary element method. *IEEE Trans. Biomed. Eng.*, 1989. **36**(10): 1038–1049.
17. van Oosterom, A., Electrocardiography, in *The Biophysics of Heart and Circulation*, J. Strackee and N. Westerhof, eds. 1993, Bristol: Institute of Physics Publication. pp. 249–256.
18. Rao, S.M. et al., A simple numerical solution procedure for statics problems involving arbitrary-shaped surfaces. *IEEE Trans. Ant. Propag.*, 1979. **AP-36**: 604–608.
19. Okon, E.E. and R.F. Harrington, The potential due to a uniform source distribution over a triangular domain. *Int. J. Numer. Meth. Eng.*, 1982. **18**: 1401–1411.
20. Kuwahara, T. and T. Takeda, An effective analysis for three-dimensional boundary element method using analytical higher order elements. *Trans. IEE Japan*, 1986. **107-A**: 275–282.
21. Kuwahara, T. and T. Tadeka, A formula of boundary integral for potential problem and its consideration. In *Proceedings of the 1st Japan-China Symposium on Boundary Element Methods*. 1987, Kyota, Japan: Pergamon Press.
22. Medina, D.E. and J.A. Liggett, Exact integrals for the three-dimensional boundary element potential problems. *Commun. Appl. Num. Anal.*, 1989. **5**: 555–561.

23. Graglia, R.D., On the numerical integration of the linear shape functions times the 3-D Green's function or its gradient on the plane triangle. *IEEE Trans. Antennas Propag.*, 1993. **41**: 1448–1455.
24. Ferguson, A.S., X. Zhang, and G. Stroink, A complete linear discretization for calculating the magnetic field using the boundary element method. *IEEE Trans. Biomed. Eng.*, 1994. **BME-41**: 455–460.
25. Munck, J.C.D., A linear discretization of the volume conductor boundary integral equation using analytically integrated elements. *IEEE Trans. Biomed. Eng.*, 1992. **BME-39**: 986–990.
26. Geselowitz, D.B., On the magnetic field generated outside an inhomogeneous volume conductor by internal sources. *IEEE Trans. Magn.*, 1970, **MAG-6**: 346–347.
27. Zhou, H. and A. van Oosterom, Mesh refinement and accuracy of numerical solutions. In Engineering solutions to current health care problems. *Proceedings of the 15-th Annual International Conference of the IEEE Engineering in Medicine and Biology Society.* 1993, Piscataway: IEEE Publishing Services.
28. Fairweather, G. and A. Karageorghis, The method of fundamental solutions for elliptic boundary value problems. *Adv. Comput. Math.*, 1998, **9**: 69–95.
29. A. van Oosterom, Closed-form analytical expressions for the potential fields generated by triangular monolayers with linearly distributed source strength. *Med Biol Eng Comput.* 2012, **25**: 1–9.

45

Principles of Electrocardiography

45.1 Introduction 45-1
45.2 Physiology 45-4
45.3 Instrumentation 45-5
    Applications
45.4 Conclusions 45-10
References 45-10
Further Information 45-11

Edward J. Berbari
Indiana University–Purdue
University, Indianapolis

45.1 Introduction

The electrocardiogram (ECG) is the recording of the electrical activity generated by the heart on the body surface. It was originally observed by Waller in 1889 [1] using his pet bulldog as the signal source and the capillary electrometer as the recording device. In 1903 Einthoven [2] improvised the technology by using the string galvanometer as the recording device and employing human subjects with a variety of cardiac abnormalities. Einthoven is chiefly responsible for introducing some concepts still in use today, including the labeling of the various waves, defining some of the standard recording sites using the arms and legs, and developing the first theoretical construct whereby the heart is modeled as a single time-varying dipole. We also owe the "EKG" acronym to Einthoven writing in German where the root word "cardio" is spelled with a "k."

To record an ECG waveform, a differential recording between two points on the body are made. Traditionally each differential recording is referred to as a lead. Einthoven defined three leads numbered with the Roman numerals I, II, and III. They are defined as:

$$I = V_{LA} - V_{RA}$$
$$II = V_{LL} - V_{RA}$$
$$III = V_{LL} - V_{LA}$$

where RA = right arm, LA = left arm, and LL = left leg. Because the body is assumed to be purely resistive, at ECG frequencies, the four limbs can be thought of as wires attached to the torso. Hence, lead I could be recorded from the respective shoulders without a loss of cardiac information. Note that these are not independent and the following relationship II = I + III holds.

For 30 years the evolution of the ECG proceeded when F.N. Wilson [3] added concepts of a "unipolar" recording. He created a reference point by tying the three limbs together and averaging their potentials so that individual recording sites on the limbs or the chest surface would be differentially recorded with the same reference point. Wilson extended the biophysical models to include the concept of the

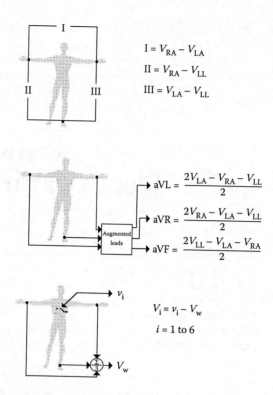

$$I = V_{RA} - V_{LA}$$
$$II = V_{RA} - V_{LL}$$
$$III = V_{LA} - V_{LL}$$

$$aVL = \frac{2V_{LA} - V_{RA} - V_{LL}}{2}$$
$$aVR = \frac{2V_{RA} - V_{LA} - V_{LL}}{2}$$
$$aVF = \frac{2V_{LL} - V_{LA} - V_{RA}}{2}$$

$$V_i = \nu_i - V_w$$
$$i = 1 \text{ to } 6$$

FIGURE 45.1 The 12-lead ECG is formed by the three bipolar surface leads: I, II, and III; the augmented Wilson terminal referenced limb leads: aVR, aVL, aVF; and the Wilson terminal referenced chest leads: V_1, V_2, V_3, V_4, V_5, and V_6.

cardiac source enclosed within the volume conductor of the body. He erroneously thought that the central terminal was a true zero potential. However, from the mid-1930s until today the 12 leads composed of the 3 limb leads, 3 leads in which the limb potentials are referenced to a modified Wilson terminal (the augmented leads [4]), and 6 leads placed across the front of the chest and referenced to the Wilson terminal form the basis of the standard 12-lead ECG. Figure 45.1 summarizes the 12-lead set. These sites are historically based, have a built in redundancy, and are not optimal for all cardiac events. The voltage difference from any two sites will record an ECG, but it is these standardized sites with the massive 90-year collection of empirical observations that has firmly established their role as the standard. Figure 45.2 is a typical or stylized ECG recording from lead II. Einthoven chose the letters of the alphabet from P–U to label the waves and to avoid conflict with other physiologic waves being studied at the turn of the century. The ECG signals are typically in the range of ±2 mV and require a recording bandwidth of 0.05–150 Hz. Full technical specification for ECG equipment has been proposed by both the American Heart Association [5] and the Association for the Advancement of Medical Instrumentation [6].

There have been several attempts to change the approach for recording the ECG. The vector cardiogram used a weighted set of recording sites to form an orthogonal *XYZ* lead set. The advantage here was minimum lead set but in practice it gained only a moderate degree of enthusiasm among physicians. Body surface mapping refers to the use of many recording sites (>64) arranged on the body so that isopotential surfaces could be computed and analyzed over time. This approach still has a role in research investigations. Other subsets of the 12-lead ECG are used in limited mode recording situations such as the digitally stored ambulatory ECG (usually 2 leads) or in intensive care monitoring at the bedside (usually 1 or 2 leads) or telemetered within regions of the hospital from patients who are not confined to bed (1 lead). The recording electronics of these ECG systems have followed the typical evolution of modern instrumentation, for example, vacuum tubes, transistors, ICs, and microprocessors.

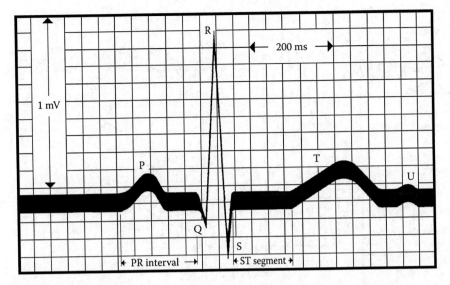

FIGURE 45.2 This is a stylized version of a normal lead II recording showing the P wave, QRS complex, and the T and U waves. The PR interval and the ST segment are significant time windows. The peak amplitude of the QRS is about 1 mV. The vertical scale is usually 1 mV/cm. The time scale is usually based on millimeter per second scales with 25 mm/s being the standard form. The small boxes of the ECG are 1×1 mm^2.

The application of computers to the ECG for machine interpretation was one of the earliest uses of computers in medicine [7]. Of primary interest in the computer-based systems was the replacement of the human reader and the elucidation of the standard waves and intervals. Originally this was performed by linking the ECG machine to a centralized computer via phone lines. The modern ECG machine is completely integrated with an analog front end, a 12–16-bit A/D converter, a computational microprocessor, and dedicated I/O processors. These systems compute a measurement matrix derived from the 12-lead signals and analyze this matrix with a set of rules to obtain the final set of interpretive statements [8]. Figure 45.3 shows the ECG of a heartbeat and the types of measurements that might be made on each of the component waves of the ECG and used for classifying each beat type and the subsequent cardiac rhythm. The depiction of the 12 analog signals and this set of interpretive statements form the final output with an example shown in Figure 45.4. The physician will over-read each ECG and modify or correct those statements that are deemed inappropriate. The larger hospital-based system will record these corrections and maintain a large database of all ECGs accessible by any combination of parameters, for example, all men, above 50 years, with an inferior myocardial infarction.

There are hundreds of interpretive statements from which a specific diagnosis is made for each ECG, but there are only about five or six major classification groups for which the ECG is used. The first step in analyzing an ECG requires the determination of the rate and rhythm for the atria and ventricles. Included here would be any conduction disturbances either in the relationship between the various chambers or within the chambers themselves. Then one would proceed to identify features that would relate to the presence or absence of scarring due to a myocardial infarction. There may also be evidence of acute events occurring that would occur with ischemia or an evolving myocardial infarction. The ECG has been a primary tool for evaluating chamber size or enlargement, but one might argue that more accurate information in this area would be supplied by noninvasive imaging technologies.

More recently, a high-resolution (HR) ECG has been developed whereby the digitized ECG is signal averaged to reduce random noise [9,10]. This approach, coupled with postaveraging high-pass filtering,

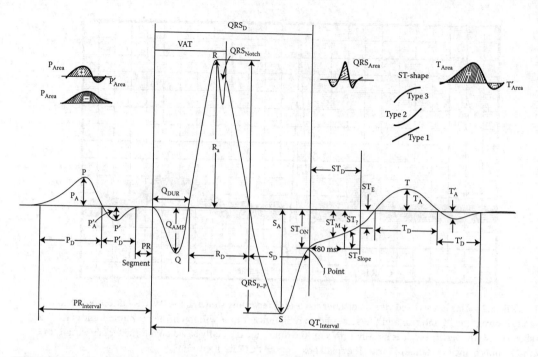

FIGURE 45.3 The ECG depicts numerous measurements that can be made with computer-based algorithms. These are primarily durations, amplitudes, and areas. (Courtesy of the Hewlett Packard Co., Palo Alto, CA.)

is used to detect and quantify low-level signals (1.0 μV) not detectable with standard approaches. This computer-based approach has enabled the recording of events which are predictive of future life-threatening cardiac events [11,12].

45.2 Physiology

The heart has four chambers, the upper two chambers are called the atria and the lower two chambers are called the ventricles. The atria are thin-walled, low-pressure pumps that receive blood from venous circulation. Located in the top right atrium are a group of cells which act as the primary pacemaker of the heart. Through a complex change of ionic concentration across the cell membranes (the current source) an extracellular potential field is established which then excites neighboring cells and a cell-to-cell propagation of electrical events occur. Because the body acts as a purely resistive medium these potential fields extend to the body surface [13]. The character of the body surface waves depends upon the amount of tissue activating at one time and the relative speed and direction of the activation wave front. Therefore, the pacemaker potentials which are generated by a small tissue mass are not seen on the ECG. As the activation wave front encounters the increased mass of atrial muscle, the initiation of electrical activity is observed on the body surface and the first ECG wave of the cardiac cycle is seen. This is the P wave and it represents activation of the atria. Conduction of the cardiac impulse proceeds from the atria through a series of specialized cardiac cells (the A–V node and the His–Purkinje system), which again are too small in total mass to generate a signal large enough to be seen on the standard ECG. There is a short relatively isoelectric segment following the P wave. Once the large muscle mass of the ventricles is excited, a rapid and large deflection is seen on the body surface. The excitation of the ventricles causes them to contract and provides the main force for circulating blood to the organs of the body. This large wave appears to have several components. The initial downward deflection is called the Q wave, the initial upward deflection is the R wave, and the

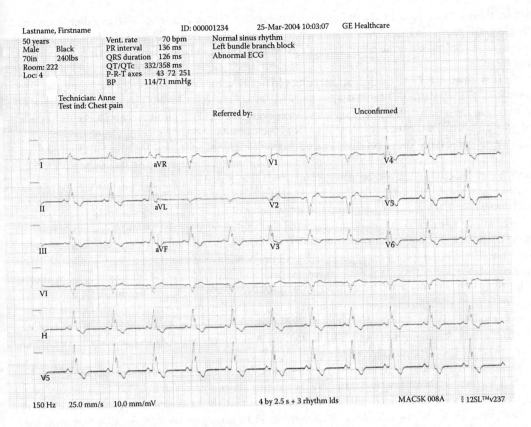

FIGURE 45.4 This is an example of an interpreted 12-lead ECG. A 2.5 s recording is shown for each of the 12 leads. The bottom trace is a continuous 10 s rhythm strip of lead II. Patient information is given in the top area, below which is printed the computerized interpretive statements. (Courtesy of GE Healthcare Technologies, Waukesha, WI.)

terminal downward deflection is the S wave. The polarity and actual presence of these three components depends upon the position of the leads on the body as well as a multitude of abnormalities that may exist. In general, the large ventricular waveform is generically called the QRS complex regardless of its makeup. Following the QRS complex is another relatively short isoelectric segment. After this short segment the ventricles return to their electrical resting state and a wave of repolarization is seen as a low-frequency signal called the T wave. In some individuals a small peak occurs at the end or after the T wave and is called the U wave. Its origin has never been fully established but is believed to be a repolarization potential.

45.3 Instrumentation

The general instrumentation requirements for the ECG have been addressed by professional societies through the years [5,6]. Briefly they recommend a system bandwidth between 0.05 and 150 Hz. Of great importance in ECG diagnosis is the low-frequency response of the system because shifts in some of the low-frequency regions, for example, the ST segment, have critical diagnostic value. While the heart rate may only have a 1 Hz fundamental frequency, the phase response of typical analog high-pass filters are such that the system corner frequency must be much smaller than the 3 dB corner frequency where only the amplitude response is considered. The system gain depends upon the total system design. The typical ECG amplitude is ±2 mV and if A/D conversion is used in a digital system, then enough gain to span the only 20% of the A/D converter's dynamic range is needed. This margin allows for recording abnormally large signals as well as accommodating base line drift if present and not corrected.

To first obtain an ECG the patient must be physically connected to the amplifier front end. The patient/amplifier interface is formed by a special bioelectrode that converts the ionic current flow of the body to the electron flow of the metallic wire. These electrodes typically rely on a chemical paste or gel with a high ionic concentration. This acts as the transducer at the tissue–electrode interface. For short-term applications the use of silver-coated suction electrodes or "sticky" metallic foil electrodes are used. Long-term recordings, such as the case for the monitored patient, require a stable electrode/tissue interface and special adhesive tape material surrounds the gel and an Ag^+/Ag^+Cl electrode.

At any given time, the patient may be connected to a variety of devices, for example, respirator, blood pressure monitor, temporary pacemaker, and so on, some of which will invade the body and provide a low-resistance pathway to the heart. It is essential that the device does not act as a current source and inject the patient with enough current to stimulate the heart and cause it to fibrillate. Some bias currents are unavoidable at the system input stage and recommendations are that these leakage currents be less than 10 μA per device. In recent years, there has been some controversy regarding the level of allowable leakage current. The Association for the Advancement of Medical Instrumentation [5] has written its standards to allow leakage currents as high as 50 μA. Studies [14,15] have shown that there may be complex and lethal physiological response to 60 Hz currents as low as 32 μA. In light of the reduced standards these research results were commented on by members of the American Heart Association Committee on Electrocardiography [16].

There is also a 10 μA maximum current limitation due to a fault condition if a patient comes in contact with the high-voltage side of the AC power lines. In this case, the isolation must be adequate to prevent 10 μA of fault current as well. This mandates that the ECG reference ground not be connected physically to the low side of the AC power line or its third ground wire. For ECG machines the solution has typically been to AM modulate a medium-frequency carrier signal (400 kHz) and use an isolation transformer with subsequent demodulation. Other methods of signal isolation can be used but the primary reason for the isolation is to keep the patient from being part of the AC circuit in the case of a patient to power line fault. In addition, with many devices connected in a patient-monitoring situation it is possible that ground loop currents will be generated. To obviate this potential hazard a low-impedance ground buss is often installed in these rooms and each device chassis will have an external ground wire connected to the buss. Another unique feature of these amplifiers is that they must be able to withstand the high-energy discharge of a cardiac defibrillator.

Older-style ECG machines recorded one lead at a time, then evolved to three simultaneous leads. This necessitated the use of switching circuits as well as analog weighting circuits to generate the various 12 leads. This is usually eliminated in modern digital systems by using an individual single-ended amplifier for each electrode on the body. Each potential signal is then digitally converted and all of the ECG leads can be formed mathematically in software. This would necessitate a 9-amplifier system. By performing some of the lead calculations with the analog differential amplifiers this can be reduced to an 8-channel system. Thus only the individual chest leads V_1 through V_6 and any two of the limb leads, for example, I and III, are needed to calculate the full 12-lead ECG. Figure 45.5 is a block diagram of a modern digital-based ECG system. This system uses an amplifier per lead wire and a 16-bit A/D converter, all within a small lead wire manifold or amplifier lead stage. The digital signals are sent via a high-speed link to the main ECG instrument. Here, the embedded microprocessors perform all of the calculations and a hard copy report is generated (Figure 45.4). Note that each functional block has its own controller and the system requires a sophisticated real-time operating system to coordinate all system functions. Concomitant with the data acquisition is the automatic interpretation of the ECG. These programs are quite sophisticated and are continually evolving. It is still a medical/legal requirement that these ECGs be over-read by the physician.

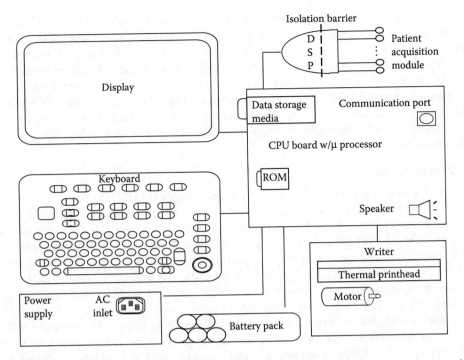

FIGURE 45.5 This is a block diagram of microprocessor-based ECG system. (Courtesy of GE Healthcare Technologies, Waukesha, WI.)

45.3.1 Applications

Besides the standard 12-lead ECG, there are several other uses of ECG recording technology which rely on only a few leads. These applications have had a significant clinical and commercial impact. The following are brief descriptions of several ECG applications that are aimed at introducing the reader to some of the many uses of the ECG.

45.3.1.1 The Ambulatory ECG

The evolution of the ambulatory or Holter ECG has an interesting history and its evolution closely followed both technical and clinical progress. The original, analog tape-based, portable ECG resembled a fully loaded backpack and was developed by Dr. Holter in the early 1960s [17], but was soon followed by more compact devices that could be worn on the belt. The original large-scale clinical use of this technology was to identify patients who developed heart block transiently and could be treated by implanting a cardiac pacemaker. This required the secondary development of a device which could rapidly play back the 24 h of tape-recorded ECG signals and present to the technician or physician a means of identifying periods of time where the patient's heart rate became abnormally low. The scanners had the circuitry to not only playback the ECG at speeds 30–60 times real time, but to detect the beats and display them in a superimposed mode on a cathode ray tube (CRT) screen. In addition, an audible tachometer could be used to identify the periods of low heart rate. With this playback capability came numerous other observations such as the identification of premature ventricular beats (PVBs), which led to the development of techniques to identify and quantify their number. Together with the development of antiarrhythmic drugs a coupling was formed between pharmaceutical therapy and the diagnostic tool for quantifying PVBs. ECG tapes were recorded before and after drug administration and the drug efficacy was measured by the reduction of the number of PVBs. The scanner technology for detecting and quantifying these arrhythmias was originally implemented with analog hardware but soon advanced to computer technology as it became economically feasible. Very sophisticated algorithms were developed based on pattern recognition techniques and were sometimes implemented with high-speed specialized numerical processors as the tape playback speeds became several hundred times real time [18]. Unfortunately this approach using the ambulatory ECG for identifying and treating cardiac arrhythmias has been on the decline as the rationale of PVC suppression was found to be unsuccessful for decreasing cardiac mortality. However, the ambulatory ECG is still a widely used diagnostic tool and modern units often have built-in microprocessors with considerable amounts of random access memory. Here, the data can be analyzed on line with large segments of data selected for storage and later analysis with personal computer-based programs.

45.3.1.2 Patient Monitoring

The techniques for monitoring the ECG in real time were developed in conjunction with the concept of the coronary care unit or CCU. Patients were placed in these specialized hospital units to carefully observe their progress during an acute illness such as a myocardial infarction or after complex surgical procedures. As the number of beds increased in these units it became clear that the highly trained medical staff could not continually watch a monitor screen and computerized techniques were added which monitored the patient's rhythm. These programs were not unlike those developed for the ambulatory ECG and the high-speed numerical capability of the computer was not taxed by monitoring a single ECG. The typical CCU would have 8–16 beds and hence the computing power was taken to its limit by monitoring multiple beds. The modern units have the central processing unit (CPU) distributed within the ECG module at the bedside, along with modules for measuring many other physiological parameters. Each bedside monitor would be interconnected with a high-speed digital line, for example, Ethernet, to a centralized computer used primarily to control communications and maintain a patient database.

45.3.1.3 HR Electrocardiography

HR capability is now a standard feature on most digitally based ECG systems, or as a stand-alone microprocessor-based unit [19]. The most common application of the HRECG is to record very low level (1.0 µV) signals which occur after the QRS complex but are not evident on the standard ECG. These "late potentials" are generated from abnormal regions of the ventricles and have been strongly associated with the substrate responsible for a life-threatening rapid heart rate (ventricular tachycardia). The typical HRECG is derived from three bipolar leads configured in an anatomic XYZ coordinate system. These three ECG signals are then digitized at a rate of 1000–2000 Hz per channel, time aligned via a real-time QRS correlator, and summed in the form of a signal average. Signal averaging will theoretically improve the signal-to-noise ratio by the square root of the number of beats averaged. The underlying assumptions are that the signals of interest do not vary, on a beat-to-beat basis, and that the noise is random. Figure 45.6 has four panels depicting the most common sequence for processing the HRECG to measure the late potentials. Panel (a) depicts a 3 s recording of the XYZ leads close to normal resolution. Panel (b) was obtained after averaging 200 beats and with a sampling frequency of 10 times as that shown in panel (a). The gain is also five times greater. Panel (c) is the high-pass filtered signal using a partially time-reversed digital filter having a second-order Butterworth response and a 3 db corner frequency of 40 Hz [12]. Note the appearance of the signals at the terminal portion of the QRS complex. A common method of analysis, but necessarily optimal, is to combine the filters XYZ leads into a vector magnitude, $(X^2 + Y^2 + Z^2)^{1/2}$. This waveform is shown in panel (d). From this waveform several parameters have been derived such as total QRS duration, including late potentials, the RMS voltage value of the terminal 40 ms, and the low-amplitude signal (LAS) duration from the 40 µV level to the end of the late potentials. Abnormal values for these parameters are used to identify patients at high risk of ventricular tachycardia following a heart attack.

45.3.1.4 His Bundle Electrocardiography

ECG can be directly recorded from the heart surface as in a modern electrophysiology (EP) study where the evaluation of the heart relies on both the body surface ECG and direct recordings obtained from

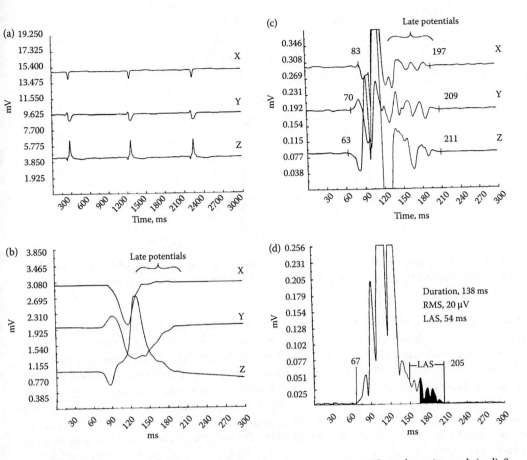

FIGURE 45.6 The signal processing steps typically performed to obtain a HRECG are shown in panels (a–d). See text for a full description.

within the heart using electrode catheters. Such catheters are introduced into a leg or arm vein or artery and advanced, under fluoroscopic control, into the interior of one of the four chambers of the heart. An electrode catheter is an insulated set of wires bundled within a polyurethane sheath. The diameters of these catheters range from about 1.0 to 2.5 mm. As many as 16 wires may be in the total assembly with ring electrodes, exposed on the outer surface of the catheter, attached to each internal wire. In addition, there are usually structural internal wires used to stiffen the catheter. With a proper controller at the rear of the catheter a trained operator can flex the catheter in a loop of almost 180°. Together with the torsional properties of the catheter almost every point within the heart can be probed for electrical events. Direct contact recordings are called electrograms to distinguish them from body surface ECGs.

Figure 45.7 shows an example of a His bundle recording. The top two traces are leads II and V_6 of the ECG and the bottom trace is the voltage difference from two electrodes on the indwelling electrode catheter. This internal view of cardiac activation combined with the His bundle electrogram has been referred to as His bundle electrocardiography [20]. Atrial activation on the catheter recording is called the "A" deflection and ventricular activation called the "V" deflection. The His bundle potential is the central "H" deflection. Since the catheter is located very close to the His bundle and AV node, it is assumed that the A deflection arises from the atrial muscle tissue close to the AV node. When combined with the surface lead information a number of new intervals can be obtained. These are the PA, AH, and HV intervals. The PA interval is a measure of atrial muscle activation time, the AH interval is a measure of AV nodal activation time, and the HV interval is a measure of the ventricular conduction system activation time.

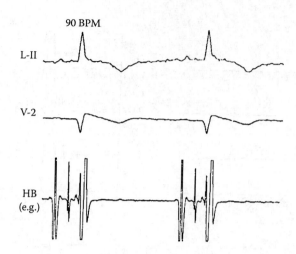

FIGURE 45.7 The top two traces are ECG leads II and V-2 and the bottom trace is a bipolar catheter recording, properly positioned inside the heart, showing the His Bundle deflection (HB), and intracardiac atrial (A) and ventricular (V) activity.

The modern electrophysiological evaluation, or EP study, may involve as many as 64 individual recordings within the heart. In addition, current can be passed through these electrodes to stimulate the heart. A variety of atrial and ventricular stimulation protocols can be used, which then allows the cardiac electrophysiologist to identify pathways and mechanisms involved in most forms of arrhythmias. Besides this diagnostic function, it is now possible to locate abnormal structures or regions of the heart that are critical to arrhythmogenesis. By passing high-energy radio frequency waves through one or more of the internal electrodes it is possible to cauterize or ablate the suspect tissue without causing any widespread injury to the rest of the heart. In many forms of arrhythmias this ablation therapy can produce a cure for the patient.

In addition to the EP study and ablation therapy internal electrodes are the primary form of signal recording for both the cardiac pacemaker and implantable defibrillator. These devices both sense cardiac activation from permanent indwelling catheters and deliver energy to the heart through them. In the case of the cardiac pacemaker these are low-level shocks which maintain the patient's heart rhythm. In the case of the implantable defibrillator the device will monitor the patient's rhythm until a serious or life-threatening arrhythmia occurs and then a high-energy pulse will be delivered in order to convert the rhythm back to normal. Both devices rely heavily on continuous monitoring of the cardiac signals obtained from internal catheter recordings using sophisticated implanted microprocessors and accurate means of signal detection and analysis.

45.4 Conclusions

The ECG is one of the oldest, instrument-bound measurements in medicine. It has faithfully followed the progression of instrumentation technology. Its most recent evolutionary step, to the microprocessor-based system, has allowed patients to wear their computer monitor or provided an enhanced, HRECG, which has opened new vistas of ECG analysis and interpretation. The intracardiac ECG also forms the basis of modern diagnostic EP studies and therapeutic devices, such as the pacemaker and implantable defibrillator.

References

1. Waller A.D. On the electromotive changes connected with the beat of the mammalian heart, and the human heart in particular. *Philos. Trans. B*, 180: 169, 1889.

2. Einthoven W. Die galvanometrische Registrirung des menschlichen Elektrokardiogramms, zugleich eine Beurtheilung der Anwendung des Capillar-Elecktrometers in der Physiologie. *Pflugers Arch. ges. Physiol.* 99: 472, 1903.
3. Wilson F.N., Johnston F.S., and Hill I.G.W. The interpretation of the falvanometric curves obtained when one electrode is distant from the heart and the other near or in contact with the ventricular surface. *Am. Heart J.* 10: 176, 1934.
4. Goldberger E. A simple, indifferent, electrocardiographic electrode of zero potential and a technique of obtaining augmented, unipolar, extremity leads. *Am. Heart J.* 23: 483, 1942.
5. Bailey J.J., Berson A.S., Garson A., Horan L.G., Macfarlane P.W., Mortara D.W., and Zywietz C. Recommendations for standardization and specifications in automated electrocardiography: Bandwidth and digital signal processing: A report for health professionals by an ad hoc writing group of the committee on electrocardiography and cardiac electrophysiology of the Council on Clinical Cardiology, American Heart Association. *Circulation* 81: 2, 730–739, 1990.
6. *Safe Current Limits for Electromedical Apparatus: American National Standard, ANSI/AAMI ES1–1993.* Arlington, VA: Association for the Advancement of Medical Instrumentation; 1993.
7. Jenkins J.M. Computerized electrocardiography. *CRC Crit. Rev. Bioeng.* 6: 307, 1981.
8. Pryor T.A., Drazen E., and Laks M. (Eds.), *Computer Systems for the Processing of Diagnostic Electrocardiograms.* IEEE Computer Society Press, Los Alamitos, CA, 1980.
9. Berbari E.J., Lazzara R., Samet P., and Scherlag B.J. Noninvasive technique for detection of electrical activity during the PR segment. *Circulation* 48: 1006, 1973.
10. Berbari E.J., Lazzara R., and Scherlag B.J. A computerized technique to record new components of the electrocardiogram. *Proc. IEEE* 65: 799, 1977.
11. Berbari E.J., Scherlag B.J., Hope R.R., and Lazzara R. Recording from the body surface of arrhythmogenic ventricular activity during the ST segment. *Am. J. Cardiol.* 41: 697, 1978.
12. Simson M.B. Use of signals in the terminal QRS complex to identify patients with ventricular tachycardia after myocardial infarction. *Circulation* 64: 235, 1981.
13. Geselowitz D.B. On the theory of the electrocardiogram. *Proc. IEEE* 77: 857, 1989.
14. Swerdlow C.D., Olson W.H., O'Connor M.E. et al. Cardiovascular collapse caused by electrocardiographically silent 60 Hz intracardiac leakage current: Implications for electrical safety. *Circulation* 99: 2559–2564, 1999.
15. Malkin R.A. and Hoffmeister B.K. Mechanisms by which AC leakage currents cause complete hemodynamic collapse without inducing fibrillation. [see comment]. *J. Cardiovasc. Electrophysiol.* 12: 1154–1161, 2001.
16. Laks M.M., Arzbaecher R., Geselowitz D., Bailey J.J., and Berson A. Revisiting the question: Will relaxing safe current limits for electromedical equipment increase hazards to patients? *Circulation* 102: 823–825, 2000.
17. Holter N.J. New method for heart studies: Continuous electrocardiography of active subjects over long periods is now practical. *Science* 134: 1214–1220, 1961.
18. Ripley K.L. and Murray A. (Eds.), *Introduction to Automated Arrhythmia Detection*, IEEE Computer Society Press, Los Alamitos, CA, 1980.
19. Berbari E.J. and Steinberg J.S. *A Practical Guide to High Resolution Electrocardiography.* Futura Publishers, Armonk, NY, 2000.
20. Scherlag B.J., Samet P., and Helfant R.H. His bundle electrogram: A critical appraisal of its uses and limitations. *Circulation* 46: 601–613, 1972.

Further Information

A Practical Guide to the Use of the High-Resolution Electrocardiogram, Edward J. Berbari and Jonathan S. Steinberg, Eds., Armonk, NY: Futura Publishers, 2000.

Cardiac Electrophysiology: From Cell to Bedside, 4th ed., D.P. Zipes and J. Jalife, Eds., Philadelphia: W.B. Saunders & Co., 2004.

Comprehensive Electrocardiology: Theory and Practice in Health and Disease, Vols. 1–3, P.W. Macfarlane and T.D. Veitch Lawrie, Eds., England: Pergamon Press, 1989.

Medical Instrumentation: Application and Design, 3rd ed., J.G. Webster, Ed., Boston: Houghton Mifflin, 1998.

46

Electrodiagnostic Studies

46.1 Introduction 46-1
46.2 Anatomy 46-1
46.3 Physiology 46-4
46.4 EMG and Force Generation 46-5
46.5 Pathology 46-6
46.6 Instrumentation 46-7
46.7 EDX Study 46-9
46.8 Motor Nerve Conduction 46-9
46.9 Sensory Nerve Conduction 46-11
46.10 Needle EMG 46-11
46.11 Single Fiber and Macro EMG 46-14
46.12 Evoked Potentials 46-16
46.13 Somatosensory Evoked Potential 46-16
46.14 Brainstem Auditory Evoked Response 46-17
46.15 Visual Evoked Potential 46-18
46.16 Engineering in EDX 46-19
References 46-19

Sanjeev D.
Nandedkar
Natus Medical Inc.

46.1 Introduction

Neuromuscular disease is suspected when a patient complains of abnormal sensation (numbness, tingling, and pain), weakness, or difficulty with movements (e.g., tremor and foot drop). Electrodiagnostic (EDX) studies have been used successfully over the last six decades to identify or to refute a neuromuscular pathology to explain the patient symptoms (Dumitru et al., 2002). The EDX studies are often performed in conjunction with other diagnostic procedures such as imaging (MRI, x-ray), blood work (biochemistry), nerve or muscle biopsy, and so on. The EDX studies offer many advantages. The EDX studies are relatively noninvasive, the study can be repeated easily, the cost of procedures is relatively low, and the study characterizes the "function" of the neuromuscular system. Imaging studies reveal the structure and thus help the overall assessment of the patient condition. In this chapter, we will review the physiologic basis and principles of EDX studies, and discuss the contributions of biomedical engineers in this exciting field of neurophysiology. The study of brain using electroencephalograph (EEG) is discussed in a separate chapter.

46.2 Anatomy

The EDX study is often described as an extension of the patient's medical history and physical examination. It is essential to understand the anatomy and the physiology of the neuromuscular system to plan and interpret the test results.

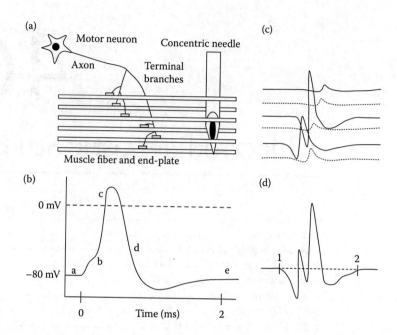

FIGURE 46.1 Schematic of MU and MUP. (a) The MU shows muscle fibers in a longitudinal view. A cross-sectional view is shown in Figure 46.3. (b) The resting and action potential in intracellular space are illustrated. (c) The extracellular AP of all muscle fibers shows variation in amplitude and arrival time at the electrode. The concentric needle tip is better seen in Figure 46.9. (d) The sum of all muscle fiber APs is the MUP. Markers 1 and 2 indicate the beginning and end of the MUP. The time difference between these points is the MUP duration. The number of phases is obtained by adding 1 to the number of baseline crossings. Hence, this MUP has five phases. (Copyright Nandedkar Productions LLC, 2010.)

A muscle is made of thousands of cells, called muscle fibers. They are organized into functional entities called motor units (MUs). An MU consists of all muscle fibers innervated by one motor neuron (MN) (Figure 46.1a). The MN is located in the spinal cord (Figure 46.2), and is also called the lower MN. The upper MN is located in the brain. The nerve fiber from the lower MN exits from a small opening between the disks separating the vertebrae. All nerve fibers exiting such an opening form the so-called root (Figure 46.2). The root is described by its anatomic location in the spinal cord, for example, the C5 root contains fibers exiting the spinal cord at the C5 level. The nerve fibers from different roots combine and separate to form distinct bundles (trunk, division, cord) and finally the individual nerve (Figure 46.2). A nerve supplies many different muscles. Note that a muscle is innervated by a single nerve and has multiple roots. Also, a nerve consists of fibers (or axons) from many roots. The lesion of individual roots or nerves will give a corresponding pattern of weakness in the muscles innervated by them.

A nerve fiber begins at the MN and upon reaching the muscle divides into many branches to connect with individual muscle fibers. The contact is called the "end-plate" or "neuromuscular junction" (Figure 46.1a). In most muscles, there is only one end-plate per muscle fiber. In large muscles such as the biceps or the tibialis anterior, the MU muscle fibers are distributed randomly over a roughly circular territory (Figure 46.3a) with 5–10 mm diameter. Most fibers are separated from other fibers of the same MU by a few hundred micrometers. There is no tendency to form groups. The fiber diameter varies slightly among different fibers of the MU. The mean muscle fiber diameter is 50–60 μm. The MU size refers mainly to the number of muscle fibers in the MU. A muscle has MUs of different sizes. The small MUs are fatigue resistant and are activated first. Large MUs have more fibers and have larger territory (Figure 46.3b). This gives them the same "fiber density (FD)" as the smaller MUs. The larger MUs are activated when a higher force is required and they fatigue easily.

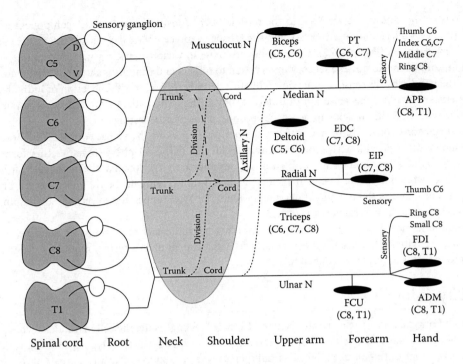

FIGURE 46.2 Illustration of the beginning of motor nerve fibers in the spinal cord and their path to reach different muscles in the upper limb. All nerves and muscles are not shown. The sensory innervation to fingers is shown. The dorsal and ventral roots are indicated by "D" and "V." The shaded area is called the brachial plexus. The knowledge of this anatomic structure is essential to plan and interpret the EDX procedures. (Copyright Nandedkar Productions LLC, 2010.)

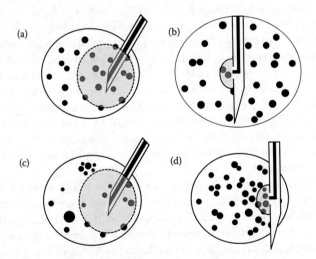

FIGURE 46.3 Cross section of a motor unit shown schematically. A single fiber electrode is superimposed on the MU cross section in (b) and (d). The shaded semicircular area near the recording tip represents the recording territory. The concentric needle (a, c) records from a much larger circular recording area. In both types of recordings, the needle is placed close to fibers of the MU. (a) A normal small MU contains fibers distributed randomly in a roughly circular territory. (b) A normal large MU. The MU in (a) is shown after (c) myopathy and (d) reinnervation (neuropathy). Note the significant difference in MU architecture that will affect the MUP waveform (shown in Figure 46.10). (Copyright Nandedkar Productions LLC, 2010.)

The axons connecting the lower MNs to the muscle fibers constitute the "motor" component of a nerve. Most nerves also contain sensory axons. The sensory axon cell body lies outside the spinal cord in the sensory ganglion (Figure 46.2). Their axons terminate in various sense organs, for example, for touch, sight, sound, and so on. The sensory innervation to fingers and thumbs is shown in Figure 46.2. Note that the hand receives sensory innervation by different nerves and roots. The lesion of individual roots or nerves will affect the sensation in different digits. Thus, the patient symptoms and physical examination will allow the clinician to select the appropriate nerves for testing.

The sensory axons convey information from the periphery toward the spinal cord and the brain, while the motor axons provide activation to the muscles located in the periphery. Together, they form a feedback system that allows a smooth coordination of muscular activity. Note that the motor fibers form the ventral root while the sensory fibers make up the dorsal root (Figure 46.2). The roots, nerves, and muscles are considered as the peripheral nervous system. The MNs (upper and lower) and their spinal connections make up the central nervous system.

The "autonomic" nervous system is responsible for other neuromuscular functions, for example, respiration and circulation, that occur subconsciously. The assessment of this system requires a different battery of tests that is beyond the scope of this chapter.

46.3 Physiology

The nerve and muscle cells are electrically "active." In their "resting" state, the cell maintains a voltage difference of 80 mV across the cell membrane, the intracellular being negative (Figure 46.1b-a). If the cell depolarizes, that is, the intracellular potential increases from −80 to −50 mV (Figure 46.1b-b), an action potential (AP) is generated. It begins by opening the voltage-dependent sodium channels in the membrane, causing a flux of sodium ions from the extracellular space to the intracellular space. The intracellular space becomes positive with respect to the extracellular space by roughly 30 mV (Figure 46.1b-c). The sodium channels then close while potassium channels open. The movement of potassium ions from the intracellular space to the extracellular space (Figure 46.1b-d) restores the cell to its normal state (Figure 46.1b-e). This event lasts for only a millisecond or two. The depolarization also spreads along the muscle or nerve fiber, causing the propagation (or conduction) of the AP. The initial depolarization of the cell membrane to produce the AP occurs via the release of neurotransmitters such as acetylcholine. The cell membrane can also be depolarized by applying an external electrical or magnetic field. This forms the basis for the nerve (or muscle) stimulation to perform conduction studies.

The nerve fibers are surrounded by an insulating tissue called myelin (Figure 46.4). The myelin is absent at the "node of Ranvier." Owing to the low impedance at the exposed region, the nerve can depolarize easily at the node. The net effect is that the AP "jumps" from one node to another in contrast to a smooth propagation seen in muscle fibers. This mechanism, called "saltatory" conduction, gives a higher velocity in nerve fibers (30–60 m/s) than in muscle fibers (2–6 m/s). The larger the fiber diameter, the higher is the conduction velocity.

The voluntary muscle activity begins by the depolarization of the MN. A nerve AP is generated and it propagates from the neuron to the periphery along the axon. When the nerve AP arrives in the endplate, the neurotransmitter "acetylcholine (Ach)" is released from the nerve ending. The Ach diffuses to the muscle membrane and causes its depolarization. The muscle fiber AP propagates from the endplate to the tendons (Figure 46.1c). Its passage activates the contractile elements of the fiber, causing it to twitch and generate a force. Thus, every time the MN discharges, all fibers of that MU respond by producing a mechanical twitch and their AP. The sum of APs of all fibers in the MU is the motor unit potential (MUP) (Figure 46.1d).

The EDX recordings are made in extracellular space. The relationship between intracellular AP (ICAP) and extracellular AP (ECAP) has been investigated using mathematical models and computer simulations (Plonsey, 1964; Andreassen and Rosenfalck, 1981; Henneberg and Plonsey, 1994; Henneberg and Roberge, 1997). The ECAP has a triphasic waveform that is quite different from the ICAP. When

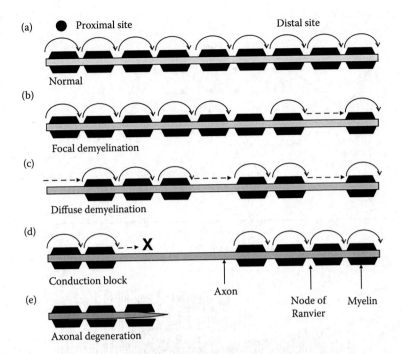

FIGURE 46.4 A normal axon (a) and its structural changes with pathology (b–e). Curved arrows indicate the saltatory conduction of AP from one node to the next. The conduction block is indicated by "X." The distal and proximal stimulation sites are shown to match abnormalities shown in Figure 46.7. (Copyright Nandedkar Productions LLC, 2010.)

the ICAP approaches the recording electrode, the electromyograph records a positive voltage (Figure 46.1c). This, by convention in EMG, produces a downward deflection on the instrument display. The main spike of the ECAP occurs when the ICAP passes the electrode. When the ICAP moves away from the electrode, the terminal positive phase is seen.

The amplitude of the ECAP decreases with the distance between the fiber and the recording electrode (Figure 46.1c). The rate of decline depends on the size of the recording surface. Small electrodes (e.g., single fiber needle) have a high rate of amplitude decline and allow "selective" recording from muscle fibers near the electrode tip (Figure 46.3b,d). Large recording surface (e.g., concentric needle) has a slower radial decline of amplitude. Hence, they can record from a much larger portion of the muscle (Figure 46.3a,c). Using electrodes of different sizes, one can obtain complementary information about the changes in MU with pathology and disease progression.

46.4 EMG and Force Generation

The MU twitch from a single MN discharge lasts only for a short period of time (<100 ms in most muscles). To maintain a constant force, the MN discharges in a recurrent manner. This continuous discharge is recognized from a corresponding MUP discharge on the EMG display (Figure 46.5). When the discharge rate (also called the firing rate) of the MU increases, the twitch from successive contractions will combine to produce a higher force. This mechanism of increasing the force is called "frequency modulation." Additional force is also generated by activating another MU. In EMG recordings, one can observe MUP discharges of that MU. The process of increasing the force by the activation of additional MUs is called "recruitment." All muscles use a combination of these two strategies to provide and maintain the desired force.

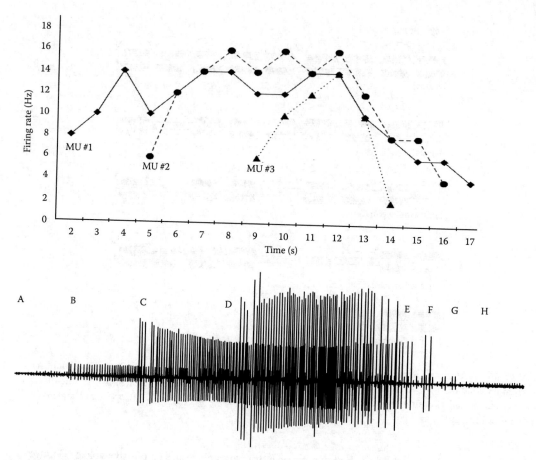

FIGURE 46.5 Concentric needle EMG recording in the biceps muscle of a normal subject when the force of contraction was increased gradually. The recruitment of MUs is easily recognized by their larger-amplitude MUP. A: Baseline, B: First MU is recruited. C: Second MU is recruited. D: Third MU is recruited. E: Third MU stops. F: Second MU stops. G: First MU stops. H: Baseline. The inserted diagram of firing rates shows a parallel change (increase or decrease) with force in all MUs. (Copyright Nandedkar Productions LLC, 2010.)

The MU recruitment is governed by their size. At rest, the EMG signal contains the baseline (Figure 46.5A). At slight effort, a small MU begins to discharge (Figure 46.5B). When the force of contraction is increased, its firing rate increases. With further increase in the force, a new MU is recruited (Figure 46.5C). Additional force is generated by increasing the firing rate of both MUs and then a third MU is recruited (Figure 46.5D). The process continues as necessary. The MUs recruited later are larger in size. When the subject relaxes, the firing rate of the MUs reduces. The MUs stop discharging in the reverse order of recruitment, that is, the large late-recruited MUs stop first, and the early-recruited MUs stop later (Figure 46.5E, F, G, H). This orderly process of activation and deactivation of the MUs is called the "size principle." The parallel increase or decrease in the firing rate of the MUs is called the "central drive" for the activation of the lower MN by the central nervous system (DeLuca et al., 1982).

46.5 Pathology

The neuromuscular diseases are classified using the primary site of the lesion. In "myopathy," the defect is in the muscle (Figure 46.3b). The main disease process is the loss of muscle fibers. In addition, the muscle fiber diameter variability is increased; some fibers become atrophic while others become hypertrophic. The hypertrophic muscle fibers may split into a cluster of smaller fibers. Examples of such diseases are the different types of dystrophies.

The MN disease can occur by the loss of MNs or by changes in their excitability. The loss of excitation will cause weakness, while hyperexcitability will cause spasticity. Polio and amyotrophic lateral sclerosis (ALS, also known as Lou Gehrig's disease) are examples of MN disease causing the death of the neuron.

The lesions of nerve, called "neuropathy," are very common. If the nerve lesion occurs at the root, it is called radiculopathy. Most patients describe this condition as a "pinched nerve in the neck or the back." A lesion affecting a single nerve is called a "mononeuropathy," while a polyneuropathy affects many nerves. The nerve lesion, from an EDX perspective, can occur in three principal ways (Figure 46.4). In demyelination, the myelin surrounding the nerve fiber is lost. It can be focal due to nerve compression (e.g., carpal tunnel syndrome, Figure 46.4b) or diffuse (e.g., due to diabetes, Figure 46.4c). Despite demyelination, the fiber can conduct the AP. The propagation velocity is however reduced. If demyelination is significant, the nerve fiber may become inexcitable. The segment distal (i.e., toward the periphery) and proximal (i.e., toward the spinal cord) to the site of the lesion can be normal. This is called the conduction block (Figure 46.4d). The conduction block can reverse and has a good prognosis. Axonopathy refers to the loss and the degeneration of nerve fibers (Figure 46.4e). This is the most severe form of the nerve lesion. We emphasize that this classification of nerve injury is slightly different from its classical description based on histological neural assessment by Sunderland (1991).

When an MN dies or the nerve fiber degenerates, the muscle fibers from that MU can no longer participate in voluntary contraction. These "denervated" muscle fibers receive terminal axon branches from the surviving MUs. As a result, one observes focal grouping of muscle fibers instead of their random distribution (Figure 46.3d). Also, the MU size is increased. The compensatory reinnervation can be adequate such that the patient may not have weakness despite significant (up to 50%) loss of MUs.

The diseases of the neuromuscular junction also cause weakness. Examples of this disease type are myasthenic gravis or the botulinum toxin poisoning.

46.6 Instrumentation

The main components of an electromyograph are a high-quality amplifier, an electrical stimulator, and a suitable display device. In the past, oscilloscopes were used for signal display. Modern systems use personal computers to digitize the signals and to display them on the computer screen. They also have the ability to store the recordings, apply signal processing algorithms to reduce the noise, perform automated analysis of waveforms, and so on.

A differential amplifier is used for signal recordings. This requires three recording electrodes: active, reference, and ground (Figure 46.6a). The amplifier measures the voltage difference between the potentials recorded by the active and reference electrodes. The ground electrode is necessary to reduce the noise. A system can have many amplifiers (called "channels") to allow recording from several sites at the same time. This is necessary for evoked potential studies. Most routine EMG and nerve conduction studies require only one channel. The differential amplification allows the system to magnify the physiologic potential while minimizing the ambient noise that is common to the active and reference input. The common mode rejection ratio of modern amplifiers exceeds 100 decibels. They also have an input impedance in excess of 100 MΩ.

The amplifiers also contain analog high-pass and low-pass filters to reduce the noise. An analog-to-digital convertor is used to sample the signals. The sampling frequency varies among different applications. In most cases, the bandpass filter settings are 10 Hz to 10 kHz. Hence, a sampling rate of 50 kHz is quite adequate. The modern systems also use digital filtering to further attenuate the noise.

The electrical stimulator is used to apply a depolarizing electrical field to the nerves. It can be programmed to deliver a pulse of constant voltage or constant current output. The output is varied by the user in the range of 0–400 V, or 0–100 mA. The duration of the pulse is also changed from 0.02 to 1 ms, as necessary. The stimulator has two pins: anode (positive pole) and cathode (negative pole). For the

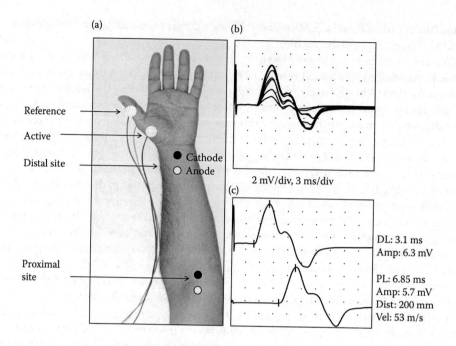

FIGURE 46.6 Median motor nerve conduction study. (a) The recording electrodes and stimulation sites are shown. The ground electrode placed on hand dorsum is not seen. (b) The change in distal CMAP with increasing stimulus intensity is shown. (c) The distal (top trace) and proximal (bottom trace) CMAPs have similar shape but the proximal CMAP has lower amplitude. (Copyright Nandedkar Productions LLC, 2010.)

nerve stimulation, the cathode is placed on the skin surface over the stimulation site (Figure 46.6a). The negative field in the extracellular space reduces the potential difference across the cell membrane, that is, it is depolarized and generates an AP under the cathode.

When the stimulus is delivered, the system acquires and displays one sweep of activity (Figure 46.6b). In this manner, the signals seen on the screen are time locked to the stimulation. The stimulus currents spread instantaneously to the recording electrodes though the skin and the fat tissue. This is recorded as the "stimulus" artifact at the beginning of the trace. The artifact is followed by the nerve or muscle response. The position of the anode is usually adjusted to minimize the stimulus artifacts.

The needle EMG signals are displayed in a free-running sweep mode. The sweep duration is usually 10 ms per division on the display grid. The sensitivity (also called gain) is adjusted as necessary (50–1000 μV/division). The signals are also assessed from their sound on an audio monitor. Experienced EMGers rely heavily on the EMG sound to adjust the needle position and to interpret different types of potentials.

The neurophysiologic potentials are best recorded using two strategies. First, the ambient noise should be reduced. Fluorescent lights give less noise than incandescent lights. The electrode cables act as an antenna and record the noise. Hence, their length should be no longer than necessary (usually <3 ft). If a longer cable is needed, it should be shielded. One should unplug all other equipments in the examination room. Using a dedicated circuit for the EDX system also helps to reduce power line frequency interference. The recording electrode cables should be directed away from any source of electromagnetic radiation, for example, power cords, computer terminals, and other electronic devices.

The second strategy is to ensure that electrodes have a good contact with the patient. The skin surface should be cleaned using water or alcohol swabs. In some instances, the dry layer of dead skin cells should be removed using a mild abrasive. Conductive gel should be used to enhance the contact with the skin surface. Electrodes may be secured using an adhesive tape. When the signal amplitude is very low, one should check and reduce the impedance to less than 5 kΩ. Furthermore, the impedance of active and reference electrodes should be similar. Large difference in electrode impedance will effectively reduce the common mode rejection and yield noisy recordings.

The EDX system should be safe for the patient and the operator. The instrument must be connected to an electrical outlet that is properly grounded. This will provide a low resistance path for the leakage current. When intramuscular electrodes are used, they should be disposed properly to avoid any cross infection. Some electrodes (e.g., single fiber) are very expensive and may be reused. The electrode manufacturer can describe the proper methods for resterilization.

46.7 EDX Study

The primary objective of the EDX study is to locate the site of the lesion (nerve, muscle, neuromuscular junction, etc.). In addition, one would like to assess the severity and time course (acute versus chronic), and possibly make a prognosis. The EDX physician reviews patient history and performs a physical examination to assess abnormal sensation, weakness, and movement. This allows the formulation of a differential diagnosis, that is, a set of conditions that can explain the patient symptoms. Next, a set of tests are performed to confirm or refute different conditions in the differential diagnosis. We will not discuss the strategy of test selection, and describe only the principles of these procedures.

46.8 Motor Nerve Conduction

In the motor nerve conduction study (MNCS), surface electrodes are used to record the activity from a muscle innervated by the tested nerve. Figure 46.6a illustrates the setup for a median motor NCS. The "active" recording surface is over the belly of abductor pollicis brevis (APB) muscle, and a "reference" electrode is placed distally over the thumb. The first stimulation site for the median nerve is at the wrist where the nerve is quite superficial. At minimal stimulus intensity, the electrical field is insufficient to depolarize any nerve fibers. Hence, no response is registered. When the intensity is increased, some axons in the nerve will be stimulated (i.e., they will adequately depolarize to generate the AP). Their APs will propagate to the muscle and activate the muscle fibers innervated by them. One may recognize a small twitch and a concomitant low-voltage electrical response on the display. When the intensity is increased, more nerve fibers will be stimulated and the response will become larger (Figure 46.6b). One continues to increase the intensity until the amplitude (i.e., signal voltage) is maximized. This indicates that all nerve fibers are stimulated. To ensure that the response is maximal, the intensity is increased further by 10–20% and the resulting potential is accepted for analysis. The signal is a sum of MUP of all MUs in the muscle and is called the "compound muscle action potential (CMAP)" (Figure 46.6c). In motor nerve conduction studies, the recording electrode is placed over the end-plate zone of the muscle. Since there is no approaching volley of APs, the CMAP does not have an initial positive phase. An initial negative (i.e., upward) deflection is used as an indication of proper electrode placement.

The CMAP is characterized by its "latency" and "amplitude." The latency is the time from stimulation (i.e., beginning of sweep) to the onset of the response. The amplitude is the voltage difference between the negative (i.e., upward) peak and the baseline. In Figure 46.6c, the onset and the peak are indicated by the two vertical tick marks. The latency reflects the propagation velocity while the amplitude reflects the number of nerve and muscle fibers contributing to the response. The latency at the wrist is called the "distal latency (DL)." In addition, one can also measure the duration and area under the negative peak. Although the surface EMG recording is mainly a low-frequency signal (<1 kHz), the bandpass filter settings for MNCS are 3 Hz to 10 kHz. Increasing the high-pass setting to even 20 Hz will significantly reduce the CMAP amplitude.

Next, the nerve is stimulated at the elbow (Figure 46.6c, bottom trace). The latency of this response is called the "proximal latency (PL)." In anatomic descriptions, a distal site is farther away from the spinal cord. The distance between the elbow and the wrist stimulation sites is measured with a measuring tape and is used to compute the conduction velocity as follows:

$$\text{Velocity (m/s)} = \text{distance}/(\text{proximal latency} - \text{distal latency})$$

In the above formula, latency is measured in milliseconds and distance in millimeters. As indicated earlier, the nerve fibers have different diameters and hence different conduction velocities. Hence, their APs reach the muscle at different times with respect to stimulation. The onset of CMAP reflects the propagation in the fastest axons. The difference in the arrival time of the fastest and slowest conducting axons is called "temporal dispersion." When the dispersion is less, the MUPs are almost synchronous and their sum, that is, CMAP, has a high amplitude. The temporal dispersion will be more with a longer distance between the stimulation and recording sites. The CMAP amplitude decreases due to "misalignment" of individual MUPs. This is called "phase cancelation" and can give a 10–20% amplitude drop on proximal stimulation (Figure 46.6c).

The type and site of the nerve lesion can be characterized by stimulating the nerve at many sites. In Figure 46.7, waveforms with different types of pathology (Figure 46.4) are compared. The top two traces are recorded from the distal and the proximal sites in a normal nerve (Figure 46.4a). In Figure 46.7b, there is a focal lesion causing a slow conduction distal to both stimulating sites (Figure 46.4b). Hence, the DL and PL are increased. However, the conduction velocity is normal, indicating a normal nerve between the two stimulation sites. In Figure 46.7c, the reduced amplitude indicates an axon loss (Figure 46.4e). The proximal stimulation appears to produce no response. But changing the gain and sweep shows that the response is significantly delayed, that is, reduced conduction velocity (Figure 46.7d). The slow conduction in the distal and proximal segments indicates a diffused demyelinating process as well (Figure 46.4c). There is a significant change in the CMAP waveform due to the increased temporal dispersion. In Figure 46.7e, the amplitude is much smaller at the proximal site but there is no change in the waveform. This indicates a conduction block between the distal and proximal stimulation sites (Figure 46.4d).

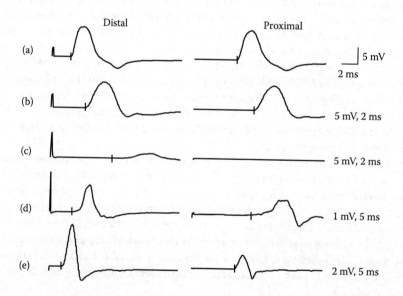

FIGURE 46.7 The CMAP waveforms at distal and proximal stimulation sites in various pathologies are compared with normal responses. See the text for details of (a)–(e). (Copyright Nandedkar Productions LLC, 2010.)

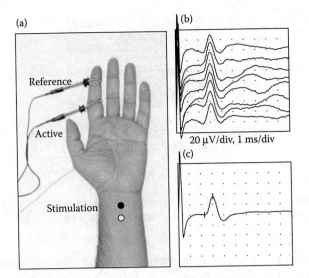

FIGURE 46.8   Median sensory nerve conduction study. (a) The antidromic method shows ring electrodes used for recording the response. The ground electrode, placed on hand dorsum, is not seen. (b) The response to individual stimuli shows a time-locked response and also background noise. (c) Averaging these responses gives a SNAP with stable baseline. (Copyright Nandedkar Productions LLC, 2010.)

46.9 Sensory Nerve Conduction

The sensory nerve conduction study (SNCS) is also performed in a similar manner. In Figure 46.8a, the nerve is stimulated at the wrist and the response is recorded over the index finger. The signal recorded at the supramaximal intensity is called the "sensory nerve action potential (SNAP)" (Figure 46.8c). This response is recorded from nerve fibers that are fewer in number compared to the number of muscle fibers stimulated in an MNCS. Therefore, the SNAP amplitude is much smaller (typically 5–100 μV). To reduce the noise, the bandpass filter settings are often set at 20 Hz to 2 kHz. On successive stimulations, the response is time locked to the stimulus while the noise is random (Figure 46.8b). Hence, averaging many responses helps reduce the baseline noise in SNAP (Figure 46.8c). Because of poor signal-to-noise ratio, it is difficult to assess the onset of SNAP. The latency of the negative peak is used for analysis. The SNCS is usually performed using a short distance between the stimulation and recording sites. A longer distance gives a much smaller SNAP amplitude. In the above method, the nerve AP propagated from the wrist to the finger, which is opposite of the natural direction of sensory nerve AP propagation (from digit toward wrist). Hence, this is called the "antidromic" technique. In "orthodromic" technique, one uses distal stimulation (e.g., digit II) and records the response proximally (e.g., over the wrist). Both methods are widely used in the EMG laboratory. In pathology, the conduction velocity is reduced and gives an increased SNAP latency. The loss of sensory axons and/or increased temporal dispersion give a reduced amplitude.

46.10 Needle EMG

The routine needle EMG study is performed using a concentric (CN) or monopolar (MN) electrode (Figure 46.9). The CN is made by inserting a metal wire through a hollow metal cylinder (called cannula). The tip of the assembly is ground to expose an elliptical recording surface (the core). The monopolar needle is an insulated metal wire that is ground to expose a cone-shaped recording surface. A surface electrode is used as a reference electrode. A ground electrode is also placed on the tested limb. The low-pass filter frequency is set to 10 kHz while the high-pass frequency is set to 10–20 Hz.

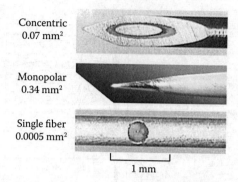

Concentric
0.07 mm²

Monopolar
0.34 mm²

Single fiber
0.0005 mm²

|— 1 mm —|

FIGURE 46.9 The geometry and construction of different needle EMG electrodes. Note the significant difference in their recording surface. The difference in the recording territory is shown in Figure 46.3. (Copyright Nandedkar Productions LLC, 2010.)

The needle EMG study has four steps. First, the needle is moved briskly into the tested muscle. The mechanical irritation causes a burst of sharp electrical potentials, called "insertional activity (IA)" (Figure 46.10, top row). The normal IA stops almost immediately after the needle movement stops (left trace). In pathology, the IA may be increased. After the needle movement stops, one can observe a sustained electrical activity (middle trace). This indicates an "unstable" muscle fiber membrane. In a wasted muscle, the IA is reduced. One observes a slow deflection of baseline without any sharp potentials following the needle movement (right trace).

In the second step, the patient is instructed to relax the tested muscle while holding the needle steady to observe the "spontaneous activity (SA)" (Figure 46.10, second row). In normal muscles one observes a quiet baseline, that is, no SA. If the needle is in the end-plate area, one may record sharp and irregularly discharging spikes. These are "end-plate spikes" and are considered normal (left trace). In pathology, SA may be seen as a single muscle fiber AP discharges in various configurations (e.g., fibrillation and positive sharp wave) (middle trace), or MUP discharges in various patterns (fasciculations, myokymia, etc.) (right trace). Abnormal SA is usually a nonspecific observation as it can be seen in patients with myopathy and neuropathy.

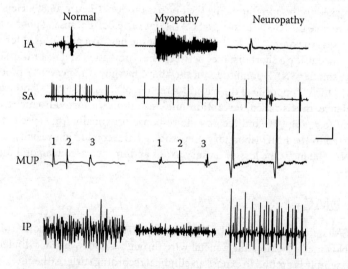

FIGURE 46.10 EMG recordings in normal subjects and patients with pathology. The amplitude calibration is 100 μV for IA, SA; 200 μV for MUPs; and 1000 μV for IP. The time calibration is 100 ms for IA, SA, and IP, and 10 ms for MUPs. See the text for details. (Copyright Nandedkar Productions LLC, 2010.)

In the third step, the patient contracts the tested muscle slightly to activate a few MUs. One observes that their MUP discharges on the screen. The needle position is manipulated to bring the electrode close to the muscle fibers of the active MU (Figure 46.3). When this is achieved, the EMG signal has a "crisp" sound that is rich in high frequencies. The signal amplitude also increases and the positive to the negative peak (i.e., down to up deflection) rise time is reduced. Examples of such recordings are shown in the third row of Figure 46.10. Individual MUPs are indicated by numbers. The peak-to-peak amplitude, duration, and overall shape are assessed. The duration best differentiates neuropathy from myopathy. The amplitude is increased in neuropathy. The waveform is polyphasic (more than four phases) in myopathy or neuropathy.

Finally, the patient increases the force to the maximal effort to activate all MUs, and the interference pattern (IP) is recorded (Figure 46.10, bottom row). In normal subjects, the MU activity completely obscures the baseline to give a "full pattern" (left trace). Patients with myopathy activate many MUs even at a slight effort. This is described as "increased" or "early" recruitment of MUs. At maximal effort, the IP has a full pattern with reduced amplitude (middle trace). In neuropathy, the baseline is not filled due to MU loss. The signal amplitude is also higher, indicating higher MUP amplitude (right trace). The recruitment is described as "reduced," indicating fewer MUs discharging for the level of effort.

The above patterns on MUP and IP abnormalities are seen in moderately affected muscles. In severely weak muscles, the MUP abnormalities may have features of neuropathy and myopathy (e.g., increased amplitude and reduced duration). Such recordings can be challenging for assessment.

In needle EMG examination, the shape of the MUP is assessed by visual inspection. Changes in MUP parameters can be useful to assess mild abnormalities, and to differentiate neuropathy from myopathy. However, the process of identifying and analyzing MUPs was tedious and time consuming. It took 30 min or more to record 20 MUPs from one tested muscle. With access to signal processing technology, it is now possible to decompose the EMG signal into constituent MUPs (Figure 46.11). The principle of analysis is quite simple. An MUP waveform repeats at a fairly constant rate in the EMG epoch. Most algorithms (McGill et al., 1985) filter the EMG signal to enhance the spike components. An amplitude level is used to detect and to break down the signal in spikes containing sharp and

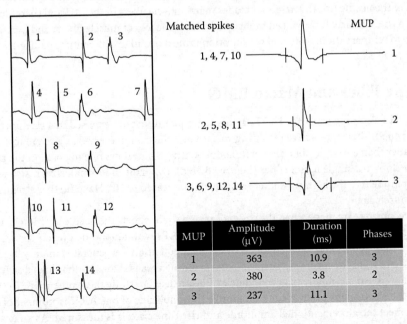

MUP	Amplitude (μV)	Duration (ms)	Phases
1	363	10.9	3
2	380	3.8	2
3	237	11.1	3

FIGURE 46.11 Schematic of the multimotor unit analysis. See the text for details. (Copyright Nandedkar Productions LLC, 2010.)

high-amplitude EMG spikes. Template-matching algorithms are used to identify spikes that repeat in the EMG signal. Averaging such spikes yields the MUP. In Figure 46.11, one can recognize 14 spikes. Furthermore, the first spike matched spikes 4, 7, and 10. Because this spike repeats in the signal, it is considered as MUP. These spikes are averaged to obtain the MUP and to measure its amplitude, duration, area, phases, and so on. In a similar manner, two other MUPs are detected in this recording. The spike labeled 13 did not match any other MUP. Hence, it was not used for analysis. Careful observation shows that this spike was not a single MUP waveform but rather a superimposition of MUP 1 and MUP 2. One such algorithm, called multimotor unit analysis (Nandedkar et al., 1995), has been used successfully in EMG laboratories for more than 15 years. It allows the clinician to record and analyze 20 different MUPs in less than 5 min.

Techniques such as multimotor unit analysis focus on recognizing the waveform for its measurement. When the MUP is corrupted by other MUPs (e.g., spike 13 in Figure 46.11), it makes no significant effort to resolve that template. Hence, some MUP discharges may not be identified. This can give an incorrect instantaneous firing rate. The objective of the precision decomposition technique is to study the MU firing rate. DeLuca and coworkers (1982) used a special needle to register three channels of EMG activity. By comparing the MU activity on each channel, they were able to identify the majority of the MUP discharges even at moderate effort and despite superimposition. Their studies have demonstrated the so-called central drive to the MUs (Figure 46.3). This should be useful to study the upper MN lesions that are not adequately assessed using the routine EDX methods.

Computer simulations (Nandedkar, 2002) indicate that MUP measurements provide complementary information about the MU architecture (Figures 46.3 and 46.10). The CN MUP amplitude is defined mainly by fibers within 0.5 mm of the needle tip, and especially by the size and distance of the closest muscle fiber. Therefore, it is increased following reinnervation in neuropathy. It may also increase due to hypertrophy in some patients with myopathy. The number of phases in the MUP is defined by the temporal dispersion of APs of muscle fibers within 1 mm of the active recording surface. When the dispersion increases, the MUP becomes polyphasic. In myopathy, this results from increased variability of fiber diameter. In neuropathy, polyphasic MUPs result from slow conduction in atrophic muscle fibers and newly formed terminal axon branches. The MUP duration is defined by muscle fibers that are within 2.5 mm of the needle tip. This region includes many muscle fibers of the MU and therefore helps study changes in the MU size. It is reduced in myopathy from the loss of muscle fibers, and increased in neuropathy due to reinnervation. Note that the duration is most useful to differentiate neuropathy from myopathy (Figure 46.3a,c).

46.11 Single Fiber and Macro EMG

The single fiber (SF) electrode consists of a 25 μm diameter platinum wire exposed in a side port of the cannula (Figure 46.9). This is the active recording surface and the cannula serves as a reference. The SF electrode is smaller than a muscle fiber diameter (about 50 μm). This allows one to position the recording surface very close to a single muscle fiber (Figure 46.3b,d). By virtue of its small size, it also records a very-high-amplitude AP. The high-pass filter frequency is increased to 500 Hz to further attenuate the APs of distant muscle fibers.

The SFEMG recordings are made when the patient exerts a slight effort. The needle position is manipulated to obtain high-amplitude APs with a short rise time. APs with amplitude greater than 200 μV and rise time less than 300 μs are accepted for analysis. Such potentials are generated mainly by muscle fibers within 300 μm from the recording surface. This recording area is shown by the shaded semicircle in Figure 46.3b and d. An amplitude trigger and delay line are used to study these potentials. In the FD measurements, the electrode is positioned to maximize the amplitude of one AP. The number of time-locked APs that meet the aforementioned amplitude and rise time criteria is measured. As an example, the electrode position shown in Figure 46.3b would yield a single muscle fiber AP (Figure 46.12a), while the position in Figure 46.3d will give five time-locked APs (Figure 46.12b). One counts the number of

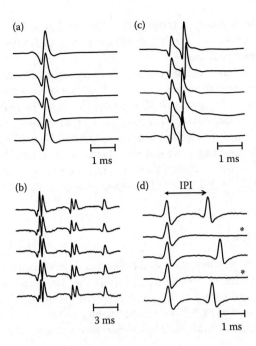

FIGURE 46.12 SFEMG recordings. (a) Single muscle fiber AP. (b) Five time-locked APs are recorded from a reinnervated MU. The MU architecture corresponding to traces in (a) and (b) is shown in Figures 46.3b and d, respectively. (c) Normal jitter (40 μs). (d) Increased jitter (180 μs) with blocking. (Copyright Nandedkar Productions LLC, 2010.)

such time-locked potentials from 20 sites in the tested muscle. The average of this measurement is called fiber density. In pathology, FD is increased due to the reorganization of muscles in the MU (Figure 46.3b versus d).

When a recording contains discharges of an AP pair (Figure 46.12c,d), the time between the APs varies from one discharge to another. This is called "jitter." To analyze this variability, the needle position is adjusted to obtain two (or more) APs. The time interval between the APs, called "interpotential interval (IPI)" is used to compute the "mean consecutive difference (MCD)"

$$MCD = \frac{\left|IPI_2 - IPI_1\right| + \left|IPI_3 - IPI_2\right| + \cdots + \left|IPI_N - IPI_{N-1}\right|}{N-1}$$

where N is the number of discharges. The terms "jitter" and "MCD" are often used as synonyms. In pathology, the MCD is increased compared to the normal. In more severe diseases, one of the APs may be missing in some discharges (Figure 46.12d, traces indicated by *). This is called "blocking." In patient studies, one records MCD from 20 different AP pairs in the tested muscle. Normal limits are defined for the mean MCD and also for individual MCD values. A study is considered abnormal when the mean jitter is increased and/or when three or more jitter values are abnormal.

The SFEMG is most sensitive to study the abnormalities of neuromuscular transmission (Stalberg et al., 2010). It is also technically challenging. The APs used for FD or jitter analysis are generated by muscle fibers that are less than 300 μm from the recording electrode. Signals will be lost even with a slight needle movement. One needs to practice the technique under supervision to feel comfortable with the quality of results and appreciate the pitfalls and errors. The operator should also take time to study the software necessary to analyze the SFEMG recordings. It often takes 30 min (or more) for experienced electromyographers to complete the jitter study in one muscle. The EDX instrument needs a high sampling rate to estimate IPI changes of just a few microseconds. Jitter analysis is usually an "option" among different software packages.

The Macro EMG electrode is a modified SF needle with the cannula insulated except for the distal 15 mm of the shaft. The SF recording surface is located at the center of the exposed part. The SFEMG recording is used to identify the discharges of one MU and the time-locked signals recorded by the cannula are averaged to obtain the "Macro MUP." The Macro MUPs are recorded from 20 different MUs and median values of amplitude and are used for analysis. Macro EMG is used mainly in research.

The SF or Macro EMG needles are expensive and reused after sterilization. The use of reusable electrodes is now banned in many countries. Hence, there is a great interest in using disposable concentric electrodes for jitter analysis. Stalberg and Sanders (2009) have described the guidelines and limitations of using this approach.

46.12 Evoked Potentials

The routine motor and sensory nerve conduction studies can detect nerve pathology distal to the stimulation site. Proximal and central lesions can be studied using the "late responses," but they are usually not very sensitive. The evoked potential (EP) studies record the nerve AP as it propagates from the periphery to the cortex (Chiappa, 1983). The EP studies may be broadly divided into three types: somatosensory evoked potential (SEP), brain stem auditory evoked response (BAER), and visual evoked potential (VEP).

The EP signals have much smaller amplitude than signals recorded in EMG or NCV studies, 0.5–10 μV in most cases. Hence, it is important to minimize the background noise and interference. One should clean the skin surface at the recording sites to remove any dirt and dead skin cells. An abrasive paste is used for this purpose. Electrolytic conductive gel is used when applying the electrode. The electrode impedance is measured, and it should be low (<5 kΩ) and similar on all electrodes. When the electrical stimulation is used, one should also reduce the impedance at the stimulation site. High impedance would require higher voltage to obtain the desired response and it will be quite painful for the patient.

The EP signals have very low amplitude and they cannot be recognized in the background noise, interference, EMG, or EEG activity. However, the signals are time locked to the stimulus. By averaging these time-locked responses, the signal-to-noise ratio is improved. Because the signals are very small, one must perform two or more independent averages to demonstrate the reproducibility of responses. The number of sweeps range from 100 to over 2000 depending upon the type of recording and patient pathology. A single modality of EP study can easily take 20–30 min. Hence, the patient should be in a comfortable position to reduce any movement and EMG artifacts. Most of the recording sites in an EP study are over the cortex. The positions (e.g., Cz, Fz, O1, and C3) are described by the so-called "10–20" system. It is beyond the scope of this review to describe them.

46.13 Somatosensory Evoked Potential

The technique of SEP is illustrated using a median nerve study (Figure 46.13). The nerve is stimulated at the wrist at an intensity level greater than the sensory perception threshold. A slight twitch of thumb may be observed. Recording electrodes are placed over the sensory cortex (channel 1), cervical spine at the C5 level (channel 2) and the Erb's point (channel 3). The Erb's point on the opposite side is used as a reference electrode in many channels. When the nerve AP arrives at the electrode, a positive (P) or negative (N) peak is registered. It is labeled using its typical latency from the stimulus. Thus, the N9 response, recorded at the Erb's point, is a negative (upward) peak with an expected latency of 9 ms. The absolute latencies and interpeak latency differences are used for analysis. In pathology, the latency is increased, indicating slow conduction. Interpeak latencies allow the localization of the lesion.

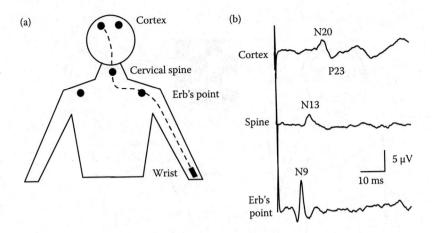

FIGURE 46.13 (a) Schematic illustration of the median SEP recording technique. (b) Recordings from a normal subject. (Copyright Nandedkar Productions LLC, 2010.)

The N13 potential is registered when APs pass through the spinal cord at the C5 level. The difference between N13 and N9 peaks represents the time of AP propagation in the most proximal part of the nerve, that is, the roots. This latency difference should be abnormal in root lesions, that is, radiculopathy. The N20 peak represents the AP arrival at the cortex. The time difference between N20 and N13 peaks is called the central conduction time. This will be increased in demyelinating central nervous system diseases such as multiple sclerosis. The SEP recordings test the integrity of the nerve from the periphery to the cortex. Hence, it is used for monitoring purposes in spinal cord surgery. A sudden increase in latency or drop in amplitude alerts the surgeon of a possible compromise of the neural pathways.

46.14 Brainstem Auditory Evoked Response

In the BAER study, an auditory stimulus is delivered via shielded headphones (Figure 46.14a). The study begins by measuring the hearing threshold of the tested ear. An intensity level 60–70 decibels (dB) above the hearing threshold is used for testing. The stimulus is described as a "click"-like sound that contains low and high frequencies. Modern instruments can deliver other types of auditory stimuli, for example, tones of different frequency. The auditory stimulus delivered on the tested side is "conducted" through the skull to the opposite side and heard faintly. To mask this effect, a white noise sound is given to the opposite side, that is, untested ear. The white noise intensity is typically 40 dB less than the test stimulus level.

A two-channel montage is used with recording electrodes placed behind the ears and over the mastoid process. A reference electrode is placed over the center of the skull (i.e., Cz position). The filter settings are 30–3000 Hz. The stimulus is given at a rate of 10–11 clicks per second. One requires several hundred, sometimes more than 1000, stimuli to obtain a good-quality average.

The BAER has a complex waveform with five or six negative peaks, called "waves." Wave I is recorded from the side of stimulation and represents the response of the auditory nerve. The remaining waves occur from deeper structures in the brain. They are registered on both channels and are called "far field potentials." As in SEP, one analyzes the absolute latencies and interpeak latencies (Wave I–Wave III, Wave III–Wave V). The amplitude of Wave I and Wave V may also be measured. The BAER is useful to study the lesions of the auditory nerve (e.g., acoustic neuroma) and the brain stem.

The BAER is also useful to test hearing. One method is to measure the Wave I latency and amplitude change when the stimulus intensity is reduced. Another method is to measure the hearing threshold using tones of difference frequencies. The absolute values and side-to-side differences are assessed.

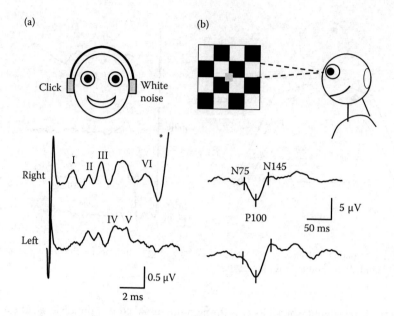

FIGURE 46.14 (a) The technique of BAER shown schematically. The waves IV and V are better recognized on the lower trace recorded from the opposite side. Near the end of the recording, a high-amplitude muscle artifact (indicated by *) is seen. (b) Illustration of the visual EP technique. Two trials show a reproducible response. (Copyright Nandedkar Productions LLC, 2010.)

46.15 Visual Evoked Potential

In the VEP study, the recording electrodes are placed over the occipital lobe of the cortex (Figure 46.14b). The stimulus is a checker board pattern that reverses the black and white squares. The pattern is shown on a cathode ray tube (CRT). The patient sits in front of the CRT at a distance such that a single check produces a 1° angle from the eye. The untested eye is covered with a patch and the patient is instructed to focus at the center of the screen, indicated by a small colored dot or square (called "fixation"). The VEP is a low-frequency signal and the bandpass filters are set at 1–100 Hz. The pattern is reversed twice every second. Signal averaging is used to extract the response from the background activity.

The VEP signal is much larger in amplitude compared to other EP recordings. Hence, a good signal is usually obtained in less than 200 stimuli. The response has a triphasic appearance with negative peaks at 75 ms (N75) and 140 ms (N140), and a positive peak at 100 ms (P100) latency. The latency of P100 peak and its amplitude are used for analysis. In pathology (e.g., multiple sclerosis), the latency is increased and the amplitude reduced. Side-to-side comparisons are also performed to assess abnormality.

The VEP pattern could be shown using an LCD screen. However, the refresh rate of the LCD may be slow and will not give a fast reversal of the pattern. Although this defect is not seen visually, the VEP does give a longer P100 latency even in normal subjects. Proper recordings also require the patient to focus on the "fixation" point on the screen. Staring at the pattern can be difficult for many subjects. Gazing elsewhere can give poor-quality waveforms. Hence, the operator administering the test must watch the patient and encourage them to focus on the screen. The waveforms are also affected by the contrast and brightness of the CRT and the illumination in the room. Each laboratory should develop its own "normal" values and then leave the CRT settings untouched. If this is not possible, one should test a few healthy subjects to ensure that results on the instrument are consistent with those reported in the literature.

46.16 Engineering in EDX

Biomedical engineers have made major contributions to make EDX a powerful diagnostic tool. The most obvious change is seen in instrumentation. Modern systems are portable and lightweight. This allows the physician to perform studies outside the EDX laboratory, for example, in intensive care unit, and satellite clinics The quality of amplifiers has improved, making it possible to record low-amplitude SNAPs. Signal averagers are available to improve the signal-to-noise ratio. The test settings (e.g., filters and amplifier gain) are loaded automatically to reduce technical errors. Test protocols can be defined for different diagnoses to ensure that the necessary tests are performed. Modern systems allow vast amount of data storage so that the signals can be saved and reviewed. Algorithms are developed to reduce the stimulation artifacts. It is possible to make more measurements, manually or automatically, than just 20 years ago. The patient data is saved in databases that can be analyzed for research. Patient reports can be uploaded to the hospital information system and made available for remote review.

Computer simulations have given us a better understanding of the EDX recordings. Note that the MUP measurements give complementary information about the MU architecture. By studying the changes in each measurement, one can get a better understanding of the underlying pathophysiology. Using a combination of different recording techniques (e.g., SFEMG and Macro EMG), one can study disease progression (Nandedkar and Stalberg, 2008).

Engineers have made significant contributions to signal measurements. Automatic methods such as MMA have reduced the time of quantitative MUP analysis by 70–80%. Marking algorithms in conduction studies have reduced the time of study, and improved the reproducibility of measurements.

The needle EMG recordings are uncomfortable for patients. Surface EMG signals do not offer the resolution to detect single muscle fiber potentials. Hence, they are not sensitive for diagnostic purpose. However, it would be of great interest to use surface EMG to perform follow-up studies to investigate disease progression (Merletti et al., 1985).

The EP studies are time consuming due to the large number of responses that must be averaged to obtain an acceptable signal-to-noise ratio. It would be of interest to develop better estimation methods for quicker and more reliable identification of EP signals. It will significantly reduce the patient discomfort. In intraoperative monitoring (IOM), this will give an earlier indication of any neural compromise during surgery.

The EDX study can generate a high volume of data. The clinician sorts the results of the conduction studies, needle EMG, and other tests to identify the underlying pathology. It would be of interest to develop "artificial intelligence" systems to support and aid this process (e.g., Pine et al., 2010). Such a system can not only aid the diagnosis but also suggest additional tests to increase the confidence in the test procedure. Such algorithms can also be used for teaching purposes. Biomedical engineers will continue to play an important role in developing future EMG systems that offer better signal quality, faster processing and measurement, knowledge databases, and rules for signal interpretation.

References

Andreassen S, Rosenfalck A: Relationship of intracellular and extracellular action potentials of skeletal muscle. *CRC Crit Rev Bioeng*, 1981; 16:267–306.

Chiappa K: *Evoked Potentials in Clinical Medicine*. Raven Press, New York, 1983.

DeLuca CJ, LeFever RS, McCue MP, Xenakis AP: Behavior of human motor units in different muscles during linearly varying contractions. *J Physiol*, 1982; 329:113–128.

Dumitru D, Amato A, Zwarts M: *Electrodiagnostic Medicine*. Hanley & Belfus Inc, Philadelphia, 2002.

Henneberg, K, Plonsey, R: Spatial and frequency domain ring source models for the single muscle fiber action potential. *Med Biol Eng Comput*, 1994; 32:27–34.

Henneberg, K, Roberge, FA: Simulation of propagation in a bundle of skeletal muscle fibers: Modulation effects of passive fibers. *Ann Biomed Eng*, 1997; 25:29–45.

McGill KC, Cummins KL, Dorfman LJ: Automatic decomposition of the clinical electromyogram. *IEEE Trans Biomed Eng*, 1985; BME-32:470–477.

Merletti R, Biey D, Biey M, Prato O, Orusa A: On-line monitoring of the median frequency of the surface EMG power spectrum. *IEEE BME*, 1985; 32:1–7.

Nandedkar SD: Models and simulations in electromyography. *Muscle Nerve*, 2002; Supplement 11:S46–S54.

Nandedkar SD, Barkhaus PE, Charles A: Multi-motor unit action potential analysis (MMA). *Muscle Nerve*, 1995; 18:1155–1166.

Nandedkar SD, Stalberg EV: Quantitative measurements and analysis in electrodiagnostic examination: Present and future. *Future Neurol*, 2008; 3:745–764.

Pine LJ, Stashuk DW, Bow SG, Doherty TJ: Probabilistic muscle characterization using DQEMG: Application to neuropathic muscle. *Muscle Nerve*, 2010; 41:18–31.

Plonsey R: Volume conduction fields of action currents. *Biophys J*, 1964; 4:317–328.

Stalberg E, Trontelj J, Sanders D: *Single Fiber EMG*. (Third edition). Edshagen Publishing House, Fiskebackskil, Sweden, 2010.

Stalberg EV, Sanders DB: Jitter recordings with concentric needle electrodes. *Muscle Nerve*, 2009; 40:331–339.

Sunderland S: *Nerve Injuries and Their Repair: A Critical Appraisal*. Churchill Livingstone, Edinburgh, 1991.

47

Principles of Electroencephalography

47.1 Historical Perspective 47-1
47.2 EEG Recording Techniques 47-2
47.3 Use of Amplitude Histograms to Quantify the EEG 47-4
    Mean • Standard Amplitude • Skewness • Kurtosis
47.4 Frequency Analysis of the EEG 47-7
47.5 Nonlinear Analysis of the EEG 47-8
Defining Terms 47-11
References 47-12
Further Information 47-12

Joseph D. Bronzino
Trinity College

Electroencephalograms (EEGs) are recordings of the minute (generally less than 300 µV) electrical potentials produced by the brain. Since 1924, when Hans Berger reported the recording of rhythmic electrical activity from the human scalp, analysis of EEG activity has been conducted primarily in clinical settings to detect gross pathologies and epilepsies and in research facilities to quantify the central effects of new pharmacologic agents. As a result of these efforts, cortical EEG patterns have shown to be modified by a wide range of variables, including biochemical, metabolic, circulatory, hormonal, neuroelectric, and behavioral factors. In the past, interpretation of the EEG was limited to visual inspection by an electroencephalographer, an individual trained to qualitatively distinguish normal EEG activity from localized or generalized abnormalities contained within relatively long EEG records. This approach left clinicians and researchers alike buried in a sea of EEG paper records. The advent of computers and the technologies associated with them has made it possible to effectively apply a host of methods to quantify the EEG changes. With this in mind, this chapter provides a brief historical perspective followed by some insights regarding EEG recording procedures and an in-depth discussion of the quantitative techniques used to analyze alterations in the EEG.

47.1 Historical Perspective

In 1875, Richard Caton published the first account documenting the recording of spontaneous brain electrical activity from the cerebral cortex of an experimental animal. The amplitude of these electrical oscillations was so low (i.e., in the microvolt range) that Caton's discovery is all the more amazing because it was made 50 years before suitable electronic amplifiers became available.

In 1924, Hans Berger of the University of Jena in Austria carried out the first human EEG recordings using metal strips pasted to the scalps of his subjects as electrodes and a sensitive galvanometer as the recording instrument. Berger was able to measure the irregular, relatively small electrical potentials (i.e., 50–100 µV) coming from the brain. By studying the successive positions of the moving element of the galvanometer recorded on a continuous roll of paper, he was able to observe the resultant patterns in these brain waves as they varied with time. From 1924 to 1938, Berger laid the foundation for many of the present applications of electroencephalography. He was the first to use the word *electroencephalogram* in describing these brain potentials in humans. Berger also noted that these brain waves were not entirely random but instead displayed certain periodicities and regularities. For example, he observed that although these brain waves were slow (i.e., exhibited a synchronized pattern of high amplitude and low frequency, <3 Hz) during sleep, they were faster (i.e., exhibited a desynchronized pattern of low amplitude and higher frequency, 15–25 Hz) during waking behaviors. He suggested, quite correctly, that the brain's activity changed in a consistent and recognizable fashion when the general status of the subject changed, as from relaxation to alertness. Berger also concluded that these brain waves could be greatly affected by certain pathologic conditions after noting a marked increase in the amplitude of these brain waves recorded during convulsive seizures. However, despite the insights provided by these studies, Berger's original paper, published in 1929, did not excite much attention. In essence, the efforts of this remarkable pioneer were largely ignored until similar investigations were carried out and verified by British investigators.

It was not until 1934, however, when Adrian and Matthews published their classic paper verifying Berger's findings that the concept of "human brain waves" was truly accepted and the study of EEG activity was placed on a firm foundation. One of their primary contributions was the identification of certain rhythms in the EEG, for example, a regular oscillation at approximately 10–12 Hz recorded from the occipital lobes of the cerebral cortex, which they termed the "alpha rhythm." This alpha rhythm was found to disappear when a subject displayed any type of attention or alertness or focused on objects in the visual field. The physiologic basis for these results, the "arousing influence" of external stimuli on the cortex, was not formulated until 1949, when Moruzzi and Magoun demonstrated the existence of pathways widely distributed through the central reticular core of the brainstem that were capable of exerting a diffuse-activating influence on the cerebral cortex. This "reticular activating system" has been called the brain's response selector because it alerts the cortex to focus on certain pieces of incoming information, while ignoring others. It is for this reason that a sleeping mother will immediately be awakened by her crying baby or the smell of smoke and yet, ignores the traffic outside her window or the television playing in the next room. (*Note:* For the interested reader, an excellent historical review of this early era in brain research is provided in a fascinating text by Brazier (1968).)

47.2 EEG Recording Techniques

Scalp recordings of spontaneous neuronal activity in the brain, identified as the EEG, allow the measurement of potential changes over time between a signal electrode and a reference electrode. Compared with other biopotentials, such as the electrocardiogram (ECG), the EEG is extremely difficult for an untrained observer to interpret, partially as a result of the spatial mapping of functions onto different regions of the brain and electrode placement. Recognizing that some standardization was necessary, the International Federation in Electroencephalography and Clinical Neurophysiology adopted the 10–20 electrode placement system. In addition to the standard 10–20 scalp array, electrodes to monitor eye movement, ECG, and muscle activity are essential for the discrimination of different vigilance or behavioral states (Bronzino, 1984; Kondraski, 1986; Smith, 1986).

Any EEG system consists of electrodes, amplifiers (with appropriate filters), and a recording device. The instrumentation required for recording EEG activity can be simple or elaborate. (*Note:* Although the discussion presented in this section is for a single-channel system, it can be extended to simultaneous multichannel recordings simply by multiplying the hardware by the number of channels required. In cases that do not require true simultaneous recordings, special electrode selector panels can minimize hardware requirements.)

Commonly used scale electrodes consist of Ag–AgCl disks, 1–3 mm in diameter, with long flexible leads that can be plugged into an amplifier. Although a low-impedance contact is desirable at the electrode–skin interface (<10 kΩ), this objective is confounded by hair and the difficulty of mechanically stabilizing the electrode. Conductive electrode paste helps obtain low impedance and keep the electrodes in place. Often, a contact cement (collodion) is used to fix small patches of gauze over the electrodes for mechanical stability, and leads are usually taped to the subject to provide some strain relief. Slight abrasion of the skin is sometimes used to obtain lower electrode impedance, but this can cause slight irritation and sometimes infection (as well as pain in sensitive subjects).

For long-term recordings, as in seizure monitoring, electrodes present major problems. Needle electrodes, which must be inserted into the tissue between the surface of the scalp and the skull, are sometimes useful. However, the danger of infection increases significantly. Electrodes with self-contained miniature amplifiers are somewhat more tolerant because they provide a low-impedance source to interconnecting leads, but they are expensive. Despite numerous attempts to simplify the electrode application process and to guarantee long-term stability, no single method has been widely accepted.

Instruments are available for measuring impedance between electrode pairs. The procedure is recommended strongly as a good practice, since high impedance leads to distortions that may be difficult to separate from actual EEG signals. In fact, electrode impedance monitors are built into some commercially available EEG devices. Note that standard direct current (DC) ohmmeters should not be used since they apply a polarizing current that can result in a buildup of noise at the skin–electrode interface.

From carefully applied electrodes, signal amplitudes of 1–10 μV can be obtained. Considerable amplification (gain = 10^6) is required to bring the signal strength up to an acceptable level for input to recording devices. Because of the length of electrode leads and the electrically noisy environment where recordings commonly take place, differential amplifiers with inherently high input impedance and high common-mode rejection ratios are essential for high-quality EEG recordings.

In some facilities, special electrically shielded rooms minimize environmental electrical noise, particularly 60 Hz alternating current (AC) line noise. Since much of the information of interest in the EEG lies in frequency bands below 40 Hz, low-pass filters in the amplifier can be used to greatly reduce 60 Hz noise. For attenuating AC noise when the low-pass cutoff is above 60 Hz, many EEG amplifiers employ a notch filter specific only for frequencies in a narrow band centered around 60 Hz.

When trying to eliminate or minimize the effect of 60-Hz sources, it is sometimes useful to use a dummy source, such as a fixed 100-kΩ resistor attached to the electrodes. By employing a dummy source as one of the input signals, the output of the differential amplifier represents only contributions from interfering sources. If noise can be reduced to an acceptable level (at least by a factor of 10 less than EEG signals), it is likely that uncontaminated EEG records can be obtained.

Different types of recording instruments obtain a temporary or permanent record of the EEG. The most common recording device is a pen or chart recorder (usually multichannel), which is an integral part of most commercially available EEG instruments. Recordings are on a long sheet of continuous paper (from a folded stack) fed past the moving pen at one of several selectable constant speeds. Paper speed is selected according to the monitoring situation at hand: slow speed (10 mm/s) for observing the spiking characteristically associated with seizure activity and faster speeds (up to 120 mm/s) to identify the presence of individual frequency bands in the EEG.

In addition to (or instead of) a pen recorder, the EEG may be recorded on a multichannel frequency-modulated (FM) analog tape recorder. During such recordings, a visual output device such as an oscilloscope or video display is often used to allow visual monitoring of signals.

Sophisticated FM tape recording and playback systems allow clinicians to review long EEG recordings over a greatly reduced time compared with that required to flip through stacks of paper or to observe recordings in real time. Such systems take advantage of time-compensation schemes, whereby a signal recorded at one speed can be played back at a faster speed. The ratio of playback to recording speed is known, so the appropriate correction factor can be applied to played-back data generating a properly scaled video display. A standard ratio of 60:1 is often used. Thus, a trained clinician can review each minute of real-time EEG in 1 s. The display is scrolled at a high rate horizontally across the display screen. Features of such instruments allow the clinician to freeze a segment of EEG on the display and to slow down or accelerate tape speed from the standard playback as needed. A vertical "tick" mark is usually displayed at periodic intervals by one channel as a time mark to provide a convenient timing reference. Computers also can be used as recording devices. In such systems, one or more channels of analog EEG signal are repeatedly sampled at a fixed time interval (sampling interval), and each sample is converted into a digital representation by an analog-to-digital (A/D) converter. The A/D converter is interfaced to a computer system so that each sample can be saved in the computer's memory. The resolution of the A/D converter is determined by the smallest amplitude that can be sampled. This is determined by dividing the voltage range of the A/D converter by 2 raised to the power of the number of bits of the A/D converter. For example, an A/D converter with a range of ±5 V and 12-bit resolution can resolve sample amplitudes as small as ±2.4 mV. Appropriate matching of amplification and A/D converter sensitivity permits resolution of the smallest signal while preventing clipping of the largest signal amplitudes.

A set of such samples, acquired at a sufficient sampling rate (at least twice the highest-frequency component of interest in the sampled signal), is sufficient to represent all the information in the waveform. To ensure that the signal is band-limited, a low-pass filter with a cutoff frequency equal to the highest frequency of interest is used. Since physically realizable filters do not have ideal characteristics, the sampling rate is usually set to twice the cutoff frequency of the filter or more. Furthermore, once converted to digital format, digital filtering techniques can be used.

Online computer recordings are only practical for short-term recordings or for situations in which the EEG is immediately processed. This limitation is primarily due to storage requirements. For example, a typical sampling rate of 128 Hz yields 128 new points per second that require storage. For an 8-s sample, 1024 points are acquired per channel recorded. A 10-min recording period yields 76,800 data points per channel. Assuming 12-bit resolution per sample, one can see that the available computer memory quickly becomes a significant factor in determining the length (in terms of time) as well as the number of channels of EEG activity to be acquired in real time by the computer.

Further data processing can consist of compression for more efficient storage (with associated loss of total information content), as in the use of compressed spectral arrays, determination of a reduced features set, including only data needed for quantification, as in evoked response recordings, or feature extraction and subsequent pattern recognition, as in automated spike detection during monitoring for epileptic seizure activity.

In addition to the information available from spontaneous EEG activity, the brain's electrical response to sensory stimulation is also important. Owing to the relatively small amplitude of a stimulus-evoked potential compared with that of spontaneous EEG potentials, the technique of signal averaging is often used to enhance the characteristics of stimulus-evoked responses. Stimulus averaging takes advantage of the fact that the brain's electrical response is time locked to the onset of the stimulus, while non-evoked, background potential changes are randomly distributed in time. Consequently, the averaging of multiple stimulus-evoked responses results in the enhancement of the time-locked activity, while the average random background activity approaches zero. The result is an evoked response that consists of a number of discrete and replicable peaks that occur, depending on the stimulus and recording parameters, at predictable latencies associated with the onset of stimulation.

47.3 Use of Amplitude Histographs to Quantify the EEG

In general, the EEG contains information regarding changes in the electrical potential of the brain obtained from a given set of recording electrodes. These data include the characteristic waveforms with accompanying variations in amplitude, frequency, phase, and so on, as well as the brief occurrence of electrical patterns, such as spindles. *Any analysis procedure cannot simultaneously provide information regarding all these variables.* Consequently, the selection of any analytical technique will emphasize changes in one particular variable at the expense of the others. This observation is extremely important if one is to properly interpret the results obtained using a given technique.

In the computation of amplitude distributions of the EEG, for example, successive EEG amplitudes must be measured and ordered into specific amplitude classes, or *bins*. The amplitude histogram that results from this process is often a symmetrical, essentially Gaussian distribution. The primary characteristics of the Gaussian distribution are summarized simply by specifying its mean and standard deviation, since the higher control moments of the distribution, such as skewness and kurtosis, are equal to zero. However, in non-Gaussian distributions, the measures of skewness and kurtosis assume nonzero values and can be used to characterize that particular amplitude distribution. The four primary statistical measures used to characterize an EEG amplitude histogram include the mean, standard amplitude, skewness, and kurtosis.

47.3.1 Mean

Since the sum of (positive and negative) EEG potential is usually on the order of a few microvolts when the analysis time is not too short, the mean is essentially a constant, although of small value. Any shifts in values of the mean, therefore, are indicative of changes in potential that are of technical origin, such as amplifier drifts, and the like.

47.3.2 Standard Amplitude

The variance of the EEG amplitude distribution is directly related to the total power of the EEG. For example, a flat EEG will provide low variance values, while a widely oscillating EEG will yield high variance values. To avoid confusion and use units that are more familiar to electroencephalographers, the term *standard amplitude* is often used.

47.3.3 Skewness

The degree of deviation from the symmetry of a normal or Gaussian distribution is measured by skewness. This third central moment of the amplitude histogram has a value of zero when the distribution is completely symmetrical and assumes some nonzero value when the EEG waveforms are asymmetrical with respect to the baseline (as is the case in some characteristic sleep patterns, murhythms, morphine spindles, barbiturate spiking, etc.). In general, a nonzero value of the skewness index reflects the presence of monophasic events in the waveform. The following methods can be used to obtain the measure of skewness:

Moment coefficient of skewness:

$$S_{Kmc} = \frac{\sum_{i=1}^{N} (x_i - \bar{x})^3 / N}{\left[\sum_{i=1}^{N} (x_i - \bar{x})^2 / N\right]^{3/2}} \tag{47.1}$$

Pearson's second coefficient of skewness:

$$S_{K_{2c}} = \frac{3(\bar{x}\ \text{median})}{SD} \tag{47.2}$$

Centile index of skewness:

$$S_{K_{cent}} = \frac{\text{Number of points} > \bar{x}}{N} \tag{47.3}$$

47.3.4 Kurtosis

The *kurtosis* measure reveals the peakedness or flatness of a distribution. A kurtosis value greater than that of a normal distribution means that the distribution is leptokurtic, or simply more peaked than the normal curve. A value less than that of a normal distribution indicates a flatter distribution. In clinical electroencephalography, when analyzing EEGs with little frequency and amplitude modulation, one observes negative values of kurtosis. High positive values of kurtosis are present when the EEG contains transient spikes, isolated high-voltage wave groups, and so on. The following methods can be used to obtain the measure of kurtosis:

Moment coefficient of kurtosis:

$$K_{mc} = \frac{\sum_{i=1}^{N} (x_i - \bar{x})^4 / N}{\left[\sum_{i=1}^{N} (x_i - \bar{x})^2 / N \right]^2} - 3 \tag{47.4}$$

Centile index of kurtosis:

$$K_{cent} \frac{\text{Number of patients such that } |x_i - \bar{x}| > \text{standard amplitude}}{N} \tag{47.5}$$

A normal distribution will have a value of 0.5 for this measure.

Figure 47.1 illustrates the sensitivity of these measures in analyzing the effect of systemic (IP) administration of morphine sulfate (30 mg/kg) on the cortical EEC. It will be noted that the skewness measure changes abruptly only immediately after the morphine injection, when the EEG was dominated by the appearance of spindles. However, the index of kurtosis characterizes the entire extent of the drug effect from onset to its return to baseline.

The central moments of the EEC amplitude histogram, therefore, are capable of (1) characterizing the amplitude distributions of the EEG and (2) quantifying alterations in these electrical processes brought

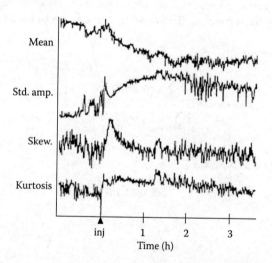

FIGURE 47.1 Plot of the indices of the amplitude distribution, that is, the mean, standard amplitude, skewness, and kurtosis, of the EEG recorded from a rat prior to and for 3 h following intraperitoneal injection of morphine sulfate (30 mg/kg). *Arrow (inj)* indicates time of injection.

about by pharmacologic manipulations. In addition, use of the centile index for skewness and kurtosis provides a computer-efficient method for obtaining these measures in real time.

47.4 Frequency Analysis of the EEG

In early attempts to correlate the EEG with behavior, analog frequency analyzers were used to examine single channels of EEG data. Although disappointing, these initial efforts did introduce the use of frequency analysis to the study of gross brain wave activity. Although *power spectral analysis*, that is, the magnitude square of the Fourier transform, provides a quantitative measure of the frequency distribution of the EEG, it does so, as mentioned earlier, at the expense of other details in the EEG such as the amplitude distribution and information concerning the presence of specific EEG patterns.

The first systematic application of power spectral analysis by general-purpose computers was reported in 1963 by Walter; however, it was not until the introduction of the *fast Fourier transform (FFT)* by Cooley and Tukey in 1965 that machine computation of the EEG became commonplace. Although an individual FFT is ordinarily calculated for a short section of EEG data (e.g., from 1 to 8 s), such signal segmentation with subsequent averaging of individual modified periodograms has been shown to provide a consistent estimator of the power spectrum. An extension of this technique, the compressed spectral array, has been particularly useful for evaluating EEG spectra over long periods of time. A detailed review of the development and use of various methods to analyze the EEG is provided by Bronzino (1984) and others (Barlow, 1993; Dempster, 1993). Figure 47.2 provides an overview of the computational processes involved in performing spectral analysis of the EEG, that is, including computation of

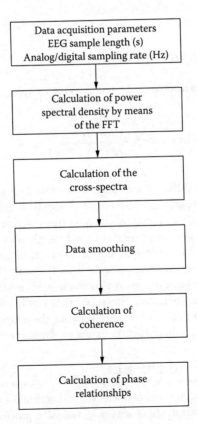

FIGURE 47.2 Block diagram illustrating the steps involved in a conventional (linear) spectral analysis of EEG activity.

auto- and *cross-spectra*. It is to be noted that the power spectrum is the *autocorrelellogram*, that is, the correlation of the signal with itself. As a result, the power spectrum provides only magnitude information in the frequency domain; it does not provide any data regarding phase. The power spectrum is computed by Equation 47.6, where $X(f)$ is the Fourier transform of the EEG signal.

$$P(f) = R_e^2[X(f)] + I_m^2[X(f)] \tag{47.6}$$

Power spectral analysis not only provides a summary of the EEG in a convenient graphic form but also facilitates statistical analysis of EEG changes that may not be evident on simple inspection of the records. In addition to absolute power derived directly from the power spectrum, other measures calculated from absolute power have been demonstrated to be of value in quantifying various aspects of the EEG. Relative power expresses the percentage contribution of each frequency band to the total power and is calculated by dividing the power within a band by the total power across all bands. Relative power has the benefit of reducing the intersubject variance associated with absolute power that arises from subject differences in skull and scalp conductance. The disadvantage of relative power is that an increase in one frequency band will be reflected in the calculation by a decrease in other bands; for example, it has been reported that directional shifts between high and low frequencies are associated with changes in cerebral blood flow and metabolism. Power ratios between low (0–7 Hz) and high (10–20 Hz) frequency bands have been demonstrated to be an accurate estimator of changes in cerebral activity during these metabolic changes.

Although the power spectrum quantifies activity at each electrode, other variables derivable from the FFT offer a means of quantifying the relationships between signals recorded from multiple electrodes or sites. Coherence (which is a complex number), calculated from the cross-spectrum analysis of two signals, is similar to cross-correlation in the time domain.

The cross-spectrum is computed by

$$\text{Cross-spectrum} = X(f)Y^*(f) \tag{47.7}$$

where $X(f)$ and $Y(f)$ are Fourier transforms and * indicates the complex conjugate.

Coherence is calculated by

$$\text{Coherence} = \frac{\text{Cross-spectrum}}{\sqrt{PX(f) - PY(f)}} \tag{47.8}$$

The *magnitude squared coherence (MSC)* values range from 1 to 0, indicating maximum and no synchrony, respectively. The temporal relationship between two signals is expressed by the phase angle, which is a measure of the lag between two signals of common frequency components or bands.

Since coherence is a complex number, the phase is simply the angle associated with the polar expression of that number. MSC and phase then represent measures that can be employed to investigate interactions of cerebral activity recorded from separate brain sites. For example, short (intracortical) and long (corticocortical) pathways have been proposed as the anatomic substrates underlying the spatial frequency and patterns of coherence. Therefore, discrete cortical regions linked by such fiber systems should demonstrate a relatively high degree of synchrony, while the temporal difference between signals, represented by the phase measure, quantifies the extent to which one signal leads another.

47.5 Nonlinear Analysis of the EEG

As mentioned earlier, the EEG has been studied extensively using signal-processing schemes, most of which are based on the assumption that the EEG is a linear, Gaussian process. Although linear analysis schemes are computationally efficient and useful, they only utilize information retained in the autocorrelation function (i.e., the second-order cumulant). Additional information stored in higher-order cumulants is therefore ignored by the linear analysis of the EEG. Thus, while the power spectrum provides the energy distribution of a stationary process in the frequency domain, it cannot distinguish nonlinearly coupled frequency from spontaneously generated signals with the same resonance.

There is evidence showing that the amplitude distribution of the EEG often deviates from Gaussian behavior. It has been reported, for example, that the EEG of humans involved in the performance of mental arithmetic tasks exhibits significant non-Gaussian behavior. In addition, the degree of deviation from Gaussian behavior of the EEG has been shown to depend on the behavioral state, with the state of slow-wave sleep showing less Gaussian behavioral than quiet waking, which is less Gaussian than rapid eye movement (REM) sleep (Ning and Bronzino, 1989a,b). Nonlinear signal-processing algorithms such as bispectral analysis are therefore necessary to address non-Gaussian and nonlinear behavior of the EEG to better describe it in the frequency domain.

But what exactly is the bispectrum? For a zero-mean, stationary process $\{X(k)\}$, the bispectrum, by definition, is the Fourier transform of its third-order cumulant (TOC) sequence:

$$B(\omega_1,\omega_2) = \sum_{m=-\alpha}^{\alpha} \sum_{m=-\alpha}^{\alpha} C(m,n)e^{-j(w_1 m + w_2 n)} \tag{47.9}$$

The TOC sequence $(C(m, n))$ is defined as the expected value of the triple product

$$C(m,n) = E\{X(k)X(k+m)X(k+n)\} \tag{47.10}$$

If process $X(k)$ is purely Gaussian, then its third-order cumulant $C(m, n)$ is zero for each (m, n), and consequently, its Fourier transform, the bispectrum, $B(\omega_1, \omega_2)$ is also zero. This property makes the estimated bispectrum an immediate measure describing the degree of deviation from Gaussian behavior. In our studies (Ning and Bronzino, 1989a,b), the sum of the magnitude of the estimated bispectrum was used as a measure to describe the EEG's deviation from Gaussian behavior, that is

$$D = \sum_{(\omega_1 \omega_2)} |B(\omega_1,\omega_2)| \tag{47.11}$$

Using bispectral analysis, the existence of significant *quadratic phase coupling (QPC)* in the hippocampal EEG obtained during REM sleep in the adult rat was demonstrated (Ning and Bronzino, 1989a,b, 1990). The result of this nonlinear coupling is the appearance, in the frequency spectrum, of a small peak centered at approximately 13–14 Hz (beta range) that reflects the summation of the two theta frequency (i.e., in the 6–7 Hz range) waves (Figure 47.3). Conventional power spectral (linear) approaches are incapable of distinguishing the fact that this peak results from the interaction of these two generators and is not intrinsic to either.

To examine the phase relationship between nonlinear signals collected at different sites, the cross-bispectrum is also a useful tool. For example, given three zero-mean, stationary processes $\{x_j(n)_j = 1, 2, 3\}$, there are two conventional methods for determining the cross-bispectral relationship, direct and indirect. Both methods first divide these three processes into M segments of shorter but equal length. The direct method computes the Fourier transform of each segment for all three processes and then estimates the cross-bispectrum by taking the average of triple products of Fourier coefficients over M segments, that is

$$B_{x_1 x_2 x_3}(\omega_1,\omega_2) = \frac{1}{M} \sum_{m=1}^{M} X_1^m(\omega_1) X_2^m(\omega_2) X_3^{m*}(\omega_1 + \omega_2) \tag{47.12}$$

where $X_j^m(\omega)$ is the Fourier transform of the mth segment of $\{x_j(n)\}$, and $*$ indicates the complex conjugate.

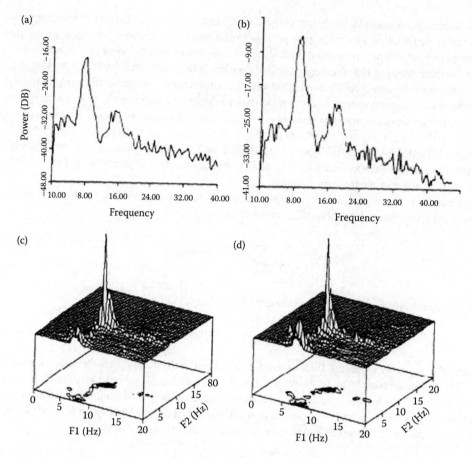

FIGURE 47.3 Plots (a) and (b) represent the averaged power spectra of 16 8-s epochs of REM sleep (digital sampling rate = 128 Hz) obtained from hippocampal subfields CA1 and the dentate gyrus, respectively. Note that both spectra exhibit clear power peaks at approximately 8 Hz (theta rhythm) and 16 Hz (beta activity). Plots (c) and (d) represent the *bispectra* of these same epochs, respectively. Computation of the bicoherence index at $f(1) = 8$ Hz, $f(2) = 8$ Hz showed significant quadratic phase coupling (QPC), indicating that the 16-Hz peak seen in the power spectra is not spontaneously generated but rather results from the summation of activity between the two recording sites.

The indirect method computes the third-order cross-cumulant sequence for all segments:

$$C_{x_1 x_2 x_3}(k,l) = \sum_{n \in \tau} x_1^m(n) x_2^m(n+k) x_3^m(n+l) \tag{47.13}$$

where τ is the admissible set for argument n. The cross-cumulant sequences of all segments will be averaged to give a resultant estimate:

$$Cx_1 x_2 x_3(k,l) = \frac{1}{M} \sum_{m=1}^{M} C_{x_1 x_2 x_3}^m(k,l) \tag{47.14}$$

The cross-bispectrum is then estimated by taking the Fourier transform of the third-order cross-cumulant sequence:

$$Bx_1 x_2 x_3(\omega_1, \omega_2) = \sum_{k=-\alpha}^{\alpha} \sum_{l=-\alpha}^{\alpha} Cx_1 x_2 x_3(k,l) e^{-j(\omega_1 k + \omega_2 l)} \tag{47.15}$$

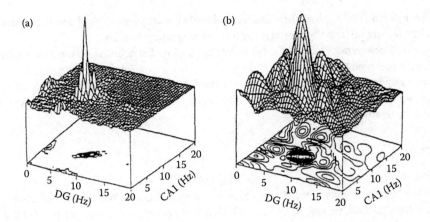

FIGURE 47.4 Cross-bispectral plots of $B_{CA1\text{-}DG\text{-}CA1}$ (ω_1, ω_2) computed using (a) the direct method and (b) the indirect method.

Since the variance of the estimated cross-bispectrum is inversely proportional to the length of each segment, computation of the cross-bispectrum for processes of finite data length requires careful consideration of both the length of individual segments and the total number of segments to be used.

The cross-bispectrum can be applied to determine the level of cross-QPC occurring between $\{x_1(n)\}$ and $\{x_2(n)\}$ and its effects on $\{x_3(n)\}$. For example, a peak at $Bx_1x_2x_3(\omega_1,\omega_2)$ suggests that the energy component at frequency $\omega_1 + \omega_2$ of $\{x_3(n)\}$ is generated due to the QPC between frequency ω_1 of $\{x_1(n)\}$ and frequency ω_2 of $\{x_2(n)\}$. In theory, the absence of QPC will generate a flat cross-bispectrum. However, owing to the finite data length encountered in practice, peaks may appear in the cross-bispectrum at locations where there is no significant cross-QPC. To avoid improper interpretation, the cross-bicoherence index, which indicates the significance level of cross-QPC, can be computed as follows:

$$bic_{x_1x_2x_3}(\omega_1,\omega_2) = \frac{Bx_1x_2x_3(\omega_1,\omega_2)}{\sqrt{P_{x_1}(\omega_1)P_{x_2}(\omega_2)P_{x_3}(\omega_1 + \omega_2)}} \tag{47.16}$$

where $P_{xj}(w)$ is the power spectrum of process $\{x(n)\}$. The theoretical value of the bicoherence index ranges between 0 and 1, that is, from nonsignificant to highly significant.

In situations where the interest is the presence of QPC and its effects on $\{x(n)\}$, the cross-bispectrum equations can be modified by replacing $\{x_1(n)\}$ and $\{x_3(n)\}$ with $\{x(n)\}$ and $\{x_2(n)\}$ with $\{y(n)\}$, that is

$$B_{xyz}(\omega_1,\omega_2) = \frac{1}{M}\sum_{m=1}^{M} X^m(\omega_1)Y^m(\omega_2)X^{m*}(\omega_1 + \omega_2) \tag{47.17}$$

In theory, both methods will lead to the same cross-bispectrum when data length is infinite. However, with finite data records, direct and indirect methods generally lead to cross-bispectrum estimates with different shapes (Figure 47.4). Therefore, like power spectrum estimation, users have to choose an appropriate method to extract the information desired.

Defining Terms

Bispectra: Computation of the frequency distribution of the EEG exhibiting nonlinear behavior.
Cross-spectra: Computation of the energy in the frequency distribution of two different electrical signals.
Electroencephalogram (EEG): Recordings of the electrical potentials produced by the brain.

Fast Fourier transform (FFT): Algorithms that permit rapid computation of the Fourier transform of an electrical signal, thereby representing it in the frequency domain.

Magnitude squared coherence (MSC): A measure of the degree of synchrony between two electrical signals at specified frequencies.

Power spectral analysis: Computation of the energy in the frequency distribution of an electrical signal.

Quadratic phase coupling (QPC): A measure of the degree to which specific frequencies interact to produce a third frequency.

References

Barlow J.S. 1993. *The Electroencephalogram.* Cambridge, MA: MIT Press.

Brazier M. 1968. *Electrical Activity of the Nervous System*, 3rd ed. Baltimore: Williams & Wilkins.

Bronzino J.D. 1984. Quantitative analysis of the EEG: General concepts and animal studies. *IEEE Trans. Biomed. Eng.* 31: 850.

Cooley J.W. and Tukey J.S. 1965. An algorithm for the machine calculation of complex Fourier series. *Math. Comput.* 19: 267.

Dempster J. 1993. *Computer Analysis of Electrophysiological Signals.* New York, NY: Academic Press.

Kondraski G.V. 1986. *Neurophysiological Measurements. Biomedical Engineering and Instrumentation*, pp. 138–179. Boston: PWS Publishing.

Ning T. and Bronzino J.D. 1989a. Bispectral analysis of the rat EEG during different vigilance states. *IEEE Trans. Biomed. Eng.* 36: 497.

Ning T. and Bronzino J.D. 1989b. Bispectral analysis of the EEG in developing rats. In *Proceedings of the Workshop Higher-Order Spectral Analysis*, Vail, CO, pp. 235–238.

Ning T. and Bronzino J.D. 1990. Autoregressive and bispectral analysis techniques: EEG applications. Special Issue on Biomedical Signal Processing. *IEEE Eng. Med. Biol. Mag.* 9: 47.

Smith J.R. 1986. Automated analysis of sleep EEG data. In *Clinical Applications of Computer Analysis of EEG and Other Neurophysiological Signals, EEG Handbook*, revised series, Vol. 2, pp. 93–130. Amsterdam: Elsevier.

Further Information

See the journals, *IEEE Transactions on Biomedical Engineering* and *Electroencephalography and Clinical Neurophysiology.*

48

Biomagnetism

48.1 Theoretical Background...48-1
    Origin of Bioelectric and Biomagnetic Signals • Measurement of the
    Biomagnetic Signals • Independence of Bioelectric and Biomagnetic
    Signals

48.2 Sensitivity Distribution of Dipolar Electric and
    Magnetic Leads 48-3
    Concepts of Lead Vector and Lead Field • Lead Fields of Leads
    Detecting the Electric and Magnetic Dipole Moments of a Volume
    Source • Independence of Dipolar Electric and Magnetic Leads

48.3 Magnetocardiography...48-7
    Selection of Source Model for MCG • Detection of the Equivalent
    Magnetic Dipole of the Heart • Diagnostic Performance of ECG and
    MCG • Technical Reasons to Use MCG • Theoretical Reasons to
    Use MCG

48.4 Magnetoencephalography...48-12
    Theoretical Aspects of MEG • Measurement Sensitivity Distribution
    of Magnetometers • Half-Sensitivity Volumes of EEG and
    MEG • Sensitivity of EEG and MEG to Radial and Tangential
    Sources • Technical Aspects of the MEG

References...48-15

Jaakko Malmivuo
Aalto University

Since the first detection of the magnetocardiogram (MCG) in 1963 by Baule and McFee (Baule and McFee, 1963), new diagnostic information from biomagnetic signals has been widely anticipated. The first recording of the magnetoencephalogram (MEG) was made in 1968 by David Cohen (Cohen, 1968), but it was not possible to record biomagnetic signals with good signal quality before the invention of the superconducting quantum interference device (SQUID) in 1970 (Zimmerman et al., 1970).

48.1 Theoretical Background

48.1.1 Origin of Bioelectric and Biomagnetic Signals

In 1819, Hans Christian Örstedt demonstrated that when an electric current flows in a conductor, it generates a magnetic field around it (Örstedt, 1820). This fundamental connection between electricity and magnetism was expressed in exact form by James Clerk Maxwell in 1864 (Maxwell, 1865). In bioelectromagnetism, this means that when electrically active tissue produces a bioelectric field, it simultaneously produces a biomagnetic field as well. Thus, the origin of both the bioelectric and the biomagnetic signals is the bioelectric activity of the tissue.

The following equations describe the electric potential field and the magnetic field of a volume source distribution $\bar{J}^i$ in an inhomogeneous volume conductor. The inhomogeneous volume conductor is represented by a piecewise homogeneous conductor where the regions of different conductivity σ are separated by surfaces S_j.

$$4\pi\sigma\,\Phi(r) = \int_v \overline{J}^i \cdot \nabla\left(\frac{1}{r}\right) dv + \sum_j \int_{S_j} (\sigma_j'' - \sigma_j')\Phi\nabla\left(\frac{1}{r}\right) \cdot dS_j \tag{48.1}$$

$$4\pi\overline{H}(r) = \int_v \overline{J}^i \times \nabla\left(\frac{1}{r}\right) dv + \sum_j \int_{S_j} (\sigma_j'' - \sigma_j')\Phi\nabla\left(\frac{1}{r}\right) \times dS_j \tag{48.2}$$

The first term on the right–hand side of Equations 48.1 and 48.2 describes the *contribution of the volume source*, and the second term describes the contribution of boundaries separating regions of different conductivity, that is, the *contribution of the inhomogeneities* within the volume conductor. These equations were developed by David Geselowitz (Geselowitz, 1967, 1970).

What we want to measure is the volume source (the first term) and what we want to eliminate is the effect of the volume conductor (the second term). This is done by optimizing the properties of the measurement lead system.

48.1.2 Measurement of the Biomagnetic Signals

The amplitude of the biomagnetic signals is very low. The strongest of them is the MCG, having amplitude on the order of 50 pT. This is roughly one-millionth of the static magnetic field of the earth. The amplitude of the MEG is roughly 1% of that of the MCG. This means that, in practice, the MEG can only be measured with the SQUID and that the measurements must be done in a magnetically shielded room. The MCG, instead, can be measured in the clinical environment without magnetic shielding.

48.1.3 Independence of Bioelectric and Biomagnetic Signals

The source of the biomagnetic signal is the *electric* activity of the tissue. Therefore, the most interesting and most important question in biomagnetism is whether the biomagnetic signals contain new information that cannot be obtained from bioelectric signals; in other words, whether the bioelectric and biomagnetic signals are fully independent or whether there is some interdependence. If the signals were fully independent, the biomagnetic measurement would possibly give about the same amount of new information as the bioelectric method. If there were some interdependence, the amount of new information would be reduced.

Helmholtz's theorem states that "A general vector field, that vanishes at infinity, can be completely represented as the sum of two independent vector fields, one that is irrotational (zero curl) and another that is solenoidal (zero divergence)" (Morse and Feshbach, 1953; Plonsey and Collin, 1961). The impressed current density $\overline{J}^i$ is a vector field that vanishes at infinity and, according to the theorem, may be expressed as the sum of two components:

$$\overline{J}^i = \overline{J}^i_F + \overline{J}^i_V \tag{48.3}$$

where the subscripts F and V denote *flow* and *vortex*, respectively. By definition, these vector fields satisfy $\nabla \times \overline{J}^i_F = 0$ and $\nabla \cdot \overline{J}^i_V = 0$. We first examine the independence of the electric and magnetic signals in the infinite homogeneous case, when the second term on the right-hand side of Equations 48.1 and 48.2, caused by inhomogeneities, is zero. The equation for the electric potential may be rewritten as

$$4\pi\sigma\,\Phi = \int_v \nabla\left(\frac{1}{r}\right) \cdot \overline{J}^i \, dv = \int_v \frac{\nabla \cdot \overline{J}^i}{r} \, dv \tag{48.4}$$

and that for the magnetic field may be written as

$$4\pi H = -\int_v \nabla\left(\frac{1}{r}\right) \times \overline{J}^i \, dv = -\int_v \frac{\nabla \times \overline{J}^i}{r} \, dv \tag{48.5}$$

Substituting Equation 48.3 into Equations 48.4 and 48.5 shows that under homogeneous and unbounded conditions, the bioelectric field arises from $\nabla \cdot \overline{J}^i_F$, which is the *flow source*, and the biomagnetic field arises from $\nabla \times \overline{J}^i_V$, which is the *vortex source*. For this reason, in the early days of biomagnetic research, it was generally believed that the bioelectric and biomagnetic signals were fully independent. However, it was soon recognized that this could not be the case. For example, when the heart beats, it produces an electric field recorded as the P, QRS, and T waves of the ECG, and it simultaneously produces the corresponding magnetic waves recorded as the MCG. Thus, the ECG and MCG signals are not fully independent.

There have been several attempts to explain the independence/interdependence of bioelectric and biomagnetic signals. Usually, these attempts discuss different detailed experiments and fail to give a satisfying general explanation. This important issue may be easily explained by considering the sensitivity distributions of the ECG and MCG lead systems, and this will be discussed in the next section.

48.2 Sensitivity Distribution of Dipolar Electric and Magnetic Leads

48.2.1 Concepts of Lead Vector and Lead Field

48.2.1.1 Lead Vector

Let us assume that two electrodes (or sets of electrodes) are placed on a volume conductor to form a lead. Let us further assume that inside the volume conductor in a certain location Q a unit dipole is placed consecutively in the x, y, and z directions (Figure 48.1a). Owing to the sources, we measure from the lead the signals c_x, c_y, and c_z, respectively. Owing to *linearity*, if instead of the unit dipoles we place in the source location dipoles that are p_x, p_y, and p_z times the unit vectors, we measure signals that are $c_x p_x$, $c_y p_y$, and $c_z p_z$, respectively.

If these dipoles are placed simultaneously to the source location, due to the principle of *superposition*, we measure from the lead a voltage that is

$$V = c_x p_x + c_y p_y + c_z p_z \tag{48.6}$$

These dipoles can be considered to be components of a dipole $\overline{p}$, that is, $\overline{p} = p_x \overline{i} + p_y \overline{j} + p_z \overline{k}$. We may understand the coefficients c_x, c_y, and c_z to be components of a vector $\overline{c}$, that is, $\overline{c} = c_x \overline{i} + c_y \overline{j} + c_z \overline{k}$. Now, we may express the lead voltage Equation 48.6 as the scalar product of the vector $\overline{c}$ and the dipole $\overline{p}$ as

$$V = \overline{c} \cdot \overline{p} \tag{48.7}$$

The vector $\overline{c}$ is a three-dimensional transfer coefficient that describes how a dipole source $\overline{p}$ at a fixed point Q inside a volume conductor influences the voltage measured from the lead and is called the *lead vector*.

The lead vector $\overline{c}$ describes what is the sensitivity of the lead to a source located at the source location. It is self-evident that for another source location the sensitivity may have another value. Thus, the sensitivity, that is, the lead vector, varies as a function of the location, and we may say that it has a certain distribution in the volume conductor. This is called the *sensitivity distribution*.

(a)

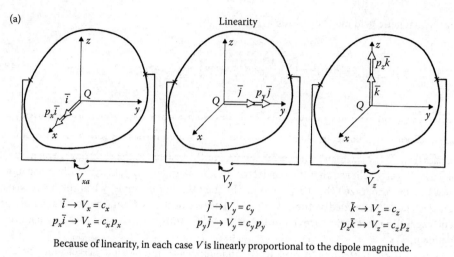

Linearity

$$\bar{i} \to V_x = c_x$$
$$p_x\bar{i} \to V_x = c_x p_x$$

$$\bar{j} \to V_y = c_y$$
$$p_y\bar{j} \to V_y = c_y p_y$$

$$\bar{k} \to V_z = c_z$$
$$p_z\bar{k} \to V_z = c_z p_z$$

Because of linearity, in each case V is linearly proportional to the dipole magnitude.

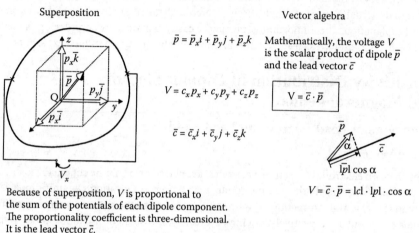

Superposition

Vector algebra

$$\bar{p} = \bar{p}_x i + \bar{p}_y j + \bar{p}_z k$$

Mathematically, the voltage V is the scalar product of dipole $\bar{p}$ and the lead vector $\bar{c}$

$$V = c_x p_x + c_y p_y + c_z p_z$$

$$\boxed{V = \bar{c} \cdot \bar{p}}$$

$$\bar{c} = \bar{c}_x i + \bar{c}_y j + \bar{c}_z k$$

$$V = \bar{c} \cdot \bar{p} = |c| \cdot |p| \cdot \cos \alpha$$

Because of superposition, V is proportional to the sum of the potentials of each dipole component. The proportionality coefficient is three-dimensional. It is the lead vector $\bar{c}$.

FIGURE 48.1 The concepts of (a) lead vector and (b) lead field. See the text for more details.

48.2.1.2 Lead Field

We may define the value of the lead vector at every point in the volume conductor. If we then place the lead vectors to the points for which they are defined, we have a field of lead vectors throughout the volume conductor. This field of lead vectors is called the *lead field* J_L. The lead field illustrates the behavior of the sensitivity in the volume conductor and is a very powerful tool in analyzing the properties of electric and magnetic leads (see Figure 48.1b).

It follows from the *principle of reciprocity*, described by Hermann von Helmholtz in 1853 (Helmholtz, 1853), that the lead field is identical to the electric current field that arises in the volume conductor if a unit current, called *reciprocal current*, I_R, is fed to the lead.

When we know the lead field $\bar{J}_L$ we can determine the signal V_L in the lead due to the volume source distribution $\bar{j}^i$. For each source element, the signal is, of course, proportional to the dot product of the source element and the lead field at the source location, as shown in Equation 48.7. The contribution of the whole volume source is obtained by integrating this throughout the volume source. Thus, the signal the volume source generates at the lead is

(b)

Field of lead vectors

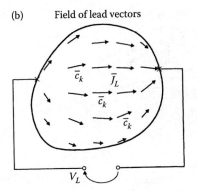

The field of the lead vectors $\bar{c}_k$ is the lead field $\bar{J}_L$

Lead voltage

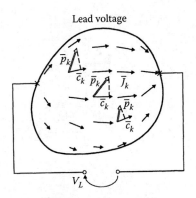

Each dipole element p_k contributes to the lead voltage by $V_k = \bar{c}_k \cdot \bar{p}_k$
The toal lead voltage is the sum of the lead voltage elements $V_L = \sum_k \bar{c}_k \cdot \bar{p}_k$

Reciprocity

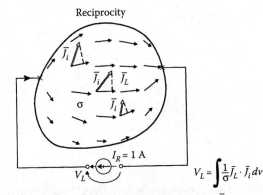

$$V_L = \int \frac{1}{\sigma} \bar{J}_L \cdot \bar{J}_i \, dv$$

Because of reciprocity, the field of lead vectors $\bar{J}_L$ is the same as the current field $\bar{J}_L$ raised by feeding a reciprocal current of 1 A to the lead.

Alternative illustration

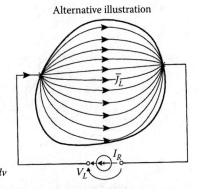

The lead field may also be illustrated with lead field current flow lines.

FIGURE 48.1 **(continued)** The concepts of (a) lead vector and (b) lead field. See the text for more details.

$$V_L = \int \frac{1}{\sigma} \bar{J}_L \cdot \bar{J}^i \, dv \tag{48.8}$$

The lead field may be illustrated either with lead vectors in certain locations in the volume conductor or as the flow lines of the distribution of the reciprocal current in the volume conductor. This is called the *lead current field*. In the latter presentation, the lead field current flow lines are oriented in the direction of the sensitivity, and their density is proportional to the magnitude of the sensitivity.

48.2.2 Lead Fields of Leads Detecting the Electric and Magnetic Dipole Moments of a Volume Source

48.2.2.1 Electric Lead

The sensitivity of a lead system that detects the electric dipole moment of a volume source consists of three orthogonal components (Figure 48.2a). Each of these is linear and homogeneous. In other words, one component of the electric dipole moment is detected when the corresponding component of all

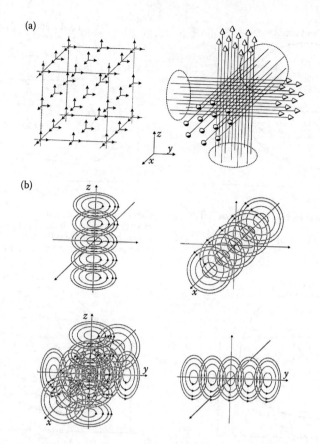

FIGURE 48.2 Sensitivity distributions, that is, lead fields of lead systems detecting (a) electric and (b) magnetic dipole moments of a volume source. The lead field of the electric lead is shown both with vectors representing the magnitude and direction of the lead field (on the left) and with lead field current flow lines (on the right). The lead field of the magnetic lead is shown with lead field current flow lines.

elements of the impressed current density $\bar{J}^i$ are detected with the same sensitivity throughout the source area.

48.2.2.2 Magnetic Lead

The sensitivity distribution of a lead system that detects the magnetic dipole moment of a volume source also consists of three orthogonal components (Figure 48.2b). Each of these has such a form that the sensitivity is always tangentially oriented around the symmetry axis (the coordinate axis). The magnitude of the sensitivity is proportional to the radial distance from the symmetry axis and is zero on the symmetry axis.

48.2.3 Independence of Dipolar Electric and Magnetic Leads

48.2.3.1 Components of the Electric Lead

The sensitivity distributions of the three components of the lead system detecting the electric dipole moment of a volume source are orthogonal. This means that none of them can be obtained as a linear combination of the two other ones. (Note that any fourth measurement having a similar linear sensitivity distribution would always be a linear combination of the three previous ones.) Thus, the sensitivity distributions, that is, the *leads*, are orthogonal and thus independent. However, because he three electric *signals* are only different aspects of the same volume source, they are not (fully) ndependent.

48.2.3.2 Components of the Magnetic Lead

The sensitivity distributions of the three components of the lead system detecting the magnetic dipole moment of a volume source are also orthogonal, meaning that none of them can be obtained as a linear combination of the two other ones. Thus, similarly, as in the measurement of the electric dipole moment, the sensitivity distributions, that is, the *leads* are orthogonal and thus independent. However, because the three magnetic *signals* are only different aspects of the same volume source, they are not (fully) independent.

48.2.3.3 Electric and Magnetic Leads

On the basis of the sensitivity distributions, we also can similarly explain the independence between the electric and magnetic signals. According to the Helmholtz's theorem, the three electric leads are orthogonal to the three magnetic leads. This means that none of these six *leads* can be obtained as a linear combination of the other five. However, the six *signals*, which they measure, are not (fully) independent because they arise from the same electrically active volume source.

48.3 Magnetocardiography

48.3.1 Selection of Source Model for MCG

In the ECG and the MCG, it is the clinical problem to solve the inverse problem, that is, to solve the source of the detected signal to obtain information about the anatomy and physiology of the source. Although the actual clinical diagnostic procedure is based on measuring certain parameters, such as time intervals and amplitudes, from the detected signal and actually not to display the components of the source, the selection of the source model is very important from the point of view of available information.

In clinical ECG, the source model is a dipole. This is the model for both the 12-lead ECG and vectorcardiography (VCG). In 12-lead ECG, the volume conductor (thorax) model is not considered, which causes considerable distortion of the leads. In VCG, only the form of the volume conductor is modeled. This decreases the distortion in the lead fields but does not eliminate it completely. Note that today the display systems used in these ECG and VCG systems do not play any role in the diagnostic procedure because the computerized diagnosis is always based on the signals, not on the display.

In selection of the source model for the MCG, it is logical, at least initially, to select the magnetic source model to be on the same theoretical level with the ECG. Only in this way is it possible to compare the diagnostic performance of these methods. It is clear, of course, that if the source model is more accurate, that is, has more independent variables, the diagnostic performance is better, but when comparing the ECG and the MCG, the comparison is relevant only if their complexity is similar (Malmivuo and Plonsey, 1995).

48.3.2 Detection of the Equivalent Magnetic Dipole of the Heart

The basic detection method of the equivalent magnetic dipole moment of a volume source is to measure the magnetic field on each coordinate axis in the direction of that axis. To idealize the sensitivity distribution throughout the volume source, the measurements must be made at a distance that is large compared with the source dimensions. This, of course, decreases the signal amplitude. The quality of the measurement may be increased considerably if bipolar measurements are used; that is, measurements are made on both sides of the source. The measurement of the magnetic field on each coordinate axis is, however, difficult to perform in the MCG due to the geometry of the human body. It would require

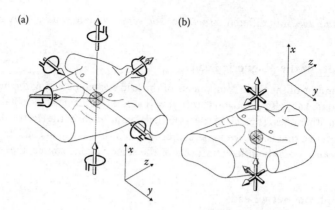

FIGURE 48.3 Measurement of the three orthogonal components of the magnetic dipole moment of the heart (a) on the coordinate axis (*xyz*-lead system) and (b) at a single location over and under the chest (unipositional lead system).

either six sequential measurements with one magnetometer (dewar) or six simultaneous measurements using six dewars (Figure 48.3).

It has been shown (Malmivuo, 1976) that all three components of the magnetic dipole can also be measured from a single location. Applying this unipositional method symmetrically so that measurements are made on both the anterior and posterior sides of the thorax at the same distance from the heart, only two dewars are needed and a very high quality of lead fields is obtained. Figure 48.4 illustrates the sensitivity distributions in nonsymmetrical and symmetrical measurements (Malmivuo and Plonsey, 1995).

48.3.3 Diagnostic Performance of ECG and MCG

The diagnostic performances of ECG and MCG were compared in an extensive study made at Tampere University of Technology (Oja, 1993). The study was made using the asymmetrical unipositional lead system, that is, making measurements only on the anterior side of the thorax. The patient material was selected, however, so that myocardial changes were located dominantly on the anterior side.

This study consisted of 290 normal subjects and 259 patients with different myocardial disorders. It was found that the diagnostic performance of ECG and MCG is about the same (83%). Diagnostic parameters were then selected from both ECG and MCG. With this combined method, called *electromagnetocardiogram* (EMCG), a diagnostic performance of 90% was obtained. This improvement in diagnostic performance was obtained without increasing the number of parameters used in the diagnostic procedure. Moreover, this improvement is significant because it means that the number of incorrectly diagnosed patients was reduced by approximately 50%.

This important result may be explained as follows: The lead system recording the electric dipole moment of the volume source has three independent leads. (This is also the case in the 12-lead ECG system.) Similarly, the lead system detecting the magnetic dipole moment of the volume source has three independent leads. Therefore, the diagnostic performances of these methods are about the same. However, because the sensitivity distributions of electric and magnetic leads are different, the patient groups diagnosed correctly with both methods are not identical.

As stated before, the electric leads are independent of the magnetic leads. If the diagnostic procedure simultaneously uses both the ECG and the MCG leads, we obtain $3 + 3 = 6$ independent leads, and the correctly diagnosed patient groups may be combined. Thus, the diagnostic performance of the combined method is better than that of either method alone. This is the first large-scale statistically relevant study of the clinical diagnostic performance of biomagnetism.

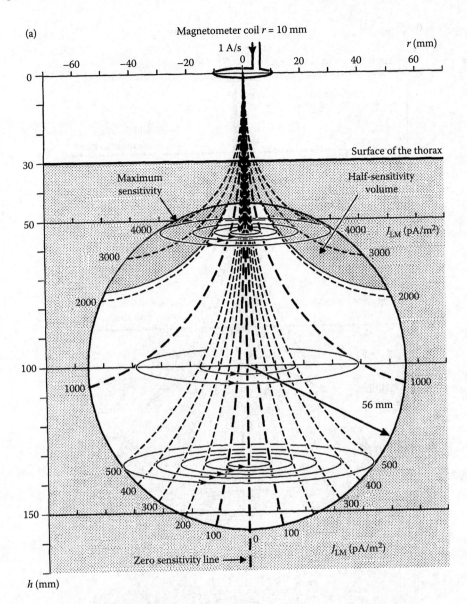

FIGURE 48.4 Sensitivity distributions in the measurement of the magnetic dipole moment of the heart. (a) Nonsymmetric and (b) symmetric measurement of the x component. (c) Symmetric measurement of the y and z components.

48.3.4 Technical Reasons to Use MCG

The technical differences between the ECG and the MCG include the MCG's far better ability to record static sources, sources on the posterior side of the heart; monitor the fetal heart; and perform electrodeless recording. As a technical drawback, it should be mentioned that the MCG instrument costs 2–3 times more. An important feature of the MCG is that, unlike the MEG instrument, owing to the stronger signal amplitude, it does not need a magnetically shielded room. This is very important because the shielded room is not only very expensive but also limits the application of the technique to a certain laboratory space.

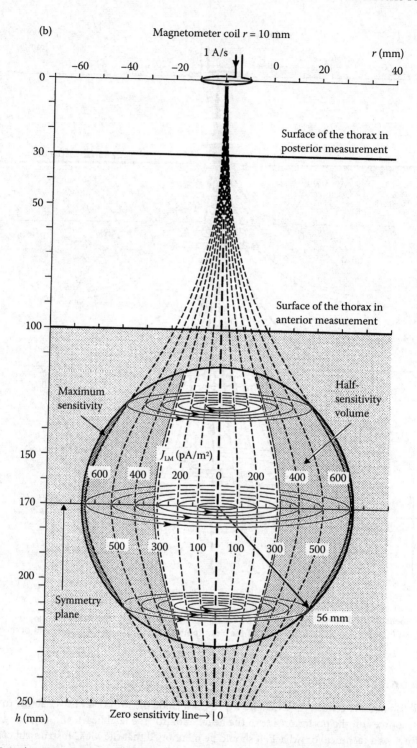

FIGURE 48.4 (continued) Sensitivity distributions in the measurement of the magnetic dipole moment of the heart. (a) Nonsymmetric and (b) symmetric measurement of the *x* component. (c) Symmetric measurement of the *y* and *z* components.

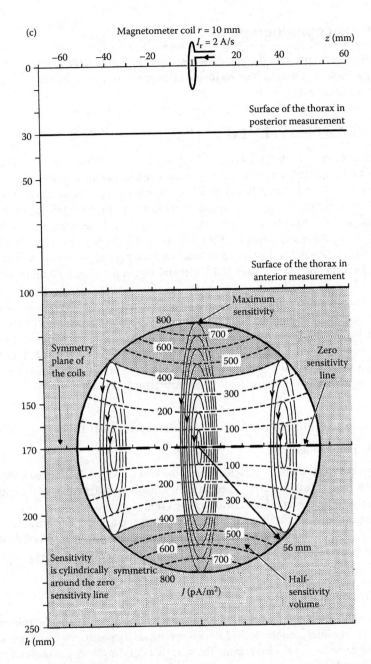

FIGURE 48.4 **(continued)** Sensitivity distributions in the measurement of the magnetic dipole moment of the heart. (a) Nonsymmetric and (b) symmetric measurement of the *x* component. (c) Symmetric measurement of the *y* and *z* components.

48.3.5 Theoretical Reasons to Use MCG

It has been shown that the MCG has clinical value and that it can be used either alone or in combination with the ECG as a new technique called the *electromagnetocardiogram* (EMCG). The diagnostic performance of the combined method is better than that of either ECG or MCG alone. With the combined method, the number of incorrectly diagnosed patients may be reduced by approximately 50%.

48.4 Magnetoencephalography

Similar to the cardiac applications, in the magnetic measurement of the electric activity of the brain, the benefits and drawbacks of the MEG can be divided into theoretical and technical ones. First, the theoretical aspects are discussed.

48.4.1 Theoretical Aspects of MEG

The two main theoretical aspects in favor of MEG are that (1) it is believed that because the skull is transparent for magnetic fields, the MEG should be able to concentrate its measurement sensitivity in a smaller region than the EEG and that (2) because the sensitivity distribution of these methods are fundamentally different, the MEG and EEG should record independent information. In the following, these issues are discussed and it will be shown that they are not true. The analysis is made using the classic spherical head model introduced by Rush and Driscoll (1969). In this model, the head is represented with three concentric spheres, where the outer radii of the scalp, skull, and brain are 92, 85, and 80 mm, respectively. The resistivities of the scalp and the brain are 2.22 Ω cm and that of the skull is 80 times higher, being 177 Ω cm.

The two basic magnetometer constructions in use in MEG are axial and planar gradiometers. In the former, both coils are coaxial, and in the latter, they are coplanar. The minimum distance of the coil from the scalp in a superconducting magnetometer is about 20 mm. The coil radius is usually about 10 mm. It has been shown (Malmivuo and Plonsey, 1995) that with this measurement distance, decreasing the coil radius does not change the distribution of the sensitivity in the brain region. In the following, the sensitivity distribution of these gradiometer constructions is discussed.

48.4.2 Measurement Sensitivity Distribution of Magnetometers

48.4.2.1 Axial Magnetometer

In a cylindrically symmetrical volume conductor model, the lead field flow lines are concentric circles and do not cut the discontinuity boundaries. Therefore, the sensitivity distribution in the brain area of the spherical model equals that in an infinite, homogeneous volume conductor.

Figure 48.5 illustrates the sensitivity distribution of an axial magnetometer. The thin solid lines illustrate the lead field flow lines. The dashed lines join the points where the sensitivity has the same value, being thus so-called isosensitivity lines. The half-sensitivity volume (see below) is represented by the shaded region.

48.4.2.2 Planar Gradiometer

Figure 48.6 illustrates the sensitivity distribution of a planar gradiometer. Again, the thin solid lines illustrate the lead field flow lines, and the dashed lines represent the isosensitivity lines. The half-sensitivity volume is represented by the shaded region. The sensitivity of the planar gradiometer is concentrated under the center of the two coils and is mainly linearly oriented.

48.4.3 Half-Sensitivity Volumes of EEG and MEG

To indicate the magnetometer's ability to concentrate its sensitivity to a small region, the concept of *half-sensitivity volume* has been defined (Malmivuo et al., 1977). This concept means the region in the source area (brain) where the detector sensitivity is one-half or more from the maximum sensitivity. The smaller the half-sensitivity volume, the better is the detector's ability to focus its sensitivity to a small region.

In magnetocardiography, it is relevant to detect the magnetic dipole moment of the volume source of the heart and to make the sensitivity distribution within the heart region as independent of the

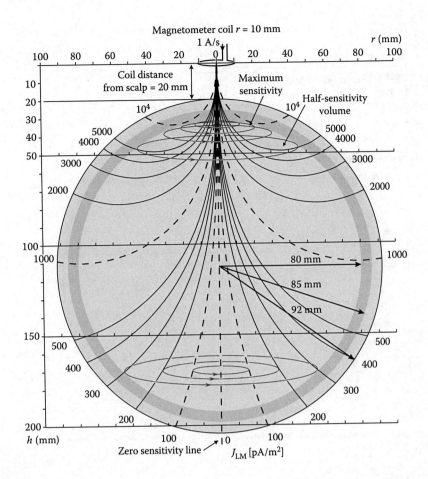

FIGURE 48.5 Sensitivity distribution of the axial magnetometer in measuring the MEG.

position in the axial direction as possible. In magnetoencephalography, however, the primary purpose is to detect the electric activity of the cortex and to localize the regions of certain activity.

The half-sensitivity volumes for different EEG and MEG leads as a function of electrode distance and gradiometer baselines are shown in Figure 48.7. The minimum half-sensitivity volume is, of course, achieved with the shortest distance/baseline. For three- and two-electrode EEG leads, the half-sensitivity volumes at 1° of electrode distance are 0.2 and 1.2 cm³, respectively. For 10 mm radius planar and axial gradiometer MEG leads, these volumes at 1° of coil separation (i.e., 1.6 mm baseline for axial gradiometer) are 3.4 and 21.8 cm³, respectively (Malmivuo et al., 1997).

Short separation will, of course, also decrease the signal amplitude. An optimal value is about 10° of separation. Increasing the separation to 10° increases the EEG and MEG signal amplitudes to approximately 70–80% of their maximum value, but the half-sensitivity volumes do not increase considerably from their values at 1° of separation.

It is now generally known that the EEG has better ability to focus its sensitivity to a small region in the brain than the MEG (Liu et al., 2002). At about 20–30° of separation, the two-electrode EEG lead needs slightly smaller separation to achieve the same half-sensitivity volume as the planar gradiometer. The sensitivity distributions of these leads are, however, very similar. Note that if the sensitivity distributions of two different lead systems, whether they are electric or magnetic, are the same, they detect exactly the same source and produce exactly the same signal. Therefore, the planar gradiometer and two-electrode EEG lead detect very similar source distributions.

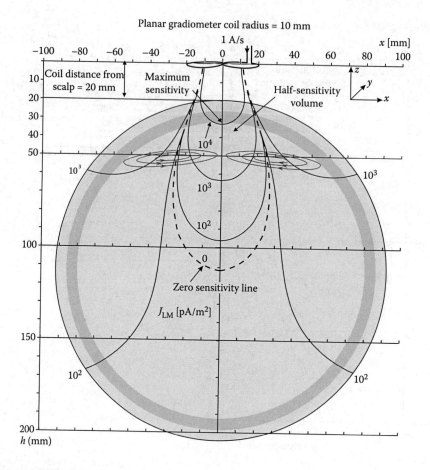

FIGURE 48.6 Sensitivity distribution of the planar gradiometer.

48.4.4 Sensitivity of EEG and MEG to Radial and Tangential Sources

The three-electrode EEG has its maximum sensitivity under that electrode, which forms the terminal alone. This sensitivity is mainly directed radially to the spherical head model. With short electrode distances, the sensitivity of the two-electrode EEG is directed mainly tangentially to the spherical head model. Thus, with the EEG, it is possible to detect sources in all three orthogonal directions, that is, in the radial and in the two tangential directions, in relation to the spherical head model.

In the axial gradiometer MEG lead, the sensitivity is directed tangentially to the gradiometer symmetry axis and thus also tangentially to the spherical head model. In the planar gradiometer, the sensitivity has its maximum under the center of the coils and is directed mainly linearly and tangentially to the spherical head model. The MEG lead fields are oriented tangentially to the spherical head model everywhere. This may be easily understood by recognizing that the lead field current does not flow through the surface of the head because no electrodes are used. Therefore, the MEG can only detect sources oriented in the two tangential directions in relation to the spherical head model.

48.4.5 Technical Aspects of the MEG

The MEG instrumentation is one to two orders of magnitude more expensive than the EEG instrumentation. First, the detector system, due to the needed superconducting instrumentation, is complicated

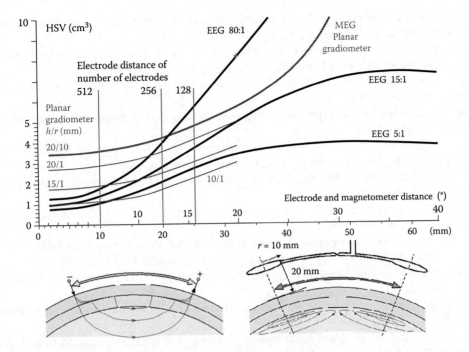

FIGURE 48.7 Half-sensitivity volumes of different EEG leads (dashed lines) and MEG leads (solid lines) as a function of electrode distance and gradiometer baseline, respectively.

and expensive. Second, owing to the small amplitude of the signal, MEG has to be measured in a magnetically shielded room. In addition to the cost of the room, it restricts the measurements to be done in the specially equipped laboratory space. Because the MEG signal is similar to the EEG signal, the data acquisition systems are similar in technology and cost.

Application of the MEG instrumentation is fast, because no electrodes are needed. The measurement dewar is placed on the head of the patient and the measurement may start. On the other hand, the patient has to keep the head in static position during the whole measurement period, which may be stressing.

Owing to the tangential orientation of the MEG lead fields, with the most advantageous MEG measurement systems it is possible to record the MEG from the fetus, because the measurement is not restricted by the *vernix caseosa*. This is the waxy substance under the skin of the fetus having high electric resistivity and which prevents the measurement of the fetal EEG.

Note: This chapter was written to the first edition of this handbook and updating of the information has been only partial. Though everything in this chapter is correct, the discipline has developed a lot during the past 20 years. Therefore the readers are advised to refer also to more modern sources of information. The review article (Malmivuo, 2012) well covers the topic of this chapter and its information is up to date.

References

Baule GM, McFee R. 1963. Detection of the magnetic field of the heart. *Am. Heart J.* 55(7):95.

Cohen D. 1968. Magnetoencephalography: Evidence of magnetic fields produced by alpha–rhythm currents. *Science* 161:784.

Geselowitz DB. 1967. On bioelectric potentials in an inhomogeneous volume conductor. *Biophys. J.* 7(1):1.

Geselowitz DB. 1970. On the magnetic field generated outside an inhomogeneous volume conductor by internal current sources. *IEEE Trans. Magn.* MAG–6(2):346.

Helmholtz HLF. 1853. Ueber einige Gesetze der Vertheilung elektrischer Ströme in körperlichen Leitern mit Anwendung auf die thierisch–elektrischen Versuche. *Ann. Physik Chemie* 89:211.

Liu AK, Dale AM, Belliveau JW. 2002. Monte Carlo simulation studies of EEG and MEG localization accuracy. *Hum. Brain Mapp.* 16:47–62.

Malmivuo, J. 2012. Comparison of the properties of EEG and MEG in detecting the electric activity of the brain. *Brain Topogr.* 25:1–19.

Malmivuo J, Plonsey R. 1995. *Bioelectromagnetism: Principles and Applications of Bioelectric and Biomagnetic Fields.* New York, Oxford University Press (www.bem.fi/book).

Malmivuo J, Suihko V, Eskola H. 1997. Sensitivity distributions of EEG and MEG measurements. *IEEE Trans. Biomed. Eng.* 44(3):196–208.

Malmivuo JA. 1976. On the detection of the magnetic heart vector: An application of the reciprocity theorem. *Acta Polytechn. Scand.* 39:112.

Maxwell J. 1865. A dynamical theory of the electromagnetic field. *Phil. Trans. R. Soc. (Lond.)* 155:459.

Morse PM, Feshbach H.1953. *Methods of Theoretical Physics, Part I.* New York, McGraw-Hill.

Oja OS. 1993. Vector Magnetocardiogram in Myocardial Disorders, MD thesis, University of Tampere, Medical Faculty.

Örstedt HC.1820. Experimenta circa effectum conflictus electrici in acum magneticam. *J. F. Chem. Phys.* 29:485.

Plonsey R, Collin R.1961. *Principles and Applications of Electromagnetic Fields.* New York, McGraw-Hill.

Rush S, Driscoll DA. 1969. EEG–electrode sensitivity: An application of reciprocity. *IEEE Trans. Biomed. Eng.* BME–16(1):15.

Zimmerman JE, Thiene P, Hardings J. 1970. Design and operation of stable rf biased superconducting point–contact quantum devices. *J. Appl. Phys.* 41:1572.

49

Electrical Stimulation of Excitable Tissue

49.1 Introduction 49-1
49.2 Fundamental Principles of Electrical Stimulation....................49-2
 Anatomy and Physiology • Electric Fields in Volume Conductors
49.3 Membrane-Electric Field Interaction..49-6
 Activation of Myelinated Axons • Effect of Polarity of Applied
 Stimulus • Effect of the Space Constant of the Axon
49.4 Electrode–Tissue Interface..49-10
 Effect of Stimulation Waveform on Threshold
49.5 Stimulation of Excitable Tissue 49-14
 Stimulation of Brain Tissue • Stimulation of the Peripheral
 Nerve • Stimulation of Muscle Tissue • Stimulation of Cardiac
 Tissue • Magnetic Stimulation of Excitable Tissue
49.6 Conclusion 49-15
Acknowledgment...49-15
References..49-15

Dominique M.
Durand
*Case Western Reserve
University*

49.1 Introduction

Two of the most vital organs in the body, the brain/nervous system and the heart, are composed of excitable tissues. Patients with disorders in either of these organs can have severe deficits such as cardiac arrythmias or epilepsy. Although rehabilitation and neural regeneration can provide some improvement [1,2], the degree of restoration of the normal function of these organs has been limited. Electrical stimulation of cardiac tissue has been particularly successful to restore the function in the heart with implanted pacemakers, and functional electrical stimulation (FES) of the nervous system can provide functional restoration to neurologically impaired individuals. By placing electrodes within the excitable tissue and passing a current through these electrodes, it is possible to activate pathways in the brain as well as in the cardiac and skeletal muscles.

Neural prostheses refer to applications for which electrical stimulation is used to replace a previously lost or damaged neural function. Electrical stimulation has been applied to restore the neural function in several neural systems (see References 3 and 4). The most successful neural prosthesis is the cochlear prosthesis. Electrical stimulation of the auditory nerves can restore hearing in deaf patients [5]. Other applications include phrenic nerve stimulation for patients with high-level spinal cord injury to generate diaphragm contractions and can restore ventilation [6,7], and for electrical stimulation of the visual cortex [8] or the retina [9] to restore vision and stimulation of upper/lower extremities [10]. There are also several applications of electrical stimulation in the brain such as deep brain stimulation that is therapeutic instead of being restorative. Neuromodulation has been applied in various places through deep brain electrodes such as thalamic nuclei to decrease tremor in patients with Parkinson's disease [11,12] or vagus nerve stimulation for seizure frequency reduction in patients with epilepsy [13].

The stimulation of the cardiac tissue has generated significant therapeutic benefits. A cardiac pacemaker is a stimulator capable of restoring the normal rhythm of the heart in patients suffering from cardiac disorders such as arrhythmia and heart block [14]. The sophistication of pacemakers has increased dramatically in recent years. Starting from the simple asynchronous (free running) to the synchronous (synchronized to the patient's heartbeat) for patients with incomplete heart block, rate-responsive pacemakers (the frequency of pacing varies with the metabolic demand) and pacemakers with defibrillators have been released.

Electrical excitation results from the interaction between extracellular electric fields and cellular membrane as described by the cable equation (see the review by Roth [15]). The interaction can be analyzed by determining the voltages and electric fields generated by the electrode using the solution of Maxwell equations. The relationship between the applied extracellular field and the transmembrane voltage is described by the source term in the cable equation and is derived below (Section 49.2). The effect of the waveform of the stimulation pulse, the electrochemistry taking place at the electrode interface, and the tissue damage are also reviewed (Section 49.3). In the last section (Section 49.4), the stimulation of the neural tissue is emphasized and the stimulation of various other excitable tissues such as skeletal muscles and cardiac tissue are discussed.

49.2 Fundamental Principles of Electrical Stimulation

49.2.1 Anatomy and Physiology

Axonal excitation by applied current is effected when the transmembrane current generated by the electrode depolarizes the membrane sufficiently to activate the sodium channels located in high density within the cell membrane. Once activated, the sodium current will further increase until the membrane reaches an unstable fixed point. This is the point at which a full action potential (~100 mV) will develop. Once started, the action will propagate unattenuated either along the nerve fibers or the cardiac tissue.

Although the dynamics of membrane channels play a major role in the excitation properties of excitable cells, the sodium channels are almost completely closed at the resting potential. Therefore, the passive properties of the membrane contribute significantly to the determination of the membrane voltage along the axons and to the site of the excitation. The transmembrane voltage is the difference between the intracellular voltage and the extracellular voltage. This extracellular voltage is generated by the current of the electrode and can be estimated with a reduced set of Maxwell equations, the quasi-static formulation.

49.2.2 Electric Fields in Volume Conductors

Although the volume conductor clearly contains material with a high dielectric constant (e.g., cell membrane), its capacitive properties can be neglected when the frequency is below 10 kHz [16]. Similarly, the inductive properties can be neglected at these low frequencies. Therefore, the volume conductor surrounding the neural excitable tissue can be assumed to be purely resistive with a resistivity varying between 50 and 500 $\Omega \cdot$ cm in most applications. The resistivity of the volume conductor can vary at different locations or in different directions and is defined at each point of the volume by a resistivity tensor. If the resistivity is the same in all directions, the volume is isotropic. If the resistivity is the same at all points of the volume, then the volume is homogeneous. A simpler form of the Maxwell equations can be derived for this type of volume conductor and its applications.

49.2.2.1 Quasi-Static Formulation of Maxwell Equations

For frequencies under 10 kHz, both the capacitive and inductive properties can be neglected and a simplified set of equations can be used to calculate the voltage and current in volume conductors [16]:

Conservation of charge

$$\nabla \cdot \mathbf{J} = 0 \tag{49.1}$$

Gauss's law

$$\nabla \cdot \mathbf{E} = \rho/\varepsilon \tag{49.2}$$

Ohm's law for conductors

$$\mathbf{J} = \sigma\mathbf{E} \tag{49.3}$$

Electric field

$$\mathbf{E} = -\nabla V \tag{49.4}$$

where $\mathbf{E}$ is the electric field (V/m) defined as the gradient of the scalar potential V, $\mathbf{J}$ is the current density (mA/m^2), the conductivity (inverse of resistivity) in S/m, ρ is the charge density in C/m^3, and ε is the permittivity of the medium (F/m).

49.2.2.2 Equivalence between Dielectric and Conductive Media

The current density $\mathbf{J}$ at any point is the sum of a source term $\mathbf{J}_s$ and an ohmic term $\mathbf{J}_\Omega$

$$\mathbf{J} = \mathbf{J}_\Omega + \mathbf{J}_s = \sigma\mathbf{E} + \mathbf{J}_s \tag{49.5}$$

Using Equation 49.1:

$$\nabla \cdot \mathbf{J} = \nabla \cdot (\sigma\mathbf{E}) + \nabla \cdot \mathbf{J}_s = 0 \tag{49.6}$$

Assuming a homogeneous volume conductor, $\nabla \cdot (\sigma\mathbf{E}) = \sigma (\nabla \cdot \mathbf{E})$; therefore

$$\nabla \cdot \mathbf{E} = -\nabla \cdot \mathbf{J}_s/\sigma \tag{49.7}$$

Since $\mathbf{E} = -\nabla V$

$$\nabla^2 V = \nabla \cdot \mathbf{J}_s/\sigma = -I_v/\sigma \tag{49.8}$$

where I_v is a volume source current in A/m^3 and ∇^2 is the Laplacian operator. The volume current I_v can be calculated from the knowledge of the distribution of sources in the volume conductor. This equation is the equivalent of the Poisson equation derived for dielectrics [17]:

$$\nabla^2 V = -\rho/\varepsilon \tag{49.9}$$

Using the following equivalence:

$$\rho \Leftrightarrow I_v$$

$$\varepsilon \Leftrightarrow \sigma$$

The solution of the Poisson equation for dielectric problems can be applied to the calculation of the current and voltage distribution in volume conductors.

49.2.2.3 Monopole Point Source

For the monopole source, the current density **J** at any point in the medium located at a distance r from the source can be obtained simply and is equal to the total current crossing a spherical surface with radius r divided by the surface area

$$\mathbf{J} = \frac{I}{4\pi r^2}\mathbf{u_r} \tag{49.10}$$

where $\mathbf{u_r}$ is the unit radial vector and r is the distance between the electrode and the measurement point. The electric field is then obtained from Equation 49.3:

$$\mathbf{E} = \frac{I}{4\pi\,\sigma\,r^2}\mathbf{u_r} \tag{49.11}$$

The electric field is the gradient of the potential. In spherical coordinates

$$\mathbf{E} = -\frac{dV}{dr}\mathbf{u_r} \tag{49.12}$$

The potential at point P measured with a reference electrode located at infinity is

$$V = \frac{I}{4\pi\sigma r} \tag{49.13}$$

Both the current density **J** and the electric field **E** have a radial distribution with an amplitude inversely proportional to the square of the distance to the source. The potential decay is inversely proportional to the distance. At $r = 0$, the potential goes to infinity and this singularity can be eliminated if the electrode is modeled as a sphere with a radius a. Equation 49.13 is then valid on the surface of the electrode $r = a$ and for $r > a$ [18].

Assuming the medium to be homogeneous and linear, using superposition, Equation 49.13 can be generalized to n monopolar electrodes with a current I_i located at a distance r_i from the recording point. The voltage is then given by

$$V = \frac{1}{4\pi\sigma}\sum_i \frac{I_i}{r_i} \tag{49.14}$$

For an axon located in the volume conductor at a distance d from the source I_s (Figure 49.1a), the voltage along the axon is given by the following equation and is plotted in Figure 49.1b ($d = 1$ cm and $I_s = 1$ mA):

$$V = \frac{I_s}{4\pi\sigma\sqrt{d^2 + x^2}} \tag{49.15}$$

The longitudinal component of the electric field (E_x) is biphasic and is plotted in Figure 49.1c.

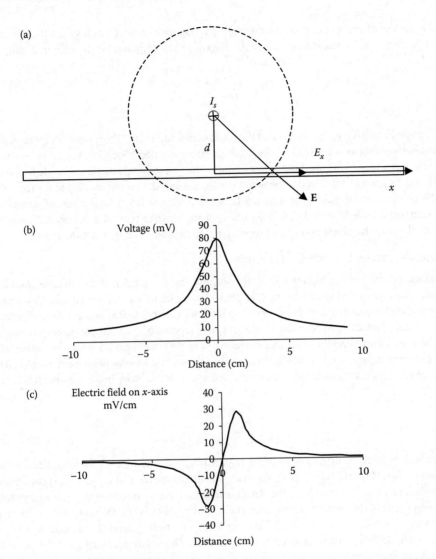

FIGURE 49.1 Electrical stimulation of a fiber. (a) An electrode is located at a distance d from the axon and an anodic stimulus is applied to the electrode. The current flows outside and inside the axon generating depolarization of the membrane. Action potentials are generated underneath the electrode and propagate both orthodromically and antidromically. The fiber is activated by the longitudinal component (E_x) of the electric field **E**. Extracellular voltage (b) and electric field (c) generated by 1 mA and measured along an axon located at 1 cm from the electrode (resistivity of the medium is assumed to be 100 $\Omega \cdot$ cm).

49.2.2.4 Bipolar Electrodes and Dipoles

Using Equation 49.14, it is possible to calculate the voltage generated by a current source and a current sink separated by a known distance d. The potential at point P (assuming that the voltage reference is at infinity) is given by

$$V = \frac{I}{4\pi\sigma}\left(\frac{1}{r_1} - \frac{1}{r_2}\right)$$

(49.16)

where r_1 and r_2 are the distances between the measuring point and the electrodes. When the distance d between the two electrodes is small compared to the distance r, the equation for the potential reduces to

$$V = \frac{I d \cos\theta}{4\pi\sigma r^2} \tag{49.17}$$

where θ is the angle between the dipole axis and the point of measurement. There is an equipotential line ($\theta = 0$) passing between the two electrodes. Therefore, an axon or a nerve located along this line (transverse excitation) has a very high threshold for excitation. The voltage generated by a dipole is inversely proportional to the square of the distance between the source and the recording site. Since the voltage decays rapidly compared to a monopole, the dipole is a much more selective method of stimulation. However, the current threshold for a dipole is significantly higher than that for monopoles. The ratio of the monopole voltage to the dipole voltage is proportional to r/d and d is much smaller than r.

49.2.2.5 Inhomogenous Volume Conductors

Biological volume conductors are highly inhomogenous and the complexity of the volume conductors requires in most cases numerical solutions using finite element or finite boundary methods. However, the effect of the boundary between two layers of various conductivities can be studied in a simple configuration. Consider two volume conductors with conductivities σ_1 and σ_2 separated by an infinite plane. A monopolar electrode is placed in region 1 and the potentials are recorded in the same region. Solving for the boundary conditions at the interface, it can be shown that the inhomogenous volume conductor can be replaced by a homogenous volume conductor by adding a mirror current source with an amplitude equal to [18]

$$I' = \frac{\sigma_1 - \sigma_2}{\sigma_1 + \sigma_2} I \tag{49.18}$$

The voltage is then given by Equation 49.14 for region 1 only. In the case where layer 1 is a volume conductor such as the body and layer 2 is air ($\sigma_2 = 0$), the mirror source I' is equal to I. If the stimulation electrode is located at the interface, the zero-current boundary condition is satisfied by simply doubling the amplitude of the current. Similarly, if the recording electrode is located on the surface, the zero-conductivity layer will double the size of the recorded potentials. If layer 2 is a perfect conductor ($\sigma_2 = \infty$), the current density must be normal at the boundary. The condition is satisfied if $I' = -I$. This image theory is applicable only in simple cases but can be useful to obtain approximations when the distance between the recording electrode and the surface of discontinuity is small thereby approximating an infinite surface [19].

49.3 Membrane-Electric Field Interaction

The interaction between the extracellular voltage and axons can be studied with a simple passive membrane model (Figure 49.2a). The membrane resistance is modeled as the rest conductance of the sodium, potassium, and leakage channels using compartmental analysis [20]. The current flowing from the outside to the inside of the cell increases the voltage across the membrane and causes hyperpolarization. When the current flows from the inside to the outside, the membrane is depolarized [21] (Figure 49.2).

A quantitative analysis of the interaction between electric fields and the neural tissue can be derived by combining the passive membrane model with the extracellular voltage (V_e) generated by stimulating electrodes. The model makes several assumptions [22]. Assuming that the presence of the fiber does not affect the extracellular voltage, the extracellular voltage can be calculated using the equations previously derived. A passive electrical model of the axon can be built and the circuit can be solved using numerical methods for compartmental analysis [23]. These methods have been analyzed using neuronal

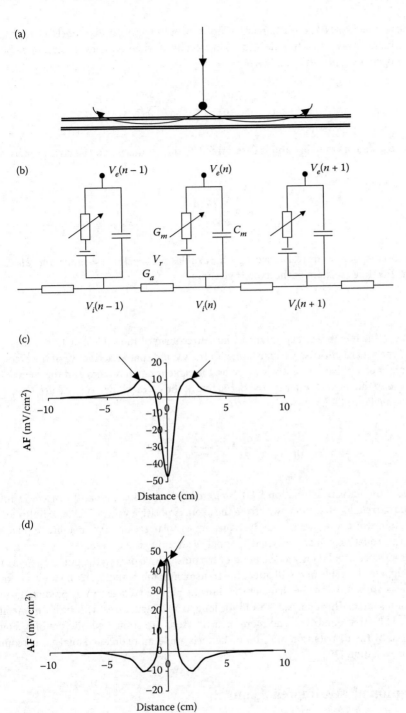

FIGURE 49.2 Activating function for the electrical stimulation of a fiber. (a) The current lines generated by an anode enter the axon underneath the electrode. The current leaves the fibers in the distal regions. (b) Electrical model of the membrane and axonal component of the fibers. (c) Activating function for an anode. The maximum positive value of the function shows the location of depolarization (excitation) of the fiber and is indicated by the two arrows. (d) For a cathode, the maximum value of the activating function is at the origin and is much greater that that in (c). Therefore, cathodes have a lower threshold than anodes.

simulation packages such as Neuron [24]. Each compartment in Figure 49.2b models a length Δx of the cell. Applying Kirchoff's law at each node and taking the limit when Δx goes to zero, one obtains the following inhomogenous cable equation [25,26]:

$$\lambda^2 \frac{\partial^2 V_m}{\partial x^2} - \tau_m \frac{\partial V_m}{\partial t} - V_m = -\lambda^2 \frac{\partial^2 V_e}{\partial x^2} \tag{49.19}$$

λ is the space constant of the fiber and is determined by the geometric and electric properties of the axon

$$\lambda = \frac{1}{2}\sqrt{\frac{R_m d}{R_a}} \tag{49.20}$$

where R_m is the specific membrane resistance, R_a is the axoplasmic specific resistance, and d is the diameter of the axon. The time constant of the axon is given by

$$\tau_m = R_m C_m \tag{49.21}$$

where C_m is the specific membrane capacitance. The source term of the cable equation is negative and is the product of the square of the space constant with the second spatial derivative of the extracellular voltage. At the onset of a pulse ($t = 0$), the voltage on the cable is equal to zero and the change in voltage is proportional to the second-order spatial derivative of the extracellular voltage also known as the activating function $\mathbf{AF}(x,t)$ [27]:

$$\frac{\partial V_m}{\partial t} = \frac{\lambda^2}{\tau_m} \frac{d^2 V_e}{dx^2}\bigg|_{t=0} = \frac{\lambda^2}{\tau_m} \mathbf{AF}(x,0) \tag{49.22}$$

The amplitude of the activating function $f(x,0)$ is plotted in Figure 49.2c for a 10-μm axon stimulated by a 1-mA anodic current located 1 cm away from the axon. A positive value of $\mathbf{AF}(x,0)$ indicates membrane depolarization while a negative value indicates hyperpolarization. The membrane polarization calculated from this equation can be predicted by simply examining the current flow pattern in and out of the axon. This analysis is valid only at the onset of the pulse, since during the pulse, currents will be distributed throughout the cable and will affect the transmembrane potential [28]. However, for short pulses, these effects are small and the shape of the transmembrane voltage can be predicted using the activation function source. This analysis is valid for long axonal structures with uniform membrane. However, when cell bodies, dendrites, and more realistic axons are simulated, the site of excitation is strongly influenced by the distribution of sodium channels and a more detailed analysis is required to predict the site of excitation [29].

49.3.1 Activation of Myelinated Axons

The cable equation derived above needs to be modified for myelinated fibers since the presence of myelin sheath around the axon forces the current to flow in and out of the membrane only at the nodes of Ranvier. Therefore, the action potential also jumps from node to node (saltatory conduction). The interaction between myelinated fibers and applied fields can be described using the model shown in Figure 49.1a with R_m and C_m replaced by R_n and C_n. In this simple model, the myelin sheath is assumed to have infinite resistance. Therefore, R_n and C_n represent the membrane resistance and capacitance only at the node of Ranvier

$$R_n = \frac{R_n^s}{\pi dl} \quad C_n = C_n^s \pi dl \tag{49.23}$$

where R_n^s and C_n^s are the specific membrane capacitance and resistance at the node, d is the inner fiber diameter, l is the width of the node, and L is the internodal distance. The resistance between nodes (R_a) is modeled by $R_a = (4R_a^s L/\pi d^2)$, where R_a^s is the axoplasmic specific resistance and L is the internodal length. The cable equation for a myelinated nerve can be derived using Kirchoff's law:

$$\frac{R_n}{R_a}\Delta^2 V_m - R_n C_n \frac{\partial V_m}{\partial t} - V_m = -\frac{R_n}{R_a}\Delta^2 V_e \tag{49.24}$$

Δ^2 is the second difference operator ($\Delta^2 V = V_n^{-1} - 2V_n + V_n^{+1}$) and R_a represents the resistance between two nodes. The source term for this equation ($-(R_n/R_a)\Delta^2 V_e = -(R_n^s/R_a^s)(d/4lL)\Delta^2 V_e$) is not explicitly dependent on the axon diameter since both l (10 μm) and d/L (0.0007) are nearly constant. However, since the distance between the node increases with the diameter of the fiber, the second-order difference does indeed depend on the diameter of the axons.

49.3.2 Effect of Polarity of Applied Stimulus

The activation of axons is determined by the amplitude of the membrane depolarization. The polarity of the membrane polarization can be predicted directly from the sign of the activating function (positive sign indicates depolarization). This activation function is plotted in Figure 49.2 and it is clear from the figure that the membrane depolarization (see arrows) generated by the cathode is greater than the depolarization generated from the anode (Figure 49.2c and d). Also note that the polarity of the stimulus affects the location of the excitation. Cathodic excitation will produce excitation directly under the cathode whereas anodic excitation will produce excitation at two sites located away from the anode (see arrows in Figure 49.2d). However, the location of excitation also depends on the largest density of sodium channels. For example, anodic stimulation of cortical pyramidal cells has a lower threshold than cathodic stimulation when applied to the surface of the brain.

49.3.3 Effect of the Space Constant of the Axon

The equivalent voltage source of the cable equation is proportional to the square of the space constant λ. λ^2 is proportional to the diameter of the fiber in Equation 49.20 for unmyelinated fibers and to the square of the diameter for myelinated fibers [19]. Therefore, in both cases, V_{eq} is higher for fibers with larger diameter and therefore, large-diameter fibers have a lower threshold. Since λ^2 is also dependent on the electrical properties of the axons, it is then possible to predict that fibers with a larger membrane resistance or lower axoplasmic resistance will also have lower thresholds.

49.3.3.1 Recruitment Order of Fibers

The physiological recruitment order by the central nervous system (CNS) is to first recruit the small fibers followed by large fibers. As previously indicated, electrical stimulation recruits large fibers first. Therefore, electrical stimulation produces a recruitment order opposite to the physiological recruitment order and this effect is known as the reverse recruitment order. Several techniques have been developed to recruit small fibers before large fibers. The first technique uses anodal block whereby axons activated under the cathode are blocked when passing underneath the anode. This blocking effect requires a long pulse (about 400 μs) to maintain the hyperpolarization of the membrane. By decreasing the amplitude of the current, the small-diameter fibers are first released from the anodic block. A further reduction of the amplitude activates the larger fibers [29], restoring a normal recruitment order. Another more recent technique places an array of contact along the nerve. When the contact separation of the electrodes is equal to the internodal distance of the fiber of a given diameter, the activation function for that fiber is reduced and the fiber does not fire [30]. By adjusting the polarity and the electrode distance, it is possible to reverse the recruitment order of the nerve activation.

49.4 Electrode–Tissue Interface

At the interface between the electrode and the tissue, the charge carrier must change between electrons in the metal and ions in the tissue. This exchange is carried out by chemical reactions that can modify the chemical milieu around the electrode, produce neural damage, and change the impedance. Moreover, the shape of the waveform can influence the threshold for activation as well as the corrosion of the electrode.

49.4.1 Effect of Stimulation Waveform on Threshold

49.4.1.1 Strength-Duration Curve

It has been known for a long time that it is the time change in the applied current and not the continuous application of the external stimulus that can activate excitable tissue. Direct currents (DC) cannot excite and even in small amplitudes, they can cause significant tissue damage. It has also been observed experimentally that the relationship between the pulse width and the amplitude suggests that it is the total charge injected, which is the important parameter. The relationship between the amplitude and the width of a pulse required to bring an excitable tissue to the threshold is shown in Figure 49.3a. The amplitude of the current threshold stimulus (I_{th}) decreases with increasing pulse width (W) and can be modeled by the following relationship [30]:

$$I_{th} = \frac{I_{rh}}{1 - \exp(-W/T)} \tag{49.25}$$

The minimum current amplitude required to cause excitation is known as the rheobase current (I_{rh}). T is the membrane time constant of the axon if the axon is stimulated intracellularly. For extracellular stimulation, T is a time constant that takes into account the extracellular space resistance. The relationship between current amplitude and pulse width can also be derived theoretically using the cable equation by assuming that the total charge on the cable for excitation is constant [31]. The pulse width required to excite the tissue with an amplitude equal to twice the rheobase current is known as the chronaxie (T_{ch}) and is equal to 0.693 T. This strength-duration curve can also be modeled by the following simpler equation:

$$I_{th} = I_{rh}[1 + (T_{ch}/W)]$$

49.4.1.2 Charge-Duration Curve

The threshold charge-injected $Q_{th} = I_{th} \times W$ is plotted in Figure 49.3b and increases with the pulse width.

$$Q_{th} = \frac{I_{rh}W}{1 - \exp(-W/T)} \tag{49.26}$$

The increase in the amount of charge required to fire the axon with increasing pulse width is due to the fact that for long pulse duration, the charge is distributed along the cable and does not participate

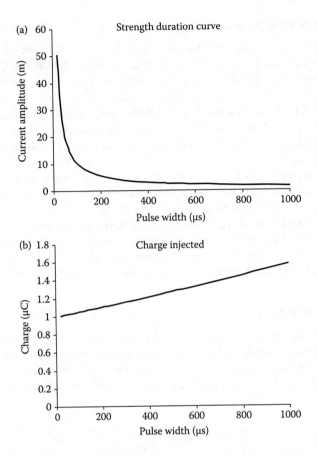

FIGURE 49.3 Strength-duration (a) and charge-duration (b) curves for the excitation of neurons. The time constant, chronaxie, and rheobase currents are 1 ms, 0.7 ms, and 1 mA, respectively.

directly in raising the membrane voltage at the excitation site. The minimum amount of charge Q_{min} required for stimulation is obtained by taking the limit of Q_{th} in Equation 49.33 when W goes to zero and is equal to $I_{rh} \times T$. In practice, this minimum charge can be nearly achieved by using narrow, current pulses. Short pulses have other advantages; they increase the spatial selectivity of stimulation [32] and fiber diameter selectivity [33].

49.4.1.3 Anodic Break

The excitation generated by cathodic current threshold normally takes place at the onset of the pulse. However, long-duration, subthreshold cathodic or anodic current pulses have been observed experimentally to generate excitation at the end of the pulse. This effect has been attributed to the voltage sensitivity of the sodium channel. The sodium channel is normally partially inactivated at rest. However, when the membrane is hyperpolarized during the long-duration pulse, the inactivation of the sodium channel is completely removed. Upon termination of the pulse, an action potential is generated since the inactivation gate has a slow time constant relative to the activation time constant and cannot recover fast enough [34]. This effect can be observed with an anodic or cathodic pulse since both can generate hyperpolarization. The anodic break can be prevented by avoiding abrupt termination of the current. The pulse shapes with slow decay phases such as exponential and trapezoidal decay shapes have been successfully used [35].

49.4.1.4 Electrochemistry of Stimulation

The conduction in a metal is carried by electrons, whereas in the tissue, the current is carried by ions. Although capacitive mechanisms have been explored, capacitive electrodes capable of storing enough charge for stimulation have not yet been developed. Therefore, most electrical stimulation electrodes rely on the Faradaic mechanisms at the interface between the metal and the tissue. Faradaic mechanisms require that oxidation and reduction take place at the interface [36]. Faradaic stimulation mechanisms can be divided into reversible and nonreversible mechanisms. Reversible mechanisms occur at or near the electrode potential and include oxide formation and reduction, and hydrogen plating. Irreversible mechanisms occur when the membrane is driven far away from its equilibrium potential and include corrosion, hydrogen, or oxygen evolution. These irreversible processes can cause damage to both the electrode and the tissue since they alter the composition of the electrode surface and can generate toxic products with pH changes in the surrounding tissue. During charge injection, the electrode potential is modified by an amount related to the charge density (total charge divided by the surface area). To maintain the electrode potential within regions producing only minimal irreversible changes, this charge density must be kept below maximum values [37]. The maximum charge density allowed depends on the metal used for the electrode, the stimulation waveform, the type of electrode used, and the location of the electrode within the body.

49.4.1.5 Stimulation Waveform

The common biphasic waveforms for stainless steel or platinum use a cathodic pulse followed by an anodic phase. An example of a square balanced biphasic waveform is shown in Figure 49.4 and can be easily implemented using a capacitor and switches. This waveform ensures that the charge is balanced since a capacitor is inserted in series with the tissue to be stimulated and the charge injected

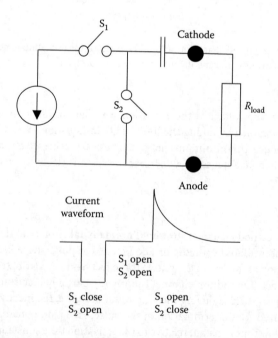

FIGURE 49.4 Method for generating biphasic cathodic-first stimulation waveform. S_1 is closed and a square negative pulse is generated through the load. S_1 is then opened and when S_2 is closed, the charge stored in the capacitor is discharged and produces the anodic phase.

s then reversed by discharging the capacitor [38]. Biphasic cathodic-first waveforms have a higher threshold than monophasic waveforms since the maximum depolarization induced by the cathodic pulse is decreased by the following anodic pulse [34]. A delay can also be added between the cathodic and anodic phase as shown in Figure 49.4. However, the time delay can also prevent adequate charge reversal and can be dangerous to the electrode and the tissue. An alternative method is to decrease the maximum amplitude of the anodic phase but to increase its length. This waveform can also be damaging to the electrode since the charge is not reversed fast enough following the cathodic pulse. The various waveforms have been ranked for their effect on tissue damage, corrosion, and threshold of activation [19,36]. The shape of the waveforms can also be optimized to minimize energy consumption [72,73].

49.4.1.6 Electrode Damage

Corrosion of the electrode is a major concern since it can cause pitting, metal dissolution, and tissue damage. Corrosion occurs at the anodic phase of the stimulation during oxidation. Therefore, by using cathodic, monophasic, or cathodic-first biphasic waveforms, corrosion can be avoided or minimized. The monophasic anodic waveform must be avoided since it will cause corrosion. Since for most applications, cathodic stimulation has a lower threshold than anodic stimulation (see Figure 49.2), the monophasic cathodic waveform has been a preferred stimulation waveform as it minimizes both the current to be injected and the corrosion. However, since the current flows only in one direction, the chemical reactions at the interface are not reversed and the electrode is driven into the irreversible region potentially generating tissue damage. A biphasic waveform will avoid both corrosion and tissue damage if the electrode potential is maintained within a reversible region [36].

49.4.1.7 Tissue Damage

A successful restoration of function with electrical stimulation requires that the activation of the excitable tissue be carried out without causing damage. Tissue damage has been divided into two categories: passive and active. Passive damage refers to surgical trauma and the lack of biocompatibility. Active damage is associated with the effect of current passing through the electrode such as physiological and electrochemical processes [39].

Surgical access to the implant site can cause significant trauma involving stretching or compression of the tissue. Postsurgical trauma can also trigger compression injury by swelling of the tissue in the presence of electrodes. Moreover, damage to the vascularization of the tissue can induce hypoxic damage. Although mechanical damage can occur, the recovery of function and normal histology has been observed [40].

The biocompatibility of the material implanted within the tissue also controls the response of the tissue. Both the metal electrode and the insulation material can contribute to the foreign tissue response. This response consists of inflammation and encapsulation of the foreign material by a layer of collagen. This layer forms 3–4 weeks following the implant and usually remains thin (about 75 μm) unless a relative movement of the implant and the tissue is allowed.

A likely cause of tissue damage is at the interface between the electrode and the tissue. The electrodes operating in the irreversible region can cause significant tissue damage since these processes can modify the pH of the surrounding tissue and generate toxic products. Balanced biphasic waveforms are preferred since the second phase can completely reverse the charge injected into the tissue. The waveforms that have the most unrecoverable charge are the most likely to induce tissue damage. The fact that electrical stimulation can cause damage directly by overdriving the tissue was obtained from experiments reporting a lesser amount of damage when the activity in the peripheral nervous system was blocked by lidocaine [41]. The mechanisms underlying this effect are still unclear but could include damage to the blood–nerve barrier, ischemia, or a large metabolic demand on the tissue, leading to changes in ionic concentration such as calcium and potassium both intra- and extracellularly.

49.5 Stimulation of Excitable Tissue

49.5.1 Stimulation of Brain Tissue

Electrodes can be placed on the surface of the brain and directly into the brain to activate the CNS pathways. The experiments with the stimulation of electrode arrays made of platinum and placed on the surface of the brain indicate that damage was produced for charge density between 50 and 300 $\mu C/cm^2$, but that the total charge/phase was also an important factor and should be kept below 3 μC [42,43]. The intracortical electrodes with a small surface area can tolerate a charge density as high as 1600 $\mu C/cm^2$ provided that the charge/phase remains below 0.0032 μC [44]. More recently, studies have shown that prolonged stimulation by electrode cortical arrays can significantly decrease the excitability of the neural tissue [45].

49.5.2 Stimulation of the Peripheral Nerve

The electrodes used with peripheral nerves are varied and include extraneural designs, such as the spiral cuffs or helix electrode [46] with electrode contacts directly on the surface of the nerve or intraneural designs placing electrode contacts directly inside the nerve [47,48]. Intraneural electrodes can cause significant damage since electrodes are inserted directly into the nerve through the perineurium but have excellent selectivity. Extraneural electrodes are relatively safe since the designs such as the spiral [49] or the helix [41], both round designs that are self-sizing, allow swelling without compression. However, the selectivity of a round electrode design is not as high as it could be since it is difficult to excite fascicles in the middle of the electrode without first activating axons located in the periphery [50]. New electrode designs aimed at producing selective stimulation by recruiting only small portions of the nerve have been proposed [51,52]. An electrode array has been designed to place electrodes directly into the nerve through the epineurium and the perineurium [53]. Another design takes advantage of the plasticity of the nerve and reshapes the nerve cross section into a flatter configuration. With this flat-interface nerve electrode (FINE) design, electrodes can be placed close to the fascicles without damaging the perineurium [40,54]. The damage in the peripheral nerve stimulation can be caused by the constriction of the nerve as well as neuronal hyperactivity and irreversible reactions at the electrode [55].

49.5.3 Stimulation of Muscle Tissue

The muscle tissue can be best excited by electrodes located on the nerve innervating the muscle [56]. However, for some applications, electrodes can be placed directly on the surface of the skin (surface stimulation, [57]), directly into the muscle (intramuscular electrode, [58]), or on the surface of the muscle (epimysial electrode, [59]). The current thresholds are higher when compared to nerve stimulation unless the electrode is carefully placed near the point of entry of the nerve [38]. Stainless steel is often used for these electrodes and is safe below 40 $\mu C/cm^2$ for coiled wire intramuscular electrodes [60].

49.5.4 Stimulation of Cardiac Tissue

The stimulation of the cardiac tissue differs in several respects from the stimulation of the nervous system. Nerve stimulation must be localized to stimulate only a single nerve or a single fascicle. In contrast, the stimulation of the heart in any appropriate region will activate the whole heart through the syncytium. Therefore, the electrode design is simpler and the timing or the pulses are of crucial importance to provide appropriate contraction patterns and to avoid the set of parameters (timing and amplitude) that can cause fibrillation (vulnerable window). Since all cells in the heart are similar in shape and size, the stimulation system does not need to consider issues dealing with fiber diameter recruitment and fatigue. Most electrodes are placed in the endocardium with a reference located on the stimulator. This monopolar stimulation can generate excitation by inducing intracellular voltage (V_m) that depends on the size of the electrode, the conductivity, the current, and the space constant. An approximate formula for the relationship between intracellular voltage V_m (mV) and extracellular current I_a (mA) is given by [61]:

$$V_m = 34 \times I_a$$

49.5.5 Magnetic Stimulation of Excitable Tissue

Time-varying magnetic fields can induce electric fields in the conducting media. Although the conductivity of the biological tissue is much lower than that of metals, it is still a good conductor. Moreover, because the conductivity is so much lower than in a metal, the magnetic field can easily penetrate within an excitable tissue such as the brain or the heart tissue. The varying magnetic field B can then induce an electric field E inside the tissue. The cable equation for magnetic stimulation is similar to the equation for electrical stimulation [62]:

$$\lambda^2 \frac{\partial^2 V_m}{\partial x^2} - \tau_m \frac{\partial V_m}{\partial t} - V_m = \lambda^2 \frac{\partial Ex}{\partial x}$$

This equation is very similar to that obtained for electrical stimulation and indicates that the nerve is excited by the first spatial derivative of the component of the electric field longitudinal with the axon. The mechanism of action of the magnetic stimulation shares similarities with electrical stimulation [63]. However, there are several important differences [64] that are not reviewed in this chapter.

49.6 Conclusion

Electrical stimulation of an excitable tissue has been highly successful as indicated by the broad application of devices such as the cardiac pacemaker and cochlear prostheses. Yet, it is also clear that the potential for these stimulation devices has not been realized. The neurotechnology industry reports revenues of $143.1 billion in 2009 [65]. Cardiac applications are also increasing rapidly as well as combined cardiac and neural applications. The challenge for researchers is to design better electrodes that can (1) be integrated within the tissue and (2) provide a functional interface with the excitable tissue. Recent advances in technology have made it possible to interface directly with the brain [66]. Yet, the mechanical and material properties of the electrodes are still not adequate for long-term implants. In the peripheral nervous system, new designs capable of intimate contact between the nerve and the electrodes has been shown to be selective for fascicle stimulation [53,67,68] and for recording [69,70]. This ability of placing the electrode closer to axons also allows fiber diameter selectivity [71] for improving the recruitment order of the nerve fibers. Yet, applications such as the neural control of an artificial limb, for example, would require that electronic circuits be embedded in these electrodes to reduce the number of leads. Therefore, this area of neural engineering has a great potential for new discoveries to help patients suffering from a wide range of disorders such as spinal injury, epilepsy, or stroke.

Acknowledgment

This work was supported by NIH grant # NS32845-10.

References

1. Grill, W.M., McDonald, J.W., Peckham, P.H., Heetderks, W., Kocsis, J., and Weinrich M., At the interface: Convergence of neural regeneration and neural prostheses for restoration of function. *J Rehabil Res Dev*, 2001. 38(6): 633–9.
2. McDonald, J.W. and Sadowsky, C., Spinal-cord injury. *Lancet*, 2002. 359(9304): 417–25.

3. Hambrecht, F.T., Neural prostheses. *Annu Rev Biophys Bioeng*, 1979. 8: 239–67.
4. Grill, W.M. and Kirsch, R.F., Neuroprosthetic applications of electrical stimulation. *Assist Technol*, 2000. 12(1): 6–20.
5. Clark, G.M., Tong Y.C., and Patrick, J.F., *Cochlear Prostheses.* Churchill Livingstone, Edinburgh, New York, 1990.
6. Glenn, W.W., Hogan, J.F., Loke, J.S., Ciesielski, T.E., Phelps, M.L., and Rowedder, R., Ventilatory support by pacing of the conditioned diaphragm in quadriplegia. *N Engl J Med*, 1984. 310(18): 1150–5.
7. Schmit, B.D. and Mortimer, J.T., The effects of epimysial electrode location on phrenic nerve recruitment and the relation between tidal volume and interpulse interval. *IEEE Trans Rehabil Eng*, 1999. 7(2): 150–8.
8. Brindley, G.S. and Lewin, W.S., The sensations produced by electrical stimulation of the visual cortex. *J Physiol*, 1968. 196(2): 479–93.
9. Chader, G.J., Weiland, J., and Humayun, M.S., Artificial vision: Needs, functioning, and testing of a retinal electronic prosthesis. *Prog Brain Res*, 2009. 175: 317–32.
10. Kilgore, K.L., Hoyen, H.A., Bryden, A. M., Hart, R.L., Keith, M.W., and Peckham, P. H., An implanted upper-extremity neuroprosthesis using myoelectric control. *J Hand Surg Am*, 2008. 33(4): 539–50.
11. Dostrovsky, J.O. and Lozano, A.M., Mechanisms of deep brain stimulation. *Mov Disord*, 2002. 17 (3): S63–8.
12. Andrews, R.J., Neuro modulation: Advances in the next five years. *Ann N Y Acad Sci*, 2010. 1199: 204–11.
13. George, M.S., Nahas, Z., Bohning, D.E., Kozel, F.A., Anderson, B., Chae, J.H., Lomarev, M., Denslow, S., Li, X., and Mu, C., Vagus nerve stimulation therapy: A research update. *Neurology*, 2002. 59(4): S56–61.
14. Greatbatch, W. and Selignman, L., *Pacemakers. Encyclopedia of Medical Devices and Instrumentation*, John Wiley and Sons, New York, 1988.
15. Roth, B.J., Mechanisms for electrical stimulation of excitable tissue. *Crit Rev Biomed Eng*, 1994. 22(3–4): 253–305.
16. Plonsey, R., *Bioelectric Phenomena.* McGraw-Hill, New York, 1969.
17. Kraus, J.D., *Electromagnetics.* McGraw-Hill, New York, 1973.
18. Nunez, N., *Electric Fields in the Brain.* Oxford Press, New York, 1981.
19. Durand, D.M., *Electrical Stimulation of Excitable Tissue. Handbook of Biomedical Engineering.* 1: pp. 17.1–17.22. CRC Press, Boca Raton, ed: J.D. Bronzino, 2000.
20. Rall, W., Core conductor theory and cable properties of neurons. *Handbook of Physiology: The Nervous System I.* (Chapter 3): pp. 39–96. American Physiological Society, Bethesda, 1979.
21. Ranck, J.B., Which elements are excited in electrical stimulation of mammalian central nervous system: A review. *Brain Res*, 1975. 98: 417–40.
22. McNeal, D.R., Analysis of a model for excitation of myelinated nerve. *IEEE Trans Biomed Eng*, 1976. 23(4): 329–37.
23. Koch, C., *Methods in Neural Modeling*, MIT Press, Cambridge, MA 1989.
24. Hines, M., Efficient computation of branched nerve equations. *Int J Biomed Comput*, 1984. 15(1): 69–76.
25. Altman, K.W. and Plonsey, R., Development of a model for point source electrical fiber bundle stimulation. *Med Biol Eng Comput*, 1988. 26(5): 466–75.
26. Rattay, F., Analysis of models for extracellular fiber stimulation. *IEEE Trans Biomed Eng*, 1989. 36(7): 676–82.
27. Rattay, F., *Electrical Nerve Stimulation, Theory, Experiments and Applications.* Springer-Verlag, New York, 1990.
28. Warman, E.N., Grill, W.M., and Durand D., Modeling the effects of electric fields on nerve fibers: Determination of excitation thresholds. *IEEE Trans Biomed Eng*, 1992. 39(12): 1244–54.
29. McIntyre, C.C. and Grill, W.M., Excitation of central nervous system neurons by nonuniform electric fields. *Biophys J*, 1999. 76(2): 878–88.

30. Lapicque, L., *Recherches Quantitatives Sur l'excitation Electrique Des Nerfs Traites*. 1907.

31. Jack, J.J.B., Noble, D., and Tsien, R.W., *Electrical Current Flow in Excitable Cells*. Clarendon Press, Oxford, 1983.

32. Grill, W.M. Jr. and Mortimer, J.T., The effect of stimulus pulse duration on selectivity of neural stimulation. *IEEE Trans Biomed Eng*, 1996. 43(2): 161–6.

33. Gorman, P.H. and Mortimer, J.T., The effect of stimulus parameters on the recruitment characteristics of direct nerve stimulation. *IEEE Trans Biomed Eng*, 1983. 30(7): 407–14.

34. Mortimer, J.T., *Electrical Excitation of Nerve. Neural Prostheses Fundamental Studies*, The University of Michigan, eds: W.F. Agnew and D.B. McCreery, 1990: pp. 67–84.

35. Fang, Z.P. and Mortimer, J.T., Selective activation of small motor axons by quasi-trapezoidal current pulses. *IEEE Trans Biomed Eng*, 1991. 38(2): 168–74.

36. Robblee, L.S. and Rose, T.L., *Electrochemical Guidelines for Selection of Protocols and Electrode Materials for Neural Stimulation. Neural Prostheses Fundamental Studies*, The University of Michigan, eds: W.F. Agnew and D.B. McCreery, 1990.

37. Shannon, R.V., A model of safe levels for electrical stimulation. *IEEE Trans Biomed Eng*, 1992. 39(4): 424–6.

38. Mortimer, J.T., *Motor Prostheses. Handbook of Physiology—The Nervous System*. 3: pp. 155–87, American Physiological Society, Bethesda, 1981.

39. McCreery, D.B. and Agnew, W.F., *Mechanisms of Stimulation Induced Neural Damage and Their Relation to Guidelines for Safe Stimulation. Neural Prostheses Fundamental Studies*, The university of Michigan, eds: W.F. Agnew and D.B. McCreery, 1990.

40. Tyler, D.J. and Durand, D.M., Chronic response of the rat sciatic nerve to the flat interface nerve electrode. *Ann Biomed Eng*, 2003. 31(6): 633–42.

41. Agnew, W.F. and McCreery, D.B., Considerations for safety with chronically implanted nerve electrodes. *Epilepsia*, 1990. 31(2): S27–32.

42. Pudenz, R.H., Bullara, L.A., and Talalla, A., Electrical stimulation of the brain. I. Electrodes and electrode arrays. *Surg Neurol*, 1975. 4(1): 37–42.

43. Pudenz, R.H., Bullara, L.A., Dru, D., and Talalla, A., Electrical stimulation of the brain. II. Effects on the blood–brain barrier. *Surg Neurol*, 1975. 4(2): 265–70.

44. Agnew, W.F., Yuen, T.G., McCreery, D.B., and Bullara, L.A., Histopathologic evaluation of prolonged intracortical electrical stimulation. *Exp Neurol*, 1986. 92(1): 162–85.

45. McCreery, D.B., Agnew, W.F., and Bullara, L.A., The effects of prolonged intracortical microstimulation on the excitability of pyramidal tract neurons in the cat. *Ann Biomed Eng*, 2002. 30(1): 107–19.

46. Naples, G.G., Mortimer, J.T., and Yuen, T.G.H., Overview of peripheral nerve electrode design and implantation, in *Neural Prostheses: Fundamental Studies*, W.F. Agnew and D.B. McCreery, eds. 1990, Prentice Hall: Englewood Cliffs, NJ, pp. 107–45.

47. Nannini, N. and Horch, K., Muscle recruitment with intrafascicular electrodes. *IEEE Trans Biomed Eng*, 1991. 38(8): 769–76.

48. Rutten, W.L., van Wier, H.J., and Put, J.H., Sensitivity and selectivity of intraneural stimulation using a silicon electrode array. *IEEE Trans Biomed Eng*, 1991. 38(2): 192–8.

49. Naples, G.G., Mortimer, J.T., Scheiner, A., and Sweeney, J.D., A spiral nerve cuff electrode for peripheral nerve stimulation. *IEEE Trans Biomed Eng*, 1988. 35(11): 905–16.

50. Choi, A.Q., Cavanaugh, J.K., and Durand, D.M., Selectivity of multiple-contact nerve cuff electrodes: A simulation analysis. *IEEE Trans Biomed Eng*, 2001. 48(2): 165–72.

51. Veraart, C., Grill, W.M., and Mortimer, J.T., Selective control of muscle activation with a multipolar nerve cuff electrode. *IEEE Trans Biomed Eng*, 1993. 40(7): 640–53.

52. Tyler, D.J. and Durand, D.M., A slowly penetrating interfascicular nerve electrode for selective activation of peripheral nerves. *IEEE Trans Rehabil Eng*, 1997. 5: 51–61.

53. Branner, A., Stein, R.B., and Normann, R.A., Selective stimulation of cat sciatic nerve using an array of varying-length microelectrodes. *J Neurophysiol*, 2001. 85(4): 1585–94.

54. Tyler, D.J. and Durand, D.M., Functionally selective peripheral nerve stimulation with a flat interface nerve electrode. *IEEE Trans Neural Syst Rehabil Eng*, 2002. 10(4): 294–303.

55. McCreery, D.B., Agnew, W.F., Yuen, T.G., and Bullara. L.A., Damage in peripheral nerve from continuous electrical stimulation: Comparison of two stimulus waveforms. *Med Biol Eng Comput*, 1992. 30(1): 109–14.

56. Popovic, D., Gordon, T., Rafuse, V.F., and Prochazka, A., Properties of implanted electrodes for functional electrical stimulation. *Ann Biomed Eng*, 1991. 19(3): 303–16.

57. Myklebust, J.B., Cusick, J.F., Sances, A.J., and Larson S.J., *Neural Stimulation.* CRC Press, Boca Raton, FL, 1985.

58. Caldwell, C.W. and Reswick, J.B., A percutaneous wire electrode for chronic research use. *IEEE Trans Biomed Eng*, 1975. 22(5): 429–32.

59. Grandjean, P.A. and Mortimer, J.T., Recruitment properties of monopolar and bipolar epimysial electrodes. *Ann Biomed Eng*, 1986. 14(1): 53–66.

60. Mortimer, J.T., Kaufman, D., and Roessman, U., Intramuscular electrical stimulation: Tissue damage. *Ann Biomed Eng*, 1980. 8(3): 235–44.

61. Malmivuo, J. and Plonsey, R., *Bioelectromagnetism.* Oxford University Press, Oxford, 1995.

62. Basser, P.J., Wijesinghe, R.S., and Roth, B.J., The activating function for magnetic stimulation derived from a three-dimensional volume conductor model. *IEEE Trans Biomed Eng*, 1992. 39(11): 1207–10.

63. Roth, B.J. and Basser, P.J., A model of the stimulation of a nerve fiber by electromagnetic induction. *IEEE Trans Biomed Eng*, 1990. 37(6): 588–97.

64. Nagarajan, S.S., Durand, D.M., and Hsuing-Hsu, K., Mapping location of excitation during magnetic stimulation: Effects of coil position. *Ann Biomed Eng*, 1997. 25(1): 112–25.

65. Casey, L., NeuroInsight. http://www.neuroinsights.com/neurotech2010release.html, 2010.

66. Donoghue, J.P., Connecting cortex to machines: Recent advances in brain interfaces. *Nat Neurosci*, 2002. 5: 1085–8.

67. Leventhal, D.K. and Durand, D.M., Chronic measurement of the stimulation selectivity of the flat interface nerve electrode. *IEEE Trans Biomed Eng*, 2004. 51(9): 1649–58.

68. McDonnall, D., Clark, G.A., and Normann, R.A., Selective motor unit recruitment via intrafascicular multielectrode stimulation. *Can J Physiol Pharmacol*, 2004. 82(8–9): 599–609.

69. Lawrence, S.M., Dhillon, G.S., Jensen, W., Yoshida, K., and Horch, K.W., Acute peripheral nerve recording characteristics of polymer-based longitudinal intrafascicular electrodes. *IEEE Trans Neural Syst Rehabil Eng*, 2004. 12(3): 345–8.

70. Yoo, P.B. and Durand, D.M., Selective fascicular recording of the hypoglossal nerve using a multicontact nerve cuff electrode. *Ann Biomed Eng*, 2003. 32: 511–19.

71. Lertmanorat, Z. and Durand, D.M., A novel electrode array for diameter-dependent control of axonal excitability: A simulation study. *IEEE Trans Biomed Eng*, 2004. 51(7): 1242–50.

72. Jezernik, S., Sinkjaer, T., and Morari, M., Charge and energy minimization in electrical/magnetic stimulation of nervous tissue. *J Neural Eng*, 2010. 7(4): 04600.

73. Wongsarnpigoon, A. and Grill, W.M., Energy-efficient waveform shapes for neural stimulation revealed with a genetic algorithm. *J Neural Eng*, 2010. 7(4): 046009–20.

V

Neuroengineering

Daniel J. DiLorenzo
University of Texas Medical Branch

50 **History and Overview of Neural Engineering** *Daniel J. DiLorenzo*
and Robert E. Gross 50-1
Background • Neural Augmentation (Neural Prostheses) • Neuromodulation •
References

51 **Theory and Physiology of Electrical Stimulation of the Central Nervous**
System *Warren M. Grill* 51-1
Introduction • Generation of Potentials in CNS Tissues • Response of Neurons
to Imposed Extracellular Potentials • From Cell to Circuit: Construction of Models
of CNS Neurons • Sites of Action Potential Initiation in CNS Neurons • Excitation
Properties of CNS Stimulation • Summary • Acknowledgments • References

52 **Transcutaneous FES for Ambulation: The Parastep System** *Daniel Graupe* 52-1
Introduction and Background • Parastep System • Patient Admissibility,
Contraindications, and Training • Walking Performance and Medical and Psychological
Benefits Evaluation Results • Regulatory Status • Concluding Comments • References

53 **Comparing Electrodes for Use as Cortical Control Signals: Tines, Wires,**
or Cones on Wires—Which Is Best? *Philip R. Kennedy* 53-1
Brief Description of the Neurotrophic Electrode and Its Neural Signals • Identification
of the Action Potentials Recorded from the NE • Functionality of the Action Potentials
Recorded from the NE • Plasticity Was Demonstrated for Single APs But Not Attempted
with LFPs • Misconceptions Regarding the Neurotrophic Electrode • Difficulties and
Disadvantages with the NE • Acknowledgments • References

54 **Development of a Multifunctional 22-Channel Functional Electrical**
Stimulator for Paraplegia *Ross Davis, T. Johnston, B. Smith, R. Betz,*
T. Houdayer, and A. Barriskill 54-1
Introduction • Historical Aspect • Neural Engineering Clinic: Two Male Subjects •
Experience at Shriners Hospitals for Children • Conclusion • Acknowledgments •
References

55 An Implantable Bionic Network of Injectable Neural Prosthetic Devices: The Future Platform for Functional Electrical Stimulation and Sensing to Restore Movement and Sensation *J. Schulman, P. Mobley, J. Wolfe, Ross Davis, and I. Arcos*... 55-1
Introduction • Evolution of the Implantable BION Devices • Battery-Powered BION System for Functional Electrical Stimulation and Sensing • Applications • References

56 Visual Prostheses *Robert J. Greenberg*... 56-1
Acknowledgment • References

57 Interfering with the Genesis and Propagation of Epileptic Seizures by Neuromodulation *Ana Luisa Velasco, Francisco Velasco, Marcos Velasco, Bernardo Boleaga, Mauricio Kuri, Fiacro Jiménez, and José María Núñez*..................... 57-1
Introduction • Electrical Stimulation of the Centromedian Thalamic Nuclei • Results • Electrical Stimulation of the Hippocampus • Study Design • Results • Neuromodulation of the Supplementary Motor Area • Conclusion • References

58 Transcranial Magnetic Stimulation of Deep Brain Regions *Yiftach Roth and Abraham Zangen*.. 58-1
Introduction • Basic Principles of TMS • Deep TMS Coils: Design Principles • A Coil for Stimulation of Deep Brain Regions Related to Mood Disorders: Simulations and Phantom Measurements • TMS of Deep Brain Regions: Evidence for Efficacy of the H-Coil • TMS of Deep Prefrontal Regions • References

50

History and Overview of Neural Engineering

50.1 Background...50-1
The Early History of Electrical Stimulation of the Nervous System
50.2 Neural Augmentation (Neural Prostheses)...............................50-3
Origins of the Field of Neural Prostheses • Neural Augmentation:
Motor Prostheses • Neural Augmentation: Sensory Prostheses
50.3 Neuromodulation..50-8
Chronic Electrical Stimulation of the Nervous System for Functional
Disorders • Early Development of Deep-Brain Stimulation
for Psychiatric Disorders and Pain • The Dawn of Deep-Brain
Stimulation for Movement Disorders • The Efforts toward
Neurostimulation for Epilepsy • Current State of the Art of
Neurostimulation
References..50-12

Daniel J. DiLorenzo
University of Texas Medical Branch
NeuroVista Corporation
DiLorenzo Biomedical, LLC

Robert E. Gross
Emory University

50.1 Background

Recent years have witnessed remarkable advances in the development of technology and its practical applications in the amelioration of neurological dysfunction. This encompasses a wide variety of disorders, and their treatment has been the purview of different, partially overlapping, medical and scientific specialties and societies. As a result of these advances, three somewhat independent and longstanding fields with unique origins—stereotactic and functional neurosurgery, neuromodulation, and functional electrical stimulation (FES)—are experiencing increasing convergence and overlap, and the distinctions separating them are beginning to blur.

Stereotactic and functional neurosurgery—which takes its origins at the beginning of neurosurgery in the late nineteenth century, but which as a society dates to the 1940s—has mainly concerned itself with the surgical treatment of nervous system conditions that manifest as disordered function, including movement disorders (Parkinson's disease, tremor, dystonia), pain, epilepsy and psychiatric illnesses. In the first part of the last century, the surgical treatment of these disorders usually involved ablation of nervous tissue, but this has almost completely been supplanted by the advent of electrical neurostimulation. Other modalities within the purview of stereotactic and functional neurosurgery include pharmacological and biological therapies that are delivered via surgical techniques.

Neuromodulation broadly involves alteration of the function of the nervous system. The International Neuromodulation Society was established in the 1990s and dedicated itself to the treatment of nervous system disorders—mostly pain and spasticity—with implantable devices, including pumps and stimulators. However, with the advances in the field, this society has broadened its scope to include implantable devices used to treat disorders of sensory and motor functions of the body. This society has been driven by both anesthesiologists and neurosurgeons, but has mainly been clinical in its purview.

FES has pertained mostly to the restoration of upper and lower limb function (after injury and ischemia), bowel, bladder and sexual function, and respiratory function. This field, represented by the International Functional Electrical Stimulation Society, also is interested in auditory and visual prostheses, and has—in contrast to the two other societies—a distinctly engineering bias, limited as it has been to electrical stimulation.

It is quite clear that each of these areas has strong overlap, both clinically as well as technologically. While one or the other may have been more clinical or basic in its scientific approach, with the progress in both technology development and its translation into the clinic, these distinctions are becoming increasingly blurred. Advances in functional neurosurgery have been driven by clinical empiricism and advances in pathophysiological understanding of the target disorders, but also by technological advancement (e.g., the development of the stereotactic frame, and then frameless image guidance stereotactic technology, and the development of implantable neurostimulation systems). Neuromodulation—based as it is on the use of implantable devices—has been driven by technical and pharmacological innovation coupled to increased understanding of neurophysiology and the pathophysiological manifestations in states of disease. Finally, FES has mostly been an undertaking driven by engineering technology, since from the outset the goals have been restoration of motor function using controlled electrical stimulation. Clinical application has always been the long-term objective, and with the current synergy of technological innovation and increasing clinical experimentalism (e.g., motor prosthesis trials for spinal cord injury) the field is making great strides.

The technology that is a main driver behind each of these overlapping disciplines can be coined "Neural Engineering." Although this domain might seem like a relatively recent innovation, a view into the historical underpinnings of neuromodulation in the eighteenth century reveals that in fact from the start, technological innovation and neuromodulation developed hand in hand, and some of this pioneering foundation building of the last several centuries might reasonably be called neural engineering.

50.1.1 The Early History of Electrical Stimulation of the Nervous System

The use of electricity for therapeutic purposes can arguably be said to date back even to the use of amber and magnetite in jewelry around 9000 BC [1]. The use of the torpedo fish or electric eel was advocated by Scribonius Largus—one of the first Roman physicians in the first millennium—for the treatment of headache and gout [2]. The patient would apply the fish to the painful region until numb (but not too long) [3]. Its use continued into the sixteenth century by which time the indications were broadened to include melancholy, migraine, and epilepsy.

By the seventeenth century electricity was identified as a form of energy and primitive devices to induce electric current were developed. The first electrostatic generator was constructed in 1672, but electrical sparks from a modified electrostatic generator were first used therapeutically to treat paralysis in 1744 [3] (the first example of neural engineering?) In 1745 in Leyden the capacity of an electrified glass jar and tin foil—the Leyden jar—to store electrical charge was inadvertently discovered when its discharge caused a physiological effect so severe that the experimenter took two days to recover [4]. Electricity and the nervous system were intricately associated early on because the most sensitive electrical detector at the time was in fact the nervous system. The new phenomenon was quickly embraced by the medical field, and "cures" of paralysis and other ailments rapidly proliferated, yielding many fantastic books from "electrotherapists" such as John Wesley the divine [3,4]. By 1752, even Benjamin Franklin was using it, to treat a 24-year-old woman with convulsions [5], and various palsies, but he at least was not convinced of any persistent benefits from the electrical treatments [4].

Albrecht von Haller felt that nerves and muscles were sensitive to the effects of electrical current, but he and others did not believe that electricity played a role in normal functioning [6]. In 1791, Galvani published his famous experiments in which he induced muscular contractions in frog leg muscle using a metallic device constructed of dissimilar metals [7]. He reasoned that the electrical current was being "discharged" from the muscle, a view which was countered by Volta who felt that the electrical current lowed from the dissimilar metals [8] and which led him to develop the voltaic bimetallic pile—the first battery—based on this insight [9]. Electrophysiological experiments using voltaic piles to generate "Galvanic current" rapidly proliferated, including important experiments by Aldini—Galvani's nephew—who was interested in, among other things, the therapeutic applications of galvanism [6] (more examples of neural engineering). His particular interest was in "reanimation" especially following near-drowning, and this work included electrically stimulating both animals and men—the latter following the not infrequent hangings and decapitations [10]. He was successful at provoking muscular contractions of the somatic musculature, but was disappointed that he could not get similar results with the heart [6]. In fact, Aldini was likely the first to induce facial muscle contractions with direct brain electrical stimulation in both oxen and human cadavers, predating Fritsch and Hitzig's influential work by many years [11]. A particularly dramatic demonstration on a hanged criminal in England garnered widespread lay coverage, possibly contributing to the inspiration behind the *Frankenstein* myth [6]. He also used the voltaic piles to treat "mental disorders" including depression—a precursor to electroconvulsive therapy—after first applying the pile safely to his own head [10].

The next major advance arose from Faraday's invention of the first electric generator in 1831, which induced alternating or "Faradic current" by rotating wires inside a magnetic field. Dubois-Reymond in 1848 demonstrated that the time-varying nature of faradic current was important in efficient stimulation, and he formulated an early expression of the strength–duration curve relating the threshold for activating the neuromuscular system to the intensity and duration of the current pulse [3]. G. B. Duchenne—regarded as the father of "electrotherapy"—established it as a separate discipline ("De l'Electrisation localisee," 1855) [3]. He used faradic current applied through moistened electrode pads, preferring it to galvanic current because of its warming properties. In 1852 he stimulated the facial nerve for palsy [12]. With Duchenne's influence and the proliferation of induction coils and batteries, therapeutic electrical stimulation spread widely. By 1900, according to McNeal, most physicians in the United States had an "electrical machine" for the treatment of a plethora of ailments—many neurological, including pain. Many different and interesting devices were constructed, for use in every part of the body (literally), including the "hydroelectric bath" (not recommended!) [3]. Called the "Golden Age of Medical Electricity," the close of the nineteenth century would only be eclipsed by the close of the following century in the proliferation of the use of electricity in medical therapeutics.

Fritsch and Hitzig [11] are said to have been the first to stimulate the cortex in living animals, and systematic mapping of cerebro-cortical function was described in animals by Ferrier [13]. The first time the human brain was directly stimulated in an awake patient was in 1878 by Barthlow, who introduced a stimulating needle into a patient's brain through an eroding scalp and skull tumor [14]. Low-amplitude faradic current elicited contralateral muscle contractions and an unpleasant tingling feeling, initiating the field of cerebral localization using electrical stimulation. Cushing observed the effects of intraoperative faradic stimulation in 1909 [15], and Foerster's intraoperative work in the 1930s influenced Wilder Penfield, culminating in Penfield and Jasper's seminal publication of *Functional Anatomy of the Human Brain* in 1954 [16].

50.2 Neural Augmentation (Neural Prostheses)

50.2.1 Origins of the Field of Neural Prostheses

The field of neural prostheses encompasses the set of technologies relevant to the restoration of neurological and neuromuscular function, and this includes both motor prostheses and sensory prostheses. The early motor work focused on technologies for restoration of limb motor function, these having clinical relevance to the treatment of both paralyzed and amputee patients. Over the last several decades, as microelectronic and microfabrication technologies have progressed, sensory prostheses have reached the state of practicality, and cochlear implants have become a standard of care in the treatment of sensorineural deafness. Research and commercialization efforts continue in remaining areas, including restoration of the motor and sensory functions of the limbs, motor functions of the bladder, bowel, and diaphragm, and sensory functions, including tactile, visual, and vestibular.

In the 1950s, a human study showing sound perception arising from electrode implantation inspired researchers across the world to investigate the possibility of a cochlear prosthesis, which, after several decades of development in academia and industry, became the first FDA-approved neural prosthesis [17].

The Neural Prosthesis Program, launched in 1972 and spearheaded by F. Terry Hambrecht, MD, brought funding, focus, and coordination to the multidisciplinary effort to develop technologies to restore motor function to paralyzed individuals. The initial efforts were in electrode–tissue interaction, biomaterials and neural interface development, cochlear and visual prosthesis development, and control of motor function using implanted and nonimplanted electrodes.

In his 1980 UC Davis PhD thesis, David Edell demonstrated chronic recording from peripheral nerves using a multichannel micromachined silicon regeneration electrode array [18,19]. This was a major achievement, as it proved that chronic recording from the nervous system was possible. Furthermore, his silicon-based implant was proof of concept that biocompatible recording interfaces could be made from silicon using existing etching and microfabrication technology—and could therefore be made to incorporate electrodes, preamplifiers, processing, memory, and telemetry elements on the same silicon substrate, implanted in the nervous system.

50.2.2 Neural Augmentation: Motor Prostheses

50.2.2.1 Neuromuscular Stimulation for Control of Limb Movement

Liberson and coworkers are credited as being the first to utilize FES to restore the functional control of movement to a paralyzed limb [20]. They treated over 100 hemiplegic patients with foot drop using a transistorized stimulator and conductive rubber electrodes placed on the skin overlying the peroneal nerve. A switch under the sole triggered stimulation during the swing phase of gait, causing contraction of the tibialis anterior and dorsiflexion of the foot [21]. All patients were reported to have received some benefit, but acceptance was limited by skin irritation from the electrode, need for precise electrode placement, hassle in applying the device compared to functional benefit, and electrode lead breakage, Liberson termed this "functional electrotherapy"; however, this term did not gain widespread acceptance; rather, "functional electrical stimulation," coined by Moe and Post, did [22].

Long and Masciarelli, intrigued by Liberson's lower extremity work, devised a system for upper extremity functional restoration in high cervical quadriplegic patients [23]. Using FES-controlled finger extension, via extensor digitorum stimulation, coupled with spring-loaded thumb and finger flexion, the device enabled control of grasp in the paralyzed limb. Though patients tolerated it very well, it did not gain widespread clinical acceptance.

Peckham and colleagues at Case Western Reserve University used chronic percutaneous stimulation of forearm muscles to provide hand grasp, including both palmar and lateral prehension and release, in C5 quadriplegic patients [24]

Restoration of some form of assisted gait in spinal cord-injured patients has been the focus of several research groups. In 1960, Kantrowitz reported the use of surface stimulation of quadriceps and gluteal muscles to effect rising and standing for several minutes from a sitting position in a paraplegic patient [25]. In 1973, Cooper reported bilateral implantation of the femoral and sciatic nerves in a T11–12 paraplegic and claimed ambulation of up to 40 ft using a walker for balance assistance [26].

Using implanted stimulators and electrodes on the femoral nerves bilaterally, Brindley was able to achieve in a paraplegic arising from a sitting position and limited gait assisted with elbow crutches but not requiring a walker, braces, or other support [27]. Several more sophisticated devices followed. Kralj et al. described a 4–6-channel skin surface electrode FES systems in which patients ambulated with the assistance of parallel bars or a roller walker [28,29]. At MIT in 1990, DiLorenzo and Durfee implemented a computer-controlled 4-channel skin surface electrode FES system with bilateral quadricep

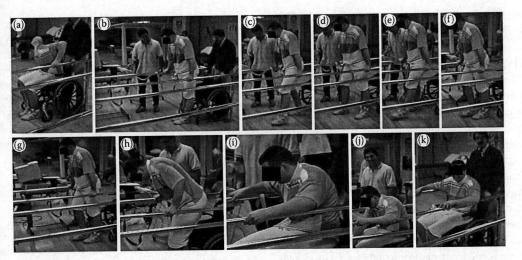

FIGURE 50.1 Series of still images from 4-channel FES gait sequence performed by author (DJD) at MIT in 1990. (a) Subject bracing to stand, (b) standing under FES control with computer-controlled stimulator on the far left (L to R: author DJD, subject, Allen Wiegner, PhD), (c) first step, (d) second step, (e) third step, (f) fourth step, (g) preparing to sit, (h) sitting down, (i) seated in wheelchair after walking, (j) repositioning feet, (k) smiling.

stimulation and peroneal nerve-withdrawal reflex stimulation and achieved 60 ft of handrail balance-assisted gait in a thoracic spinal cord-injured patient [30] and developed adaptive closed-loop controllers which compensated for time-varying muscle performance, including gain changes due to muscle fatigue [31,32]. Figure 50.1 shows a sequence of still frames from a gait sequence using this 4-channel surface FES configuration [30]. Convinced of the greater potential for clinical efficacy and market success with implanted technologies, DiLorenzo pursued related implanted FES work [30,33–36], and Goldfarb and Durfee continued this line of surface FES work to include a long-legged brace with a computer-controlled friction brake, for improved energy efficiency and control [37].

Marsolais reported improved motor function in patients with intramuscular stainless-steel electrodes implanted in the quadriceps, hip flexors, extensors, and abductors [38]. Though significant motor torque improvement was achieved in some of these patients, all of whom had some motor function pre-implantation, patients required supervision for ambulation.

Dan Graupe extended the surface FES technology developed by Lieberson and Kralj to include a patient borne and controlled system [39,40]. Graupe then commercialized this technology for clinical use as the ParaStep system. The history of the field of FES for ambulation and the commercialization of ParaStep is described in more detail in the chapter by Graupe in this volume.

The first generation of implanted FES systems for upper extremity functional restoration were developed at Case Western Reserve University and Cleveland Veterans Affairs Medical Center for the restoration of hand grasp to patient with cervical spinal cord injury [41]. This system allowed the paraplegic patient to control hand grasp on an otherwise paralyzed limb by generating movement commands using contralateral shoulder movements. This technology was commercialized by NeuroControl Corporation, which was founded by Hunter Peckham, PhD, Ronald Podraza, and colleagues at Case Western Reserve University in Cleveland, Ohio. NeuroControl received FDA approval in 1997 to market the grasp restoration device, known as the FreeHand System.

50.2.2.2 Chronically Implanted Neuroelectric Interfaces (Recording Arrays)

50.2.2.2.1 Basic Neuroscience

Separate but concurrent research efforts by many investigators in basic neurophysiology were making significant advancements in developing an understanding of how cortical and spinal neural systems control motor function. Extensive research on control of movement by hundreds of neuroscientists has revealed correlations between parameters of limb movement and neural activity in many motor centers, including the primary motor cortex, premotor and supplementary motor cortex, cerebellum, and spinal cord.

The motor cortex was the first area to undergo detailed quantitative study of neuronal activity during whole-arm reaching movements in an awake behaving primate [42]. Georgopoulos et al. [42] first demonstrated a relation between neural cell activity and movement direction. They found that cell firing rates are directionally sensitive in a graded manner, that is, the firing rate is maximal in a so-called preferred direction, and the firing rate tapers off gradually as the direction of movement deviates from this preferred direction. In 1984, Georgopoulos et al. [43] demonstrated the presence of cells in both primary motor cortex and in area 5 the firing rates of which correlate linearly with position of the hand in two-dimensional space. Subsequent work expanded this knowledge to include additional movement parameters and limb movement in three-dimensional space [44–48].

Later research, beginning in the 1990s focused on control using neural signals, in both nonhuman primate and human subjects, lending credence to the notion that sufficient information may be extracted from neural signals to be used as a control signal for a prosthetic system. Schwartz extended this work and characterized neural firing patterns associated with limb movement in three-dimensional space [46] and with Taylor and Tillary developed a real-time adaptive prediction algorithm with which a primate was able to control robot arm movement [49]. Donoghue et al. [50] pursued similar lines of research and characterized patterns of behavior from large populations of cells. DiLorenzo showed evidence for the presence of real-time motor feedback error signals in the primate motor cortex, suggesting the presence of feedforward and feedback signals in primary motor cortex [51]. Using the 100-channel intracortical array developed by Richard Normann, Donoghue characterized additional information content in correlations between neuronal activity [52]. Using wire electrode arrays, Nicolelis also characterized real-time prediction of limb trajectory using neural ensembles, and in collaboration with Srinivasan showed remote control of robot movement by a nonhuman primate [53].

50.2.2.3 Initial Application to Humans

Kennedy and Bakay demonstrated human 2-D control of cursor movement by a paralyzed human patient using the cone neurotrophic electrode [54–56]. This novel electrode facilitates regeneration of neural processes into an insulating glass cone where a stable electrical and mechanical interface forms, providing a long-term high signal-to-noise ratio. In 1987, Kennedy founded neural signals to develop the cone electrode for clinical use; however, the company has refocused its direction on the commercialization of a less-invasive EMG-driven system for locked-in patients.

A spinout from Donoghue's and Normann's research efforts, Cyberkinetics Neurotechnology Systems, Inc., has demonstrated in pilot studies human control of cursor movement using a 4×4 mm 96-channel intracortical microelectrode array chronically implanted into the primary motor cortex [57]. As of this writing, they have demonstrated the ability to record over 6 months post-implantation.

50.2.3 Neural Augmentation: Sensory Prostheses

50.2.3.1 Sensory Stimulation: Auditory (Cochlear Implant)

Auditory prostheses, which provide patterned stimulation of the eighth cranial nerve, were the first commercially available sensory neural prosthesis. As of this writing, it is the only approved sensory prosthesis; however, visual prostheses are already in clinical trials and are likely to be available in the not too distant future.

An experiment published in 1957 by Djourno and Eyries is credited with inspiring the development of the cochlear implant [17]. Paris otologist C. Eyries, and neurophysiologist A. Djourno implanted wires in the inner ear of a deaf patient and were able to elicit sensations of sound with electrical stimulation. This experiment was reproduced in 1964 by Doyle et al. in Los Angeles [58].

Inspired by this 1957 Djourno article, William House, MD joined with Jack Urban, president of an electronics company, in Los Angeles to develop a cochlear implant, and they published results on their first patients in 1973 [59]. Working with investigators at the House Ear Institute, founded by his brother Howard House, MD, also an otolaryngologist, William House pioneered the development of the single-channel cochlear implant and achieved its approval by the FDA [60].

Blair Simmons of Stanford University first evaluated multichannel cochlear stimulation, placing 4 wires into the auditory nerve [61]. Several years later, Dr. Robin Michelson, an otolaryngologist at the University of California San Francisco (UCSF), implanted a multichannel cochlear implant placed in the scala tympani [62]. Michael Merzenich, also of UCSF, led the research and development of this and subsequent multichannel cochlear implants [63]. Al Mann founded Advanced Bionics' Corporation in 1993, licensed the UCSF cochlear implant technology, and recruited Joe Schulman, PhD and Tom Santogrossi to develop this technology into the CLARION cochlear implant [64–67].

In parallel with developments in the United States, in Melbourne, Australia, Graeme Clark initiated a large and extremely productive clinical and research program at the University of Melbourne in Australia [68–71]. The implants developed under Clark are manufactured by Cochlear Ltd., a subsidiary of Nucleus Pty. Ltd. in Sydney, and Cochlear has the largest worldwide population of implanted patients, with over 65,000 patients having been implanted with the Nucleus worldwide [72].

In 1975, Ingeborg and Erwin Hochmair began development of a multi-channel cochlear implant, which was implanted in Vienna 2 years later [73,74]. They continued development of the device for nearly a decade and in 1989 founded MED-EL, which has since become the third major manufacturer of cochlear implants.

There are several factors that have contributed to the success of the cochlear implant. (1) Well-developed foundation of basic science, particularly in the area of auditory neurophysiology. (2) Focused and coordinated research programs and funding, including that of the NIH Neural Prosthesis Program. (3) Clinician champions who were active in the research and facilitated its clinical acceptance as early adopters themselves and as thought leaders. (4) Cochlear anatomy, including the tonotopic arrangement of sensory receptors and their protection by a bony encasement, facilitating stable chronic neuroelectric interfacing. Because of this surgically accessible anatomy, an electrode array may be placed and press chronically against a rigid surface while being in close proximity to neural cells, without the risk of damage to or migration through soft neural tissues. This neural interfacing problem is a major hurdle in the development of visual, somatosensory, and motor prostheses, which generally must interface directly with soft neural tissues, which are subject to perpetually changing forces and displacements.

50.2.3.2 Sensory Stimulation: Visual

The restoration of vision has captivated the imagination of man since biblical times. Now, after four decades of modern research, beginning with the stimulation of the visual cortex by Giles Brindley in 1966 [75], visual prostheses are making the transition from basic science research to commercialization. William Dobelle, PhD achieved similar results using cortical stimulation to evoke phosphenes in 1974 [76,77], and he was a pioneer in the drive to commercialize the visual cortex prosthesis. In 1983, he acquired Avery Labs, a manufacturer of electrodes for brain stimulation. From this and other ventures he derived funds to advance his vision prosthesis research and development efforts at the Dobelle Institute, located in Portugal. An excellent historical review is provided in this volume by Greenberg (Figure 50.2).

50.2.3.3 Sensory Stimulation: Tactile

Electrocutaneous nerve stimulation was discovered in 1745 by von Kleist who described a shock from an electrostatically charged capacitor [79]. Studies published by von Frey in 1915 [80] and Adrian in 1919 [81] demonstrated the spectrum of sensations elicited by electrocutaneous stimulation, ranging

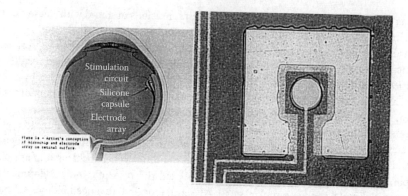

FIGURE 50.2 Example of an early microfabricated Pt–Ir bipolar electrode for acute preclinical experimentation in retinal stimulation built in 1991 by author (DJD). Retinal implant: Microelectrode array for retinal activation fabricated on flexible substrate for adherence to retinal curvature: Schematic implanted eye (left), photo-micrograph of 1 of 10 bipolar gold electrode pairs with 25 μm inner electrode (right). (From DiLorenzo, D.J., Unpublished data on microfabricated multichannel electrode array for retinal stimulation, 1991, Massachusetts Institute of Technology.)

from vibration to prickling and stinging pain. In 1966, Beeker described an artificial hand with electrocutaneous feedback of thumb contact pressure. Initial results, although qualitative, were positive [82]. In 1977, Schmidl reported that electrocutaneous sensory feedback of grip strength improved control of an experimental hand. He found electrocutaneous feedback to be less susceptible to adaptation than vibrotactile feedback [83]. In 1979, Shannon showed that electrocutaneous feedback on the skin above the median nerve is used to encode gripping force in a myoelectrically controlled prosthesis, patients reported an improved level of confidence when using the prosthesis [84].

In 1974 at Duke University, Clippinger implanted a sensory feedback system incorporating an electrode pair to stimulate the median nerve. He provided a frequency modulated signal which transmitted gripping force at the terminal hook. Patients were able to perceive grip force as well as object consistency [85]. In 1977, Clippinger reported a system using implanted electrodes to provide afferent sensory feedback for upper extremity amputees [86]. The same year, he reported that postoperative stimulation of the sciatic nerve by lower-extremity prosthesis offered the additional benefit of postoperative pain reduction, and in 1982, he reported 6-year success in a lower-extremity amputee using sciatic nerve stimulation to transmit heel strike force and leg structure bending moment on a single channel [87]. No further work on implanted sensory feedback prostheses is published by Clippinger.

In 1995 at MIT, DiLorenzo and Edell demonstrated functionality of a chronically implanted multichannel intrafascicular peripheral electrode array in an animal model using behavioral and neurophysiological recording, including eye blink reflexes and somatosensory-evoked potentials. These studies demonstrated the functionality of sensory afferent fibers following transaction as well as the functionality of a chronically implanted intrafascicular stimulating neuroelectric interface [33–35,78]. Horch et al. have developed percutaneous flexible microwires for intrafascicular stimulation of neural tissue [88–90].

50.3 Neuromodulation

50.3.1 Chronic Electrical Stimulation of the Nervous System for Functional Disorders

The early history of the use of electrical stimulation of the nervous system was limited to the acute setting because of the lack of availability of implantable stimulators for chronic use. The first progress in this regard was in the area of cardiac pacing—which only recently has come to be viewed, rightfully, as neuromodulation. Although Aldini was motivated to "reanimate" the heart with galvanic stimulation [6], the first success was by Albert Hyman who used faradic stimulation to resuscitate the heart in animals and apparently some patients as well, after cardiac arrest [3]. It was not until 1952 that an artificial pacemaker was successfully used by Paul Zoll, and in 1958, a chronic pacemaker was used for 96 days (although it had to be wheeled around on a table!) [91]. An implantable device that had to be charged through the skin was implanted the next year in Sweden [92], followed by a radio-frequency coupled pacemaker [93,94], and the first fully implantable, self-powered device was implanted in 1960 [95].

50.3.2 Early Development of Deep-Brain Stimulation for Psychiatric Disorders and Pain

The availability of implantable pacemakers paved the way for their use in treating nervous system disorders of "function," including movement disorders (tremor, Parkinson's disease, dystonia), pain, epilepsy and psychiatric disorders. Until this time, a common procedure in the 1950s was subfrontal leucotomy for various psychiatric indications, and in fact Spiegel and Wycis developed their stereotactic frame mainly for use in this surgery. J. Lawrence Pool at the Neurological Institute at Columbia University was the first to reason that electrical stimulation might provide a nondestructive, reversible alternative to ablative procedures, in this case for psychiatric indications. He had previously—in 1945—implanted the first patient with an induction coil for stimulating the femoral nerve for paraparesis (the first example of true FES) [96] and in 1948 he placed a silver electrode in the caudate nucleus of a patient with Parkinson's disease afflicted with intractable depression, coupled to a permanent mini induction coil placed in the skull. His intent was to activate the caudate with electrical stimulation (although his reasoning is not made clear), and indeed he reported that the patient had some benefits from daily stimulation (with an external primary coil?) for 8 weeks, but a wire broke and therapy was discontinued. Pool also implanted a psychotic patient in 1948 with a cingulate gyrus stimulator.

Neural ablation within the pain-mediating pathways of the brain and spinal cord was the standard treatment for deafferentation (neuropathic) or cancer-related (nociceptive) pain, which was refractory to medical treatment. Thus the nonablative treatment of pain was advanced when in 1954, R. G. Heath at Tulane reported pain relief in schizophrenic patients following electrical stimulation of the septal nuclei via a stereotactic approach (first done in 1950) [97], and similar results were reported by Pool using Heath's technique in a patient treated exclusively for pain (with an externalized electrode wire) [98]. In his 1954 monograph, Pool reported that "focal electrical stimulation of deep midline frontal lobe structures is a new technique that is now being used more and more frequently" [98, p. 457], which apparently included both himself and Heath in patients with psychiatric disease and/or pain. By this time, Spiegel and Wycis were also implanting chronic electrodes for stimulation, through a stereotactic approach [99]. However, there were as yet no reports of the use of chronic stimulation for the treatment of movement disorders. In the 1960s, levo-dopa for the treatment of Parkinson's disease arrived, and virtually eliminated—for the next several decades—the surgical treatment of Parkinson's disease, except for severe tremor. Moreover, by this time, public outcry eliminated the surgical treatment of psychiatric disorders, which, although mainly directed against leucotomy and lobotomy, also included electrical brain stimulation. Thus, the next advances occurred exclusively in the treatment of pain.

By 1960 Heath and colleagues were stimulating the septal nuclei for pain (without concurrent psychiatric disorder), and in 1961 Mazars and colleagues introduced the sensory thalamus as a target with the idea that stimulation of the deafferented neurons in the thalamus following amputation or stroke, for example, would relieve neuropathic pain [100,101]. In these and other reports of brain stimulation for pain (septal region [102]; caudate [103]), only acute stimulation through externalized wires was used. However, Glenn pioneered the use of his RF-coupled device—first introduced for cardiac pacing in 1959 [94]—to pace the phrenic nerve in a paralyzed patient in 1963 [104]. Shortly thereafter, Sweet and Wepsic [105] implanted an RF stimulator to suppress pain in the peripheral nervous system, and it was used in the first dorsal column stimulator implantation in 1967 by Shealy [106], based on the Melzack and Wall "gate control" theory of pain transmission in the spinal cord [107]. In 1982 at Duke, Nashold, Walker, and Mullen demonstrated a technique for intraoperatively mapping peripheral nerve bundles in order to accurately place electrodes on individual fasiculi to relieve chronic limb pain [108].

Pursuing an anatomically more central approach, Hosobuchi and colleagues [109] reported successful chronic stimulation of the sensory thalamus for facial pain in 1973, and this was followed by chronic stimulation of sensory thalamus by Mazars [110] and of other regions as well. Notable among these is the periventricular gray region which—based on the findings of analgesia induced by electrical stimulation in the rat by Reynolds [111]—was chronically stimulated in patients in 1973 by Hosobuchi and colleagues [112] and Richardson and Akil [113,114]. Ultimately, the fully implantable battery-powered stimulator was developed for cardiac pacing [95] and then adapted for use in the treatment of pain [14].

50.3.3 The Dawn of Deep-Brain Stimulation for Movement Disorders

The earliest use of chronic therapeutic stimulation for movement disorders appears to be that of Bechtereva and colleagues in the erstwhile USSR. They implanted 24–40 electrodes in 4–6 bundles into the "thalamic—striopallidal nuclei" for patients with hyperkinesias as a result of Parkinson's disease, torsion dystonia, and other causes [115,116]. Benefits of intermittent stimulation were seen for as long as 3 years, although no implantable stimulator was used. Other early results were from electrical stimulation of sensory thalamus [110,117] or centromedian-parafascicular complex (CM/Pf) [118] for thalamic deafferentation pain, when improvements in the often associated dyskinesia were noted. Another avenue was that of Cooper and colleagues in the 1970s [119], who stimulated the anterior lobe of the cerebellum to treat various movement disorders, including spasticity and dystonia. Davis and colleagues performed cerebellar stimulation on 316 patients between 1974 and 1981 for spastic motor disorders with good success [120].

By the 1970s, when Parkinson's disease was mostly being treated pharmacologically, the usual indication for stereotactic surgery in movement disorders was tremor and hyperkinesias (e.g., in dystonia), and the preferred operation was thalamotomy of the ventral intermediate (Vim) nucleus. It had long been appreciated that acute high frequency, but not low-frequency electrical stimulation of Vim led to immediate tremor arrest, which was used as a final check prior to radiofrequency ablation [121,122]. The first chronic stimulator implantations directed at movement disorders per se were by Mundinger in 1975 [123]. Brice and McClellan [124] implanted DBS leads in the subthalamic region (a common site for subthalamotomy at the time) in three patients for severe intention tremor resulting from multiple sclerosis. The latter paper is of special interest in that it anticipates by decades the idea of a contingent, on-demand system. Andy [125] implanted nine patients with stimulating electrodes in the thalamus, but concluded that the likely target was CM/Pf.

At about the same time in 1987, Benabid [126,127] and Seigfried [128] began implanting deep-brain stimulators into Vim of the thalamus for tremor from PD and essential tremor. Benabid's report of his large series of Vim stimulators in 1996 [129], followed shortly thereafter by the North American series [130] brought international attention to the field of electrical brain stimulation. The field came full circle as a result of other important trends. The limitations and complications of levo-dopa treatment for PD began to become apparent by the 1980s, and as a result Laitinen—a student of Leksell, a leader in functional neurosurgery in the 1950s during which time pallidotomies were carried out—began to revisit ablative surgery for PD. His influential report in 1992 of the results of pallidotomy refocused attention on the surgical treatment of PD [131]. With a large experience by then in DBS, Siegfried carried out the first implantation of a stimulator electrode into the posteroventral internal globus pallidus for PD in 1992 [132]. The next advance resulted from new insights into the pathophysiology of PD: the report of DeLong and colleagues of the amelioration of experimental PD in nonhuman primates by the ablation of the subthalamic nucleus, whose glutamatergic driving actions on the globus pallidus internus was elucidated [133]. Benabid then targeted this novel region for deep-brain stimulation in 1993 (the subthalamic region, including white matter projections, had been the target for "subthalamotomies," but never before had the subthalamic nucleus per se been targeted because of concerns over the development of hemiballism) [134].

50.3.4 The Efforts toward Neurostimulation for Epilepsy

In the 1950s, Cooke [135] and Dow [136] described their work in rats and primates showing that stimulation of the cerebellum had effects on the electroencephalogram and the frequency of seizures. On this basis, in 1973 Cooper and colleagues reported the use of chronic cerebellar stimulation in patients with epilepsy. They also reported benefits for spasticity [119]. Unfortunately, several subsequent clinical series were unable to replicate Cooper's results with epilepsy [137]. Also in the 1970s, Chkhenkeli reported preliminary results of stimulating the caudate nucleus for epilepsy (followed in 1997 by a larger series) (Chkhenkeli and Chkhenkeli, 1997).

On the basis of the idea that anterior nucleus of the thalamus (ANT) has widespread connections with and therefore possible modulatory effects on the cortex, Cooper also investigated and reported the results of stimulation of the anterior nucleus of the thalamus for epilepsy [138]. Also around that time Mirski and Fisher began providing experimental evidence for a role of the anterior nucleus in epilepsy [139,140], and that electrical stimulation can mitigate seizure activity [141]. This has provided the impetus to revisit this target for epilepsy [142,143], and current trials are underway. Meanwhile, Velasco reported that DBS of the centromedian nucleus (CM)—an intralaminar nucleus with widespread connections to the striatum and cortex—reduced seizure frequency in medically refractory patients [144]. Although not replicated in a limited clinical trial [145], results continue to be good for generalized epilepsy [12].

Also during the 1980s, the groups of Gale [146] and Moshe [147] independently began to report a role for the basal ganglia in regulating seizures. These and other lines of investigation paved the way for two small clinical series involving electrical stimulation of the subthalamic nucleus [148,149] which, although providing mixed results, have led to a larger clinical trial currently underway.

As early as the 1960s, the role of electrical stimulation of vagal nerve afferents on the electroencephalogram was appreciated [150]. This observation led Jacob Zabara, a physiologist at Temple University, to investigate the effect of vagal afferent stimulation on seizures in animal models [151,152]. These preclinical findings were the basis for launching Cyberonics, founded by Jacob Zabara and Reese S. Terry Jr. in 1987, which developed an implantable vagus nerve stimulator (VNS). Cyberonics conducted trials of vagal nerve stimulation for epilepsy in human patients beginning in 1988 [153,154] and achieved clinical approval for its use as an adjuvant therapy in 1997.

In the 1990s, Lesser discovered the phenomenon of afterdischarges in the cortex, following electrical stimulation; and he found that subsequent electrical stimulation can terminate these afterdischarges [155].

In 1997, Robert Fishell founded NeuroPace to develop an implant that applies the principle of afterdischarge termination to the treatment of seizures. In 2001, NeuroPace licensed seizure detection technology developed by Brian Litt, PhD, Frank Fisher and Ben Pless were recruited as CEO and CTO of NeuroPace and as of this writing, the company is in clinical trials for its Responsive Neurostimulator (RNS) device.

In the 1990s, DiLorenzo designed a closed-loop neuromodulation technology, and in 2002 he founded NeuroBionics Corporation. In 2003 and 2004, while a neurosurgical resident he assembled a team and venture financing term sheets to launch the company. In 2004, after a nationwide search, he recruited several executives from Northstar Neuroscience to join the company which was renamed BioNeuronics and subsequently NeuroVista Corporation; and as of this writing the company has begun human trials of an implanted seizure prediction and advisory system.

Several trials of deep-brain stimulation are currently underway. In addition, direct electrical stimulation of the epileptic focus in the cortex or hippocampus, in some cases coupled to contingent and others to closed-loop stimulation algorithms, are being examined by a number of investigators.

50.3.5 Current State of the Art of Neurostimulation

Electrical stimulation of the central, peripheral, and autonomic nervous systems has reached the point of standard clinical practice for an expanding list of indications. New indications are under active investigation, such as Tourette's syndrome [156] and cluster headache [157]. Vagal nerve stimulation is routinely performed for epilepsy but deep-brain stimulation and cortical stimulation are actively being studied. As a nondestructive alternative, electrical stimulation is spurring a judicious resurgence of psychosurgery for obsessive–compulsive disorder (internal capsule, nucleus accumbens) and depression (same targets as for OCD, plus vagus nerve and area 25 [158]), from which a large number of patients are disabled and treatment resistant. The treatment of pain continues to lag behind even though it was one of the earliest indications for DBS studies. Spinal cord stimulation is frequently performed for various types of peripheral pain, as is peripheral nerve stimulation. Motor cortex stimulation is under active investigation for neuropathic deafferentation pain (as well as for movement disorders [159] and for rehabilitation after stroke [160]).

In addition to advancing the field through expanding indications, technological and scientific advances are promising to increase effectiveness in certain settings. Most promising is the development of closed-loop strategies for the treatment of the epilepsies, and perhaps other disorders (recall the early work of Brice and McClellan [124] with tremor, discussed above). The ability to detect and/or predict [161] seizures is being capitalized on to tailor stimulation or other neuromodulatory interventions. This promises to increase effectiveness, and decrease cellular injury, adaptation or habituation, and to decrease battery drain. Other advances may include new electrode designs and stimulation strategies aimed at optimizing activation (or inhibition) of selected neural elements, such as axons over cell bodies. This work will be advanced by increasing understanding of the mechanisms of neurostimulation, which has lagged behind empirical, clinically based progress. Of course, progress in battery technology, including rechargeability and miniaturization, will increase long-term ease-of-use and tolerability of neurostimulation devices. With the more sophisticated neurostimulators on the drawing board and in development at several companies, the battery lifetime becomes an even more important issue than in first-generation devices.

At the turn of the twentieth century, the remarkable results seen with deep-brain stimulation in movement disorders (historically, the last indication for which it was tried) have led to the great resurgence in the use of electrical stimulation for the treatment of a wide variety of neurological disorders. Not since the turn of the nineteen century has interest in this therapy been so widespread. The difference, hopefully, is that we are now also in the age of evidence-based medicine so that the seemingly striking benefits of electrical neuromodulation have been and will continue to be subjected to objective standards of evaluation and that the enormous potential neural engineering holds will be responsibly harnessed for the patient's best interest.

References

1. Velasco, F., Neuromodulation: An overview. *Arch Med Res*, 2000. **31**(3): 232–236.
2. Largus, S., *Compositiones medicae. Joannes Rhodius recensuit, notis illustrauit, lexicon scriboniaum adiecit.* 1655, P. Frambotti: Patavii.
3. McNeal, D.R., 2000 years of electrical stimulation, in *Functional Electrical Stimulation*, F.T. Hambrecht and J.B. Reswick, Editors. 1977, Marcel Dekker: New York. pp. 3–33.
4. Chaffe, E. and R. Light, A method for remote control of electrical stimulation of the nervous system. *Yale J Biol Med*, 1934. 7: 83.
5. Evans, C., *Medical Observations and Inquiries by a Society of Physicians in London*. 1757. I: 83–86.
6. Parent, A., Giovanni Aldini: From animal electricity to human brain stimulation. *Can J Neurol Sci*, 2004. **31**: 576–584.
7. Galvani, L., De viribus electricitatis in motu musculari, commentarus. *De Bononiensi Scientiarum et Artium Instituto atque Academia*, 1791. 7: 363–418.

8. Volta, A., Account of some discoveries made by Mr. Galvani from Mr. Alexander Volta to Mr. Tiberius Cavallo. *Philos Trans Roy Soc*, 1793. **83**: 10–44.

9. Volta, A., On the electricity excited by the mere contact of conducting substances of different kinds. *Philos Trans*, 1800. **90**: 403.

10. Aldini, J., *Essai théorique et expérimental sur le galvanisme, avec une série d'expériences faites devant des commissaires de l'Institut national de France, et en divers amphithéâtres anatomiques de Londres.* 1804, Paris: Fornier Fils.

11. Fritsch, G. and E. Hitzig, Über die elektrische Erregbarkeit des Grosshirns. *Archiv Anat Physiol wissenschaftl Med*, 1870. **37**: 300–322.

12. Velasco, M. et al., Acute and chronic electrical stimulation of the centromedian thalamic nucleus: Modulation of reticulo-cortical systems and predictor factors for generalized seizure control. *Arch Med Res*, 2000. **31**(3): 304–15.

13. Ferrier, D., The localization of function in the brain. *Proc. R. Soc. Lond.*, 1873. **22**: 229.

14. Davis, R., Chronic stimulation of the central nervous system, in *Textbook of Stereotactic and Functional Neurosurgery*, P.L. Gildenberg and R.R. Tasker, Editors. 1998, McGraw-Hill: New York. p. 963.

15. Cushing, H., Faradic stimulation of postcentral gyrus in conscious patients. *Brain*, 1909. **32**: 44–53.

16. Penfield, W. and H.H. Jasper, *Epilepsy and the Functional Anatomy of the Human Brain.* 1954, Boston: Little, Brown and Co.

17. Djourno, A. and C.H. Eyries, Prothese auditive par excitation electrique a distance du nerf sensoriel a l'aide d'un bobinage inclus a demeure. *La Presse Medicale*, 1957. **65**: 1417.

18. Edell, D., A peripheral nerve information transducer for amputees: Long-term multichannel recordings from rabbit peripheral nerves. *IEEE Trans Biomed Eng*, 1986. **33**(2): 203–214.

19. Edell, D.J., *Development of a chronic neuroelectronic interface*, 1980, PhD thesis, U.C. Davis, Davis, CA.

20. Liberson, W.T. et al., Functional electrotherapy: Stimulation of the peroneal nerve synchronized with the swing phase of the gait of hemiplegic patients. *Arch. Phys. Med. Rehabil.*, 1961. **42**: 101–105.

21. Liberson, W.T., Functional neuromuscular stimulation: Historical background and personal experience, in *Functional Neuromuscular Stimulation: Report of a Workshop.* April 27–28, 1972, M.A. LeBlanc, Editor. 1972: Washington, DC, pp. 147–156.

22. Moe, J.H. and H.W. Post, Functional electrical stimulation for ambulation in hemiplegia. *Lancet*, 1962. **82**: 285–288.

23. Long, C. and V. Masciarelli, An electrophysiological splint for the hand. *Arch. Phys. Med. Rehabil.*, 1963. **44**: 449–503.

24. Peckham, P.H., J.T. Mortimer, and E.B. Marsolais, Controlled prehension and release in the C5 quadriplegic elicited by functional electrical stimulation of the paralyzed forearm musculature. *Ann. Biomed. Eng.*, 1980. **8**: 369–388.

25. Kantrowitz, A., *Electronic Physiologic Aids: A Report of the Maimonides Hospital.* 1960: Brooklyn, NY, pp. 4–5.

26. Cooper, E.B., W.H. Bunch, and J.H. Campa, Effects of chronic human neuromuscular stimulation. *Surg. Forum*, 1973. **24**: 477–479.

27. Brindley, G.S., Polkey, C.E., and D.N. Ruston, Electrical splinting of the knee in paraplegia. *Paraplegia*, 1978. **16**: 434–441.

28. Bajd, T. et al., The use of a four-channel electrical stimulator as an ambulatory aid for paraplegic patients. *Phys. Therapy*, 1983. **63**(7): 1116–1120.

29. Kralj, A. et al., Gait restoration in paraplegic patients: A feasibility demonstration using multichannel surface electrode FES. *J. Rehab. R & D*, 1983. **20**(1): 3–20.

30. DiLorenzo, D.J. and W.K. Durfee, *Unpublished data on 4-channel surface FES for gait restoration*, 1990, Massachusetts Institute of Technology.

31. Durfee, W.K. and D.J. DiLorenzo. Linear and nonlinear approaches to control of single joint motion by functional electrical stimulation. In *Proceedings of the 1990 American Control Conference*, San Diego, CA. 1990.

32. Durfee, W.K. and D.J. DiLorenzo, Sliding mode control of FNS knee joint motion. *Abstracts of the First World Congress of Biomechanics*, 1990. **2**: 329.

33. DiLorenzo, D.J. et al. Chronic intraneural electrical stimulation for prosthetic sensory feedback, in *IEEE EMBS 1st International Conference on Neural Engineering*. 2003. Capri Island, Italy: IEEE.

34. DiLorenzo, D.J. et al. Multichannel intraneural electrical stimulation for prosthetic sensory feedback, in *Society for Neuroscience Annual Meeting*. 1997. New Orleans, LA.

35. DiLorenzo, D.J. et al. Multichannel intraneural electrical stimulation for prosthetic sensory feedback. In *Congress of Neurological Surgeons Annual Meeting*. 1997. New Orleans, LA.

36. DiLorenzo, D.J., Cortical technologies: Innovative solutions for neurological disease, 1999. Masters thesis, Massachusetts Institute of Technology, MIT Sloan School of Management: Management of Technology (MOT) Program, Cambridge, Massachusetts, 72pp.

37. Goldfarb, M. and W.K. Durfee, Design of a controlled-brake orthosis for FES-aided gait. *IEEE Trans. Rehab. Eng.*, 1996. **4**(1): 13–24.

38. Marsolais, E.B. and R. Kobetic, Functional walking in paralyzed patients by means of electrical stimulation. *Clin. Orthopaed. Relat. Res.*, 1983(175): 30–36.

39. Graupe, D. et al. EMG-controlled electrical stimulation. in *Proc. IEEE Frontiers of Eng. & Comp. in Health Care*. 1983. Columbus, OH.

40. Graupe, D. and K.H. Kohn, *Functional Electrical Stimulation for Ambulation by Paraplegics*. 1994, Malabar, FL: Krieger Publishing Co.

41. Keith, M.W. et al., Implantable functional neuromuscular stimulation in the tetraplegic hand. *J. Hand Surg.*, 1989. **14A**: 524–530.

42. Georgopoulos, A.P. et al., On the relations between the direction of two-dimensional arm movements and cell discharge in primate motor cortex. *J. Neurosci.*, 1982. **2**(11): 1527–1537.

43. Georgopoulos, A.P., R. Caminiti, and J.F. Kalaska, Static spatial effects in motor cortex and area 5: Quantitative relations in a two-dimensional space. *Exp. Brain Res.*, 1984. **54**(3): 446–454.

44. Caminiti, R. et al., Shift of preferred directions of premotor cortical cells with arm movements performed across the workspace. *Exp. Brain Res.*, 1990. **83**(1): 228–232.

45. Kalaska, J.F. et al., A comparison of movement direction-related versus load direction-related activity in primate motor cortex, using a two-dimensional reaching task. *J. Neurosci.*, 1989. **9**(6): 2080–2102.

46. Schwartz, A.B., R.E. Kettner, and A.P. Georgopoulos, Primate motor cortex and free arm movements to visual targets in three-dimensional space. I. Relations between single cell discharge and direction of movement. *J. Neurosci.*, 1988. **8**(8): 2913–2927.

47. Georgopoulos, A.P., R.E. Kettner, and A.B. Schwartz, Primate motor cortex and free arm movements to visual targets in three-dimensional space. II. Coding of the direction of movement by a neuronal population. *J. Neurosci.*, 1988. **8**(8): 2928–2937.

48. Kettner, R.E., A.B. Schwartz, and A.P. Georgopoulos, Primate motor cortex and free arm movements to visual targets in three-dimensional space. III. Positional gradients and population coding of movement direction from various movement origins. *J. Neurosci.*, 1988. **8**(8): 2938–2947.

49. Taylor, D.M., S.I. Tillary, and A.B. Schwartz, Direct cortical control of 3D neuroprosthetic devices. *Science*, 2002. **296**: 1828–1832.

50. Hatsopoulos, N.G. et al., Information about movement direction obtained from synchronous activity of motor cortical neurons. *Proc. Natl. Acad. Sci. USA*, 1998. **95**(26): 15706–15711.

51. DiLorenzo, D.J., *Neural correlates of motor performance in primary motor cortex*, 1999, PhD thesis, Massachusetts Institute of Technology, Department of Mechanical Engineering, Cambridge, MA, 104pp.

52. Maynard, E.M. et al., Neuronal interactions improve cortical population coding of movement direction. *J. Neurosci.*, 1999. **19**(18): 8083–8093.

53. Wessberg, J. et al., Real-time prediction of hand trajectory by ensembles of cortical neurons in primates. *Lett. Nat.*, 2000. **408**: 361–365.

54. Kennedy, P.R., The cone electrode: A long-term electrode that records from neurites grown onto its recording surface. *J. Neurosci. Methods*, 1989. **29**: 181–193.

55. Kennedy, P.R. and R.A. Bakay, Restoration of neural output from a paralyzed patient by a direct brain connection. *Neuroreport*, 1998. **9**(8): 1707–1711.

56. Kennedy, P.R. et al., Direct control of a computer from the human central nervous system. *IEEE Trans. Rehab. Eng.*, 2000. **8**(2): 198–202.

57. Saleh, M. et al. Case study: Reliability of multi-electrode array in the knob area of human motor cortex intended for a neuromotor prosthesis application. In *ICORR—9th International Conference on Rehabilitation Robotics*. 2005. Chicago, IL.

58. Doyle, J.H., J.B. Doyle, and F.M. Turnbull, Electrical stimulation of eighth cranial nerve. *Arch. Otolaryng.-Head Neck Surg.*, 1964. **80**: 388.

59. House, W.F. and J. Urban, Long term results of electrode implantation and electronic stimulation of the cochlea in man. *Ann. Otol., Rhinol. Laryngol.*, 1973. **82**: 504.

60. House, W.F. and K.I. Berliner, Safety and efficacy of the House/3M cochlear implant in profoundly deaf adults. *Otolaryngol. Clin. North America*, 1986. **19**: 275.

61. Simmons, F.B. et al., Auditory nerve: Electrical stimulation in man. *Science*, 1965. **148**: 104.

62. Michelson, R.P., Electrical stimulation of the human cochlea: A preliminary report. *Arch. Otolaryngol.—Head Neck Surg.*, 1971. **93**: 317.

63. Merzenich, M.M., D.N. Schindler, and M.W. White, Feasibility of multichannel scala tympani stimulation. *Laryngoscope*, 1974. **84**: 1887.

64. Kessler, D.K., The CLARION multi-strategy cochlear implant. *Ann. Otol., Rhinol. Laryngol.—Suppl.*, 1999. **177**: 8–16.

65. Schindler, R.A. and D.K. Kessler, The UCSF/Storz cochlear implant: Patient performance. *Am. J. Otol.*, 1987. **8**(3): 247–255.

66. Schindler, R.A., D.K. Kessler, and H.S. Haggerty, Clarion cochlear implant: phase I investigational results.[see comment][erratum appears in Am J Otol 1993 Nov;14(6):627]. *Am. J. Otol.*, 1993. **14**(3): 263–272.

67. Schindler, R.A. et al., The UCSF/Storz multichannel cochlear implant: Patient results. *Laryngoscope*, 1986. **96**(6): 597–603.

68. Clark, G.M., A surgical approach for a cochlear implant: An anatomical study. *J. Laryngol. Otol.*, 1975. **89**(1): 9–15.

69. Clark, G.M. et al., The University of Melbourne—Nucleus multi-electrode cochlear implant. *Adv. Oto-Rhino-Laryngol.*, 1987. **38**: V–IX.

70. Clark, G.M. and R.J. Hallworth, A multiple-electrode array for a cochlear implant. *J. Laryngol. Otol.*, 1976. **90**(7): 623–627.

71. Clark, G.M., R.J. Hallworth, and K. Zdanius, A cochlear implant electrode. *J. Laryngol. Otol.*, 1975. **89**(8): 787–792.

72. Cochlear Limited. *Cochlear Limited Corporate Website*. [Corporate Website] 2005 [cited 2005 July 18, 2005]. Available from: http://www.cochlear.com/.

73. Burian, K. et al., Designing of and experience with multichannel cochlear implants. *Acta Oto-Laryngol.*, 1979. **87**(3–4): p. 190–5.

74. Burian, K. et al., Electrical stimulation with multichannel electrodes in deaf patients. *Audiology*, 1980. **19**(2): 128–36.

75. Brindley, G.S. and W.S. Lewin, The sensations produced by electrical stimulation of the visual cortex. *J. Physiol.*, 1968. **196**(2): 479–493.

76. Dobelle, W.H. and M.G. Mladejovsky, Phosphenes produced by electrical stimulation of human occipital cortex, and their application to the development of a prosthesis for the blind. *J. Physiol.*, 1974. **243**(2): 553–576.

77. Dobelle, W.H. et al., "Braille" reading by a blind volunteer by visual cortex stimulation. *Nature*, 1976. **259**(5539): 111–112.

78. DiLorenzo, D.J., *Unpublished data on microfabricated multichannel electrode array for retinal stimulation*, 1991, Massachusetts Institute of Technology.

79. Canby, E.T., *A History of Electricity*. 1962, New York: Hawthorne Books. p. 21.

80. Frey, V.M., Physiological experiments on the vibratory sensation [German]. *Z. Biol.*, 1915. **65**: 417–427.

81. Adrian, E.D., The response of human sensory nerves to currents of short duration. *J. Physiol. (London)*, 1919. **53**: 70–85.

82. Beeker, T.W., J. During, and A. Den Hertog, Technical note: Artificial touch in a hand prosthesis. *Med. Biol. Eng.*, 1967. **5**: 47–49.

83. Schmidl, H., The importance of information feedback in prostheses for the upper limbs. *Prosth. Orthot. Int.*, 1977. **1**: 21–24.

84. Shannon, G.F., A myoelectrically-controlled prosthesis with sensory feedback. *Med. Biol. Eng. Comput.*, 1979. **17**: 73–80.

85. Clippinger, F.W., A sensory feedback system for an upper-limb amputation prosthesis. *Bull. Prosthet. Res.*, 1974. **BPR 10–22**: 247–258.

86. Clippinger, F.W., in *Textbook of Surgery: The Biological Basis of Modern Surgical Practice*, D.C.e. Sabiston, Editor. 1977, W.B. Saunders: Philadelphia. pp. 1582–1594.

87. Clippinger, F.W., Afferent sensory feedback for lower extremity prosthesis. *Clin. Orthop.*, 1982. **169**: 202–206.

88. Malmstrom, J.A., T.G. McNaughton, and K.W. Horch, Recording properties and biocompatibility of chronically implanted polymer-based intrafascicular electrodes. *Ann. Biomed. Eng.*, 1998. **26**(6): 1055–1064.

89. McNaughton, T.G. and K.W. Horch, Metallized polymer fibers as leadwires and intrafascicular microelectrodes. *J. Neurosci. Methods*, 1996. **70**(1): 103–110.

90. Lawrence, S.M. et al., Long-term biocompatibility of implanted polymer-based intrafascicular electrodes. *J. Biomed. Mater. Res.*, 2002. **63**(5): 501–506.

91. Furman, S. and J.B. Schwedel, An intercardiac pacemaker for Stokes-Adams seizures. *N. Engl. J. Med.*, 1959. **261**: 943–948.

92. Senning, A., Implantable cardiac pacemaker. *Mal. Cardiovasc.*, 1963. **4**: 503–512.

93. Glenn, W.W. et al., Total ventilatory support in a quadriplegic patient with radiofrequency electrophrenic respiration. *N. Engl. J. Med.*, 1972. **286**(10): 513–516.

94. Glenn, W.W. et al., Remote stimulation of the heart by radiofrequency transmission. Clinical application to a patient with Stokes-Adams Syndrome. *N. Engl. J. Med.*, 1959. **261**: 948–951.

95. Chardack, W.M., A.A. Gage, and W. Greatbatch, A transistorized, self-contained, implantable pacemaker for the long-term correction of complete heart block. *Surgery*, 1960. **48**(654).

96. Pool, J.L., Nerve stimulation in paraplegic patients by means of buried induction coil. Preliminary report. *J. Neurosurg.*, 1946. **3**: 192.

97. Heath, R.G., *Studies in Schizophrenia: A Multidisciplinary Approach to Mid Brain Relationships.* 1954, Cambridge, MA: Harvard University Press.

98. Pool, J.L., Psychosurgery in older people. *J. Am. Geriatr. Soc.*, 1954. **2**(7): p. 456–66.

99. Spiegel, E.A. and H.T. Wycis, Chronic implantation of intracerebral electrodes in humans, in *Electrical Stimulation of the Brain*, D.E. Sheer, Editor. 1961, Austin, TX: University of Texas Press, pp. 37–44.

100. Mazars, G., L. Merienne, and C. Ciolocca, Intermittent analgesic thalamic stimulation. Preliminary note. *Rev Neurol (Paris)*, 1973. **128**(4): 273–279.

101. Mazars, G.J., Intermittent stimulation of nucleus ventralis posterolateralis for intractable pain. *Surg Neurol*, 1975. **4**(1): 93–95.

102. Gol, H., Relief of pain by electrical stimulation of the septal area. *J. Neurol. Sci.*, 1967. **5**: 115–120.

103. Ervin, F.R., C.E. Brown, and V.H. Mark, Striatal influence on facial pain. *Conf. Neurol.*, 1966. **27**: 75–86.

104. Glenn, W.W. et al., Diaphragm pacing by radiofrequency transmission in the treatment of chronic ventilatory insufficiency. Present status. *J. Thorac. Cardiovasc. Surg*, 1973. **66**(4): 505–520.

105. Sweet, W. and J. Wepsic, Control of pain by focal electrical stimulation for suppression. *Arizona Med.*, 1969. **26**: 1042–1045.
106. Shealy, C.N., J.T. Mortimer, and J.B. Reswick, Electrical inhibition of pain by stimulation of the dorsal columns: Preliminary clinical report. *Anesth. Analg.*, 1967. **46**(4): 489–491.
107. Melzack, R. and P.D. Wall, Pain mechanisms: A new theory. *Science*, 1965. **150**(699): 971–979.
108. Mullen, J.B., C.F. Walker, and B.S. Nashold, Jr., An electrophysiological approach to neural augmentation implantation for the control of pain. *J. Bioeng.*, 1978. **2**(1–2): 65–67.
109. Hosobuchi, Y., J.E. Adams, and B. Rutkin, Chronic thalamic stimulation for the control of facial anesthesia dolorosa. *Arch Neurol.*, 1973. **29**(3): 158–161.
110. Mazars, G., L. Merienne, and C. Cioloca, [Use of thalamic stimulators in the treatment of various types of pain]. *Ann Med Interne (Paris)*, 1975. **126**(12): 869–871.
111. Reynolds, D.V., Surgery in the rat during electrical analgesia induced by focal brain stimulation. *Science*, 1969. **164**: 444–445.
112. Hosobuchi, Y., J.E. Adams, and R. Linchitz, Pain relief by electrical stimulation of the central gray matter in humans and its reversal by naloxone. *Science*, 1977. **197**(4299): 183–186.
113. Richardson, D.E. and H. Akil, Pain reduction by electrical brain stimulation in man. Part 2: Chronic self-administration in the periventricular gray matter. *J. Neurosurg.*, 1977. **47**(2): 184–194.
114. Richardson, D.E. and H. Akil, Pain reduction by electrical brain stimulation in man. Part 1: Acute administration in periaqueductal and periventricular sites. *J. Neurosurg.*, 1977. **47**(2): 178–183.
115. Bechtereva, N.P. et al., Therapeutic electrostimulation of deep brain structures. *Vopr Neirokhir.*, 1972. **1**: 7–12.
116. Bechtereva, N.P. et al., Method of electrostimulation of the deep brain structures in treatment of some chronic diseases. *Confin Neurol*, 1975. **37**(1–3): 136–140.
117. Mazars, G., L. Merienne, and C. Cioloca, Control of dyskinesias due to sensory deafferentation by means of thalamic stimulation. *Acta Neurochir. Suppl. (Wien)*, 1980. **30**: 239–243.
118. Andy, O.J., Parafascicular-center median nuclei stimulation for intractable pain and dyskinesia (painful-dyskinesia). *Appl. Neurophysiol.*, 1980. **43**(3–5): 133–144.
119. Cooper, I.S. et al., Chronic cerebellar stimulation in cerebral palsy. *Neurology*, 1976. **26**(8): 744–53.
120. Davis, R. et al., Update of chronic cerebellar stimulation for spasticity and epilepsy. *Appl. Neurophysiol.*, 1982. **45**(1–2): 44–50.
121. Hassler, R. et al., Physiological observations in stereotaxic operations in extrapyramidal motor disturbances. *Brain*, 1960. **83**: 337–350.
122. Jurko, M.F., O.J. Andy, and D.P. Foshee, Diencephalic influence on tremor mechanisms. *Arch. Neurol.*, 1963. **9**: 358–362.
123. Mundinger, F. and H. Neumuller, Programmed stimulation for control of chronic pain and motor diseases. *Appl. Neurophysiol.*, 1982. **45**(1–2): 102–111.
124. Brice, J. and L. McLellan, Suppression of intention tremor by contingent deep-brain stimulation. *Lancet*, 1980. **1**(8180): 1221–1222.
125. Andy, O.J., Thalamic stimulation for control of movement disorders. *Appl. Neurophysiol.*, 1983. **46**(1–4): 107–111.
126. Benabid, A.L. et al., Combined (thalamotomy and stimulation) stereotactic surgery of the VIM thalamic nucleus for bilateral Parkinson disease. *Appl. Neurophysiol.*, 1987. **50**(1–6): 344–346.
127. Benabid, A.L. et al., Long-term suppression of tremor by chronic stimulation of the ventral intermediate thalamic nucleus. *Lancet*, 1991. **337**(8738): 403–406.
128. Siegfried, J., Therapeutical neurostimulation—Indications reconsidered. *Acta Neurochir. Suppl. (Wien)*, 1991. **52**: 112–117.
129. Benabid, A.L. et al., Chronic electrical stimulation of the ventralis intermedius nucleus of the thalamus as a treatment of movement disorders. *J. Neurosurg.*, 1996. **84**(2): 203–214.
130. Koller, W. et al., High-frequency unilateral thalamic stimulation in the treatment of essential and parkinsonian tremor. *Ann. Neurol.*, 1997. **42**(3): 292–299.

131. Laitinen, L.V., A.T. Bergenheim, and M.I. Hariz, Leksell's posteroventral pallidotomy in the treatment of Parkinson's disease. *J. Neurosurg.*, 1992. **76**(1): 53–61.

132. Siegfried, J. and B. Lippitz, Bilateral chronic electrostimulation of ventroposterolateral pallidum: A new therapeutic approach for alleviating all parkinsonian symptoms. *Neurosurgery*, 1994. **35**(6): 1126–1129; discussion 1129–1130.

133. Bergman, H., T. Wichmann, and M.R. DeLong, Reversal of experimental parkinsonism by lesions of the subthalamic nucleus. *Science*, 1990. **249**(4975): 1436–1438.

134. Benabid, A.L. et al., Acute and long-term effects of subthalamic nucleus stimulation in Parkinson's disease. *Stereotact. Funct. Neurosurg.*, 1994. **62**(1–4): 76–84.

135. Cooke, P.M. and R.S. Snider, Some cerebellar influences on electrically-induced cerebral seizures. *Epilepsia*, 1955. **4**: 19–28.

136. Dow, R.S., A. Fernandez-Guardiola, and E. Manni, The influence of the cerebellum on experimental epilepsy. *Electroencephalogr. Clin. Neurophysiol.*, 1962. **14**: 383–398.

137. Krauss, G.L. and R.S. Fisher, Cerebellar and thalamic stimulation for epilepsy. *Adv Neurol*, 1993. **63**: 231–245.

138. Upton, A.R. et al., Suppression of seizures and psychosis of limbic system origin by chronic stimulation of anterior nucleus of the thalamus. *Int. J. Neurol.*, 1985. **19–20**: 223–230.

139. Mirski, M.A. and J.A. Ferrendelli, Interruption of the mammillothalamic tract prevents seizures in guinea pigs. *Science*, 1984. **226**(4670): 72–74.

140. Mirski, M.A. and J.A. Ferrendelli, Anterior thalamic mediation of generalized pentylenetetrazol seizures. *Brain Res.*, 1986. **399**(2): 212–223.

141. Mirski, M.A. et al., Anticonvulsant effect of anterior thalamic high frequency electrical stimulation in the rat. *Epilepsy Res.*, 1997. **28**(2): 89–100.

142. Hodaie, M. et al., Chronic anterior thalamus stimulation for intractable epilepsy. *Epilepsia*, 2002. **43**(6): 603–608.

143. Kerrigan, J.F. et al., Electrical stimulation of the anterior nucleus of the thalamus for the treatment of intractable epilepsy. *Epilepsia*, 2004. **45**(4): 346–354.

144. Velasco, F. et al., Electrical stimulation of the centromedian thalamic nucleus in the treatment of convulsive seizures: A preliminary report. *Epilepsia*, 1987. **28**(4): 421–430.

145. Fisher, R.S. et al., Placebo-controlled pilot study of centromedian thalamic stimulation in treatment of intractable seizures. *Epilepsia*, 1992. **33**(5): 841–851.

146. Gale, K., Mechanisms of seizure control mediated by gamma-aminobutyric acid: role of the substantia nigra. *Fed. Proc.*, 1985. **44**(8): 2414–2424.

147. Moshe, S.L. and B.J. Albala, Nigral muscimol infusions facilitate the development of seizures in immature rats. *Brain Res.*, 1984. **315**(2): 305–308.

148. Benabid, A.L. et al., Deep brain stimulation of the corpus luysi (subthalamic nucleus) and other targets in Parkinson's disease. Extension to new indications such as dystonia and epilepsy. *J. Neurol.*, 2001. **248**(Suppl 3): III37–III47.

149. Loddenkemper, T. et al., Deep brain stimulation in epilepsy. *J. Clin. Neurophysiol.*, 2001. **18**(6): 514–532.

150. Chase, M.H., M.B. Sterman, and C.D. Clemente, Cortical and subcortical patterns of response to afferent vagal stimulation. *Exp. Neurol.*, 1966. **16**(1): 36–49.

151. Zabara, J., Time course of seizure control to brief, repetitive stimuli. *Epilepsia*, 1985. **28**: 604.

152. Zabara, J., Control of hypersynchronous discharge in epilepsy. *Electroencephalogr. Clin. Neurophysiol.*, 1985. **61**: 162.

153. Penry, J.K. and J.C. Dean, Prevention of intractable partial seizures by intermittent vagal stimulation in humans: Preliminary results. *Epilepsia*, 1990. **31**(Suppl 2): p. S40–3.

154. Uthman, B.M. et al., Treatment of epilepsy by stimulation of the vagus nerve. *Neurology*, 1993. **43**(7): 1338–1345.

155. Lesser, R.P. et al., Brief bursts of pulse stimulation terminate afterdischarges caused by cortical stimulation. *Neurology*, 1999. **53**(9): 2073–2081.

156. Visser-Vandewalle, V. et al., Chronic bilateral thalamic stimulation: A new therapeutic approach in intractable Tourette syndrome. Report of three cases. *J. Neurosurg.*, 2003. **99**(6): 1094–1100.

157. Franzini, A. et al., Stimulation of the posterior hypothalamus for treatment of chronic intractable cluster headaches: First reported series. *Neurosurgery*, 2003. **52**(5): 1095–1099; discussion 1099–1101.

158. Mayberg, H.S. et al., Deep brain stimulation for treatment-resistant depression. *Neuron*, 2005. **45**(5): 651–660.

159. Pagni, C.A., S. Zeme, and F. Zenga, Further experience with extradural motor cortex stimulation for treatment of advanced Parkinson's disease. Report of 3 new cases. *J. Neurosurg. Sci.*, 2003. **47**(4): 189–193.

160. Brown, J.A. et al., Motor cortex stimulation for enhancement of recovery after stroke: case report. *Neurol. Res.*, 2003. **25**(8): 815–818.

161. Litt, B. and J. Echauz, Prediction of epileptic seizures. *Lancet Neurol.*, 2002. **1**(1): 22–30.

51

Theory and Physiology of Electrical Stimulation of the Central Nervous System

51.1 Introduction 51-1
51.2 Generation of Potentials in CNS Tissues 51-2
51.3 Response of Neurons to Imposed Extracellular Potentials 51-4
51.4 From Cell to Circuit: Construction of Models of CNS
Neurons 51-5
51.5 Sites of Action Potential Initiation in CNS Neurons 51-5
51.6 Excitation Properties of CNS Stimulation 51-7
Strength–Duration Relationship • Current–Distance Relationship •
Effect of Stimulus Polarity and Stimulus Waveform on CNS
Stimulation • Indirect Effects of Extracellular Stimulation
51.7 Summary 51-12
Acknowledgment 51-12
References 51-12

Warren M. Grill
Duke University

51.1 Introduction

Electrical stimulation is a widespread method to study the form and function of the nervous system and a technique to restore function following disease or injury. The central nervous system (CNS) includes the brain and spinal cord (Figure 51.1). Both the spinal cord and the brain include regions primarily populated by cell bodies (somas) of neurons, and termed gray matter for its color, and regions primarily populated by axons of neurons, and termed white matter. The diversity of neuronal elements and complexity of the volume conductor make understanding the effects of stimulation more challenging in the case of CNS stimulation than in the case of peripheral stimulation. Specifically, it is unclear, in many cases, what neuronal elements (axons, cell bodies, presynaptic terminals; Figure 51.1) are activated by stimulation (Ranck, 1975). Further, it is unclear how targeted neural elements can be stimulated selectively without coactivation of other surrounding elements. This chapter presents a review of the properties of CNS stimulation as required for rational design and interpretation of therapies employing electrical stimulation.

Electrical stimulation has been used to determine the structure of axonal branching (Jankowska and Roberts, 1972), examine strength of connections between neurons, and determine the projection patterns of neurons (Lipski, 1981; Tehovnik, 1996). Examples of application of CNS stimulation from treatment of neurological disorders include the treatment of pain by stimulation of the brain (Coffey, 2001) and spinal cord (Cameron, 2004), treatment of tremor and the motor system symptoms of Parkinson's disease (Gross

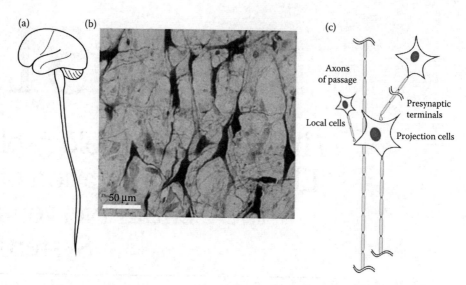

FIGURE 51.1 Structure of the CNS. (a) The CNS includes the brain and the spinal cord. (b) The gray matter of the CNS contains the cell bodies of neurons as well as the dendritic and axonal processes. (c) When an electrode is placed within the heterogeneous cellular environment of the CNS it is unclear which neuronal elements are affected by stimulation.

and Lozano, 2000), as an experimental treatment for epilepsy (Velasco et al., 2001; Hodaie et al., 2002), as well as a host of other neurological disorders (Gross, 2004). In addition, CNS stimulation is being developed for restoration of including hearing by electrical stimulation of the cochlear nucleus (Otto et al., 2002) and for restoration of vision (Brindley and Lewin, 1968; Schmidt et al., 1996; Troyk et al., 2003).

A nerve cell or a nerve fiber can be artificially stimulated by depolarization of the cell's membrane. The resulting action potential propagates to the terminal of the neuron leading to release of neurotransmitter that can impact the postsynaptic cell. The passage of current through extracellular electrodes positioned near neurons creates extracellular potentials in the tissue. The resulting potential distribution can result in an outward flowing transmembrane current and depolarization. Alternately, extracellular potentials may modulate or block ongoing neuronal firing depending on the magnitude, distribution, and polarity of the potentials.

The objective of this chapter is to present the biophysical basis for electrical stimulation of neurons in the CNSs. The focus is on using fundamental understanding of both the electric field and its effects on neurons to determine the site of neuronal excitation or modulation in the CNS where electrodes are placed among heterogeneous populations of neuronal elements, including cells, axons, and dendrites.

51.2 Generation of Potentials in CNS Tissues

Passage of current through tissue generates potentials in the tissue (recall Ohm's law: $V = IR$). The potentials are dependent on the electrode geometry, the stimulus parameters (current magnitude), and the electrical properties of the tissue. For example, the potential generated by a monopolar point source can be determined analytically using the relationship $V_e(r) = I/(4\pi\sigma r)$ where I is the stimulating current, σ is the conductivity of the tissue medium (Table 51.1), and r is the distance between the electrode and the measurement point. The point source model is a valid approximation for sharp electrodes with small tips (McIntyre and Grill, 2001). Larger electrodes are typically used for chronic stimulation of the CNS, and the spatial distribution of the potentials in the tissue differs from those produced by a point source electrode (Figure 51.2). Examples of the spectrum of electrode types used for CNS stimulation (and recording) are shown in Figure 51.3.

TABLE 51.1 Electrical Conductivity of CNS Tissues

Tissue Type	Electrical Conductivity (S/m)	Reference
Dura	0.030	Holsheimer et al. (1995)
Cerebrospinal fluid	1.5; 1.8	Crile et al. (1922); Baumann et al. (1997)
Gray matter	0.20	Ranck (1963); Li et al. (1968); Sances and Larson (1975)
White matter		Anisotropic
Transverse		
	0.6	Ranck and BeMent (1965) (cat dorsal columns)
	1.1	Nicholson (1965) (cat internal capsule)
Longitudinal		
	0.083	Ranck and BeMent (1965)
	0.13	Nicholson (1965)
Encapsulation tissue	0.16	Grill and Mortimer (1994)

The extracellular potentials generated by the passage are dependent on the electrical properties of the tissue. The electrical properties of peripheral nerves are both inhomogeneous and anisotropic (Table 51.1), and the distribution of potentials within the nerve will depend strongly on the nerve and electrode geometries. In general, biological conductivities have a small reactive component (Eisenberg and Mathias, 1980; Ackman and Seitz, 1984), and thus a relatively small increase in conductivity at higher frequencies (Ranck, 1963, Nicholson, 1965, Ranck and BeMent, 1965).

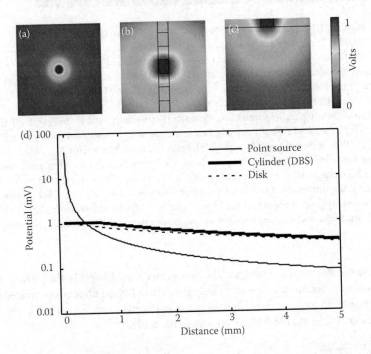

FIGURE 51.2 Electric fields generated by passage of current in CNS tissue. The first step in determining the response of CNS neurons to extracellular stimulation is to calculate the electric potentials generated in the tissue by passage of current through the electrode. Potentials produced by passage of current into a homogenous region of the CNS ($s = 0.2$ S/m) using a point source electrode (a) a cylindrical electrode (b) as used for deep-brain stimulation, and a disk electrode (c) as used for epidural or cortical surface stimulation. (d) Although a simple analytical solution exists for the potentials generated by a point source electrode, they differ substantially from the potentials generated by larger cylindrical or disk electrodes.

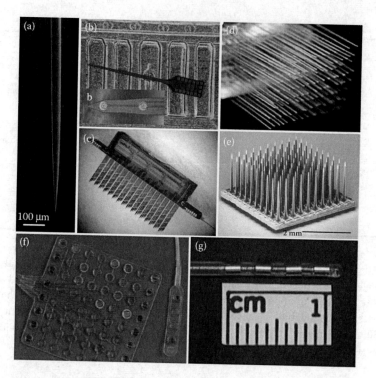

FIGURE 51.3 Electrodes for CNS stimulation. (a) Single iridium microwire electrode developed at Huntington Medical Research Institutes that can be used for extracellular recording from single units or extracellular microstimulation of small populations of neurons. (Adapted from McCreery DB et al. *IEEE Trans Biomed Eng* 1997; 44(10):931–939.) (b) Multisite silicon microprobe developed at the University of Michigan and higher magnification view (b) of two electrode sites near the tip. (Images courtesy of J.F. Hetke, University of Michigan.) (c) Three-dimensional assembly of multisite silicon microprobes (Bai et al., 2000). The array is four probes, 256 sites on 400 μm centers in 3D. There are 16 parallel stimulating channels (16 sites active at any time) with off-chip current generation. The array is fed by a 7-lead ribbon cable at a data rate of up to 10 Mbps. It operates from ±5 V supplies. (Image courtesy of K.D. Wise, University of Michigan.) (d) Arrays of up to 128 microwires enable simultaneous extracellular recording from multiple single neurons. Each wire is 50 μm diameter stainless steel, insulated with Teflon. (Adapted from Nicolelis MAL et al. *Proc Natl Acad Sci, USA* 2003; 100:11041–11046.) (e) Multielectrode silicone array developed at the University of Utah. (Adapted from Normann RA et al. *Vision Res* 1999; 39(15):2577–2587.) (f) Subdural grid and strip electrode arrays used for cortical stimulation and recording (PMT Corporation, Chanhassen, MN). (g) Quadrapolar electrode used for deep-brain stimulation (Medtronic Inc., Minneapolis, MN).

Spatial variations in the electrical properties of the tissue can cause changes in the patterns of activation (Grill, 1999). In most cases, to calculate accurately the extracellular potentials generated by extracellular stimulation requires a numerical solution using a discretized model, for example, with the finite element method (e.g., Veltink et al., 1989; McIntyre and Grill, 2002).

51.3 Response of Neurons to Imposed Extracellular Potentials

As described in the previous section, the distribution of extracellular potentials is dependent on the electrode geometry, the electrical properties of the extracellular tissue, and the stimulation amplitude. The effect of the potentials on neurons is dependent on the nerve cell type, its size and geometry, as well as the temporal characteristics of the stimulus. During stimulation of peripheral nerves it is clear that it is the axons in the vicinity of the electrodes that are activated. However, the CNS contains a heterogeneous population of neuronal elements including local cells projecting locally around the electrode as well as those projecting away from the region of stimulation, axons passing by the electrode, and presynaptic terminals projecting onto neurons in the region of the electrode (Figure 51.1c). Effects of stimulation can be mediated by activation of any or all of these elements and include both direct effects of stimulation of postsynaptic elements, as well as indirect effects mediated by electrical stimulation of presynaptic terminals that mediate the effects of stimulation via synaptic transmission.

From this complexity arise two principal questions during stimulation of the CNS (Grill and McIntyre, 2001): What neuronal elements are activated by extracellular stimulation? and how can targeted elements be stimulated selectively? Computational modeling provides a powerful tool to study extracellular excitation of the CNS neurons. The volume of tissue stimulated, both for fibers and cells, and how this changes with electrode geometry, stimulus parameters, and the geometry of the neuronal elements is quite challenging to determine experimentally. Using a computer model enables these parameters to be examined under controlled conditions, and enables determination of the effects of stimulation on all the different neural elements around the electrode simultaneously. Computational modeling of the effects of extracellular stimulation on neurons involves a two-step approach. The first step is to calculate the electric potentials generated in the tissue by passage of current through the electrode. The second step is to determine the effect(s) of those potentials on the surrounding neurons.

51.4 From Cell to Circuit: Construction of Models of CNS Neurons

Electrical circuits are used to model the electrical behavior of neurons. These electrical-equivalent circuits, often referred to as cable models, represent the neuron as a series of cylindrical elements. Each cylinder is in turn replaced by a "compartment," representing the neuronal membrane, and a resistor representing the intracellular space. Thus, the model becomes a series of membrane compartments, connected by resistors. Each compartment is itself an electrical circuit that includes a capacitor representing the membrane capacitance of the lipid bilayer, resistors representing the ionic conductances of the transmembrane proteins (ion channels), and batteries representing the differences in potential (Nernst potential) arising from ionic concentration differences across the membrane. The process of constructing an equivalent electric circuit model of a CNS neuron is illustrated in Figure 51.4.

The values of circuit elements can be readily calculated from the geometry of the neurons and the specific values of neuron electrical properties. Consider a cylindrical representation of a segment of neuronal element, with diameter d and length l (Figure 51.4e). If we cut and "unroll" the cylinder, then the membrane resistance, R_m, can be calculated as:

R_m = specific membrane resistance/area of segment = $r_m/\pi * l * d$, where typical values for the specific membrane resistance are from 1000 to 5000 Ω cm². The membrane resistance is nonlinear, where the value of the membrane resistance depends on the voltage across the membrane (transmembrane potential). Further, separate elements (typically calculated as conductances) are used to represent the transmembrane paths for different ionic species, and the model of a patch of membrane includes several of these in parallel (Figure 51.4e). Similarly, the membrane capacitance, C_m, can be calculated as: C_m = specific membrane capacitance * area of segment = $c_m/\pi * l * d$, where typical values of the specific membrane capacitance are from 1 to 2 μF/cm². The intracellular resistance, R_i, can be calculated as: R_i = intracellular resistivity * segment length/cross-sectional area of segment = $\rho_i * l/(\pi * (d/2)^2)$, where typical values of the intracellular resistivity are from 50 to 400 Ω cm.

51.5 Sites of Action Potential Initiation in CNS Neurons

The response of a cable model, representing a CNS neuron, to extracellular electrical stimulation is shown in Figure 51.5. The transmembrane potential as a function of time, in different segments of the

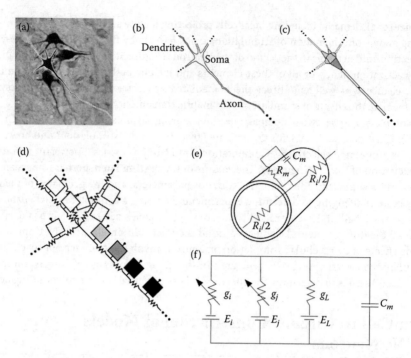

FIGURE 51.4 Construction of models of CNS neurons. (a) Examples of stained neurons in the CNS. (b) The morphology of stained neurons can be reconstructed in three dimensions. (c) The morphology is then converted into a series of equivalent cylindrical elements. (d) The cylindrical elements are subsequently replaced by electrical equivalent circuits with resistive elements representing the intracellular space, and compartmental models representing the membrane. (e) Each cylindrical segment includes a representation of the membrane and the intracellular space and the values of the equivalent circuit elements can be calculated from the geometry of the cylinder and specific parameter values. (f) Each compartment model of the membrane may contain several nonlinear ionic conductances (g_i, g_j) and linear ionic conductance (g_L) representing various ionic channels in the membrane, batteries representing the Nernst potential arising from the difference in concentration of ions on the inside and outside of the membrane (E_i, E_j, E_L), and a capacitor (C_m) representing the capacitance arising from the lipid bilayer of the cell.

neuron, is shown for a cathodic electrode positioned over the axon (Figure 51.5a), for a cathodic electrode positioned over the cell body (Figure 51.5b), and for an anodic electrode positioned over the cell body (Figure 51.5c).

During stimulation over the axon with a cathodic current the axon is depolarized immediately beneath the electrode, and hyperpolarized in regions lateral to the electrode (arrowheads Figure 51.5a). Action potential initiation occurs in the most depolarized node of Ranvier, immediately beneath the electrode (arrow) and then propagates in both directions.

The response of a CNS neuron is more complex. With both cathodic and anodic stimuli delivered through an electrode placed 1 mm above the cell body, action potential initiation occurred in the axon, even though the electrode is positioned directly over the soma. With 0.1 ms duration cathodic stimuli action potential initiation occurred at the second node of Ranvier from the cell body (arrow), and with 0.1 ms duration anodic stimuli action potential initiation occurred in the third node of Ranvier from the cell body (arrow). During the cathodic stimulus pulse, the node of Ranvier where action potential initiation occurred was hyperpolarized by the stimulus (arrowhead). Following termination of the stimulus, the cell body and dendritic tree discharged through the axon, leading to action potential initiation (McIntyre and Grill, 1999). This finding in a computational model is consistent with contemporary in vitro results from the cortex (Nowak and Bullier, 1998a,b). Thus, with cathodic stimuli action potential

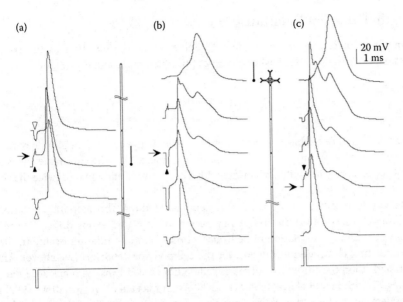

FIGURE 51.5 Action potential initiation by extracellular stimulation in CNS neurons by cathodic and anodic stimuli. Each trace shows transmembrane voltage as a function of time for different sections of the neuron. (a) Stimulation with a monophasic cathodic stimulus pulse from an electrode positioned 1 mm over a node of Ranvier of the axon. Depolarization occurs in the node directly beneath the electrode (solid arrowhead) and hyperpolarization occurs in the adjacent nodes of Ranvier (open arrowhead). Action potential initiation occurs in the node of Ranvier directly under the electrode (arrow) and the action potential propagates in both directions. (b) During threshold stimulation with an electrode positioned 1 mm over the cell body, action potential initiation occurs at a node of Ranvier of the axon. With cathodic stimuli (duration 0.1 ms) action potential initiation occurred at the second node of Ranvier from the cell body (arrow). (c) With anodic stimuli (duration 0.1 ms) action potential initiation occurred in the third node of Ranvier from the cell body (arrow).

initiation occurred in a part of the neuron that was hyperpolarized by the stimulus, and this indirect mode of activation increases the threshold for activation of local cells with cathodic stimuli. Conversely, with anodic stimuli, the site of action potential initiation was at the node that was most depolarized by the stimulus (arrowhead). These position-dependent thresholds are reflected in exciting populations of neurons, as well (see below).

51.6 Excitation Properties of CNS Stimulation

The finding that action potential initiation occurs in the axon has several important implications for CNS stimulation. First, since excitation occurs in the axon there is little difference in the extracellular chronaxie times for excitation of local cells and excitation of passing axons (see Section 51.6.1). Therefore, chronaxie time is not a sensitive indicator of the neuronal element that is activated by extracellular stimulation (Miocinovic and Grill, 2004). Second, since action potential initiation occurs at some distance from the site of integration of synaptic inputs, the effects of coactivation of presynaptic fibers may be less than expected and the axon may still fire even when the cell body is hyperpolarized, for example, by inhibitory synaptic inputs (see Section 51.6.4). Therefore, extracellular unit recordings of cell body firing may not accurately reflect the output of the neuron (Grill and McIntyre, 2001; McIntyre et al., 2004). Finally, the difference in the mode of activation of local cells by cathodic stimuli and anodic stimuli is the basis for the difference in threshold between cathodic and anodic stimuli (see Section 51.6.3).

51.6.1 Strength–Duration Relationship

The stimulus amplitude necessary for excitation, I_{th}, increases as the duration of the stimulus is decreased. The strength–duration relationship describes this phenomena and is given by

$$I_{th} = I_{th}[1 + T_{ch}/PW]$$

where the parameter I_{rh} is the rheobase current, and is defined as the current amplitude necessary to excite the neuron with a pulse of infinite duration, and the parameter T_{ch} is the chronaxie and is defined as the pulse duration necessary to excite the neuron with a pulse amplitude equal to twice the rheobase current.

Measurements with intracellular stimulation have demonstrated that the temporal excitation characteristics, including chronaxie (T_{ch}) and refractory period, of cells and axons differ (Figure 51.6a). However, during extracellular stimulation of neurons, action potential initiation occurs in the axon, even with the stimulating electrode positioned over the cell body or dendrites (see above). Although with intracellular activation the chronaxies of many cell bodies exceed 1 ms, with extracellular activation they are below 1 ms (Stoney et al., 1968; Ranck, 1975; Asanuma et al., 1976; Swadlow, 1992) and lie within the ranges determined for extracellular activation of axons (Ranck, 1975; Li and Bak, 1976; West and Wolstencroft, 1983). For stimulation of cortical gray matter, the mean T_{ch} for *intracellular* stimulation of cells (15 ms) was substantially longer than T_{ch} for *extracellular* stimulation of axons (0.27 ms), the mean T_{ch} for *extracellular* stimulation of local cells (0.38 ms) was comparable to that for extracellular stimulation of axons (Nowak and Bullier, 1998a). Further, during extracellular stimulation the chronaxies measured with extracellular stimulation were dependent on a number of factors other than the neuronal element that was stimulated (Miocinovic and Grill, 2004). The chronaxies of different neuronal elements determined with extracellular stimulation overlap and do not enable unique determination of the neuronal element stimulated.

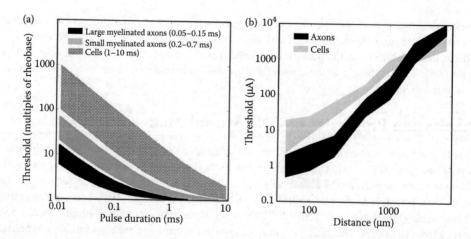

FIGURE 51.6 Properties of CNS stimulation. (a) The strength–duration relationship describes the amplitude required for stimulation as a function of the stimulation pulse duration. Strength duration curves for intracellular stimulation of different neural elements were constructed from data summarized in Ranck (1976). (b) The current–distance relationship describes the threshold intensity required for stimulation as a function of the distance between the electrode and the neuron. Current–distance curves for axons and cells were constructed from data summarized in Ranck (1976).

51.6.2 Current–Distance Relationship

The current required for extracellular stimulation of neurons, threshold, I_{th}, increases as the distance between the electrode and the neuron, r, increases. This is described by the current–distance relationship (Stoney et al., 1968):

$$I_{th}I_R + k \cdot r^2$$

where the offset, I_R, determines the absolute threshold and the slope, k, determines the threshold difference between neurons at different distances from the electrode. Current–distance relationship for excitation of axons and cells in the CNS have been measured in a large number of preparations, and current–distance curves for these two populations are summarized in Figure 51.6b.

51.6.3 Effect of Stimulus Polarity and Stimulus Waveform on CNS Stimulation

During excitation of axons in the peripheral nervous system different stimulus polarities produce changes in the threshold as well as changes in the site of action potential initiation, and similar, but more pronounced effects occur during CNS stimulation. Figure 51.7 shows the results of a computational

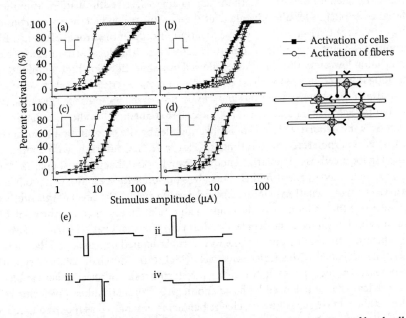

FIGURE 51.7 Effect of stimulus polarity and waveform on excitation of populations of local cells and passing axons. (a–d) Input–output curves from a population model containing 50 passing axons and 50 local cells randomly positioned around a point source stimulating electrode. The curves are the percent of neurons (passing axons, local cells) activated as a function of the stimulation amplitude for excitation with (a) 0.2 ms duration monophasic cathodic pulses, (b) 0.2 ms duration monophasic anodic pulses, (c) anodic phase first biphasic symmetric pulses (0.2 ms per phase), and (d) cathodic phase first biphasic symmetric pulses (0.2 ms per phase). (Modified from McIntyre CC, Grill WM. *Ann Biomed Eng* 2000; 28:219–233.) (e) Examples of asymmetric charge balanced biphasic pulses. Cathodic-phase first (i) and anodic-phase first pseudo-monophasic pulses have a low-amplitude second phases and exhibit excitation properties similar to monophasic cathodic and anodic stimuli, respectively. Novel asymmetric pulses that manipulate neuronal excitability via a sub-threshold first that also balances charge that also provides charge balancing. The anodic prepulse (0.2 ms) followed by a cathodic stimulus phase (0.02 ms) enables preferential excitation of passing axons, while a cathodic prepulse (1.0 ms) followed by an anodic stimulus pulse (0.1 ms) enables preferential excitation of local cells. (Adapted from McIntyre CC, Grill WM. *Ann Biomed Eng* 2000; 28:219–233.)

study to determine which neuronal elements are activated by extracellular stimulation in the CNS. A model including populations of local cells and axons of passage, randomly positioned around a point source stimulating electrode, was used to compare activation of local cells to activation of passing fibers with different stimulation waveforms (McIntyre and Grill, 2000). Using cathodic pulses the threshold for activation of passing axons was less than the threshold for activation of local neurons, and when 70% of the axons were activated approximately 10% of the local cells were also activated. When using anodic pulses, the threshold for activation of local cells is less than the threshold for activation of passing axons, and when the stimulus amplitude that activated 70% of the local cells also activated 25% of the passing axons. The basis for this effect can be understood by comparing action potential initiation in local cells using cathodic and anodic stimuli described above.

To prevent possible degradation of the stimulating electrode(s) or damage to the tissue, chronic stimulation is conducted with biphasic stimulus pulses (Lilly et al., 1955; Robblee and Rose, 1990). The response of passing axons and local cells to symmetric biphasic pulses is shown in Figure 51.7c and d. Using either anodic-phase first or cathodic-phase first pulses, the threshold for activation of passing axons was less than the threshold for activation of local neurons, and the relative selectivity for axons was lower with either pulse than with monophasic cathodic pulses.

These results and previous experimental evidence demonstrates that different neuronal elements have similar thresholds for extracellular stimulation (Roberts and Smith, 1973; Gustafsson and Jankowska, 1976) and illustrates the need for design of methods that enable selective stimulation. Stimulus waveforms can be designed explicitly to take advantage of the nonlinear conductance properties of neurons and thereby increase the selectivity between activation of different neuronal elements. Biphasic asymmetrical stimulus waveforms capable of selectively activating either local cells or axonal elements consist of a long duration low-amplitude pre-pulse followed by a short duration high-amplitude stimulation phase. The long duration pre-pulse phase of the stimulus is designed to create a sub-threshold depolarizing pre-pulse in the nontarget neurons and a hyperpolarizing pre-pulse in the target neurons (Grill and Mortimer, 1995; McIntyre and Grill, 2000) Recall that during cathodic stimulation, the site of excitation in axons is the depolarized node of Ranvier, while the site of excitation in local cells is a node of Ranvier that is hyperpolarized by the stimulus (Figure 51.5). Conversely, with anodic stimuli, the site of excitation in local cells is a depolarized node of Ranvier, and that the most polarized node of passing axons is hyperpolarized by the stimulus. Thus, the same polarity pre-pulse will produce opposite polarization at the sites of excitation in local cells and passing axons. The effect of this subthreshold polarization is to decrease the excitability of the nontarget population and increase the excitability of the target population via alterations in the degree of sodium channel inactivation (Grill and Mortimer, 1995). Therefore, when the stimulating phase of the waveform is applied neuronal population targeted for stimulation will be activated with greater selectively (McIntyre and Grill, 2000). Asymmetrical charge-balanced biphasic cathodic phase first stimulus waveforms result in selective activation of local cells, while asymmetrical charge-balanced biphasic anodic phase first stimulus waveforms result in selective activation of fibers of passage. Further, charge balancing is achieved as required to reduce the probability of tissue damage and electrode corrosion. Note that these prepulse waveforms differ from the pseudo-monophasic waveforms used in some stimulators in that the low-amplitude long-duration phase of the waveform precedes rather than follows the high-amplitude short-duration phase of the waveform (Figure 51.7e).

51.6.4 Indirect Effects of Extracellular Stimulation

The thresholds for excitation of presynpatic terminals and subsequent indirect effects on local neurons (mediated by synaptic transmission) are similar to thresholds for direct effects (mediated by stimulus current) during extracellular stimulation (Figure 51.8a) of spinal cord motoneurons (Gustaffson and Jankowska, 1976), rubrospinal neurons (Baldissera et al., 1972), and corticospinal neurons (Jankowska

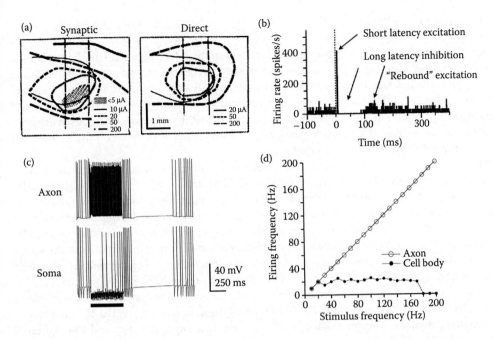

FIGURE 51.8 CNS stimulation results in direct effects and indirect effects on CNS neurons. (a) Two-dimensional maps of thresholds for indirect (synaptic) and direct activation of neurons in the red nucleus. (From Baldissera F, Lundberg A, and Udo M. *Exp Brain Res* 1972; 15:151–167.) (b) Complex polyphasic changes in the firing rate of a cortical neuron in response to extracellular stimulation. (From Butovas S, Schwarz C. *J Neurophysiol* 2003; 90(5):3024–3039.) (c) Transmembrane potential in the axon (top trace) and cell body (bottom trace) of a model thalamocortical neuron before, during (black bar at bottom), and after extracellular stimulation. (From McIntyre CC et al. *J Neurophysiol* 2004; 91:1457–1469.) Extracellular stimulation results in simultaneous inhibition of the cell body, as a result of activation of presynaptic terminals and subsequent indirect effects, and excitation of the axon, as a result of direct action potential initiation in a node of Ranvier. (d) Firing rate in the cell body and axon during extracellular stimulation of a model thalamocortical neuron. (Modified from McIntyre CC et al. *J Neurophysiol* 2004; 91:1457–1469.) The firing rate in the cell body is lower that that in the axon, as a result of simultaneous indirect synaptic effects on the soma, and direct excitation of the axon.

et al., 1975). Further, the chronaxie of presynaptic terminals (~0.14 ms in the frog spinal cord, Tkacs and Wurster, 1991; 0.06–0.54 ms in the rat subthalamic nucleus, Hutchison et al., 2002) is comparable to that of passing axons, and thus effects may be attributed to activation of passing axons when in fact they arise from activation of presynaptic elements. These "indirect" effects of stimulation must be considered when electrodes are placed within the heterogeneous environment of the CNS. During extracellular stimulation, release of inhibitory and/or excitatory neurotransmitters from presynaptic terminals can result in complex poly-phasic changes in the firing rate of postsynaptic neurons (Figure 51.8b) (Butovas and Schwarz, 2003) and modulate the threshold for excitation of the postsynaptic neuron (Swadlow, 1992; McIntyre and Grill, 2002). Thus, indirect effects mediated by synaptic transmission may alter the direct effects of stimulation on the postsynaptic cell. Further, antidromic propagation of action potentials originating from activation of axon terminals can lead to widespread activation or inhibition of targets distant from the site of stimulation through axon collaterals. However, recall that action potential initiation occurs at some distance from the soma, where integration of synaptic inputs occurs, and thus the axon may be excited even when the cell body is hyperpolarized (Figure 51.8c). Therefore, extracellular unit recordings of firing in the soma may not accurately reflect the output of the neuron (Figure 51.8d) (Grill and McIntyre, 2001; McIntyre et al., 2004).

51.7 Summary

This chapter described electrical activation of neurons within the CNS. Electrical stimulation is used to study the form and function of the nervous system and a technique to restore function following disease or injury. The successful application of electrical stimulation to treat nervous system disorders as well as interpretation of the results of stimulation requires understanding of the cellular level effects of stimulation. Quantitative models provide a means to understand the response of neurons to extracellular stimulation. Further, accurate quantitative models provide powerful design tools that can be used to engineer stimuli that produce a desired response.

The fundamental properties of excitation of CNS neurons were presented with a focus on what neural elements around the electrode are activated under different conditions. During CNS stimulation action potentials are initiated in the axons of local cells, even for electrodes positioned over the cell body. The threshold difference between cathodic and anodic stimuli arises due to differences in the mode of activation. Anodic stimuli cause depolarization of the axon and excitation via a "virtual cathode," while cathodic stimuli cause hyperpolarization at the site of excitation and the action potential is initiated during repolarization. The threshold for activation of presynaptic terminals projecting into the region of stimulation is often less than or equal to the threshold for direct excitation of local cells, and indirect effects mediated by synaptic transmission may alter the direct effects of stimulation on the postsynaptic cell. The fundamental understanding provided by this analysis enables rational design and interpretation of studies and devices employing electrical stimulation of the brain or spinal cord.

Acknowledgment

The research carried out in Dr. Grill's laboratory and the preparation of this chapter were supported by NIH Grant R01 NS-40894.

References

Ackman, JJ, Seitz, MA. Methods of complex impedance measurement in biologic tissue. *CRC Crit Rev Biomed Eng* 1984; 11:281–311.

Asanuma H, Arnold A, Zarezecki P. Further study on the excitation of pyramidal tract cells by intracortical microstimulation. *Exp Brain Res* 1976; 26:443–461.

Bai Q, Wise KD, Anderson DJ. A high-yield microassembly structure for three-dimensional microelectrode arrays. *IEEE Trans Biomed Eng* 2000 Mar;47(3):281–289.

Baldissera F, Lundberg A, Udo M. Stimulation of pre- and postsynaptic elements in the red nucleus. *Exp Brain Res* 1972; 15:151–167.

Baumann SB, Wozny DR, Kelly SK, Meno FM, The electrical conductivity of human cerebrospinal fluid at body temperature. *IEEE Trans Biomed Eng* 1997 Mar;44(3):220–223.

Brindley GS, Lewin WS. The sensations produced by electrical stimulation of the visual cortex. *J Physiol* 1968; 196:479–493.

Butovas S, Schwarz C. Spatiotemporal effects of microstimulation in rat neocortex: A parametric study using multielectrode recordings. *J Neurophysiol* 2003 Nov; 90(5):3024–3039.

Cameron T. Safety and efficacy of spinal cord stimulation for the treatment of chronic pain: A 20-year literature review. *J Neurosurg* 2004; 100(3 Suppl):254–267.

Coffey RJ. Deep brain stimulation for chronic pain: Results of two multicenter trials and a structured review. *Pain Med* 2001; 2:183–192.

Crile, GW, Hosmer, HR, Rowland, AF. The electrical conductivity of animal tissues under normal and pathological conditions. *Am J Physiol* 1922; 60:59–106.

Eisenberg, RS, Mathias, RT. Structural analysis of electrical properties of cells and tissues. *CRC Crit Rev Biomed Eng* 1980; 4:203–232.

Grill WM. Modeling the effects of electric fields on nerve fibers: Influence of tissue electrical properties. *IEEE Trans Biomed Eng* 1999; 46:918–928.

Grill WM, McIntyre CC. Extracellular excitation of central neurons: Implications for the mechanisms of deep brain stimulation. *Thalamus Relat Systems* 2001; 1:269–277.

Grill WM, Mortimer JT. Electrical properties of implant encapsulation tissue. *Annals Biomed Eng* 1994; 22:23–33.

Grill WM, Mortimer JT. Stimulus waveforms for selective neural stimulation. *IEEE Eng Med Biol* 1995; 14:375–385.

Gross RE. Deep brain stimulation in the treatment of neurological and psychiatric disease. *Expert Rev Neurother* 2004; 4:465–478.

Gross RE, Lozano AM. Advances in neurostimulation for movement disorders. *Neurol Res* 2000; 22:247–258.

Gustafsson B, Jankowska E. Direct and indirect activation of nerve cells by electrical pulses applied extra-cellularly. *J Physiol* 1976; 258:33–61.

Hodaie M, Wennberg RA, Dostrovsky JO, Lozano AM. Chronic anterior thalamus stimulation for intrac-table epilepsy. *Epilepsia* 2002; 43:603–608.

Holsheimer J, Struijk JJ, Tas NR. Effects of electrode geometry and combination on nerve fibre selectivity in spinal cord stimulation. *Med Biol Eng Comput* 1995; 33:676–682.

Hutchison WD, Chung AG, Goldshmidt A. Chronaxie and refractory period of neuronal inhibition by extracellular stimulation in the region of rat STN. Program No. 416.3. 2002 Abstract Viewer/Itinerary Planner CD-ROM, Society for Neuroscience, Washington, DC.

Jankowska E, Padel Y, Tanaka R. The mode of activation of pyramidal tract cells by intracortical stimuli. *J Physiol* 1975; 249:617–636.

Jankowska E, Roberts WJ. An electrophysiological demonstration of the axonal projections of single spi-nal interneurones in the cat. *J Physiol* 1972; 222:597–622.

Li CL, Bak A. Excitability characteristics of the A- and C-fibers in a peripheral nerve. *Exp Neurol* 1976; 50:67–79.

Li C-H, Bak AF, Parker LO. Specific resistivity of the cerebral cortex and white matter. *Exp Neurol* 1968; 20:544–557.

Lilly JC, Hughes JR, Alvord EC Jr, Galkin TA. Brief noninjurious electric waveform for stimulation of the brain. *Science* 1955; 121:468–469.

Lipski J. Antidromic activation of neurones as an analytic tool in the study of the central nervous system. *J Neurosci Methods* 1981; 4:1–32.

McCreery DB, Yuen TG, Agnew WF, Bullara LA. A characterization of the effects on neuronal excitability due to prolonged microstimulation with chronically implanted microelectrodes. *IEEE Trans Biomed Eng* 1997 Oct; 44(10):931–939.

McIntyre CC, Grill WM. Excitation of central nervous system neurons by nonuniform electric fields. *Biophys J* 1999; 76:878–888.

McIntyre CC, Grill WM. Selective microstimulation of central nervous system neurons. *Ann Biomed Eng* 2000; 28:219–233.

McIntyre CC, Grill WM. Finite element analysis of the current-density and electric field generated by metal microelectrodes. *Annals of Biomedical Engineering* 2001; 29(3):227–235.

McIntyre CC, Grill, WM. Extracellular stimulation of central neurons: Influence of stimulus waveform and frequency on neuronal output. *J Neurophysiol* 2002; 88:1592–1604.

McIntyre CC, Grill WM, Sherman DL, Thakor NV. Cellular effects of deep brain stimulation: Model-based analysis of activation and inhibition. *J Neurophysiol* 2004; 91:1457–1469.

Miocinovic S, Grill WM. Sensitivity of temporal excitation properties to the neuronal element activated by extracellular stimulation. *J Neurosci Methods* 2004; 132:91–99.

Nicholson PW. Specific impedance of cerebral white matter. *Exp Neurol* 1965; 13:386–401.

Nicolelis MAL, Dimitrov D, Carmena JM, Crist R, Lehew G, Kralik JD, Wise SP. Chronic, multisite, multielecrode recording in macaque monkeys. *Proc Natl Acad Sci, USA* 2003; 100:11041–11046.

Normann RA, Maynard EM, Rousche PJ, Warren DJ. A neural interface for a cortical vision prosthesis. *Vision Res* 1999 Jul;39(15):2577–2587.

Nowak LG, Bullier J. Axons, but not cell bodies, are activated by electrical stimulation in cortical gray matter. I. Evidence from chronaxie measurements. *Exp Brain Res* 1998a; 118:477–488.

Nowak LG, Bullier J. Axons, but not cell bodies, are activated by electrical stimulation in cortical gray matter. II. Evidence from selective inactivation of cell bodies and axon initial segments. *Exp Brain Res* 1998b; 118:489–500.

Otto SR, Brackmann DE, Hitselberger WE, Shannon RV, Kuchta J. Multichannel auditory brainstem implant: Update on performance in 61 patients. *J Neurosurg* 2002, 96:1063–1071.

Ranck JB Jr. Analysis of specific impedance of rabbit cerebral cortex. *Exp Neurol* 1963; 7:153–174.

Ranck JB Jr., BeMent SL. The specific impedance of the dorsal columns of the cat: An anisotropic medium. *Exp Neurol* 1965; 11:451–463.

Ranck JB Jr. Which elements are excited in electrical stimulation of mammalian central nervous system: A review. *Brain Res* 1975; 98:417–440.

Robblee LS, Rose TL. Electrochemical guidelines for selection of protocols and electrode materials for neural stimulation. In: *Neural Prostheses: Fundamental Studies*, Edited by Agnew, WF and McCreery DB, Prentice-Hall, Englewood Cliffs, NJ, 1990; pp. 25–66.

Roberts WJ, Smith DO. Analysis of threshold currents during microstimulation of fibers in the spinal cord. *Acta Physiol Scand* 1973; 89:384–394.

Sances A, Jr. Larson SJ. Impedance and current density studies. In: *Electroanesthesia: Biomedical and Biophysical Studies*; Edited by Sances A and Larson SJ, Academic Press, NY, 1975, pp. 114–124.

Schmidt EM, Bak MJ, Hambrecht FT, Kufta CV, O'Rourke DK, Vallabhanath P. Feasibility of a visual prosthesis for the blind based on intracortical microstimulation of the visual cortex. *Brain* 1996; 119:507–522.

Stoney SD Jr, Thompson WD, Asanuma H. Excitation of pyramidal tract cells by intracortical microstimulation: Effective extent of stimulating current. *J Neurophys* 1968; 31:659–669.

Swadlow HA. Monitoring the excitability of neocortical efferent neurons to direct activation by extracellular current pulses. *J Neurophysiol* 1992; 68:605–619.

Tehovnik EJ. Electrical stimulation of neural tissue to evoke behavioral responses. *J Neursci Methods* 1996; 65:1–17.

Tkacs NC, Wurster RD. Strength-duration and activity-dependent excitability properties of frog afferent axons and their intraspinal projections. *J Neurophysiol* 1991; 65:468–476.

Troyk P, Bak M, Berg J, Bradley D, Cogan S, Erickson R, Kufta C, McCreery D, Schmidt E, Towle V. A model for intracortical visual prosthesis research. *Artif Organs* 2003; 27:1005–1015.

Velasco F, Velasco M, Jimenez F, Velasco AL, Marquez I. Stimulation of the central median thalamic nucleus for epilepsy. *Stereotact Funct Neurosurg* 2001; 77:228–232.

Veltink PH, Van Veen BK, Struijk JJ, Holsheimer J, Boom HBK. A modeling study of nerve fascicle stimulation. *IEEE Trans Biomed Eng* 1989; 36(7):683–692.

West DC, Wolstencroft JH. Strength–duration characteristics of myelinated and non-myelinated bulbospinal axons in the cat spinal cord. *J Physiol* 1983; 337:37–50.

52

Transcutaneous FES for Ambulation: The Parastep System

52.1 Introduction and Background 52-1
   Historical Background • Brief Review of FES Systems for
   Ambulation by Paraplegics
52.2 Parastep System 52-3
   System's Electric Charge and Charge Density Parameters • System
   Parameters and Design
52.3 Patient Admissibility, Contraindications, and Training 52-12
   Patient Admissibility Criteria • Contraindications • Patient
   Training
52.4 Walking Performance and Medical and Psychological
   Benefits Evaluation Results 52-14
   Walking Performance Data • Evaluation Results on Medical
   Benefits of Walking with the Parastep System • Psychological
   Outcome Evaluation Results
52.5 Regulatory Status 52-17
52.6 Concluding Comments 52-17
References 52-18

Daniel Graupe
*University of Illinois at
Chicago*

52.1 Introduction and Background

52.1.1 Historical Background

Functional electrical (neuromuscular) stimulation, denoted as FES (or FNS), has its origins in Luigi Galvani's experiment on electrically exciting a frog's leg in the 1780s as described by him in "De Viribus Electricitatis in Motu Muscular" (1791), which despite some faults due to the state of scientific knowledge at its time, can be shown to lay the foundation to two great disciplines, electrical engineering and neurophysiology [1].

The first demonstrated modern application of FNS to a human patient for functional movements of extremities was reported by Lieberson in 1960 [2] in the case of a hemiplegic patient, whereas the first application to a paraplegic patient is that by Kantrowitz [3].

Unbraced short-distance ambulation by transcutaneous FNS of a complete paraplegic was first described in 1980 by Kralj et al. [4].

In early 1982, the first patient-controlled ambulation for a complete paraplegic as necessary for independent ambulation was achieved by Graupe et al. [5–7], employing EMG (electromyograph) control. A manually controlled system, known as the Parastep FNS system was tested from 1982 and received FDA approval in 1994 to become the first FNS ambulation system to be so approved and to be commercially available for use by individuals beyond research environments.

The systems of Graupe et al. [5,7] employ a walker for balancing support. It was commercialized by Sigmedics, Inc. (founded for this purpose in 1987) as the Parastep system (Parastep-I system) and was the first (and still is the only) FES ambulation system to have received FDA approval in 1994 [8] and approval by Medicare/Medicaid for reimbursement in 2003 [9,10].

In parallel, work was carried out since the early 1980s on percutaneous FNS, especially at Case Western Reserve University [11,12] in Vienna, Austria [13], and in Augusta, Maine [14].

FNS as discussed above is applicable for traumatic complete (or near-complete as far as sensation, leg extension, and hip flexion are concerned) upper-motor-neuron thoracic-level paraplegics. To date, approximately 1000 such patients are or have been able to ambulate over short distances with the FDA-approved Parastep system. They have been trained in over 20 hospitals or rehabilitation centers in the United States and in Europe, with no known detrimental effects. These patients can ambulate independently between 20 and several hundred meters (some up to 1 mile) without sitting down. The number of complete paraplegic patients who ambulate with implanted (percutaneous) electrodes is very small—about a dozen. The latter patients must undergo surgery (often of several hours) and they require occasional repeat surgery to correct electrode breakage or slippage, which are still unresolved problems. They also experience infections at the sites of electrode penetration through the skin. Consequently, at the present state of implantation, and noting the performance of the transcutaneous Parastep FNS users, it appears that for some time to come, the transcutaneous approach will be the more common one, and not just due to it being the only one available outside the research lab. It is for these reasons and since it is the only system for which there exists a body of independent source published material on clinical experience and data collection that this chapter concentrates on the Parastep ambulation system. Still, for the completeness of this chapter, a very brief discussion on some of the other major ambulation systems is presented.

52.1.2 Brief Review of FES Systems for Ambulation by Paraplegics

A very brief discussion on some of the other major FES ambulation systems is presented here.

1. *Noninvasive (transcutaneous) FES systems*: The only other transcutaneous FES system (but for the Parastep) or both standing and ambulation that has been used outside their inventors' laboratory is the *Ljubljana FES system*, which is based on the work of Kralj et al. [15,16] and which emanated from that group's earlier pioneering work [4] on FES (related to the still earlier work of Lieberson et al. [2] concerning hemiplegia). The bench model of the Ljubljana system was the first to achieve ambulation via FES by a complete thoracic-level paraplegic [4]. Its principles are similar to those of the Parastep system in their purpose and in their general function, which can, in part, already be found in the principles of the earlier Ljubljana work on hemiplegia and in Lieberson's work. It differs from the Parastep system in that it was not designed to maximize walking distance and it also differs in its control and in its channel coordination (to result in a bulkier system than the Parastep system). Its patient-borne version is usually a four-channel system. Its signal generation is essentially a two-channel signal generator, such that the four-channel system is a double two-channel system. The Ljubljana system is not yet commercially available (at least, not outside the use in research programs, mainly in Europe) and is presently not FDA-approved. No independent multipatient ambulation performance studies and statistics and no multipatient medical evaluations or psychological evaluations were published on that system.

   Other noninvasive (transcutaneous) FES systems for standing and ambulation, apart from the Ljubljana system and the Parastep system, are essentially all *bench devices*, as developed in various research laboratories for the purpose of their own research (see References 17 and 18, and the Stanmore system of Phillips et al. [19]). Whereas all FES ambulation systems can be and are used for *standing*, there are several transcutaneous FES systems for standing alone (see References 20 and 21, and the Odstock standing system of Taylor et al. [22]). These are obviously limited in scope and are not within the main theme of this review. None is commercially available.

2. *Hybrid FES-long-leg brace ambulation systems:* Hybrid FES-long-leg-brace or FES-body-brace systems, which combine transcutaneous FES with a long-leg brace or with a body brace for standing and ambulation by paraplegics, have been developed since the 1970s ([8,23,24], Solomonow et al. [the Louisiana State University (LSU) system] [25]). These systems are also intended for upper-motor-neuron (thoracic-level) LSI. They represent a regression from FES since they give up one of the major goals of FES ambulation, namely, patient's independence. Since hybrid systems use a body brace or long-leg braces, they are far heavier and far more cumbersome than, say, the 10.5 ounce Parastep. They require 30 min to don and a long time to doff, requiring help from an able-bodied person in donning and in doffing the system. This also affects patient compliance and regular use of the system, while the system's weight reduces ambulation distances [25].

3. *Implanted FES ambulation systems:* As stated earlier in this section, research on implanted FES for standing and ambulation has been carried out in parallel with the work on transcutaneous noninvasive FES, the latter being the subject of the present review. It is however important for the completeness of this review to comment briefly on implanted FES.

Work on both invasive FES and noninvasive FES started in the late 1970s and early 1980s. Also, the first applications to thoracic-level complete traumatic paraplegic were reported for both approaches in the early 1980s [4–6,11,13]. Also, both approaches are based on the fundamental user by Lieberson et al. [2]. However, invasive methods, both *percutaneous* [11,13] and fully implanted systems [26], always involve a major surgery in contrast to the noninvasive transcutaneous methods on which this review concentrates. It is not just the surgery (and its cost). Furthermore, so far, all noninvasive methods encounter loss of contact of electrodes, wire breakage, and sometimes even tearing of nerve fibers. Such occurrences then require resurgery. Fully implanted FES [27] does not encounter infections at locations where wires penetrate the skin as it happens with percutaneous methods. (In fully implanted systems, a radio-frequency [RF] receiver is implanted that receives RF signals through the skin, from a transmitter attached above the skin and the received RF is rectified to provide electric power.) All invasive systems require some kind of patient control from a nonimplanted device, as do noninvasive systems. Also, all invasive systems require similar patient training and muscle strengthening. Of course, an implanted device requires no electrode placement each morning and removal each evening. However, with the Parastep system, donning time is 5–8 min for a trained user and doffing time is 3–4 min. Connection and disconnection of the FES control device and, in percutaneous systems, connection of wires to the implanted electrodes from outside, also takes a few minutes. It is therefore not surprising that the Parastep system was the first and is still the only FES system for standing and ambulation that has received (1994) FDA approval and is commercially available. We note that there are presently some 600 users of the Parastep and it is used both at home and at workplace. In contrast, there are presently only a few (in the order of a dozen) users of even the most advanced percutaneous system (based on Marsolais work and that of his colleagues in Cleveland, as mentioned above), whereas the fully implanted system is not yet complete to allow out-of-clinic ambulation.

We comment that the work on implanted FES has resulted in great advances in implantation techniques and materials that are of value in situations where there is no alternative to implantation (unlike the case of FES for standing and ambulation). However, the difficulties in implanted systems are still with us and they will always require surgery.

52.2 Parastep System

52.2.1 System's Electric Charge and Charge Density Parameters

The FNS consists of sequences (trains) of electrical impulses that are applied transcutaneously so that the stimulation reaches the peripheral motor neurons at selected sites. Stimulation serves only to trigger action potentials (APs) at these motor units. The resultant APs produced in the motor neurons

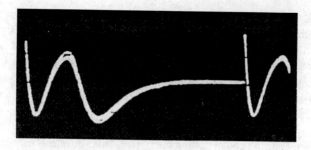

FIGURE 52.1 Action potential in response to stimulation at a quadriceps stimulated site.

concerned, in response to these triggers (stimulation impulses), subsequently cause contraction of muscle fibers that are associated with these motor neurons [27,28] (see Figure 52.1).

Comment: This AP is a summation of many synchronous APs produced in response to a stimulation signal. It is recoded by surface electrodes at the stimulation site. The sharp peak at the beginning of each AP is an artifact of the stimulus.

52.2.1.1 Parameters of Stimulation Signals and Safety Standard Constraints

The stimulation trains that are employed are trains of impulses of 120–150 μs in duration (width) and their rate is 20–25 pulses/s. The pulse duration above is selected to be as low as possible while still allowing full contractions [27,29]. This is necessitated by considerations of minimizing the electrical charge density applied to the stimulation site for the patient's safety: it, therefore, also minimizes battery power, to result in a compact lightweight portable system (Figure 52.2). The system is powered by a 9.6 VDC battery pack consisting of 8 AA or AAA Ni-Cad rechargeable batteries, to power the stimulator and its computer.

The maximal current per pulse is limited [27] in our system to 0.3 A = Io. As per the 1985 ANSI standard, Section 3.2.2.2 of the Association for Advancement of Medical Instrumentation and the American National Standard Institute [30], the stimulation should be limited to below 10 mA average current. Hence, stimuli of $T = 150$ μs duration (pulse width) at $f = 24$ pulses/s result in an average current I_{ave} of

$$I_{ave} = Io \times T \times f \tag{52.1}$$

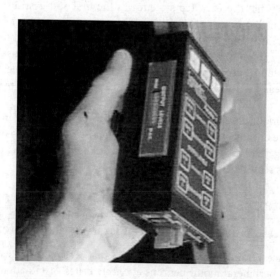

FIGURE 52.2 The parastep unit.

namely, $0.3 \times 24 \times 0.00015 = 0.00108$ A or 1.08 mA, as is well below the ANSI limit. Another critical ANSI parameter is that of maximal electrical charge per pulse of 75 μC/pulse. The Parastep system's maximal output electrical charge value is given by

$$Q = IoT \tag{52.2}$$

or 0.3×0.00015 C = 45 μC = Q. Thus, the current density I_{ave}/S for electrodes is 1.75×3.75 in.^{2} (namely, $S = 40$ cm$^2 = 4000$ mm^2). The current density in the case of the Parastep system is therefore

$$I_{ave}/S = 0.00108/4000 \text{ A/mm}^2 = 0.25 \text{ μC/mm}^2 \tag{52.3}$$

which is well below the ANSI limit of 10 μC/mm^2.

52.2.2 System Parameters and Design

The Parastep system is based on a single microprocessor [27,29], which is its main component and where the stimulation signals of all channels are shaped and controlled and where synchronization between channels is performed for the four different stimulation operational menus. The microprocessor generates and shapes trains of stimulation pulses that are multiplexed and directed by the algorithm imbedded in that microcomputer to six output channels, which are individually controlled by the microcomputer, in response to menu selection by the patient to avoid robot-like movements. Channel separation is performed by a timing program, which is passed from the microcomputer to an array of microcomputer-controlled optoisolators and then appropriately amplified, thus providing the system's outputs to 12 surface electrodes that are attached to the skin at appropriate placements. These skin electrodes are self-adhesive and are reusable for 14 days. They are to be attached by the patient himself in the morning and removed each evening or as desired at locations that the patient has been taught to remember. The stimulator unit weighs 7.6 ounces (Figure 52.2), excluding a battery pack of six AA 1.5 V rechargeable alkaline (or eight rechargeable NiMH) batteries to allow at least 60 min of standing or walking [27]. The system is shown in Figures 52.3 and 52.4.

The same microchip also controls optic isolation chips to allow using a single power amplifier for all channels. This allows the Parastep to employ six stimulation channels (12 electrodes) rather than the

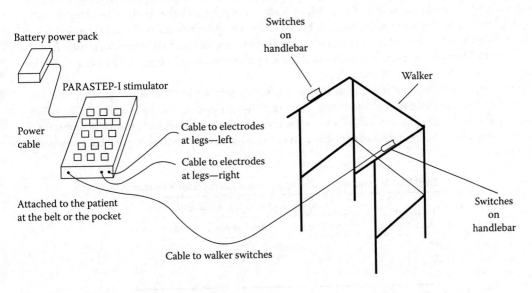

FIGURE 52.3 Parastep system with battery pack and walker.

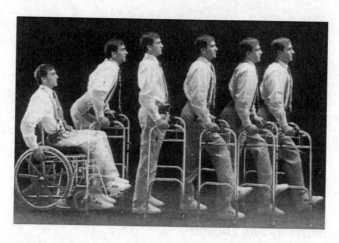

FIGURE 52.4 Parastep system in use during walk by paraplegic patient.

usual four stimulation channels and to integrate them to reduce the system's weight, while facilitating full patient control of all channels. Furthermore, it facilitates considerable battery power savings. The additional two stimulation channels (at the paraspinals for trunk stability) play a major role in enhancing standing time, ambulation distances, and speeds as compared with four-channel systems.

52.2.2.1 Pulse Width and Pulse Repetition Rate (Frequency)

Pulse durations (widths) are set to be of 120–150 μs [27]. Higher durations are undesirable and unnecessary. Higher pulse width speeds up the rate of muscle fatigue and therefore reduces the maximal ambulation distance (see Table 52.1) and the maximal time a patient can stand or walk via FES. It also sends into the body more electrical charge than is needed and requires higher battery power and hence higher battery weight.

The interpulse repetition rate (frequency) is set higher than the average pulse rate in the able-bodied individual, but is still kept as low as possible (22–24 pulses/s) to reduce the rate of fatigue (see Table 52.1). It is determined by considerations of fatigue, tetanization, and force (note that while standing or walking, the body weight dampens vibrations considerably). At even lower frequencies, muscle vibrations are observed that are no more dampened and that may affect the patient's balance when standing or walking. Higher frequencies also imply that a higher electrical charge enters the body and requires higher battery power and heavier batteries. Furthermore, higher pulse rates speed up the rate of muscle fatigue to reduce the duration and range of ambulation. Both pulse widths and rates, while constant, can be adjusted if necessary (see Figure 52.5).

Therefore, a combination of a short pulse duration, low stimulation levels, and low pulse rate is essential to reduce muscle fatigue, thus extending walking distance (walking time) per walk [5]. The consequences of lower battery power needs, of lower system weight, and of the resultant effect on compactness are of course also significant for a patient-borne system and for user friendliness, especially, in a body-borne system.

TABLE 52.1 Stimulation Frequency versus Rate of Muscle Fatigue

Stimulation Frequency (Hz)	% Drop in Isometric Moment at Ankle Joint		
	After 10 min	After 20 min	After 30 min
20	<2	<2	3
30	4	14	40
50	17	53	71

Pulse duration: 300 μs throughout.

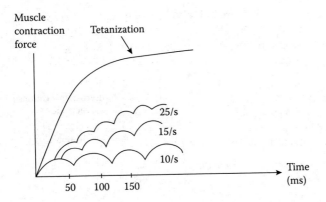

FIGURE 52.5   Muscle contraction force versus stimulation rate and time.

52.2.2.2 Menus for Pulse Shaping and Synchronization

Pulse-amplitude shaping is a major aspect of the pulse shaping algorithm and it is the subject of four different menus within that algorithm. The menus are patient selectable, through touch of finger-touch switches located on the Parastep's walker or on the Parastep's elbow-support canes. The menus are those for standing up, for right step, for left step, and for sitting down (see Figure 52.6). Pulse-amplitude shaping is dynamic and varies for each of the six stimulation channels and as per each menu, as does the distribution of output signal to each output channel [5,11]. The time variation of the pulse amplitudes in each menu and per each channel, as in Figure 52.6, is therefore unique and is based on considerations of the executions of the given menu's function (say, taking a right step) and of doing so safely, efficiently, and smoothly.

52.2.2.3 Stimulation Sites

The stimulation electrodes are self-adhesive electrodes (12 in total), placed at six stimulation sites [27], two electrodes per site, as follows: two over the right quadriceps and two over the left quadriceps, to stimulate knee extension; two over the common peroneal nerve right and left (to activate dorsi-flexion and to elicit a hip flexion reflex via sensory neural feedback). Finally, two electrodes are placed over the right paraspinals at the right and two at the left, for upper-trunk stability in patients with lesions at T7 or higher (to be placed approximately 1 in. below the level of start of sensation, but not too close to the heart). Patients with spinal cord injury (SCI) lesions at lower levels will have electrodes placed over the

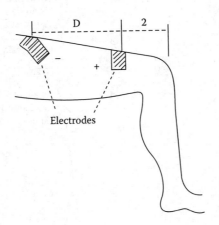

FIGURE 52.6   Placement of quadriceps stimulation electrodes (right leg, lateral side view).

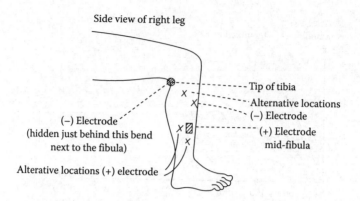

FIGURE 52.7 Placement of peroneal nerve electrodes (to elicit step via hip flexion reflex).

gluteus medius and maximus for improved stability, whereas patients with lesions at T-1 0 or lower usually do not require paraspinal stimulation at all (Figures 52.6 through 52.8). We comment that improved trunk stability affects not just patient safety but also helps to reduce fatigue, thus improving ambulation performance and appearance (which is not just an esthetic aspect but also a psychological one).

As shown in Figure 52.8, alternatives to the peroneal nerve placements are possible in some cases (see Chapter 7 of Reference 5). These alternatives involve other branches of the sciatic nerve, which trigger the hip flexion reflex.

The number of channels (of electrode pairs) to be used is a matter of trade-off. Obviously, with more channels, more muscle groups (at below the SCI lesion) can contract. However, when increasing the

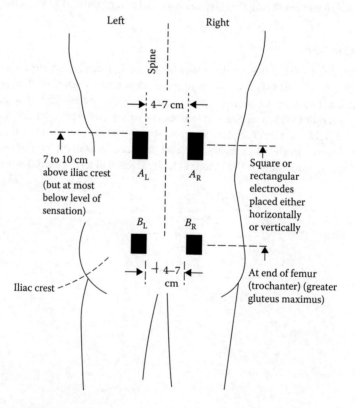

FIGURE 52.8 Paraspinal electrodes placement (patient's back).

number of channels, say from six to eight, the patient must place (every morning) 16 electrodes instead of 12 and for a paraplegic patient this involves a lot of additional effort and time. Furthermore, the six channels that are stimulated by the Parastep system, as discussed above, are the ones that are the easiest to be reached by the user and the ones where there is the greatest tolerance in terms of error in the placement's localization, while additional sites will require more care in exact placement. It is our experience that with more than six channels, most patients will soon stop using the system. Hence, human factor considerations imply to limit the system to the most important functions (channels) as far as performance is concerned. The resulting performance, as discussed later in this chapter (Section 52.5), appears to justify this choice and to result in a rather smooth walk that can be viewed in a 15-min movie of a walk of a complete thoracic-level paraplegic using the Parastep system (see http://www.ece. uic.edu/~graupe).

52.2.2.4 Sequencing-Control Menus for Stimulation Signals

Pulse-amplitude shaping is a major aspect of the pulse-shaping algorithm and it is the subject of four different menus within that algorithm. The menus are patient selectable, through touch of finger-touch switches located on the Parastep's walker or on the Parastep's elbow-support canes. The menus are those for standing up, for right step, for left step, and for sitting down (see Figure 52.9). Pulse-amplitude shaping is dynamic and varies for each of the six stimulation channels and per each menu, as does the distribution of output signal to each output channel [6,27]. The time variation of the pulse amplitudes in each menu and per each channel, as in Figure 52.9, is therefore unique and is based on considerations of the executions of the given menu's function (say, taking a right step), and of doing so safely, efficiently, and smoothly.

The stimulation signals are sequenced at the system's microcomputer chip as in Figure 52.9, where the envelope patterns of the stimulation impulses (and not the individual pulses) are illustrated. This pattern is automatically sequenced by the stimulator's computer to give a ramp increase of impulse levels for stand-up to be followed by a lower constant level while the patient is standing, both being applied to the right and left quadriceps electrodes and to the right and left paraspinal/gluteal electrodes. When a left step menu is selected, either manually or through above-lesion (chest-level) EMG (as described later), then the stimulation is stopped at the left quadriceps and paraspinals/gluteus while at the same time the common peroneal nerve is being stimulated to elicit a step. This lasts for a fixed duration of

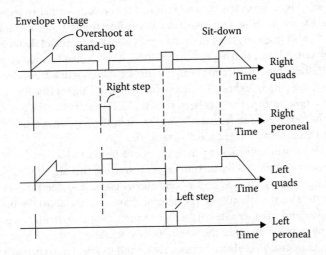

FIGURE 52.9 Synchronization scheme of envelopes of stimulation signals at various channels. (*Note:* Broken vertical lines divide between the four Parastep menus. Paraspinal signal envelopes correspond in shape to quadriceps channels except for peaks.)

$T = 0.4$–1.0 s, as is preselected for the convenience of the patient. At the end of this period T, the stimulation to the left common peroneal stops and the left quadriceps and left paraspinals/gluteus are stimulated. However, during the step period, the level of stimulation at the right quadriceps is automatically increased by the sequencing program to compensate for the fact that the full body weight is borne by the right leg over that period. If a right step is selected, then the same menu is employed, with a reversal of roles of right and left. When a sit-down menu is selected, the sequencing program first triggers an audible and a visual warning to allow the patient to abort the sit-down if he is not ready to sit and to allow some time for the patient to reach a chair and to comfortably sit down. Also, at that time, the stimulation to the quadriceps is increased to compensate for possible weakening of the quadriceps that may have caused the patient to decide to sit.

The microchip also controls optic isolation chips to allow using a single power amplifier for all channels. This allows the Parastep to employ six rather than the usual four stimulation channels and to integrate them to reduce system weight, while facilitating full patient control of all channels. Furthermore, it facilitates considerable further battery power savings. The additional two stimulation channels (at the paraspinals, for trunk stability) play a major role in enhancing standing time, ambulation distances, and speeds as compared to four-channel systems.

The control of the FES is performed by the stimulation signal's sequencing program of the Parastep's microcomputer, while the selection of menus of that program is performed either manually (as in the Parastep commercial system) or via an above-lesion EMG-control algorithm for menu selection [5,7,29].

52.2.2.5 Finger-Touch Menu Selection

Menu-selection finger-touch switches [27,29] are located on the walker's handlebars for easy finger reach while normally holding the walker (or cane). They require only a light single and quick (short) finger touch without changing the hand position on the bars. The adaptation and learning of balancing and of menu selection (only two menus during walking; of right and of left step, activated at the right or the left handlebar) is very easy and fast. Only finger-touch selection is available in the commercial Parastep system.

52.2.2.6 Above-Lesion EMG-Controlled Menu Selection

While the commercial Parastep system employs only manual touch buttons for menu selection, the laboratory Parastep system, which was tested on 14 patients at Michael Reese Hospital, Chicago, Illinois, also allowed for above-lesion surface-EMG (electromyographic) menu selection with good results [7,27,29]. However, menu-selection EMG control was not incorporated in the commercial system (and is not covered by its FDA approval), since training is far lengthier and requires the donning of four more electrodes (for EMG pickup). This was felt to greatly limit the number of users. We comment that the EMG electrode placement is much more critical than that of placing the stimulation electrodes themselves.

The above-lesion EMG-based menu selections employ surface-EMG signals from electrodes placed at above-lesion locations on the patient's chest. The thus-obtained EMG signal (see Figure 52.8) serves to map a pattern of upper-trunk posture that has been shown [5,7,27] to predict the intended body function, corresponding to the four menus above (stand, left step, right step, and sit menus), with an accuracy of better than 99.8%. In this case, no finger controls are needed.

We emphasize that the relevant information from the above-lesion EMG signal is *not* based on the EMG level (power) but on the whole stochastic time-series pattern of that signal [27,29]. Therefore, the patient does not have to produce a specific upper-body above-lesion (shoulder) movement to select a particular menu. The patient's natural walk and the natural changes in the above-lesion muscles, as are needed to move the walker and to otherwise balance when intending a particular step (or to stand up or to sit down), causes dynamic changes in the whole EMG stochastic pattern. These pattern changes are then recognized in the microchip's algorithm as a command to select a particular menu (from the menus above). In this way, the above-lesion EMG control differs from others that require unnatural pulling of shoulders or of arms to produce an EMG-based command. Such intentional and unnatural movements divert the patient's concentration and yield an unnatural walk.

The mapping of the upper-trunk posture considers the above-lesion EMG signal, denoted as $y(k)$, to satisfy a pure autoregressive (AR) time-series model [7,29]:

$$y(k) = a(1)y(k-1) + a(2)y(k-2) + \cdots + a(n)y(k-n) + w(k) \qquad (52.4)$$

where k is discrete time, such that $k = n+1, n+2, n+3, \ldots$, and $w(k)$ denotes a discrete white-noise process.

We comment that both under finger-touch control (menu selection) and under EMG menu selection, the direction of step (and hence, of a walk) is determined by the shoulder movement of the patient as naturally performed when intuitively moving the walker to any desired direction.

52.2.2.7 Stimulation Signal's Level Control

The stimulation level is adjusted at the Parastep's microcomputer chip, in accordance to either the patient's single finger-touch menu switching command or t in response to an above-lesion EMG signal from the patent's chest that is interpreted in the same microchip.

52.2.2.8 Finger-Touch Force Level Control

The degree of the recruitment of motor neurons determines the contraction force exerted by the muscle fibers that are associated with these neurons [27,29]. The degree of recruitment is, in turn, dependent on the level of the stimulation signal when the motor neurons are triggered by FES stimuli. In the commercial Parastep, the stimulation level is controlled by the touch buttons at the left- and right-hand sides of the walker. Each finger touch raises the level by a single increment. Out of the 10 possible level increments that are color marked, most patunts use one of the three lowest levels to start their walk, to minimize the rate of fatigue. During a half-hour walk, a patient will usually have to adjust the FES level only 2–3 times by a single discrete increment. The range of levels can be factory-set to suit special needs (patients).

52.2.2.9 Below-Lesion Response-EMG FES Level Control

Alternatively, in the Parastep lab system tried at Michael Reese Hospital, a below-lesion surface-EMG stimulation-level control, denoted as response-EMG-level control, was successfully tested on some patients [27,29].

Obviously, in complete upper-motor-neuron paraplegics (thoracic-level SCI patients), no EMG occurs below the level of the lesion, since the lower-extremity neurons do not fire. However, under FES, APs arise at the stimulated motor neurons. These produce APs similar to those in nonimpaired situations. Furthermore, since any stimulation electrode-pair activates many hundreds of motor neurons simultaneously, all resultant APs are fully synchronized and appear as one very strong AP due to this combined and synchronized firing (see Figure 52.1). This is in contrast to the surface-EMG above the lesion, which results from unsynchronized firing of hundreds of neurons. Furthermore, the resulting response-EMG increases with the degree of recruitment. It can thus serve to detect the progression of fatigue and serve to adjust the stimulation levels accordingly. The commercial system uses only finger-touch level control, since the reliability in the calibration of relations between response-EMG level (and shape) against desired FES stimuli strength (to counter the fatigue) is still not sufficiently reliable. It is also not covered by the Parastep's FDA approval. However, when using optoisolators, the stimulation electrodes can simultaneously serve as response-EMG electrodes. This is due to the very short duration of the Parastep's stimulus in relation to the duration of a single AP (which is given by the stimulation of low pulse rate used by the Parastep system).

52.2.2.10 Peripheral Equipment

The Parastep FES system uses a walker (see Figures 52.3 and 52.4), or in a few cases, a pair of elbow-support (Canadian) canes [27,29]. Walkers are employed in all other FES ambulation systems, invasive or not. Walkers (or elbow-support canes) serve mainly for balance. Walkers carry (in the Parastep system) only 5% or less of body weight in trained FES users during standing and are crucial during the standing-up mode. Their balancing role is due to the fact that complete SCI paraplegics have no sensation (in addition to having no motor functions below their lesion). Hence, indirect sensation coming through their arms and hands, while holding the walker's handlebars, lets the users sense the ground to provide a certain psychological security. It thus allows the users to balance their body by slight shoulder and arm movements to balance better during standing and walking. The users are able to easily and rather naturally change the direction of walking, at will, through shoulder positioning by which they turn their steps. One major function of the walker is during the stand-up phase from a seated position. The patient then gets up with the arms leaning on the walker. All these reasons indicate the crucial role of walkers toward achieving independent standing and walking.

The Parastep system is described in further detail in Graupe and Kohn [27,28].

52.3 Patient Admissibility, Contraindications, and Training

52.3.1 Patient Admissibility Criteria

The cardiovascular status of the patients must be good. Hence, the criteria for a patient to be admitted to train and to use the Parastep standing/ambulation system are as follows [7,27,29]:

1. The patient must be in good general health and with a complete traumatic spinal cord lesion at levels no higher than C-7 and no lower than T-12.
2. Intact lower motor units (lumbar level L-1 and below).
3. Must have a complete/near-complete SCI lesion that does not allow the patient to stretch his/her knees for standing up and where the patient has no substantial sensation (pain) of the stimuli.
4. Surgery/wound following SCI must have healed, as determined by the surgeon.
5. Stable ortho-neuro-metabolic systems.
6. No recent history of long bone stress fractures, osteoporosis, or severe hip or knee joint disease. A bone density test is advisable in case of women over 40 years of age or patients who are many years (10 or more) beyond the date of injury. The author had a patient 40 years postinjury, who had no problem and was accepted to the FES ambulation program.
7. No history of cardiac or respiratory problems.
8. Adequate trunk stability so that once quadriceps are stimulated, the patient can hold his upper trunk upright while supporting himself with a walker.
9. The patient demonstrates appropriate muscle contractions in response to stimulation (absence of such response usually implies some lesions below T-12).
10. Standing tolerance: The patient has adequate fatigue tolerance to practice and perform standing and walking functions after initial training.
11. Balance and trunk control (at least when paraspinals are stimulated).
12. The patient must have adequate hand and finger control or VOICE control to manipulate the system controls. Future systems may circumvent the need for finger control via speech recognition to allow patients lacking hand/finger control to use the system.
13. Sufficient upper body and arm strength to lift oneself up to the walker for a second or two without stimulation and to grasp the chair when stimulation is stopped for any reason.
14. No severe scoliosis.
15. No irreversible contractures.
16. No morbid obesity.
17. The patient is not pregnant.
18. Motivation: The patient demonstrates and expresses appropriate desire and commitment to the training program.

Also, the interference of the stimulation signal with an electronic cardiac pacemaker must be avoided.

52.3.2 Contraindications

Once the admission criteria of Section 52.3.1 are followed, no contraindications are known to the author from his personal observations or training experience with approximately 100 patients. Also, none are known to have been reported in the literature.

52.3.3 Patient Training

The author's experience of over 23 years of working with patients and of observing Parastep training programs outside his own training program in the use of the Parastep FES system for standing indicates that once the patient satisfies the criteria as above, the patient is able to stand and to ambulate, if trained properly. Distances and speed vary widely and even distances (and speeds) well below the averages mentioned in this chapter may be a major achievement for some patients, depending on their general health, level of lesion, age, and any other limitations they may have. The author had trained a 62-year-old T-3/T-4 complete paraplegic patient (gunshot wounds) who was in the wheelchair for 40 years and never been stimulated. This patient stood up in his first session and took 12 steps in his third 1-h session. Motivation is the definite key factor and this also implies family/friends' and (and physician's) encouragement and support. Family/friends' support is crucial. This should not just be verbal, but also in terms of helping the candidate stand/walk at home after or between training sessions by walking next to him/her to be able to prevent the patient from a possible fall, and moving (sharp) obstacles out of the way. The patient should have at least one strong armchair (possibly a metal chair) with arm rests at an adequate height for the patient to be able to get up and sit down independently of the walker. Some patients do initially need help in placing the lower paraspinal or gluteus electrodes on the skin. It is very advisable that a family member or friend should observe at least part of one training session. The skin electrodes need be replaced once every 2 weeks (or less, if contact to skin is inadequate). Bad electrodes or broken electrode connectors are the main reasons for stimulation failure.

Training programs vary widely and so do their respective results. This author is familiar with Parastep training programs that involve 5–6 h a day of supervised training for 5 or 10 consecutive days, of Parastep programs of one hourly session every week or every 2 weeks for over 1 year, of Parastep programs of three 1-h sessions a week for 11 weeks (Klose et al. [31], the University of Miami program), and of Parastep programs of 2 h per day, 5 days a week for over 4 months (Cerrel-Bazo et al. [32], the Vicenza program, Italy). Since all these programs use the same FES system (the Parastep system), only the performance results shed a light on their efficiency. However, they differ widely in cost and in the required commitment of time by the patient. Therefore, the decision on which kind of program to attend is usually not a matter of choice.

Regardless of the training program, it is of utmost importance that the patient complements each supervised training session with after-hour home exercise of at least 15 min (many programs require much more).

In almost all training programs, training starts with reconditioning and strengthening of the muscles involved and also of arm muscles. First, the quadriceps muscles, which are those that are the most involved in stand-up and in standing require strengthening. Treadmill exercises in walking are often used. In many programs, monitoring of heart rate and of blood pressure is done during treadmill training. Parallel-bar standing and walking are sometimes used at the initial stages, during a muscle-strengthening phase. But parallel-bar exercise does not help in learning to rely on and to balance oneself with the walker and may therefore be counterproductive. Muscle strengthening while seated is a very major part of the home exercise throughout training, but takes place only in the first or second supervised sessions. It is psychologically most important to make a patient stand up, even for 20–30 s (as long as it is safe) even in the first session. This and taking of the first few steps (even 2 or 3) early on are great motivators. Hence, the first step should be taken after the patient can stand safely (with a walker) for about 3 min. Eventually, training and muscle strengthening should aim at standing for 10 min or more and walking for as long as is possible. These sessions should start with treadmill standing and walking. At the last stages of training, patients should be taught to fall, by sudden power shutdown (they will learn to avoid an actual fall through proper use of walker). They will also learn to lift themselves up from the ground with no help, to walk on rough ground, and on reasonable slopes. They will train in getting in and out of a car unaided. The most advanced T-9 to T-12 patients can then train on using elbow-support cane.

Continuous walking after the end of training on a near-daily basis for at least 45 min a day (not necessarily in one session per day) is essential for progress and for improved performance.

The first training session must involve getting sufficient quadriceps contraction to lift each leg while the patient is in a seated position. Psychologically and motivationally, it is desired that the patient gets up (to a walker, not to parallel bars) in the first or second session. However, this should not defer rigorous muscle strengthening in future sessions (actually, until the end of the training program). For best results, daily (5 days/week) training of 1–2 h/day, followed by home exercises, yields far better outcomes at the end of training than a 3 h/week program and even more, if the whole training program is condensed over only 1–2 weeks. Still, whatever the training program, if after the completion of training, the patient continues to walk daily for 30–45 min, he will continue improving and his performance will equal the best program (of course, considering his individual status, lesion level, age, and general health).

Home exercising while undergoing training should be done when the patient stimulates while seated—except when, later in training (and with the trainer's explicit permission), the patient is permitted to take a walker home and stands/takes steps *while* an able-bodied person is close at hand.

52.4 Walking Performance and Medical and Psychological Benefits Evaluation Results

52.4.1 Walking Performance Data

Walking distances covered by Parastep users vary with the individual user's level of injury, training, learned skills, and physical condition. Distance walked will vary and increase with practice and training. Individual goals are established for each user by the physical therapist. Studies conducted in different clinical settings reported distances walked by individual users ranging from a few feet to over a mile at a time, with the average distance being around 1450 ft (450 m/walk) for fully trained patients in certain training programs [32,33].

Performance is influenced by the training program, but mostly by how rigorously the patient continues to actively stand and walk with the FES system after the end of training. Improvements in performance will be very noticeable 1 or 2 years after the end of formal training. Approximately 5% of the Parastep users known to the author (from several U.S. training programs) can ambulate 1 mile per walk on occasions (usually 1 year or more after the end of formal training). The author expects this to be the case too for the Vicenza (Italy) training program.

The Miami Project to Cure Paralysis of the University of Miami reports average ambulation distances for Parastep users of 115 m/walk at a mean pace of 5 m/min at the end of the training program of 33 sessions over 11 weeks [31]. For the Parastep training program of daily sessions over 4 months at the Centro di Rehabilitazione di Villa Margherita in Argugnano, Vicenza, Italy, an average distance of 444 m per walk was reported, at a mean speed of 14.5 m/min and with mean daily walk time of 90 min [32]. See also Chaplin [33]. These performance differences are very significant.

Still, there is no reason to assume that persistent FES users in the 11-week program cannot do as well as those in the 4-month program at 1 year after the end of training. However, continuous use may be higher for patients whose performance at the end of training is considerably higher. This is the author's experience in his own (once weekly over 1-year program). The Vicenza program reports zero dropout

TABLE 52.2 Ambulation Performance Results (Parastep Users)

	Average Distance	
Average Speed	m/Walk	m/min
Approximately 85 sessions daily over 4 months; Vicenza [32]	444.3	14.5
32 sessions; 3/week, 12 weeks; University of Miami [31]	115	5.0

14–39 months after the end of training [32]. The author is not aware of other training programs with similar results.

We comment that the averages given are for patients whose SCI lesion levels are more or less evenly distributed between T-1 and T-12. Usually, the performance is better if the LSI lesion is lower (toward T-12). However, motivation and persistence often make up for the level of lesion. Still, patients who for various medical or age reasons cannot walk more than 10 m (per walk) at the end of training should still continue exercising since the benefits of the FES exercise are more than just a matter of distance or speed, as is discussed later. Kralj et al. [15] give the general utilization statistics on the Ljubljana FES system for performance tests carried out by its developers.

However, these do not include performance data or medical or psychological patient evaluation on that system. The data given here on the Parastep system are from independent centers (University of Miami Medical School and the Vicenza Rehabilitation Center, Italy) that are not connected with the system's manufacturers or its developers.

Table 52.2 provides further ambulation performance data.

A 14-min video of complete thoracic-level paraplegic patients, while walking with the Parastep system, is shown in www.ece.uic.edu/~graupe.

52.4.2 Evaluation Results on Medical Benefits of Walking with the Parastep System

The benefits of using the Parastep system go well beyond the benefits in the ability to walk, as discussed in Section 52.4.1. Medical and psychological evaluations that were published on Parastep users show several medical and psychological benefits to walking with the Parastep. These are discussed in this and in the next section. Most important medically is the major improvement in circulation at below the level of the SCI lesion. We discuss the medical and physiological evaluation results here, while the psychological evaluation outcomes are summarized in Section 52.4.3.

1. *Lower-extremity blood flow:* A study performed as a part of the Miami Project, to Cure Paralysis of the Departments of Neurological Surgery and of Orthopedics and Rehabilitation of the University of Miami, authored by Nash et al. [34] and involving 12 Parastep users, reports an average increase of lower-extremity blood inflow volume f 56% (from 417 to 650 mL/min) after 12 weeks (32 sessions) of Parastep training. Dr. Cerrel-Bazo reported (verbally) to this author similar improvements (at the Vicenza program in Italy). It is noted that, after paralysis due to thoracic-level SCI, blood flow to the lower extremities decreases considerably, with detrimental subsequent effects on kidney function and eventual cardiovascular effects. Hence, such an improvement is of major significance.

2. *Other cardiovascular effects:* The above 12-patient study at the Miami Project of the University of Miami [34] has shown that the average resting heartbeat of Parastep users decreased from 70.1 (prior to FES training) to 63.2 (posttraining). Also, the Common Femoral Artery cross-sectional area increased by 50%, from 0.36 cm^2 (pretraining) to 0.48 cm^2 (post-FES training).

3. *Physiological responses to peak arm ergometry:* A study on physiological responses by 15 Parastep users [27] to peak-arm ergometry exercises has shown that the average time to fatigue has improved from 15.3 min prestart of FES training to 19.2 min after 33 sessions of training. Also, the peak workload increased from 48.1 to 60 W. Oxygen uptake at peak-arm ergometry increased from 20.02 mL/kg/min pretraining to 23.01 mL/kg/min posttraining, while the respiratory exchange ratio dropped from 1.26 pretraining to 1.18 posttraining, to indicate an improvement in all these parameters. The patients (12 men, 3 women) ranged in age from 21 to 45 years, in years from injury from 0.7 to 8.8, and in body weight from 52.6 to 83.5 kg.

4. *Muscle mass:* A significant increase (10–22%) in circumference was measured on Parastep users after 3–6 months of training at the University of Illinois/Michael Reese Hospital training program in Chicago [5].

5. *Spasticity:* Spasticity is common to all SCI patients with upper-motor lesions. In the authors experience in 19 years of observing well over 100 patients training with or using the Parastep system, almost all patients who complained of spasticity commented on either considerable or some improvement in spasticity. This improvement was usually observed after the first 2–3 training sessions. Usually, the higher the degree of spasticity, the greater was the improvement that was reported. This improvement was often reported as one of the reasons for participating in the FES program. The improvement in spasticity is important with regard to the detrimental effect of medications (Baclofen, Valium, Lioresal) on alertness and fatigue as medication doses can then be reduced in many cases [5].

6. *Bone density:* Practically all paraplegics suffer from reduced bone density. This happens right after injury and may be aggravated when the patient does not put weight on the legs. One of the Parastep patients in the author's program recorded a 50% bone density prior to training (but no bone injuries) with no improvement after 1 year though he continued to walk and reached 1 mile/walk. The only study published till now (Needham-Shropshire et al. [36]) does not show any improvement in bone density due to FES ambulation. However, this study refers to the end of 11 weeks of training. No study exists on patients who have consistently walked via FES for several years.

7. *Pressure ulcers (decubitus ulcers):* Almost all paraplegics suffer from decubitus ulcers. However, all but one patient at the author's FES program (at Michel Reese Hospital, Chicago) had no occurrence of a new ulcer while regularly using FES. Improved blood circulation at below the lesion is most likely the cause for this [27]. The exception was due to a cut from a sharp object.

The medical and physiological evaluation data are summarized in Table 52.3.

TABLE 52.3 Medical and Physiological Evaluation Data (Parastep Users)

	Pre-FES Training (Average)	Post-FES Training (Average)	
Lower-extremity blood flow	417 mL/min	650 mL/min (improvement)	12 patient data/University of Miami [34]
Heart rate	70.1	63.2 (improvement)	12 patients/Miami [34]
Time to fatigue (at peak-arm ergometry test)	15.3 min	19.2 min (improvement)	15 patients/Miami [35]
Peak workload heart rate (peak-arm ergometry test)	188.5	183.1 (improvement)	15 patients/Miami [35]
Oxygen uptake (peak-arm ergometry test)	20 mL/kg/min	23 mL/kg/min (improvement)	15 patients/Miami [35]
Spasticity		Usually improvement, especially for very spastic pretraining	Michael Reese Hospital, Chicago [6,27,29]
		Training, where no significant change was reported	

TABLE 52.4 Psychological Evaluation Results: Parastep Users

	Pre-FES Training (Average)	Post-FES Training (Average)	
Physical self-concept (TSCS scores)	43.2 TSCS	52 TSCS (improvement)	15 patients/Miami [37]
Depression scores (BDI scores)	8.8 BDI	5.4 BDI (improvement)	15 patient data [37]

52.4.3 Psychological Outcome Evaluation Results

1. *Psychological evaluation results—self-concept scores:* A study on 14 Parastep users after 11 weeks of training at the Miami program [37] concerning physical self-concept using the Tennessee Self-Concept Scale (TSCS), compares TSCS scores before the beginning of Parastep training against the score at the end of the 11-week program. It shows that the average TSCS score improved in a statistically significant manner from 44.3 to 52.0. Furthermore, all patients with a score below 50 prior to FES training have improved, whereas no patient with an initial score above 50 dropped to below 50.

2. *Psychological observations—depression scores:* The same study [37] as in Section 52.4.3 reports on comparing Beck depression inventory (BDI) scores for measuring depression before and after 11 weeks of Parastep training. BDI scores of below 9 refer to no depression and scores below 18 to mild depression, whereas scores from 18 to 29 point to moderate depression. The results of the study show that all five patients who were initially at the mild or moderate depression score levels (one was initially even beyond the moderate range) did improve significantly. The patient who was initially beyond the moderate depression range (31 BDI score) improved to 24 (mild depression range). One of the two patients, who were initially in the moderate range, improved to the low-mild range and the other to the no-depression range. All patients who were initially in the low-depression range stayed in that range.

The psychological evaluation results, as in the present section, are summarized in Table 52.4.

52.5 Regulatory Status

The Parastep-I functional neuromuscular (electrical) system (referred to throughout this chapter as the Parastep system) for standing and for ambulation by thoracic-level paraplegics received FDA approval on April 20, 1994 [8]. It was the first and is still the only noninvasive FES ambulation system to have received FDA approval. Furthermore, effective April 1, 2003, the Centers for Medicare and Medicaid Services (CMS) made a National Coverage Determination extending coverage to the Parastep-I system for qualifying Medicare beneficiaries. Specific healthcare common procedure coding system (HCPCS) codes have been assigned to cover costs associated with both the acquisition of the Parastep-I equipment [9] and for the physical therapy training services Parastep-I [10]. Medicare covers approximately 80% of equipment acquisition costs. Following the CMS example, most major medical insurers in the United States have already amended their policies to cover the Parastep system. The Parastep's manufacturer, Sigmedics, Inc. of Fairborn, Ohio, physical therapy training services has set up its own Patient Case Management Department for the purpose of facilitating the insurance reimbursement process.

52.6 Concluding Comments

This chapter discusses the Parastep system, which is the first and still the only FDA-approved transcutaneous (noninvasive) FES system for ambulation by complete or near-complete thoracic-level paraplegics. It describes what this system can already do for the thoracic-level (complete) paraplegic patient in noninvasive FES. It gives concrete data from many studies on how that system performs. It also discusses its design, operation, admission criteria, contraindications, and training.

We thus conclude that a totally noninvasive FES for independent standing and mobility is already a reality for complete upper-motor-neuron thoracic-level traumatic paraplegics. Furthermore, it is commercially available and it received (2003) approval for reimbursement by the CMS that regulates Medicare and Medicaid reimbursements policies in the United States and subsequently, by practically all medical insurance companies in the United States. Training programs for that system exist in many hospitals and rehabilitation centers. As was discussed above, upon completion of 4 months of daily training, the ambulation distances for the Parastep system were reported to average 444 [32] or 115 m/walk in a 33-session 11-week program [31]. Medical benefits have been documented, in terms of greatly increased blood flow to the lower extremities [34], reduced spasticity [29], reduced incidence of decubiti [27], increased thigh circumference [27], and of psychological benefits (improved self-concept and depression scores) [37].

However, even 10 years after the FDA approval of such a noninvasive FES system and 2 years after the reimbursement was approved by Medicare, Medicaid, and by most insurers, there is still great ignorance in the paraplegics community about the availability of such a system and of its performance and benefits. In Reference 38, a statement by a patient is quoted (made in a recent symposium of prospective FES users, funded by the Whitaker Foundation), that "in 3 to 4 different rehabilitation facilities and (having) talked to over 200 patients…none of them ever mentioned FES." These indicate ignorance, regarding the role of the FES in paraplegia, among physicians involved in caring for paraplegics, and among the (physical and occupational) therapists and other related staff.

The consensus of the symposium above (and which agrees with what this author repeatedly hears from patients) was that desire to stand upright independently and to ambulate even short distances is the prime desire of paraplegics but long-term compliance and long-term use of FES is a problem. However, the circulatory benefits and the other medical and psychological benefits should play an important role, for patients, for physicians, and for insurance companies involved.

All this does not detract in any way from the urgent need to repair the spinal cord through regeneration. Neither the Parastep nor any other FES approach can substitute for this, since FES does not heal. It is an aid, just like eyeglasses or a hearing aid. It is hoped that regeneration will be a reality for human SCI patients. In the meantime, a realistic aid does exists that is already FDA-approved and reimbursable. It can always be and will be improved, but its performance even now is usually pretty good.

References

1. Galvani, L. 1791, *Commentary on the Effect of Electricity on Muscular Motion*, Translated by R.M. Green 1953, Elizabeth Licht Publishing Co., Cambridge, MA.
2. Lieberson, W.T., Holmquest, H.J., Scott, D., and Dow, H. 1961, Functional electrotherapy stimulation of the swing phase of the gait in hemiplegic patients, *Arch. Phys. Med. Rehabil.*, 42: 101–105.
3. Kantrowitz, A. 1960, *A Report of the Maimonides Hospital*, Brooklyn, NY, pp. 4–5.
4. Kralj, A., Bajd, T., and Turk, R. 1980, Electrical stimulation providing functional use of paraplegic patients muscles, *Med. Prog. Technol.*, 7: 3.
5. Graupe, D., Kralj, A., and Kohn, K.H. 1982, Computerized signature discrimination of above-lesion EMG for stimulating peripheral nerves of complete paraplegics, *Proceedings of the IFAC Symposium Prosthetics Control*, Columbus, OH, March.
6. Graupe, D., Kohn, K.H., Basseas, S., and Naccarato, E. 1983, EMG-controlled electrical stimulation, *Proceedings of IEEE Frontiers of Eng. & Comp. in Health Care*, Columbus, OH.
7. Graupe, D., Kohn, K.H., Basseas, S., and Naccarato, E. 1984, Electromyographic control of functional electric stimulation in selected paraplegics, *Orthopedks*, 7: 1134–1138; Graupe, D. 1989, EMG pattern analysis for patient-responsive control of FES in paraplegics, *IEEE Trans. Biomed. Eng.*, 36: 711–719.

8. FDA approval P900038 1994, http://www.fda.gov/cdrh/pma94.html, April 20.

9. Centers for Medicare and Medicaid Services (CMS), Code K0600 (Parastep-I equipment acquisition), http://www.cms.hhs.gov/coverage, 2003.

10. Centers for Medicare and Medicaid Centers (CMS), Code 97116 (physical training services with Parastep-I), http://www.cms.hhs.gov/coverage, 2003.

11. Marsolais, E.B. and Kobetic, R. 1983, Functional walking in paralyzed patients by means of electrical stimulation, *Clin. Orthop.*, **175**: 30–36.

12. Marsolais, E.B. and Kobetic, R. 1986, Implantation techniques and experience with percutaneous intramuscular electrodes in the lower extremities, *J. Rehabil. Res. Dev.*, **23**(3): 1–8.

13. Holle, J., Frey, M., Gruber, H., Kern, H., Stoehr, H., and Thoma, H. 1984, Functional electrostimulation of paraplegics, experimental investigations and first—clinical experience—with an implantable stimulation device, *Orthopedks*, **7**: 1145–1155.

14. Davis, R., Kuzma, J., Patrick, J., Heller, J.W., McKendry, J., Eckhouse, R., and Emmons, S.E. 1992, Nucleus FES-22 stimulator for motor function in a paraplegic subject, *Proceedings of the RESNA International Conference*, June 6–11.

15. Kralj, A. and Bajd, T. 1989, *Functional Electrical Stimulation: Standing and Walking After Spinal Cord Injury*, CRC Press, Boca Raton, FL.

16. Kralj, A., Turk, R., Bajd, T., Stafancic, M., Sarvin, R., Benko, H., and Obreza, P. 1993, FES utilization statistics for 94 patients, *Proceedings of the Ljubljana FES Conference*, Ljubljana, Slovenia, pp. 79–81.

17. Popovic, D. 1986, Control methodology for gait restoration, *Proceedings of the 8th Annual Conference of IEEE Engineering in Medical and Biological Society*, Dallas-Ft. Worth, TX, pp. 675–678.

18. Mayagoitia, R.E., Phillips, G.F., and Martinez, L.M. 1993, Mexican programmable eight channel surface stimulator, *Proceedings of the Ljubljana FES Conference*, Ljubljana, Slovenia, pp. 169–170.

19. Phillips, G.F., Adler, J.R., and Taylor, S.J.G. 1993, A portable stimulator for surface FES, *Proceedings of the Ljubljana FES Conference*, Ljubljana, Slovenia, pp. 166–168.

20. Jaeger, R. 1986, Design and simulation of closed-loop electrical stimulation orthoses for restoration of quiet standing in paraplegia, *J. Biomech.*, 825.

21. Kralj, A., Bajd, T., Turk, R., and Benko, H. 1989, Paraplegic patients standing by functional electrical stimulation, *Digest 12th International Conference of Medical Biology Engineering*, Jerusalem, Israel. Paper 59.3.

22. Taylor, P.N., Ewins, D.J., and Swain, I.D. 1993, The odstock closed-loop FES standing system—Experience in clinical use, *Proceedings of the Ljubljana FES Conference*, Ljubljana, Slovenia, pp. 97–100.

23. Tomovic, R., Vukobratovic, M., and Vodovnik, L. 1973, Hybrid actuators for orthotic systems—Hybrid assistive system, *Proceedings of the International Symposium on External Conference Human Extremities*, Dubrovnik, Yugoslavia, p. 73.

24. Andrews, B.J. and Bajd, T. 1984, Hybrid orthoses for paraplegics, *Proceedings of the International Symposium on External Control Human Extremities*, Dubrovnik, Yugoslavia, p. 55.

25. Solomonow, M., Best, R., Aguilar, E., Cetzee, T., D'Ambrosia, R., and Rarrata, R.V. 1997, Reciprocating gait orthosis powered with electrical muscle stimulation (RGO-2), *Orthopedics*, pp. 315–324 (Part 1); pp. 411–418 (Part 2).

26. Davis, R., MacFarland, W., and Emmons, S. 1994, Initial results of the nucleus FES-22 stimulator implanted system for limb movement in paraplegia, *Stereotat. Funct. Neurosurg.*, **63**: 192–197.

27. Graupe, D. and Kohn, K.H. 1994, *Functional Electrical Stimulation for Ambulation by Paraplegics*, Krieger Publishing Co., Malabar, FL.

28. Graupe, D. and Kohn, K.H. 1998, Functional neuromuscular stimulator for short-distance ambulation by certain thoracic-level spinal-cord-injured paraplegics, *Surg. Neurol.*, **36**: 202–207.

29. Graupe, D. and Kohn, K.H. 1997, Transcutaneous functional neuromuscular stimulation of certain traumatic complete thoracic paraplegics for independent short-distance ambulation, *Neurol. Res.*, **19**: 323–333.

30. Association for Advancement of Med Instrumentation/Amer. Nat. Standard Inst.: American National Standard for Transcutaneous Nerve Stimulators, *AINSllAAMI NS4* 0 1985, Arlington, VA, Approved: May 20, 1986.

31. Klose, K.J., Jacobs. P.L., Broton, J.G., Guest, R.S., Needham-Shopshire, B.M., Lebwohl, N., Nash, M.S., and Green. B.A. 1997, Evaluation of a training program for persons with SCI paraplegia using the Parastep-I ambulation system, Part 1: Ambulation performance and anthropometric measures, *Arch. Phys. Med. Rehabil.*, **78**: 789–793.

32. Cerrel-Bazo, H.A., Rizetto, A., Pauletto, D., Lucca, L., and Caldana, L. 1997, Assisting paraplegic individuals to walk by means of electrically induced muscle contraction: Gait performance and patient compliance, Session 91, Paper 66, *Eighth World Congress of the International Rehabilitation Medicine Association*, Kyoto, Japan.

33. Chaplin, E. 1995, Functional neuromuscular stimulation for mobility in people with spinal cord injuries. The Parastep I system, *J. Spinal Cord Med.*, **19**: 99–105.

34. Nash, M.S., Jacobs, P.L., Montalvo, P.M., Klose, K.J., Guest, R.S., and Needham-Shropshire, B.M. 1997, Evaluation of a training program for persons with SCI paraplegia using the Parastep-I ambulation system, Part 5: Lower extremity blood flow and hypermic responses to occlusion are augmented by ambulation training, *Arch. Phys. Med. Rehabil.*, **78**: 808–814.

35. Jacobs, P.L., Nash, M.S., Klose, K.J., Guest, R.S., Needham-Shropshire, B.M., and Green, B.A. 1997, Evaluation of a training program for patients with SCI paraplegia using the parastep-I ambulation system, Part 2: Effects on physiological responses of peak arm ergometry, *Arch. Phys. Med. Rehabil.*, **78**: 794–798.

36. Needham-Shropshire, B.M., Broton, G.J., Klose, K.J., Lebwohl, N., Guest, R.S., and Jacobs, P.L. 1997, Evaluation of a training program for persons with SCI paraplegia using the Parastep-I ambulation system, Part 3: Lack of effect on bone mineral density, *Arch. Phys. Med. Rehabil.*, **78**: 799–803.

37. Guest, R.L., Klose, K.J., Needham-Shropshire, B.M., and Jacobs, P.L. 1997, Evaluation of a training program for persons with SCI paraplegia using the Parastep-I ambulation system, Part 4: Effects on physical self-concept and depression, *Arch. Phys. Med. Rehabil.*, **78**: 804–807.

38. Kilgore, K.L., Scherer, M., Bobblit, R., Dettloff, J., Dombrowski, D.M., Goldbold, N., Jatich, J.W. et al. 2001, Neuroprosthesis Consumers' Forum: Consumer priorities for research directions, *Veterans Administration—J. Rehabil. Res. Develop.*, 655–660.

53

Comparing Electrodes for Use as Cortical Control Signals: Tines, Wires, or Cones on Wires—Which Is Best?

53.1 Brief Description of the Neurotrophic Electrode and Its Neural Signals 53-4

53.2 Identification of the Action Potentials Recorded from the NE 53-7
Identification of APs

53.3 Functionality of the Action Potentials Recorded from the NE 53-7
Subjects Drove a Cursor in 2D for Communication Using Single Action Potentials and LFPs

53.4 Plasticity Was Demonstrated for Single APs But Not Attempted with LFPs 53-9
Directionality Was Detected in Single APS and LFPs • LFPs Were Used to Drive Simulated Cyber Digits

53.5 Misconceptions Regarding the Neurotrophic Electrode 53-14
Limited Number of Units per Contact and per Electrode

53.6 Difficulties and Disadvantages with the NE 53-15

Acknowledgments 53-15

References 53-15

Philip R. Kennedy
Neural Signals Inc

In the fields of neural prosthetics and neural engineering, there are several viable contenders for the prize of best long-term electrode to access cortical control signals for the restoration of communication and movement in humans. These contenders can be classified into three main groups. The first group includes those who have developed millimeter-sized tines or pins that are driven into the cortex and provide signals for months and sometimes years [1,3,4,6]. The second group produces flexible wires that are inserted into the cortex and provide signals also for months and sometimes years [5]. The third type of electrode is also a wire configuration but allows for the growth of the brain's neuropil into the hollow glass tip of the electrode that envelops the wires. Robust signals have been recorded for years from this neurotrophic electrode (NE) [3,4,6,11]. Thus, these electrodes can be classified into (a) those that protrude toward neurons (tines and wires) and (b) the NE that welcomes the neurites into its tip and thus fuses with the neuropil.

The holy grail of all these efforts is the restoration of movement to the paralyzed, control of robot arms, communication with computers, and restoration of speech to the mute. For example, quadriplegics need use of their limbs, and cortical control of functional neuromuscular stimulation devices would appear to be one answer to this need. These systems, though they provide access to cortical control signals, may not alone restore movement to those with spinal cord injury. Instead, I suspect these recording technologies will be hybridized with spinal cord regeneration efforts to restore movement to those paralyzed by spinal cord injuries. Similarly, for amputees, robotic technologies will be wed with cortical and peripheral control signal technologies for successful control of artificial limbs, as is envisioned by some DARPA projects. With respect to speech restoration, the technologies available in speech recognition and other decoding paradigms and integrated circuit paradigms will be instrumental in developing a speech prosthesis.

Herculean efforts have been expended by all workers in this field to provide single-unit recordings in the belief that the precision and speed needed for the control of digits is found only in the firing patterns of cortical single units recorded from primates. While not doubting this conclusion, less precise control may be sufficient for some prosthetic applications. An example of less precision is found in local field potential recordings (LFPs), which are simply an aggregate of single-unit recordings. These LFPs may prove very useful as prosthetic controllers [1,8,12,14]. Furthermore, this chapter will conclude with the hypothesis that not only precision but plasticity too may be the unique (and very necessary) feature available from single-unit recordings, which is not present in LFPs. In recent years, advances in analysis techniques in the frequency domain have strongly suggested that gamma band activity might be used as a cortical control signal.

First, let us look more closely at these three electrode categories and discuss the pros and cons. Conflict of interest statement: Yes, it is true that this author is the developer of the NE. Nevertheless, I will try to be as impartial as I can and assess the facts as published and known to me. Table 53.1 summarizes electrode similarities and differences. I apologize in advance if any worker in this field is underrepresented.

The first three investigators use tine-type electrodes that are either the 100-pin array (Utah or Blackrock array devised by Dick Norman), and used by Donoghue and colleagues [15], or the Michigan probe used by Schwartz's group [16]. Anderson and colleagues use their version of the array [1]. Nicholelis et al.

TABLE 53.1   Characteristics of Electrodes

	Tines	Tines	Tines	Wires	Neurotrophic
Investigators	Anderson	Donoghue	Schwartz	Nicholelis	Kennedy
1-Longevity	1+ years	5+ years	1+ years	3+ years	5+ years human
2a-Stability	Poor	Poor	Poor	Poor	Yes
2b-Functional stability	Yes	Yes	Yes	Yes	Yes
3-Plasticity	Yes	Yes	Yes	Yes	Yes
4-Directionality	2D	2D	3D	2D	2D
5-Force	N/T	N/T	N/T	Yes	N/T
6-LFPs	Yes	N/T	N/T	N/T	Yes
7-Gamma band	Yes	Yes	Yes	Yes	Yes
8-Single units/contact	1–2	1–2	1–2	1–2	15
9-Multi units/contact	1–2	1–2	1–2	1–2	Over 15
9-Single units/electrode	40	100–40	40	100++	31
10-EMG-related	N/T	N/T	N/T	N/T	Yes
11-Stimulation	Yes	Yes	Yes	Yes	No

N/T = Not tested.

use microwires devised by them [5]. Kennedy is the only one to use the NE so far [3,4,6,9,11,13]. Let us take these characteristics point by point.

1. *Longevity* is of prime importance in a chronic electrode that is to be implanted in a young adult human for a lifetime that can extend beyond 50 years. Clearly, the NE is ahead in this respect so far [4,6,11], though recent reports from Donoghue's lab show a few signals enduring for a few years [15] with enduring function for 5 years [2]. In all animal and human subjects, the signals from the NE continued until the preparation was destroyed or the subject died. The NE has endured in two humans for over 4 years and continues in one subject for over 5 years [4,6].

2. *Stability* of signal is of great importance too. This is difficult to assess over long time periods, especially if the subject is totally paralyzed because in that case, there is no behavior or electro-myographic (EMG) activity available for correlation. Stability has been shown in the NE [3,4,6,9–11,13] and to some extent in all others. One can argue, however, that stable single units may not be of great importance now with the advent of electrocorticographic (ECog) and LFP recordings. Because the ECog and LFP signals are inherently more stable, the loss of a few single units may not matter to the overall quality of the LFP. Nevertheless, there is no firm evidence of that yet, so sta-bility still remains important. In addition, the concept of functional stability may be important. Functional stability implies that functional relationships remain stable even when single units do not. Presumably, other single units that remain active take on the function of the "lost" single unit. All electrodes can claim functional stability but the question then becomes "for how long?"

3. *Plasticity* is one important feature of single units that is probably not available from ECog or LFPs. It should be easier to train one unit than an unruly classroom of poorly correlated units! The expec-tation is that perhaps any unit recorded from anywhere in the brain can be trained to control a spe-cific output. If this plasticity expectation is to be fulfilled, however, there must be *a priori* stability of the unit. Without stability and longevity, repeated sessions of retraining would be required. So far, the NE is unique in achieving the goals of plasticity, stability, and longevity [4,6,9,11].

4. *Directionality* has been tested by all investigators and found to be present. Schwartz and col-leagues are the only ones to have shown directionality in three dimensions using a virtual reality environment [16]. In these trials, the cursor was driven under the influence of the single units into all eight corners of the virtual cube space. In addition, seven-dimensional control of a robotic arm has been demonstrated by this group (Velliste et al.). There does not seem to be any overwhelming reason why other electrode configurations should be deficient in this task. Directionality with the NE was achieved without resorting to the firing rate, but was deduced from the initial direction of depolarization of the action potentials [10].

5. *Force* has been tested by the Nicholelis group who found that force and direction can be controlled by the monkey [5]. This feature has not been tested by others. Again, there is no overwhelming reason why force relationships could not be found with other electrode configurations.

6. *Local field potentials* have been studied by Anderson et al. [1], Kennedy et al. [8,12], and Leuthardt [14] and found to be useful. Anderson's group found that LFPs indicate cognitive state of the monkey and has also indicated directionality. The Kennedy group also found directionality within the LFPs [11], and in addition, used them to control a cursor and a cyber hand on the computer monitor. The subject was able to flex the cyber digits under control of the LFPs with reasonable speed [11]. Again, there is no overwhelming reason why other electrode configurations should be deficient in record-ing LFPs. In fact, it may minimize the impact of unit instability inherent in other electrodes and thus improve their functional stability and hence, longevity. ECog, like LFP, recordings in recent years has shown remarkable improvement in its ability to identify functional relationships [14].

7,8. *Units per contact and per electrode* have been presented by all authors. Tines and wires usually have only a few units, but have many tines or wires, thus providing a large number of units overall. For example, the Blackrock array is a 10×10 array and initially has one or two units per tine. This makes the processing of the signal outputs per electrode relatively straightforward, but implies that a large number of electrodes are needed to provide many signals. On the other hand, the NE has 5–20 signals per electrode and up to 19 in one subject and 31 in another [4,6], which means that fewer electrodes are required. The processing of these signals using spike sorting technologies is complicated but very achievable with today's systems [4,6,11]. The NE advantage is that fewer electrodes, and hence, implantable amplifiers, are needed.

9. *Relatedness to EMG activity* EMG activity has been studied by the Kennedy group in one almost paralyzed subject. They found that EMG was related to movement onsets, and poorly related to single-unit recording, though fairly well related to LFP onsets [in prep]. Other electrode signals have been related to EMG activity [14]. Though interesting, these results are not essential to the success of any of the electrodes. After all, the subjects to be implanted will be paralyzed *a priori*. Furthermore, there is no overwhelming reason why other electrode configurations should be deficient in this task.

10. Stimulation of the underlying cortex can be achieved by all electrodes except the NE. The NE is not designed for stimulation. Its design constraints do not preclude it from being used as a stimulation electrode. Tests cannot be carried out in humans for technical reasons (no implantable stimulating electronics, subjects are paralyzed) and ethical reasons (implants are allowed only to provide communication with the external world). In animal studies, stimulation was attempted and no response, such as limb movement, was seen. It would have been surprising if a response was seen because the NE contains a limited number of axons within its tip (as discussed later), and stimulation with conventional electrodes affects a large number of neurons (with or without passing fibers) to produce a measurable response. If it can never be shown to produce a response with stimulation, then it has the disadvantage of being used only for recording.

Let us now look more closely at the evidence for some functional advantages of the NE in humans. Disadvantages will be enumerated and discussed at the end of this section. Published data have shown the following:

1. Subjects drove a cursor in 2D for communication using single action potentials (APs) and LFPs [10,11].
2. Plasticity was demonstrated for single APs, but was not attempted with LFPs [10,11].
3. Directionality was detected in single APs [10,11] and LFPs [12].
4. LFPs were used to drive simulated cyber digits [12].
5. In a speech task, APs identified about half the 39 English phonemes [4]. In this same subject, APs were used in a paradigm involving real-time production of vowels. An 80% success rate was achieved after several months of training [4].

53.1 Brief Description of the Neurotrophic Electrode and Its Neural Signals

First, let us understand the unusual configuration of the NE. Figure 53.1 illustrates the salient features of the NE. Reference 16 has full details. The glass tip is 1–2 mm in length with a 50 μm diameter at the lower end where the neurites grow in. The upper end is about 300 μm wide to allow at least two wires to enter. They are held in place by methylmethacrylate glue. The wire ends are usually 500 μm from each other and from each end of the glass. The amplifier is connected to the wires. Because the ingrown neurites become myelinated, the neural signals recorded should be considered APs (see histology discussion later). The APs shown have opposite initial depolarization directions. This is because the amplifier has fixed polarity with positive and negative wires. So, axons close to one wire will have initial AP depolarizations opposite in direction to the AP depolarizations recorded at the other wire. This has important implications for directionality as discussed later.

A brief description of implantation techniques is required. Prior to surgery, localization of an active cortical site is essential, and this is achieved using functional MRI. An example of active areas is shown

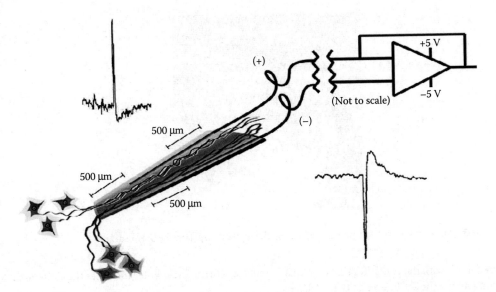

FIGURE 53.1 Neurotrophic Electrode consists of a glass tip that is 50 microns and a few hundred microns at the upper end. The teflon insulated, 2 mil gold wires glued are inside with ethyl cyanoacrylate. The gold wire tips are cut transversely. The wires are coiled for strain relief and connected in a bipolar mode to the amplifiers. The neurons grow processes inside over a few weeks and stabilize over three months. Those myelinated axons close to one wire (top left) will depolarize in the opposite direction to those myelinated axons near the other wire (bottom right).

in red in Figure 53.2. The subject imagines movement of digits, for example, and the scanner detects this as blood flow changes. This has been described previously [4,6]. All subjects undergo fMRI prior to implantation to localize the implantation target.

The implantation target is chosen based on stereotaxic 3D guidance using a system such as the Stealth navigation system (Medtronic, Minneapolis, MN). Figure 53.3 shows the white pointer wand that is

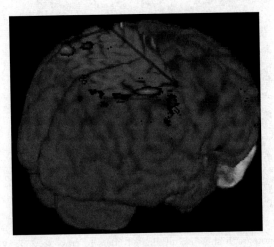

FIGURE 53.2 3D representation of the active areas in a functional MRI of the patient producing silent speech.

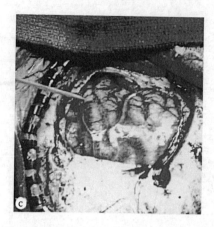

FIGURE 53.3 Surgical site with the pointer indicating the implant target on the brain surface.

registered in 3D with the computer that contains the subject's MRI. The pointer indicates the active area by moving it over the active area of the fMRI.

Histological processing has shown that there are myelinated neurites inside the cone tip of the electrode as shown in this electron microscopic image as shown in Figure 53.4. The tissue contains normal neuropil except for the lack of neurons [9,13]. There are myelinated neurites, axo-dendritic synapses, blood vessels, and dendroglial cells, but no microglial scavenger cells, no gliosis, and no neurons. Our interpretation is that the neurons sprouted neurites that grew into the cone tip and became myelinated. Thus, the NE records APs from axons, and because there are usually many axons close together, we appear to be recording compound APs when the firing rates are high. Stable [1] and long-lasting [5] signals have persisted in two subjects for over 4 years, with durations limited by the deaths of the subjects from their underlying diseases. A more recent subject is now in his 6th year of postimplantation recording, with promising data [4,6].

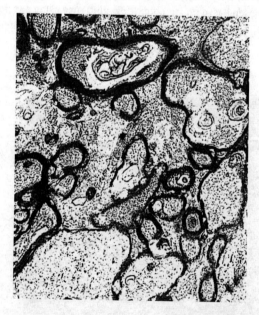

FIGURE 53.4 Histological photograph showing myelinated fibers in cross section. Width of photograph is approximately 100 microns.

53.2 Identification of the Action Potentials Recorded from the NE

53.2.1 Identification of APs

Single units or action potentials (APs) are probably very important for the precision and speed of a neural prosthetic. In addition, for some basic studies, APs are essential. Therefore, we have gone to great trouble to separate the APs from the multiunit activity. This is a difficult task and requires detailed information on the cluster cutting process to convince the skeptical reader that it is possible.

The system we use is NeuraLynx's Spike Sort program. First, the data are stabilized by removing the low-frequency components with a 300 Hz filter setting. Artifacts are removed as described in Reference 17. Threshold crossings above and below the continuous data stream are used to trigger a 1-ms data sample at 32 kHz. The time of the threshold crossing is logged as a timestamp. The system then measures the user set parameters such as peak, valley, and spike width and decides into which category the spike falls. The time it takes to perform these calculations is irrelevant to the timestamp. The calculations are performed at the level of the input buffer, not the CPU. Other methods such as template matching take the data and timestamp them with the width of the spike. In the Neuralynx paradigm, the timestamp is not affected by the cluster decision. There is a user set time of 264 μs during which the system cannot trigger another timestamp. This is implemented to avoid spikes too close together that could not be realistically distinguished. Thus, spikes can be detected that are at least 0.25 ms apart.

This has significant implications for the interpretation of interspike interval histograms (ISIHs). With the retrigger time (or dead time) being a quarter ms, there will be a necessary quarter ms initial gap in the ISIH. Thus, any gap more than a quarter ms implies a single unit. An example of an ISIH analysis is shown in Figure 53.5a. Note that some units have slow firing rates so that the "gap" is artificially prolonged. The fast-firing units in the bottom row have small gaps less than 1 ms. In contrast, multiunits have no gaps, as shown in Figure 53.5b, or a gap if the units are very slow firing (left panel, second from top). The physiological aspects of the different rate APs are discussed in a recent publication [7]. Briefly, the fast-firing APs are likely interneurons, whereas the slow-firing APs are probably corticospinal tract APs originating from Betz cells.

53.3 Functionality of the Action Potentials Recorded from the NE

53.3.1 Subjects Drove a Cursor in 2D for Communication Using Single Action Potentials and LFPs

Subject JR was the world's first cyborg because he was the first to control a computer directly with his brain [10,11]. Our first subject MH only provided binary signals and did not demonstrate the control of a computer. JR was implanted on March 24, 1998 and by mid-summer, he was controlling the cursor [9]. We thresholded his signals and separated them into large- and small-amplitude APs. One set drove the cursor in the horizontal, and the large units drove the cursor in the vertical direction. The firing rate of the APs was directly proportional to the cursor movement above a user-determined threshold firing. The gain of firing rate to cursor velocity was also user determined but held fixed during trials. Results of testing on postimplantation days 120, 121, and 122 demonstrated that within five trials he could control the cursor as shown in Figure 53.5c. The cursor was placed at the top left of the screen, and he had to move it across and down the screen as quickly as possible, thus forcing him to fire the large units that drove the cursor vertically downward.

When asked to drive the cursor to a particular icon about halfway across the screen, he succeeded quite well as shown in Figure 53.6 for day 243. Target 4 (on the ordinate) was the requested target that he hit repeatedly after initial inaccurate hitting of target 3 for five trials. Gaps between bars indicate rest

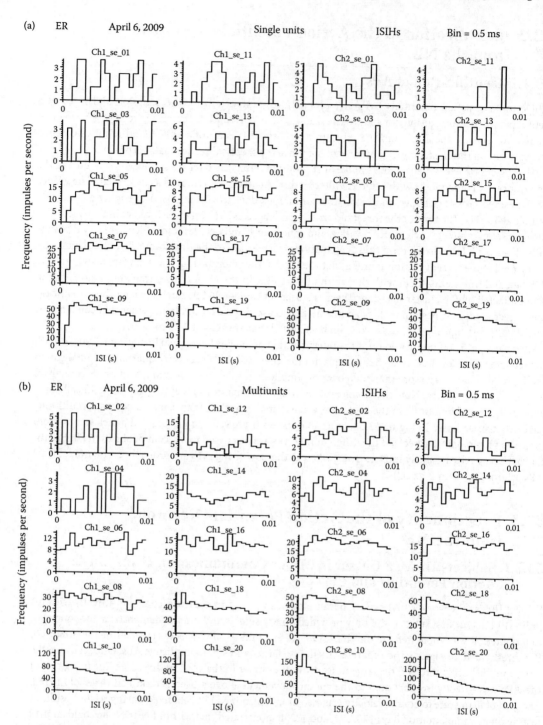

FIGURE 53.5 (a) Identification of single units using interspike interval histograms is shown here where there is a 1 ms (or less) gap between the unit firing and zero. Compare this with the multi-unit data in (b) where there is no gap. These data are only valid for the fast firing APs in the lower part of the figure. These data were recorded five years after implantation. (b) Identification of multi-units. See legend for figure (a). (c) Subject JR moves the cursor across and down the screen to a target in the lower left of the screen. After the fourth trial, the cursor is moved within a few seconds, showing a learning curve.

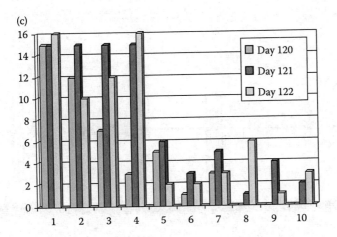

FIGURE 53.5 (continued) (a) Identification of single units using interspike interval histograms is shown here where there is a 1 ms (or less) gap between the unit firing and zero. Compare this with the multi-unit data in (b) where there is no gap. These data are only valid for the fast firing APs in the lower part of the figure. These data were recorded five years after implantation. (b) Identification of multi-units. See legend for figure (a). (c) Subject JR moves the cursor across and down the screen to a target in the lower left of the screen. After the fourth trial, the cursor is moved within a few seconds, showing a learning curve.

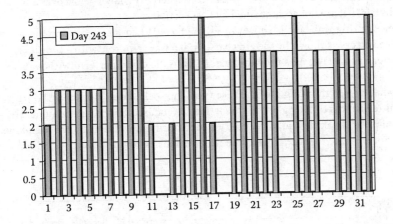

FIGURE 53.6 Subject JR moves the cursor to a target at position 4. The gaps are where he took a rest.

periods. Thus, subject JR demonstrated cursor control in two dimensions even before it was demonstrated in monkeys [11].

53.4 Plasticity Was Demonstrated for Single APs But Not Attempted with LFPs

In JR, we implanted area 4, hand representation, as determined by the functional MRI. We realized that he was moving facial muscles, specifically eyebrow movements, to produce neural activations. We preferred of course that he use neural activity that was not related to face or other residual movements. We asked JR not to use face movements of any kind during cursor driving. He appeared to comply with this request. To ensure that he did not move, we placed electrodes over his eyebrows to measure the

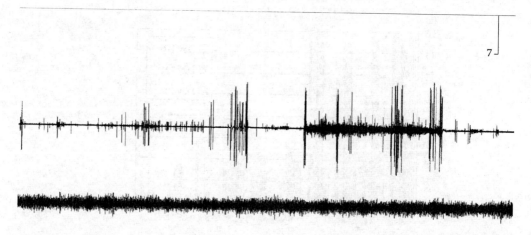

FIGURE 53.7 Single units are shown firing on the top line and the silent forehead EMG is shown below. Note that even though he was firing the single units, the EMG did not fire.

EMG activity. This activity would have driven the cursor in the vertical direction. This would have upset his performance in a task that required him to move horizontally to hit icons. Thus, he had to maintain relaxation of his eyebrow muscles. The neural activity that drove the cursor is shown in Figure 53.7 with the target icon entry point on the right above, and the EMG activity shown below over a 10-s timebase. Note the neural bursts that are not accompanied by EMG activity.

His performance during this task is shown in Figure 53.8. When he tried to perform too quickly (<20 s), he produced errors as shown by the gray bars. Trial 5 was error free with a time of 22 s, whereas trials 3 and 4 performed in 11 or 12 s produced errors. Thus, he could perform without activating his face muscles.

When asked what he was thinking during these trials, he spelled out "nothing" [11]. However, the next day, he admitted he was thinking of the cursor. He was focused on the cursor alone. He was driving the cursor simply by thinking about it. Thus, we concluded that what had once been *hand-related cortex was now cursor-related cortex*. This is the first demonstration of plasticity in human cortical recording.

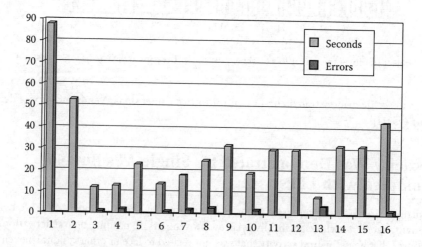

FIGURE 53.8 These data trials indicate that when he moved slowly (light gray) he made few errors, but when he moved quickly, he made some errors (dark gray).

53.4.1 Directionality Was Detected in Single APS [10,11] and LFPs [12]

In other electrode configurations, directionality is detected by the firing rate of a neuron in a specific direction [15,16], for example Figure 53.9. With the NE however, directionality is independent of firing rate. Instead, it is determined by the initial depolarization direction of the action potential as shown in Figure 53.10. We noted that individual action potentials can be discrete depolarizations in positive or negative directions or can appear to be a single biphasic unit (last unit in sequence) (Figure 53.9), which is in reality the near overlap of positive and negative depolarizations.

Deflections in one direction are shown in the upper panel of Figure 53.10, where virtually all action potentials have initial deflections in the negative or downward direction at rest. The subject JR was then requested to think of moving the cursor in the horizontal direction and all APs were thresholded above and below the baseline to drive the cursor. JR saw the cursor moving horizontally. The lower panel of Figure 53.10 shows the resulting AP directions, namely, upward or positive, that drove it horizontally. Thus, the initial direction of depolarization allows the detection of directionality.

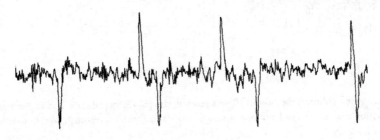

FIGURE 53.9 Single units firing slowly, one from one wire and the other from the second wire. The unit on the far right is when the units fired together, one overlapping the other.

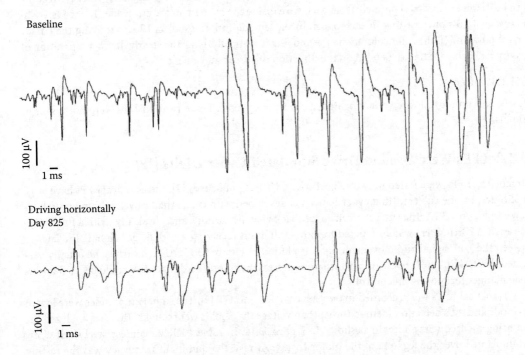

FIGURE 53.10 The upper line demonstrates baseline firing with the deflections driving in one direction (downward). The lower line demonstrates the reversal of the firing direction when driving horizontally.

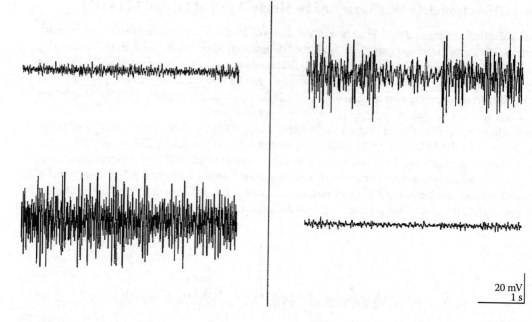

FIGURE 53.11 On the left column, the subject JR was moving the panel horizontally, and in the right column vertically. Across the top are recordings from one wire, and across the bottom, recordings from a different wire. Note the crossed relationship.

Directionality was also detected during LFP recordings as shown in Figure 53.11. In these recordings, LFPs were recorded separately from each wire inside the cone tip of the electrode. The wires are in the rows with 5 s of recording in each panel. In the left column, the subject JR was moving the cursor horizontally, and in the right column, he was moving it vertically. Note the clearly distinct separation of activity for each wire that depended on the direction of cursor movement.

53.4.1.1 Force

Clearly, we cannot test force relationships in paralyzed people. Force relationships were not tested in animals.

53.4.2 LFPs Were Used to Drive Simulated Cyber Digits [12]

Intracortical LFPs were tested in two subjects JR and TT as published [12]. Intracortical LFPs have large amplitudes. In one subject, JR, a cyber hand was developed with digits that moved with firing rate as shown in Figure 53.12. The subject received feedback visually, aurally, and physically (with a finger tap) with each AP firing. He was instructed to move a digit on receiving a verbal "go" signal. The latency between the "go" signal and movement onset is plotted in Figure 53.13. After six trials, he usually performed this task in under 5 s. This performance improvement indicated that LFPs could be used in this crude manner for movement control.

Extracortical LFPs were recorded in two subjects, RR and GT [8]. The signal amplitudes were low in this mode and thus detection methods other than voltage thresholds were sought. Thus, we analyzed the data using the frequency domain as shown in Figure 53.14. In subject RR, a stainless-steel skull screw was implanted over the leg area of the motor cortex. At rest, the dominant frequency was the resting 8 Hz (alpha waves) and a 16–20 Hz signal. During attempted (and very slight) foot movements, the 8-Hz

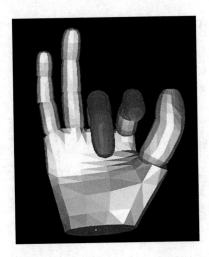

FIGURE 53.12 Cyber hand with digits was developed and the digits moved under the control of single units by subject JR.

signal shifted lower and the lowest frequency increased in amplitude near 2 Hz. Changes such as these can provide a binary switch signal. In this subject, this binary output was used to operate a light switch as published [8].

Thus, LFPs can be used as binary outputs and for controlling crude movements.

In a speech task, APs identified about half the 39 English phonemes [4]. In this same subject, APs were used in a paradigm involving real time production of vowels. An 80% success rate was achieved after several months of training [4].

These results have been published recently [4,6]. In this subject (ER), an 80% success rate was achieved when the subject was producing vowels in a center out task. The vowel, "uh" was used as the center and four other vowels, "iy," "oo," "aa," and "ih" were the targets in a two-dimensional formant frequency space task. This is a major step in developing a speech prosthesis. A second step is controlling consonant production. A third step, vocalization onset, would help immensely in decoding paradigm efficiency in these mute subjects.

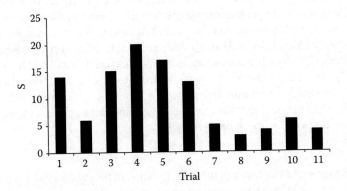

FIGURE 53.13 The 11 trials demonstrate that after 6 trials he could control the digit movements.

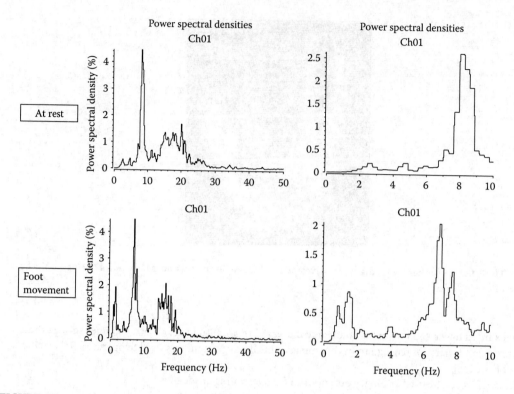

FIGURE 53.14 Power analysis in subject RR, shows the resting alpha peak (upper row) that dropped lower to about 7 Hz during very slight foot movements (lower row).

53.5 Misconceptions Regarding the Neurotrophic Electrode

53.5.1 Limited Number of Units per Contact and per Electrode

One of the misconceptions about the NE is that only one or two can be implanted and thus only one or two signals can be obtained. It is true that only a few can be implanted, and that is due to the bulk of the implanted electronics, not the electrode. Once the electronics can be further miniaturized, many electrodes can be implanted. Even with one electrode, however, recent off-line analysis of human recorded data has revealed as many as 19 units from one electrode in subject JR. In the recent subject ER, 20 single units are still being recorded 5 years after implantation. The results on the speech prosthesis were obtained 4–5 years after implantation, and could not have been obtained with unstable units.

These large numbers of units per electrode are in sharp contrast to other electrodes where about one, maybe two, units are recorded at each electrode tip. With 100 tines on the Cyberkinetic's probe, this is indeed impressive [15]. Over time, however, this number drops to 40% or less of tines that continue to record unit activity. Furthermore, each unit varies due to micromovements, so the stability of units is questionable and difficult to provide control. Nevertheless, recent results 1000 days after implantation describe a subject operating a communication device [2].

53.5.1.1 Stimulation

Attempts at microstimulation in rats through the NE implanted in the leg area did not produce movement. Evoked movements would have been surprising because only a few tens of axons could have been stimulated and usually an observable movement of a leg in response to stimulation would be produced in response to a large area of stimulated neurons and passing axons. Increasing the stimulating current was not an option due to the danger of electrolytically destroying the axons inside the electrode tip. All other electrodes, whether wires or tines, have provided stimulation safely. Thus, for stimulation, other electrode configurations are preferred. Nevertheless, it should be possible to use the NE for stimulation in carefully designed studies.

53.6 Difficulties and Disadvantages with the NE

1. Accurate histological reconstruction of recorded units is not possible due to the destruction inherent in placing it in the cortex and the trophic changes that take place as the tissue grows into the cone tip. This is not, however, of importance in neural prosthetics where functionality is paramount.
2. Manufacture of the electrode at present is difficult and requires many months of practice.
3. Implantation of the electrode is also difficult and requires much practice by someone with micro-surgical skills.
4. There is a delay of 3 or 4 months before the tissue has grown in and signals stabilize.
5. Replacement of the electrode in the exact same area would hardly produce the same signals unless many months passed to allow healing and reconstitution of the tissue.
6. Training time may be prolonged since plastic changes may be needed to produce useful function.

For successful usage of the NE, skill in manufacture and implantation is required. The delay in signal acquisition of 3 months is surely tolerable for someone who requires a lifetime of use. Replacement is unnecessary if it continues recording as studies strongly suggest. Training time, again, is hardly a problem when used for the lifetime of the subject.

We will allow the reader to judge for themselves as to who the eventual winner will be because I cannot be considered unbiased! The LFPs discussed so far may allow other electrodes to produce useful signals even though they may not be able to retain single units over the required lifetime of the subject. LFPs may prove adequate when crude control is needed, but will hardly prove adequate for *precise* control. Only time and effort will tell which electrode and recording technique will be instrumental in providing cortical control of prosthetic devices.

Acknowledgments

This work is supported by the NIH, NINDS, Neural Prostheses Program, grant no. 2 R44 NS36913-02. It is also supported by Neural Signals Inc internal funds.

Financial disclosure: The author PK may derive some financial gain from the commercialization of the Neurotrophic Electrode. USA patent number 4,852,573 and Speech patent number 2,275,035_B2.

References

1. Andersen RA, Buneo CA, Intentional maps in posterior parietal cortex. *Annu Rev Neurosci.* 2002; 25:189–220
2. Bacher D, Stavisky, SD, Simeral D, Donoghue JP, Hochberg LR, Use of a general purpose communication interface by an individual with tetraplegia in the brain Gate2 clinical trial. Society for Neuroscience Abstract 899.8, San Diego, November 2010.
3. Bartels J, Andreasen D, Ehirim P, Mao H, Seibert S, Wright EJ, Kennedy PR. Neurotrophic electrode: Method of assembly and implantation into human motor speech cortex. *J Neurosci Methods.* 2008 Sep 30; 174(2):168–176. Epub 2008 July 10.
4. Brumberg JS, Nieto-Castanon A, Kennedy PR, Guenther FH. Brain-computer interfaces for speech communication. *Speech Commun.* 2010 Apr 1;52(4):367–379.

5. Carmena JM, Lebedev MA, Crist RE, O'Doherty JE, Santucci DM, Dimitrov DF, Patil PG, Henriquez CS, Nicholelis MAL Learning to control a brain-machine interface for reaching and grasping by primates. *PloS Biol.* 2003; 1(2):193

6. Guenther FH, Brumberg JS, Wright EJ, Nieto-Castanon A, Tourville JA, Panko M, Law R et al. A wireless brain-machine interface for real-time speech synthesis. *PLoS One.* 2009 Dec 9; 4(12):e8218

7. Kennedy P, Andreasen D, Bartels J, Ehirim P, MacLean G, Mao H, Velliste M, Wichmann T, Wright EJ. Making the lifetime connection between brain and machine for restoring and enhancing function. *Proceedings of the International Conference on Brain Computer Interfacing,* to be published *in Proceedings in Brain Research,* 2011.

8. Kennedy P, Andreasen D, Ehirim P, King B, Kirby T, Mao H, Moore MM. Using human extra-cortical local field potentials to control a switch. *J Neural Eng.* 2004; 1:63–71. FDA approval number: G960032/S10, Brain to computer interfacing device.

9. Kennedy P. A long-term electrode that records from neurites grown onto its recording surface. *J Neurosci Methods.* 1989; 29:181–193.

10. Kennedy PR, King B. Dynamic interplay of neural signals during the emergence of cursor related cursor in a human implanted with the neurotrophic electrode. Chapter 7 in *Neural Prostheses for Restoration of Sensory and Motor Function.* Eds. Chapin J and Moxon, K. CRC Press, Boca Raton, FL, 2001.

11. Kennedy PR, Bakay RA, Moore MM, Adams K, Goldwaithe J, Direct control of a computer from the human central nervous system. *IEEE Trans Rehabil Eng.* 2000; 8(2):198.

12. Kennedy PR, Kirby MT, King B, Mallory A, Adams K, Moore MM, Computer control using human cortical local field potentials. *IEEE Trans Neural Syst Rehabil Eng,* accepted 2004.

13. Kennedy, PR, Mirra S, Bakay, RAE, The cone electrode: Ultrastructural studies following long-term recording. *Neurosci Lett.* 1992; 142:89–94.

14. Leuthardt EC, Schalk G, Wolpaw JR, Ojemann JG, Moran DW. A brain-computer interface using electrocorticographic signals in humans. *J Neural Eng.* 2004; 1:63–71.

15. Serruya MD, Hatsopoulos NG, Paninski L, Fellows MR, Donoghue JP, Instant neural control of a movement signal. *Nature* 2002; 416:141

16. Taylor DM, Tillery SI, Schwartz AB, Direct cortical control of 3D neuroprosthetic devices. *Science* 2002; 7(296):1829–1832.

54

Development of a Multifunctional 22-Channel Functional Electrical Stimulator for Paraplegia

Ross Davis
Florida Institute of Technology

T. Johnston
Shriners Hospital for Children

B. Smith
Shriners Hospital for Children

R. Betz
Shriners Hospital for Children

T. Houdayer
Neural Engineering Clinic

A. Barriskill
Neopraxis Pty. Ltd.

54.1 Introduction 54-1
54.2 Historical Aspect 54-2
54.3 Neural Engineering Clinic: Two Male Subjects 54-3
    Nucleus FES22 Stimulating System • Praxis FES24-A System • Praxis FES24-B System
54.4 Experience at Shriners Hospitals for Children 54-6
    Upright Mobility
54.5 Conclusion 54-10
Acknowledgments 54-10
References 54-10

54.1 Introduction

The authors' aim has been to develop a generic functional electrical stimulation (FES) implant for the restoration of functions in spinal cord-injured (SCI) paraplegic individuals, the functions or modes of which can be matched to an individual's requirements: upright functional mobility, pressure relief and lower extremity exercise, and bladder and bowel control [1–6]. In addition, for bladder control, less invasive surgical procedures were proposed to avoid posterior conus rhizotomy, and sacral laminotomy to access the sacral nerve roots for stimulation [7,8]. It was hoped that this system would offer more functions and less surgery to patients with a cost–benefit ratio. This approach was termed "Multi-Functional."

Simple locomotor functions can complement the use of a wheelchair and can be helpful in overcoming obstacles to wheelchair access, especially doorsteps and unadapted bathroom facilities. In addition, being able to stand up to reach objects and perform prolonged manual tasks would be convenient for many workplace and home situations [3–5]. Five paraplegic volunteers (two at the Neural Engineering Clinic (NEC) in Augusta, ME and three at the Shriners Hospital for Children (SHC) in Philadelphia, PA) have participated in this device's evolution.

During 1983, R.D. (NEC) became aware of the possibilities of modifying and using the 22-channel cochlear implant technology (Cochlear Ltd., Lane Cove, N.S.W., Australia) as the basis for an implantable FES system for the restoration of multiple functions in SCI paraplegics.

The state of FES in paraplegia has been extensively reviewed [1–5]. These SCI individuals are unable to move their lower extremities or control bladder and bowel function. They must regularly self-catheterize (~3–6 times per day). Secondary medical problems are prone to occur, such as pressure sores, osteoporosis, muscular atrophy in the lower limbs, muscle spasticity, deep-vein thrombosis, cardiovascular disease, and depression. Although considerable FES achievements have been made, there has yet to be developed a safe, practical FES system for these multiple functions that is completely independent of the laboratory and is an energy-efficient mobility aid for prolonged use at home and in the workplace. The reason lies in the fact that FES is addressing complex problems requiring not only interdisciplinary knowledge from muscle and nerve physiology and electrical stimulation technology but also the implementation of biomechanical and control principles [6].

Other reasons that limit clinical application may also be significant, for example, cost–benefit considerations (especially for implanted systems). Although spinal injury results in the loss of multiple physiological systems, neural implants to date have been developed to restore only specific functions. An approach was proposed to develop a generic FES implant, the functions or modes of which can be matched to an individual patient's requirements. In addition, less invasive surgical procedures were proposed to avoid the posterior conus rhizotomies and sacral laminectomy associated with the existing implanted bladder implants [7,8].

Since 1984, three FES implant models have evolved from the Cochlear's technology and its subsidiary: Neopraxis Pty. Ltd. The initial Nucleus FES-22 stimulator was implanted in 1991 after animal and human studies, and with the U.S. Food and Drug Administration's approval (IDE# G87014) and Institutional Review Board (IRB) approval in 21-year-old paraplegic subject (ASIA: T10).

54.2 Historical Aspect

In 1984, the Veterans Administration (VA) funded the initial animal studies at the Togus VA Medical Center (Augusta, ME). These were aimed at determining what changes would be required to use a modified cochlear implant with a maximum pulse output of 4.3 mA and 0.4 ms pulse width to be suitable for FES use in humans. An initial decision was taken to utilize epineurally placed electrodes (2.5-mm-diameter platinum disks) in preference to epimysial or intramuscular electrodes because it was known that the stimulation currents would be lower and that there would be less movement of the electrodes. To determine exactly how low the stimulation currents would be and to determine the stimulation sites, initial anesthetized rabbits studies were conducted [9]. The threshold found for each branch of the split sciatic nerves was 0.1–0.2 mA at 0.2 ms with 50 pps. The maximal stimulation was achieved usually between 0.5 and 1.0 mA. Simultaneous dorsiflexion of both paws as well as cocontraction in the anterior and posterior muscle groups could be achieved.

At the Togus VA Medical Center, with the approval of the IRB and volunteer patients undergoing lower extremity amputation, stimulation studies were carried out at 0.2 ms pulse duration with 20 pps frequency, with a portable, battery-operated, and calibrated constant-current unit (Cordis Corp., Miami, FL, Model 910 A). The pulse amplitudes for producing maximal stimulation and contraction in the largest of the nerves (medial sciatic) ranged from 0.6 to 2.5 mA, which falls well within the range of the Cochlear receiver-stimulating unit to be used [9,10]. Using the *Color Atlas of Human Anatomy, First Edition* edited by R. M. H. McMinn and R. T. Hutchings (Yearbook Medical Publishers, Inc., Chicago, IL), whose dissections were reproduced as life-size photographs, allowed measurements of the diameters to be made at different points along the nerves. These measurements were in relatively close agreement with the amputated nerve diameters of the nine volunteer patients [10].

54.3 Neural Engineering Clinic: Two Male Subjects

54.3.1 Nucleus FES22 Stimulating System

As a first device, the FES22 stimulator was only intended to provide its recipient with enhanced mobility functions. During 1985, Roger Avery (Custom Med Laboratories, Durham, NH) started work on the design and manufacture for the implantable leads and electrodes. Because of the need for higher output currents, it was also necessary to design a new transmitter coil capable of delivering the higher power. To make each of the 22-output channels individually available, a circular epoxy housing was designed with 22 sockets around the perimeter (Figure 54.1a) with the diameter of the housing being determined by the diameter of the coil. During November/December 1991, the Nucleus FES-22 system was implanted in subject A (21-year-old male paraplegic subject; ASIA: A T10) in three sessions at the Kennebec Valley Medical Center (now Maine General Medical Center), Augusta, ME. The receiver–stimulator was placed subcutaneously at the lower right anterior intercostal margin with 11 connecting leads subcutaneously tunneled to the right and another 11 subcutaneously tunneled to the left hip areas. Following this, 2.5-mm-diameter platinum disk electrodes were placed epineurally on the individual branches of the right and left femoral nerves by suturing the silicone elastomer ring around each electrode to the connective tissues on each side of the nerve branches. In the second and third procedures, electrodes were attached over gluteal, posterior tibial, peroneal, and sciatic nerves bilaterally [11]. A total of 20 electrodes were implanted epineurally, with one electrode placed subcutaneously in a Teflon bag in each of the femoral triangles, as the spare lead.

Six weeks following surgery (January 1992), the FES-22 system did produce threshold and maximal muscle contractions as tested in all 20 channels. At the second testing session in February 1992, the implanted system did not function properly owing to a suspected electrostatic damage in the implant, resulting in the loss of seven channels. Hardware and software changes were made allowing the remaining 15 channels to work. In December 1992, the 15 channels were retested for threshold and maximal muscle contractions; the multivariate analysis did not show any change with time or body side, but a significant effect was seen with the electrode locations [12].

Subject A exercised his lower extremity muscles at home using a personal computer (PC) to control the implanted stimulator. In January 1997, he was provided with a battery-operated external portable conditioning system ($19 \times 11 \times 6$ cm), which he uses at home and at work sitting in his wheelchair. The exercise protocol stimulates the right and left knee extensors and ankle plantar/dorsiflexors alternately 4 s on/4 s off, for a total of 20 min. After the muscles have been conditioned, dynamometric testing (isometric mode) has shown that the implanted FES stimulation produces bilateral knee extension torque of 45–55 Nm at 30° and 65 Nm at 60° of the knee flexion. C.S. exercises at least 3 days a week, and finds if he does not do so, the spasticity in the lower extremities increases.

(a) Nucleus FES-22   (b) Praxis FES-24A

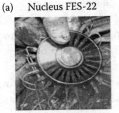 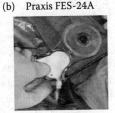

Implanted 1991   Implanted 1998

FIGURE 54.1 (a) The first 22-channel RF FES System (Nucleus FES-22) implanted in Subject A in 1991. (b) The second developed RF FES-24A Praxis System, implanted in Subject B in 1998.

The laboratory PC-based FES-22 system implements a 10 ms duty-cycle state machine for open- and closed-loop control for use in the prolonged standing mode. The controller is divided into three phases: (1) open-loop "sit-to-stand," (2) closed-loop stand, and (3) closed-loop "stand-to-sit." To initiate standing up and sitting down, the subject uses a remote switch on a hand glove. The sensors used for closed-loop control are electrogoniometers across both knees, which respond to a 10° knee buckle, and accelerometers attached to the back at T6 level.

A controlled Nucleus FES-22 stimulation to the motor nerves of the quadriceps and gluteal muscles has resulted in uninterrupted standing for over 60 min [12]. This has been achieved by use of the bilateral knee-angle goniometer sensors with the Andrews stabilizing anterior floor reaction orthosis (AFRO), which is an ankle–foot brace. With the knee goniometers sensing for a 10° buckle, the stimulator would come "ON" to correct the buckle; usually, this occurred between 3% and 8% of the standing time. On recovery, the automatic switch "OFF" occurs when the knee flexion has returned to less than 5°. Otherwise, lower extremity muscle activation is not required to maintain the upright posture [13].

54.3.2 Praxis FES24-A System

In 1998, Cochlear Ltd. formed a subsidiary company, Neopraxis Pty. Ltd., which decided to build on the knowledge gained from the FES22 implant and to produce the Praxis FES22A system. This system was designed to provide multiple functions, bladder and bowel control, enhanced mobility, and seated pressure relief, to provide recipients with a cost-effective device that addresses their most important needs.

54.3.2.1 Bladder Control

The traditional bladder stimulator, Finetech-Brindley stimulator, and now, the "Vocare" (NeuroControl Corp., Cleveland, OH) operates by stimulating the sacral anterior roots [8]. This system has two primary drawbacks, which the Praxis system was designed to eliminate: (a) posterior sacral rhizotomies are done, via a laminectomy, to achieve an areflexive bladder with increased capacity and (b) a sacral laminectomy is done to access the anterior sacral roots for fitting cuff-type electrodes. The rhizotomy procedure eliminates reflex erection in male recipients. Further, Creasey [8] states that "a patient who has the rhizotomies but does not use the implant (stimulator) would therefore be expected to become more constipated."

In August 1998, the Praxis FES24-A stimulator (Figure 54.1b) was developed by Neopraxis Pty. Ltd. and implanted in subject B (35-year-old male paraplegic subject; ASIA: A, T10). Eighteen channels were used for stimulating individual nerves or branches for muscle contractions and limb movements, including exercise, pressure relief, standing, and stepping. The electrodes implanted for epineural stimulation were 10 thin flexible platinum cuffs (Flexi-Cuff) that were sized, cut, and sutured closed with at least twice the diameter of the encircled nerve. The other eight electrodes were 3-mm-diameter, platinum buttons that were placed on the epineurium. Each button has an attached Dacron mesh surround that was sutured to the adjacent connective tissue on each side of the nerve.

Three channels for bilateral sacral root stimulation (S2–4) for bladder control (bowel control and erection, if possible) were provided. Sacral-root stimulation was achieved by three pairs of linear polarization resistance (LPR) electrodes (10 mm long, solid platinum tubing of 1.0 mm diameter) inserted into the external sacral foramina in a lateral direction to follow and to stimulate the nerve roots epidurally. Further, one channel was connected to an epidural spinal cord-stimulating electrode (Pisces Quad: Medtronic Inc., Minneapolis, MN) for conus medullaris modulation of the spastic bladder and bowel reflexes.

54.3.2.2 Praxis System Clinical Results

For a year prior to his implantation, subject B was able to stand without knee bracing using a combination of the Andrews' AFRO and closed-loop skin surface of FES applied directly over the femoral nerves, 2–3 cm below the inguinal ligament. With closed-loop control of the stimulation, he would typically

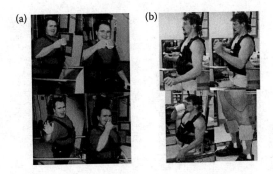

FIGURE 54.2   Prolonged standing (1 h): controlled FES + Andrews' AFO.

stand uninterrupted for 30 min, and up to 70 min. With training, subject B did achieve the "C" posture and stood with the stimulation "OFF" for more than 50% of the standing time [14]. In December 1997, muscle strength tests done on the Biodex dynamometer (isometric mode) showed that surface stimulation of the right quadriceps (femoral nerve) was capable of eliciting 50 Nm of knee extension at 30° of the knee flexion and 45 Nm at 45° [13–15].

After implantation of the Praxis FES 24-A system in August, 1998, subject B carried out an FES exercise routine, which stimulated three separate sequences (quadriceps group, buttocks and posterior thigh group, and ankle group), each running initially for 5 min and extending to 15 min over a 2-week period. Each muscle in the sequence would be stimulated sequentially for 4 s on and off. F.R. found that daily stimulation decreased his muscle spasms and spasticity level.

When standing with the implanted system, he was able to perform a variety of one-handed tasks, including reaching for and holding a 2.2 kg object at arm's length. These tasks were achieved while in the "C" posture with closed-loop activation to the lower extremity muscles and with balance maintained by the other upper extremity muscles (15; Figure 54.2b).

54.3.2.3 Bladder Results

On September 4, 1998, in the Urodynamic Testing Laboratory, subject 2 had his sacral roots (S3 and 4) bilaterally stimulated intermittently. This showed that on 3 occasions the bladder contracted with recorded pressures between 45 and 50 cm of water. On December 14, 1998, urodynamic testing again showed consistent results from S3 and 4 sacral root stimulation producing three sustained bladder contractions with pressures of 40–55 cm of water and urination (Figure 54.3) with each stimulation pattern (5 s on/5 s off, 20 Hz, eight bursts). On April 2, 1999, urodynamic testing was repeated with two bladder reflex activations from each pattern of stimulation (5 s on/5 s off, 20 Hz, 8–14 bursts). Pressures of 50–70 cm of water were recorded.

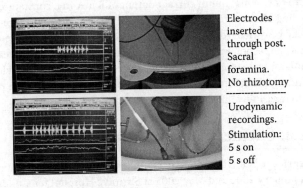

Electrodes inserted through post. Sacral foramina. No rhizotomy

Urodynamic recordings. Stimulation: 5 s on 5 s off

FIGURE 54.3   SCI: Bladder voiding: Bilateral S3 + 4 stimulation.

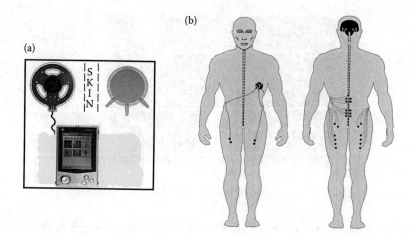

FIGURE 54.4 (a) The external parts of the Praxis FES24B System with the control unit and surface applied antenna over the implanted Receiver-stimulator. (b) The Radio-stimulator with the connecting 22 leads to the electrodes on nerves and spinal cord conus.

In April 1999, the internal FES24-A unit's connecting wire between the internal antenna and the stimulator module broke as a result of F.R.'s repeated bending at the waist [15]. The receiver/stimulator unit was removed in 1999, as F.R. complained of discomfort from the two connectors under the abdominal skin. The network of leads and electrodes were left for a possible replacement of the newly designed system.

54.3.3 Praxis FES24-B System

This third iteration system: FES24-B system (Figure 54.4), which eliminates this internal wire breakage possibility consists of

- A body-worn controller "Navigator" capable of executing a wide variety of software control strategies
- A skin surface stimulator "ExoStim" to mimic an implant and to provide simple exercise functions prior to implantation
- Sensor packs incorporating accelerometers and a gyroscope to provide feedback information to control strategies
- A new implant receiver/stimulator was based on the latest cochlear implant control integrated circuit (IC), the "CIC3"
- A range of implantable electrode leads suitable for the system's multiple functions

The FES24-B system provides a maximum current output of 8 mA in a constant-current mode. The stimulation is achieved using biphasic (negative and positive phases, closely charge-matched) current pulses. The pulse widths can be varied from 25 to 500 µs and a per-channel pulse frequency of 0–400 Hz on each of the 22 channels can be obtained, which were designed as cathodes whereas the rear surface plate of the receiver/stimulator was connected to be the anode. The stimulator provides real-time data telemetry functions, including the ability to measure the impedance of the current path through each electrode and the ability to transmit voltage measurements from each electrode [16].

54.4 Experience at Shriners Hospitals for Children

Three males with paraplegia, aged 18, 21, and 21 years, underwent surgical implantation of the Praxis FES24-B system between January 2002 and May 2003 at Shriners Hospital for Children, Philadelphia. Eighteen epineural electrodes (Table 54.1) were implanted for upright mobility in all three subjects and

TABLE 54.1   Muscles Implanted per Channel of Stimulation

Muscle(s)
Posterior adductor magnus
Biceps femoris—long head* or short head**
Gluteus maximus
Gluteus medius, minimus, and tensor fascia lata
Vastus lateralis and vastus intermedius
Vastus medialis and vastus lateralis
Tibialis anterior and extensor digitorum longus
Gastrocnemius, soleus, and flexor hallucis longus
Iliopsoas***

* Subjects 1 and 2, ** subject 3, ***subjects 2 and 3.

three pairs of bifurcated linear pararadicular electrodes were placed extradurally on the bilateral S2, S3, and S4 mixed nerve roots for bladder and bowel function in the first two subjects.

54.4.1 Upright Mobility

Four weeks postimplantation, the subjects participated in 4 weeks of strengthening and conditioning of the implanted muscles followed by 17–22 weeks in which the focus was on programming of the upright mobility strategies and training for their functional use. The goals included the achievement of the transitions between sitting and standing, swing through and/or reciprocal gait with a walker or crutches, and prolonged standing. For the reciprocal gait, the swing was achieved through stimulation to the iliopsoas, biceps femoris, and/or the tibialis anterior to create a flexor withdrawal response. Additional training goals include advanced activities, such as ascending and descending stairs (Figure 54.5a) and the achievement of subject-specific goals (Figure 54.5b). Bilateral ankle–foot orthoses were worn for all upright mobility activities.

Following training, the data were collected for a variety of mobility activities, including transitions between sitting and standing, a short (6 m) and a long (6 min) walk, ascending and descending stairs,

    (a)   (b)

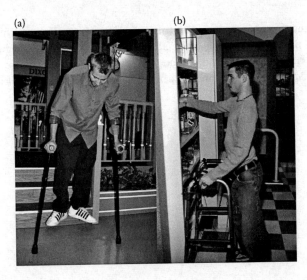

FIGURE 54.5   Two subjects using the Praxis system for functional activities. (a) Subject 2 uses forearm crutches to descend stairs. (b) Subject 3 reaches for items on a shelf using a walker to support himself with one upper extremity.

and maneuvering in an inaccessible bathroom stall. All subjects chose to use a swing-through gait pattern for the tested activities, except subject 2 who chose a reciprocal pattern for ascending stairs only. Subjects 1 and 3 each used a walker with wheels to perform the mobility activities and subject 2 used forearm crutches. None of the subjects required physical assistance to complete the activities. Subjects 1 and 3 required supervision for all tested activities, and subject 2 was independent for all activities except stairs where he required supervision. The data for ascending and descending stairs were not collected for subject 1 as the activity was felt to be unsafe for him. Several activities could not be performed by subject 3 secondary to complaints of shoulder pain related to poor scapular muscle control.

54.4.1.1 Bladder and Bowel

Neuromodulation was attempted with subject 1 and acute suppression of reflexive bladder contractions during bladder filling was observed. When using stimulation to both S3 nerve roots throughout the day, this subject maintained a catheterized schedule (every 6 h) comparable to that used when he took anticholinergic medication. This suggested that neuromodulation may have helped to suppress reflexive bladder activity on a daily basis as during the control period (without the neuromodulation or medication) he catheterized more frequently, on an average of every 4 h. The ability to improve bowel evacuation was examined in subject 2, using two different stimulation paradigms: low-frequency electrical stimulation (20 Hz, 350 μs, 8 mA) and a combination of low frequency and high frequency (500 Hz, 350 μs, 8 mA). The daily use of electrical stimulation appeared to cause a reduction in the time to complete defecation by 40% with the first stimulation strategy and by 60% with the second strategy.

Despite numerous attempts with varying stimulation parameters to the sacral nerve roots, neither subject could obtain detrusor pressures sufficient to provide voiding with stimulation. Both subjects continued to catheterize for bladder emptying.

54.4.1.2 Electrode Stability

Three of the 52 electrodes placed for lower extremity stimulation experienced changes in the responses of the muscles. One of these was due to a disconnection at the connector site between the implant and the electrode lead. This was repaired and the electrode continued to function without further problems. The remaining two electrodes (biceps femoris and tibial nerve) were not replaced, as they did not impact the function for the subjects involved.

54.4.1.3 Sensors

Closed-loop standing using sensor packs incorporating accelerometers and a gyroscope was attempted with subject 1. The sensor packs were attached externally on the thigh and the calf (Figure 54.6) to detect the position of the knee while standing. Stimulation would decrease until a change in the knee joint angle was detected, at which time stimulation would again increase to prevent a knee buckle.

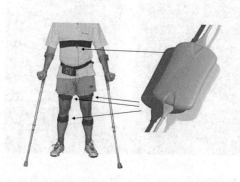

FIGURE 54.6 Sensor packs used for closed-loop standing.

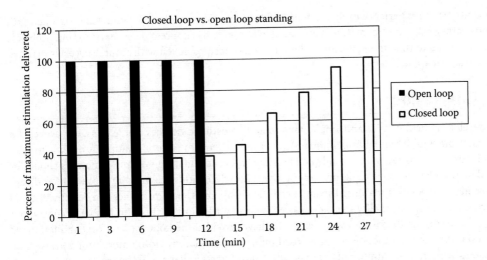

FIGURE 54.7 Using open-loop control, the stimulation remained at 100% for 12 min of standing after which the subject's muscles were too fatigued for him to remain upright. Using closed-loop control, the stimulation could be maintained at a lower level, increasing over time as needed. With closed-loop control, the standing time was more than doubled to 27 min.

Figure 54.7 demonstrates the use of the sensors for closed- loop feedback to the right quadriceps muscles during quiet standing. Using closed-loop control, the subject was able to stand with less stimulation to the quadriceps than what he had been using while standing with open-loop control. He was also able to stand for a longer period of time before the muscle fatigued, requiring him to sit. The algorithm for increasing and decreasing stimulation to the quadriceps did not create any balance disturbances for this subject.

54.4.1.4 Complications

54.4.1.4.1 *Follow-Up of the First Two Implanted at the NEC Site, Subjects (A and B)*

In 2002, subject A accidentally cut his left foot, which was treated superficially. In 3–4 days, his left lower extremity was swollen with an infection, which was immediately treated with intravenous antibiotics for 2 weeks. The swelling resolved, but 6 weeks later, the tissues around the Nucleus FES-22 system were swollen and inflamed. After 3 days of I.V. antibiotics, the implanted system was explanted taking as much time as when it was implanted. The most difficult part was finding and dissecting the small 2.5-mm platinum electrodes and their silastic backing. He recovered well without further complications.

In 2001, subject B was experiencing intermittent pain in the T7-8 vertebra at the postfractured site; after conservative treatment failed, the spine was fused in this area. By that time, he was ready for implanting the Praxis FES24-B stimulator in 2003; the Neopraxis Company was closed by Cochlear Ltd. However, he was offered the stimulator for implantation, but without further support by the company, he decided not to continue and have the leads and electrodes removed.

At the SHC site, during the training period, subject 2 sustained a stress fracture of the left proximal first metatarsal, which he believed happened when his left leg experienced greater impact at initial contact due to his poor control of swing for that step. The subject was immobilized for 6 weeks in a soft boot after which he was able to return to training without further problems. At the end of June 2002, subject 1 sustained an abrasion near his ankle and antibiotics were started once this was reported. Then, at the beginning of August 2002, he began experiencing high fevers and complained of heat and inflammation around one of his surgical incisions. Despite treatment with intravenous antibiotics, this subject continued to experience problems with inflamed incisions, some of which resulted in open skin and fluid drainage. Antibiotic treatment appeared to temporarily suppress these reactions but problems continued. Owing to this, the majority of the system has been removed with future surgeries planned to remove the remainder.

54.5 Conclusion

In the developing field of FES and implantable neural prosthetic devices, there has been a need for reliable and safe, multichannel implantable stimulating systems to restore multiple functions in neurologically impaired patients. In paraplegic individuals, the stimulating systems' functions should be designed to modulate spasticity and precisely activate individual muscles for joint movement and control of bladder and bowel functions. The more channels available, the more nerves can be activated and the more modes of functionality can be restored. Our contribution to this aim has been continuous since 1983, and the two Praxis FES systems [11–16] have provided the hope for a new rehabilitation aid for the restoration of the function in spinal cord injury paraplegia. Providing more functions with an FES system with a greater number of channels introduced new challenges to the subjects and research teams, including the need for multiple surgical procedures, new surgical approaches to placing electrodes, increased risk of infection, and greater hospitalization and rehabilitation time. Importantly, these challenges are being addressed through multiple research efforts [17] at various centers.

Acknowledgments

Our thanks to Cochlear Ltd. and Neopraxis Pty. Ltd. for making these studies possible. Our sincere thanks to our many collaborators at NEC: S.E. Emmons, J. McKendry, R. Eckhouse, A. Delehunty, and W. MacFarland; and at SHC: M.J. Mulcahey, B. Benda, G. Creasey, and M. Pontari.

References

1. Kralj A, Bajd T. *Functional Electrical Stimulation: Standing and Walking after Spinal Cord Injury.* CRC Press, Boca Raton, FL, 1989.
2. Davis R. International functional electrical stimulation society: The development of controlled neural prostheses for functional restoration. *Neuromod*, 2000; 3:1–5.
3. Agarwal S, Triolo RJ, Kobetic R, Miller M, Bieri C, Kukke S, Rohde L, Davis JA. Long-term user perceptions of an implanted neuroprosthesis for exercise, standing, and transfers after spinal cord injury. *J Rehabil Res Dev*, 2003; 40(3):241–252.
4. Bonaroti D, Akers J, Smith BT, Betz RR, Mulcahey MJ. Comparison of functional electrical stimulation to long leg braces for upright mobility for children with complete thoracic level spinal injuries. *Arch Phys Med Rehab*, 1999; 80:1047–1053.
5. Johnston TE, Betz RR, Smith BT, Mulcahey MJ. Implanted functional electrical stimulation: An alternative for standing and walking in pediatric spinal cord injury. *Spinal Cord*, 2003; 41(3):144–152.
6. Bajd T, Jaeger R. FES for movement restoration. *BAM*, 1994; 4:228–229.
7. Brindley G. The first 500 patients with sacral anterior root stimulator implants: General description. *Paraplegia*, 1994; 32:795–805.
8. Creasey G. Managing bladder, bowel and sexual function after spinal cord injury. *Handbook of Neuro-Urology*, Rushton D. (ed). Marcel Dekker, New York, 1994, pp. 233–251.
9. Davis R, Eckhouse J, Patrick J, Delehunty A. Computerized 22 channel stimulator for limb movement. *Appl Neurophysiol*, 1987; 50:444–448.
10. Davis R, Eckhouse J, Patrick J, Delehunty A. Computer-controlled 22-channel stimulator for limb movement. *Acta Neurochir*, 1987; 39:117–120.

11. Davis R, Kuzma J, Patrick J, Heller J, McKendry J, Eckhouse J, Emmons S. Nucleus FES-22 stimulator for motor function in a paraplegic subject. *RESNA Int*, Toronto, Canada, June 6–11, 1992; 228–229.
12. Davis R, MacFarland W, Emmons S. Initial results of the Nucleus FES-22-implanted stimulator for limb movement in paraplegia. *Stereotact Funct Neurosurg*, 1994; 63(1–3):192–197.
13. Davis R, Houdayer T, Andrews B, Emmons S, Patrick P. Paraplegia: Prolonged closed-loop standing with implanted nucleus FES-22 stimulator and Andrews foot–ankle orthosis. *Stereotact Funct Neurosurg*, 1997; 69:281–287.
14. Davis R, Houdayer T, Andrews B, Barriskill A. Prolonged closed-loop functional electrical stimulation and Andrews ankle–foot orthosis. *Artif Organs*, 1999; 23:418–420.
15. Davis R, Houdayer T, Andrews B, Barriskill A, Parker S. Paraplegia: Implantable Praxis24-FES system and external sensors for multi-functional restoration. *Proceedings of the 5th Annual Conference on International Functional Electrical Stimulation Society*, Aalborg, Denmark, June 18–21, 2000; pp. 35–38.
16. Davis R, Patrick J, Barriskill A. Development of functional electrical stimulators utilizing cochlear implant technology. *Med Electron Phys*, 2001; 23:61–68.
17. Schulman J, Mobley P, Wolfe J, Voelkel A, Davis R, Arcos I. An implantable bionic network of injectable neural prosthetic devices: The future platform for functional electrical stimulation and sensing to restore movement and sensation. In DiLorenzo DJ and Bronzino JD (eds). *Neuroengineering*. CRC Press, Boca Raton, FL, 2008; 18:1–16.

55

An Implantable Bionic Network of Injectable Neural Prosthetic Devices: The Future Platform for Functional Electrical Stimulation and Sensing to Restore Movement and Sensation

J. Schulman
Alfred Mann Foundation for Scientific Research

P. Mobley
Alfred Mann Foundation for Scientific Research

J. Wolfe
Alfred Mann Foundation for Scientific Research

Ross Davis
Florida Institute of Technology

I. Arcos
Alfred Mann Foundation for Scientific Research

55.1 Introduction 55-1
55.2 Evolution of the Implantable BION Devices 55-2
55.3 Battery-Powered BION System for Functional Electrical Stimulation and Sensing 55-4
55.4 Applications 55-13
References 55-15

55.1 Introduction

Functional electrical stimulation (FES) is a rehabilitation technique for the restoration of lost neurological function, resulting from conditions such as stroke, spinal cord injury, cerebral palsy, head injuries, and multiple sclerosis. FES utilizes low-level electrical current applied in programmed patterns to different nerves or reflex centers in the central nervous system to produce functional movements. The stimulation may be triggered by a single switch (open-loop) or from sensor(s) or neuronal activity (closed-loop).

While FES has been used successfully to pace the heart[1] and to restore hearing[2] in the past, it has not been widely adopted as a means of reanimating paralyzed limbs that result from stroke and spinal cord injury (SCI). It is estimated by the U.S. National Institutes of Health (NIH) that there are more than 600,000 people who experience a stroke each year in the United States, with an associated comprehensive cost of $43 billion per year.[3] Of the more than 4 million stroke survivors alive today, many experience permanent impairments of their ability to move, think, understand and use language, or speak—losses that compromise their independence and quality of life. Furthermore, stroke risk increases with age, and as the American population is growing older, the number of persons at risk for experiencing a stroke is increasing. There are also estimated to be 250,000 Americans living with spinal cord injuries with 10,000–12,000 new spinal cord injuries reported every year in the United States. The cost of managing the care of SCI patients approaches $4 billion each year.[4]

The potential of FES to restore function in these areas has been largely unfulfilled mostly due to the limitations of the FES devices currently available. FES could also be used in limb loss applications to reduce phantom pain and to restore the functional movement of prosthetic limbs. In 2000/2001, about 130,000 lower-limb amputations were performed each year in the United States.[5,6]

An optimal FES system should have the following fundamental characteristics. It should (1) provide both stimulating and sensing capabilities, (2) be fully implantable, (3) be minimally invasive, (4) have real-time communication capability, (5) allow a practically unlimited number of stimulation and sensing channels, and (6) function without external equipment or interconnected leads between components.

This chapter describes a network of wireless implantable microstimulators/microsensors, also known as battery-powered BION®[*] (BIOnic Neuron) devices for functional electrical stimulation and sensing (FES-BPB system). This new platform was designed to overcome the limitations of the current FES technology by providing

1. Microdevices that can be programmed to be either stimulators or sensors for use in closed-loop applications
2. Minimally invasive implantation procedures to reduce labor-intensive surgery and associated patient risks and to provide rapid recovery
3. Wireless bidirectional communications and telemetry to all stimulators and sensors, which eliminates the use of both transcutaneous leads (which are susceptible to infection), and surface applied coils and stimulators
4. Real-time communication between the stimulators, sensors, and control unit, to maintain continuous closed-loop control
5. Flexibility and functional expandability since there are no leads and each implant has a full complement of programmable stimulators and sensors
6. A large number of channels, which allows the same system to be used for a variety of applications without interference in the same patient
7. Self-powered operation using rechargeable batteries to power the implantable devices. External equipment (e.g., power antennas) are only needed during battery recharging
8. Wireless sensors capable of measuring biopotentials, angle, position, pressure, temperature, and permanent magnet fields

55.2 Evolution of the Implantable BION Devices

In 1988, J. Loeb proposed and W.J. Heetderks showed mathematically that the concept of a wireless network of injectable microstimulators powered by an external antenna/coil was possible.[7] It was thought that these microstimulators would eliminate many of the problems associated with the use of percutaneous electrodes, since they do not incorporate leads. J.H. Schulman, G.E. Loeb, and P.R. Troyk, under support contracts from the U.S. NIH (contract N01-NS-9-2327), the Alfred Mann Foundation (AMF, Santa Clarita, CA), and the Canadian Network for Neural Regeneration and Functional Recovery, developed an injectable, glass-enclosed microstimulator (Figure 55.1) that is powered and controlled by an external alternating magnetic field generated by a coil connected to a control unit. This first 255-channel stimulating system, later called the radio-frequency (RF) BION device, allowed instantaneous control of stimulation pulse amplitude, frequency, pulse width, pulse position timing, and pulse charge-recovery current.[8]

AMF continued to develop and improve the wireless RF BION device. As a result of these efforts, a second-generation RF BION device, which incorporates a ceramic case, an output capacitor, and Zener

---

[*] BION is a registered trademark of the Advanced Bionics Corporation, a Boston Scientific company.

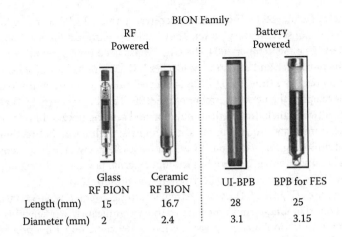

FIGURE 55.1 Evolution of the BION devices. It shows four BIONS to the same scale.

diodes to protect the device against electrostatic discharges, was developed (Figure 55.1).[9] These RF BION devices are currently being used or have been used in several clinical studies being conducted by AMF and its affiliated organizations, the Alfred Mann Institute (University of Southern California, Los Angeles, CA) and Advanced Bionics Corporation (Santa Clarita, CA). As of September 2004, 33 patients have been implanted with RF BION devices for the treatment of urinary incontinence, obstructive sleep apnea, pain associated with shoulder subluxation, knee osteoarthritis, forearm contracture, and foot drop applications.[10–13]

While the wireless RF BION device eliminates the need for the leads associated with the percutaneous electrodes, it requires the patient to wear an external coil during use, to transmit power and data to the implanted device. To both improve the patient acceptance of this technology and increase the reliability of the system, it was necessary to eliminate the need to constantly use an external coil to power and control the device. Thus, the idea for a battery-powered BION device (hereinafter BPB) was conceived at the AMF.

AMF developed, with guidance from Jet Propulsion Lab (JPL), a small cylindrical lithium ion rechargeable battery. A new company (Quallion, Inc.) was formed and financed by Alfred Mann to manufacture and improve these unique highly reliable batteries. Today, these batteries can be safely recharged if discharged to 0 V and are expected to operate for over 10 years. These batteries were designed specifically for the BPB (Figure 55.2).

AMF licensed the BPB technology to Advanced Bionics Corp., which designed and implemented the first BPB (stimulator only) for urinary incontinence (referred to as the UI–BPB). This was the first BION

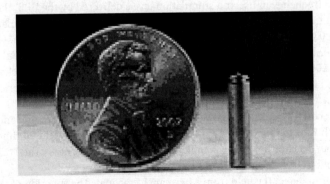

FIGURE 55.2 Quallion battery for the BPB.

to have two-way telemetry (Figure 55.1). The telemetry receiver in this UI-BPB turns on for a very short time interval every 1.5 s, to conserve battery power. Thus, rapid synchronization for limb control is not feasible with the UI-BPB. As of September 2004, the UI-BPB has been implanted in 35 patients for the treatment of urinary incontinence and migraine headaches.[14] Owing to its lack of sensing capabilities and slow communication response time, the UI-BPB is not well suited for FES applications.

AMF is currently developing the next generation of the BPB. This BPB (Figure 55.1) allows the creation of a wireless FES network, including both stimulation and sensing in each BPB for fully implantable closed-loop applications; data processing for sensed signals; high-speed bidirectional telemetry; wireless oscilloscope monitoring for fitting purposes, via back telemetry of voltage-sensed signals; a rechargeable battery (enabling prolonged operation without external power); and capability of communications with over 850 BPBs simultaneously (effectively 100 communications/s).[15]

The ceramic BION devices (Figure 55.1) use an extremely strong zirconia with 3% yttrium ceramic case. The FDA pointed out that long-term immersion in water significantly weakens this ceramic (Joe Schulman, personal communication). Over a 3-year period, AMF came up with a process to improve the longevity of this ceramic. Today, accelerated life testing has shown that this ceramic will retain 80% of its strength after 80 years of soaking in saline solution.[16-18]

55.3 Battery-Powered BION System for Functional Electrical Stimulation and Sensing

The FES-BPB system is a wireless, multichannel network of separately implantable battery-powered BION devices that can be used for both stimulation and sensing. The system is composed of a master control unit (MCU), a clinician's programmer, a recharging subsystem (charger and coil), and BPBs. Additional equipment, dissolvable suture material, and surgical insertion tools (used only during the implantation procedure) are also part of the system. The FES-BPB system can be set up for use in two configurations: fitting mode and stand–alone mode. A block diagram of the FES-BPB system is shown in Figure 55.3.

The MCU is the communication and control hub for the FES-BPB system. The MCU transmits commands to and receives data from all the BPBs and the recharging subsystem. There are two versions contemplated for the MCU packaging: (1) an external MCU, which will be outside the body and have a few controls accessible to the patient, and (2) an implantable MCU, which will be implanted in a convenient location in the body. The implantable MCU version will have a small patient control unit (PCU).

The clinician's programmer consists of software loaded on a computer that allows the clinician to configure and test the FES-BPB system for each patient.

The recharging subsystem (charger and coil) is used when the rechargeable battery of the BPB needs to be recharged. The charging process requires the placement of the coil close to the area on the patient's body where the BPB is implanted. Recharging is mandatory when the battery of the BPB is low. Depending on the frequency of use and stimulation levels delivered by the BPB, the battery could potentially run down in 1–8 days. Under normal stimulation conditions (nerve stimulation of 1–2 mA pulse amplitude, 15–100 μs pulse width, and 20 pulses per second), charging for about 5–20 min per day is required to charge the battery. The BPB maximum stimulation capability (20 mA pulse amplitude at 14 V compliance with 200 μs pulse width and 125 pulses per second) can rapidly discharge the battery in a very short time and would result in the need to recharge the battery for longer periods of time and much more frequently.

The external charger coil transmits only power to the implanted devices. Charging and battery status are transmitted by each BPB to the MCU. Each BPB can accept a charging field 20 times the nominal field to recharge, without overheating. Upon completion of the charging process, the MCU then issues a stop-charging command to the charger.

The BPB has a sensor to detect the field from a permanent magnet. The function of the magnet is to hold the stimulation off. This is a safety feature in case the BPB is stimulating in an undesired manner

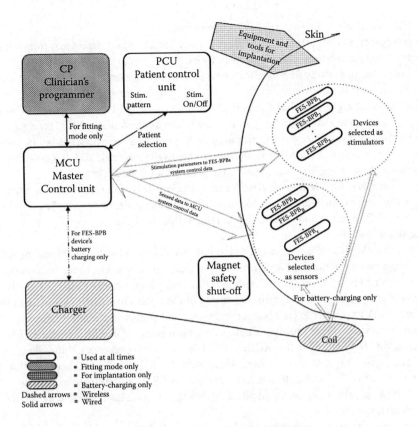

FIGURE 55.3   Functional electrical stimulation and sensor system (FES-BPB).

and the patient does not have access to his control unit. When the magnet is positioned on the patient's body over the area where the BPB is implanted, a magnetic sensor inside the BPB detects the external magnetic field and holds the stimulation off. When the magnet is removed, the stimulation turns back on. This is the default mode of the magnetic detector. Other modes can be programmed during fitting.

The BPB implantation is performed in a minimally invasive procedure and is accomplished using a combination of specially designed insertion tools and commercially available items.

The functional description of the FES-BPB system components is presented here:

1. Master control unit

   The MCU is the communication and control hub for the FES-BPB system. The MCU transmits commands to and receives data from each one of up to a total of 850 BPBs in the system within one-hundredth of a second. When the patient uses the FES-BPB system (stand-alone mode), the MCU coordinates the activity of the BPBs by receiving data from implanted devices programmed as sensors, transmitting stimulation commands, and monitoring the overall system status. It also serves as the basic user interface for the patient, providing system ON/OFF control and alarms, as well as program selection and limited parameter control. During fitting, the MCU acts as a conduit between the clinician's programmer and the rest of the system, enabling the transparent setup of each BPB and the coordination needed among BPBs to implement the desired functional movement.

   The MCU also manages the recharging subsystem. The charger communicates with the system in the same manner that the BPBs do, and it can be turned ON/OFF or checked for correct operation via the MCU.

The MCU contains the following safety mechanisms:

- An emergency STOP button on the external MCU, which when depressed, immediately issues a "stop stimulation" command to all BPBs.
- During recharging, if any BPB overheats or overcharges and cannot protect itself, it would communicate this information to the MCU, which would issue a "stop charging" command to the charger and alert the patient. If an external MCU is being used, it would produce a sound to alert the patient. In the case where an implantable MCU is being used, the MCU would send a command to the BPBs to produce a specific stimulation pattern to alert the patient and would also communicate with the external PCU, if it is within the communication range. The PCU would then generate an audible alert.

The MCU also stores patient usage data for the clinician. This data can be used to verify compliance and to analyze the stimulation and sensing parameters of each session. The approximate location of each BPB in the body is also maintained in this database.

2. Software and firmware

The software for the FES-BPB system is divided into two components. One component is the clinician's programmer application, which runs on a laptop computer. The other component is the firmware running on the MCU. The PC with the clinician's programmer interfaces with the MCU via a serial communication link. During the fitting of the system to a particular patient, the two components work in concert to facilitate measurement and storage of the stimulation and sensor calibration parameters. Once these parameters have been gathered in a fitting session, the essential information can be stored in the MCU, so that the MCU can operate in a stand-alone mode to facilitate the desired functional movement. Ultimately, the MCU will modulate the stimulation output in response to the information it receives from the BPBs programmed as sensors.

The clinician's programmer uses a graphical interface that contains screens to perform the following essential functions:

- Gather basic personal information for the patient, including information about the location in the body of his/her BPBs
- Establish the stimulation range for each implanted BPB and allow selection of the stimulation parameters
- Specify the details of the activity sequences that will be involved in the FES algorithm
- Gather the trigger information that will be used to generate transitions between activity sequences in response to the sensor inputs
- Compose the finite-state machine functions that will drive a routine and download the complete program to the MCU for either immediate execution or later use

3. Battery-powered BION device (BPB)

The BPB is a battery-powered microdevice that is capable of both delivering electrical stimulation and acting as a general-purpose sensor for recording biopotential signals, pressure, distance, or angle between two BPBs and temperature. The following sections describe the functional building blocks of the BPB, battery, and packaging. The specifications of the BPB are provided in Table 55.1, Section 6. Figure 55.4 shows the internal components of the BPB and Figure 55.5 shows a cross section of an assembled BPB.

The BPB has the following subsystems:

3.1 Stimulation

The BPB is a single-channel, constant-current, charge-balanced stimulator. The stimulation output is capacitance-coupled, which also prevents direct connection between the battery or battery-generated DC voltages and the tissue. Stimulation pulse amplitude, width, and frequency can be independently adjusted. In addition, triggering events can cause the stimulation to be delivered continuously or in a pulse burst, which can be ramped up and/or down with a variety of start/stop times.

TABLE 55.1   Battery-Powered BION Device Specifications

1. **Physical**

Implant weight	0.6 g		
Implant length with eyelet++ and diameter	$25~mm_{max}$ length/$3.15~mm_{max}$ diameter		
Electrodes area	5.2 sq. mm (0.008 sq. in.) stimulation electrode		
	12.8 sq. mm (0.019 sq. in.) return electrode		
Case materials	Yttria-stabilized zirconia; titanium 6Al4V alloy		
Electrode material	Iridium		

2. **Stimulation parameters**

Pulse amplitude	5 µA to 20 mA in 3.3% exponential steps (255 levels)		
Pulse width	7.6–1953 µs in 7.6 or 15.2 µs steps		
Pulse frequency	1–4096 pps		
Stimulation control response time	10.6 ms maximum		
Capacitor recharge current	10–500 µA		
Compliance voltage	Up to 14 V automatically adjusted		
Stimulation output capacitor	4 µF		
Delay to start from a trigger	0–42.4 h in 15.6 ms, 125 ms, 2 s, 1 min, 10 min steps		
Burst On/Off time	Min	Max	Step
Range 1	0.031 s	0.9996 s	0.0156 s
Range 2	0.25 s	8.00 s	0.125 s
Range 3	4 s	128 s	2 s
Range 4	2 min.	64 min.	1 min.

3. **Sensors**

Temperature	16°–50°C with 0.3% accuracy
Magnetic field to trigger shut off	10.0 Gauss threshold
Goniometry (number of frequency channels)	8
Range	1–20 cm
Repeatable accuracy error	Less than 1% for 1–10 cm
Pressure (range)	Readout = AC-coupled. 300–900 mm-Hg absolute
Accuracy	±10 mm-Hg
Biopotential sensing (amplification)	10, 30, 100, 300, 1000
Low frequency roll-off	1, 10, 30, 100, 300 Hz
High frequency roll-off	300, 1 K, 3 K, 10 K Hz
Notch filter	50 or 60 Hz
Input referred noise	5 µVrms

4. **Communication**

Number of implants per patient	Up to 850 at 10 ms
ID, MCU/BPB	27/30 bits
Bandwidth	5 MHz
Sense-to-stimulate delay	10.6 ms maximum
Frequency band	100–500 MHz
MCU to BPB data rate 15 bits/6 µs	(15-bits data + 16-bits FEC)/6 µs
BPB to MCU data rate 8 bits/5 µs	(8-bits data + 8-bits FEC)/5 µs
Data streaming (oscilloscope mode)	39.8 K samples/s × 3 channels (8-bit resolution)

5. **Charging**

Frequency of charging field	127 kHz
Excessive magnetic field permissible	20 times nominal

continued

TABLE 55.1   (continued) Battery-Powered BION Device Specifications

6.	Battery: Lithium ion rechargeable, hermetically sealed	
	Battery length and diameter	13 mm length, 2.5 mm diameter
	Battery weight	0.21 g
	Battery capacity	3.0 mAh, 10 mWh
	Cell voltage range	3.0–4.0 V (3.6 V nom.)
	Battery life	Nominally 10 years (usage dependent)

FEC = Forward error correction.

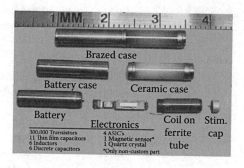

FIGURE 55.4   Battery-powered BION internal components.

3.2 Communication

The bidirectional propagated wave RF communication between the MCU and the BPBs is established through a dipole antenna (Figure 55.5). This link operates at a frequency in the band 100–500 MHz, using Quad phase modulation with a 5 MHz bandwidth. The BPB communication module includes a crystal-controlled transmitter, receiver, and digital processing unit that synchronizes with and processes the MCU transmissions. The digital processing unit in the BPB also corrects small numbers of errors in the received data, decodes the MCU commands, and generates the responses to the MCU, including the reporting of higher numbers of communication errors that cannot be mathematically corrected. In this latter situation, the MCU would resend the message.

The communication protocol between the MCU and BPBs is shown in Figure 55.6. The timing of the frame is completely controlled by the MCU and every BPB will synchronize to its MCU's clock.

The header and trailer fields are used for frame synchronization and for carrying frame control data intended for all BPBs and/or for other MCUs. When an MCU detects another MCU, the one with the higher ID number shifts the time slots of all the BPBs it is controlling,

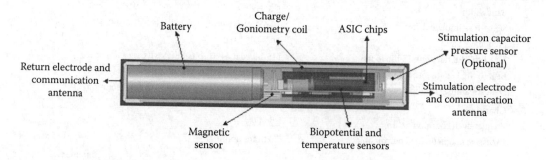

FIGURE 55.5   Battery-powered BION device cross section.

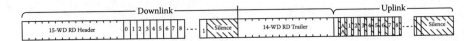

FIGURE 55.6 MCU: BPB communication protocol.

to avoid communication interference. Once the MCU assigns the time slots for the downlink and uplink data packets to each one of the BPBs in the net, each BPB turns on its receiving or transmitting circuitry for only a few microseconds at the assigned times in each frame to save battery. The downlink data packets contain stimulation and/or sensing control data and forward error correction (FEC) bits to correct up to 4- or 5-bit errors. Bit errors beyond that number are reported to the MCU, which will then resend the message. If some messages are vital, the message would be sent twice or the value would be sent back to the MCU for the MCU to verify and authorize the command. Uplink data packets are transmitted by each of the BPBs and are used to carry information to the MCU (e.g., sensed data). The FEC in the uplink data packet only corrects 1- or 2-bit errors.

3.3 Power (battery and charging)

The main power source for the BPB is a 10 mWh rechargeable lithium ion battery that allows the implanted device to operate as a stand-alone stimulator/sensor. Its special nonflammable lithium ion chemistry provides long life and permits the voltage to go to zero and be recovered safely without damage to the battery. The recharge process is achieved via a low frequency (127 kHz) magnetic link with an external coil worn or placed nearby when charging. Assuming continuous stimulation pulses at 20 pps with 100 μs pulse width and 2 mA pulse amplitude into a 2 kΩ load, the battery of a BPB selected as a stimulator will provide 100 h of continuous operation. For a BPB selected as a sensor, the battery will also provide 100 h of continuous operation.

The lithium ion battery is specified to have a cycle life of 2000 cycles for a standard charge/discharge cycle, which is a fairly deep discharge of the battery before recharge occurs. The nominal stimulation/sensing requirements in many applications are such that the battery would not be discharged to the standard low level (if recharged daily). Thus, the 2000 cycles represent a lifetime of over 10 years if the battery is recharged daily.

3.4 Safety

The BPB includes the following safety features:

- A miniature magnetic sensor that detects the magnetic field from an external magnet and holds off the stimulation if, for some reason, it needs to be turned off.
- A temperature sensor that communicates with the charger, via the MCU, to terminate charging, if appropriate and disconnects the battery when the temperature rises above a predetermined threshold.
- Battery safety circuitry that protects the battery from overvoltage, overdischarge, and overcharging.
- BPBs can protect themselves from magnetic fields in excess of 20 times the field necessary for maximum charging and, for a short time, for fields in excess of 50 times the field for maximum charging. This short time is more than sufficient for the BPB to send a message to the MCU to turn off the charger and to alert the patient of the risk.

3.5 Biopotential sensing, data display, and data analysis

The biopotential function is implemented to record neural or muscular electrical signals (EMG signals). Biopotential sensing is accomplished using a low-noise amplifier and band–pass filter circuit, followed by a digital postprocessing circuit. The amplifier is adjustable from a gain of 10 to a gain of 1000. The low-frequency setting of the band–pass filter is adjustable from below 1 to 300 Hz. The high-frequency setting is adjustable from 300 Hz to 10 kHz. Input referred noise is less than 5 μVrms (20 μV peak).

3.5.1 Data display: Oscilloscope mode

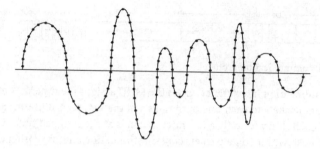

FIGURE 55.7   Biopotential sensing module, oscilloscope display mode.

During fitting, the analog signal from the amplifier/filter section can be digitized and transmitted from the BPB to the MCU to the clinician's programmer screen at a rate of 40,000 samples per second. This "oscilloscope mode" (Figure 55.7) can be used when evaluating the placement of the BPB and during fitting, but it is not suitable for long-term use due to its high power demands.

3.5.2 Data analysis

The analog output of the biopotential sensor also passes to a programmable window detection circuitry that can be set by the clinician to (1) count pulses that fall within (or above or below) the set thresholds (Figure 55.8, left), or (2) rectify and integrate the sensed signal (Figure 55.8, right). (1) Counting pulses: The neuronal pulses that occur are accumulated every 10 ms and relayed to the MCU. (2) Rectify and integrate: Every 10 ms, if required, the circuit can rectify the amplitude of the biopotential sensor's analog output and sum up the average rectified signal. An output between 0 and 255 will be generated, indicating the average energy occurring every 10 ms.

3.6 Pressure sensing

Some BPBs will be fabricated with a pressure transducer mounted at one end. The initial version of this sensor is about 3 mm in diameter and is sensitive to pressures along the axial dimension of the BPB. Future versions will be sensitive to lateral pressure, and may be mounted remotely from the BPB. The present full-scale absolute pressure range is 400–900 mm-Hg. This signal can be read out either AC- or DC-coupled. When DC-coupled, it reads the absolute pressure. Since ambient pressure varies with altitude changes, this offset can be accounted for by placing a reference sensor of the same type in the MCU, then subtracting off this baseline.

3.7 Angle/position sensing (goniometry)

The same internal coil that is used to receive the magnetic field to charge the BPB battery, may also be programmed as a transmitter in any selected BPB or as a receiver in another selected BPB. The goniometry function is implemented using one BPB as a transmitter, and the other BPB as a receiver. The BPB programmed as a receiver, detects and measures the

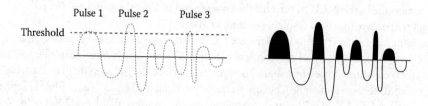

FIGURE 55.8   Data analysis with the BPB biopotential sensing module. Left: Counting pulses above threshold line. Right: Rectify and integrate neural signal.

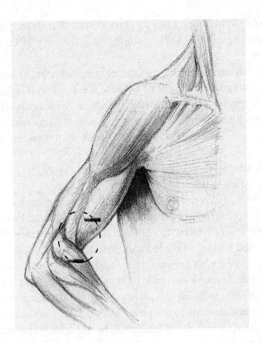

FIGURE 55.9 Use of BPBs for distance/angle measurements.

signal strength of the received signal (Figure 55.9). The distance between two BPBs is derived from the intensity of the received magnetic field, which falls off approximately with the cube of the distance between the devices.

There are eight different programmable transmitter–receiver frequencies available for goniometry use. The eight frequencies are clustered around 127 kHz. This permits eight parallel goniometry systems consisting of one transmitter and any number of receivers. There is no limit on the number of BPB receivers that can process the signal strength to give distance measurements (from each of the transmitters). Each BPB receiver is able to send back a measurement 100 times per second. A goniometry pair (transmitter–receiver) can be used to measure distances between 1 and 20 cm.

3.8 Temperature sensing

An internal temperature sensor is incorporated as an additional safety mechanism to guard against overheating of the BPB and to provide temperature data to patients, such as certain quadriplegics who do not sense temperature. The sensor is accurate to within one-third degree Celsius and is operable over the range from 16°C to 50°C. In the event a significant temperature rise is detected, the BPB can be shut down and/or communication with the MCU can be made to initiate appropriate external action (such as shutting down the charging field, if present). Readings are taken once per second and can be read by the MCU.

4. Recharging subsystem (charger and external coil)

The charger produces a 127 kHz signal that generates a magnetic field in the charging coil. The MCU communicates with the charger to indicate when to turn on a charging field. The MCU interrogates each BPB to determine which BPB is going to be charged and when the BPB is fully charged. The MCU determines which BPBs are not being charged and indicates to the patient where the coil has to be moved to charge those BPBs. If the charger is coupled to several coils but can only power one coil at a time, the MCU can then cause the charger to switch coils so the uncharged BPBs can be charged. The MCU can also determine the state of the charge in each BPB and can initially select the most discharged devices to be charged first.

The recharging subsystem includes a temperature sensor that stops the recharging process if the external coil temperature adjacent to the patient skin, rises over 41°C.

5. Magnet

The patient can stop stimulation by placing an external magnet near the location of the implanted device(s). A neodymium magnet is being used because it is small and lightweight, and because it produces a very strong magnetic signal. The default mode of this magnet is to hold the stimulation off when the magnet is positioned on the patient's body, over the area where the BPB is implanted. When the magnet is removed, the stimulation turns back on. Other magnet control modes are available.

6. FES-BPB system specifications

7. Minimally invasive procedure to implant BPBs

To implant a BPB, a minimally invasive procedure is followed. The implantation procedure can be done in a clean procedure room, where the patient's implant sites can be surgically cleansed and draped with sterile towels and covered with adherent sterile plastic drapes. The implant physician scrubs his/her forearms and hands, is gowned and gloved, and wears a cap and mask.

The implantation (insertion) tools are shown in Figure 55.10. Under local anesthesia, a 5-mm skin incision is made. A sterile probe electrode (0.71 mm OD; insulated except at the tips, Figure 55.10) connected to an external stimulator is directed into the tissues to excite and find the target nerve/motor-point. With adjustments to the probe electrode, the optimal target muscle contraction is located. A customized introducer (dilator plus sheath) is then slid over the probe electrode. Stimulation with the probe electrode is repeated to ensure a similar optimal response and correct location. The probe electrode and dilator are then withdrawn, leaving the sheath in position.

The BPB has a dissolvable suture attached to the return electrode. The BPB's stimulation electrode end is inserted into the sheath and gently pushed by the ejection tool to the sheath tip so that only the BPB stimulation electrode end protrudes. From the ejection tool tip, saline is infused into the sheath to allow the anodal end of the BPB to have electrical connection to the tissues through small holes in the distal sheath. The BPB is activated to test and confirm its optimal position relative to the target nerve/motor-point. By withdrawing the sheath over the ejection tool, the BPB is deposited into the tissues (Figure 55.11). The sheath and the ejection tool are then removed.

The BPB is retested to confirm that the optimal response is achieved. If this position is not satisfactory in regard to the responses to stimulation or recording, then the BPB can be retrieved by pulling on the suture attached to the BPB (Figure 55.12) and then reinserted. The emerging sutures are cut at the subcutaneous tissue level, and the wound is then closed.

The implanted BPB is tested 1 week after implantation to confirm that the responses are still adequate. If an inadequate response is observed, the wound could be reopened and the BPB retrieved by pulling on the sutures. A new BPB could then be reinserted to obtain proper response.

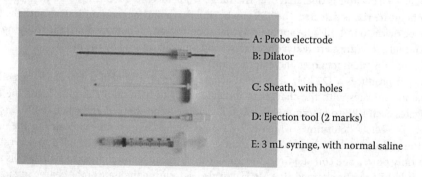

A: Probe electrode

B: Dilator

C: Sheath, with holes

D: Ejection tool (2 marks)

E: 3 mL syringe, with normal saline

FIGURE 55.10 BPB implantation tools.

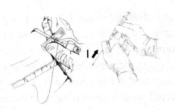

FIGURE 55.11 BPB implantation technique.

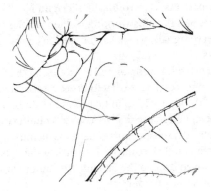

FIGURE 55.12 Retrieval of BPB.

55.4 Applications

The different functions of the BPB (as a stimulator, biopotential signal sensor, goniometry sensor, pressure or temperature sensor) and the availability of multiple BPBs in one patient (up to 850 BPBs) gives the clinician many opportunities to restore neurological function, especially in poststroke syndrome, spinal cord injury, cerebral palsy, multiple sclerosis, traumatic brain injury, and for limb sensing in amputees to control fitted prostheses.

Take, for example, the case where a paralyzed upper extremity is implanted with multiple BPBs placed near motor-points or nerves of muscles in the arm, forearm, and hand. It will be possible to trigger sequential functional muscle actions to extend the arm and forearm, and open the hand to grasp an object. The limits of each functional action can be controlled from implanted BPBs working as goniometry sensors, measuring the angles of the elbow (see Figure 55.9) and wrist and implanted BPBs working as pressure sensors, measuring the pressure at the finger tip (Figure 55.13).

The reverse of this extension can be similarly achieved using this stimulating and sensing system to bring the grasped object, for example, to the mouth. Similar closed-loop controls of stimulation could be used in

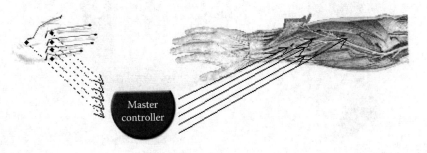

FIGURE 55.13 BPBs measuring pressure in fingers.

the lower extremities for standing and ambulation. For partially paralyzed extremities, sensing of the muscle activities using BPBs would act as triggers to other BPBs to stimulate the motor-points of these muscles, thus augmenting the total action. Goniometry sensors would add the closed-loop controls to reduce or stop the actions. This approach could be used to augment swallowing, bladder control, and respiration.

Where pressure points need to be monitored, for example, at the heel (as a trigger for improving walking on stroke patients) or buttock (to avoid pressure sores) or hand (to detect the grasping of an object), BPB devices placed in these sites can measure the pressure and either trigger motor-point functional stimulation to activate muscles or stop a functional stimulation sequence.

8. FES-BPB system in amputee patients: Controlling artificial limbs

For amputee patients (Figure 55.14), BPBs working as biopotential sensors, are inserted in the "stump" to pick up motor nerve signals, which can be used to control the movement of the artificial limb flexible components.

9. Cortical interface device: A cortical stimulator and sensor using the BPB system technology

Individuals with spinal cord injury or disease that limits control over voluntary motion or sensing may be able to regain some of the ability of voluntary motion by monitoring the motor cortex and feeding back sensed response signals to the sensory cortex. Voluntary motion is expressed as neural activity in the motor cortex. The sensory cortex depends on muscle spindles and other sensors to help control the limb movement. By feeding back signals to the sensory cortex, the psychological use of the limb would be given back to the patient. The motor cortex signals can also be used to control wheel chairs and other helpful devices.

The miniaturized components developed for the BPB are used to create a cortical interface device (CID) with multiple stimulation and sensing electrodes within a single implantable package (Figure 55.15). The CID has the capability of monitoring up to several hundred electrodes that can be implanted or positioned in the motor cortex, sensory cortex, or a combination of both. The CID system consists of a base unit implanted in the skull, underneath the scalp, and one or several electrode arrays placed on the sensory or motor cortices.

The CID is equivalent to a group of 64 BPBs in its communication ability. It also includes an additional switching matrix that allows any amplifier to sense voltages either unipolar or bipolar from any two electrodes. The CID base unit dimensions and internal components are shown in Figure 55.16. The CID is constructed with the same technology developed for the BPB. It contains the same electronics as those used in the BPB as far as the communication, charging, power management, biopotential sensing, and stimulation modules are concerned. A CID base unit contains

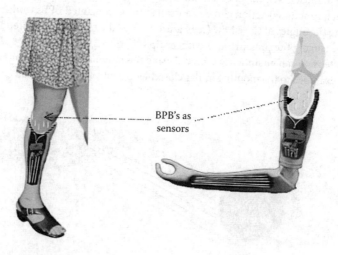

BPB's as
sensors

FIGURE 55.14 Use of BPBs in amputee patients.

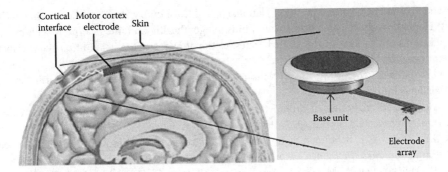

FIGURE 55.15 Cortical interface device.

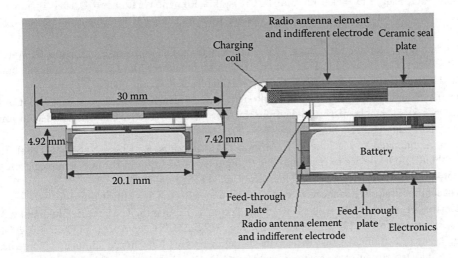

FIGURE 55.16 Cortical interface device. Left: Dimensions. Right: Cross section.

64 biopotential sensing modules attached to one or more electrode arrays. The battery used in the CID provides 50 mAh at 3.6 V.

The electrode arrays could be configured for sensing or stimulating purposes. The sensing electrode array includes signal processing capabilities by using the same electronics as those in the biopotential sensing module in the BPB. The stimulating electrode array contains the same stimulation electronics as those in the BPB stimulation module. The CID contains a powerful microprocessor to analyze the signals from the motor cortex and to reduce the data to 64 eight-bit messages that the MCU can use to control up to 64 muscles.

References

1. Heart Disease and Stroke Statistics—2004 Update, American Heart Association.
2. http://www.bionicear.com/support/clinical_papers/supp_research_demo2.html, http://www.bionicear.com/support/clinical_papers/supp_research_demo1.html, http://www.bionicear.com/printables/Bilateral.pdf, http://www.nidcd.nih.gov/health/hearing/coch_moreon.asp, http://www.cochlear.com/896.asp.
3. Stroke Testimony before the House Committee on Energy and Commerce Subcommittee on Health. NINDS opening statement to the House Committee on Energy and Commerce Subcommittee on Health, June 6, 2002. http://www.ninds.nih.gov/about_ninds/2002_stroke_testimony.htm#background

4. Facts and Figures at a Glance. May 2001. National Spinal Cord Injury Statistical Center. Spinal Cord Injury: Hope through Research http://www.ninds.nih.gov/health_and_medical/pubs/sci.htm

5. Complications of Diabetes in the United States. National Diabetes Statistics. http://www.diabetes.niddk.nih.gov/dm/pubs/statistics/

6. Amputee Statistics (SAMPLE) from National Database http://rehabtech.eng.monash.edu/techguide/als/Stats.htm

7. Heetderks, W.J. RF powering of millimeter- and submillimeter-sized neural prosthetic implants. *IEEE Trans. Biomed. Eng.* 35, 323–327, 1988.

8. Loeb, G.E., Zamin, C.J., Schulman, J.H., Troyk, P.R. Injectable microstimulator for functional electrical stimulation. *Med. Biol. Eng Comput.* 29, NS13–NS19, 1991.

9. Arcos, I., Davis, R., Fey, K., Mishler, D., Sanderson, D., Tanacs, C., Vogel, M.J., Wolf, R., Zilberman, Y., Schulman, J. Second-generation microstimulator. *Artif. Organs* 26, 228–231, 2002.

10. Dupont, A.C., Bagg, S.D., Baker L., Chun S., Creasy, J.L., Romano C., Romano, D. et al. Therapeutic electrical stimulation with BIONS: Clinical trial report. *Proc. IEEE-EMBS Conference* (Houston, TX, 2002).

11. Richmond, F.J.R., Dupont, A.C., Bagg, S.D., Chun, S., Creasy, J.L., Romano, C., Romano, D., Waters, R.L., Wederich, C.L., Loeb, G.E. Therapeutic electrical stimulation with BIONs to rehabilitate shoulder and knee dysfunction. *Proc. IFESS Conference* (Ljubljana, Slovenia, 2002).

12. Buller, J.L., Cundiff, G.W., Noel, K.A., VanRooyen, J.A., Leffler, K.S., Ellerkman, R.M., Bent, A.E. RF BION™: An injectable microstimulator for the treatment of overactive bladder disorders in adult females. *European Association of Urology* (Feb 2002).

13. Misawa, A., Shimada Y., Matsunaga, T., Aizawa, T., Hatakeyama, K., Chida, S., Sato, M. et al. The use of the RF BION device to treat pain due to shoulder subluxation in chronic hemiplegic stroke patient—A case report. *Proc. IFESS Conference* (United Kingdom, 2004).

14. E-mail communication, Advanced Bionics Corporation, a Boston Scientific Company.

15. Schulman, J. H., Mobley, J. P., Wolfe, J., Regev, E., Perron, C.Y., Ananth, R., Matei, E., Glukhovsky, A., Davis, R.. Battery powered BION FES network. *Proc. IEEE-EMBS Conference* (San Francisco, 2004).

16. Jiang, G., Fay, K., Schulman, J. In-Vitro and in-vivo aging tests of BION® micro-stimulator. Biomedical Engineering Department, University of Southern California, Los Angeles, CA. *7th Annual Fred S. Grodins Graduate Research Symposium*, March 2003.

17. Jiang, G., Purnell, K., Schulman, J. Accelerated life tests and in-vivo tests of 3Y-TZP ceramics. *Materials & Processes for Medical Devices Conference, Proc.* 2003.

18. Jiang, G., Mishler, D., Davis, R., Mobley, P., Schulman, J. Ceramic to metal seal for implantable medical device. Biomed. Eng. Dept. USC, Los Angeles, CA. *Proc. 8th Annual F. Grodins Graduate Research Symposium*, pp. 92–92, March 2004.

56

Visual Prostheses

Robert J. Greenberg
Second Sight Inc.

Acknowledgment...56-5
References..56-5

The possibility of restoring vision to blind patients using electricity began with the discovery that an electric charge delivered to a blind eye produces a sensation of light. This discovery was made by LeRoy in 1755.[1] However, it was not until 1966 that the first human experiments in this field began with Giles Brindley's experiments with electrical stimulation of the visual cortex.[2] He used 180 cortical surface electrodes that were able to perceive spots of light called "phosphenes" but they were ill defined and could not be combined to make an image. This did fail to produce useful vision in these patients. Similar experiments by William Dobelle in 1974 essentially produced the same results.[3,4]

Since these early experiments, efforts have been underway to produce penetrating arrays of electrodes that offer the possibility of more closely spaced electrodes and therefore, higher-resolution cortical devices.[5–8] Richard Normann (University of Utah) has micromachined 100 electrodes out of silicon, which were primarily used for recording in the sensory cortex of animals.[5] Another group at the University of Michigan led by Ken Wise has also produced micromachined penetrating electrodes for recording.[6] In the 1990s, an effort at the National Institute of Health (NIH) headed by Terry Hambrecht made an array of 38 penetrating microelectrodes, which were implanted in a patient and yielded separable phosphenes at electrode placements closer than that had been produced with surface electrodes.[7,8] Electronics for an implantable cortical prosthesis are being developed (with 1024 channels) at the Illinois Institute of Technology by Philip Troyk (personal communication).

While the cortical-stimulation approaches have made progress, it has been hampered by the physiology. The processing that has occurred by the time the neural signals have reached the cortex is greater than the more distal sites such as the retina. This results in more complex phosphenes being perceived by the patient. The surgery and the implanted prosthesis do provide risks such as intracranial hemorrhage to a blind patient who has an otherwise normal brain. These factors and the lack of availability of implantable electronics have limited the clinical application of these devices.

The limitations of the cortical approach encouraged several groups in the United States over the last 10 years to explore the possibility of producing vision in patients with an intact optic nerve with damaged photoreceptors from stimulating the retina.[9–15] The likely candidate diseases are retinitis pigmentosa (RP) or age-related macular degeneration (AMD). It is difficult to determine exactly how many patients are blinded by these diseases since patients often stop seeing their ophthalmologist after being told there is nothing that can be done. However, estimates of legal blindness in the Western (developed world) run as high as 300,000 people with RP and 3,000,000 people with AMD. 1.2 million people are afflicted (but not yet blind) with RP worldwide and 10 million people are afflicted with AMD in the United States alone.[16]

There have emerged two major approaches to retinal stimulation—epiretinal and subretinal. In the epiretinal approach, electrodes are placed on top of the retina to produce phosphenes. In the subretinal approach, photodiodes are implanted underneath the retina and are used to generate currents, which stimulate the retina. The epiretinal approach has been pursued by a team at the Johns Hopkins University led by Eugene de Juan and Mark Humayun[9,15] and another approach has been pursued at Harvard/MIT Centers led by Joseph Rizzo and John Wyatt.[10] Recently, Rizzo and Wyatt have decided to pursue the subretinal approach. Second Sight, a privately held company in Sylmar, CA is developing a chronically implantable epiretinal prosthesis. Six patients have been implanted with a first-generation device containing 16 electrodes and a 60-electrode second-generation device should be implanted in patients soon. Patients with the first device have shown the ability to read large letters, locate objects, and detect the direction of motion of objects and light. They have also shown the ability to discriminate multiple levels of gray. The second-generation device is expected to work even better. The subretinal approach has been pursued by the Chow brothers in Chicago—one an ophthalmologist and the other an engineer—who have formed a company called Optobionics (Chicago, IL).[14] They implanted 10 patients in an initial feasibility study that showed some temporary subjective improvements in vision that Optobionics believes was caused by a secondary neurotrophic effect and not direct stimulation by the implant and, more recently, they have implanted 20 additional patients at three centers with better vision than the first group. Subretinal and epiretinal implants are also being pursued in Germany by large groups led by Eberhart Zrenner[11] and Rolf Eckmiller,[12] respectively. Two companies have been formed in Germany by these individuals as well. There is also a group in Japan at Nagoya University led by Tohru Yagi. This group is primarily focused on cultured neuron preparations (personal communication).

Finally, there is a group at the Neural Rehabilitation Engineering Laboratory in Brussels, Belgium led by Claude Veraart who has implanted a nerve cuff electrode with four electrodes around the optic nerve of a blind patient. That patient is able to identify which quadrant she sees a phosphene.[17] Recently, a second patient has been implanted with an eight-channel device. The new device was implanted inside the ocular orbit and has not performed as well as the first implant.

On February 19, 2000, the inaugural symposium of the Alfred Mann Institute-University of Southern California (AMI-USC) titled, "Can We Make the Blind See?—Prospects for Restoring Vision to the Blind" was held. The lecturers included Dean Baker, director of the AMI-USC; Gerald Loeb, an FES (functional electrical stimulation) researcher at the AMI-USC; Dean Bok, a retinal physiologist from UCLA (University of California, Los Angeles); retinal prosthesis researchers—Robert Greenberg, Mark Humayun, Joseph Rizzo, John Wyatt, and Alan Chow; cortical prosthesis researchers—Richard Normann and Philip Troyk; and Dana Ballard, a visual psychophysicist from the University of Rochester.

Dr. Baker provided the welcome and Dr. Loeb gave a brief history of neural prosthetics. Dr. Bok's talk highlighted biological approaches to inherited retinal degenerations, which result in photoreceptor loss. He chose to talk about two genes (rhodopsin and retinal degeneration slow (RDS)) whose mutations cause a form of autosomal-dominant inherited blindness—RP.[18] He discussed the biological approaches of these diseases. Specifically, he described the work by Matthew LaVail, William Hauswirth, and Al Lewin Laboratories where subretinal injections were performed in transgenic rats carrying one of the rhodopsin mutations (P23H). By injecting viral-vectored ribozymes for the selective destruction of mutant mRNA produced by the P23H mutation, there was a dramatic arrest in the photoreceptor degeneration. Dr. Bok also spoke about his own work with Matthew LaVail and William Hauswirth laboratories where a viral-vectored secreted form of ciliary neurotrophic factor (CNTF) was injected subretinally. When tested with transgenic rats containing an RDS mutation (peripherin P216 L), the photoreceptor loss was again slowed (Figure 56.1).

After Dr. Greenberg gave a brief introduction to retinal prosthetics, Mark Humayun spoke about the epiretinal prosthesis efforts at the Johns Hopkins University.[9,15] He spoke about recent experiments of intraocular electrical stimulation in RP and AMD patients. Under local anesthesia, different stimulating electrodes were inserted through the eye wall and positioned over the surface of the retina. The data from the 10 most recently tested patients were reported. These awake patients reported simple forms in response to pattern electrical stimulation of the retina. A nonflickering perception was created with stimulating frequencies between 40 and 50 Hz. The stimulation threshold was also dependent on the targeted retinal area (higher in the extramacular region).

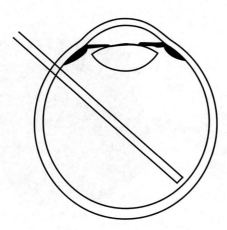

FIGURE 56.1 Experimental protocol for intraocular patient testing at the Johns Hopkins Medical Center.

Next, Joseph Rizzo and John Wyatt spoke about the work at the Massachusetts Eye and Ear Infirmary and the Massachusetts Institute of Technology (MEEI-MIT).[10] They reported tests on six humans tested intraocularly similar to the tests performed at the Johns Hopkins Medical Center. Using microfabricated electrode arrays placed in contact with the retina, five patients blinded from RP and one volunteer with normal vision were tested. The normal volunteer was having their eye enucleated because of a cancer. Their most significant results included: (1) safe contact of the retina with a microfabricated array, (2) determination of strength–duration curves in two volunteers, and (3) creation of visual percepts with crude form. In the best cases, the volunteers were able to distinguish two spots of light when two electrodes separated by roughly 2° of visual angle were driven. The thresholds reported exceed the accepted charge-density limits for chronic neural stimulation for the electrodes used. It was suggested that the quality of these results would improve with a chronically implantable prosthesis.

Alan Chow from Optobionics spoke about his Artificial Silicon Retina™(ASR).[14] ASRs are semiconductor-based silicon chip microphotodiode arrays (microscopic solar cells) designed to be surgically implanted into the subretinal space. The arrays are approximately 2–3 mm in diameter, 50–75 μm thick. Dr. Chow reported a successful electrical stimulation of normal animal retinas.

Robert Greenberg spoke about "Second Sight" and its mission of producing a chronically implantable retinal prosthesis. "Second Sight" has chosen a retinal prosthesis approach over the cortical approach because of concerns of patient safety even though the cortical approach has the potential to treat the largest number of blind patients (since it does not require the patients to have an intact retina or an optic nerve). Second Sight has also chosen the epiretinal approach (see Figure 56.2) over the subretinal approach because of the belief that the photodiodes used by Dr. Chow and Dr. Zrenner will not be able to produce enough electrical energy to stimulate abnormal human retinas.

Richard Normann from the University of Utah spoke about his electrode arrays that have been used to record both acute and chronic electrophysiological recordings from various brain structures in monkeys, cats, and rats.[5] The standard array is a 4.2-mm square grid with 100 silicon microelectrodes, 1.0 mm long and a spacing of 0.4 mm (see Figure 56.3). Dr. Normann also spoke about his new Utah slant array (USA) electrodes that have been used to record from the peripheral nerve.

Philip Troyk from the Illinois Institute of Technology spoke about the issues of implantable hardware. One issue raised was that the next-generation neuroprostheses will be 5–10 times denser, electrically and physically than current neuroprosthetic devices. Dr. Troyk discussed the need for heat dissipation by implanted prosthetics, particularly eye-mounted devices. The data were presented where a suspended-carrier closed-loop Class-E transcutaneous magnetic link was used to generate data-transmission rates of over 1 Mbit/s with a 5 MHz carrier.[19] Dr. Troyk also pointed out that the

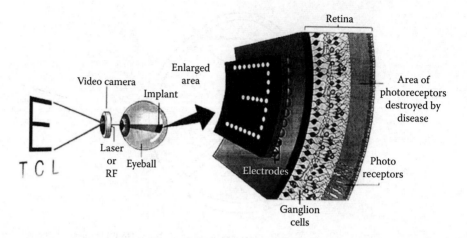

FIGURE 56.2 Concept for an epiretinal prosthesis.

stimulation strategies to produce usable sight are still unknown. When reliable implantable hardware systems become available, testing can begin to devise efficacious image-to-stimulation transformations. It is important that the implantable hardware developed at this phase does not restrict the nature of the stimulation sequences from the standpoint of amplitude, pulse–width, frequency, and temporal modulation.

Then, Dana Ballard from the University of Rochester discussed the visual representations that affect sensorimotor task performance.[20] The volunteers were shown videos of a simulated driving environment and their eye movements were monitored. By tracking saccadic eye movements, inferences can be drawn by describing the underlying cortical processing.[21]

Finally, a panel discussion was convened where the relative merits of the different approaches to visual prosthetics were debated. The session ended with a general consensus that visual prostheses are technically feasible and that chronically implanted devices and clinical testing are a necessary next step to assess the efficacy.

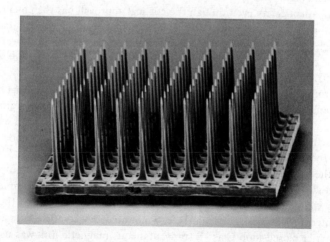

FIGURE 56.3 Penetrating cortical electrode array designed by Richard Normann's laboratory.

Acknowledgment

This chapter resulted from the inaugural symposium of the Alfred E. Mann Institute for Biomedical Engineering at the University of Southern California, Los Angeles, California on February 19, 2000. The Alfred E. Mann Institute for Biomedical Engineering at the University of Southern California (AMI-USC) was established with a $150 million donation by Mr Mann to the University and has as its goal the transfer of university research to the public sector for the benefit of patients.

References

1. Clausen, J. Visual sensations (phosphenes) produced by AC sine wave stimulation. *Acta Physiol. Neurol. Scand. Suppl.* 94:1–101, 1955.
2. Brindley, G. and Lewin, W. The sensations produced by electrical stimulation of the visual cortex. *J. Physiol. (London)* 196:479–93, 1968.
3. Dobelle, W.H. and Mladwovsky, M.G. Phosphenes produced by electrical stimulation of human occipital cortex and their application to the development of a prosthesis for the blind. *J. Physiol.* 243:553–76, 1974.
4. Dobelle, W.H., Mladejovsky, M.G., Evans, J.K., Roberts, T.S., Girvin, J.P. "Braille" reading by a blind volunteer by visual cortex stimulation. *Nature* 259:111–12, 1976.
5. Rousche, P.J. and Normann, R.A. Chronic recording capability of the Utah intracortical electrode array in cat sensory cortex. *J. Neurosci. Methods* 82(1):1–15.
6. Hoogerwerf, A.C. and Wise, K.D. A three-dimensional microelectrode array for chronic neural recording. *IEEE Trans. Biomed. Eng.* 41(12):1136–46.
7. Bak, M., Girvin, J.P., Hambrecht, F.T., Kuftar, C.V., Loeb, G.E., Schmidt, E.W. Visual sensations produced by intracortical microstimulation of the human occipital cortex. *Med. Biol. Eng. Comp.* 28:257–59, 1990.
8. Schmidt, E.M., Bak, M.J., Hambrecht, F.T., Kufta, C.V., O'Rourke, D.K., Vallabhanath, P. Feasibility of a visual prosthesis for the blind based on intracortical microstimulation of the visual cortex. *Brain* 119 (2):507–22, 1996.
9. Humayun, M.S., deJuan, E., Dagnelie, G., Greenberg, R.J., Propst, R., Phillips, D.H. Visual perception elicited by electrical stimulation of retina in blind humans. *Arch. Ophthalmol.* 114:40–46, 1996.
10. Wyatt, J. and Rizzo, J. Ocular implants for the blind. *IEEE Spectr.* 33(5): 47–53, 1996.
11. Zrenner, E., Miliczek, K.D., Gabel, V.P., Graf, H.G., Guenther, E., Haemmerle, H., Hoeffinger, B. et al. The development of subretinal microphotodiodes for replacement of degenerated photoreceptors. *Ophthalmic Res.* 29(5):269–80, 1997.
12. Eckmiller, R. Learning retina implants with epiretinal contacts. *Ophthalmic Res.* 29:281–89, 1997.
13. Greenberg, R.J. Analysis of electrical stimulation of the vertebrate retina—Work towards a retinal prosthesis (thesis) Johns Hopkins University, Baltimore, MD, 1998.
14. Chow, A.Y. and Peachey, N.S. The subretinal microphotodiode array retinal prosthesis. *Ophthalmic Res.* 30(3):195–8, 1998.
15. Humayun, M.S., deJuan, E., Weiland, J.D., Dagnelie, G., Katona, S., Greenberg, R., Suzuki, S. Pattern electrical stimulation of the human retina. *Vision Res.* 39:2569–76, 1999.
16. Davis, R. Future possibilities for neural stimulation. In *Textbook of Stereotactic and Functional Neurosurgery*, McGraw-Hill, New York, NY, Chapter 217, pp. 2064–66, 1997.
17. Veraart, C., Raftopoulos, C., Mortimer, J.T., Delbeke, J., Pins, D., Michaux, G., Vanlinerde, A., Parrini, S., Wanet-Defalque, M.C. Visual sensations produced by optic nerve stimulation using an implanted self-sizing spiral cuff electrode. *Brain Res.* 813(1):181–6, 1998.
18. Kedzierski, W., Bok, D., Travis, G.H. Transgenic analysis of RDS/peripherin N-glycosylation: Effect on dimerization, interaction with rom1, and rescue of the RDS null phenotype. *J. Neurochem.* 72(1):430–8, 1999.

19. Troyk, P.R. and Schwan, M.A. Closed-loop class E transcutaneous power and data link for microimplants. *IEEE Trans. Biomed. Eng.* 39(6):589–99, 1992.
20. Smeets, J.B., Hayhoe, M.M., Ballard, D.H. Goal-directed arm movements change eye–head coordination. *Exp. Brain Res.* 109(3):434–40, 1996.
21. Ballard, D.H., Hayhoe, M.M., Li, F., Whitehead, S.D. Hand–eye coordination during sequential tasks. *Philos. Trans. R Soc. Lond. B Biol. Sci.* 337(1281):331–9, 1992.

57

Interfering with the Genesis and Propagation of Epileptic Seizures by Neuromodulation

Ana Luisa Velasco
Mexico City General Hospital

Francisco Velasco
Mexico City General Hospital

Marcos Velasco
Mexico City General Hospital

Bernardo Boleaga
CTScanner de México

Mauricio Kuri
CTScanner de México

Fiacro Jiménez
Mexico City General Hospital

José María Núñez
Mexico City General Hospital

57.1	Introduction	57-1
57.2	Electrical Stimulation of the Centromedian Thalamic Nuclei	57-2
	Patient's Selection • Correct Targeting • Periodic Monitoring of the Reliability of ESCM on a Long-Term Follow-Up	
57.3	Results	57-5
57.4	Electrical Stimulation of the Hippocampus	57-5
57.5	Study Design	57-8
	Chronic Stimulation Parameters	
57.6	Results	57-9
57.7	Neuromodulation of the Supplementary Motor Area	57-10
57.8	Conclusion	57-11
	References	57-12

57.1 Introduction

Epilepsy is a medical condition that is very frequent around the world. It is estimated that 1% of the population suffers from epilepsy. From these patients, only 70% are controlled with antiepileptic medication. The other 30% of patients may benefit from surgical intervention. The use of chronic stimulation of the brain, the so-called neuromodulation, has been shown to be a reliable procedure in the control of epileptic seizures. In 1970, the first totally implantable stimulating systems were available (Rise, 2000). On the basis of the work of Cooke and Snider (1955), Cooper et al. (1978) used cerebellar stimulation to control different varieties of epileptic seizures.

Our group has worked on three deep-brain stimulation procedures according to the type of epileptic seizures: (1) stimulation of the centromedian (CM) nucleus of the thalamus in the control of intractable generalized seizures and atypical absences of the Lennox–Gastaut syndrome (LGS) (Velasco et al., 1987, 1989, 1993a,b, 1995, 2000a,b, 2002), (2) stimulation of the hippocampus for the control of mesial temporal lobe seizures (Velasco et al., 2000c–e, 2001b), and (3) stimulation of the supplementary motor area for motor seizures initiated in this zone (unpublished data).

57.2 Electrical Stimulation of the Centromedian Thalamic Nuclei

Although electrical stimulation of the centromedian (ESCM) has been used in cases of difficult-to-control seizures with multifocal onset in the frontal and temporal lobes, as well as in cases of seizures with no evidence of focal onset such as LGS, it has proven to have its best result in the latter.

The role of midline and intralaminar thalamic nuclei in the genesis and propagation of epileptic attacks was proposed long ago on the basis of clinical observations (Penfield and Jasper, 1954). Although the controversy on the anatomical initiation of the epileptic attacks remains, there seems to be an agreement that the thalamocortical interactions are essential in the development of most of them (Pollen et al., 1963, Gloor et al., 1977, Quesney et al., 1977, Avoli et al., 1983, Steriade 1990, Velasco et al., 1991).

The decision to stimulate the CM was based on the idea to interfere with the thalamocortical interactions and thus stop either the genesis or the propagation of the seizures. In 1984, our group performed the first ESCM trial on a 12-year-old male who had severe atypical absences refractory to high levels of antiepileptic medication. The CM was chosen as a target because of its relatively large size and close relationship to the conventional stereotaxic landmarks and because the CM is an intralaminar nucleus that forms a part of the nonspecific reticular–thalamocortical system that transmits and integrates the cerebral inputs of the generalized seizures (Jasper and Droogleever-Fortuyn, 1947, Hunter and Jasper, 1949, Gloor et al., 1977). Since then, several types of seizures were included in the protocol of ESCM (Velasco et al., 1993a). The best results were obtained in patients with generalized seizures of the LGS (associated with 2 Hz spike-wave complexes and mental deterioration). Other forms of seizures, particularly those with focal origins (as in temporal lobe seizures), are not significantly improved by ESCM to a lesser extent (Velasco et al., 2000b). However, secondary tonic–clonic generalization is relieved suggesting that ESCM interferes with the propagation mechanisms of focally initiated epileptic activity.

The ESCM procedure has been refined progressively by increasing the number of treated patients and lengthening the follow-up period. Our group has also defined better a number of predictor factors that must be taken into account to achieve a good outcome. There are three main predictor factors that must be taken into account to achieve a good outcome: (1) selection of responding patients, (2) verifying the correct deep brain stimulation (DBS) implantation based on the definition of the stereotaxic coordinates of the CM optimal effective areas and neurophysiological characterization of the targeted area, and (3) performing periodic monitoring of the reliability of ESCM on a long-term follow-up (Velasco et al., 2000b, 2001a).

57.2.1 Patient's Selection

In this chapter, we analyze the last 13 patients with LGS selected from patients of the Epilepsy Surgery Clinic of the General Hospital of Mexico on the basis of having a generalized difficulty to control seizures of the LGS. They underwent ESCM with the idea to correlate seizure type, stereotaxic targeting, and neurophysiological responses with the final outcome of the patient. The LGS is one of the severest forms of childhood epilepsy. It is characterized by drug-resistant generalized seizures, the most characteristic being the tonic and atonic seizures, atypical absences, myoclonic attacks, episodes of nonconvulsive, and tonic *status epilepticus*. The peak onset is known to be between 1 and 7 years of age. It is usually preceded by other types of seizure disorders, especially infantile spasms. LGS is accompanied by severe mental deterioration as it progresses. From the electroencephalogram (EEG) standpoint, the diagnosis is based upon the presence of slow spike-wave complexes (<2.5 cps) and bursts of rapid (10 Hz) rhythms during slow sleep. The overall prognosis is very severe; 90% of the patients are mentally retarded and 80% continue to have seizures through adulthood (Aicardi, 1994). The selected patients had either secondary LGS with stable or nonprogressive diseases (birth trauma, postencephalitic sequelae, cortical dysplasia, and stable tuberous sclerosis) or primary LGS with no demonstrable lesion in the magnetic resonance imaging (MRI).

57.2.2 Correct Targeting

To have the optimal results with ESCM, it is of extreme importance to have good patient selection combined with adequate target localization. The latter should be obtained from two points of view: stereotaxic (defined with ventriculography and MRI) and neurophysiological definition.

57.2.2.1 Ventriculographic Definition of CM Target

Surgical technique: Under general anesthesia, electrodes (Medtronic Model 3387 DBS lead Medtronic, Inc., Minneapolis, MN) are stereotactically placed in both the left and the right CM nuclei through a coronal incision and bifrontal burr holes made at a distance of 10–15 mm at each side of the midline at the level of the coronal suture. The CM localization is accomplished by air ventriculography. This method allows us to demonstrate the anterior (AC) and posterior (PC) commissures of the third ventricle with remarkable precision. Two lines are drawn, the AC–PC line and the vertical line perpendicular to the PC (VPC). The target point for the electrode tip was a distance 10 mm from the midline and the intersection of the AC–PC line with the VPC (Velasco et al., 1989, 2000b).

Electrodes are fixed to burr holes using a plastic ring and silastic ring caps (Medtronic). The position of the contacts along the trajectory of the electrode is plotted on the sagittal and frontal sections of the Schatenbrand and Bailey (1959) according to the standardization technique described elsewhere (Velasco et al., 1975).

The optimal targets for seizure arrest are located in the basolateral portion of the CM that corresponds to the parvocellular portion; this is an area of maximal neuronal population (Mehler, 1996) (Figure 57.1). The best antiepileptic results are located as follows: LAT = 10.0 ± 2.0 mm from the midline, H = from 2.0 to 7.0 mm above the AC–PC line, and AP = from 3.0 to 5.0 mm in front or PC–VPC intersection. Since the CM is a large nucleus with several subdivisions, it is important to point out that the electrode contacts used for stimulation in patients with good outcome are positioned in the ventrolateral or parvocellular part of the CM considered by anatomists as the core of the CM nucleus of Luys that is surrounded by denser fiber connections ascending from the brain stem to terminate in other nuclei of the thalamus (Mehler, 1996).

57.2.2.2 MRI Confirmation of the CM Target

Electrodes are left externalized to confirm their position by MRI. The scans are performed using 1.5 T Edge equipment software version 9.3 (Marconi Medical Systems, Cleveland, Ohio), using T2-weighted fast spin-echo sequence (echo time 11 ms, repetition time 4070 ms, field of view 16.0 cm, and 256 × 256

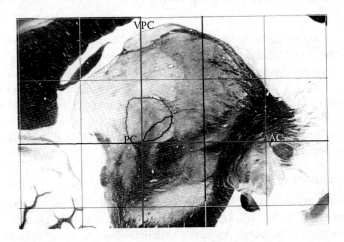

FIGURE 57.1 Optimal targets for seizure arrest located in the basolateral portion of the CM.

matrix). The sections are oriented parallel and perpendicular to the AC–PC line for axial and frontal views, and parallel to the midsagittal plane for sagittal sections (Velasco et al., 2000b, 2002).

57.2.2.3 Neurophysiological Confirmation of the CM Target

Stimuli are delivered by a Grass S8 stimulator and the isolation unit is attached to the patient by means of a Tektronix clock recovery unit (CRU) and a comparative 10 kΩ resistor to monitor the voltage (V), current flow (μA), and impedance (kΩ) of the stimulated contacts within the brain tissue (Velasco et al., 1993a).

The electrical incremental and desynchronizing responses are elicited by unilateral electrical stimulation through adjacent electrode contacts (where the cathode was always the lower contact). Stimuli consist of 5–30 s trains of monophasic square pulses of 1.0 ms duration and 6–60 Hz frequency. The analysis of the scalp distribution of the incremental spike-wave and desynchronizing electro-cortical responses is made from EEG recordings taken from fronto-polar (FP2, FP1), frontal (F4, F3), central (C4, C3), parietal (P4, P3), occipital (O2, O1), fronto-temporal (F8, F7), and anterior temporal (T4, T3) referred to as ipsilateral ears (A2, A1) (sensitivity = 10 μA/cm, time constant = 0.35 s, and paper speed = 15 mm/s).

Low-frequency (6/s), threshold (4–5 V = 320–400 μA) unilateral stimulation of CM elicits incremental responses with the typical waxing and waning profiles. The incremental responses produced by this stimulation procedure along the CM or other structures are described elsewhere (Velasco et al., 1996). Although there are three types of incremental responses that may be elicited, type A points the best place to obtain the optimum antiepileptic effect. They are recruiting-like responses elicited by the stimulation of the caudal–basal portions of CM (parvocellular CM close to the nonspecific mesencephalic structures, such as the mesencephalic *tegmentum* tract). They consist of monophasic negative potentials with a latency of 20 ms and a peak latency of 30–35 ms (Figure 57.2a). Suprathreshold type A responses show a bilateral regional scalp distribution with maximal amplitude at the frontal region ipsilateral to the stimulated side (Figure 57.2b) (Velasco et al., 1996).

Unilateral high-frequency (60/s) threshold and suprathreshold stimulation of the caudal–basal and central CM elicits a regional EEG desynchronization consisting of an increased frequency of the EEG activity superimposed on a slow negative shift. It also shows a bilateral regional scalp distribution with maximal amplitude at the frontal region ipsilateral to the stimulated side (Figure 57.2c) (Velasco et al., 1996).

57.2.3 Periodic Monitoring of the Reliability of ESCM on a Long-Term Follow-Up

Incremental responses, EEG desynchronization, and slow negative shifts may be useful as biological responses for monitoring the efficiency of the ESCM, particularly when the stimulating electrodes are internalized subcutaneously and the physical characteristics of the electrical stimuli cannot be monitored any longer (Velasco et al., 1995). In view of the patient's lack of subjective sensations and the long latency of the antiepileptic effects of ESCM, the reliability of ESCM is questionable. The use of 10 or 60/s and 6 V (800 μA) transcutaneous activation of CM with the Medtronic internalized pulse generator (IPG) by Medtronic, Inc., Minneapolis and the recording of scalp incremental responses, EEG desynchronization, and slow negative shifts is advisable.

57.2.3.1 Chronic Stimulation Parameters

The parameters recommended for ESCM are as follows: 2 h of daily stimulation sessions. The stimulus consists of 1 min trains of Lilly pulses with an interstimulus interval of 4 min, alternating the right and the left CM. Such trains consist of a 130 Hz frequency, with individual pulses of 450 μs in duration and amplitude of 400–600 μA.

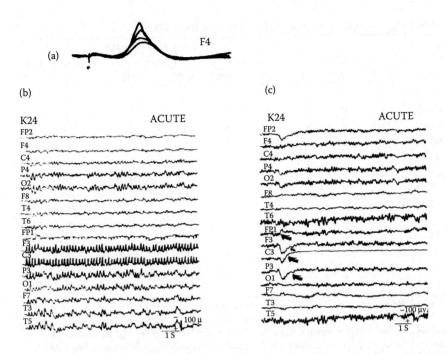

FIGURE 57.2 Neurophysiological confirmation of the CM target. (a) Type A recruiting-like responses elicited by the stimulation of the caudal–basal portions of CM. They consist of monophasic negative potentials with a latency of 20 ms and a peak latency of 30–35 ms. (b) Low-frequency (6/s) stimulation elicits suprathreshold type A responses showing a bilateral regional scalp distribution with maximal amplitude at the frontal region ipsilateral to the stimulated side. (c) Unilateral high-frequency (60/s) threshold and suprathreshold stimulation of the caudal–basal and central CM elicits a regional EEG desynchronization consisting of an increased frequency of the EEG activity superimposed on a slow negative shift with a bilateral regional scalp distribution with maximal amplitude at the frontal region ipsilateral to the stimulated side.

57.3 Results

ESCM produces a significant reduction in the number of primary and secondary generalized tonic-clonic seizures, atypical absences of the LGS, and also the number of interictal generalized slow spike-wave complexes.

As said above, the results depend on both the seizure type and correct target selection. Note that the patients with excellent result (i.e., 100% improvement) had generalized seizures, correct stereotaxic placement, and electrophysiological responses. All patients who had less than 80% seizure improvement had other seizure type (i.e., LC who had residual complex partial seizures) and/or incorrect target selection according to either anatomic (stereotaxic) or physiological parameters (Table 57.1).

57.4 Electrical Stimulation of the Hippocampus

In the Epilepsy Surgery Clinic of the General Hospital of Mexico, 70% of patients referred for surgery have complex partial seizures arising from the hippocampal formation; other series have reported a similar referral number (Wieser et al., 1993, Williamson et al., 1993). Resective surgery of the epileptic focus yields very good results (Engel, 1987, Velasco et al., 2000c); nevertheless, there are cases that escape this surgical possibility, that is, patients with bilateral hippocampal foci or patients with epileptic focus located near eloquent areas for speech and memory (usually the left side). These latter patients cannot be operated upon because it would mean having severe neurological impairment particularly related to

TABLE 57.1 Predictors of Seizure Relief Obtained after ESCM

Initials	Seizure Type			Stereotactic Placement		Electrophysiological Placement		Final Improvement (%)
	GTC	AA	CXP	RCM	LCM	RCM	LCM	
GA	Y	Y	N	C	C	C	C	100
MAM	Y	Y	N	C	C	C	C	100
AMP	Y	Y	N	C	I	C	C	95
MS	Y	Y	N	C	C	C	C	95
MAPR	Y	Y	N	C	I	C	C	95
JM	Y	Y	N	C	C	C	C	91
JS	Y	Y	N	C	C	C	C	89
IM	Y	Y	N	C	C	C	C	87
LC	Y	Y	Y	C	C	I	I	80
EGV	Y	Y	N	C	C	C	I	70
DC	N	Y	N	C	I	C	C	58
JR	Y	Y	N	C	I	I	I	53
LVAP	N	Y	N	C	C	I	I	30

Source: From Velasco et al., submitted for publication.

Note: All patients had generalized tonic–clonic seizures (GTC), atypical absences (AA), and only LC also had complex partial seizures (CXP). Correct (C) and incorrect (I) stereotaxic and electrophysiological parameters are shown. Note that all patients with a seizure improvement of 100% had generalized seizures and correct target-localization parameters.

short-term memory. These patients are candidates for neuromodulating procedures. Unfortunately, our experience with ESCM pointed out that CM is not the place to stimulate in patients with complex partial seizures originating in the temporal lobe. On the other hand, animal experiments showed that the application of an electrical stimulus to the amygdala or hippocampus following the kindling stimulus produces a significant and long-lasting suppressive effect on seizures (Weiss et al., 1995). For these reasons, we decided to perform a preliminary study in 10 patients with nonlesional temporal lobe epilepsy in whom intracranial electrodes were implanted (either subdural basotemporal grid or hippocampal electrodes) for the detection of the epileptic foci (Velasco et al., 2000c). The study consisted of performing subacute hippocampal stimulation (SAHCS) trial of 2–3 weeks duration once the epileptic focus was located and before performing the temporal lobectomy. Two patients had bilateral hippocampal depth electrodes implanted to determine the lateralization of the epileptic focus and eight had unilateral subdural electrode grids on the pial surface of the basotemporal cortex to determine the precise site and extent of the focus (Figure 57.3). In all patients, antiepileptic drugs were discontinued for 72 h before SAHCS initiation. Thereafter, SAHCS was applied for a minimum of 16 days. SAHCS was bipolar and between continuous electrode contacts (cathode attached to the most anterior contact) and consisted of continuous stimulation with biphasic Lilly pulses (130 Hz frequency, 450 µs in duration, and amplitude of 200–400 µA). The reliability of SAHCS was determined by the daily measurement of voltage, impedance, and current flow at the intracerebral contacts by means of externalized electrode systems (Velasco et al., 1993a).

To evaluate the antiepileptic effects of SAHCS on temporal lobe epileptogenesis, the number and type of clinical seizures per day and the number of interictal negative EEG spikes at the epileptic focus per 10 s were evaluated. At the completion of the clinical and EEG studies, SAHCS was discontinued, the electrodes were removed, and an anterior temporal lobectomy was performed ipsilateral to the epileptic focus and SAHCS. Biopsies of the mesial and lateral temporal lobes were fixed in 10% formaldehyde buffer solution, embedded in paraffin, and cut in serial coronal sections of 10 µm thickness and perpendicular to the fascia dentata, taken every 1000 µm and stained with hematoxylin–eosin for perikaryon

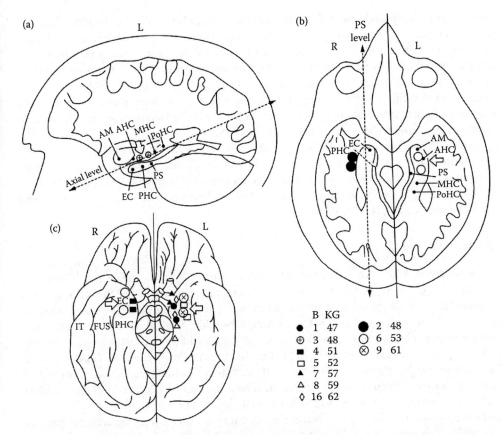

FIGURE 57.3 Diagrams showing the position of the depth and subdural electrode contacts for SAHCS. (a) and (b) show parasagittal and axial sections and (c) shows basotemporal cortex, all of them showing the position of the stimulation contacts in different patients (indicated by different symbols at the right bottom corner). The arrows indicate sites where SAHCS produced evident and fast antiepileptic responses. AHC, MHC, and PoHC: anterior, middle, and posterior hippocampus; AM: amygdala; PS: presubiculum; PHC, EC, FUS, and IT: parahippocampal, entorhinal, fusiform, and inferior temporal gyri. (From Velasco A.L. et al. *Arch Med Res*, 2000d, 31:316–328.)

and with Gomori's technique used for the collagen. A histopathological analysis of the temporal lobe tissue was performed under light microscope by comparing the contiguous hippocampal tissue at the stimulated versus nonstimulated tissues.

In seven patients in whom stimulation sites were located within the hippocampal formation and gyrus, there was an evident antiepileptic response. Both complex partial and secondary generalized tonic–clonic seizures were abolished after 6 days of continuous stimulation and interictal EEG spikes were significantly reduced from days 4 to 11 of SAHCS. The most evident and fastest antiepileptic responses were found in five patients in whom the stimulation contacts were located either at the anterior pes-hippocampus near the amygdala or at the anterior parahippocampal gyrus near the entorhinal cortex. Three patients did not respond, two of them responded when SAHCS was accidentally interrupted, and the other patient responded when the stimulated contacts were located at the white matter lateral to the hippocampus.

Histopathological analysis of the hippocampal tissues revealed abnormalities due to depth electrode penetration or lesion due to the foreign body electrodes. However, no histopathological differences were found between stimulated and nonstimulated hippocampal tissues. Therefore, the SAHCS effect does not appear to depend on a lesional process but rather to a functional blockage of the hippocampus.

During this preliminary study, we took advantage of this ethically permissible situation and studied some basic mechanisms underlying the beneficial therapeutic effect on seizures due to hippocampal stimulation (Velasco et al., 2000d,e, 2001a,b). Such studies suggest that the antiepileptic effect of hippocampal stimulation is due to an inhibition mechanism, that is, increased threshold and decreased duration of the afterdischarges induced by acute hippocampal stimulation, depression of the paired pulse hippocampal recovery cycles, single-photon emission computed tomography (SPECT) hypoperfusion, and autoradiographic increase of the benzodiazepine receptor binding in the stimulated hippocampal tissue (Cuéllar-Herrera et al., 2004).

On the basis of these results, we decided to proceed with a long-term hippocampal stimulation protocol to demonstrate that chronic hippocampal stimulation (CHCS) may produce a sustained antiepileptic effect without undesirable effects on language and memory. Up to now, we have stimulated eight patients on a long-term basis, but we will only take into consideration those six patients who have a follow-up period of at least 1 year (1–4 years).

57.5 Study Design

The candidates were selected from patients of the Epilepsy Surgery Clinic of the General Hospital of Mexico on the basis of having difficulty to control temporal lobe seizures. All of them underwent a careful clinical history with special emphasis on the seizure type (complex partial seizures), adequate antiepileptic medication with adequate blood levels, four serial EEGs, magnetic resonance, SPECT, neuropsychological exam, and psychiatric evaluation. All of them had bilateral hippocampal transitory eight contact-depth electrodes (SD 8P, Ad Tech Medical Instrument Co., Racine, WI, USA) implanted to be able to assess the epileptic foci. Two of them had bilateral independent hippocampal foci and the other four patients were selected on the basis of having their hippocampal focus on the dominant hemisphere, with neuropsychological evidence of verbal memory situated here.

Once the precise epileptic focus was defined, the transitory electrodes were replaced by four contact-depth brain stimulation electrodes (3789 DBS and IPG by Medtronic, Inc, Minneapolis, MN) (Figure 57.4) and were connected to an independent IPG system that was placed in a subcutaneous subclavicular pocket on each side. The target of the electrode contacts was the site of maximal interictal

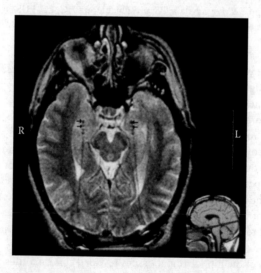

FIGURE 57.4 MRI axial view of patient KG67 showing the placement of bilateral DBS electrodes and the position of the four contacts along the hippocampus. The arrows indicate the contacts used for ESHC. (From Velasco F. et al. *Electrical Stimulation for Epilepsy*. London: Taylor & Francis Health Sciences, 2003, pp. 287–300.)

nd ictal activities. All antiepileptic drugs were withdrawn to avoid any possible interference with the *n*euromodulation procedure (Velasco et al., 2000e) and were replaced with phenytoin.

57.5.1 Chronic Stimulation Parameters

The parameters recommended for ESHC are as follows: daily stimulation sessions with 1 min trains *o*f Lilly pulses with an interstimulus interval of 4 min. Such trains consist of a 130 Hz frequency, with *i*ndividual pulses of 450 μs in duration and amplitude of 400–600 μA. In those patients with bilateral *e*lectrodes, the stimulation has the same characteristics but the stimulation alternates the right and the *l*eft hippocampus.

57.6 Results

In analyzing the antiepileptic effect of ESHC, the six patients were divided into two distinct groups: three patients had normal MRIs and the other three had ipsilateral hippocampal sclerosis. The best results were obtained in the first group with normal MRIs. The antiepileptic effect was evident since the stimulation started and the patients were seizure free after the first 3–6 months of stimulation. Our longest follow-up period is on patient KG67 who had bilateral hippocampal stimulation, and has now been seizure free for 4 years. Patient KG101 is under left hippocampal stimulation and has been seizure free for 15 months and the most recent patient KG109 also has left hippocampal stimulation and has been seizure free for a year. The neuropsychological tests in all of them became normal after 6 months of stimulation (Figure 57.5a).

The patients who constitute the second group have unilateral left mesial temporal sclerosis. Patient KG71 had bilateral epileptic foci. Even though he had a 75% seizure reduction, he persisted with auras

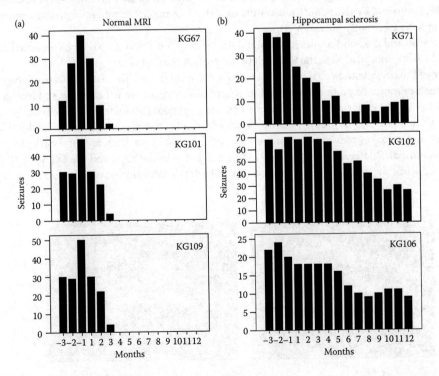

FIGURE 57.5 Seizure reduction per month in six patients with ESHC. The graphs show a 3-month baseline period, stimulation started at the 4th month (arrow), and after that, a 12-month stimulation follow-up. (a) Three patients with normal MRI. (b) Three patients with left hippocampal sclerosis.

during the 10 months follow-up. Unfortunately, he had to undergo explantation because of skin erosion. Patient KG102 had 60% seizure improvement that could be observed very slowly and took 9 months to reach its actual seizure number (follow-up of 20 months). KG106 has only had 50% seizure improvement after 1-year stimulation (Figure 57.5b). In all the patients of this group, there has only been a slight improvement in the neuropsychological tests. The three patients in this group improved only slightly in their memory tests after more than 6 months stimulation.

Even though these are preliminary results, we may say that stimulating the hippocampal epileptic focus is effective in the control of mesial temporal lobe seizures. The best cases are those who have normal MRI, in whom seizure control can be achieved up to 100%. This result is of extreme importance because these patients with intractable seizures and normal MRI are the ones that are excluded as candidates for temporal lobectomy and are left with no other alternative. Patients with mesial temporal lobe sclerosis do not do so well and their follow-up shows only 50–75% seizure reduction. If the patient has temporal sclerosis and the seizures are starting within the sclerotic hippocampus, lobectomy could be risked. Patients with bilateral hippocampal foci and unilateral sclerosis should be considered for neuromodulation since they could have better results and the risk of having residual seizures after unilateral lobectomy is high.

57.7 Neuromodulation of the Supplementary Motor Area

The supplementary motor area (SMA) plays a crucial role in movement organization, basically in the sequential timing and planning of motor tasks (Morris, 1993). It is located in the mesial surface of the superior frontal gyrus.

In contrast with temporal lobectomy that yields great benefit for patients with complex partial seizures originating in the hippocampus, ablation of the SMA renders limited results and is associated with a high incidence of neurological deficit, impacting the patients' quality of life (Mihara et al., 1996, Olivier, 1996, Smith and King, 1996). These results have limited surgery in patients who show no evolving lesions or with apparently normal MRI.

For this reason and the good results we obtained stimulating the hippocampal foci, we started a new project for the neuromodulation of the SMA. Here, we present the first case:

A 17-year-old male was studied. He started seizing at 14 years of age. The seizures were characteristic supplementary motor ones, that is, brief, with abrupt posturing of the left arm and sudden version of the head to the left, with preserved consciousness and occasional secondary tonic–clonic seizures. He had up to 10 seizures a day, 80% of them being released by sound. Conduct abnormalities with perseverance and verbal aggressiveness were present. EEG showed frontal parasagittal epileptic activity. MRI was normal. Bilateral 20 contact grids were implanted in the right and the left SMA (Figure 57.6a). Anti-epileptic drugs (AEDs) were tapered and daily-depth recording was performed for epileptic

(a)

(b)

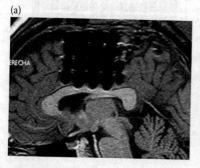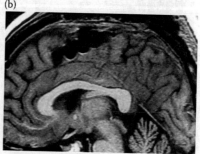

FIGURE 57.6 MRI sagittal images showing the electrode position. (a) A diagnostic 20-contact grid on the right hemisphere. (b) A definite four-contact electrode position. Contacts 2 and 3 where the epileptic focus was located are currently being stimulated.

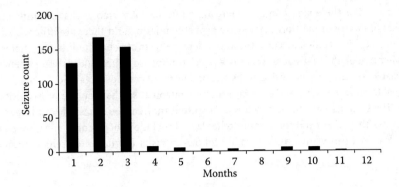

FIGURE 57.7 Graph shows seizure occurrence; months 1, 2, and 3 show the baseline period. The arrow indicates SMA chronic stimulation onset. Note the important seizure reduction that occurs during neuromodulation.

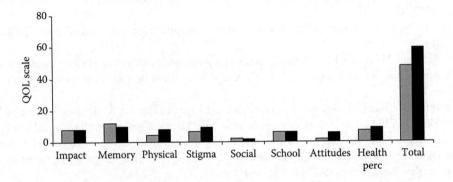

FIGURE 57.8 QOL scale shows in grey bars the patient's baseline and black bars show the results after 9 months stimulation. Note the increase after chronic neuromodulation.

focus location. Ictal EEG activity showed a mesial focus located in the right SMA. The patient reinitiated AEDs. The grids were explanted and replaced by a four-contact electrode for chronic stimulation (Resume, Medtronic Inc.) connected to a DBS system (Figure 57.6b). Stimulation was started with the following parameters: bipolar continuous stimulation of 130 Hz, 3.0 V (350 μA).

The follow-up showed immediate decrease in seizure occurrence and now, this effect has been maintained for 9 months (Figure 57.7). Quality of life (QOL) scale has improved too (Figure 57.8). No adverse effects have been reported up to now.

57.8 Conclusion

Neuromodulation constitutes an innovative neurosurgical technique in the treatment of difficult-to-control seizures. The stimulation should be targeted according to the seizure type: ESCM for generalized seizures and ESHC for mesial temporal lobe epilepsy. Neuromodulation is a method that has several advantages: it is nonlesional, with reversible effect when turned off, does not interfere with the functioning eloquent areas, and even improves neuropsychological performance. Unfortunately, it has some disadvantages: neurostimulating systems are expensive, they need periodic follow-up visits to verify that they are functioning adequately, and the stimulators have to be exchanged when the batteries wear off that imply a surgical procedure. Probably, the most important disadvantage is the skin erosion due to the stimulating system that often leads to explantation mainly in young children.

Challenges remain. For the epileptologists, there are a number of variables that are influencing the antiepileptic effect of neurostimulation that we are probably missing and there are other seizure types as well that are subject to be studied to know the antiepileptic effects of neuromodulation, that is, occipital or frontal epilepsy. For the engineers, there is a need to improve neuromodulation systems so that they are less invasive (so, they are not rejected by the patients and can be implanted in small children), include rechargeable batteries, and maybe even remote controlled so that the use of extension cables is discontinued. The systems have to be at a low cost so that they can be accessed by a larger number of epileptic patients. They also need to be more reliable and include user-friendly software so that the patient can check it by himself to avoid so many follow-up visits to guarantee reliable functioning.

References

Aicardi, J.: *Lennox–Gastaut Syndrome in Epilepsy in Children*, 2nd ed. New York: Raven Press, 1994, pp. 44–66.

Avoli, M., Gloor, P., Kostopoulus, G., Gutman, J.: An analysis of penicillin-induced generalized spike and wave discharges using simultaneous recordings of cortical and thalamic single neurons. *J Neurophysiol*, 1983, 50:819–837.

Cooke, R.M., Snider, R.S.: Some cerebellar influences on electrically induced cerebral seizures. *Epilepsia*, 1955, 4:19–28.

Cooper, I.S., Rickland, M., Amin, I., Cullinan, T.: A long term follow up study of cerebellar stimulation for the control of epilepsy. In: Cooper, I., (ed). *Cerebellar Stimulation in Man*. New York: Raven Press, 1978, pp. 19–27.

Cuellar-Herrera, M., Velasco, M., Velasco, F., Velasco, AL., Jiménez, F., Orozco, S., Briones, M., Rocha, L.; Evaluation of GABA system and cell damage in parahippocampus of patients with temporal lobe epilepsy showing antiepileptic effects alter subacute electrical stimulation. *Epilepsia*, 2004, 45:459–466.

Engel, J. Jr.: Outcome with respect to epilepsy seizures. In: Engel, J. Jr., (ed.) *Surgical Treatment of the Epilepsies*. New York: Raven, 1987, pp. 553–569.

Gloor, P., Quesney, L.F., Zumstein, H.: Pathophysiology of generalized penicillin seizures in the cat. The role of cortical and subcortical structures. II. Topical application of penicillin to the cerebral cortex and to sucortical structures. *Electroencephalogr Clin Neurophysiol*, 1977, 48:79–94.

Hunter, J., Jasper, H.H.: Effects of thalamic stimulation in unanesthetized animals. The arrest reaction and petit mal-like seizures activation patterns and generalized convulsions. *Electroenceph Clin Neurophysiol*, 1949, 11:305–324.

Jasper, H.H, Droogleever-Fortuyn, J.: Experimental studies of the functional anatomy of petit mal epilepsy. *Res Public Assoc Nerv Ment Dis*, 1947, 26:272–298.

Mehler, R.W.: Further notes of the centromedian nucleus of Luys. In: Purpura, D.P., Yahr, M.D., (eds.). *The Thalamus*. New York: Columbia University Press, 1996, pp. 102–111.

Mihara, T., Inoue, Y., Seino, M.: Surgical strategies for patients with supplementary sensorimotor area epilepsy. The Japanese experience. *Adv Neurol*, 1996, 70:405–414.

Morris, H.: Supplementary motor seizures. In: Morris, H., (ed.) *The Treatment of Epilepsy, Principles and Practice*. 2nd ed. New York: Lea & Febirger, 1993, pp. 541–546.

Olivier, A.: Surgical strategies for patients with supplementary sensorimotor area epilepsy. The Montreal experience. *Adv Neurol*, 1996, 70:429–443.

Penfield, W., Jasper, H.: *Epilepsy and the Functional Anatomy of the Human Brain*. Boston: Little Brown, 1954, pp. 566–596.

Pollen, D.A., Perot, P., Reid, K.H.: Experimental bilateral spike and wave from thalamic stimulation in relation to the level of arousal. *Electroencephalogr Clin Neurophysiol*, 1963, 15:459–473.

Quesney, L.F., Gloor, P., Kratzemberg, E., Zumstein, H.: Pathophysiology of generalized penicillin seizures in the cat. The role of cortical and subcortical structures. I. Systemic application of penicillin. *Electroencephalogr Clin Neurophysiol*, 1977, 42:640–655.

Rise, M.T.: Instrumentation for neuromodulation. *Arch Med Res*, 2000, 34:237–247.

Schatenbrand, G., Bailey, P.: *Introduction to Stereotaxis with an Atlas of the Human Brain*. George Thieme Verlog, Stuttgart, 1959.

Smith, J.R., King, D.W.: Surgical strategies for patients with supplementary sensorimotor area epilepsy. The medical college of Georgia experience. *Adv Neurol*, 1996, 70: 415–427.

Steriade, M.: Spindling, incremental thalamo-cortical responses and spike-wave like epilepsy. In: Avoli, M., Gloor, P., Kustopoulus, G., Naquet, R., (eds.) *Generalized Epilepsy: Neurobiological Approaches*. Boston: Birkhouser 1990, pp. 161–180.

Velasco, A.L., Boleaga, B., Brito, F., Jiménez, F., Gordillo, J.L., Velasco, F., Velasco, M.: Absolute and relative predictor values of some non-invasive and invasive studies for the outcome of anterior temporal lobectomy. *Arch Med Res*, 2000c, 31:62–74.

Velasco, A.L., Velasco, M., Velasco, F., Ménes, D., Gordon, F., Rocha, L., Briones, M., Márquez, I.: Subacute and chronic electrical stimulation of the hippocampus on intractable temporal lobe seizures. *Arch Med Res*, 2000d, 31:316–328.

Velasco, F., Velasco, A.L., Velasco, M., Rocha, L., Ménes, D.: Electrical stimulation of the epileptic focus in cases of temporal lobe seizures. In: Lüders, H.O., (ed). *Electrical Stimulation for Epilepsy*. London: Taylor and Francis Health Sciences , 2003, pp. 287–300.

Velasco, F., Velasco, M., Alcalá, H.: The electrical stimulation of the thalamus. In: Kutt, H., Resor, S.R., (eds.) *Advances in Neurology. Medical Treatment of Epilepsy*. New York: Marcel Decker, 1989, pp. 677–780.

Velasco, F., Velasco, M., Jiménez, F., Velasco, A.L., Brito, F., Rise, M., Carrillo-Ruiz, J.D.: Predictors in the treatment of difficult to control seizures by electrical stimulation of the centromedian thalamic nucleus. *Neurosurgery*, 2000b, 47:295–305.

Velasco, F., Velasco, M., Jiménez, F., Velasco, AL., Rojas, B., Pérez, M.L.: Centromedian nucleus stimulation for epilepsy: Clinical, electroencephalographic and behavioral observations. *Thalamus Relat Syst*, 2002, 34:1–12.

Velasco, F., Velasco, M., Machado, J.P.: A statistical outline of the subthalamic target for the arrest of tremor. *Appl Neurophysiol*, 1975, 38:38–46.

Velasco, F., Velasco, M., Ogarrio, C., Fanghänel, F.: Electrical stimulation of the centromedian thalamic nucleus in the treatment of convulsive seizures. A preliminary report. *Epilepsia*, 1987, 28:421–430.

Velasco, F., Velasco, M., Velasco, A.L., Jimenez, F.: Effect of chronic electrical stimulation of the centromedian thalamic nuclei on various intractable seizure patterns: I. Clinical seizures and paroxysmal EEG activity. *Epilepsia*, 1993a, 34:1052–1064.

Velasco, F., Velasco, M., Velasco, AL., Jimenez, F., Rise, M.: Electrical stimulation of the centromedian thalamic nucleus in control of seizures: Long-term studies. *Epilepsia*, 1995, 36:63–71.

Velasco, F., Velasco, M., Velasco, A.L., Ménez, D., Rocha, L.: Electrical stimulation for epilepsy 1. Stimulation of hippocampal foci. *Stereotact Funct Neurosurg*, 2001b, 77:223–227.

Velasco, M., Velasco, F., Alcalá, H, Dávila, G., Díaz de León, A.E.: Epileptiform EEG activities in the centromedian thalamic nuclei in children with intractable generalized seizures of the Lennox–Gastaut syndrome. *Epilepsia*, 1991, 32:310–321.

Velasco, M., Velasco, F., Velasco, A.L.: Centromedian thalamic and hippocampal electrical stimulation for the control of intractable epileptic seizures. *Clin Neurophysiol*, 2001a, 18:1–15.

Velasco, M., Velasco F., Velasco, A.L., Boleaga, B., Jiménez, F., Brito, F., Márquez, I.: Subacute electrical stimulation of the hippocampus blocks intractable temporal lobe seizures and paroxysmal EEG activities. *Epilepsia*, 2000e, 41:158–169.

Velasco, M., Velasco, F., Velasco, A.L., Jiménez, F., Brito, F., Márquez, I.: Acute and chronic electrical stimulation of the centromedian thalamic nucleus: Modulation of reticulo-cortical systems and predictor factors for generalized seizure control. *Arch Med Res*, 2000a, 31:304–315.

Velasco, M., Velasco, F., Velasco, A.L., Jimenez, F., Márquez, I., Rojas, B.: Electrocortical and behavioral responses produced by acute electrical stimulation of the human centromedian thalamic nucleus. *Electroenceph Clin Neurophysiol*, 1996, 102:461–471.

Velasco, M., Velasco, F., Velasco, A.L., Velasco, G., Jimenez, F.: Effect of chronic electrical stimulation of the centromedian thalamic nuclei on various intractable seizure patterns: II. Psychological performance and background activity. *Epilepsia*, 1993b, 34:1065–1074.

Weiss, S.B.R., Li, X.L., Rosen, J.B., Li, H., Heynen, T.: Post R.M. quenching: Inhibition of development and expression of amygdala kindled seizures with low frequency stimulation. *Neuroreport*, 1995, 4:2171.

Wieser, H.G., Engel, J. Jr., Williamson, P.D., Babb, T.L., Gloor, P.: Surgically remediable temporal lobe syndromes. In: Engel, J. Jr., (ed.) *Surgical Treatment of the Epilepsies*. New York: Raven, 1993, pp. 49–63.

Williamson, P.D., French, J.A., Thadani, V.M.: Characteristics of medial temporal lobe epilepsy II. Interictal and ictal scalp electroencephalography, neuropsychological testing, neuroimaging, surgical results and pathology. *Ann Neurol*, 1993,34:781–787.

Transcranial Magnetic Stimulation of Deep Brain Regions

58.1 Introduction 58-1
58.2 Basic Principles of TMS 58-2
58.3 Deep TMS Coils: Design Principles 58-4
58.4 A Coil for Stimulation of Deep Brain Regions Related to
      Mood Disorders: Simulations and Phantom Measurements ... 58-6
      Methods • Results
58.5 TMS of Deep Brain Regions: Evidence for Efficacy
      of the H-Coil 58-13
      Methods • Results • Discussion
58.6 TMS of Deep Prefrontal Regions 58-18
      Comparison of Electric Field Distributions
References 58-23

Yiftach Roth
Sheba Medical Center

Abraham Zangen
*Weizmann Institute
of Science*

58.1 Introduction

Transcranial magnetic stimulation (TMS) is a noninvasive technique used to apply brief magnetic pulses to the brain. The pulses are administered by passing high currents through an electromagnetic coil placed upon the scalp that can induce electrical currents in the underlying cortical tissue, thereby producing a localized axonal depolarization. Neuronal stimulation by TMS was first demonstrated in 1985 (Barker et al., 1985), when a circular coil was placed over a normal subject vertex and evoked action potentials from the abductor digiti minimi. Since then, this technique has been applied to studying nerve conduction, excitability, and conductivity in the brain and peripheral nerves, and to studying and treating various neurobehavioral disorders, primarily mood disorders (Kirkcaldie et al., 1997; Wassermann and Lisanby, 2001).

The ability of the TMS technique to elicit a neuronal response has until recently been limited to the brain cortex. The coils used for TMS (such as round or a figure-of-eight coils) induce stimulation in the cortical regions mainly just superficially under the windings of the coil. The intensity of the electric field drops dramatically deeper in the brain as a function of the distance from the coil (Maccabee et al., 1990; Tofts, 1990; Tofts and Branston, 1991; Eaton, 1992). Therefore, to stimulate deep brain regions, a very high intensity would be needed. Such intensity cannot be reached by standard magnetic stimulators, using the regular figure-of-eight or circular coils. The stimulation of regions at a depth of 3–4 cm, such as the leg motor area, may be achieved using coils such as the double-cone coil (Terao et al., 1994, 2000; Stokic et al., 1997), which is a larger figure of eight with an angle of about 95° between the two wings. However, the intensity needed to stimulate the deeper brain regions effectively would stimulate cortical regions and facial nerves over the level that might lead to facial pain and facial and cervical muscle contractions, and may cause epileptic seizures and other undesirable side effects.

This chapter describes the principles and the design of TMS coils for deep brain stimulation. The construction of such coils should simultaneously meet several goals:

1. High-enough electric field intensity in the desired deep brain region that will surpass the threshold for neuronal activation
2. High percentage of electric field in the desired deep brain region relative to the maximal intensity in the cortex
3. Minimal aversive side effects during stimulation such as pain and activation of facial muscles

58.2 Basic Principles of TMS

The TMS stimulation circuit consists of a high-voltage power supply that charges a bank of capacitors, which are then rapidly discharged via an electronic switch into the TMS coil to create the briefly changing magnetic field pulse. A typical circuit is shown in Figure 58.1, where low-voltage alternating current (ac) is transformed into high-voltage direct current (dc), which charges the capacitors. A crucial component is the thyristor switch, which has to traverse very high current at a very short time of 50–250 μs. The cycle time depends on the capacitance (typically 10–250 μF) and on the coil inductance (typically 10–30 μH). The typical peak currents and voltages are 5000 A and 1500 V, respectively.

Most TMS stimulators produce a biphasic pulse of electric current. During the discharge cycle, the TMS circuit behaves like an RCL (i.e., resistance, capacitance, and inductance) circuit, and the current I is given by

$$I(t) = \frac{V}{wL} \exp(-\alpha t) \sin(wt) \tag{58.1}$$

where $\alpha = R/2\,L$, $w = \sqrt{(LC)^{-1} - \alpha^2}$, and R, C, and L are the total values of the resistance, capacitance, and inductance, respectively, in the circuit. The inductance is mainly the coil inductance, but there is an additional contribution from the cables, and the resistance includes contributions from the thyristor and the coil.

Biologically, the most relevant parameter for neuronal activation is the induced electric field, which is proportional to the rate of change of the current (dI/dt). The brief strong current generates a time-varying magnetic field B. An electric field E is generated at every point in space with the direction perpendicular to the magnetic field and with an amplitude proportional to the time rate of change of the vector potential A(r).

The vector potential A(r) in position r is related to the current in the coil I by the expression

$$A(r) = \frac{\mu_0 I}{4\pi} \int \frac{dl'}{|r - r'|} \tag{58.2}$$

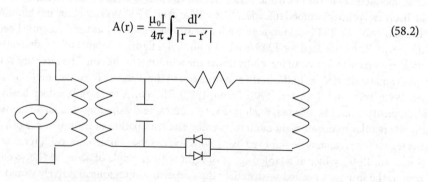

FIGURE 58.1 Typical magnetic stimulation circuit, including high-voltage transformer, capacitor, resistor, thyristor trigger, and stimulating coil.

where $\mu_0 = 4\pi \times 10^{-7}$ Tm/A is the permeability of free space, the integral of dl` is over the wire path, and ` is a vector indicating the position of the wire element. The magnetic and electric fields are related to the vector potential through the expressions

$$B_A = \nabla \times A \tag{58.3}$$

$$E_A = \frac{\partial A}{\partial t} \tag{58.4}$$

The only quantity that is changing with time is the current I. Hence, the electric field E_A can be written as

$$E_A = \frac{-\mu_0 \partial I}{4\pi \partial t} \int \frac{dl'}{|r - r'|} \tag{58.5}$$

Since the brain tissue has conducting properties, while the air and skull are almost complete insulators, the vector potential will induce the accumulation of electric charge at the brain surface. This charge is another source for the electric field, which can be expressed as

$$E_\Phi = -\nabla \Phi \tag{58.6}$$

where Φ is the scalar potential produced by the surface electrostatic charge.

The total field in the brain tissue E is the vectorial sum of these two fields:

$$E = E_A + E_\Phi \tag{58.7}$$

The influence of the electrostatic field E_Φ is in general to oppose the induced field E_A and consequently to reduce the total field E. The amount of surface charge produced and hence the magnitude of E_Φ depend strongly on the coil configuration and orientation. This issue will be elaborated in the following sections.

Figure 58.2 demonstrates the electric field pulse produced by a figure-of-eight coil, as measured by a two-wire probe in a brain phantom filled with saline solution at physiological concentration. In repetitive TMS (rTMS), several such pulses are administered in a train of between 1 and 20 Hz.

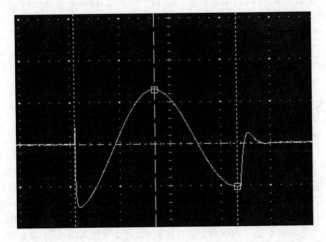

FIGURE 58.2 The induced electric field of a figure-of-eight coil versus time over a TMS pulse cycle. The timescale is 100 μs.

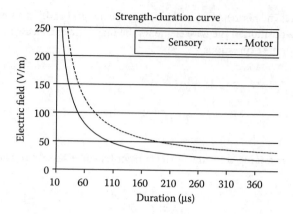

FIGURE 58.3 Neural strength–duration curve depicting the stimulation threshold versus duration.

This electric field produces an action potential in excitable neuronal cells, which might result in the activation of neuronal circuits when applied above a certain threshold. The neuronal response depends not only on the electric field strength but also on the pulse duration, through a strength–duration curve of the form

$$E_{th} = b(1 + c/\tau) \tag{58.8}$$

where E_{th} is the threshold electric field required to induce the neuronal response and τ is the duration of the field that was above this threshold. The biological parameters determining the neural response are the threshold at infinite duration, termed the rheobase (b, measured in V/m), and the duration at which the threshold is twice the rheobase, termed the chronaxie (c, in μs). The motor and sensory curves as reported by Bourland et al. (1996) are shown in Figure 58.3. These curves should be treated as illustrative only, since the chronaxie and rheobase depend on many biological and experimental factors, such as whether the nerves are myelinated or not (hence the peripheral and cortical parameters should be different), or the train frequency in rTMS, which in general reduces the threshold for stimulation.

As shown by Heller and Van Hulstein (1992), the three-dimensional maximum of the electric field intensity will always be located at the brain surface, for any configuration or superposition of the TMS coils. It is possible, however, to considerably increase the depth penetration and the percentage of electric field intensity in deep brain regions, relative to the maximal field at the cortex. The next section will outline the construction principles for efficient deep brain stimulation, and the following sections will demonstrate several examples of TMS coils designed to accomplish this goal.

58.3 Deep TMS Coils: Design Principles

While the activation of peripheral nerves depends mainly on the derivative of the electric field along the nerve fiber (Maccabee et al., 1993), the most relevant parameter for the activation of brain structures seems to be the electric field intensity (Amassian et al., 1992; Thielscher and Kammer, 2002). In both cases, however, physiological studies indicate that optimal activation occurs when the field is oriented in the same direction as the nerve fiber (Durand et al., 1989; Roth and Basser, 1990; Basser and Roth, 1991; Brasil-Neto et al., 1992; Mills et al., 1992; Pascual-Leone et al., 1994; Niehaus et al., 2000; Kammer et al., 2001). Hence, to stimulate deep brain regions, it is necessary to use coils in such an orientation that they will produce a significant field in the preferable direction to activate the neuronal structures or axons under consideration.

In light of these findings, the geometrical features of each specific design are mainly dependent on two goals:

1. The location and size of the deep brain region or regions intended to be activated
2. The preferred direction or directions we want to stimulate

The design of a specific coil is dictated by these goals. Nevertheless, all deep TMS coils have to share the following important features:

1. *Base complementary to the human head.* The part of the coil close to the head (the base) must be optimally complementary to the human skull at the desired region. In some coils, the base may be flexible and is able to receive the shape of an individual patient, and in other coils, it may be more robust, namely, arcuated in a shape that fits the average human skull at the desired region. In the last case, there may be few similar models designed to fit smaller and larger heads.
2. *Proper orientation of stimulating coil elements.* The coils must be oriented such that they will produce a considerable field in a direction tangential to the surface, which should also be the preferable direction to activate the neurons under consideration. That is, the wires of the coils are directed in one or more directions, which results in a preferred activation of neuronal structures oriented in these particular directions. In some cases, there is one preferred direction along the length or width axis, and in other cases, there are two preferred directions along both the length and width axes.
3. *Summation of electrical impulses.* The induced electric field in the desired deep brain regions is obtained by optimal summation of electric fields, induced by several coil elements with a common direction, located in different places around the skull. The principle of summation may be applied either in time or in space, or in a combination of both. The main types of summation are listed below:
   a. *One-point spatial summation.* In this type of summation, the coil elements, carrying current in the desired direction, are placed in various locations around the head, in such a configuration so as to create a high electric field intensity in a specific deep brain region, which is simultaneously a high percent of the maximal electric field at the brain cortex.
   b. *Morphological line spatial summation.* The goal of this summation is to induce the electric field at several points along a certain neuronal structure. This line should not be straight and may have a complex bent path. The application of diffusion tensor imaging (DTI) in magnetic resonance imaging (MRI) for fiber tracking is an evolving field, which may significantly improve the efficacy of the TMS treatment. If, for example, we know the path of a certain axonal bundle, a coil shall be designed in a configuration that will produce a significant electric field at several points along the bundle. This configuration may enable the induction of an action potential in this bundle, while minimizing the activation of other brain regions. For example, the TMS coil may be activated with an intensity that will induce the subthreshold electric field at most brain regions, which will not induce an action potential, while the induction of the subthreshold field along the desired path may induce an action potential in this bundle, thus increasing the specificity of the TMS treatment.
   c. *Temporal summation.* The various coil elements may be stimulated consecutively and not simultaneously. As shown in Figure 58.3, the neuronal activation threshold depends on both the electric field intensity and the stimulation duration. The TMS coil may be designed in such a configuration that the various elements are scattered around the desired region or path, so that passing a current in each element will produce a significant field at the desired deep brain region. In such a case, the coil may be stimulated consecutively, so that at each time period, only a certain element or a group of elements are activated. This way, in the desired deep brain region, a significant electric field will be induced at all time periods, while in more cortical regions, a significant field will be induced mainly at certain periods, when the proximate coil elements are activated. This will enable the stimulation of the deep brain structure while minimizing the stimulation of other brain regions, and specifically of the cortical regions.

A detailed study into the neural response to trains with interpulse intervals of milliseconds (instead of hundreds of milliseconds as in rTMS) will aid in refining this technique.

4. *Minimization of radial components.* Coil construction is meant to minimize wire elements carrying current components that are nontangential to the skull. The electrical field intensity in the tissue to be stimulated and the rate of decrease of the electrical field as a function of distance from the coil depend on the orientation of the coil elements relative to the tissue surface. It has been shown that coil elements that are nontangential to the surface induce the accumulation of surface charge, which leads to the cancelation of the perpendicular component of the induced field at all points within the tissue, and the reduction of the electrical field in all other directions. At each specific point, the produced electric field is affected by the lengths of the nontangential components and their distances from this point. Thus, the length of the coil elements that are not tangential to the brain tissue surface should be minimized. Furthermore, the nontangential coil elements should be as small as possible and should be placed as far as possible from the deep region to be activated.

5. *Remote location of return paths.* The wires leading the currents in a direction opposite to the preferred direction (the return paths) should be located far from the base and the desired brain region. This enables higher absolute electric field in the desired brain region. In some cases, the return paths may be in the air, namely, far from the head. In other cases, a part of the return paths may be adjacent to a different region in the head, which is distant from the desired brain region.

6. *Shielding.* Feature 5 enables the possibility of screening. Since the return paths are far from the main base, it is possible to screen all or part of their field, by inserting a shield around them or between them and the base. The shield is composed of a material with high magnetic permeability, capable of inhibiting or diverting a magnetic field, such as mu metal, iron, or steel core. Alternatively, the shield is composed of a metal with high conductivity, which can cause electric currents or charge accumulation that may oppose the effect produced by the return portions.

Specific deep TMS coils for stimulating different deep brain regions are described in the following sections.

58.4 A Coil for Stimulation of Deep Brain Regions Related to Mood Disorders: Simulations and Phantom Measurements

Accumulating evidence suggests that the nucleus accumbens plays a major role in mediating reward and motivation (Self and Nestler, 1995; Schultz et al., 1997; Breiter and Rosen, 1999; Ikemoto and Panksepp, 1999; Kalivas and Nakamura, 1999). Functional MRI and positron emission tomographic studies showed that the nucleus accumbens is activated in cocaine addicts in response to cocaine administration (Lyons et al., 1996; Breiter et al., 1997). Other brain regions are also associated with reward circuits, such as the ventral tegmental area, amygdala, and medial prefrontal, cingulate, and orbitofrontal cortices (Breiter and Rosen, 1999; Kalivas and Nakamura, 1999). Moreover, neuronal fibers connecting the medial prefrontal, cingulate, or orbitofrontal cortex with the nucleus accumbens may have an important role in reward and motivation (Jentsch and Taylor, 1999; Volkow and Fowler, 2000). The nucleus accumbens is also connected to the amygdala and the ventral tegmental area. Therefore, the activation of these brain regions may affect the neuronal circuits mediating reward and motivation. In rats and monkeys, and even in humans, electrical stimulation of the median forebrain bundle is rewarding, and when a stimulating electrode is inserted into various parts of that bundle (including the ventral tegmental area, the median prefrontal cortex, and the nucleus accumbens septi), compulsive self-stimulation can be obtained (Jacques, 1999; Milner, 1991). The new coil (termed the *Hesed coil*) is designed to effectively stimulate deeper brain regions without increasing the electrical field intensity in the superficial cortical regions. Numeric simulations and phantom measurements of the total electrical field produced by the Hesed coil inside a homogeneous spherical volume conductor are presented and compared with the results from a circular coil in different orientations and from the double-cone coil. The drop of the electrical field in the brain as a function of the distance from he new coil is much slower compared with the previous coils. It is hoped that such a coil can stimulate deeper regions such as the nucleus accumbens and the fibers connecting the medial prefrontal or cingulate cortex with the nucleus accumbens. The activation of these fibers may induce reward, and chronic treatment may have antidepressant properties or may serve as a new strategy against drug addiction.

58.4.1 Methods

58.4.1.1 Numerical Simulations

The simulations were conducted using a Mathematica program (Wolfram, 1999). The head was modeled as a spherical homogeneous volume conductor with a radius of 7 cm. The induced and electrostatic fields at a specific point inside the spherical volume were computed for several coil configurations, using the method presented by Eaton (1992), and the total electric fields in the x, y, and z directions were calculated.

The vector potential A and scalar potential Φ can be expanded in terms of spherical harmonic functions up to N order. After enforcing the boundary conditions at the sphere boundary, the final expressions for the total electric field in the three Cartesian directions are

$$E_j = E_{Aj} + E_{\Phi j} \quad j = x, y, z \tag{58.9}$$

where the induced field in each direction is given by

$$E_{Aj} = -\frac{\mu_0 \partial I}{\partial t} \sum^{N} \sum^{l} r^l \, Y_{lm}(\theta, \varphi) \, C_{lm}^j \quad j = x, y, z \;\; l = 0 \;\; m = -l \tag{58.10}$$

where $Y_{lm}(\theta, \varphi)$ are the spherical harmonic functions, r, θ, and φ are the spherical coordinates of the point inside the conductive sphere where the electric field is calculated (see Figure 58.4), and C_{lm}^j are j-components of the integration over the coil path

$$C_{lm}^j = \int_{coil} \frac{Y_{lm}^*(\theta', \varphi' \phi) \, dlj}{(2l + 1) \, r'^{l+1}} \quad j = x, y, z \tag{58.11}$$

where * means complex conjugate, r', θ', and φ' are the spherical coordinates of the coil element (Figure 58.4), and dlj is the j component of the differential element of the coil.

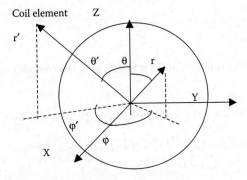

FIGURE 58.4 The relation between the spherical coordinate system and the Cartesian coordinate system in which the field components at every point were calculated. R is the radius vector to the point inside the sphere where the field is computed, and r' is the vector of the differential coil element on which the integration is performed.

The electrostatic fields in x, y, and z directions are given by

$$E_{\Phi x} = -\sin(\theta)\cos(\phi) \sum_{l=1}^{N+1} \sum_{m=-l}^{l} V_{lm} \, l \, r^{l-1} \, Y_{lm}(\theta,\phi) +$$

$$\cos(\theta)\cos(\phi) \sum_{l=1}^{N+1} \sum_{m=-l}^{l} V_{lm} r^{l-1} \tfrac{1}{2}[\exp(i\phi) \, \sqrt{((l-m+1)(l+m))} \, Y_{1,m-1}(\theta,\phi) -$$

$$\exp(-i\phi) \, \sqrt{((l+m+1)(l-m))} \, Y_{1,m+1}(\theta,\phi)] +$$

$$\sin(\phi) \sum_{l=1}^{N+1} \sum_{m=-l}^{l} V_{lm} \, r^{l-1} \, im \, Y_{lm}(\theta,\phi) \tag{58.12}$$

$$E_{\Phi y} = -\sin(\theta)\sin(\phi) \sum_{l=1}^{N+1} \sum_{m=-l}^{l} V_{lm} \, l \, r^{l-1} \, Y_{lm}(\theta,\phi) +$$

$$\cos(\theta)\sin(\phi) \sum_{l=1}^{N+1} \sum_{m=-l}^{l} V_{lm} \, r^{l-1} \tfrac{1}{2}[\exp(i\phi) \, \sqrt{((l-m+1)(l+m))} \, Y_{1,m-1}(\theta,\phi) -$$

$$\exp(-i\phi) \, \sqrt{((l+m+1)(l-m))} \, Y_{1,m+1}(\theta,\phi)] -$$

$$\cos(\phi) \sum_{l=1}^{N+1} \sum_{m=-l}^{l} V_{lm} \, r^{l-1} \, im \, Y_{lm}(\theta,\phi) \tag{58.13}$$

$$E_{\Phi z} = -\cos(\theta) \sum_{l=1}^{N+1} \sum_{m=-l}^{l} V_{lm} \, l \, r^{l-1} \, Y_{lm}(\theta,\phi) -$$

$$\sin(\theta) \sum_{l=1}^{N+1} \sum_{m=-l}^{l} V_{lm} \, r^{l-1} \tfrac{1}{2}[\exp(i\phi) \, \sqrt{((l-m+1)(l+m))} \, Y_{1,m-1}(\theta,\phi) -$$

$$\exp(-i\phi) \, \sqrt{((l+m+1)(l-m))} \, Y_{1,m+1}(\theta,\phi)] \tag{58.14}$$

where $i = \sqrt{-1}$ and V_{lm} is a complex function of the integrals over the coil path C_{lm}^{j}:

$$V_{lm} = -\frac{\mu_0 \partial I}{1 \, \partial t}(\sqrt{[(l+m-1)(l+m)/(2l+1)(2l-1)]} \, 0.5 \, (C_{l-1,m-1}^{y} \, i - C_{l-1,m-1}^{x}) +$$

$$\sqrt{[(l-m-1)(l-m)/(2l+1)(2l-1)]} \, 0.5 \, (C_{l-1,m+1}^{y} \, i + C_{l-1,m+1}^{x}) +$$

$$\sqrt{[(l-m)(l+m)/(2l+1)(2l-1)]} \, C_{l-1,m}^{z}) \tag{58.15}$$

The simulations were performed using 10th-order approximation. The summations in Equations 58.10 through 58.15 were computed up to $N = 10$. The convergence rate depends on the distance from the coil elements and on coil configuration, and in general, is faster for more remote points. For the new coil design, the convergence rate was faster than for the circular coil. For points close to the coils (up to 1.5 cm), the induced field was corrected by the exact formula (Equation 58.5). For more remote points, the error was less than 1%. In all the calculations, the rate of current change was taken as 10,000 A/100 μs. The field is given in volts per meter.

58.4.1.2 Measurements of the Electrical Field Induced in a Phantom Brain

The electrical field induced by the new coil and the double-cone coil (Magstim; Whitland, UK) was measured in a saline solution placed in a hollow glass model of the human head (15 × 17 × 20 cm; Cardinal Industries, Inc., Milwaukee, WI, USA), using a two-wire probe. The distance between the noninsulated edges of the two wires of the probe was 14 mm. The voltage measured divided by the distance between the wire edges gives the induced electrical field figure. Stimulation was delivered using the Magstim Model 200 stimulator at 100% power level. The coils were placed on the glass surface and the electrical field was measured in numerous points within the saline solution.

58.4.2 Results

The simulations revealed that, in general, the presence of the accumulating surface charge induced by coil configurations having a radial current component changes the total field in a nontrivial way. The presence of an electrostatic field not only reduces the total field at any point but also leads to significant reduction in the percentage of the total field in depth, relative to the total field at the surface. Moreover, both the total field and the percentage relative to the surface at any specific point depend on their distance from the nontangential coil elements.

The basic concept of the new coil design is to generate summation of the electrical field in depth by inducing electrical fields at different locations around the surface of the head, all of which have a common direction. Such an approach increased the percentage of electrical field induced in depth, relative to the field in the surface regions. In addition, because a radial component had a dramatic effect on the percentage of the electrical field in depth, an effort was made to minimize the overall length of the nontangential coil elements and to locate them as distant as possible from the deep region to be activated. This region simulated the location of the nucleus accumbens. The calculations for several coil configurations were made and the optimal configuration (termed the *Hesed coil*) was compared with the standard circular coils and with the double-cone coil. We compare the simulation results of the field distribution of the Hesed coil design (Figure 58.5), of a double-cone coil, and of a circular coil oriented perpendicular (Figure 58.6a) and parallel (Figure 58.6b) to the head. Figure 58.5 shows the coil design when applied on the human head. The coil contains several strips (e.g., 26 in Figure 58.5) attached to the head, all connected serially, and having wires that induce stimulation in the desired direction. This desired direction is the anteroposterior direction in the example shown in Figure 58.5 (z direction). For each strip, there is a return path wire having the current component at the opposite direction (z direction), located 5 cm above the head. These return paths are located at the top edges of four fans, to remove the currents flowing through them away from the deep regions of the head. The specific design of the fans is meant to reduce the inductance of the coil. The fans are connected to the frame near strips 7, 9, 18, and 20 (see Figure 58.5). These loci were chosen to remove the return paths as much as possible from the deep brain region to be activated most effectively. The only wires with currents that have radial components are those connecting the strips that are attached to the head with their return paths, along the sides of the fans. An optimized coil would have a flexible frame allowing all elements of the coil that are touching the head to be tangential to the head surface (see Figure 58.5).

In the calculations of the field produced by the Hesed coil design, we assumed that the only coil elements carrying current components that are not tangential to the surface are the wires connecting the return paths with the strips that are attached to the head (along the fans). This is a plausible assumption

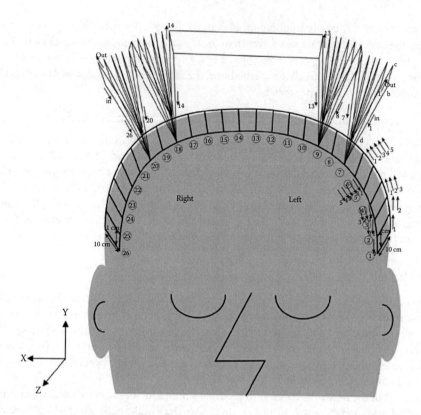

FIGURE 58.5 The Hesed coil shape when applied over the human head. The same coil can be placed around the forehead to stimulate nerve fibers in the superoinferior direction. The only elements that produce an electrical field in the z direction are the 26 strips attached to the head (numbered 1–26), where the current is in the +z direction, and the 26 return paths at the edges of the fans where the current is in the –z direction.

in the realistic case, where the coil is attached to the skull. In the human head, the cerebral spinal fluid is approximately parallel to the skull everywhere and it can be assumed that the conductive properties of the cerebral spinal fluid are similar to those of the brain. The electrostatic field resulting from the contribution of the nontangential elements was calculated for each point and subtracted from the induced field of the coil. To obtain maximal efficacy, given the limitations of the stimulator and the need for a specific range of the coil inductance (15–25 μH), the average lengths of the strips were taken as 8 cm. The simulations were made for strips of length 9 cm over one hemisphere and of 7 cm over the other hemisphere (to obtain a slight preference for one hemisphere stimulation and to have the opportunity to reach the stimulation threshold only in one hemisphere). The wires connecting the head strips to their return paths (the nontangential elements) were taken as 5 cm long. The locations of the strips were determined to fit the human head, as in Figure 58.5. Hence, the distances of strips 13 and 14 from the sphere center were taken as approximately 6 cm; strips 3 and 24 were located approximately 7 cm from the sphere center. For the orientation shown in Figure 58.5, the maximal total field in the anteroposterior direction (z direction) was produced at the cortex near the center of strips 1 and 26 at the sides. The field at the top of the head was reduced considerably because of the influence of the return paths and of the nontangential wires along the sides of the fans.

Figure 58.7 shows the induced (Figure 58.7a) and the total (Figure 58.7b) fields in the z direction (E_z, defined in Figure 58.6) of a one-turn 5.5-cm-diameter circular coil placed perpendicular and parallel to a 7-cm-radius spherical volume conductor, as a function of the distance from the coil edge. The fields were calculated along the line connecting the sphere center to the coil point closest to the surface (line

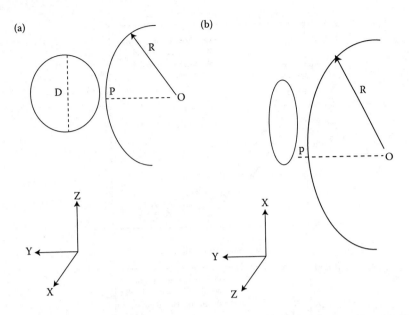

FIGURE 58.6 (a) A circular coil with diameter D placed perpendicular to the head surface. The head is modeled as a sphere with a radius R = 7 cm. The coil has a current component in the y direction, which is perpendicular to the head, and a component in the z direction, which is completely parallel to the head surface only at the attachment point p. (b) A circular coil with diameter D placed tangential to the head surface. The coil has current components in the x and z directions, which are completely parallel to the head surface only at the attachment point p.

o–p in Figure 58.6). It is clear that the reduction in the total field resulting from charge accumulation is much larger when the coil is oriented perpendicular to the surface (Figure 58.7). In addition, a comparison was made with the induced and the total fields of one winding from the new Hesed coil, including strip 1 with its connection to the return path and its return path itself (and taking strips of length 5.5 cm). The simulations show that although the induced field of the strip is slightly larger than that of a circular coil with similar dimensions (see Figure 58.7), the difference in the total field is much larger (see Figure 58.7). This results from the fact that the field reduction due to electrostatic charge accumulation in the case of the winding of strip 1 is very small because the only elements carrying radial current components are the wires along paths a–b and c–d (see Figure 58.5), which are a relatively small fraction of the winding length, and are distant from the points under consideration. The induced and the total fields in the z direction (Ez) resulting from the entire Hesed coil compared with the double-cone coil are shown in Figure 58.8. The field of the Hesed coil is computed along the line from strip 26 (where it is maximal) to the sphere center. The field of the double-cone coil is computed along the line from the junction at the coil center (where it is maximal) to the sphere center. Although the double-cone coil produces a much larger induced field than the Hesed coil (see Figure 58.8a), the rate of decay of the effective total field with distance is much smaller for the Hesed coil (see Figure 58.8b). Hence, at a depth of 6 cm, the total electrical field of the Hesed coil is already a little larger than that of the double-cone coil (see Figure 58.8b).

Figure 58.9 shows the z component of the electrical field as a function of distance, relative to the field at a distance of 1 cm, for the Hesed coil, a double-cone coil with 14 cm diameter for each wing, and the 5.5-cm-diameter circular coil oriented tangential and perpendicular to the head surface. The field produced by the Hesed coil at a depth of 6 cm is approximately 35% of the field at a depth of 1 cm near the middle of strip 26 (where the field induced by the Hesed coil is highest throughout the brain). The field produced by the double-cone coil at a depth of 6 cm is only about 8% of the field 1 cm from the coil. The field produced by the 5.5-cm-diameter circular coil at this depth is less than 2% of the field 1 cm from

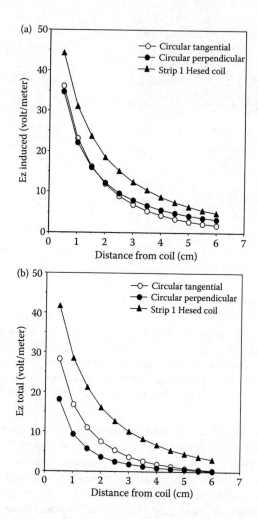

FIGURE 58.7 Induced (a) and total (b) electrical field in the z direction plotted as a function of distance from a one-turn circular coil of 5.5 cm diameter placed tangential or perpendicular to the head surface. In addition, the induced and total fields of the winding of the Hesed coil connected to strip 1 (see Figure 58.2) is shown for the case of the strip of length 5.5 cm.

the coil. For a larger circular coil, the percentage of the field in depth is somewhat higher, but is still smaller than that of the double-cone coil (data not shown).

The actual measurements of the electrical fields in a phantom brain using the first manufactured version of the Hesed coil and a double-cone coil basically confirmed our theoretical calculations. Both coils produced slightly lower fields at any point in the phantom brain compared with the theoretical calculations. However, this was more evident in the case of the Hesed coil, and the percentage of the field in depth relative to the surface was slightly lower compared with our calculations. The results for the total field and the percentage in depth are presented in Figure 58.10.

It is clear that the total field induced by the double-cone coil, using the maximal output of the stimulator (10,000 A/100 μs) produces a markedly greater electrical field up to 6 cm depth, compared with the Hesed coil (see Figure 58.10a), but the percentage in depth is markedly greater when the Hesed coil is used (see Figure 58.8).

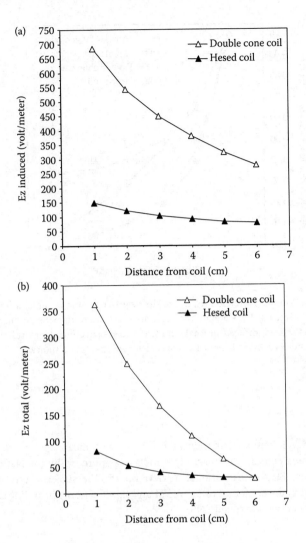

FIGURE 58.8 Induced (a) and total (b) electrical fields in the z direction plotted as a function of distance for the double-cone coil and the Hesed coil. The electrical fields were calculated for a six-turn double-cone coil with a diameter of 14 cm for each wing, an opening angle of 95°, and a central linear section of 3 cm, and for the Hesed coil with strip lengths of 9 cm over the right hemisphere and of 7 cm over the left hemisphere. The field of the Hesed coil is computed along the line from strip 26 (where Ez is maximal) to the sphere center. The field of the double-cone coil is computed along the line from the central linear section (where Ez is maximal) to the sphere center.

58.5 TMS of Deep Brain Regions: Evidence for Efficacy of the H-Coil

The biological efficacy of the H-coil was tested (Zangen et al., 2005) using the motor threshold as a measure of a biological effect. The rate of decrease of the electric field as a function of distance from the coil was measured by gradually increasing the distance of the coil from the skull and measuring the motor threshold at each distance. A comparison was made to the figure-8 coil.

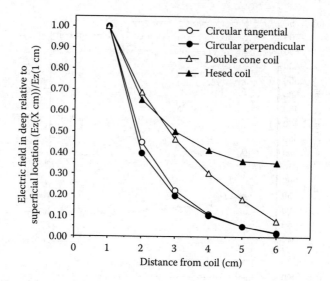

FIGURE 58.9 Electrical field in the z direction relative to the field 1 cm from the coil as a function of distance. The data are presented for the Hesed coil, the double-cone coil, and the 5.5-cm-diameter circular coil oriented tangential and perpendicular to the head surface. The total electrical field at each point along the line from the point of maximal Ez to the sphere center was divided by the Ez value calculated at a 1 cm distance.

58.5.1 Methods

58.5.1.1 Subject

Six healthy, right-handed volunteers (four men and two women, mean age 36 years, range 25–45 years) gave written informed consent for the study, which was approved by the National Institute of Neurological Disorders and Stroke Institutional Review Board. The subjects were interviewed and examined by a neurologist and were found to be free of any significant medical illness or medications known to affect the central nervous system (CNS).

58.5.1.2 TMS Coils

The TMS coils used in this study were a specific version of the H-coil and a figure-of-eight coil. The H-coil version used in this study allows a comfortable placement on the hand motor cortex. The theoretical considerations and design principles of the H-coils are explained in our previous study (Roth et al., 2002). In short, the coil is designed to generate summation of the electric field in a specific brain region by locating coil elements at different locations around this region, all of which have a common current component that induce the electric field in the desired direction (termed +z direction). In addition, since a radial component has a dramatic effect on the electric field magnitude and on the rate of decay of the electric field with distance, the overall length of coil elements that are nontangential to the skull should be minimized, and these elements as well as coil elements having the current component in the opposite direction (−z direction) should be located as distant as possible from the brain region to be activated.

The H-coil version used in this study is shown in Figure 58.11. The coil has 10 strips carrying a current in a common direction (+z direction) and are located around the desired motor cortex site (segments A–B and G–H in Figure 58.11). The average length of the strips is 11 cm. The only coil elements having radial current components are those connected to the return paths of five of the strips (segments C–I and J–F in Figure 58.1). The length of these wires is 8 cm. The return paths of the other five strips are placed on the head at the contralateral hemisphere (segment D–E in Figure 58.11). The wires connecting

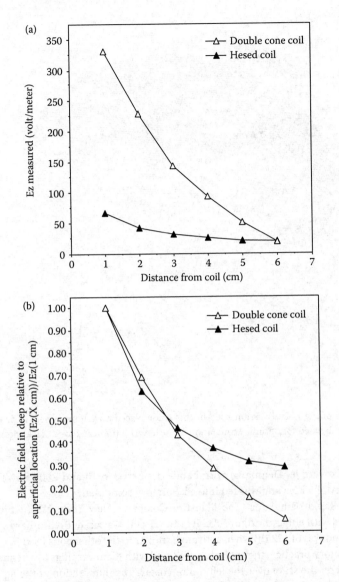

FIGURE 58.10 Measurements of the electrical field induced by the Hesed coil and the double-cone coil in a phantom brain. The electrical field induced in the z direction (a) and the electrical field in the z direction *relative* to the field 1 cm from the coil (b) are plotted as functions of the distance from the coil. For both coils, the data show the measurements along the line from the point where the maximal Ez value is obtained (as described earlier) for the sphere center.

between the strips and the return paths (segments B–C and F–A in Figure 58.11) are on average 9 cm long. The H-coil was compared to a standard commercial Magstim figure-of-eight coil with internal loop diameters of 7 cm.

58.5.1.3 Experimental Setup

The subjects were seated with the right forearm and hand supported. Motor-evoked potentials (MEPs) of the right abductor pollicis brevis (APB) muscle were recorded using silver–silver chloride surface electrodes. The subjects were instructed to maintain muscle relaxation throughout the study. Electromyogram (EMG) amplitude was amplified using a conventional EMG machine (Counterpoint,

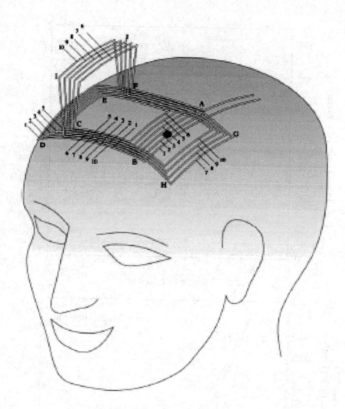

FIGURE 58.11 Sketch of the H-coil version used in this study placed on a human head. The coil orientation shown in the figure is designated for optimal stimulation of the left APB (indicated by a black spot).

Dantec Electronics, Skovlunde, Denmark) with band-pass between 10 and 2000 Hz. The signal was digitized at a frequency of 5 kHz and was fed into a laboratory computer.

A Magstim Super Rapid stimulator (The Magstim Company, New York, NY), which produces a biphasic pulse, coupled with either the figure-8 coil or the H-coil, was used. Preliminary studies showed the H-coil to have a loudness of 122 dB when activated, similar to the other coils used in our laboratory. As the standard laboratory practice, the subjects were fitted with foam earplugs to attenuate the sound.

The coil was placed on the scalp over the left motor cortex. The intersection of the figure-8 coil was placed tangentially to the scalp with the handle pointing backward and laterally at a 45° angle away from the midline. Thus, the current induced in the neural tissue was directed approximately perpendicular to the line of the central sulcus and therefore was optimal for activating the corticospinal pathways trans-synaptically (Brasil-Neto et al., 1992; Kaneko et al., 1996). Similarly, the H-coil was placed on the scalp with the handle pointing backward in such a way that the centers of the strips cover the motor cortex and in such a direction that the current induced in the neural tissue would be perpendicular to the line of the central sulcus. With a slightly suprathreshold stimulus intensity, the stimulating coil was moved over the left hemisphere to determine the optimal position for eliciting MEPs of maximal amplitudes (the "hot spot"). The optimal position of the coil was then marked on the scalp to ensure coil placement throughout the experiment. The resting motor threshold was determined to the nearest 1% of the maximum stimulator output and was defined as the minimal stimulus intensity required to produce MEPs of >50 μV in ≥5 of the 10 consecutive trials at least 5 s apart.

The coils were held in a stable coil holder, which could be adjusted at different heights above the "hot spot" on the scalp. The resting motor threshold was determined at different distances above the scalp, using increments of 0.5 cm.

58.5.1.4 Safety Measurements

Since the H-coil was not used in the previous clinical TMS studies, we asked the subjects to report any side effects, including pain, anxiety, or dizziness, and we performed cognitive and hearing tests before and after the TMS session. For the cognitive testing, we used the CalCap computer program to test immediate and delayed memories as described previously (Wassermann et al., 1996).

58.5.2 Results

None of the six subjects who participated in the study reported any significant side effects after the TMS session. We did not find any change in cognitive or hearing abilities in these six subjects. A slight and short-lasting headache was reported by one out of the six subjects. In a different experiment done subsequently, not reported in this chapter, we used the H-coil to deliver single or paired pulses at 1 Hz during 20 s at five different locations on the scalp in three additional subjects. The third of these subjects experienced some hearing loss in his left ear, a 30 dB loss at 4000 Hz that has been stable for 10 months and appears to be permanent. The ear protection had fallen out transiently during the study.

The percentage of stimulator output required for APB activation by each coil is plotted in Figure 58.12 as a function of distance from the "hot spot" on the scalp. It can be seen that the efficacy of the H-coil at large distances from the scalp was significantly greater as compared to the figure-8 coil. When using the maximal stimulation power output, the figure-8 coil can be effective (reach stimulation threshold) up to 2 cm away from the coil, while the H-coil can be effective at 5.5 cm away from the coil. Moreover, the rate of decay of effectiveness as a function of the distance from the coil is much slower in the H-coil relative to the figure-8 coil (Figure 58.12).

58.5.3 Discussion

The findings confirm our theoretical calculations and phantom brain measurements (Roth et al., 2002) indicating the ability of the H-coil to stimulate brain structures at a large distance from the

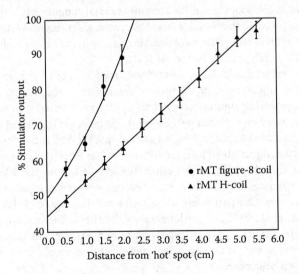

FIGURE 58.12 Intensity needed for APB stimulation at different heights above the scalp. The resting motor threshold of the APB was measured at different distances above the "hot spot" when using either the H-coil or the figure-8 coil. The percent of stimulator power needed to reach the resting motor threshold versus the distance of the coil from the "hot spot" on the skull is plotted. The points represent means and standard deviations (SDs) of six healthy volunteers.

coil. The comparison between the TMS coils demonstrated a significantly improved depth penetration, and a much slower rate of decay of effectiveness as a function of the distance from the coil, when using the H-coil relative to the regular figure-8 coil. This indicates that when stimulating deep brain regions by using the H-coil, the cortical stimulation is not much higher for the same activation in depth.

The H-coil produces a summation of the electric field from several coil elements carrying current in the same direction. In contrast, the electric field of the figure-8 coil is produced by a concentrated region in the center of the coil. In addition, the relative fraction of the figure-8 field that is produced by coil elements that are nontangential to skull surface is much larger than in the H-coil. These two reasons lead to the fact that although the figure-8 field is more focal, it has more significant reduction both in the absolute field magnitude at any point and in the percentage of the deep region field relative to the field at the surface.

According to our calculations and phantom brain measurements (Roth et al., 2002), the field induced in cortical regions by the H-coil is much lower than that of the double- cone coil. Therefore, it is likely that the excitation threshold can be reached at 4–6 cm using the H-coil without inducing pain and other side effects.

It should be emphasized that although the structure stimulated in this study was in the motor cortex, and the medium between the coils and the "hot spot" was mainly air, the rate of decay within the brain itself should be very similar. This is a delicate point that should be elaborated. The electric conductivity of the brain is much greater than that of air. In conductive materials such as the brain, the radial current components of the coil would lead to charge accumulation on the surface of the brain, which would cause a decrease of the field at any point inside the brain. Hence, the rate of decay of the electric field with distance would be faster in the brain than that measured in air. Nevertheless, the field distribution inside the brain is *independent* of the location of the interface between the conductive and insulating media (Tofts, 1990; Branston and Tofts, 1990; Eaton, 1992). As a result, the rate of decay within the brain when attaching the coil to the skull would be similar to that measured in this study, where the coil was raised above the skull. Small changes are expected due to the fact that the coil configuration relative to the skull is somewhat different when it is raised. The H-coil is designed to minimize the radial current components when attached to the scalp; hence, the amount of radial components may be slightly different and may be probably larger when the H-coil is raised above the scalp. Therefore, the advantage of the H-coil as compared to the figure-8 coil, in terms of the rate of decay of the field as a function of distance, may be even greater when the coils are attached to the scalp.

Although the H-coil has a remarkable ability to penetrate into deeper brain regions, due to the slower decay of the electric field as a function of distance, none of the subjects in the present study reported any side effects and cognitive or hearing abilities were not affected. Nevertheless, it should be emphasized that subjects in the present study experienced only 20–30 single pulses at intensities greater than those needed for minimal APB activation (when looking for the hot spot for APB activation) and that the rest of the pulses were given just at the minimal level for APB activation when the coil was placed either on the scalp or at different heights above the scalp. Future studies will address the safety and efficacy of the H-coil when used in higher doses. As we have reported, one subject has experienced some hearing loss in a subsequent experiment. Our past safety studies have not demonstrated that hearing loss is to be expected (Pascual-Leone et al., 1992). As the loudness of the H-coil does not appear different from other coils, this result may be due in part to particularly sensitive hearing in this subject and lapse in the hearing protection. However, as we did caution before, the event does emphasize the need in all TMS studies to take care to protect hearing.

58.6 TMS of Deep Prefrontal Regions

The medial prefrontal and orbitofrontal regions are known to be associated with reward circuits. The H1 and H2 coils are designed to stimulated deep prefrontal structures, with minimal undesired side effects such as pain, motor stimulation, and facial muscles activation. The coils are wounded with a double 14 American wire gauge (AWG)-insulated copper wire winded into several windings, connected in series. The detailed illustration of the wiring pattern of H1 is shown in Figure 58.13 and of H2 is shown in Figure 58.14.

The effective part of the H1 coil, in contact with the patient's scalp, has a shape of half a donut, with 14 strips of 7–12 cm length (Figure 58.13). These strips produce the most effective field of the coil, and are oriented in an anterior–posterior axis. The 14 strips are distributed above the prefrontal cortex of the left hemisphere, with a separation of 1 cm between them. Three strips (8–10 in Figure 58.13) are elongated toward the forehead and their continuations pass in the left–right direction along the orbitofrontal cortex (segments I–J, 8–10 in Figure 58.13), with a separation of 1 cm between them. The return paths of strips 1–7 are attached to the head in the right hemisphere (segments D–E, 1–7 in Figure 58.13), with a separation of 0.8 cm between them. The return paths of strips 8–14 are remote 7 cm from the head (segments M–G, 8–14 in Figure 58.13), with a separation of 0.3 cm between them.

The frame of the inner rim of the half-donut is flexible to fit the variability in human skull shape.

The paths of the 14 windings of the H1 coil are shown in Figure 58.13. The windings of strips 1–7 traverse the path A–B–C–D–E–F–G–H–A. The windings of strips 8–10 traverse the path A–I–J–K–L–M–G–H–A. The windings of strip 11–14 traverse the path A–N–L–M–G–H–A.

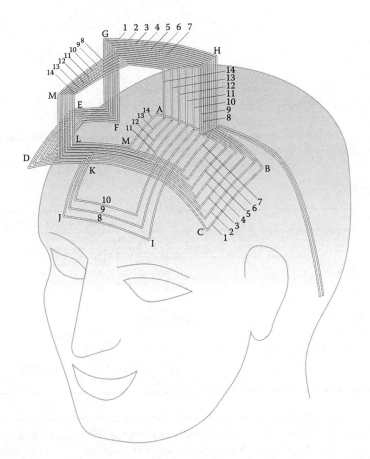

FIGURE 58.13 Sketch of the H1 coil near a human head. The coil orientation shown in the figure is designated for the activation of structures in the prefrontal cortex, in the anterior–posterior direction.

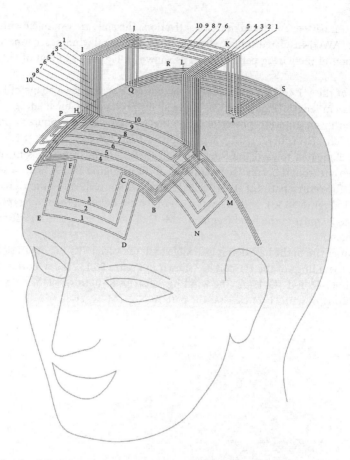

FIGURE 58.14 Sketch of the H2-coil near a human head. The coil orientation shown in the figure is designated for the activation of structures in the prefrontal cortex, in the lateral–medial direction.

H1-Coil Specifications

Number of Windings	4 Wire Loops, Including Strips and Return Paths
Strips length	Strips 1–7, 11–14:7 cm
	Strips 8–10:10–12 cm
Main induced field direction	Anterior–posterior axis
Strips separation	1 cm (typical)
Connecting cable	2 ± 0.5 m
Coil inductance (including cable)	30 ± 1 μH
Maximum magnetic field strength	3.2 T
Maximum electric field strength of 0.5 cm from the coil	200 V/m
Wire size (circular section of copper)	Two 14 AWG insulated wires in parallel
Wire length	750 cm

Figure 58.14 shows a diagram of the H2 coil, which is designed to stimulate deep brain regions and fit the human head. The effective part of the coil, in contact with the patient's scalp, has a shape of half a donut, with 10 strips of 14–22 cm length (Figure 58.14). These strips produce the most effective field of the coil, and are oriented in a right–left direction (lateral–medial axis). Three strips pass in front of the forehead along the orbitofrontal cortex (1–3 in Figure 58.14), with separation of 1 cm between them.

seven strips pass above the forehead along the prefrontal cortex (4–10 in Figure 58.14), with a separation of 0.8 cm.

The paths of the 10 windings are shown in Figure 58.3. The windings of strips 1–3 traverse the path A–B–C–D–E–F–G–H–I–J–Q–R–S–T–K–L–A. The winding of strip 4 traverses the path A–B–G–H–I–J–Q–R–S–T–K–L–A. The winding of strip 5 traverses the path A–M–N–B–G–O–P–H–I–J–Q–R–S–T–K–L–A. The windings of strips 6–7 traverse the path A–M–N–B–G–O–P–H–I–J–K–L–A. The windings of strips 8–9 traverse the path A–B–G–H–I–J–K–L–A. The winding of strip 10 traverses the path A–H–I–J–K–L–A.

H2-Coil Specifications

Number of Windings	10 Wire Loops, Including Strips and Return Paths
Strips length	14–22 cm
Main induced field direction	Lateral–medial axis
Strips separation	0.8 cm (typical)
Connecting cable	2 ± 0.5 m
Coil inductance (including cable)	25 ± 1 µH
Maximum magnetic field strength	3.0 T
Maximum electric field strength of 0.5 cm from the coil	190 V/m
Wire size (circular section of copper)	Two 14 AWG insulated wires in parallel
Wire length	800 cm

58.6.1 Comparison of Electric Field Distributions

The electric field distribution produced by H1 and H2 coils was measured in a brain phantom with general dimensions of $23 \times 19 \times 15$ cm, which was filled with 0.9% weight per volume of saline. To determine the output of the coil at depth, the induced electric field was measured using a two-wire probe. The distance between the ends of the two wires of the probe was measured to be 12.7 ± 0.2 mm. The voltage measured divided by the distance between the wires gives the induced electric field value. The two coils were compared to a standard Magstim figure-8 coil with an internal loop diameter of 7 cm and a Magstim double-cone coil. The double-cone coil is considered to be able to stimulate deeper brain regions compared to other coils (Terao et al., 1994, 2000; Stokic et al., 1997).

The depth penetration of the coils was tested by measuring the electric field along the up–down line (z axis) beneath the center of the most effective part of the coil, at 100% output of Magstim Rapid stimulator. In H1, the most effective part was under strip 8 (under the third strip of A–I, the eighth segment in Figure 58.13), where the probe is oriented in an anterior–posterior direction (y axis). In H2, the most effective part was the center of strip 5 (center of C–F, the fifth segment in Figure 58.14), where the probe is oriented in a lateral–medial direction (x axis). In the double-cone coil and in the figure-8 coil, the most effective part was the junction at the coil center, where the probe is oriented in an anterior–posterior direction (y axis). The plots of the total electric field as a function of distance are shown in Figure 58.15.

Figure 58.16 shows the electric field as a function of distance, relative to the field at a distance of 1 cm, for the four coils.

It can be seen that the total electric field induced by the double-cone coil and by the figure-8 coil, using the maximal output of the stimulator, is markedly greater than the field produced by the H1 and H2 at short distances of 1–2 cm. Yet, at distances of above 5 cm, the fields of the H1 and H2 coils become greater due to their much slower rate of decay. From Figure 58.16, it can be seen that the percentage in depth for the H-coils is greater than the other two coils already at a distance of 2 cm, and this advantage of the H-coils becomes more prominent with increasing distance. By comparing the two H-coils, it can be seen that H1 produces slightly smaller absolute field magnitude, but a larger percentage in depth, relative to H2. The fields produced by the H1 and H2 at 6 cm depth are about 63% and 57% of the field

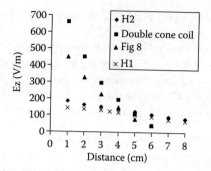

FIGURE 58.15 Phantom measurements of the electric field in the z direction (up–down direction), plotted as a function of distance, for H1 and H2 coils, the double-cone coil, and the figure-8 coil.

1 cm from the coil, respectively, while the fields of the double-cone coil and the figure-8 coil attenuate to 8–10% at this distance.

The stimulation of brain structures at 3–4 cm depth with the double-cone coil are painful since a much higher field is induced at superficial cortical areas and at the facial muscles. To reach the stimulation threshold at 5–8 cm depth, a much higher intensity would be needed that would increase pain and the risk for other side effects such as convulsions. The total field induced by the H1 and H2 coils, even at the maximal power output, will be 3–4 times lower than the double cone in cortical regions. The H1 and H2 fields at 5–6 cm depth are not much smaller than their fields in the cortex and are greater than the double-cone coil field at that depth. Therefore, it is likely that the excitation threshold can be reached at 6–7 cm using the H-coils, without the induction of pain and other side effects. The percentage of the electric field in depth produced by the standard figure-8 coils is similar to the double-cone coil, but the absolute field magnitude is much smaller. Therefore, the figure-8 coil would not only cause greater side effects but also could not reach the stimulation threshold in depth, even at the maximal power output.

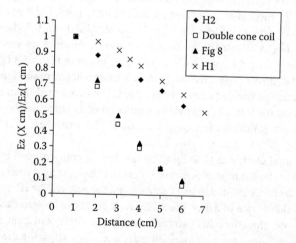

FIGURE 58.16 Electric field relative to the field 1 cm from the coil, as a function of distance, for the H1 and H2 coils, the double-cone coil, and the figure-8 coil, according to the phantom brain measurements.

References

Amassian VE, Eberle L, Maccabee PJ, and Cracco RQ. Modeling magnetic coil excitation of human cerebral cortex with a peripheral nerve immersed in a brain-shaped volume conductor: The significance of fiber bending in excitation. *Electroenceph Clin Neurophysiol* 1992; 85:291–301.

Barker AT, Garnham CW, and Freeston IL. Magnetic nerve stimulation—The effect of waveform on efficiency, determination of neural membrane time constants and the measurement of stimulator output, in magnetic motor stimulation: Basic principles and clinical experience. *Electroenceph Clin Neurophysiol* 1991; Suppl 43:227–237.

Barker AT, Jalinous R, and Freeston IL. Non-invasive magnetic stimulation of the human motor cortex. *Lancet* 1985; 1:1106–1107.

Basser PJ, and Roth BJ. Stimulation of a myelinated nerve axon by electromagnetic induction. *Med Biol Eng Comput* 1991;29:261–268.

Bohning DH. Introduction and overview of TMS physics. In *Transcranial Magnetic Stimulation in Neuropsychiatry*, p 13.

Bourland JD, Nyenhuis JA, Noe WA, Schaefer JD, Foster KS, and Geddes LA. Motor and sensory strength–duration curves for MRI gradient fields, in *Proceedings of the International Society of Magnetic Resonance Medicine, 4th Scientific Meeting and Exhibit*, New York, 1996; p 1724.

Branston NM, and Tofts PS. Magnetic stimulation of a volume conductor produces a negligible component of induced current perpendicular to the surface. *J Physiol (Lond)* 1990;423:67.

Brasil-Neto JP, Cohen LG, Panizza M, Nilsson J, Roth BJ, and Hallett M. Optimal focal transcranial magnetic activation of the human motor cortex: Effects of coil orientation, shape of the induced current pulse, and stimulus intensity. *J Clin Neurophysiol* 1992; 9:132–136.

Breiter HC, Gollub RL, Weisskoff RM, Kennedy DN, Markis N, Berke JD, Goodman JM et al. Acute effects of cocaine on human brain activity and emotion. *Neuron* 1997; 19:591–611.

Breiter HC, and Rosen BR. Functional magnetic resonance imaging of brain reward circuitry in the human. *Ann N Y Acad Sci* 1999; 877:523–547.

Cohen D, and Cuffin BN. Developing a more focal magnetic stimulator. Part I: Some basic principles. *J Clin Neurophysiol* 1991; 8:102–111.

Cohen LG, Roth BJ, Nilsson J, Dang N, Panizza M, Bandinelli S, Friauf W. Effects of coil design on delivery of focal magnetic stimulation. Technical considerations. *Electroencephal Clin Neurophysiol* 1990; 75:350–357.

Durand D, Ferguson AS, and Dalbasti T. Induced electric fields by magnetic stimulation in non-homogeneous conducting media. *IEEE Eng Med Biol Soc, 11th Annual International Conference*, Seattle, WA, 1989; 6:1252–1253.

Eaton H. Electric field induced in a spherical volume conductor from arbitrary coils: Application to magnetic stimulation and MEG. *Med Biol Eng Comput* 1992; 30:433–440.

Heller L and Van Hulstein DB. Brain stimulation using electromagnetic sources: Theoretical aspects. *Biophys J* 1992; 63:129–138.

Ikemoto S, and Panksepp J. The role of nucleus accumbens dopamine in motivated behavior: A unifying interpretation with special reference to reward-seeking. *Brain Res Rev* 1999; 31:6–41.

Jacques S. Brain stimulation reward: "Pleasure centers" after twenty five years. *Neurosurgery* 1999; 5:277–283.

Jentsch JD, and Taylor JR. Impulsivity resulting from frontostriatal dysfunction in drug abuse: Implications for the control of behavior by reward-related behaviors. *Psychopharmacology* 1999; 146:373–390.

Kalivas PW, and Nakamura M. Neural systems for behavioral activation and reward. *Curr Opin Neurobiol* 1999; 9:223–227.

Kammer T, Beck S, Thielscher A, Laubis-Herrmann U, and Topka H. Motor thresholds in humans. A transcranial magnetic stimulation study comparing different pulseforms, current directions and stimulator types. *Clin Neurophysiol* 2001; 112:250–258.

Kaneko K, Kawai S, Fuchigami Y, Morita H, and Ofuji A. The effect of current direction induced by transcranial magnetic stimulation on the corticospinal excitability in human brain. *Electroencephalogr Clin Neurophysiol* 1996; 101:478–482.

Kirkcaldie MT, Pridmore SA, and Pascual-Leone A. Transcranial magnetic stimulation as therapy for depression and other disorders. *Aust N Z J Psychiatry* 1997; 31:264–272.

Lyons D, Friedman DP, Nader MA, and Porrino LJ. Cocaine alters cerebral metabolism within the ventral striatum and limbic cortex of monkeys. *J Neurosci* 1996; 16:1230–1238.

Maccabee PJ, Amassian VE, Eberle VE, and Cracco RQ. Magnetic coil stimulation of straight and bent amphibian and mammalian peripheral nerve *in vitro*: Locus of excitation. *J Physiol* 1993; 460:201–219.

Maccabee PJ, Eberle L, Amassian VE, Cracco RQ, Rudell A, and Jayachandra M. Spatial distribution of the electric field induced in volume by round and figure "8" magnetic coils: Relevance to activation of sensory nerve fibers. *Electroenceph Clin Neurophysiol* 1990; 76:131–141.

Mills KR, Boniface SJ, and Schubert M. Magnetic brain stimulation with a double coil: The importance of coil orientation. *Electroenceph Clin Neurophysiol* 1992; 85:17–21.

Milner PM. Brain–stimulation reward: A review. *Can J Psychol* 1991; 45:1–36.

Niehaus L, Meyer BU, and Weyh T. Influence of pulse configuration and direction of coil current on excitatory effects of magnetic motor cortex and nerve stimulation. *Clin Neurophysiol* 2000; 111:75–80.

Pascual-Leone A, Cohen LG, Brasil-Neto JP, and Hallett M. Non-invasive differentiation of motor cortical representation of hand muscles by mapping of optimal current directions. *Electroenceph Clin Neurophysiol* 1994; 93:42–48.

Pascual-Leone A, Cohen LG, Shotland LI, Dang N, Pikus A, Wassermann EM, Brasil-Neto JP, Valls-Sole J, and Hallett M. No evidence of hearing loss in humans due to transcranial magnetic stimulation. *Neurology* 1992; 42:647–651.

Ren C, Tarjan PP, and Popovic DB. A novel electric design for electromagnetic stimulation: The slinky coil. *IEEE Trans Biomed Eng* 1995; 42:918–925.

Roth BJ, and Basser PJ. A model of the stimulation of a nerve fiber by electromagnetic radiation. *IEEE Trans Biomed Eng* 1990; 37:588–597.

Roth BJ, Cohen LG, Hallet M, Friauf W, and Basser PJ. A theoretical calculation of the electric field induced by magnetic stimulation of a peripheral nerve. *Muscle Nerve* 1990; 13:734–741.

Roth Y, Zangen A, and Hallett M. A coil design for transcranial magnetic stimulation of deep brain regions. *J Clin Neurophysiol* 2002; 19:361–370.

Ruhonen J, and Ilmoniemi RJ. Focusing and targeting of magnetic brain stimulation using multiple coils. *Med Biol Eng Comput* 1998; 38:297–301.

Schultz W, Dayan P, and Montague PR. A neural substrate of prediction and reward. *Science* 1997; 275:1593–1599.

Self DW, and Nestler EJ. Molecular mechanisms of drug reinforcement and addiction. *Annu Rev Neurosci* 1995; 18:463–495.

Stokic DS, McKay WB, Scott L, Sherwood AM, and Dimitrijevic MR. Intracortical inhibition of lower limb motor-evoked potentials after paired transcranial magnetic stimulation. *Exp Brain Res* 1997; 117:437–443.

Terao Y, Ugawa Y, Hanajima R et al. Predominant activation of I1-waves from the leg motor area by transcranial magnetic stimulation. *Brain Res* 2000; 859:137–146.

Terao Y, Ugawa Y, Sakai K, Uesaka Y, and Kanazawa I. Transcranial magnetic stimulation of the leg area of motor cortex in humans. *Acta Neurol Scand* 1994; 89:378–383.

Thielscher A, and Kammer T. Linking physics with physiology in TMS: A spherical field model to determine the cortical stimulation site in TMS. *Neuroimage* 2002; 17:1117–1130.

Tofts PS. The distribution of induced currents in magnetic stimulation of the brain. *Phys Med Biol* 1990; 35:1119–1128.

Tofts PS, and Branston NM. The measurement of electric field, and the influence of surface charge, in magnetic stimulation. *Electroenceph Clin Neurophysiol* 1991; 81:238–239.

Volkow ND, and Fowler JS. Addiction, a disease of compulsion and drive: Involvement of the orbitofrontal cortex. *Cereb Cortex* 2000; 10:318–325.

Wassermann EM, Grafman J, Berry C, Hollnagel C, Wild K, Clark K, and Hallett M. Use and safety of a new repetitive transcranial magnetic stimulator. *Electroencephalogr Clin Neurophysiol* 1996; 10:412–417.

Wassermann EM, and Lisanby SH. Therapeutic application of repetitive transcranial magnetic stimulation: A review. *Clin Neurophysiol* 2001; 112:1367–1377.

Watson D, Clark LA, and Tellegen A. Development and validation of brief measures of positive and negative effect: The PANAS scales. *J Pers Soc Psychol* 1988; 54:1063–1070.

Zangen A, Roth Y, Voller B, and Hallett M. Transcranial magnetic stimulation of deep brain regions: Evidence for efficacy of the H-coil. *Clin Neurophysiol.*2005; 116(4):775–779.

Zimmermann KP, and Simpson RK. "Slinky" coils for neuromagnetic stimulation. *Electroencephalogr Clin Neurophysiol* 1996; 101:145–152.

Index

A

AA-PEAs, *see* Amino-acid-based PEAs (AA-PEAs)
AA-PEEA, *see* Amino-acid-based poly(ether ester amide) (AA-PEEA)
AA-UPEAs, *see* Unsaturated poly(ester amide) s (AA-UPEAs)
AB, *see* Amyloid-beta (AB)
Abductor pollicis brevis (APB), 46-9, 58-15
ABM, *see* Agent-based models (ABM)
Above-lesion EMG-controlled menu selection, 52-10 to 52-11
ABS copolymers, *see* Acrylonitrile–butadiene–styrene copolymers (ABS copolymers)
AC, *see* Alternating current (AC); Anterior commissures (AC); Auditory cortex (AC)
Accelerometry, 12-4
Accommodation, 4-2
Acetabular fossae, 10-15; *see also* Hip
Acetabulum, 30-20
Acetol, 36-17
Acetylcholine (Ach), 46-4; *see also* Electrodiagnostic studies (EDX studies)
Ach, *see* Acetylcholine (Ach)
ACL, *see* Anterior cruciate ligament (ACL)
Acrylic polymer, 30-10; *see also* Biomaterial polymers
Acrylonitrile–butadiene–styrene copolymers (ABS copolymers), 30-11
Actin
    fibers, 25-3
    and integrin binding, 23-7
Action potential (AP), 3-2, 38-2, 38-8 to 38-9, 42-2, 42-21, 46-4, 52-3, 53-7; *see also* Electrodiagnostic studies (EDX studies); Electrophysiology; Membrane models
    in excitable cell, 42-2
    functionality, 53-7 to 53-9
    initiation sites, 51-5 to 51-7
    nerve, 46-4
    recorded from NE, 53-7
    refractory period, 42-3

Action potentials and membrane currents, 38-9; *see also* Electrophysiology
    excitation phase, 38-11
    patch action potential, 38-10
    recovery phase, 38-11
    resting phase, 38-9
    stimulation phase, 38-9
Action potential wave forms, 38-11; *see also* Electrophysiology
    end repolarization, 38-13
    excitation phase, 38-13
    recovery phase, 38-13
    resting phase, 38-12
    stimulation phase, 38-12 to 38-13
Active process, 24-10
    hair bundle transduction process, 24-12
    outer hair cell electromotility, 24-11 to 24-12
AD, *see* Alzheimer's disease (AD)
Adaptive methods, 43-15; *see also* Computer modeling and simulation
    energy norms, 43-17 to 43-18
    potential field approximation, 43-16
    sequence convergence, 43-17
A/D converter, *see* Analog-to-digital converter (A/D converter)
Addition polymerization, 30-20
Adenosine diphosphate (ADP), 26-1
Adenosine monophosphate (AMP), 26-2
Adenosine triphosphate (ATP), 20-7, 26-1, 27-1, 27-2, 39-2
ADH, *see* Antidiuretic hormone (ADH)
Adhesion
    kinetic models, 23-11
    state diagram, 23-9
    junction proteins, 41-4
ADP, *see* Adenosine diphosphate (ADP)
Adverse reaction to metal debris (ARMD), 37-14
Aerobic threshold, 26-5
Aerobic training, 27-7 to 27-8
AFM, *see* Atomic force microscopy (AFM)
AFRO, *see* Anterior floor reaction orthosis (AFRO)
Agent-based models (ABM), 20-11

Age-related macular degeneration (AMD), 56-1
Agranulocytes, 1-2
Airway
    architecture, 7-4
    classification and dimensions, 7-3
    remodeling, 7-14
Alanine (Ala), 33-18
Albumin, 1-2
    -coated surfaces, 30-14
ALCAP ceramic, *see* Aluminum–calcium–
        phosphorous oxide ceramic
        (ALCAP ceramic)
Aldosterone, 2-18
Aliphatic polycarbonates, 32-9
Allysine, 33-18
ALOPEX system, 3-8
    inverse pattern-recognition scheme, 3-9
α-parameter, *see* Womersley number
Alpha rhythm, 47-2; *see also* Electroencephalography
        (EEG)
Alternating current (AC), 47-3, 58-2
Alumina, 29-3 to 29-5, 29-26; *see also* Bioinert
        bioceramics
    calcined, 29-4
    property, 29-5
Aluminum–calcium–phosphorous oxide ceramic
        (ALCAP ceramic), 29-13; *see also*
        Biodegradable ceramics
Alveolar ventilation, 7-7
Alveoli, 7-2 to 7-4, 7-20
Alzheimer's disease (AD), 3-12; *see also* Parkinson's
        disease (PD)
    antioxidant-rich diet, 3-13
    changes in brain, 3-13
    visual-evoked potentials, 3-13
Amacrine cells, 4-3
Amalgam, 28-19
Ambient temperature and pressure (ATP), 7-9
Amblyopia, 4-6
Ambulation performance, 52-15
American Society of Testing and Materials (ASTM),
        28-2
Amidediols, 32-12; *see also* Nonaliphatic polyester-type
        biodegradable polymers
Amino-acid-based PEAs (AA-PEAs), 32-12; *see also*
        Nonaliphatic polyester-type biodegradable
        polymers
    biodegradation of Phe-based, 32-17
    chemical structure, 32-13, 32-16
    drug-eluting AA-PEA fibrous membranes, 32-20
    inflammatory response, 32-19
    physical forms, 32-18, 32-19
    synthesis of pendant functional, 32-15
    via Z-amino acid-NCA, 32-16
Amino-acid-based poly(ether ester amide) (AA-PEEA),
        32-16 to 32-17; *see also* Amino-acid-based
        PEAs (AA-PEAs)

AMP, *see* Adenosine monophosphate (AMP)
Amplitude histograms, 47-4; *see also*
        Electroencephalography (EEG)
    amplitude distribution indices, 47-6
    kurtosis, 47-6 to 47-7
    mean, 47-5
    skewness, 47-5
    standard amplitude, 47-5
Amyloid-beta (AB), 3-12
Anaerobic glycolysis, 26-2
Anaerobic threshold, 26-5, 26-10
Analog-to-digital converter (A/D converter), 47-4
Analytical models, 25-4
Aneurysm, 17-9, 36-17; *see also* Arterial
        macrocirculatory hemodynamics
Angiogenesis, 20-6, 20-11, 20-12; *see also*
        Microvascular blood flow mechanics
Angle of anteversion, 10-15; *see also* Hip
Ankle joint, 10-2; *see also* Joint-articulating surface
        motion
    angle variation tibia and empirical axis, 10-6
    articulating surface geometry, 10-2 to 10-3
    inclination variations in subtalar joint axis, 10-8
    joint contact, 10-3
    morphometry of, 10-4
    ratio of contact area to joint area, 10-5
    rotation axes, 10-3, 10-6, 10-7
    talocalcaneal joint contact area, 10-5
    3D characteristics, 10-3
Ankle joint replacement, 37-16
Anode, 28-19
Anodic break, 49-11
ANT, *see* Anterior nucleus of the thalamus (ANT)
Antagonist muscle, 3-3
Anterior commissures (AC), 57-3
Anterior cruciate ligament (ACL), 33-17
Anterior floor reaction orthosis (AFRO), 54-4
Anterior nucleus of the thalamus (ANT), 50-11
Anteroventral CN (AVCN), 5-7
Anthropomorphic test devices (ATD), 13-10
Antidiuretic hormone (ADH), 1-11, 2-18
Antifacilitation, 3-5
Aortic root, 16-3; *see also* Aortic valve
Aortic valve, 16-3; *see also* Cardiac biomechanics;
        Heart valve dynamics
    aortic root, 16-3, 16-6
    bicuspid, 16-10
    congenital malformations, 16-9
    disease and treatment, 16-8 to 16-10
    excised porcine, 16-4
    fluid dynamics, 16-7 to 16-8
    function, 16-6 to 16-8
    leaflet dynamics, 16-6 to 16-7
    mechanical response of, 16-6
    pressure and flow curve for, 16-2
    vs. pulmonic valve, 16-11
    rheumatic fever, 16-9

sinuses of Valsalva, 16-3
stained, 16-5
stenosis, 16-8
structure, 16-3 to 16-6
three-directional velocity vectors, 16-8
velocity profiles of, 16-9
Apatite, 8-20
APB, *see* Abductor pollicis brevis (APB)
API, *see* Application program interface (API)
Apolipoprotein E (apoE), 3-12
Apoptosis, 3-12
Apparent density, 8-9, 33-15, 33-18
Apparent viscosity, 20-3, 20-12; *see also* Microvascular
    blood flow mechanics
Application program interface (API), 43-20
Arches of Corti, 24-4
Arcuate zone, 24-3, 24-4
Area 17, 4-4
Area expansivity modulus, 21-11
Area V1, 4-4 to 4-7
Arginine (Arg), 33-18
ARMD, *see* Adverse reaction to metal debris
    (ARMD)
Arterial circulation, 17-1; *see also* Arterial
    macrocirculatory hemodynamics
Arterial macrocirculatory hemodynamics, 17-1
    arterial impedances, 17-5, 17-6, 17-8
    blood vessel walls, 17-1 to 17-2
    flow characteristics, 17-2 to 17-3
    hemodynamic values, 17-3
    input impedance, 17-7
    Moens–Korteweg relationship, 17-4
    pathology, 17-9
    pressure wave velocities in arteries, 17-4, 17-8
    reflection coefficient, 17-5
    turbulence, 17-3
    vascular dimensions in dog, 17-2
    velocity profiles, 17-9
    wave propagation, 17-4 to 17-9
    Womersley number, 17-3
Arterioles, 20-3 to 20-4; *see also* Microvascular blood
    flow mechanics
Artery, 36-17
Arthritis, 11-15; *see also* Biotribology
Articular cartilage, 9-1; *see also* Cartilage
Articular cartilage mimetics, 35-8
Artificial circulatory support, 36-10
Artificial Silicon Retina™ (ASR), 56-3
Artificial skins, 36-28; *see also* Percutaneous
    implants
ASA, *see* Average spinal acceleration (ASA)
Aspartic acid (Asp), 33-18
ASR, *see* Artificial Silicon Retina™ (ASR)
ASTM, *see* American Society of Testing and Materials
    (ASTM)
ATD, *see* Anthropomorphic test devices (ATD)
Atelocollagen, 33-4, 33-18; *see also* Collagen

Atherosclerosis, 17-9, 17-10, 36-17; *see also* Arterial
    macrocirculatory hemodynamics
Atomic force microscopy (AFM), 20-2, 23-4
ATP, *see* Adenosine triphosphate (ATP); Ambient
    temperature and pressure (ATP)
Atrioventricular node (AV node), 1-12
ATS valve, 36-17
Auditory cortex (AC), 5-1, 5-12, 5-13
Auditory hair cells, 25-1
Auditory research, 24-1
Auditory system
    auditory cortex, 5-12, 5-13
    basilar membrane, 5-4
    bat cortex, 5-12
    central auditory system, 5-5
    cochlear amplifier, 5-4
    cochlear nuclei, 5-7 to 5-9
    dorsal nucleus LL, 5-11
    ear anatomy, 5-1 to 5-4
    eustachian tube, 5-2
    gamma-amino-butyric acid, 5-12
    human cortex, 5-13 to 5-14
    inferior colliculi, 5-11 to 5-12
    inner hair cells, 5-6
    isofrequency laminae, 5-8
    medial geniculate, 5-12
    monaural, 5-3
    nuclei of lateral lemniscus, 5-11
    organ of corti, 5-5
    outer hair cells, 5-3
    pathologies, 5-14 to 5-15
    peripheral auditory system, 5-1 to 5-2
    peristimulus time histogram, 5-7, 5-9
    response-field maps, 5-10
    scala media, 5-3
    scala tympani, 5-3
    scala vestibule, 5-3
    spike discharge patterns, 5-9 to 5-11
    superior olivary complex, 5-11
    tympanic membrane, 5-2
Austenitic stainless steels, 28-2; *see also* Stainless
    steels
Autoclaving, 36-17
Autocorrelellogram, 47-8; *see also*
    Electroencephalography (EEG)
Autonomic nervous system, 1-12
Autoregulation, 2-10
AVCN, *see* Anteroventral CN (AVCN)
Average spinal acceleration (ASA), 14-3
Averaging operation, 3-6
Avogadro's principle, 7-9
Axial magnetometer, 48-12; *see also*
    Magnetoencephalography (MEG)
    sensitivity distribution of, 48-13
Axons, 3-2; *see also* Nervous system
    axonal excitation, 49-2
    axon time constant, 49-8

B

Back scattered scanning electron microscopy (BSEM), 8-18
Baroreceptors, 26-3, 26-10
Basal ganglia, 3-11
Basal labyrinth, 2-14
Basilar membrane (BM), 5-1, 5-4, 24-2, 24-4
Basophils, 1-2
Bat cortex, 5-12
Battery-powered BION device (BPB), 55-6; *see also* Implantable Bionic neural prosthetic devices
    applications, 55-13 to 55-15
    device specifications, 55-7 to 55-8
    for distance/angle measurements, 55-11
    for FES, 55-4
    implantation tools, 55-12
    internal components, 55-8
    system components, 55-5 to 55-6, 55-8 to 55-12
BC, *see* Blunt criterion (BC)
BCG, *see* Biconjugate gradient (BCG)
Bed sore, *see* Pressure sore
Bell–Magendie law, 3-3
Bell's model, 23-8
Below-lesion response-EMG FES level control, 52-11
Beta dispersion, 40-3; *see also* Electrical conductivity of tissues
Biconjugate gradient (BCG), 43-15
Bicuspid aortic valve, 16-10; *see also* Aortic valve
Bidomain, 40-11
Bifurcation law, 20-6; *see also* Microvascular blood flow mechanics
Binocular convergence, 4-5, 4-10
Bioactive ceramics, 29-16; *see also* Ceramic biomaterials
    ceravital, 29-19 to 29-20
    examples of, 29-17
    glass ceramics, 29-16 to 29-19
    uses of, 29-17
Bioceramic manufacturing techniques, 29-23; *see also* Ceramic biomaterials
    using additives, 29-23 to 29-24
    drip casting technique, 29-24
    gel casting, 29-23
    hard tissue replacement, 29-23 to 29-24, 29-25
    hydroxyapatite synthesis method, 29-24 to 29-25
    injection molding, 29-23
    stress shielding, 29-23
    tissue integration, 29-24, 29-25
    wet chemistry-based methods, 29-23
Bioceramics, 29-1; *see also* Bioactive ceramics; Biodegradable ceramics; Ceramic biomaterials
Biocompatibility, 30-20
Biocoral, 29-13; *see also* Biodegradable ceramics

Biodegradable ceramics, 29-8; *see also* Bioactive ceramics; Calcium phosphate; Ceramic biomaterials
    ALCAP ceramics, 29-13
    coralline, 29-13 to 29-14
    examples, 29-10
    ferric–calcium–phosphorous oxide ceramics, 29-15, 29-16
    tricalcium phosphate ceramics, 29-14
    uses of, 29-11
    zinc–calcium–phosphorous oxide ceramics, 29-14 to 29-15
    zinc–sulfate–calcium–phosphate ceramics, 29-15
Biodegradable polymers, 30-13, 32-1; *see also* Biofunctional hydrogels; Biomaterial polymers; Glycolide/lactide-based polyesters; Nonaliphatic polyester-type biodegradable polymers; Silk; Synthetic polymer biodegradation
    advantages, 32-1
    aliphatic biodegradable polyesters, 32-11, 32-24 to 32-27
    commercially significant, 32-2
    commercial uses, 32-2 to 32-3
    P4HB vs. synthetic aliphatic polyesters, 32-4
    supercritical carbon dioxide sterilization, 32-27 to 32-29
    synthetic absorable polymers, 32-3
    3HB co-monomers effect on P4HB copolymer, 32-4
    types, 32-2
Biodegradation, 32-1, 32-29
Bioelectricity, 38-2; *see also* Electrophysiology
Biofunctional hydrogels, 35-1, 35-10 to 35-11
    application, 35-1, 35-2
    articular cartilage mimetics, 35-8
    biofunctionality, 35-3, 35-7
    cell adhesion peptides, 35-4
    cell-mediated degradation, 35-6
    cellular adhesion, 35-3 to 35-5
    design, 35-9 to 35-10
    enzyme-degradable peptide, 35-6
    fibroblast for substrate rigidity, 35-9
    functional vessel formation, 35-5
    growth factors and signaling molecules, 35-5 to 35-6
    in situ gelation, 35-3
    laser-based photomodification, 35-10
    laser scanning lithography, 35-10
    PEG-based, 35-7
    photolithography, 35-9
    polymeric materials, 35-2 to 35-3
    properties, 35-8 to 35-9
    synthetic hydrogels, 35-2
Bioglass, 29-18; *see also* Glass ceramics
Bioinert bioceramics, 29-2; *see also* Carbons; Ceramic biomaterials
    alumina, 29-3 to 29-5

relatively, 29-2 to 29-3
uses of, 29-4
zirconia, 29-5
Biomagnetism, 48-1; *see also* Magnetocardiogram
  (MCG); Magnetoencephalography (MEG);
  Sensitivity distribution
  bioelectric and biomagnetic signal, 48-1 to 48-3
  electric lead, 48-5 to 48-7
  electric potential equation, 48-2
  lead current field, 48-5
  lead field, 48-4 to 48-5
  lead vector, 48-3, 48-4
  magnetic lead, 48-6
  magnetic potential equation, 48-3
  reciprocity, 48-4
Biomaterial polymers, 30-8; *see also* Polymeric
  biomaterials
  biodegradable polymers, 30-13
  fluorocarbon polymers, 30-11 to 30-12
  polyacetal, 30-12
  polyamides, 30-11
  polycarbonate, 30-13
  polyesters, 30-11
  polyethylene, 30-9 to 30-10
  polymethylmethacrylate, 30-10
  polypropylene, 30-10
  polysulfone, 30-12
  polyurethanes, 30-12
  polyvinylchloride, 30-8 to 30-9
  PS and copolymers, 30-10 to 30-11
  rubbers, 30-12
Biomaterials, 30-20; *see also* Collagen; Silk
  properties, 31-5
Biomechanical response of body, 14-1
Biomedical device development, 36-23; *see also*
  Nonblood-interfacing implants
Biomedical polymers, 30-2; *see also* Polymeric
  biomaterials
Biomer, 36-17
BioModels database, 20-12
Bioprostheses, 36-17
BioPSE, 43-20 to 43-22; *see also* Software for bioelectric
  field problems
Biotribology, 11-1; *see also* Joint lubrication; Tribology
  and arthritis, 11-15 to 11-18
  degenerative joint disease, 11-16
  lubricants used, 11-19
  osteoarthritis–tribology connections, 11-17
  tribological aspects of synovial lubrication, 11-17
Biphasic cathodic-first stimulation waveform, 49-12
Bipolar electrodes and dipoles, 49-5 to 49-6
BIS-GMA, *see* Bisphenol A glycidyl methacrylate
  (BIS-GMA)
Bispectra, 47-11
Bisphenol A (BPA), 32-11
Bisphenol A glycidyl methacrylate (BIS-GMA), 31-5
Blindsight, 4-9

Blood, 1-1, 17-2, 20-2; *see also* Arterial
  macrocirculatory hemodynamics; Heart;
  Microvascular blood flow mechanics; Tissue
  transport mechanics
  albumin, 1-2
  and respiratory parameter during exercise, 26-5
  basophils, 1-2
  control of blood pressure, 1-12
  distribution prioritization, 1-11
  eosinophils, 1-2
  erythrocyte, 1-1, 1-2
  fibrinogen, 1-2
  flow, 1-11, 20-6, 26-4
  globulin, 1-2
  hematocytes, 1-1, 1-2
  hematocytopoiesis, 1-1
  lactate, 20-8
  leukocyte, 1-1, 1-2
  lymphocytes, 1-2
  minerals, 1-2
  monocytes, 1-2
  neutrophils, 1-2
  oxygenators, 36-17
  plasma, 1-1, 1-2, 1-4 to 1-5
  plasma, 20-3
  pressures, 26-4
  proteins, 1-2
  serum, 1-2
  thrombocytes, 1-2
  vitamins, 1-2
Blood flow regulation, 20-9; *see also* Microcirculation
  physiome
  angiogenesis and vascular remodeling, 20-11
  local regulation, 20-10
  neurohumoral regulation, 20-9 to 20-10
  resistance vessels, 20-9
  vasomotor response coordination, 20-10 to 20-11
Blood-interfacing implants, 36-1, 36-16 to 36-17; *see
  also* Heart valve prostheses; Nonblood-
  interfacing implants; Vascular prostheses
  blood pump configuration, 36-12
  electrically driven blood pumps, 36-11
  TAHs, 36-10
  ventricular assist devices, 36-10
Blood vessels, 1-7, 17-1 to 17-2, 18-1; *see also* Arterial
  macrocirculatory hemodynamics; Blood;
  Heart
  anisotropic, 18-10 to 18-13
  arterial system, 1-8
  assumptions, 18-1
  axisymmetric deformation, 18-3 to 18-4
  capillaries, 1-10
  conducting vessels, 1-10
  cylindrical geometry of, 18-3
  distributing branches, 1-10
  equilibrium, 18-5 to 18-7
  experimental measurements, 18-5

Blood vessels (*Continued*)
  homogeneity, 18-1
  incompressibility, 18-1
  inelasticity, 18-2
  isotropic, 18-7 to 18-10
  layers, 1-10
  longitudinal distending force, 18-6, 18-9,
      18-10, 18-11
  muscular vessels, 1-10
  pressure–radius curves, 18-4, 18-9, 18-10,
      18-11
  pseudoelasticity, 18-7
  remodeling, 18-2
  resistance vessels, 1-10
  retractive force of wall, 18-5 to 18-6
  strain energy density, 18-7
  stress and strain, 18-2
  stress distribution, 18-6, 18-12
  vascular anatomy, 18-2
  venous system, 1-9
  wall tension, 18-5
Blunt criterion (BC), 14-6
BM, *see* Basilar membrane (BM)
BMP-2, *see* Bone morphogenetic protein-2
      (BMP-2)
Body temperature and pressure, saturated (BTPS),
      7-9, 7-20
Bond formation in cells, 23-10
Bone, 8-1, 37-1; *see also* Hard tissue mechanics; Joint
      replacements; Long bone repair
  bovine, 31-4
  cancellous bone, 8-2
  composition, 8-4
  conduction, 24-17
  elastic stiffness coefficients for, 8-6
  femur, 8-2
  ingrowth, 37-11
  laminar, 8-7
  loss tangent of, 8-16
  mammalian, 8-3
  mechanical testing methods, 8-9
  osteons, 8-2
  plates, 37-7
  properties, 31-5
  relaxation spectra, 8-16
  resorption, 37-19
  screws, 37-5
  structure, 8-2
  types of, 8-2
Bone cement, 30-20; *see also* Joint replacements;
      Polymethylmethacrylate (PMMA)
  fixation, 37-10 to 37-11
  fixed hip joint, 37-13
Bone morphogenetic protein-2 (BMP-2), 34-8
Bony shelf, 24-3
Bootstrap effect, 22-10; *see also* Tissue transport
      mechanics

Boundary element method (BEM), 44-1 to 44-2, 43-7,
      43-14, 43-22; *see also* Computer modeling
      and simulation
Bovine
  bone, 31-4
  heterograft, 36-17
Bowman's capsule, 2-5
Bowman's space, 2-5
BPA, *see* Bisphenol A (BPA)
BPA-carbonates, *see* Poly(BPA-carbonates)
BPB, *see* Battery-powered BION device (BPB)
Bradycardia, 1-12
Brain stem auditory evoked response (BAER), 46-16,
      46-17 to 46-18; *see also* Electrodiagnostic
      studies (EDX studies)
Brain tissue stimulation, 49-14
Branching, 30-20
Breast implants, 36-30; *see also* Nonblood-interfacing
      implants
Breathing, 7-14
Bronchi, 7-2
Bronchiolus, 7-2
Brush border, 2-12
BSEM, *see* Back scattered scanning electron
      microscopy (BSEM)
BTPS, *see* Body temperature and pressure, saturated
      (BTPS)
Bundles, 25-2
  stiffness, 25-8
Burst mode, 32-10

C

Cable theory, 40-11
Calcification, 36-17
Calcified tissue, *see* Hard tissue
Calcium, 42-8; *see also* Membrane currents
Calcium phosphate, 29-8, 29-26; *see also* Biodegradable
      ceramics
  mechanical properties of, 29-9
  physical properties of, 29-12
  polycrystalline hydroxyapatite, 29-10 to 29-12
Callus, 37-19
Calyx, 2-4
Cancellous bone, 8-2, 8-20; *see also* Bone
Cancer modeling, 23-15
Capacitance, 19-2; *see also* Venous system
Capacity, 19-3; *see also* Venous system
Capillary, 22-13
Capito-lunate (CL), 10-30
CarboMedics bileaflet valve, 36-4; *see also* Heart valve
      prostheses
Carbons, 29-5; *see also* Bioinert bioceramics
  compatibility, 29-8
  crystalline, 29-6
  elastic modulus vs. density, 29-7
  fiber-reinforcment properties, 29-8

in fluidized bed, 29-9
fracture stress vs. density, 29-7
graphite structure, 29-6
properties of, 29-7
pyrolitic, 29-8
Cardiac biomechanics, 15-1
analysis models, 15-14 to 15-15
calcium concentrations, 15-14
cardiac extracellular matrix, 15-7
cardiac geometry and structure, 15-1
cardiac pump function, 15-9
cardiac tissue structure, 15-8
EDPVR, 15-13
ejection fraction, 15-10
erectile effect, 15-13
EW, 15-12
extracellular matrix organization, 15-7 to 15-8
focal length, 15-3, 15-4
heart and body mass, 15-4
law of the Heart, 15-12
left ventricular pressure–volume loops, 15-11
muscle contractile properties, 15-13 to 15-16
muscle fiber orientations, 15-6
myocardial properties, 15-13, 15-16 to 15-20
myocardial stress effect, 15-3
myofiber architecture, 15-5 to 15-7
myofilament Ca^{2+} activation, 15-15 to 15-16
passive myocardium, 15-18
patient-specific modeling, 15-22
PVA, 15-12
relative isometric tension, 15-14
strain energy, 15-18 to 15-20
stress determinants, 15-2
stress–strain curves for myocardium, 15-17
stroke volume, 15-10
truncation factor, 15-2
ventricular collagen, 15-8
ventricular geometry, 15-2 to 15-4
ventricular hemodynamics, 15-9 to 15-10
ventricular mechanics, 15-20 to 15-22
ventricular minor-axis dimensions, 15-3
ventricular pressure–volume, 15-10 to 15-13
Cardiac cells, 42-16; *see also* Membrane models
amphibian sinus venosus and atrial cells, 42-18
to 42-19
atrial muscle, 42-17
atrioventricular node, 42-17
Purkinje fiber, 42-16
sinoatrial node, 42-17
ventricular muscle, 42-17 to 42-18
Cardiac ejection fraction, 1-7
Cardiac extracellular matrix, 15-7; *see also* Cardiac
biomechanics
Cardiac microimpedances, 41-1
electrode array, 41-5
impact, 41-4 to 41-5
literature-based data on, 41-2 to 41-4

multisite stimulation, 41-5 to 41-7
recording and stimulating site arrangement, 41-6
segmentation, 41-3
tissue model, 41-2
transmembrane and interstitial potential
distributions, 41-1
uPDs, 41-6, 41-7
Cardiac muscle, 1-12
Cardiac output (CO), 1-7
Cardiac pacemakers, 36-17
Cardiac reserve volume, 1-7
Cardiac tissue, 40-8; *see also* Cardiac biomechanics
stimulation, 49-2, 49-14 to 49-15
structure, 15-8
Cardiopulmonary bypass, 36-17
Cardiovascular adjustments, 26-3 to 26-4
Cardiovascular control, 1-11 to 1-12
Cardiovascular drift, 26-8, 26-10
Cardiovascular system, 1-1; *see also* Blood; Heart
autonomic nervous system, 1-12
AV node, 1-12
bradycardia, 1-12
cardiac muscle, 1-12
cardiovascular control, 1-11 to 1-12
endocrine system, 1-12
endothelium, 1-12
homeostasis, 1-12
inotropic, 1-12
physiologic regulation, 1-11
precapillary sphincters, 1-12
SA node, 1-13
stem cells, 1-13
tachycardia, 1-12
Carina, 7-2
Carpentier–Edwards (CE), 36-2
Carpometacarpal (CMC), 10-32
Carrying angle, 10-23, 10-24
Cartilage, 9-1, 33-7; *see also* Collagen; Soft tissues
equilibrium equations, 9-8 to 9-9
modeling, 9-7 to 9-10
properties, 9-4
stress on, 9-7
surface displacement, 9-9
Cartilage wear, 11-11; *see also* Joint lubrication
based on hydroxyproline content of debris, 11-12
collagenase-3 effect on, 11-15
device for, 11-13
friction and wear, 11-12
by sliding contact, 11-14
test device for, 11-13
Cataracts, 4-7
Catheters, 36-17
Cathode, 28-19
Cathode ray tube (CRT), 3-8, 45-7, 46-18
Cavitation bubbles (vapor cavitation), 36-17
Cavitation phenomenon, 13-1; *see also* Head
mechanics

CE, *see* Carpentier–Edwards (CE)
CEJ, *see* Dentin–cementum junction (CEJ)
Cell; *see also* Cell mechanics modeling; Cell motility;
    Rolling and adhesion
  adhesive proteins, 30-19
  crawling, 23-10, 23-12
  mechanical properties, 23-2 to 23-5
Cell mechanics modeling, 23-1; *see also* Cell; Cell
    motility; Modeling cells in disease
  atomic force microscopy, 23-4
  cell component properties, 23-5
  coarse grain triangular element model, 23-6
  electromechanical transduction, 23-15
  as liquid drop encapsulated in elastic ring, 23-8
  magnetocytometry, 23-4
  mechanoelectrical transduction, 23-14
  mechanosensitive channels, 23-14
  mechanotransduction, 23-13 to 23-14
  membrane modeling, 23-5
  membrane tethers, 23-6
  micropipette aspiration effect, 23-3 to 23-4
  modeling cellular membranes, 23-5
  nuclear properties, 23-5
  particle tracking microrheology, 23-5
Cell motility, 23-6; *see also* Cell; Cell mechanics
    modeling; Rolling and adhesion
  actin and integrin binding, 23-7
  crawling, 23-10, 23-12
  nematode cell locomotion model, 23-13
  spreading and interactions, 23-6 to 23-7
  stress fiber model, 23-7
  swimming and gliding, 23-12 to 23-13
Cellular solid, 31-2
  structures, 31-9
Center of curvature, 10-2
Center/surround receptive fields, 4-3
Central auditory system, 5-5
Central delay, 3-3
Central nervous system (CNS), 3-1, 26-1, 51-1, 58-14
  AP initiation sites, 51-5 to 51-7
  electrical conductivity of, 51-3
  neuron models, 51-5
  potential generation in, 51-2
  structure of, 51-2
Central processing unit (CPU), 45-8
Centromedian (CM), 57-1
Ceramic biomaterials, 29-1; *see also* Bioactive ceramics;
    Bioceramic manufacturing techniques;
    Biodegradable ceramics; Bioinert
    bioceramics
  deterioration of, 29-20
  fatigue life of, 29-21 to 29-22
  flexural strength after aging, 29-21
  minimum service life, 29-22 to 29-23
  properties of, 29-2
  strain vs. number of cycles to failure, 29-21
Ceramics, 29-1

Ceravital, 29-19 to 29-20; *see also* Bioactive ceramics
    Glass Ceramics, 29-18; *see also* Glass ceramics
CF, *see* Continuous frequency (CF)
CFUs, *see* Colony forming units (CFUs)
CG, *see* Conjugate gradient (CG)
cGMP, *see* Cyclic guanosine monophosphate (cGMP)
Channel open probability, 25-4
Channels, 46-7
Charge conservation, 49-3
CHCS, *see* Chronic hippocampal stimulation (CHCS)
Chemogradient surface, 30-20
Chemoreceptors, 7-20, 26-6, 26-10
Chest and abdomen impact, 14-1
  acceleration injury, 14-2 to 14-3
  biomechanical responses, 14-6 to 14-8
  compression injury, 14-4 to 14-5
  crushing injury, 14-6
  force–deflection response, 14-7
  force injury, 14-3 to 14-4
  injury criteria and tolerances, 14-2
  injury mechanisms, 14-1 to 14-2
  injury probability functions, 14-11
  injury risk assessment, 14-8 to 14-11
  injury severity, 14-4
  logist injury probability function, 14-10
  lumped-mass model of human thorax, 14-9
  soft tissue behavior, 14-5
  thoracic trauma index, 14-2
  tolerance, 14-2, 14-3, 14-9, 14-10
  viscous injury, 14-5 to 14-6
Chinchilla cochlea, 24-15; *see also* Cochlea
Chinese hamster ovaries (CHO), 30-17
CHO, *see* Chinese hamster ovaries (CHO)
Chondroitin sulfate, 33-18
Chronically implanted neuroelectric interfaces, 50-5
    to 50-6
Chronic electrical stimulation, 50-8 to 50-9
Chronic hippocampal stimulation (CHCS), 57-8
Chronic obstructive pulmonary disease (COPD), 7-14
Chronotropic, 1-12
CI, *see* Composite impedance (CI)
Ciliary neurotrophic factor (CNTF), 56-2
Circulating vasoconstrictors, 17-1; *see also* Arterial
    macrocirculatory hemodynamics
CL, *see* Capito-lunate (CL)
Clips, 36-25; *see also* Nonblood-interfacing implants
Clock recovery unit (CRU), 57-4
Closing dynamics, 36-17
CM, *see* Centromedian (CM)
CMAP, *see* Compound muscle action potential
    (CMAP)
CMC, *see* Carpometacarpal (CMC)
CN, *see* Cochlear nucleus (CN)
cNOS, *see* Constitutive NOS (cNOS)
CNS, *see* Central nervous system (CNS)
CNTF, *see* Ciliary neurotrophic factor (CNTF)
CO, *see* Cardiac output (CO)

Coarse grain triangular element model, 23-6
Cobalt–chromium alloys (CoCr alloys), 28-4; *see also*
      Metallic biomaterials
  chemical compositions of, 28-4
  elasticity modulus for, 28-6
  implant manufacturing, 28-19
  mechanical property, 28-5
  specific gravities of, 28-6
  tensile and cold work, 28-5
  types of, 28-4
COCB, *see* Crossed olivocochlear bundle (COCB)
Cochlea, 24-2
  anatomy, 24-2 to 24-3
  arcuate zone, 24-3, 24-4
  basilar membrane, 24-2, 24-4
  bony shelf, 24-3
  chinchilla, 24-15
  corti, 24-3, 24-4
  endolymphatic fluid, 24-3
  estimates for Young's modulus, 24-5
  helicotrema, 24-3
  Henson cells, 24-4
  inner sulcus, 24-4
  material properties, 24-5
  pectinate zone, 24-4
  perilymphatic fluid, 24-3
  Reissner's membrane, 24-3
  reticular lamina, 24-4
  scala media, 24-3
  scala tympani, 24-3
  scala vestibuli, 24-3
  spiral ligament, 24-3
  tectorial membrane, 24-4
Cochlear amplifier, 5-4
Cochlear mechanics, 24-1, 24-19; *see also* Active
      process; Hair cell
  active models, 24-12
  bone conduction, 24-17
  fluid viscosity, 24-9
  frequency range capability of BM, 24-6
  linear acceleration, 24-1
  multiple traveling wave modes, 24-18
  neural threshold and BM velocity, 24-16
  OHC roll-off, 24-17 to 24-18
  one-dimensional model, 24-7 to 24-8
  push-forward/pull-backward active model, 24-12
      to 24-16
  resonators, 24-5 to 24-6
  sinusoidal stereociliary displacement, 24-1
  standard straight box model, 24-2
  stiffness change, 24-18
  tectorial membrane, 24-18
  three-dimensional model, 24-9 to 24-10, 24-11
  traveling wave, 24-17
  two-dimensional model, 24-8 to 24-9
Cochlear nucleus (CN), 5-7 to 5-9
Cochlear prosthesis, 49-1

CoCr alloys, *see* Cobalt–chromium alloys (CoCr alloys)
Coding of sensory information, 3-3
Coherence, 47-8; *see also* Electroencephalography (EEG)
Collagen, 9-1, 15-7, 17-10, 33-1; *see also* Biomaterials;
      Cartilage; Collagen-based medical implant
  amino acid content of, 33-2
  atelocollagen, 33-4
  biologic properties, 33-10
  biomechanical properties, 33-7 to 33-9
  biotechnology of, 33-11
  cartilage, 33-7
  cell interaction properties, 33-10 to 33-11
  composite matrix, 33-13
  connective tissue fibers, 33-6
  denaturation temperature of, 33-7
  elastic properties of, 33-8
  electrostatic properties, 33-9 to 33-10
  fiber-forming properties, 33-10
  fibrils, 9-2
  filamentous matrix, 33-13
  formation of, 33-3
  gel matrix, 33-12
  hemostatic properties, 33-10
  immunologic properties, 33-11
  ion and macromolecular binding properties, 33-10
  isolation and purification of, 33-11
  matrix fabrication technology, 33-11 to 33-13
  mechanical properties of, 33-9
  medical applications, 33-12
  membranous matrix, 33-12
  physiochemical properties, 33-9
  porous matrix, 33-12
  protein structure, 33-2
  R&D activities, 33-17
  rich tissue properties, 33-7
  scanning electron micrograph of, 33-5
  soft tissue composition, 33-7
  solution matrix, 33-13
  stress–strain curves of, 33-7, 33-8
  structure, 33-1 to 33-6
  telopeptides, 33-4
  tissue engineering, 33-17 to 33-18
  triple helix model, 33-4
  tubular matrices, 33-13
  type I, 33-3, 33-6
  xenogeneic collagenous tissue device, 33-11
Collagenase, 33-18
Collagen-based medical implant, 33-13; *see also*
      Collagen
  apparent density, 33-15
  biocompatibility, 33-14 to 33-15
  hydrophilicity, 33-16
  in vivo stability, 33-16 to 33-17
  mechanical property, 33-15 to 33-16
  permeability, 33-16
  physical dimension, 33-15
  pore structure, 33-15

Collecting ducts, 2-5
Colloid osmotic pressure, 22-13
Colon, 6-11
Colonic slow-wave activity, 6-11 to 6-12
Colony forming units (CFUs), 32-29
Color, 4-7
    constancy, 4-10
    vision, 4-7
Complex cells, 4-5
Complex conductivity, 40-2; *see also* Electrical
        conductivity of tissues
Compliance, 7-12, 36-17
Composite biomaterials, 31-1, 31-13; *see also* Fibrous
        composites; Particulate composites; Porous
        materials
    anisotropy of composites, 31-3 to 31-4
    applications of, 31-1
    biocompatibility, 31-12 to 31-13
    bounds on properties, 31-2 to 31-3
    cross-coupling constants, 31-4
    independent elastic constants, 31-4
    morphology of, 31-2
    Reuss stiffness, 31-3
    stiffness vs. volume fraction, 31-3
    stress and strain, 31-3
    structure, 31-1 to 31-2
    triclinic crystal, 31-4
    Voigt relation for stiffness, 31-2
    Young modulus of Voigt composite, 31-2
Composite impedance (CI), 41-3; *see also* Cardiac
        microimpedances
Composite matrix, 33-13; *see also* Collagen
Compound muscle action potential (CMAP), 46-9; *see
        also* Electrodiagnostic studies (EDX studies)
Computed tomography (CT), 43-3
Computer modeling and simulation, 43-1; *see also*
        Adaptive methods; Software for bioelectric
        field problems
    boundary element method, 43-14
    electromagnetic field propagation simulation, 43-3
    finite difference method, 43-8
    finite element method, 43-9 to 43-10
    focal current source modeling, 43-6
    focal current source simulation, 43-2
    Galerkin method, 43-7 to 43-8
    implantable cardiac defibrillator simulation, 43-2
        to 43-5
    method comparison, 43-15
    model construction and mesh generation, 43-5
    numerical methods, 43-7
    problem formulation, 43-2
    solution methods and computational
        considerations, 43-14 to 43-15
Computer vision, 4-1
Condensation polymerization, 30-20; *see also*
        Polymerization
    polymers, 30-2

Conducting airways, 7-1 to 7-2
Conductivity, 40-11
Cone photoreceptors, 4-7
Congenital malformations, 16-9; *see also* Aortic valve
Conjugate gradient (CG), 43-14
Constitutive models, 9-11
Constitutive NOS (cNOS), 20-8
Continuous frequency (CF), 5-12
COPD, *see* Chronic obstructive pulmonary disease
        (COPD)
Copolymers, 30-21
Coral, 29-13 to 29-14; *see also* Biodegradable ceramics
Corona discharge apparatus, 30-16
Corrosion, 28-19
Cortical bone, 8-20; *see also* Bone
Cortical tension, 21-11
Countercurrent
    heat exchange, 26-8
    multiplication, 2-17
Coupled nonlinear oscillators, 6-5 to 6-6
Covalent
    bonding, 30-21
    bonded ceramics, 29-1
Coxa valga, 10-15; *see also* Hip
CP, *see* Creatine phosphate (CP)
CPU, *see* Central processing unit (CPU)
Creatine phosphate (CP), 26-1
Crevice corrosion, 28-19
Crimping, 36-17
Cross-bridge models, 9-10 to 9-11
Cross-coupling constants, 31-4; *see also* Composite
        biomaterials
Crossed olivocochlear bundle (COCB), 5-11
Cross-eyed, 4-6
Cross-spectrum, 47-8, 47-11; *see also*
        Electroencephalography (EEG)
CRT, *see* Cathode ray tube (CRT)
CRU, *see* Clock recovery unit (CRU)
CT, *see* Computed tomography (CT)
CTB, *see* Cytochalasin B (CTB)
Curie temperature, 28-19
Current for ionic species, 42-6; *see also* Membrane
        currents
Cutaneous circulation, 1-11
Cyanoacrylates, 36-26 to 36-27; *see also* Nonblood-
        interfacing implants
Cyclic guanosine monophosphate (cGMP), 20-8
Cytoarchitectonics, 4-4, 4-10
Cytochalasin B (CTB), 21-8
Cytoplasmic viscosity, 21-11

D

Dacron, 30-21; *see also* Vascular prostheses
    vascular graft, 36-14
DAI, *see* Diffuse axonal injury (DAI)
Dalton's law, 7-8

db, *see* Decibels (db)

DBS, *see* Deep brain stimulation (DBS)

DC effective longitudinal conductivity, 40-6; *see also* Electrical conductivity of tissues

DCP, *see* Dynamic compression plate (DCP)

Dead space, 7-20

Decibels (db), 46-17

Declarative memory, 3-9

Deep brain stimulation (DBS), 3-11
 for movement disorders, 50-10 to 50-11
 for psychiatric disorders and pain, 50-9 to 50-10

Deep brain stimulation coil, 58-6 to 58-7; *see also* Hesed coil; Transcranial magnetic stimulation (TMS)
 electrical field induced in phantom brain, 58-9
 numerical simulations, 58-7 to 58-9
 results, 58-9 to 58-13

Degenerative joint disease, 11-16

Degree of polymerization (DP), 30-4; *see also* Polymeric biomaterials

Degrees of freedom (DOF), 43-5

Dehydrohydroxylysinonorleucine (deH-HLNL), 33-18

DEJ, *see* Dentin–enamel junction (DEJ)

Delrin®, 36-17, 30-21; *see also* Polyacetal

Δpressure, *see* Pressure difference (Δpressure)

Dendrites, 3-2

Dental; *see also* Metallic biomaterials; Particulate composites
 composites, 31-5
 metals, 28-12 to 28-13

Dentin, 8-17; *see also* Hard tissue mechanics
 dentin tubuledistribution, 8-18
 elasticity, 8-18 to 8-20
 elastic modulus, 8-20
 intertubular, 8-17
 partially demineralized, 8-18
 structure and composition, 8-17 to 8-18

Dentin–cementum junction (CEJ), 8-17

Dentin–enamel junction (DEJ), 8-17

Depolarization, 42-21

Deterministic chaos, 20-4; *see also* Microvascular blood flow mechanics

DHA, *see* Dihydroxyacetone (DHA)

Dialysers, 36-17

Diffuse axonal injury (DAI), 13-2

Diffusion, 7-7, 7-20
 capacity, 7-19

Diffusion tensor magnetic resonance imaging (DTI), 15-5

Diffusion-weighted imaging (DWI), 43-24

Dihydroxyacetone (DHA), 32-20

Dimethyltrimethylene carbonate (DMTMC), 32-9

Direct current (DC), 39-2, 47-3, 58-2

Directional derivative, 39-4; *see also* Volume conductor theory

Distal convoluted tubule, 2-5

Distal latency (DL), 46-9

Divergence, 40-1; *see also* Electrical conductivity of tissues

DL, *see* Distal latency (DL)

DMPO, *see* Dorsomedial periolivary nucleus (DMPO)

DMTMC, *see* Dimethyltrimethylene carbonate (DMTMC)

DNLL, *see* Dorsal nucleus LL (DNLL)

Doctrine of specific nerve energies, 3-3

DOF, *see* Degrees of freedom (DOF)

Doppler-shifted CF (DSCF), 5-12

Dorsal nucleus LL (DNLL), 5-11

Dorsomedial periolivary nucleus (DMPO), 5-11

Dowson–Higginson expression, 11-5

DP, *see* Degree of polymerization (DP)

Drip casting technique, 29-24; *see also* Bioceramic manufacturing techniques

DSCF, *see* Doppler-shifted CF (DSCF)

D spacing, 33-18

DTI, *see* Diffusion tensor magnetic resonance imaging (DTI)

Dual-slit method, 20-2

Duramater, 36-17

DWI, *see* Diffusion-weighted imaging (DWI)

Dynamic compression plate (DCP), 37-6; *see also* Long bone repair

E

Ear and eye implants, 36-29 to 36-30; *see also* Nonblood-interfacing implants

EC, *see* Endothelial cell (EC)

ECA, *see* Electrical control activity (ECA)

ECAP, *see* Extracellular AP (ECAP)

ECG, *see* Electrocardiography (ECG)

ECM, *see* Extracellular matrix (ECM)

Edema, 20-9, 22-13

EDHF, *see* Endothelium-derived hyperpolarizing factor (EDHF)

EDPVR, *see* End-diastolic pressure–volume relation (EDPVR)

EDRF, *see* Endothelium–derived relaxing factor (EDRF)

EDV, *see* End-diastolic volume (EDV)

EDX studies, *see* Electrodiagnostic studies (EDX studies)

EEG, *see* Electroencephalography (EEG)

Effective conductivity, 40-2, 40-3; *see also* Electrical conductivity of tissues

Effective molecular diameter, 2-11

EGG, *see* Electrogastrogram (EGG)

EHL, *see* Elastohydrodynamic lubrication (EHL)

Ejection fraction, 15-10; *see also* Cardiac biomechanics

Ejection phase, 15-10; *see also* Cardiac biomechanics

Ejection ratio, *see* Cardiac ejection fraction

EKG, *see* Electrocardiogram (EKG)

Elastin, 17-10, 33-18

Elastohydrodynamic lubrication (EHL), 11-4

Elastomers, 30-6, 30-21; *see also* Polymeric
biomaterials
Elbow, 10-21; *see also* Joint-articulating surface motion
articulating surface geometry, 10-23
carrying angle, 10-23, 10-24
contact areas of articular surfaces, 10-26, 10-27
flexion and extension, 10-27
humeral–ulnar joint, 10-21
joint contact, 10-24 to 10-25
joint geometry, 10-24
rotation axes, 10-25, 10-26, 10-28
Elbow joint replacement, 37-17
Electrical activity, 42-1; *see also* Membrane models
Electrical conductivity of tissues, 40-1; *see also*
Syncytia
beta dispersion, 40-3
calculation of electrical potential, 40-1
cell suspensions, 40-2 to 40-4
complex conductivity, 40-2
DC effective longitudinal conductivity, 40-6
divergence, 40-1
effective conductivity, 40-2, 40-3 to 40-4
effective conductivity measurement, 40-7
electrical permittivity, 40-2
electric field and gradient, 40-1
extracellular voltage drop, 40-5
fiber suspensions, 40-4 to 40-8
four-electrode technique, 40-7
nerve, 40-8
one-dimensional cable theory, 40-5
one-dimensional nerve, 40-5
skeletal muscle, 40-8
transmembrane potential, 40-5
Electrical control activity (ECA), 6-3
Electrically active membrane, 38-3; *see also*
Electrophysiology
leakage channels, 38-5
mathematical model of patch, 38-5
membrane capacitance, 38-4
patches, 38-3
potassium ion channels, 38-4
sodium ion channels, 38-4 to 38-5
sodium–potassium pump, 38-4
Electrical potential calculation, 40-1; *see also* Electrical
conductivity of tissues
Electrical response activity (ERA), 6-3
Electrical stimulation, 49-2
axonal excitation, 49-2
bipolar electrodes and dipoles, 49-5 to 49-6
charge conservation, 49-3
dielectric and conductive media, 49-3 to 49-4
electric field, 49-2, 49-3
Gauss's law, 49-3
inhomogenous volume conductors, 49-6
monopole point source, 49-4 to 49-5
Ohm's law, 49-3
transmembrane voltage, 49-2

Electrical stimulation of CNS, 51-1, 51-12
AP initiation sites, 51-5 to 51-7
CNS neuron models, 51-5
current–distance relationship, 51-9
depolarizing cell's membrane, 51-2
indirect effects of stimulation, 51-10 to 51-11
neuron response to imposed potentials, 51-4 to 51-5
potential generation in CNS, 51-2 to 51-4
properties of, 51-7
stimulus polarity and waveform effect on, 51-9 to
51-10
strength–duration relationship, 51-8
Electrical stimulation of the centromedian (ESCM),
57-2; *see also* Epileptic seizure intervention
chronic stimulation parameters, 57-4
clock recovery unit, 57-4
hippocampus stimulation, 57-5 to 57-8
MRI confirmation of CM target, 57-3 to 57-4
neurophysiological confirmation of CM target, 57-4
patient's selection, 57-2
reliability, 57-4 to 57-5
seizure arrest targets, 57-3
target localization, 57-3
ventriculographic definition of cm target, 57-3
Electric field, 49-3
in volume conductors, 49-2
Electric lead, 48-5 to 48-6; *see also* Biomagnetism
Electrocardiogram (EKG), 6-9
Electrocardiography (ECG), 43-1, 45-1, 45-10, 47-2;
see also Electroencephalography (EEG);
Magnetocardiogram (MCG)
ambulatory ECG, 45-7 to 45-8
applications, 45-7
approach for recording, 45-2
bipolar catheter recording, 45-10
computer-based algorithms, 45-4
computers and, 45-3
diagnostic performance of, 48-8 to 48-9
ECG leads II and V-2, 45-10
his bundle electrocardiography, 45-8 to 45-10
HR electrocardiography, 45-8
instrumentation, 45-5 to 45-6
12-lead ECG, 45-2, 45-5
microprocessor-based ECG system, 45-7
older-style ECG machines, 45-6
patient monitoring, 45-8
physiology, 45-4 to 45-5
signal processing steps, 45-9
stylized version of normal lead II recording, 45-3
Electrochemical cell, 28-14; *see also* Metallic implant
corrosion
Electrochemistry of stimulation, 49-12
Electrode
damage, 49-13
placement, 52-7, 52-8
characteristics, 53-2 to 53-4
stability, 54-8

Electrode comparison, 53-1; *see also* Plasticity
  difficulties with NE, 53-15
  electrodes characteristics, 53-2 to 53-4
  NE misconceptions, 53-14 to 53-15
  neurotrophic electrode and neural signals, 53-4 to 53-6
  to restore movement in paralyzed, 53-2
Electrode–tissue interface, 49-10; *see also* Excitable tissue stimulation
  anodic break, 49-11
  brain tissue stimulation, 49-14
  cardiac tissue stimulation, 49-14 to 49-15
  charge-duration curve, 49-10 to 49-11
  electrochemistry of stimulation, 49-12
  electrode damage, 49-13
  excitable tissue stimulation, 49-14
  generating biphasic cathodic-first stimulation waveform, 49-12
  magnetic stimulation of excitable tissue, 49-15
  muscle tissue stimulation, 49-14
  peripheral nerve stimulation, 49-14
  stimulation waveform, 49-10, 49-12 to 49-13
  strength-duration curve, 49-10
  tissue damage, 49-13
Electrodiagnostic studies (EDX studies), 46-1, 46-9
  anatomy, 46-1 to 46-4
  axons, 46-4, 46-5
  brainstem auditory evoked response, 46-17 to 46-18
  CMAP waveforms, 46-10
  EMG and force generation, 46-5 to 46-6
  EMG recording, 46-6, 46-11 to 46-14
  EMG signals, 46-8
  engineering in, 46-19
  evoked potentials, 46-16
  instrumentation, 46-7 to 46-9
  motor nerve conduction, 46-8 to 46-11
  motor nerve fiber path, 46-3
  motor unit, 46-3
  MU and MUP, 46-2
  multimotor unit analysis, 46-13
  MU recruitment, 46-6
  myelin, 46-4
  nerve and muscle cells, 46-4
  nerve AP, 46-4
  pathology, 46-6 to 46-7
  physiology, 46-4 to 46-5
  sensory nerve conduction, 46-11
  single fiber and macro EMG, 46-14 to 46-16
  somatosensory evoked potential, 46-16 to 46-17
  visual evoked potential, 46-18
Electroencephalography (EEG), 3-14, 6-9, 46-1, 47-1, 47-11; *see also* Amplitude histograms; Electrodiagnostic studies (EDX studies); Magnetoencephalography (MEG)
  alpha rhythm, 47-2
  autocorrelellogram, 47-8
  averaged power spectra of 168-s epochs of REM sleep, 47-10
  coherence, 47-8
  cross-bispectral plots, 47-11
  cross-spectrum, 47-8
  electrodes, 47-2 to 47-3
  frequency analysis of, 47-7 to 47-8
  half-sensitivity volumes of, 48-12 to 48-13
  historical perspective, 47-1 to 47-2
  human brain waves, 47-2
  instrumentation, 47-2
  nonlinear analysis of, 47-8 to 47-11
  recording techniques, 47-2 to 47-4
  reticular activating system, 47-2
  sensitivity to radial and tangential sources, 48-14
  spectral analysis of EEG, 47-7
Electrogastrogram (EGG), 6-9 to 6-10
Electrogoniometry, 12-4
Electrohydraulic blood pump, 36-18
Electrolyte, 28-14; *see also* Metallic implant corrosion
Electromagnetocardiogram (EMCG), 48-8
Electromechanical transduction, 23-15
Electromyography (EMG), 12-2, 58-15
Electron spectroscopy for chemical analysis (ESCA), 30-17
Electrophysiology (EP), 38-1, 45-8; *see also* Action potentials and membrane currents; Action potential wave forms; Electrically active membrane; Electrocardiography; Electrophysiology; Propagation
  action potentials, 38-2, 38-8 to 38-9
  energy and resting potential, 38-6 to 38-7
  failures, 38-20
  field stimulation, 38-17 to 38-19
  Galvani experiment, 38-2
  Galvani in hindsight, 38-19
  Galvanism, 38-2
  linkages, 38-20
  magnetics, 38-19 to 38-20
  membrane stimulation, 38-7 to 38-9
  Nernst potential, 38-6
  resting potential, 38-6
Embolus, 30-21
EMCG, *see* Electromagnetocardiogram (EMCG)
EMG, *see* Electromyography (EMG)
End-diastolic pressure–volume relation (EDPVR), 15-10, 15-13
End-diastolic volume (EDV), 1-7
Endergonic reactions, 27-1
Endocrine cells, 42-16; *see also* Membrane models
  chromaffin cells, 42-16
  pancreatic β-cells, 42-16
  pituitary gonadotrophs and corticotrophs, 42-16
Endocrine system, 1-12
Endoluminal stent-grafts, 36-15 to 36-16; *see also* Vascular prostheses
Endolymphatic fluid, 24-3

Endoprosthetic reconstruction, 37-17 to 37-19
Endothelial cell (EC), 30-14, 35-4, 36-18
Endothelial NOS (eNOS), 20-8
Endothelial surface layer (ESL), 20-5
Endothelium, 1-12, 2-6, 17-10
Endothelium-derived hyperpolarizing factor (EDHF), 20-10
Endothelium–derived relaxing factor (EDRF), 20-10
End-plate, 46-2
End-systolic pressure–volume relation (ESPVR), 15-10
End-systolic volume (ESV), 1-7
End-to-end configuration, 36-18
End-to-side configuration, 36-18
Energy
    demandoptimization, 26-8
    transfer mechanics, 26-2
    transformation, 27-1, 27-2
Energy barrier in rate theory model, 42-8; *see also* Membrane currents
Engineered biofunctionality, 35-3; *see also* Biofunctional hydrogels
Engineered silk matrices, 34-4; *see also* Silk
    fibroin as 3D scaffold matrix, 34-8
    fibroin films and coatings, 34-6 to 34-7
    fibroin hydrogels, 34-10
    fibroin micro-/nanofibrous nets/mats/membranes, 34-5 to 34-6
    fibroin porous sponges, 34-8 to 34-10
    fibroin processing and applications, 34-5
    fibroin scaffolds with various pore sizes, 34-9
    silk microspheres, 34-10 to 34-11
    surface-decorated silk fibroin films, 34-7 to 34-8
Engram, 3-10
eNOS, *see* Endothelial NOS (eNOS)
Environmental scanning microscope (ESM), 11-11
Enzyme-degradable peptide substrates, 35-6
Eosinophils, 1-2
Epilepsy, 3-13, 57-1; *see also* Nervous system functions; Parkinson's disease (PD)
    pathological waveforms, 3-14
    prediction algorithms, 3-14
    types, 3-13
Epileptic seizure intervention, 57-1, 57-11 to 57-12
    ESCM, 57-2
    neuromodulation of SMA, 57-10 to 57-11
    study design, 57-8 to 57-10
EPOC, *see* Excess post-exercise oxygen consumption (EPOC)
ePTFE, *see* Expanded polytetrafluoroethylene (ePTFE)
Equivalence between dielectric and conductive media, 49-3 to 49-4
Equivalent circuit, 38-15 to 38-16
Equivalent double layer, 39-6; *see also* Volume conductor theory
ERA, *see* Electrical response activity (ERA)
Erectile effect, 15-13; *see also* Cardiac biomechanics
Erosion, 36-18

ERV, *see* Expiratory reserve volume (ERV)
Erythrocytes, 1-1, 1-2, *see* Red blood cell (RBC)
Erythropoietin, 2-18 to 2-19
ESCA, *see* Electron spectroscopy for chemical analysis (ESCA)
ESCM, *see* Electrical stimulation of the centromedian (ESCM)
ESL, *see* Endothelial surface layer (ESL)
ESM, *see* Environmental scanning microscope (ESM)
Espin, 25-3
ESPVR, *see* End-systolic pressure–volume relation (ESPVR)
Estimates for Young's Modulus, 24-5
ESV, *see* End-systolic volume (ESV)
Ethylene oxide (ETO), 32-27; *see also* Supercritical carbon dioxide sterilization
Ethylene vinyl acetate (EVA), 29-23
ETO, *see* Ethylene oxide (ETO)
Eustachian tube, 5-2
EVA, *see* Ethylene vinyl acetate (EVA)
Evoked potential (EP), 3-7, 46-16; *see also* Electrodiagnostic studies (EDX studies)
EW, *see* External work (EW)
Excess post-exercise oxygen consumption (EPOC), 26-6, 26-10
Exchange vessels, 20-7
Excitable tissue stimulation, 49-1, 49-14, 49-15; *see also* Electrical stimulation; Electrode–tissue interface; Membrane-electric field interaction
    cardiac tissue stimulation, 49-2
    cochlear prosthesis, 49-1
    neural prostheses, 49-1
Excitatory–inhibitory (E–I), 25-3
    axis, 25-4
    direction of cell, 25-3
Exercise physiology, 26-1
    aerobic threshold, 26-5
    anaerobic glycolysis, 26-2
    anaerobic threshold, 26-5, 26-10
    applications, 26-8, 26-10
    baroreceptors, 26-3, 26-10
    blood and respiratory parameter in exercise, 26-5
    blood pressures, 26-4
    cardiovascular adjustments, 26-3 to 26-4
    cardiovascular drift, 26-8, 26-10
    chemoreceptors, 26-6, 26-10
    countercurrent heat exchange, 26-8
    diverted blood flow, 26-4
    energy demand optimization, 26-8
    energy transfer mechanics, 26-2
    exercise responses, 26-9
    force by myocardial tissue, 26-4
    glycogen, 26-2
    heart functioning, 26-4
    hemoconcentration, 26-8
    maximum oxygen uptake, 26-4 to 26-6

mechanoreceptors, 26-10
muscle energetics, 26-1 to 26-2
oxygen deficit, 26-6, 26-10
oxygen uptake during exercise, 26-6
plasma volume, 26-8
respiratory responses, 26-6 to 26-7
sweating, 26-8
thermoregulatory response, 26-8
Exercise responses, 26-9
Exergonic reactions, 27-1
Expanded polytetrafluoroethylene (ePTFE), 36-16;
    see also Vascular prostheses
Expiration, 7-20
Expiratory reserve volume (ERV), 7-6
Explicit memory, *see* Declarative memory
External elastic lamina, 1-10
External work (EW), 15-12
Extracellular AP (ECAP), 46-4
Extracellular matrix (ECM), 34-5, 35-1
Extracellular path, 38-16 to 38-17
Extracellular voltage drop, 40-5; *see also* Electrical
    conductivity of tissues
Extracorporeal devices, 36-1; *see also* Heart valve
    prostheses
Eye movements, 4-9
Eyes, 4-2
Eyring rate theory models, 42-6 to 42-8; *see also*
    Membrane currents

F

Facilitation, 3-4
Factors affecting mechanical work in humans,
    27-1
    aerobic training, 27-7 to 27-8
    age effect, 27-6 to 27-7
    blood lactate, 27-8
    efficiency for hand cranking or bicycling, 27-5
    energy transformation, 27-1, 27-2
    equilibrium, 27-1
    force and aging, 27-7
    force and power output of muscle, 27-4
    force by muscles, 27-4
    gender effect, 27-8
    genetic factors, 27-8 to 27-9
    locomotion, 27-5 to 27-6
    muscular efficiency, 27-3 to 27-5
    muscular movement, 27-2
    negative work, 27-4
    optimal walking speed, 27-5
    power required for walking, running, and cycling,
        27-6
    resting muscle length, 27-4
    skeletal muscle as class 3 lever, 27-3
    stability requirement, 27-2
    strength training, 27-7, 27-8
    weight fractions for body parts, 27-2

Fahraeus effect, 20-3, 20-12; *see also* Microvascular
    blood flow mechanics
Faradaic stimulation, 49-12
Fascia lata, 36-18
Fast Fourier transform (FFT), 47-7, 47-12
Fatigue stress, 36-18
FD, *see* Fiber density (FD)
FD method, *see* Finite difference method (FD method)
Feature extractors, 3-7
FECAP ceramics, *see* Ferric–calcium–phosphorous
    oxide polyphasic ceramics (FECAP
    ceramics)
Federal Motor Vehicle Safety Standard (FMVSS),
    13-4
FEFs, *see* Forced expiratory flows (FEFs)
FEM, *see* Finite-element method (FEM)
Femoral stem, 37-12
Ferric–calcium–phosphorous oxide polyphasic
    ceramics (FECAP ceramics), 29-15, 29-16;
    see also Biodegradable ceramics
FES, *see* Functional electrical stimulation (FES)
FEVs, *see* Forced expiratory volumes (FEVs)
FFT, *see* Fast Fourier transform (FFT)
Fiber density (FD), 46-2
Fibers, 31-6, 33-18; *see also* Fibrous composites;
    Muscle
    recruitment order, 49-9 to 49-10
    architecture, 9-3
Fibrils, 8-17, 33-18
Fibrinogen, 1-2, 30-21
Fibroblast, 33-18, 36-18
Fibrochondrocyte, 33-18
Fibrosa, 16-3; *see also* Aortic valve
Fibrous composites, 31-6; *see also* Composite
    biomaterials
    carbon fiber-reinforced UHMWPE, 31-8
    carbon fibers, 31-7 to 31-9
    failure in, 31-7
    knee prostheses, 31-7
    stiffness, 31-7
Fibrous long spacing (FLS), 33-18
Fibrous membrane, 37-19
Filamentous matrix, 33-13; *see also* Collagen
Filler, 30-21
Filtration, 2-8
Fimbrin, 25-3
FINE, *see* Flat-interface nerve electrode (FINE)
Finger joint replacement, 37-17
Finger-touch force level control, 52-11
    below-lesion response-EMG FES level control,
        52-11
    peripheral equipment, 52-11 to 52-12
Finger-touch menu selection, 52-10
Finite difference method (FD method), 43-7, 43-8
    to 43-9; *see also* Computer modeling and
    simulation
Finite element analysis, 36-18

Finite-element method (FEM), 13-10, 24-2, 25-5 to
    25-6, 43-7, 43-9 to 43-10; *see also* Computer
    modeling and simulation
    application for 3D domains, 43-10 to 43-14
    Dirichlet condition, 43-14
    FE approximation, 43-12
    Green's divergence theorem, 43-13
    Neumann boundary condition, 43-13
    problem formulation, 43-12
FitzHugh–Nagumo model, 42-20; *see also* Membrane
    models
Fixation, 46-18; *see also* Electrodiagnostic studies
    (EDX studies)
Flat-interface nerve electrode (FINE), 49-14
Flow–volume curve, 7-17
Flow–volume loops, 7-18
Fluid; *see also* Nonblood-interfacing implants
    drag, 25-6
    flow stimulation, 25-6
    transfer implants, 36-31
Fluorocarbon polymers, 30-11 to 30-12; *see also*
    Biomaterial polymers
Flux equations, 42-8; *see also* Membrane currents
FM, *see* Frequency modulation (FM)
fMRI, *see* Functional magnetic resonance imaging
    (fMRI)
FMVSS, *see* Federal Motor Vehicle Safety Standard
    (FMVSS)
Foams, 31-1
Focal epilepsy, 3-13
Focal length, 15-3, 15-4
Foot off, *see* Toe off
Foot processes, 2-7
Force
    platforms, 12-4
    and power output of muscle, 27-4
    production and aging, 27-7
    resultant, 21-11
Forced expiratory flows (FEFs), 7-16
Forced expiratory volumes (FEVs), 7-16
Forced vital capacity (FVC), 7-6
Formaldehyde, 36-18
Formed elements in blood, 36-18
Forward and backward ion flux rates, 42-8; *see also*
    Membrane currents
Four-electrode technique, 40-7; *see also* Electrical
    conductivity of tissues
Fovea, 4-3
Fractional clearance, 2-11, 2-12
Fracture personality, 37-2; *see also* Long bone repair
FRC, *see* Functional residual capacity (FRC)
Free radical polymerization, *see* Addition
    polymerization
Free volume, 30-21
Frequency modulation (FM), 47-2, 50-12
Frequency range capability of BM, 24-6
Fretting, 28-18; *see also* Metallic implant corrosion

Friction, 11-12; *see also* Joint lubrication
Fringed-micelle model, 30-4, 30-6; *see also* Polymeric
    biomaterials
Functional electrical neuromuscular stimulation (FNS)
Functional electrical stimulation (FES), 50-1, 55-1; *see
    also* Battery-powered BION device (BPB);
    Electrical stimulation; Excitable tissue
    stimulation; Parastep system
    for ambulation by paraplegics, 52-2 to 52-3
    4-channel FES gait sequence, 50-5
    history, 50-2 to 50-3
    hybrid FES-long-leg brace ambulation systems,
        52-3
    implanted FES ambulation systems, 52-3
    noninvasive FES systems, 52-2
    in paraplegia, 52-2 to 52-3, 54-2
    to restore functionality, 49-1, 50-2 , 54-1
    and sensor system, 55-5
    transcutaneous, 52-1 to 52-2
Functional magnetic resonance imaging (fMRI), 3-7
Functional residual capacity (FRC), 7-6, 7-20
FVC, *see* Forced vital capacity (FVC)

G

GABA, *see* Gamma-amino-butyric acid (GABA)
Gadd Severity Index (GSI), 13-4, 13-8
Gait analysis, 12-1
    accelerometry, 12-4
    clinical example, 12-8 to 12-11
    components, 12-2
    current status, 12-11 to 12-12
    data collection protocol, 12-3
    data reduction, 12-6 to 12-8
    data reference system, 12-2 to 12-3
    dynamic EMG, 12-5 to 12-6
    electrogoniometry, 12-4
    force platforms, 12-4
    free body diagram of foot, 12-7
    fundamental concepts, 12-2
    gait cycle, 12-2
    ground reaction measurement, 12-4 to 12-5
    kinematics, 12-2
    marker-based coordinate systems, 12-6
    measurement approaches and systems, 12-3
    motion measurement, 12-4
    muscle moments, 12-8
    pathologies served by, 12-1 to 12-2
    pedobarography, 12-5
    stride and temporal parameters, 12-3 to 12-4
    toe off, 12-2
    video camera-based systems, 12-4
Galerkin method, 43-7; *see also* Computer modeling
    and simulation
Galvanic corrosion, 28-15, 28-19; *see also* Metallic
    implant corrosion
Galvanic series, 28-19

Galvani experiment, 38-2; *see also* Electrophysiology
Galvanism, 38-2; *see also* Electrophysiology
Gamma-amino-butyric acid (GABA), 5-12
Ganglion cells, 4-3
Gas constant, 42-5; *see also* Membrane currents
Gas partial pressure, 7-8 to 7-10
Gastrointestinal electrical activity, 6-3, 6-12
    colonic slow-wave activity, 6-11 to 6-12
    coupled nonlinear oscillators, 6-5 to 6-6
    ECA, ERA, and muscular contractions, 6-4
    electrogastrogram, 6-9 to 6-10
    gastric ECA slow-wave activity, 6-8 to 6-9
    hour rhythms, 6-7 to 6-8
    intercellular communication, 6-5
    migrating motility complex, 6-4
    minute rhythms, 6-6 to 6-7
    nomenclature in, 6-8
    phase-resetting phenomena, 6-5
    small intestinal MMC, 6-11
    small intestinal slow-wave activity, 6-10
Gastrointestinal system (GI system), 6-1; *see also*
        Gastrointestinal electrical activity
    colon, 6-11
    function of, 6-1
    GI tract, 6-2
    interstitial cells of Cajal, 6-1 to 6-3
    layers of GI wall, 6-3
    small intestine, 6-10
    stomach, 6-8
Gating variables, 42-6; *see also* Membrane currents
Gauss's law, 49-3
GBM, *see* Glomerular basement membrane (GBM)
Gelatin, 33-18
Gel casting, 29-23; *see also* Bioceramic manufacturing
        techniques
Gel matrix, 33-12; *see also* Collagen
Generalized epilepsy, 3-13
Generalized singular value decomposition (GSVD),
        43-5
General purpose polystyrene (GPPS), 30-10
Geometric gain, 25-4
Gerota's fascia, 2-3
GFR, *see* Glomerular filtration rate (GFR)
Glass ceramics, 29-16, 29-26; *see also* Bioactive
        ceramics
    compositions of, 29-18
    temperature–time cycle for, 29-18
    tissue–glass–ceramic bonding, 29-19
Glass transition temperature, 30-7, 30-8, 30-21
Glaucoma, 36-31; *see also* Nonblood-interfacing implants
Globulin, 1-2
Glomerular barrier surface area, 2-9 to 2-10
Glomerular basement membrane (GBM), 2-6, 2-7
Glomerular filtration rate (GFR), 2-8
Glomerular visceral epithelium, *see* Podocytes
Glomerulus, 2-5, 2-6; *see also* Kidney physiology
    endothelium, 2-6

filtration, 2-8
foot processes, 2-7
glomerular basement membrane, 2-6, 2-7
glycocalyx, 2-6
mechanical properties of, 2-7
mesangium, 2-5
nephrin, 2-7
podocin, 2-7
podocytes, 2-6, 2-7
porosity, 2-9
slit diaphragm, 2-7
tubular pole, 2-5
Glutamic acid (Glu), 33-18
Glycine (Gly), 33-18
Glycocalyx, 2-6
Glycogen, 26-2
Glycolide–lactide copolymer, 32-10; *see also* Glycolide/
        lactide-based polyesters
Glycolide/lactide-based polyesters, 32-4; *see also*
        Biodegradable polymers
    burst mode, 32-10
    ether linkage, 32-8 to 32-9
    glycolide–lactide copolymer, 32-10
    homopolymer polyesters, 32-5
    lactide polymers, 32-9 to 32-11
    Maxon, 32-7
    monocryl, 32-7
    poly(depsipeptides), 32-10
    poly(L-lactide) composition effect, 32-6
    polyester-based co-monomers, 32-6 to 32-8
Glycoprotein, 33-18
Glycosaminoglycans (GAG), 33-9, 33-18; *see also* Collagen
Goldman–Hodgkin–Katz constant field formulation,
        42-6; *see also* Membrane currents
GPPS, *see* General purpose polystyrene (GPPS)
Grafts, 30-21
Granulocytes, 1-2, 21-7
Gravimetric techniques, 19-5
Gross movement, 10-1
GSI, *see* Gadd Severity Index (GSI)
GSVD, *see* Generalized singular value decomposition
        (GSVD)
GTP, *see* Guanosine triphosphate (GTP)
Guanosine triphosphate (GTP), 20-8

H

H&E, *see* Hematoxylin and Eosin (H&E)
HA, *see* Hydroxyapatite (HA)
Habituation, 3-10
Hair bundle; *see also* Hair cell bundle mechanics; Hair
        cells
    mechanical properties of, 25-7 to 25-9
    response to stimuli, 25-9 to 25-10
    shape effect, 25-10
    stiffness, 25-8
    transduction process, 24-12

Hair cell bundle mechanics, 25-1, 25-11; *see also* Active
        process; Hair cells
    analytical models, 25-4
    bundle stiffness, 25-8
    channel open probability, 25-4
    E–I axis, 25-4
    finite element models, 25-5 to 25-6
    fluid drag, 25-6
    geometric gain, 25-4
    link structures, 25-7 to 25-8
    mechanical properties, 25-7 to 25-9
    Oseen's drag, 25-6
    response to stimuli, 25-9 to 25-10
    single-degree-of-freedom model, 25-4
    stiffness, 25-3 to 25-4
    tonotopic arrangement, 25-3
    transduction channel kinetics, 25-6 to 25-7
Hair cells, 25-1; *see also* Hair bundle; Hair cell bundle
        mechanics
    actin fibers, 25-3
    bundles, 25-2
    E–I direction of cell, 25-3
    espin, 25-3
    fimbrin, 25-3
    kinocilium, 25-1, 25-2, 25-3
    sensitiveness, 25-4
    stereocilia, 25-1, 25-2, 25-3
    stiffness, 25-3 to 25-4
    structure, 25-1 to
    tip links, 25-1, 25-2, 25-3
Hand, 10-32; *see also* Joint-articulating surface motion
    center of curvature locus, 10-35
    contact areas, 10-37
    curvature of joint articular surface, 10-35
    helical angle intersections, 10-37
    joint center of rotation, 10-38
    joint contact, 10-35 to 10-37
    MCP joint contact area, 10-36
    rotation axis, 10-37 to 10-38, 10-39, 10-40
    surface geometry, 10-32
Hangman's fractures, 13-2; *see also* Neck mechanics
Hard tissue, 8-1; *see also* Soft tissues
Hard tissue mechanics, 8-1; *see also* Bone; Dentin; Soft
        tissues
    apparent density, 8-9
    bulk modulus, 8-8
    compliance coefficients, 8-4
    elastic anisotropy characterization, 8-10 to 8-12
    elastic behavior modeling, 8-12 to 8-14
    elastic properties, 8-4 to 8-10
    equations for transverse isotropy, 8-8
    Hooke's law, 8-4
    loss modulus, 8-15
    mechanical testing methods, 8-9
    percentage compressive, 8-10 to 8-12
    percentage shear, 8-10 to 8-12
    research, 8-17

    shear modulus, 8-8
    stiffness matrix, 8-4 to 8-5, 8-8
    storage modulus, 8-15
    transformation equations, 8-8
    viscoelastic properties, 8-14 to 8-17
    wave equation, 8-6
    Young's modulus variations, 8-13
Hard tissue replacement, 28-1, 37-1; *see also* Joint
        replacements; Long bone repair; Metallic
        biomaterials; Total joint replacements
Haversian bone, 8-20; *see also* Bone
Haynes 25, 36-18
HCPCS, *see* Healthcare common procedure coding
        system (HCPCS)
HDPE, *see* High density polyethylene (HDPE)
Head injury criterion (HIC), 13-4, 13-8
Head mechanics, 13-1; *see also* Neck mechanics
    brain response, 13-3 to 13-5
    GSI, 13-8
    head injury risk curve, 13-9
    HIC, 13-8
    human surrogates of head and neck, 13-10 to 13-11
    injury mechanisms, 13-1 to 13-2
    tolerance estimates for MTBI, 13-9
    tolerance of head, 13-7 to 13-9
    Wayne state tolerance curve, 13-7 to 13-8
Head-related transfer function (HRTF), 5-3
Healthcare common procedure coding system
        (HCPCS), 52-17
Heart, 1-3, 1-6; *see also* Blood vessels; Cardiovascular
        system
    cardiac output, 1-7
    chambers, 1-6 to 1-7
    functioning, 26-4
    pulmonary circulation, 1-6
    systemic circulation, 1-6
Heart valve dynamics, 16-1; *see also* Aortic valve;
        Mitral valve (MV); Pulmonary valve;
        Tricuspid valve (TV)
Heart valve prostheses, 36-2, 36-5; *see also* Blood-
        interfacing implants
    bileaflet design, 36-3
    biological heart valves, 36-7 to 36-9
    biomaterial used in, 36-9
    caged-ball heart valve prosthesis, 36-2 to 36-3
    CarboMedics bileaflet valve, 36-4
    cavitation bubbles, 36-6
    closing dynamics of, 36-6
    homografts, 36-7
    mechanical heart valves, 36-2 to 36-7
    pitting and erosion, 36-6, 36-7
    porcine bioprosthesis, 36-8
    problems with implanted valves, 36-10
    synthetic heart valves, 36-9 to 36-10
    thromboembolic complications, 36-5
    tilting disk valve prosthesis, 36-4
    tri-leaflet heart valve prosthesis, 36-5

in United States, 36-2
xenografts, 36-7
Helical pitch, 33-18
Helicotrema, 24-3
Helmholtz's theorem, 48-2
Hematocytes, 1-1, 1-2, 21-1, 21-10; *see also* Leukocytes;
     Red blood cell (RBC)
  constitutive relations for fluid flow, 21-2
  fundamentals, 21-2
  mean shear rate, 21-3
  newtonian fluid flow equations, 21-2 to 21-3
  shear deformation rate, 21-2
  stresses and strains, 21-2
Hematocytopoiesis, 1-1
Hematoxylin and Eosin (H&E), 41-5
Hemidecussation, 4-4
Hemoconcentration, 26-8
Hemorrhagic complications, 30-14
Hemostat, 33-18
Henson cells, 24-4
Heparin, 30-14, 30-21
Hesed coil, 58-6, 58-9; *see also* Hesed coil
     efficacy; Transcranial magnetic
     stimulation (TMS)
  over human head, 58-10
Hesed coil efficacy, 58-13
  discussion, 58-17 to 58-18
  experimental setup, 58-15 to 58-16
  results, 58-17
  safety measurements, 58-17
  TMS coils, 58-14 to 58-15
Hexafluoroisopropanol (HFIP), 34-2, 34-8
HFIP, *see* Hexafluoroisopropanol (HFIP)
HH, *see* Hodgkin and Huxley (HH)
HIC, *see* Head injury criterion (HIC)
HIF1, *see* Hypoxia-inducible factor (HIF1)
High density polyethylene (HDPE), 30-9
Higher cortical centers, 4-8
High impact PS (HIPS), 30-10
High-resolution (HR), 6-9, 45-3
High-speed loading, 14-1
Hill model, 9-11, 42-19 to 42-20; *see also* Membrane
     models
Hilum, 2-4
Hindmarsh–Rose models, 42-20; *see also* Membrane
     models
Hip, 10-13; *see also* Joint-articulating surface motion
  acetabular fossae, 10-15
  anteversion angle, 10-15, 10-16
  coxa valga, 10-15
  coxa vara, 10-15
  joint contact, 10-16 to 10-17
  joint replacement, 37-12 to 37-14
  neck–shaft angle, 10-15
  pressure distribution and contact area, 10-16
  proximal femur geometry, 10-15
  resultant force, 10-17

rotation axes, 10-17 to 10-18
surface geometry, 10-15 to 10-16
HIPS, *see* High impact PS (HIPS)
Hodgkin and Huxley (HH), 42-6; *see also* Membrane
     currents; Nerve cells
  equations, 42-10
  resistor battery model, 42-5 to 42-6
Homeostasis, 1-12
Homografts, 36-7, 36-18; *see also* Heart valve
     prostheses
Horizontal cells, 4-3
Horseradish peroxidase (HRP), 34-10
Hour rhythms, 6-7 to 6-8
HR, *see* High-resolution (HR)
HRP, *see* Horseradish peroxidase (HRP)
HRTF, *see* Head-related transfer function (HRTF)
Human brain waves, 47-2; *see also*
     Electroencephalography (EEG)
Human cortex, 5-13 to 5-14
Human perception, 3-7, 3-9
Hybrid FES-long-leg brace ambulation systems, 52-3
Hydraulic permeability (Lp), 2-9
Hydrocephalus, 36-31; *see also* Nonblood-interfacing
     implants
Hydrodynamic factor, 11-5
Hydrodynamic lubrication theories, 11-4
Hydrogels, 30-21, 35-1; *see also* Biofunctional hydrogels
Hydrogen bonding, 30-21
Hydrophilicity, 33-18
Hydrophilic polymers, 35-2
Hydrophobicity, 33-18
Hydroquinone, 30-21
Hydroxyapatite (HA) , 29-26, 37-11; *see also* Joint
     replacements
  synthesis method, 29-24 to 29-25; *see also*
     Bioceramic manufacturing techniques
Hydroxylysine (Hyl), 33-18
Hydroxyproline (Hyp), 33-18
Hyp, *see* Hydroxyproline (Hyp)
Hyperacuity, 4-3
Hyperpolarization, 42-21
Hyperthermia, 28-19
Hypoxia-inducible factor (HIF1), 20-11
Hysteresis, 3-10
Hysteresivity, 7-12

I

IA, *see* Insertional activity (IA)
IC, *see* Inferior Colliculi (IC); Inspiratory capacity (IC)
ICAP, *see* Intracellular AP (ICAP)
ICC, *see* Interstitial cells of Cajal (ICC)
ICCG, *see* Incomplete Choleski conjugate gradient
     (ICCG)
ICD, *see* Implantable cardiac defibrillator (ICD)
IGF-I, *see* Insulin-like growth factor I (IGF-I)
IHCs, *see* Inner hair cells (IHCs)

ILDs, *see* Interaural level differences (ILDs)
Immunity, 28-16, 28-20; *see also* Pourbaix diagram
IM nails, *see* Intramedullary devices (IM nails)
Impedance, 17-10
Implantable bioceramics, 29-2; *see also* Ceramic
    biomaterials
Implantable Bionic neural prosthetic devices, 55-1; *see*
    also Battery-powered BION device (BPB)
    BION devices, 55-3
    evolution of, 55-2 to 55-4
Implantable cardiac defibrillator (ICD), 43-2
Implanted FES ambulation systems, 52-3
Implant manufacturing, 28-18; *see also* Metallic
    biomaterials
    Co–Cr alloys, 28-19
    stainless steels, 28-18 to 28-19
    Ti and alloys, 28-19
Implicit memory, *see* Nondeclarative memory
Incomplete Choleski conjugate gradient (ICCG), 43-15
Independent elastic constants, 31-4; *see also* Composite
    biomaterials
Inducible NOS (iNOS), 20-8
Inferior Colliculi (IC), 5-7, 5-11 to 5-12
Inflammatory cell, 33-19
Information processing, 3-4
Inhomogenous volume conductors, 49-6
Inite element models, 25-5 to 25-6
Initiator, 30-21
Injection molding, 29-23; *see also* Bioceramic
    manufacturing techniques
Injury, 14-1
Inner ear, 5-3 to 5-4, 24-1
Inner hair cells (IHCs), 5-1, 5-6
Inner sulcus (IS), 24-4, 24-18
Inorganic biodegradable polymers, 32-2; *see also*
    Biodegradable polymers
Inorganic phosphate (Pi), 26-1
iNOS, *see* Inducible NOS (iNOS)
Inotropic, 1-12
Insertional activity (IA), 46-12; *see also*
    Electrodiagnostic studies (EDX studies)
Inspiration, 7-20
Inspiratory capacity (IC), 7-6
Inspiratory reserve volume (IRV), 7-5
Institutional Review Board (IRB), 54-2
Insulin-like growth factor I (IGF-I), 34-10
Interaural level differences (ILDs), 5-11
Interaural time differences (ITDs), 5-11
Intercellular communication, 6-5
Interference pattern (IP), 46-13
Interlocking, 37-8; *see also* Long bone repair
Intermolecular crosslink, 33-19
International Neuromodulation Society, 50-1
Interpotential interval (IPI), 46-15; *see also*
    Electrodiagnostic studies (EDX studies)
Interstitial cells of Cajal (ICC), 6-1
Interstitial lamellae, *see* Haversian bone

Interstitial space, 40-11
Interstitium, 22-13
Intra-aortic balloon pumps, 36-18
Intracellular AP (ICAP), 46-4
Intracellular current flow, 38-16
Intrafibrillar volume, 33-19
Intraluminal pressure of glomerular capillary, 2-10
Intramedullary devices (IM nails), 37-7 to 37-8; *see also*
    Long bone repair
Intraocular lenses (IOLs), 36-24
Intraoperative monitoring (IOM), 46-19; *see also*
    Electrodiagnostic studies (EDX studies)
Intravenous (IV), 30-9
IOLs, *see* Intraocular lenses (IOLs)
IOM, *see* Intraoperative monitoring (IOM)
Ion channel, 42-21; *see also* Membrane currents
    kinetics, 42-6
    selectivity, 42-2
Ion exchanger, 42-8, 42-21; *see also* Membrane currents
Ionic bonding, 30-21
Ionic salts, 29-1
Ion pump, 42-8, 42-21; *see also* Membrane currents
IP, *see* Interference pattern (IP)
IPI, *see* Interpotential interval (IPI)
IRB, *see* Institutional Review Board (IRB)
IRV, *see* Inspiratory reserve volume (IRV)
Isoelectric point, 33-19
Isofrequency laminae, 5-8
Isoleucine (Ile), 33-19
Isovolumetric relaxation, 16-3
ITDs, *see* Interaural time differences (ITDs)
IV, *see* Intravenous (IV)

J

Joint-articulating surface motion, 10-1, 10-2, 10-38,
    10-40; *see also* Ankle joint; Elbow; Hand;
    Hip; Knee; Shoulder; Wrist
Joint lubrication, 11-1, 11-21 to 11-22; *see also* Cartilage
    wear; Lubrication; Synovial joints; Tribology
    cartilage-on-cartilage combination, 11-18
    experimental contact systems, 11-18 to 11-19
    hip joint forces and angular velocities, 11-20
    lubrication regime existence, 11-20 to 11-21
    recent developments, 11-21
    rheology and friction, 11-19 to 11-20
Joint replacements, 37-8; *see also* Hard tissue
    replacement; Total joint replacements
    bone cement fixation, 37-10 to 37-11
    cartilage functions, 37-9
    implant fixation methods, 37-9
    porosity types, 37-11
    porous ingrowth fixation, 37-11 to 37-12
    porous tantalum, 37-12
    total, 37-9
Joints, 10-2
Juxtaglomerular apparatus, 2-5

K

Kedem–Katchalsky equations, 20-9; *see also* Molecular transport in microcirculation
Kevlar®, 30-11, 30-21
Kidney anatomy, 2-1, 2-2; *see also* Nephron
  acid-Schiff-stained section of, 2-20
  basal labyrinth, 2-14
  brush border, 2-12
  calyx, 2-4
  cortex, 2-3
  Gerota's fascia, 2-3
  glomerulus, 2-2
  hilum, 2-4
  kidney parenchyma, 2-4, 2-5, 2-13
  medulla, 2-4
  medullary pyramids, 2-4
  papilla, 2-4
  pelvis, 2-4
  renal artery, 2-4
  renal lobe, 2-3
  renal vein, 2-4
  tubule, 2-2
  variations, 2-5
  vascular organization, 2-3, 2-4
Kidney physiology, 2-1; *see also* Glomerulus
  aldosterone, 2-18
  antidiuretic hormone, 2-18
  autoregulation, 2-10
  as blood regulator, 2-1
  countercurrent multiplication, 2-17
  effective molecular diameter, 2-11
  erythropoietin, 2-18 to 2-19
  filtration, 2-1, 2-8
  fractional clearance, 2-11, 2-12
  GFR, 2-8 to 2-9
  hydraulic permeability, 2-9
  intraluminal pressure of glomerular capillary, 2-10
  kidney function assessment, 2-19 to 2-20
  permselectivity, 2-11
  pH regulation, 2-16
  reabsorption, 2-1
  renal plasma flow, 2-8
  renin, 2-18
  renin–angiotensin hormone system, 2-10, 2-11
  secretion, 2-1
  small solutes recovery, 2-16
  sodium reabsorption, 2-15 to 2-16
  solute transport, 2-14 to 2-15
  starling's law of capillary filtration, 2-8
  surface area of glomerular barrier, 2-9 to 2-10
  tubuloglomerular feedback, 2-11
  tubulo-interstitial structure and organization, 2-12 to 2-14
  ultrafiltration coefficient, 2-10
  uptake, 2-15
  urine, 2-2

  variations, 2-5
  vitamin D metabolism, 2-19
  water reabsorption, 2-16 to 2-17
Kinematic analysis of human movement, 10-1
Kinocilial links (KL), 25-8
Kinocilium, 25-1, 25-2, 25-3
KL, *see* Kinocilial links (KL)
Knee, 10-5; *see also* Joint-articulating surface motion
  articulating surface geometry, 10-7
  contour of tibial plateau, 10-9
  distal femur, 10-9
  femoral condyle spherical radius, 10-10
  femur displacement, 10-12
  flexion angle, 10-14
  joint contact, 10-7
  patella contact areas, 10-13
  patellar facet angles, 10-11
  proximal tibia geometry, 10-10
  rotation axes, 10-10 to 10-13, 10-14
  sulcus angle, 10-11
  tibial plateau, 10-10, 10-12
  tibiofemoral contact area, 10-12
  trochlear geometry indices, 10-11
Knee joint replacement, 37-15 to 37-16
Knee prostheses, 31-7; *see also* Fibrous composites
Krogh–Erlang equation, 20-7
Krogh tissue cylinder model, 20-7, 20-12
Kurtosis, 47-6 to 47-7; *see also* Amplitude histographs

L

LAS, *see* Low-amplitude signal (LAS)
Laser Doppler anemometry, 36-18
Laser scanning lithography (LSL), 35-10
Lateral geniculate nucleus (LGN), 4-4
Lateral inhibition, 3-6 to 3-7
Lateral lemniscus (LL), 5-7
Lateral superior olive (LSO), 5-11
Law of projections, 3-3
Law of the Heart, 15-12; *see also* Cardiac biomechanics
LCP, *see* Locking compression plate (LCP)
LDPE, *see* Low density polyethylene (LDPE)
Lead; *see also* Biomagnetism
  current field, 48-5
  field, 48-4 to 48-5
  vector, 48-3, 48-4
Leaflets, 36-18
Leakage channels, 38-5; *see also* Electrically active membrane
Learning, 3-10
LEDs, *see* Light-emitting diodes (LEDs)
Left ventricular assist devices, 36-18
Lennox–Gastaut syndrome (LGS), 57-1
Leucine (Leu), 33-19

Leukocytes, 1-1, 1-2, 21-7; *see also* Hematocytes
  apparent viscosity, 21-9 to 21-10
  classification, 21-7
  cortical tension, 21-8
  Maxwell fluid model, 21-9 to 21-10
  mechanical behavior, 21-8
  power law fluid, 21-9
  pseudopodia, 21-10
  size and shape, 21-7 to 21-8
  viscous parameters of, 21-9
  white cell activation, 21-11
Lexan, 30-21
LFPs, *see* Local field potential recordings (LFPs)
LGN, *see* Lateral geniculate nucleus (LGN)
LGS, *see* Lennox–Gastaut syndrome (LGS)
L'Hopital's Rule, 42-10 to 42-11; *see also* Nerve cells
Ligaments, *see* Tendons
Light-emitting diodes (LEDs), 12-4
LINC, *see* Linker nucleoskeleton and cytoskeleton
      (LINC)
Linear acceleration, 24-1
Linear aliphatic biodegradable polyesters, 32-2, 32-6,
      32-24; *see also* Biodegradable polymers
  limitations, 32-27
  natural origin, 32-25
  nonwoven PGA matrices, 32-25
  PLLA-impregnated and annealed PGA matrix,
      32-26
  scaffold structure, 32-25
Linear alkyl groups, 32-22
Linear low density polyethylene (LLDPE), 30-9
Linear polymers, 30-5; *see also* Polymeric biomaterials
Linker nucleoskeleton and cytoskeleton (LINC), 23-5
Link structures, 25-7 to 25-8
Lipid, 33-19
Liquid vapor pressure, 36-18
LL, *see* Lateral lemniscus (LL)
LLDPE, *see* Linear low density polyethylene (LLDPE)
Local current loop, 38-15
Local field potential recordings (LFPs), 53-2
Locking compression plate (LCP), 37-6; *see also* Long
      bone repair
Locomotion, 27-5 to 27-6
Long bone repair, 37-1; *see also* Hard tissue
      replacement
  biomaterial applications in internal fixation, 37-3
  bone plates, 37-7
  bone screws, 37-5
  failure modes of internal fixation devices, 37-3
  fracture treatment, 37-2
  interlocking, 37-8
  internal and external fixation of wrist, 37-2
  intramedullary nails, 37-7 to 37-8
  metallic pin tips, 37-4
  pins, 37-4
  plates, 37-5 to 37-7
  primary healing, 37-2

  screws, 37-4 to 37-5
  secondary healing, 37-2
  total hip joint replacement, 37-2
  wires and cables, 37-3 to 37-4
Long-term depression (LTD), 5-10
Long-term potentiation (LTP)
Loop of Henle, 2-5, 2-14
Loss modulus, 8-15
Louisiana State University (LSU), 52-3
Low-amplitude signal (LAS), 45-8; *see also*
      Electrocardiography
Low density polyethylene (LDPE), 30-9
Lower-upper (LU), 43-14
Low-temperature isotropic (LTI), 29-8, 36-18
  carbon, 29-26
Low-viscosity liquids, 31-5
LSL, *see* Laser scanning lithography (LSL)
LSO, *see* Lateral superior olive (LSO)
LSU, *see* Louisiana State University (LSU)
LTD, *see* Long-term depression (LTD)
LTI, *see* Low-temperature isotropic (LTI)
LU, *see* Lower-upper (LU)
Lubricating ability, 11-10; *see also* Joint lubrication
Lubrication, 11-3, 11-18; *see also* Joint lubrication
  boundary lubrication, 11-6
  Dowson–Higginson expression, 11-5
  hydrodynamic lubrication theories, 11-4 to 11-5
  principles of, 11-3
  reduced modulus of elasticity, 11-5
  regimes of, 11-4, 11-5
  transition from hydrodynamic to boundary
      lubrication, 11-6
Lumped-parameter model, 7-12
Lung, 7-1
  perfusion, 7-7 to 7-8
  volumes, 7-5 to 7-7
Lunula, 16-3; *see also* Aortic valve
Lymph, 22-2; *see also* Tissue transport mechanics
Lymphatic endothelial microvalves, 22-9; *see also*
      Tissue transport mechanics
Lymphatic system, 22-13; *see also* Tissue transport
      mechanics
Lymphatic transport mechanics, *see* Tissue transport
      mechanics
Lymphatic vessels, 22-12; *see also* Tissue transport
      mechanics
Lymphocytes, 1-2, 21-7
Lyotropic salts, 33-10
Lysine (Lys), 33-19

M

Mach bands, 3-6
Macrophage, 33-19
Macula densa, 2-5, 2-14
Macula lutea, 4-3
Magnetic lead, 48-6; *see also* Biomagnetism

Magnetic resonance imaging (MRI), 16-8, 27-8, 43-3
Magnetic stimulation of excitable tissue, 49-15; *see also*
    Excitable tissue stimulation
Magnetocardiogram (MCG), 48-1; *see also*
    Biomagnetism; Electrocardiography (ECG)
  detection of equivalent magnetic dipole, 48-7 to
    48-8
  diagnostic performance of, 48-8 to 48-9
  source model selection for, 48-7
  technical reasons to use, 48-9
  theoretical reasons to use, 48-11
Magnetoencephalography (MEG), 43-19, 48-1; *see also*
    Biomagnetism; Electroencephalography
    (EEG)
  axial magnetometer, 48-12
  half-sensitivity volumes of, 48-12 to 48-13, 48-15
  measurement sensitivity distribution, 48-12
  planar gradiometer, 48-12
  sensitivity to radial and tangential sources, 48-14
  technical aspects of, 48-14 to 48-15
  theoretical aspects of, 48-12
Magnification, 4-5, 4-10
Magnitude squared coherence (MSC), 47-8, 47-12
Magnocellular cells (M cells), 4-4
Major sperm protein (MSP), 23-12
Malaria modeling, 23-16
MAPK, *see* Mitogen-activated protein kinases (MAPK)
Mapped clock oscillator (MCO), 6-6
Markov-state models, 42-6; *see also* Membrane
    currents
Markup languages, 20-12
Martensite, 28-20
Massachusetts Eye and Ear Infirmary and the
    Massachusetts Institute of Technology
    (MEEI-MIT), 56-3
Mass spectrometer, 7-20
Mathematical cell mechanics model, 23-7
Matrix metalloproteinases (MMPs), 35-6
Maxillofacial implants, 36-28 to 36-29; *see also*
    Nonblood-interfacing implants
Maximal oxygen consumption (VO_2max), 26-4 to
    26-6, 26-10, 27-8
Maximum radius ratio, 29-26
Maxon, 32-7; *see also* Glycolide/lactide-based
    polyesters
Maxwell fluid, 21-11; *see also* Leukocytes
  model, 21-9 to 21-10
MCD, *see* Mean consecutive difference (MCD)
M cells, *see* Magnocellular cells (M cells)
MCG, *see* Magnetocardiogram (MCG)
MCO, *see* Mapped clock oscillator (MCO)
MCP joint, *see* Metacarpophalangeal joint
    (MCP joint)
MD, *see* Morpholine 2,5-dione (MD)
Mean consecutive difference (MCD), 46-15
Mean filling pressure, 19-3; *see also* Venous system
Mean transit time (MTT), 19-4

Measurement of rebreathing pulmonary diffusing
    capacity, 7-19
Mechanical prostheses, 36-18
Mechanoelectrical transduction, 23-14
Mechanoreceptors, 7-20, 26-10
Mechanosensitive channels, 23-14
Mechanotransduction, 23-13 to 23-14
Medial geniculate, 5-12
Medial geniculate body (MGB), 5-11
Medial superior olive (MSO), 5-11
Medium-caliber blood vessels, 18-2; *see also* Blood
    vessels
Medullary pyramids, 2-4
MEEI-MIT, *see* Massachusetts Eye and Ear Infirmary
    and the Massachusetts Institute of
    Technology (MEEI-MIT)
MEG, *see* Magnetoencephalography (MEG)
Membrane
  bending modulus, 21-6, 21-11; *see also* Red blood
    cell (RBC)
  capacitance, 38-4; *see also* Electrically active
    membrane
  shear modulus, 21-11
  tethers, 23-6
  viscosity, 21-11
Membrane currents, 38-16, 42-5; *see also* Membrane
    models
  calcium as second messenger, 42-8
  circuit representation of, 42-6
  current for ionic species, 42-6
  energy barrier in rate theory model, 42-8
  Eyring rate theory models, 42-6 to 42-8
  flux equations, 42-8
  forward and backward ion flux rates, 42-8
  gas constant, 42-5
  gating variables, 42-6
  Goldman–Hodgkin–Katz constant field
    formulation, 42-6
  Hodgkin–Huxley resistor battery model, 42-5 to
    42-6
  ion channel kinetics, 42-6
  ion exchangers, 42-8
  ion pump, 42-8
  Markov-state models, 42-6
  Nernst–Planck equations, 42-5
  Nernst potential, 42-6
  synapses, 42-8
  voltage-clamp protocols, 42-6
Membrane-electric field interaction, 49-6; *see also*
    Excitable tissue stimulation
  activating function, 49-7
  activation of myelinated axons, 49-8 to 49-9
  axon space constant effect, 49-9
  axon time constant of, 49-8
  membrane polarization, 49-8
  effect of polarity of applied stimulus, 49-9
  recruitment order of fibers, 49-9 to 49-10

Membrane models, 42-1; *see also* Cardiac cells;
Membrane currents; Nerve cells; Patch
clamp method
action potential, 42-2 to 42-3
databases, 42-22
endocrine cells, 42-16
epithelial cells, 42-19
FitzHugh–Nagumo model, 42-20
Hill model, 42-19 to 42-20
Hindmarsh–Rose models, 42-20
ion channel selectivity, 42-2
lipid bilayer, 42-2
numerical methods, 42-21 to 42-22
patch-clamp data, 42-3
plant cells, 42-19
resting potential, 42-2
simplified models, 42-19
skeletal muscle cells, 42-14 to 42-15
smooth muscle, 42-19
transmembrane potential difference, 42-1 to 42-2
Membrane polarization, 49-8
Membranous matrix, 33-12; *see also* Collagen
Memory, 3-9, 3-10
Memory consolidation, 3-10
MEMS, *see* Microelectrical mechanical systems
(MEMS)
Meniscus, 33-19
Mental images, 3-7
Menus for Pulse Shaping and Synchronization, 52-7
MEPs, *see* Motor-evoked potentials (MEPs)
Mesangium, 2-5
Metacarpophalangeal joint (MCP joint), 10-35
Metal-catalyzed Haber–Weiss reaction, 32-23
Metallic biomaterials, 28-1; *see also* Cobalt–
chromium alloys (CoCr alloys); Implant
manufacturing; Metallic implant corrosion;
Stainless steels; Titanium alloys (Ti alloys)
dental metals, 28-12 to 28-13
other metals, 28-13
platinum group metals, 28-13
surface modifications of, 28-13
tantalum, 28-13
Metallic implant corrosion, 28-14; *see also* Metallic
biomaterials
corrosion of available metals, 28-18
corrosion rate and polarization curves, 28-17
to 28-18
electrochemical aspects, 28-14 to 28-16
electrochemical cell, 28-14
galvanic corrosion, 28-15
micro-corrosion cells, 28-15
potential–current density curves, 28-17
potential difference, 28-15
pourbaix diagrams in corrosion, 28-16 to 28-17
reduction reactions, 28-14
standard electrochemical series, 28-15
stress corrosion cracking, 28-18

Metalloproteinases (MMPs), 20-11
Metals, 28-1; *see also* Metallic biomaterials
Metameric color matching, 4-7
Method of fundamental solutions (MFS), 44-17
1-Methyl-4-phenyl-1,2,3,6-tetrahydropyridine
(MPTP), 3-11
MFS, *see* Method of fundamental solutions (MFS)
MGB, *see* Medial geniculate body (MGB)
MG method, *see* Multigrid method (MG method)
Microcirculation, 20-1; *see also* Blood flow regulation;
Microvascular blood flow mechanics;
Molecular transport in microcirculation;
Tissue transport mechanics
functions of, 20-7
Microcirculation physiome, 20-1; *see also*
Microcirculation
Project, 20-2
tools and methodologies, 20-11 to 20-12
Micro-computed tomography imaging (micro-CT
imaging), 24-2
Micro-corrosion cells, 28-15; *see also* Metallic implant
corrosion
micro-CT imaging, *see* Micro-computed tomography
imaging (micro-CT imaging)
Microelectrical mechanical systems (MEMS), 41-5
Microfabricated Pt–Ir bipolar electrode, 50-8
Microsaccades, 4-3
Microspectrophotometric method, 20-2
Microvascular blood flow mechanics, 20-2; *see also*
Microcirculation physiome
arteriolar and venular blood flow, 20-5 to 20-6
arterioles, 20-3 to 20-4
bifurcation law, 20-6
capillary blood flow, 20-5
deterministic chaos, 20-4
Fahraeus effect, 20-3
microvascular networks, 20-6
plasma, 20-3
platelets, 20-3
stress–strain relationship, 20-4
time-dependent vessel behavior, 20-4
venules, 20-3
viscosity, 20-3
wall mechanics, 20-3 to 20-5
Microvasculature, 20-6; *see also* Microvascular blood
flow mechanics
Microvilli-coated hard sphere covered with adhesive
spring model, 23-11
Middle temporal (MT), 4-8
Migrating motility complex (MMC), 6-4
Migrating myoelectric complex (MMC), 6-7
Mild traumatic brain injury (MTBI), 13-4
Mineralized tissue, *see* Hard tissue
Minimum service life, 29-22 to 29-23; *see also* Ceramic
biomaterials
Minute rhythms, 6-6 to 6-7
Mitogen-activated protein kinases (MAPK), 20-12

Mitral valve (MV), 16-12; *see also* Heart valve
    dynamics
    chordae tendineae, 16-15 to 16-16, 16-19
    chordal insertion pattern in, 16-13
    disease and treatment, 16-20 to 16-21
    dynamics, 16-17 to 16-18, 16-20
    explanted porcine valve, 16-20
    forces acting on, 16-17
    function, 16-17 to 16-20
    leaflets, 16-13, 16-14, 16-15, 16-18
    mechanical properties, 16-16 to 16-17
    mitral annulus, 16-14, 16-18
    papillary muscle, 16-16, 16-19 to 16-20
    pressure and flow curve for, 16-2
    structure, 16-12 to 16-17
Mitral valve closure (MVC), 15-9; *see also* Cardiac
    biomechanics
    time of, 15-10
Mitral valve opening (MVO), 15-9; *see also* Cardiac
    biomechanics
MMC, *see* Migrating motility complex (MMC);
    Migrating myoelectric complex (MMC)
MMPs, *see* Matrix metalloproteinases (MMPs)
MN, *see* Motor neuron (MN)
MNCS, *see* Motor nerve conduction study (MNCS)
Modeling cells in disease, 23-15 to 23-16
    cancer, 23-15
    malaria, 23-16
    nuclear envelope deficiency, 23-16 to 23-17
Modular segmental system, 37-18 to 37-19
Modular total hip system, 37-13
Moens–Korteweg relationship, 17-4; *see also* Arterial
    macrocirculatory hemodynamics
Mohs scale, 29-26
Molecular transport in microcirculation, 20-7; *see also*
    Microcirculation physiome
    carbon dioxide, 20-7
    exchange vessels, 20-7
    filtration and absorption, 20-9
    Kedem–Katchalsky equations, 20-9
    Krogh–Erlang equation, 20-7
    Krogh tissue cylinder model, 20-7
    nitric oxide, 20-7 to 20-8
    oxygen diffusion, 20-7
    solutes and water, 20-8 to 20-9
    solvent drag, 20-8
    Starling's law, 20-9
    symmorphosis hypothesis, 20-7
Molecular weight (MW), 30-4
Molecular weight distribution (MWD), 34-13
Monaural, 5-3
Monocryl, 32-7; *see also* Glycolide/lactide-based
    polyesters
Monocytes, 1-2
Monopole point source, 49-4 to 49-5
Morpholine 2,5-dione (MD), 32-9; *see also* Glycolide/
    lactide-based polyesters

Motion, 4-8
Motor-evoked potentials (MEPs), 58-15
Motor nerve conduction study (MNCS), 46-8, 46-9; *see
    also* Electrodiagnostic studies (EDX studies)
    conduction velocity, 46-10
    median, 46-8, 46-11
    temporal dispersion, 46-10
Motor neuron (MN), 46-2; *see also* Electrodiagnostic
    studies (EDX studies)
Motor unit potential (MUP), 46-4
Motor units (MUs), 46-2; *see also* Electrodiagnostic
    studies (EDX studies)
Moving sensor, 4-9 to 4-10
MPTP, *see* 1-Methyl-4-phenyl-1,2,3,6-
    tetrahydropyridine (MPTP)
MRI, *see* Magnetic resonance imaging (MRI)
MSC, *see* Magnitude squared coherence (MSC)
MSO, *see* Medial superior olive (MSO)
MSP, *see* Major sperm protein (MSP)
MT, *see* Middle temporal (MT)
MTBI, *see* Mild traumatic brain injury (MTBI)
MTT, *see* Mean transit time (MTT)
MTU, *see* Muscle–tendon unit (MTU)
Mulberry silkworm (*Bombyx mori*), 34-1, 34-3; *see also*
    Silk
Multifunctional 22-Channel Functional Electrical
    Stimulator, 54-1, 54-10
    bladder contractions, 54-8
    bowel evacuation, 54-8
    complications, 54-9 to 54-10
    electrode stability, 54-8
    FES in paraplegia, 54-2
    historical aspect, 54-2
    Nucleus FES22 Stimulating System, 54-3 to 54-4
    Praxis FES24-A system, 54-4 to 54-6
    Praxis FES24-B system, 54-6
    Praxis system for functional activities, 54-7
    sensor packs, 54-8
    upright mobility, 54-7 to 54-10
Multigrid method (MG method), 43-7; *see also*
    Computer modeling and simulation
Multiple traveling wave modes, 24-18
Multiscale mode, 20-11, 20-12
MUP, *see* Motor unit potential (MUP)
MUs, *see* Motor units (MUs)
Muscle, 9-2; *see also* Soft tissues
    architectural properties, 9-7, 9-8, 9-9
    constitutive models, 9-11
    contractile component, 9-11
    contraction velocity, 9-5
    cross-bridge models, 9-10 to 9-11
    contraction force vs. stimulation rate and time, 52-7
    dynamic properties, 9-6
    energetics, 26-1 to 26-2
    fiber architecture, 9-3
    force generation, 9-12
    force–length relationship, 9-5

Muscle (*Continued*)
    force predicting models, 9-10
    force–velocity relation, 9-6
    gross morphology, 9-2
    Hill model, 9-11
    material properties, 9-4 to 9-7
    modeling, 9-10 to 9-13
    moments, 12-8
    myosin protein, 9-4
    pennation angle, 9-13
    phenomenological model, 9-11
    sarcomere, 9-3 to 9-4
    skeletal muscle, 9-3
    stress, 9-5
    tissue stimulation, 49-14
Muscle–tendon unit (MTU), 9-11
Muscular efficiency, 27-3 to 27-5
Muscular movement, 27-2
MV, *see* Mitral valve (MV)
MVC, *see* Mitral valve closure (MVC)
MVO, *see* Mitral valve opening (MVO)
MW, *see* Molecular weight (MW)
MWD, *see* Molecular weight distribution (MWD)
Mycobacterium, 33-19
Myelin, 46-4
Myelinated axons, 3-2
    activation, 49-8 to 49-9
Myocardial tissue force, 26-4
Myocardium, 26-4
Myogenic, 17-10
    response, 20-12
Myoglobin-facilitated O_2 diffusion, 20-7, 20-12
Myosin protein, 9-4; *see also* Muscle

N

NA-MIC, *see* National Alliance for Medical Image
    Computing (NA-MIC)
National Alliance for Medical Image Computing
    (NA-MIC), 43-19
National Football League (NFL), 13-9
Natural polymers, 30-2; *see also* Polymeric
    biomaterials
NE, *see* Neurotrophic electrode (NE)
Neck–shaft angle, 10-15; *see also* Hip
Neck mechanics, 13-1; *see also* Head mechanics
    cervical facet capsule stretch, 13-7
    compression–extension injuries, 13-3
    compression–flexion injuries, 13-3
    hangman's fractures, 13-2
    human surrogates of head and neck, 13-10 to 13-11
    injuries involving lateral bending, 13-3
    injury mechanisms, 13-2
    loading corridor, 13-5, 13-6
    mechanical response of neck, 13-5 to 13-7
    relative displacement of C4 on C5, 13-6
    tension–extension injuries, 13-2 to 13-3

    tension–flexion injuries, 13-2
    tolerance of neck, 13-9 to 13-10
Necrosis, 37-19
Negative pressure transients, 36-18
Negative work, 27-4
Nematode cell locomotion model, 23-13
Neointima, 36-18
Neointimal hyperplasia, 36-18
Nephrin, 2-7
Nephron, 2-1 to 2-2, 2-3, 2-4 to 2-5; *see also* Kidney
    anatomy
    Bowman's capsule, 2-5
    Bowman's space, 2-5
    collecting ducts, 2-5
    distal convoluted tubule, 2-5
    juxtaglomerular apparatus, 2-5
    loop of Henle, 2-5, 2-14
    macula densa, 2-5, 2-14
    proximal convoluted tubule, 2-5
    urine, 2-5
    vasa recta, 2-14
Nernst–Planck equations, 42-5; *see also* Membrane
    currents
Nernst potential, 28-20, 38-6, 42-6; *see also* Membrane
    currents
Nerve, 3-1
Nerve cells, 42-9; *see also* Membrane models; Neuron
    abdominal ganglion R15 cell, 42-11
    cerebellar granule cells, 42-12
    chopper units, 42-11
    dopaminergic neurons, 42-12
    efferent neurons, 42-13 to 42-14
    enteric nervous system, 42-13
    fly optic lobe tangential cells, 42-13
    gastropod neuron, 42-11
    hippocampal pyramidal, 42-11
    Hodgkin–Huxley equations, 42-10
    human node of Ranvier, 42-12
    interstitial cells of cajal, 42-14
    invertebrate photoreceptor neurons, 42-13
    lamprey CNS neurons, 42-11 to 42-12
    leech heartbeat oscillator interneuron, 42-14
    L'Hopital's Rule, 42-10 to 42-11
    mammalian spinal motoneuron, 42-14
    muscle spindle primary endings, 42-13
    myelinated auditory-nerve neuron, 42-12
    myelinated Ia primary afferent neurons, 42-13
    prefrontal cortex neurons, 42-12
    primary afferents and related efferents, 42-13
    pyloric constrictor neurons, 42-14
    rabbit sciatic nerve axons, 42-12
    rate constants, 42-10
    rat mesencephalic trigeminal neurons, 42-13
    rat nodose neurons, 42-13
    retinal ganglion cells, 42-13
    retinal horizontal cells, 42-13
    sensory neurons, 42-12 to 42-13

small intestine cholinergic and adrenergic neurons, 42-14
snail RPa1 bursting neuron, 42-14
squid axon, 42-10 to 42-11
stomatogastric ganglion neurons, 42-11
sympathetic neurons, 42-13 to 42-14
thalamocortical cells, 42-12
toad myelinated neuron, 42-11
vertebrate motoneuron, 42-14
vertebrate retinal cone photoreceptors, 42-13
xenopus central pattern generator neuron, 42-14
Nerve growth factor (NGF), 34-10
Nervous system, 3-1; *see also* Epilepsy
    basal ganglia, 3-11
    dendrites, 3-2
    doctrine of specific nerve energies, 3-3
    muscle fibers, 3-2
    nerve, 3-1
    neurons, 3-2
    receptors and transducers, 3-2
    roles of, 3-2
    soma, 3-2
    synaptic junctions, 3-2
Nervous system functions, 3-3; *see also* Alzheimer's
        disease (AD); Parkinson's disease (PD)
    action potential, 3-2
    adaptation, 3-2
    adequate stimulus, 3-2
    ALOPEX system, 3-8, 3-9
    antagonist muscle, 3-3
    Antifacilitation, 3-5
    averaging operation, 3-6
    Bell–Magendie law, 3-3
    central delay, 3-3
    coding of sensory information, 3-3
    consolidation of memory, 3-10
    declarative memory, 3-9
    engram, 3-10
    facilitation, 3-4
    feature extractors, 3-7
    habituation, 3-10
    human perception, 3-7, 3-9
    hysteresis, 3-10
    information processing, 3-4
    lateral inhibition, 3-6 to 3-7
    learning, 3-10
    mach bands, 3-6
    memory, 3-9, 3-10
    mental images, 3-7
    neural networks, 3-11
    nodes of Ranvier, 3-2
    nonassociative memory, 3-10
    nondeclarative memory, 3-9
    pattern recognition, 3-7 to 3-8
    phantom limb pain, 3-15
    plasticity, 3-10
    posttetanic potentiation, 3-5

priming effects, 3-10
    reaction time, 3-3
    readable code, 3-5
    receptive field, 3-7
    receptor potential, 3-2
    reflex arc, 3-3
    representation of Information in, 3-5
    stretch error, 3-3
    temporal summation, 3-4
Neural ablation, 50-9
Neural augmentation, 50-; *see also* Neuromodulation
    human application, 50-6
    implanted neuroelectric interfaces, 50-5 to 50-6
    microfabricated Pt–Ir bipolar electrode, 50-8
    neuromuscular stimulation, 50-4to 50-5
    origins, 50-3 to 50-4
    stimulation for hearing, 50-6 to 50-7
    stimulation for touch sense, 50-7 to 50-8
    stimulation for vision, 50-7
Neural engineering, 50-1, 50-2; *see also* Neural
        augmentation; Neuromodulation
Neural networks, 3-11
Neural prostheses, 49-1, *see* Neural augmentation
Neural threshold and BM velocity, 24-16
Neuromodulation, 50-1, 57-11; *see also* Epileptic
        seizure intervention; Neural augmentation
    deep-brain stimulation, 50-10 to 50-11
    electrical stimulation, 50-8 to 50-9
    for hearing, 50-6 to 50-7
    neural ablation, 50-9
    neurostimulation, 50-11, 50-12
    for touch sense, 50-7 to 50-8
    vagal nerve stimulation, 50-12
    for vision, 50-7
Neuromuscular junction, 46-2; *see also*
        Electrodiagnostic studies (EDX studies)
Neuromuscular stimulation, 50-4 to 50-5
Neuron, 3-2
    models, 51-5
    neurostimulation for epilepsy, 50-11
    response to imposed potentials, 51-4 to 51-5
Neuronal NOS (nNOS), 20-8
Neurostimulation, 50-12
Neurotrophic electrode (NE), 53-1
    and neural signals, 53-4 to 53-6
Neutrophils, 1-2, 21-7
Newtonian, 17-10
    viscous fluid, 22-3; *see also* Tissue transport
        mechanics
NFL, *see* National Football League (NFL)
NGF, *see* Nerve growth factor (NGF)
NIH, *see* U.S. National Institutes of Health (NIH)
Nitric oxide (NO), 20-7
nNOS, *see* Neuronal NOS (nNOS)
NO, *see* Nitric oxide (NO)
Noble, 28-20
Nodes of Ranvier, 3-2

Nonaliphatic polyester-type biodegradable polymers, 32-11; *see also* Amino-acid-based PEAs (AA-PEAs); Biodegradable polymers
  AA-PEAs, 32-12 to 32-13
  amidediols, 32-12
  amino acid-based poly(ester amide) s and copolymers, 32-12 to 32-20
  poly(alkylene oxalates) and copolymers, 32-12
  poly(carbonate-acetal) s from dihydroxyacetone, 32-20 to 32-21
  polycarbonates, 32-11 to 32-12
  unsaturated AA-UPEAs, 32-14
Nonassociative memory, 3-10
Nonblood-interfacing implants, 36-23; *see also* Blood-interfacing implants; Percutaneous implants
  breast implants, 36-30
  clips, 36-25
  ear and eye implants, 36-29 to 36-30
  fluid transfer implants, 36-31
  maxillofacial implants, 36-28 to 36-29
  nonsuture fibrous and microporous implants, 36-25
  pins, 36-25
  space-filling implants, 36-30
  staples, 36-25
  surface phosphonylation, 36-33
  surgical tape, 36-25 to 36-26
  sutures, 36-23 to 36-25
  technologies, 36-32 to 36-33
  tissue adhesives, 36-26 to 36-27
Nondeclarative memory, 3-9
Noninvasive FES systems, 52-2
Nonlocal bending resistance, 21-7, 21-11; *see also* Red blood cell (RBC)
Nonsuture fibrous and microporous implants, 36-25; *see also* Nonblood-interfacing implants
NOS, *see* NO synthase (NOS)
NO synthase (NOS), 20-7
Novakill, 32-27; *see also* Supercritical carbon dioxide sterilization
NovaSterilis scCO$_2$ sterilization process, 32-27; *see also* Supercritical carbon dioxide sterilization
Nuclear envelope deficiency modeling, 23-16 to 23-17
Nuclei of Lateral Lemniscus, 5-11
Nucleus FES22 Stimulating System, 54-3 to 54-4
Number-average molecular weight, 30-4
Numerical technique, 43-5; *see also* Computer modeling and simulation
Nylon, 36-18; *see also* Polyamides

O

OA, *see* Osteoarthritis (OA)
ODE, *see* Ordinary differential equation (ODE)
OHCs, *see* Outer hair cells (OHCs)
Ohm's law, 40-11
  for conductors, 49-3

One-dimensional cable theory, 40-5; *see also* Electrical conductivity of tissues
One-dimensional model, 24-7 to 24-8
Opponent process of color vision theory, 4-7
Optic chiasm, 4-4
Optic radiations, 4-4
Optic tracts, 4-4
Optimal walking speed, 27-5
Optokinetic nystagmus, 4-9
Orbital repair materials, 36-29; *see also* Nonblood-interfacing implants
Ordinary differential equation (ODE), 23-6
Organ of Corti, 5-5, 24-3, 24-4
Orthotropic, 8-20
O*seen*'s drag, 25-6
Osseointegration, 28-9, 37-19; *see also* Titanium alloys (Ti alloys)
Osteoarthritis (OA), 11-2, 11-16; *see also* Arthritis
  tribology connections, 11-17
Osteoarthrosis, *see* Osteoarthritis
Osteolysis, 37-14, 37-19
Osteons, *see* Haversian bone
Outer hair cells (OHCs), 5-3, 24-12
  electromotility, 24-11 to 24-12
  roll-off, 24-17 to 24-18
Oxides, 29-1
Oxygen
  cost, 7-14
  deficit, 26-6, 26-10
  uptake during exercise, 26-6
Oxygenator, 30-21
Oxyhemoglobin dissociation curve (ODC), 20-12, 20-7

P

P4HB, *see* Poly-4-hydroxybyutrate (P4HB)
PAAm, *see* Polyacrylamide (PAAm)
Papilla, 2-4
Paraspinal electrodes placement, 52-8
Parastep system, 52-3, 52-17 to 52-18
  above-lesion EMG-controlled menu selection, 52-10–52-11
  with battery pack and walker, 52-5
  contraindications, 52-13
  electric charge and charge density parameters, 52-3 to 52-4
  finger-touch menu selection, 52-10
  healthcare common procedure coding system, 52-17
  muscle contraction vs. stimulation rate, 52-7
  paraspinal electrodes placement, 52-8
  patient admissibility criteria, 52-12
  patient training, 52-13 to 52-14
  peroneal nerve electrodes placement, 52-8
  pulse synchronization menus, 52-7
  pulse width and repetition rate, 52-6
  quadriceps stimulation electrode placement, 52-7

sequencing-control menus, 52-9 to 52-10
stimulation signals and safety standard constraints, 52-4 to 52-5
stimulation signal's level control, 52-11
stimulation sites, 52-7 to 52-9
system design, 52-5
during walk, 52-5
Parkinson's disease (PD), 3-11 to 3-12; *see also* Alzheimer's disease (AD); Epilepsy
Partially stabilized zirconia (PSZ), 29-24
Partial pressure, 7-8, 7-20
Particulate composites, 31-4; *see also* Composite biomaterials
  biomaterial properties, 31-5
  dental composite resins, 31-5 to 31-6
  microfilled composites, 31-6
  stiffness, 31-4
Parvocellular cells (P cells), 4-4
Passivation, 28-20
Passivity, 28-16, 28-20; *see also* Pourbaix diagram
Patch action potential, 38-10; *see also* Action potentials and membrane currents
Patch clamp method, 42-3; *see also* Membrane models
  capacitative current, 42-3
  membrane capacitance, 42-3
  membrane currents and, 42-4
  transmembrane potential difference, 42-3
  whole-cell patch-clamp configuration, 42-3
Patency, 36-18
Pathological waveforms, 3-14
Patient admissibility criteria, 52-12
Patient control unit (PCU), 55-4
Patient training, 52-13 to 52-14
Pattern recognition, 3-7 to 3-8
Pattern-recognition device (PRD), 3-8
PBMA, *see* Poly-*n*-butylmethacrylate (PBMA)
PBS, *see* Phosphate-buffered saline (PBS)
PC, *see* Posterior commissures (PC)
PCA, *see* Poly(carbonate-acetal)s (PCA)
P cells, *see* Parvocellular cells (P cells)
PCL, *see* Poly-ε-caprolactone (PCL)
PCSA, *see* Physiological cross-sectional area (PCSA)
PCU, *see* Patient control unit (PCU)
PD, *see* Parkinson's disease (PD)
PDGF, *see* Platelet derived growth factor (PDGF)
PDS, *see* Poly-*p*-dioxanone (PDS)
PE, *see* Polyethylene (PE)
PEAs, *see* Poly(ester amide)s (PEAs)
PECAM-1, *see* Platelet endothelial cell adhesion molecule (PECAM-1)
Pectinate zone, 24-4
Pedobarography, 12-2, 12-5
PEEK, *see* Polyetherether ketone (PEEK)
Peeling model, 23-11
PEG, *see* Poly(ethylene glycol) (PEG)
PEGDA, *see* Poly(ethylene glycol) diacrylate (PEGDA)
Pennation angle, 9-13

PEO, *see* Polyethyleneoxide (PEO)
PEPBO, *see* Poly(ethylene 1,4-phenylene-bis-oxyacetate) (PEPBO)
Pepsin, 33-4, 33-19
Percutaneous implants, 36-27; *see also* Nonblood-interfacing implants
  artificial skins, 36-28
  factors influencing device design, 36-27 to 36-28
Perfusion, 7-20
Pericardial prostheses, 36-18
Perilymphatic fluid, 24-3
Peripheral auditory system, 5-1to 5-2
Peripheral equipment, 52-11 to 52-12
Peripheral nerve stimulation, 49-14
Peripheral nervous system (PNS), 3-1
Peripheral resistance (PR), 1-12
Perisaccadic remapping, 4-10
Peristimulus time histogram (PSTH), 5-7, 5-9
Perixosome-proliferatoractivated-receptor-gamma coactivator 1α (PGC1α), 20-11
Permeability, 33-19
Permittivity, 40-11
Permselectivity, 2-11
PET, *see* Positron emission tomography (PET)
PFTs, *see* Pulmonary function tests (PFTs)
PG, *see* Polyglycolide (PG); Proteoglycan (PG)
PG910, *see* Polyglactin 910 (PG910)
PGA, *see* Polyglycolic acid (PGA)
PGC1α, *see* Perixosome-proliferatoractivated-receptor-gamma coactivator 1α (PGC1α)
PGI2, *see* Prostacyclin (PGI2)
Phantom limb, 3-3
Phantom limb pain (PLP), 3-15
Phase-resetting phenomena, 6-5
Phasic adaptation, 3-2
PHB, *see* Poly(β-hydroxybutyrate) (PHB)
PHEMA, *see* Polyhydroxyethyl-methacrylate (PHEMA)
Phenolalanine (Phe), 33-19
Phenomenological model, 9-11
Phosphate-buffered saline (PBS), 32-17
Phosphorylcholine, 36-31; *see also* Nonblood-interfacing implants
Photolithography, 35-9
pH regulation, 2-16
PHV, *see* Poly(β-hydroxyvalerate) (PHV)
Physiological cross-sectional area (PCSA), 9-4
Physiome, 20-12
Pi, *see* Inorganic phosphate (Pi)
Picture element (Pixel), 3-6
Pill-rolling tremor, 3-11
Pins, 36-25; *see also* Nonblood-interfacing implants
Pitting, 28-20, 36-18
Pixel, *see* Picture element (Pixel)
PL, *see* Proximal latency (PL)
PLA, *see* Poly(lactide) (PLA)

Planar gradiometer, 48-12; *see also*
  Magnetoencephalography (MEG)
  sensitivity distribution of, 48-14
Plasma, 1-1, 20-2 ; *see also* Microvascular blood flow
  mechanic; Serum
  proteins, 1-2
  volume, 26-8
Plasmin, 35-6
Plasticity, 3-10, 53-9 to 53-10; *see also* Electrode
  comparison
  directionality in APS and LFPs, 53-11 to 53-12
  LFPs for cyber digits, 53-12 to 53-14
Plasticizer, 30-21
Platelet, 20-3, 21-1, 33-19, 36-18; *see also* Thrombocytes
Platelet derived growth factor (PDGF), 20-11, 35-5
Platelet endothelial cell adhesion molecule
  (PECAM-1), 22-9
Plates, 37-5; *see also* Long bone repair
Platinum group metals, 28-13; *see also* Metallic
  biomaterials
Plethysmography, 7-18, 7-20, 19-4
Pleura, 7-5, 7-20
Plexiform, 8-20
PLGA, *see* Poly(lactide-*co*-glycolide) (PLGA)
PLLA, *see* Poly-L-lactide (PLLA)
PMA, *see* Poly(β-malic acid) (PMA)
PMMA, *see* Polymethylmethacrylate (PMMA)
Pneumotach, 7-17, 7-20
PNS, *see* Peripheral nervous system (PNS)
PNVP, *see* Poly(*N*-vinyl-2-pyrrolidone) (PNVP)
Podocin, 2-7
Podocytes, 2-6, 2-7
Point attachment model, 23-11
Poiseuille's law, 20-12
Polarity effect on applied stimulus, 49-9
Polyacetal, 30-12; *see also* Biomaterial polymers
Polyacrylamide (PAAm), 30-10; *see also* Biomaterial
  polymers
Poly(alkylene oxalates) and copolymers, 32-12; *see also*
  Nonaliphatic polyester-type biodegradable
  polymers
Polyamides, 30-11; *see also* Biomaterial polymers
Polyamino acids, 32-2; *see also* Biodegradable polymers
Poly(β-hydroxybutyrate) (PHB), 32-11
Poly(β-hydroxyvalerate) (PHV), 32-11
Poly(β-malic acid) (PMA), 32-11
Poly(BPA-carbonates), 32-11
Polycarbonate, 30-13, 32-11 to 32-12; *see also*
  Biomaterial polymers; Nonaliphatic
  polyester-type biodegradable polymers
Poly(carbonate-acetal)s (PCA), 32-20; *see also*
  Nonaliphatic polyester-type biodegradable
  polymers
  synthesis of, 32-20 to 32-21
Polycrystalline hydroxyapatite, 29-10; *see also* Calcium
  phosphate
  electrical properties of, 29-12

scanning electron micrograph, 29-12
  structure, 29-11
Poly(depsipeptides), 32-10; *see also* Glycolide/lactide-
  based polyesters
Polydioxanone (PDS), 33-19, 36-24
Poly-ε-caprolactone (PCL), 32-2, 32-11; *see also*
  Biodegradable polymers
Poly(ester amide)s (PEAs), 32-12; *see also* Nonaliphatic
  polyester-type biodegradable polymers
Polyesters, 30-11; *see also* Biomaterial polymers
Polyetherether ketone (PEEK), 36-32
Polyethylene (PE), 30-4, 30-9 to 30-10; *see also*
  Polymeric biomaterials; Biomaterial polymers
Poly(ethylene glycol) (PEG), 32-8, 35-2; *see also*
  Glycolide/lactide-based polyesters
Poly(ethylene glycol) diacrylate (PEGDA), 32-15;
  see also Nonaliphatic polyester-type
  biodegradable polymers
Polyethyleneoxide (PEO), 30-17, 32-10; *see also*
  Glycolide/lactide-based polyesters
Poly(ethylene 1,4-phenylene-bis-oxyacetate) (PEPBO),
  32-7; *see also* Glycolide/lactide-based
  polyesters
Polyethylene terephthalate (PET), 30-11, 36-24; *see also*
  Biomaterial polymers
Polyglactin 910 (PG910), 32-26
Polyglycolic acid (PGA), 32-5, 33-14, 33-19, 34-12; *see
  also* Biodegradable polymers
  FTIR spectra of PGA disks, 32-5
Polyglycolide (PG), 36-24
Poly(glycolide*co*-lactide) (PLGA), 30-13
Poly(glycolide-trimethylene carbonate) (TMC), 32-2;
  see also Biodegradable polymers
Poly(HEMA), *see* Poly(2-hydroxyethyl methacrylate)
  [Poly(HEMA)]
Poly-4-hydroxybyutrate (P4HB), 32-2; *see also*
  Biodegradable polymers
Poly(2-hydroxyethyl methacrylate) [Poly(HEMA)],
  36-27 to 36-28
Polyhydroxyethyl-methacrylate (PHEMA), 30-10, 35-2;
  see also Biomaterial polymers
Polylactic acid (PLA), 30-13, 37-2, 33-14, 33-19
Poly(lactide) (PLA), 34-12
Poly(lactide-*co*-glycolide) (PLGA), 34-12
Poly-L-lactide (PLLA), 32-8, 32-9; *see also* Glycolide/
  lactide-based polyesters
  biomedical applications, 32-11
  effect in polyglycolide, 32-6
  impregnated and annealed PGA matrix, 32-26
Polymeric biomaterials, 30-1; *see also* Polymerization;
  Biomaterial polymers
  advantages of, 30-1
  arrangements of copolymers, 30-6
  biomedical application of, 30-9
  for biomedical polymers, 30-2
  chemogradient surfaces, 30-16 to 30-20
  corona discharge apparatus, 30-16

fibroblast cell proliferation rates, 30-19
fringed-micelle model, 30-4, 30-6
gamma irradiation effect on, 30-14
growth on chemogradient PE surfaces, 30-18
number-average molecular weight, 30-4
polymer chain arrangement, 30-5
serum protein adsorption, 30-20
effect of side-chain substitution, 30-8
sterilization, 30-13 to 30-14
structural modification effect on, 30-7 to 30-8
structure, 30-4 to 30-7
surface modifications, 30-14 to 30-15
vinyl polymers, 30-6
weight average molecular weight, 30-5
Polymerization, 30-1; *see also* Polymeric biomaterials
    addition, 30-3 to 30-4
    condensation, 30-2
    monomers for, 30-3
    propagation, 30-3
Polymethylmethacrylate (PMMA), 30-10, 31-4, 37-9;
    see also Biomaterial polymers
Polymorphism, 33-19
Polymorphonuclear leukocyte, 33-19; *see also*
    Neutrophil
Poly-*n*-butylmethacrylate (PBMA), 32-19
Poly(*N*-vinyl-2-pyrrolidone) (PNVP), 35-2
Polyoxymethylene, *see* Polyacetal
Poly-*p*-dioxanone (PDS), 32-2; *see also* Biodegradable
    polymers
Polypeptide, 33-19
Polypropylene (PP), 30-10, 36-18; *see also* Biomaterial
    polymers
Polysaccharide, 33-19
Polystyrene (PS), 30-6; *see also* Polymeric biomaterials;
    Biomaterial polymers
    and copolymers, 30-10 to 30-11
Polysulfone, 30-12; *see also* Biomaterial polymers
Polytetrafluoroethylene (PTFE), 30-11, 36-2, 36-18,
    36-25; *see also* Biomaterial polymers
Polyurethanes, 30-12; *see also* Biomaterial polymers
Poly(vinyl alcohol) (PVA), 34-9, 35-2
Polyvinylchloride (PVC), 30-6, 30-8 to 30-9; *see
    also* Biomaterial polymers; Polymeric
    biomaterials
Porcine bioprosthesis, 36-8; *see also* Heart valve
    prostheses
Porosity, 2-9
Porous materials, 31-9; *see also* Collagen; Composite
    biomaterials; Joint replacements
    on bone-compatible implants, 31-11
    cellular solid structures, 31-9
    elastic collapse of elastomeric foam, 31-10
    irregular pore structure of porous coating, 31-11
    matrix, 33-12
    production, 31-12
    in soft tissue applications, 31-12
    stiffness, 31-9

strength for crushing of brittle foam, 31-10
stress–strain curve, 31-10
tantalum, 37-12
Positron emission tomography (PET), 3-7
Postcapillary oxygen transport, 20-7
Posterior commissures (PC), 57-3
Posttetanic potentiation, 3-5
Potassium channels, 38-4, 42-2; *see also* Electrically
    active membrane; Membrane models
Pourbaix diagram, 28-16, 28-20; *see also* Metallic
    implant corrosion
    for chromium, 28-16
    immunity, 28-16
    passivity, 28-16
    significance of, 28-17
PowerApps, 43-22 to 43-24; *see also* Software for
    bioelectric field problems
Power law fluid, 21-9, 21-11; *see also* Leukocytes
Power requirement, 27-6
Power spectral analysis, 47-7, 47-12; *see also*
    Electroencephalography (EEG)
PP, *see* Polypropylene (PP)
PR, *see* Peripheral resistance (PR)
Praxis system
    for functional activities, 54-7
    Praxis FES24 system, 54-4 to 54-6
PRD, *see* Pattern-recognition device (PRD)
Precapillary oxygen transport, 20-7, 20-12
Precapillary sphincters, 1-12
Premature ventricular beats (PVBs), 45-7; *see also*
    Electrocardiography
Pressure difference (Δpressure), 26-4
Pressure sore, 31-12
Pressure–volume area (PVA), 15-12
Primary healing, 37-2, 37-19; *see also* Long bone repair
Primary source, 39-7; *see also* Volume conductor theory
Primary spiral osseous lamina, 24-3
Priming effects, 3-10
Principal extension ratios, 21-11
Principle of reciprocity, 48-4; *see also* Biomagnetism
Proline (Pro), 33-19
Propagation, 30-3, 38-13; *see also* Electrophysiology;
    Polymerization
    AO and currents from two sites, 38-14
    comparative transmembrane potentials, 38-14
    equivalent circuit, 38-15 to 38-16
    extracellular path, 38-16 to 38-17
    intracellular current flow, 38-16
    membrane current, 38-16
    propagation cartoon, 38-14 to 38-15
    propagation velocity, 38-17
    of spatial relationships, 38-15
    2-and 3-dimensions, 38-17
Prostacyclin (PGI2), 20-10
Prostheses
    intervertebral disk, 37-17
    for limb salvage, 37-17 to 37-19

Protein structure, 33-2; *see also* Collagen
Proteoglycan (PG), 9-1
Proteolytic enzymes, 33-4, 33-19; *see also* Collagen
Proximal convoluted tubule, 2-5
Proximal latency (PL), 46-9
PS, *see* Polystyrene (PS)
Pseudoelasticity, 18-7; *see also* Blood vessels
Pseudopodia, 21-10; *see also* Leukocytes
PSLF, *see* Purified synovial lubricating factor (PSLF)
PSTH, *see* Peristimulus time histogram (PSTH)
Psychological observations, 52-17
Psychophysics, 4-1
PSZ, *see* Partially stabilized zirconia (PSZ)
Pulmonary circulation, 1-11, 7-4 to 7-5, 7-20,
      17-10; *see also* Arterial macrocirculatory
      hemodynamics
Pulmonary function tests (PFTs), 7-16
Pulmonary mechanics, 7-10 to 7-14
Pulmonary resistance, 7-10
Pulmonary valve, 16-11; *see also* Heart valve dynamics
    dynamics, 16-11
    leaflet vs. aortic valve leaflet, 16-11
    mechanical properties, 16-11
    structure, 16-10 to 16-11
    velocity profiles after, 16-12
Purified synovial lubricating factor (PSLF), 11-10
Pusher plate devices, 36-18
Push-forward/pull-backward active model, 24-12 to
    24-16
PVA, *see* Poly(vinyl alcohol) (PVA); Pressure–volume
    area (PVA)
PVBs, *see* Premature ventricular beats (PVBs)
PVC, *see* Polyvinylchloride (PVC)
Pyrolytic carbon, 29-8, 36-18

Q

QPC, *see* Quadratic phase coupling (QPC)
Quadratic phase coupling (QPC), 47-9, 47-12; *see also*
    Electroencephalography (EEG)
Quasistatic, 40-11

R

RA, *see* Rheumatoid arthritis (RA)
Radio-frequency (RF), 55-2
Radiopacity, 36-18
Rapid eye movement (REM), 3-11, 47-9
RBC, *see* Red blood cell (RBC)
RDS, *see* Retinal degeneration slow (RDS)
Reaction time, 3-3
Readable code, 3-5
Receptive field, 3-7, 4-10
Receptor potential, 3-2
Recessed oxygen microelectrode, 20-2
Reciprocal current, 48-4; *see also* Biomagnetism
Red blood cell (RBC), 20-2, 21-3; *see also* Hematocytes

    bending elasticity, 21-6 to 21-7
    constitutive relations for membrane, 21-6
    cytosol, 21-4
    isotropic force resultant, 21-4
    mammalian, 20-2 to 20-3
    membrane area dilation, 21-4
    membrane shear deformation, 21-4 to 21-5
    membrane shear force resultant, 21-5
    parameter values for, 21-3
    under pathological conditions, 20-6
    size and shape, 21-3 to 21-4
    sphericity, 21-3
    stress relaxation and strain hardening, 21-5 to 21-6
    temperature dependence of viscoelastic coefficients,
      21-5
    viscosity of red cell cytosol, 21-4
Redox reactions, 32-23
Reduced modulus of elasticity, 11-5
Reduction reactions, 28-14; *see also* Metallic implant
    corrosion
Reflex arc, 3-3
Refractive index, 30-21
Refractory period, 42-3, 42-21; *see also* Membrane
    models
Regulatory status, 52-17
Reissner's membrane, 24-3
Relative isometric tension, 15-14
Remodeling, 18-2; *see also* Blood vessels
Renal artery, 2-4
Renal circulation, 1-11
Renal lobe, 2-3
Renal plasma flow, 2-8
Renal vein, 2-4
Renin, 2-18
    angiotensin hormone system, 2-10, 2-11
Repeating unit, 30-21
Repetitive transcranial magnetic stimulation (rTMS),
    3-12, 58-3
Repolarization, 42-21
Resistance vessels, 20-9; *see also* Blood flow regulation
Resonators, 24-5 to 24-6
Resorbable ceramics, *see* Biodegradable ceramics
Resorbable collagen, 33-20; *see also* Collagen-based
    medical implant
Resorbable implant, 33-13; *see also* Collagen-based
    medical implant
Respiratory responses, 26-6 to 26-7
Respiratory system, 7-1, 7-2; *see also* Spirometry
    air and constituents, 7-9
    airway architecture, 7-4
    airway classification, 7-3
    airway remodeling, 7-14
    alveolar ventilation, 7-7
    alveoli, 7-2 to 7-4, 7-20
    Avogadro's principle, 7-9
    body plethysmography, 7-18
    breathing, 7-14

burst, 32-22
chemoreceptors, 7-20
compliance, 7-12
conducting airways, 7-1 to 7-2
control, 7-14 to 7-15
COPD, 7-14
Dalton's law, 7-8
dead space, 7-20
diffusion, 7-7, 7-19, 7-20
expiratory reserve volume, 7-6, 7-20
forced vital capacity, 7-6
functional residual capacity, 7-6, 7-20
gas partial pressure, 7-8 to 7-10
hysteresivity, 7-12
inspiration, 7-20
inspiratory capacity, 7-6
inspiratory reserve volume, 7-5
lumped-parameter model, 7-12
lung perfusion, 7-7 to 7-8
lungs, 7-1
lung volumes, 7-5 to 7-7
mechanical properties of lungs and thorax, 7-13
mechanoreceptors, 7-20
muscles, 7-5
oxygen cost, 7-14
partial pressure, 7-8, 7-20
perfusion, 7-20
pleura, 7-5, 7-20
pressure difference, 7-13
pulmonary circulation, 7-4 to 7-5
pulmonary function tests, 7-16
pulmonary mechanics, 7-10 to 7-14
pulmonary resistance, 7-10
rebreathing pulmonary diffusing capacity, 7-19
resistance, 7-10, 7-11
respiratory control, 7-14 to 7-15
respiratory muscles, 7-5
respiratory resistance, 7-10, 7-11
Rohrer's equation, 7-10 to 7-11
tidal volume, 7-6
total lung capacity, 7-6
ventilation volume, 7-6
ventilatory perfusion, 7-7
Response-field maps, 5-10
Responsive neurostimulator device (RNS device),
            50-11
Resting length of muscle, 27-4
Resting potential, 38-6, 42-2; *see also* Membrane
            models
Reticular activating system, 47-2; *see also*
            Electroencephalography (EEG)
Reticular lamina, 24-4
Retina, 4-2 to 4-3
Retinal degeneration slow (RDS), 56-2
Retinex theory of color vision, 4-8
Retractive force of wall, 18-5 to 18-6; *see also* Blood
            vessels

Reuss orthotropic symmetry, 8-25
Reuss transverse isotropic symmetry, 8-25
RF, *see* Radio-frequency (RF)
Rheumatic fever, 16-9; *see also* Aortic valve
Rheumatoid arthritis (RA), 11-15
RHS, *see* Right-hand side (RHS)
Right-hand side (RHS), 43-12
River of life, *see* Blood
RNS device, *see* Responsive neurostimulator device
            (RNS device)
Rohrer's equation, 7-10 to 7-11
Rolling and adhesion, 23-7 to 23-10; *see also* Cell
            mechanics modeling
    adhesion diagram, 23-9
    adhesion kinetic models, 23-11
    Bell's model, 23-8
    bond formation, 23-10
    cell as liquid drop encapsulated in elastic ring, 23-8
    cell membrane as thin inextensible membrane, 23-8
    mathematical models, 23-7
    shear rate diagram, 23-9
Rotation center, 10-2
rTMS, *see* Repetitive transcranial magnetic stimulation
            (rTMS)
Rubbers, 30-12; *see also* Elastomers; Biomaterial
            polymers

S

SA, *see* Spontaneous activity (SA)
Saccade, 4-9
SAHCS, *see* Subacute hippocampal stimulation
            (SAHCS)
SAL6, *see* Sterility assurance levels of 10-6 (SAL6)
Saltatory conduction, 46-4
Salt-linkage, 33-20
SAM, *see* Scanning acoustic microscopy (SAM)
SA node, *see* Sinoatrial node (SA node)
Sarcomere, 9-3 to 9-4; *see also* Muscle
    force generating capacity of, 9-12
    length–tension and velocity–tension relations, 9-13
SBML, *see* Systems biology markup language (SBML)
SC, *see* Scapho-capitate (SC)
Scala media (SM), 5-3, 24-3
Scala tympani (ST), 5-3, 24-3
Scala vestibule (SV), 5-3, 24-3
Scanning acoustic microscopy (SAM), 8-18
Scapho-capitate (SC), 10-30
Scapho-trapezial-trapezoid (STT), 10-30
SCI, *see* Spinal cord injury (SCI)
SCIRun, 43-20; *see also* Software for bioelectric field
            problems
SCM, *see* Succinimidyl carboxymethyl (SCM)
Screws, 37-4 to 37-5; *see also* Long bone repair
S.D, *see* Standard deviations (S.D.)
Secondary healing, 37-2, 37-19; *see also* Long bone
            repair

Secondary source, 39-6; *see also* Volume conductor theory
Second Piola Kirchhoff stress tensor, 15-18
Segment-long-spacing (SLS), 33-20
Selectivity, 42-21
Semicrystalline solid, 30-21
Sensitiveness, 25-4
Sensitivity distribution, 48-3; *see also* Biomagnetism
  of axial magnetometer, 48-13
  of lead system, 48-6
  in nonsymmetrical and symmetrical
    measurements, 48-9, 48-10 to 48-11
  of planar gradiometer, 48-14
Sensor packs, 54-8
Sensory nerve action potential (SNAP), 46-11; *see also*
    Electrodiagnostic studies (EDX studies)
Sensory nerve conduction study (SNCS), 46-11; *see also*
    Electrodiagnostic studies (EDX studies)
Sensory receptors, 3-2
Sensory transducers, 3-2
Sequencing-control menus for stimulation signals,
    52-9 to 52-10
Serum, 1-2; *see also* Plasma
Servo-null method, 20-2
Sewing rings, 36-18
SF, *see* Single fiber (SF)
SFEMG, *see* Single fiber EMG (SFEMG)
sGC, *see* Soluble guanylate cyclase (sGC)
SGCs, *see* Spiral ganglion cells (SGCs)
Shaft links (SL), 25-8
Shape memory effect (SME), 28-11, 28-20
SHC, *see* Shriners Hospital for Children (SHC)
Shear rate diagram, 23-9
Shoulder, 10-18; *see also* Joint-articulating surface
    motion
  acromion and coracoid process, 10-22
  glenohumeral contact areas, 10-20
  glenohumeral–scapulothoracic rotation, 10-20
  glenoid faces, 10-19
  humeral contact positions, 10-20
  humerus articular surface orientation, 10-18
  joint contact, 10-19 to 10-20
  joint replacement, 37-16
  motion of representative case, 10-23
  rotation axes, 10-20
  scapula rotation on thorax, 10-22
  stability ratio, 10-19
  surface geometry, 10-18 to 10-19
Shriners Hospital for Children (SHC), 54-1
Silk, 34-1, 34-14; *see also* Engineered silk matrices
  applications of, 34-11
  based bone tissue engineering, 34-11 to 34-12
  based cartilage tissue engineering, 34-12 to 34-13
  degradation, 34-13
  degummed, 34-14
  fibers, 34-1
  fibroin matrix formats, 34-5

  fibroin structure, 34-3
  hydrogels, 34-10
  immunological responses, 34-13 to 34-14
  mechanical properties of, 34-2
  protein processing, 34-3 to 34-4
  proteins source, 34-2
  silkworm, 34-3
  spheres, 34-10 to 34-11
  structure and properties, 34-1 to 34-2
  virgin, 34-13
Simple cells, 4-5
Single-capillary cannulation method, 20-2
Single-degree-of-freedom model, 25-4
Single fiber (SF), 46-14
Single fiber EMG (SFEMG), 46-14 to 46-16; *see also*
    Electrodiagnostic studies (EDX studies)
Single-nephron glomerular filtration rate (snGFR), 2-8
Single-photon emission computed tomography
    (SPECT), 57-8
Sinoatrial node (SA node), 1-13
Sinuses of Valsalva, 16-3; *see also* Aortic valve
Sinusoidal stereociliary displacement, 24-1
Skeletal muscle, 9-3; *see also* Muscle
  as class 3 lever, 27-3
  specific tension, 9-6
Skeletal muscle cells, 42-14; *see also* Membrane models
  barnacle muscle, 42-15
  frog sartorius muscle cell, 42-14 to 42-15
Skeleton, 37-1; *see also* Long bone repair
SL, *see* Shaft links (SL)
Sliding motion, 10-2
Slit diaphragm, 2-7
SM, *see* Scala media (SM)
SMA, *see* Supplementary motor area (SMA)
Small intestine, 6-10
  MMC, 6-11
  slow-wave activity, 6-10
SMCs, *see* Smooth muscle cells (SMCs)
SME, *see* Shape memory effect (SME)
SMG, *see* Supramarginal gyrus (SMG)
Smooth muscle cells (SMCs), 35-4
SNAP, *see* Sensory nerve action potential (SNAP)
SNCS, *see* Sensory nerve conduction study (SNCS)
snGFR, *see* Single-nephron glomerular filtration rate
    (snGFR)
S-nitrosothiols (SNOs), 20-8
SNOs, *see* S-nitrosothiols (SNOs)
SNS, *see* Sympathetic nervous system (SNS)
SOC, *see* Superior olivary complex (SOC)
SOD, *see* Superoxide dismutase (SOD)
Sodium; *see also* Electrically active membrane
  ion channels, 38-4 to 38-5
  potassium pump, 38-4
  reabsorption, 2-15 to 2-16
Soft tissue replacements, 36-1, 36-23; *see also* Blood-
    interfacing implants; Nonblood-interfacing
    implants

Soft tissues, 8-1, 9-1; *see also* Hard tissue mechanics;
    Muscle
  actin filament lengths, 9-10
  cartilage, 9-1
  material properties, 9-4
  modeling, 9-7 to 9-13
  tendon and ligament, 9-2
  viscoelastic behavior of, 14-5
Software for bioelectric field problems, 43-18; *see also*
    Computer modeling and simulation
  BioFEM custom interface, 43-23
  BioPSE, 43-20 to 43-22
  BioTensor PowerApp, 43-24
  PowerApps, 43-22 to 43-24
  SCIRun, 43-20
Soluble collagen, 33-20; *see also* Collagen
Soluble guanylate cyclase (sGC), 20-8
Solute transport, 2-14 to 2-15
Solution; *see also* Collagen
  casting, 36-18
  matrix, 33-13
Solvent drag, 20-8
Soma, 3-2
Somatosensory evoked potential (SEP), 46-16 to 46-17;
    see also Electrodiagnostic studies (EDX
    studies)
SOR, *see* Successive overrelaxation (SOR)
Space constant effect of axon, 49-9
Space-filling implants, 36-30; *see also* Nonblood-
    interfacing implants
Spatial frequency, 40-11
SPECT, *see* Single-photon emission computed
    tomography (SPECT)
Speech, 4-6
Sphericity, 21-3, 21-11; *see also* Red blood cell (RBC)
Spike bursts, *see* Electrical response activity (ERA)
Spike discharge patterns, 5-9 to 5-11
Spike train, *see* Action potential (AP)
Spiral ganglion cells (SGCs), 5-1
Spiral ligament, 24-3
Spirometry, 7-16
  flow–volume curve, 7-17
  flow–volume loops, 7-18
  limitations of, 7-18
  pneumotach, 7-17
  tracing, 7-16
Splenic circulation, 1-11
Spongiosa, 16-3; *see also* Aortic valve
Spontaneous activity (SA), 46-12; *see also*
    Electrodiagnostic studies (EDX studies)
SQUID, *see* Superconducting quantum interference
    device (SQUID)
ST, *see* Scala tympani (ST); Strength training (ST)
Stability; *see also* Shoulder

ratio, 10-19
  requirement, 27-2
Stainless steels, 28-2; *see also* Metallic biomaterials
  austenitic stainless steels, 28-2
  effect of cold work, 28-3
  implant manufacturing, 28-18 to 28-19
  effect of Ni and Cr contents on, 28-3
  specific gravities of, 28-6
  stainless steel wire and TiNi SMA wire springs,
    28-11
  surface modification methods, 28-2
  types, 28-2
Standard deviations (S.D.), 21-3
Standard straight box model, 24-2
Standard temperature and pressure, dry (STPD), 7-9
Staples, 36-25; *see also* Nonblood-interfacing implants
Starling–Landis equation, 22-2; *see also* Tissue
    transport mechanics
Starling's law, 20-9, 20-12, 26-4; *see also* Molecular
    transport in microcirculation
  of capillary filtration, 2-8
Starr–Edwards caged ball prostheses, 36-2; *see also*
    Heart valve prostheses
Steinmann pins, 37-4; *see also* Long bone repair
Stellite 21, 36-18
Stem cells, 1-13
Stent, 36-18
Stereocilia, 25-1, 25-2, 25-3
Stereopsis, 4-6, 4-10
Steric hindrance, 30-21
Sterility assurance levels of 10-6 (SAL6), 32-27; *see also*
    Supercritical carbon dioxide sterilization
Stiffness, 25-3 to 25-4
  change in cochlea, 24-18
Stimulation; *see also* Deep brain stimulation (DBS)
  signal's level control, 52-11
  sites, 52-7 to 52-9
Stomach, 6-8
Storage modulus, 8-15
STPD, *see* Standard temperature and pressure, dry
    (STPD)
Strabismus, 4-6
Strain energy density, 18-7; *see also* Blood vessels
Strength training (ST), 27-7, 27-8
Stress; *see also* Bioceramic manufacturing techniques;
    Metallic implant corrosion
  corrosion cracking, 28-18
  fiber model, 23-7
  shielding, 29-23, 37-19
Stressed volume, 19-2; *see also* Venous system
Stretch error, 3-3
Stroke volume (SV), 1-7, 15-10; *see also* Cardiac
    biomechanics
Structural metals, 31-8; *see also* Fibrous composites
Strut, 36-18
STT, *see* Scapho-trapezial-trapezoid (STT)
Subacute hippocampal stimulation (SAHCS), 57-6

Successive overrelaxation (SOR), 43-14; *see also* Computer modeling and simulation
Succinimidyl carboxymethyl (SCM), 35-7
Sulcus angle, 10-11
Superconducting quantum interference device (SQUID), 48-1
Supercritical carbon dioxide, 32-27, 32-29
Supercritical carbon dioxide sterilization, 32-27; *see also* Biodegradable polymers
    ETO sterilization, 32-27
    NovaSterilis scCO$_2$ sterilization process, 32-27
    supercritical carbon dioxide, 32-27, 32-29
    tensile stresses, 32-28
Superelasticity, 28-20
Superior Colliculus, 4-9
Superior olivary complex (SOC), 5-7, 5-11
Superoxide dismutase (SOD), 32-22
Supplementary motor area (SMA), 57-10
Supramarginal gyrus (SMG), 5-14
Surface
    modification, 28-2
    reactive ceramics, *see* Bioactive ceramics
    replaced hip joint, 37-13
Surgical tape, 36-25 to 36-26; *see also* Nonblood-interfacing implants
Surgical wires and cables, 37-3; *see also* Long bone repair
Sutures, 30-21; *see also* Nonblood-interfacing implants
    and suture anchors, 36-23 to 36-25
SV, *see* Scala vestibule (SV); Stroke volume (SV)
Sweating, 26-8
Symmorphosis hypothesis, 20-7; *see also* Molecular transport in microcirculation
Sympathetic nervous system (SNS), 26-3
Synapses, 3-2, 42-8; *see also* Membrane currents
Syncytia, 40-8, 40-11; *see also* Electrical conductivity of tissues
    cardiac muscle, 40-10
    to determine bidomain conductivities, 40-10 to 40-11
    effective interstitial conductivity, 40-9
    effective intracellular conductivity, 40-10
    2-dimensional syncytium, 40-9
Synovial fluid, 11-8; *see also* Joint lubrication
    LGP-I, 11-10
    lubricating ability, 11-10
    lubrication mechanisms, 11-9
    natural and normal lubrication theories, 11-8 to 11-11
    observations on lubrication theories, 11-10
    tribological aspects of, 11-17
    weeping lubrication, 11-8
Synovial joints, 11-7, *see* Synovial fluid
Synthetic absorbable sutures, 32-3; *see also* Biodegradable polymers
Synthetic polymer biodegradation, 32-21; *see also* Biodegradable polymers

free radical role in, 32-22 to 32-24
metal-catalyzed Haber–Weiss reaction, 32-23
oxygen reduction, 32-22
redox reactions, 32-23
respiratory burst, 32-22
structural factors to control polymer degradability, 32-21
superoxide role, 32-23
theoretical modeling of, 32-21 to 32-22
Synthetic polymeric materials, 30-1
Synthetic vascular grafts, 36-13; *see also* Vascular prostheses
Systemic circulation, 17-10; *see also* Arterial macrocirculatory hemodynamics
Systems biology markup language (SBML), 20-12

T

Tachycardia, 1-12
Tacticity, 30-21
TAH, *see* Total artificial heart (TAH)
Tantalum, 28-13; *see also* Metallic biomaterials
    mechanical properties of, 28-13
TCP, *see* Tricalcium phosphate (TCP)
TCPS, *see* Tissue culture-treated polystyrene (TCPS)
tDCS, *see* Transcranial direct current stimulation (tDCS)
Tectorial membrane (TM), 24-4, 24-18
Teeth properties, 31-5
Teflon®, 30-21, *see* Polytetrafluoroethylene (PTFE)
Telopeptides, 33-3, 33-4, 33-20; *see also* Collagen
Temporal dispersion, 46-10; *see also* Electrodiagnostic studies (EDX studies)
Temporal summation, 3-4
Temporary implant devices, 28-2; *see also* Metallic biomaterials
Tendons, 9-2; *see also* Soft tissues
    biomechanical properties, 9-5
    material properties, 9-4
    modeling, 9-10
Tennessee Self-Concept Scale (TSCS), 52-17
TephaFlex®, 32-2; *see also* Biodegradable polymers
TGF-β, *see* Transforming growth factor-beta (TGF-β)
TH, *see* Triquetral-hamate (TH)
Thalamus, 4-4
Thermochemical initiator, 31-5
Thermoregulatory response, 26-8
Third-order cumulant (TOC), 47-9
Thoracic trauma index, 14-2
Three-dimensional model, 24-9 to 24-10, 24-11
Threshold, 42-21
Thrombocytes, 1-2
Thromboembolic complications, 36-19
Thrombus, 36-19, 30-21
Ti alloys, *see* Titanium alloys (Ti alloys)
Tibial plateau, 10-12
Tidal volume, 7-6

Tilting disk valves, 36-19; *see also* Heart valve prostheses prosthesis, 36-4

TiNi alloys, *see* Titanium–nickel alloys (TiNi alloys)

Tip link assemblies (TLA), 25-7 to 25-8

Tip links, 25-1, 25-2, 25-3

Tissue; *see also* Metallic biomaterials; Nonblood-interfacing implants

    adhesives, 36-26 to 36-27

    compatible materials, 28-13

    damage, 49-13

    derived biomaterials; *see also* Collagen

    engineering, 29, 32-2, 33-17

Tissue culture-treated polystyrene (TCPS), 32-19

Tissue reperfusion, 20-5; *see also* Microvascular blood flow mechanics

Tissue transport mechanics, 22-1, 22-12 to 22-13; *see also* Microcirculation

    bootstrap effect, 22-10

    concepts of, 22-2

    fluid pressure, 22-3

    fluid transport, 22-5 to 22-6

    fluid velocity, 22-2

    initial lymphatic cross-sectional area, 22-11

    intraluminal lymphatic valves, 22-8

    intramuscular pressure oscillations, 22-5

    leukocyte flux, 22-13

    lymphatic architecture, 22-6 to 22-7

    lymphatic channel, 22-6

    lymphatic morphology, 22-7

    lymphatic valves, 22-8 to 22-9

    lymph flow rates, 22-12

    lymph formation, 22-9

    lymph leukocyte count, 22-13

    lymph pump mechanism, 22-10 to 22-12

    resistance, 22-3

    Starling–Landis equation, 22-2

    starling pressures and edema prevention, 22-3 to 22-4

    transcapillary filtration, 22-2 to 22-3

Titanium, 36-19

Titanium alloys (Ti alloys), 28-6; *see also* Metallic biomaterials

    cell surface interaction, 28-10

    chemical compositions of, 28-6

    implant, 28-8, 28-10, 28-19

    interface between titanium implant and bioliquid, 28-10

    mechanical properties of, 28-7, 28-8

    microstructure of, 28-8

    osseointegration, 28-9

    phase diagram of Ti–Al–V, 28-7

    properties, 28-7

    pure Ti and Ti6Al4V, 28-6

    resistance to corrosion, 28-8

    specific gravities of, 28-6

    TiNi alloys, 28-11 to 28-12

    yield strength-to-density, 28-9

Titanium implant surface, 28-8; *see also* Titanium alloys (Ti alloys)

Titanium–nickel alloys (TiNi alloys), 28-11; *see also* Titanium alloys (Ti alloys)

    chemical composition of Ni–Ti alloy wire, 28-12

    mechanical properties, 28-12

    stainless steel wire and TiNi SMA wire springs, 28-11

TLA, *see* Tip link assemblies (TLA)

TLC, *see* Total lung capacity (TLC)

TMC, *see* Poly(glycolide-trimethylene carbonate) (TMC)

TMS, *see* Transcranial magnetic stimulation (TMS)

TOC, *see* Third-order cumulant (TOC)

Toe off, 12-2

Tolerance, 14-2

Tonic adaptation, 3-2

Tonotopic arrangement, 25-3

Topographic mapping, 4-10

Total artificial heart (TAH), 36-1, 36-10 to 36-12; *see also* Blood-interfacing implants

    prototype designs of, 36-11

Total joint replacements, 37-12; *see also* Hard tissue replacement; Joint replacements

    ankle joint replacement, 37-16

    biomaterials for, 37-10

    bone cement fixed hip joint, 37-13

    elbow joint replacement, 37-17

    endoprosthetic reconstruction, 37-17 to 37-19

    femoral stem, 37-12

    finger joint replacement, 37-17

    hip joint replacement, 37-12 to 37-14

    knee joint replacement, 37-15 to 37-16

    modular segmental system, 37-18 to 37-19

    modular total hip system, 37-13

    possible combination of, 37-13

    prostheses for, 37-16, 37-17 to 37-19

    prosthetic intervertebral disk, 37-17

    shoulder joint replacement, 37-16

    surface-replaced hip joint, 37-13

    types of, 37-10

Total lung capacity (TLC), 7-6

TR, *see* Tricuspid regurgitation (TR)

Trafficking mediators, 41-4

Transcranial direct current stimulation (tDCS), 3-12

Transcranial magnetic stimulation (TMS), 58-1; *see also* Deep brain stimulation coil; Hesed coil

    circuit, 58-2

    of deep prefrontal regions, 58-18 to 58-21

    deep TMS coils, 58-4 to 58-6

    electric field distribution comparison, 58-21 to 58-22

    neural strength–duration curve, 58-4

    principles of, 58-2 to 58-4

Transduction channel kinetics, 25-6 to 25-7

Transforming growth factor-beta (TGF-β), 35-5

Transmembrane potential, 40-5; *see also* Electrical conductivity of tissues; Membrane models

    difference, 42-1 to 42-2, 42-21

Transmembrane voltage, 49-2
Transverse isotropy, 8-20
Traveling wave, 24-7, 24-17
Triangular boundary element fields, 44-1, 44-17 to
      44-18
   analysis, 44-12
   autosolid angle, 44-5 to 44-6
   BEM, 44-1 to 44-2
   double-layer, 44-12 to 44-13
   examples, 44-12
   field produced by line source, 44-3 to 44-4
   integral of $r(\lambda)$, 44-4
   monolayer, 44-13 to 44-15
   notation, 44-2
   numerical aspects, 44-12
   potential field of linearly distributed double layer,
      44-9 to 44-11
   potential field of linearly distributed monolayer,
      44-11 to 44-12
   potential field of uniform double layer, 44-4 to 44-5
   potential field of uniform monolayer, 44-6 to 44-8
   preliminaries, 44-2
   singularities, 44-15 to 44-17
Tribology, 11-2; *see also* Biotribology; Joint lubrication
   friction, 11-2
   interrelated factors affecting, 11-7
   in movable joint, 11-16
   osteoarthritis–tribology connections, 11-17
   of synovial joint lubrication, 11-17
   wear and surface damage, 11-2 to 11-3
Tricalcium phosphate (TCP), 29-26; *see also*
      Biodegradable ceramics
   ceramics, 29-14
Tricarboxylic acid (TCA), 30-13
Trichromacy, 4-7
Triclinic crystal, 31-4
Tricuspid regurgitation (TR), 16-23 to 16-24; *see also*
      Tricuspid valve (TV)
Tricuspid valve (TV), 16-21; *see also* Heart valve
      dynamics
   annulus, 16-22
   disease and treatment, 16-23 to 16-24
   papillary muscle groups, 16-22
   TR, 16-23 to 16-24
   valve dynamics, 16-22 to 16-23
   valve structure, 16-21 to 16-22
Trigones, 16-14; *see also* Mitral valve (MV)
Triquetral-hamate (TH), 10-30
Tropocollagen, 33-3, 9-1; *see also* Cartilage; Collagen
Truncated singular value decomposition (TSVD), 43-5
Truncation factor, 15-2
TSCS, *see* Tennessee Self-Concept Scale (TSCS)
TSVD, *see* Truncated singular value decomposition
      (TSVD)
Tubular matrices, 33-13; *see also* Collagen
Tubular pole, 2-5
Tubule, 2-2

Tubuloglomerular feedback, 2-11
Tubulo-interstitial structure and organization, 2-12
      to 2-14
Tunica adventitia, 1-10
Tunica intima, 1-10
Tunica media, 1-10
Turbulent stresses, 36-19
TV, *see* Tricuspid valve (TV)
Two-dimensional cell as liquid drop model, 23-11
Two-dimensional elastic ring model, 23-11
Two-dimensional model, 24-8 to 24-9
Tympanic membrane, 5-2

U

UCSF, *see* University of California San Francisco (UCSF)
Udel®, 30-22
UHMWPE, *see* Ultra-high-molecular-weight
      polyethylene (UHMWPE)
UI, *see* User interface (UI)
UL, *see* Upper lateral links (UL)
ULTI, *see* Ultra-low-temperature isotropic (ULTI)
Ultrafiltration coefficient, 2-10
Ultra-high-molecular-weight polyethylene
      (UHMWPE), 29-5, 30-9, 36-19, 37-12
Ultra-low-temperature isotropic (ULTI), 29-8
Umbilical cord vein grafts, 36-19
Unequal anisotropy ratios, 40-8; *see also* Electrical
      conductivity of tissues
University of California San Francisco (UCSF), 50-7
Unmyelinated axons, 3-2
Unsaturated poly(ester amide) s (AA-UPEAs), 32-14;
      see also Amino-acid-based PEAs (AA-PEAs)
Unstressed volume, 19-2; *see also* Venous system
Upper lateral links (UL), 25-8
Urinary incontinence, 36-31 to 36-32; *see also*
      Nonblood-interfacing implants
Urine, 2-2, 2-5
User interface (UI), 43-19
US FDA, *see* U.S. Food and Drug Administration
      (US FDA)
U.S. Food and Drug Administration (US FDA), 36-26
U.S. National Institutes of Health (NIH), 55-1

V

VA, *see* Veterans Administration (VA)
VACET, *see* Visualization and Analytics Center for
      Enabling Technologies (VACET)
Vacuum forming, 36-19
Vagus nerve stimulator (VNS), 50-11
Valence electrons, 30-22
Valine (Val), 33-20
Valvular disorders, 36-19
Valvular structures, 36-19
Vanadium steel, 28-1; *see also* Metallic biomaterials
van der Waals bonding, 30-22

Vasa recta, 2-14
Vascular compliance, 19-2; *see also* Venous system
Vascular distensibility, 19-2; *see also* Venous system
Vascular endothelial growth factor (VEGF), 20-11, 35-5
Vascular grafts, 36-19
Vascular prostheses, 36-12z; *see also* Blood-interfacing
    implants
    classification of, 36-13
    Dacron vascular graft, 36-14
    endoluminal stent-grafts, 36-15 to 36-16
    implanted biological grafts, 36-12 to 36-13
    implanted synthetic grafts, 36-13 to 36-15
    transluminally placed endovascular prostheses, 36-15
Vascular remodeling, 20-11
Vasoconstrictor, 17-10
Vasodilator, 17-10
Vasomotion, 20-4, 20-12; *see also* Microvascular blood
    flow mechanics
Vasopressin, *see* Antidiuretic hormone (ADH)
VC, *see* Viscous response (VC)
VCG, *see* Vectorcardiography (VCG)
Vectorcardiography (VCG), 48-7
VEGF, *see* Vascular endothelial growth factor (VEGF)
Venous characteristic measurement methods, 19-3; *see
    also* Venous system
    capacitance, 19-4
    compliance, 19-4
    gravimetric techniques, 19-5
    integral of inflow minus outflow, 19-5
    outflow occlusion, 19-5
    resistance, 19-3 to 19-4
Venous inertance, 19-3; *see also* Venous system
Venous resistance, 19-3; *see also* Venous system
Venous system, 19-1; *see also* Venous characteristic
    measurement methods
    capacitance, 19-2
    capacity, 19-3
    conduit characteristics of, 19-1
    mean filling pressure, 19-3
    stressed volume, 19-2
    unstressed volume, 19-2
    values, 19-5 to 19-6
    vascular compliance, 19-2
    vascular distensibility, 19-2
    venous inertance, 19-3
    venous resistance, 19-3
Ventilation, 7-20
    perfusion, 7-7
    volume, 7-6
Ventricular assist devices, 36-10; *see also* Blood-
    interfacing implants; Total artificial
    heart (TAH)
Ventricularis, 16-3; *see also* Aortic valve
Venules, 20-3; *see also* Microvascular blood flow
    mechanics
VEPs, *see* Visual-evoked potentials (VEPs)
Vergence, 4-9

Vertical line perpendicular to PC (VPC), 57-3
Very low density polyethylene (VLDPE), 30-9
Vesicoureteral reflux, 36-32; *see also* Nonblood-
    interfacing implants
Vestibular hair cells, 25-1
Vestibulo-ocular reflex, 4-9
Veterans Administration (VA), 54-2
Vicryl sutures, 32-6
Video camera-based systems, 12-4
Vinyl monomers, 30-17
Vinyl polymers, 30-6, 30-22; *see also* Polymeric
    biomaterials
Viscoelastic substance, 17-10
Viscous response (VC), 14-5
Vision system, 4-1
    accommodation, 4-2
    amacrine cells, 4-3
    amblyopia, 4-6
    area 17, 4-4
    Area V1, 4-4 to 4-7
    binocular convergence, 4-5, 4-10
    blindsight, 4-9
    cataracts, 4-7
    center/surround receptive fields, 4-3
    color, 4-7, 4-10
    complex cells, 4-5
    computer vision, 4-1
    cone photoreceptors, 4-7
    cross-eyed, 4-6
    cytoarchitectonics, 4-4, 4-10
    eyes, 4-2
    fovea, 4-3
    Ganglion cells, 4-3
    hemidecussation, 4-4
    higher cortical centers, 4-8
    horizontal cells, 4-3
    hyperacuity, 4-3
    lateral geniculate nucleus, 4-4
    macula lutea, 4-3
    magnification, 4-5, 4-10
    metameric color matching, 4-7
    microsaccades, 4-3
    motion, 4-8
    moving sensor, 4-9 to 4-10
    optic chiasm, 4-4
    optic radiations, 4-4
    optic tracts, 4-4
    optokinetic nystagmus, 4-9
    perisaccadic remapping, 4-10
    psychophysics, 4-1
    receptive field, 4-10
    retina, 4-2 to 4-3
    retinex theory of color vision, 4-8
    saccade, 4-9
    simple cells, 4-5
    speech, 4-6
    stereopsis, 4-6, 4-10

Vision system (*Continued*)
  strabismus, 4-6
  superior colliculus, 4-9
  thalamus, 4-4
  topographic mapping, 4-10
  trichromacy, 4-7
  vergence, 4-9
  vestibulo-ocular reflex, 4-9
  wall-eyed, 4-6
Visual-evoked potentials (VEPs), 3-13, 46-16, 46-18; *see also* Electrodiagnostic studies (EDX studies)
Visualization and Analytics Center for Enabling Technologies (VACET), 43-19
Visual prostheses, 56-1
  cortical-stimulation, 56-1
  effect of electric charge, 56-1
  epiretinal prosthesis, 56-4
  intraocular patient testing, 56-3
  nerve cuff electrode, 56-2
  penetrating cortical electrode array, 56-4
  photoreceptor degeneration prevention, 56-2
  retinal stimulation, 56-1to 56-2
Vitamin D metabolism, 2-19
VLDPE, *see* Very low density polyethylene (VLDPE)
VNS, *see* Vagus nerve stimulator (VNS)
VO$_2$max, *see* Maximal oxygen consumption (VO$_2$max)
Voigt orthotropic symmetry, 8-25
Voigt transverse isotropic symmetry, 8-25
Voltage clamp, 42-21; *see also* Membrane currents protocols, 42-6
Volume conductor, 40-11
Volume conductor theory, 39-1
  basic relations, 39-1 to 39-3
  conductivity values for cardiac bidomain, 39-5
  directional derivative, 39-4
  electric field, 39-2
  equivalent double layer, 39-6
  monopole and dipole fields, 39-3 to 39-4
  passive tissue properties, 39-4 to 39-5
  primary source, 39-7
  secondary double-layer source, 39-7
  secondary source, 39-6
  surface potential, 39-7
  total current density, 39-2
  volume conductor inhomogeneities effect, 39-5 to 39-7
VPC, *see* Vertical line perpendicular to PC (VPC)
Vulcanization, 30-7, 30-22

W

Walking performance, 52-14
  ambulation performance, 52-15
  data, 52-14
  depression scores, 52-17
  evaluation data, 52-16, 52-17
    medical benefits, 52-15
    psychological outcome evaluation, 52-17
Wall-eyed, 4-6
Wall tension, 18-5; *see also* Blood vessels
Water reabsorption, 2-16 to 2-17
Wayne state tolerance curve, 13-7 to 13-8; *see also* Head mechanics
Wear, 11-12; *see also* Joint lubrication
Weeping lubrication, 11-8; *see also* Lubrication; Synovial joints
Weight average molecular weight, 30-5
Weights fractions for body parts, 27-2
Wet chemistry-based methods, 29-23; *see also* Bioceramic manufacturing techniques
White blood cells, *see* Leukocytes
Whole-body tolerance, 14-3
Wolff's law, 37-19; *see also* Long bone repair
  of bone remodeling, 37-1
Womersley number, 17-3; *see also* Arterial macrocirculatory hemodynamics
Wound healing, 35-6
Wrist, 10-28; *see also* Joint-articulating surface motion
  areas of contact, 10-30
  carpal rotation, 10-33, 10-34
  contact area and load relation, 10-30
  force transmission at joints, 10-30
  forearms reconstructions, 10-32
  geometry change, 10-29
  joint contact, 10-29 to 10-30
  rotation axes, 10-31 to 10-32
  rotation center in ulnar deviation, 10-31
  surface geometry, 10-28 to 10-29

X

Xenogeneic collagenous tissue devices, 33-11; *see also* Collagen
Xenografts, 36-7, 36-19; *see also* Heart valve prostheses

Z

ZCAP ceramics, *see* Zinc–calcium–phosphorous oxide polyphasic ceramics (ZCAP ceramics)
Ziegler–Natta catalyst, 30-22
Zinc, 29-14
Zinc–calcium–phosphorous oxide polyphasic ceramics (ZCAP ceramics), 29-14; *see also* Biodegradable ceramics
Zinc–sulfate–calcium–phosphate polyphasic ceramics (ZSCAP ceramics), 29-15, 29-16; *see also* Biodegradable ceramics
Zirconia, 29-5; *see also* Bioinert bioceramics
ZSCAP ceramics, *see* Zinc–sulfate–calcium–phosphate polyphasic ceramics (ZSCAP ceramics)

T - #1048 - 101024 - C0 - 254/178/48 - PB - 9781138748071 - Gloss Lamination